Surgical Techniques in Total Knee Arthroplasty

Springer
New York
Berlin
Heidelberg
Barcelona
Hong Kong
London
Milan
Paris
Singapore
Tokyo

Giles R. Scuderi, M.D.
Insall Scott Kelly Institute
New York, New York

Alfred J. Tria, Jr., M.D.
Orthopaedic Center
of New Jersey
Somerset, New Jersey

Editors

Surgical Techniques in Total Knee Arthroplasty

With a Foreword by John N. Insall, M.D.

With 948 Illustrations

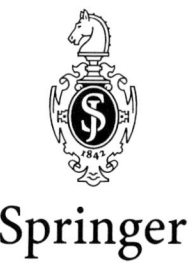

Springer

Giles R. Scuderi, M.D.
Insall Scott Kelly Institute
170 East End Avenue
New York, NY 10128
USA

Alfred J. Tria, Jr., M.D.
Orthopaedic Center of New Jersey
1527 State Highway 27, Suite 1300
Somerset, NJ 08873
USA

Cover illustration: An anteroposterior X-ray of a Legacy prosthesis total knee arthroplasty.

Library of Congress Cataloging-in-Publication Data
Scuderi, Giles R.
    Surgical techniques in total knee arthroplasty / Giles R. Scuderi,
  Alfred J. Tria.
      p.   cm.
    Includes bibliographical references and index.
    ISBN 0-387-98389-9 (hardcover : alk. paper)
    1. Total knee replacement.   2. Knee—Surgery.   3. Artificial knee.
  I. Tria, Alfred J.   II. Title.
    [DNLM: 1. Arthroplasty, Replacement, Knee—methods.   WE 870 S384s
1998]
RD561.S4 2002
617.5′820592—dc21
DNLM/DLC   98-22362

Printed on acid-free paper.

© 2002 Springer-Verlag New York, Inc.
All rights reserved. This work may not be translated or copied in whole or in part without the written permission of the publisher (Springer-Verlag New York, Inc., 175 Fifth Avenue, New York, NY 10010, USA), except for brief excerpts in connection with reviews or scholarly analysis. Use in connection with any form of information storage and retrieval, electronic adaptation, computer software, or by similar or dissimilar methodology now known or hereafter developed is forbidden.
The use of general descriptive names, trade names, trademarks, etc., in this publication, even if the former are not especially identified, is not to be taken as a sign that such names, as understood by the Trade Marks and Merchandise Marks Act, may accordingly be used freely by anyone.
While the advice and information in this book are believed to be true and accurate at the date of going to press, neither the authors nor the editors nor the publisher can accept any legal responsibility for any errors or omissions that may be made. The publisher makes no warranty, express or implied, with respect to the material contained herein.

Production coordinated by WordCrafters Editorial Services, Inc., and managed by Lesley Poliner; manufacturing supervised by Jacqui Ashri.
Typeset by Matrix Publishing Services, Inc., York, PA.
Printed and bound by Maple-Vail Book Manufacturing Group, York, PA.
Printed in the United States of America.

9 8 7 6 5 4 3 2 1

ISBN 0-387-98389-9   SPIN 10659209

Springer-Verlag   New York   Berlin   Heidelberg
A member of BertelsmannSpringer Science+Business Media GmbH

*This book is dedicated to
our mentor,
John N. Insall, M.D.*

Foreword

In my opinion, the most important factor in creating a successful total knee arthroplasty is surgical technique. The instrument systems provided for a particular implant and the information contained in the brochures will aid the surgeon in producing a handsome radiograph, but not necessarily a satisfied patient. I can recall seeing many such situations in which the result is marked by stiffness or instability, small contractures or imbalances, or "unexplained" pain—possibly related to component malposition. *Surgical Techniques in Total Knee Arthroplasty* is dedicated to reducing "minor" errors that contribute to a less than optimal arthroplasty; it contains all the information needed to obtain consistently reliable results.

While this book does not resolve all the controversies in total knee arthroplasty, it does provide insight into the subtleties of various surgical concepts and implant designs. The reader will encounter apparently disparate advice in some areas, some of which is due to honest differences in opinion and some related to the type of implant. For example, a tight flexion space is advisable when using a posterior cruciate ligament substituting prosthesis, but inappropriate for a posterior cruciate retaining design, where loss of flexion may occur. Likewise, when a surgical approach is being selected, the procedure chosen will depend on the surgeon's preference and experience.

Gil Scuderi and Fred Tria have assembled a splendid compendium of total knee techniques that deserves a place in the library of all surgeons interested in total knee arthroplasty. They are to be congratulated for their effort.

JOHN N. INSALL, M.D.
New York, New York
October 2000

Preface

Surgical Techniques in Total Knee Arthroplasty was initiated 4 years ago when we saw the need for a thorough, comprehensive text that would deliver all of the best techniques for total knee surgery in a single volume. We sought to bring together the best experts in the field and asked each author to address an area of total knee surgery with which he or she was intimately familiar. It was our plan to make the text a reference for all aspects of total knee arthroplasty. We were fortunate: Every author we contacted agreed to supply a chapter.

The sections on preoperative planning and clinical evaluation provide a good lead-in to the topic and set the present-day atmosphere of total knee arthroplasty. The costs of implants and hospitalization are a significant problem for the practicing orthopaedic surgeon, and the collection of outcome data on results of surgery will be increasingly critical in the next few years. With the variety of implant designs on the market, we are fortunate that many of the contributors are designing surgeons who review their lifetime experience with individual prosthetic designs.

With the diversity of exposure in the arthritic knee, the section on surgical approaches is comprehensive and includes chapters written by the authors who popularized the techniques. The section on correction of deformity is comprehensive on the management of soft tissues. This includes ligament releases for the varus and valgus knee, as well as management of flexion contractures. As an alternative, ligament advances are included in this section. The authors have submitted chapters that reflect their unique experience in each area.

Achieving a successful outcome goes beyond soft tissue balancing and must include orientation of the implant. Component positioning and alignment, the subject of the next section, is critical in knee arthroplasty. This section is thoroughly covered by the contributors, who describe their individual techniques and preferences. The following sections discuss methods of component fixation and patellar preparation.

The sections that follow discuss the complex issues of revision arthroplasty. The contributors describe the evaluation of the painful knee, component removal, and a step-wise technique for performing the revision arthroplasty. Specific chapters on management of bone loss, component fixation, infection, extensor mechanism dysfunction, and fractures round out the topics of revision total knee arthroplasty.

The section on special situations provides the reader with a comprehensive overview of clinical findings that may make the primary arthroplasty more complicated. These contributing experts provide us with their clinical experience.

In the final section on postoperative management, the chapters include rehabilitation, pain management, the stiff knee, and DVT prophylaxis. The authors provide surgeons with practical guidelines for these topics.

As the text developed, we broadened our goals and included a glossary of product descriptions and photographs to help identify most of the knee replacement systems in the world.

Now that the book is completed, we have had the opportunity to look back and review the entire process. We feel fortunate to have persuaded so many well-known orthopaedic surgeons to contribute to the text. We are grateful to all of them and believe that the final product is, indeed, a reflection of the combined efforts of these experts.

We have both had the honor of training with Dr. John N. Insall, who is certainly one of the leaders in the field of total knee arthroplasty, if not its founding father. With this in mind, we dedicate this text to him, our mentor.

GILES R. SCUDERI, M.D.
New York, New York

ALFRED J. TRIA, JR., M.D.
New Brunswick, New Jersey
October 2001

Contents

Foreword vii
Preface ix
Contributors xvii

Section 1   **PREOPERATIVE PLANNING** 1

1 Indications and Patient Selection 3
   STEVEN F. HARWIN

2 Preoperative Radiographic Assessment 9
   KEVIN R. MATH AND GILES R. SCUDERI

3 Cost Considerations: An Historical Perspective 19
   STEVEN STERN

Section 2   **CLINICAL EVALUATION** 29

4 Knee Scores in Total Knee Arthroplasty 31
   JOSÉ ALICEA

5 Outcomes Data Collection 39
   NORMAN A. JOHANSON

Section 3   **PROSTHETIC DESIGN** 47

6 PCL-Sparing Total Knee Arthroplasty 49
   PAUL N. SMITH AND CECIL H. RORABECK

7 Posterior Cruciate-Sacrificing Total Knee Arthroplasty 61
   P. JOHN KUMAR AND LAWRENCE D. DORR

8 The Insall-Burstein® Posterior Stabilized Condylar Knee Prosthesis ... 67
   THOMAS J. ALLARDYCE, GILES R. SCUDERI, AND JOHN N. INSALL

9 Constrained Prostheses 75
   KELLY G. VINCE

10 Meniscal-Bearing Total Knee Arthroplasty 81
   FREDERICK F. BUECHEL

11 Mensical-Bearing Knee: Principles, Technique,
   and Preliminary Results 90
   PAOLO AGLIETTI, JOHN N. INSALL, ROBERTO BUZZI, AND PETER WALKER

12 Constrained Total Knee Designs for Revision Arthroplasty 97
   JAMES RAND AND WILLIAM MARTIN

13	Unicondylar Replacement C. LOWRY BARNES AND RICHARD D. SCOTT	106

Section 4   SURGICAL APPROACHES   113

14	Medial Parapatellar Arthrotomy STEVEN H. STERN	115
15	Subvastus Approach KELLY G. VINCE	119
16	Midvastus Approach GERARD A. ENGH	127
17	The Trivector-Retaining Arthrotomy KENNETH W. BRAMLETT, WILLIAM N. HALLER III, AND WILLIAM D. KRAUSS	131
18	The Lateral Approach PETER A. KEBLISH	137
19	Quadriceps Snip KEVIN L. GARVIN	149
20	V-Y Quadricepsplasty JOHN J. CALLAGHAN AND RUSSELL E. WINDSOR	155
21	Tibial Tubercle Osteotomy LEO A. WHITESIDE	159

Section 5   PRINCIPLES OF PRIMARY TOTAL KNEE ARTHROPLASTY   163

22	The Basic Principles GILES R. SCUDERI	165
23	Draping Technique for Total Knee Arthroplasty SERGIO GOMEZ, DAVID J. YASGUR, GILES R. SCUDERI, AND JOHN N. INSALL	168

Section 6   INSTRUMENTATION   175

24	Total Knee Arthroplasty ALFRED J. TRIA, JR.	177

Section 7   CORRECTION OF DEFORMITY   187

25	Medial Release for Fixed-Varus Deformity DAVID J. YASGUR, GILES R. SCUDERI, AND JOHN N. INSALL	189
26	Lateral Release for Fixed-Valgus Deformity FRANKIE M. GRIFFIN, GILES R. SCUDERI, AND JOHN N. INSALL	197
27	Medial and Lateral Ligament Advancement KENNETH KRACKOW	205
28	Flexion Contracture in Total Knee Arthroplasty PAUL A. LOTKE AND R.G. SIMON	210
29	Correction of Combined Deformity PAOLO AGLIETTI AND ROBERTO BUZZI	216

Section 8   COMPONENT POSITION   225

30	The Epicondylar Axis for Femoral Component Rotation PASCAL L. POILVACHE	227

31	Tibial Shaft Axis for Femoral Component Rotation JAMES B. STIEHL	236
32	Alternatives for Rotational Alignment of the Femoral Component CHITRANJAN S. RANAWAT AND JOSÉ A. RODRIGUEZ	240
33	Tibial Component Position LAWRENCE S. CROSSETT AND HARRY E. RUBASH	243

Section 9   FIXATION   255

34	Cement in Primary Total Knee Arthroplasty ALFRED J. TRIA, JR.	257
35	Cementless Total Knee Arthroplasty AARON A. HOFMANN AND DAVID F. SCOTT	262
36	Hybrid Total Knee Arthroplasty MICHAEL W. BECKER	273
37	Hydroxyapatite MATTHEW J. KRAAY AND VICTOR M. GOLDBERG	277

Section 10   BONE DEFECTS   287

38	Autogenous Bone Grafting for Tibial Deficiency THOMAS P. SCULCO AND WILLIAM O'CONNOR	289
39	Bone Grafting in Primary Femoral Deficiency THOMAS P. SCULCO	295

Section 11   PATELLAR PREPARATION   299

40	Onset Patella LISA NASON AND MICHAEL A. KELLY	301
41	Inlay Technique RICHARD S. LASKIN	304
42	Rotating Patella FREDERICK F. BUECHEL	310

Section 12   EXTENSOR MECHANISM ALIGNMENT   315

43	The Intraoperative Assessment of Patellar Tracking MARK W. PAGNANO AND MICHAEL A. KELLY	317
44	Benefits and Pitfalls of Lateral Patella Release FRED D. CUSHNER AND W. NORMAN SCOTT	326
45	Proximal Patellar Realignment for Recurrent Patellar Instability JONATHAN ARCHER AND GILES R. SCUDERI	332
46	Distal Realignment for Recurrent Patellar Instability LEO A. WHITESIDE	337

Section 13   EVALUATION OF THE PAINFUL TOTAL KNEE ARTHROPLASTY   343

47	Clinical Evaluation AARON G. ROSENBERG AND RICHARD A. BERGER	345
48	Imaging of the Painful TKR KEVIN R. MATH AND ROBERT SCHEIDER	351

49	Arthroscopic Management of Problematic Total Knee Arthroplasty	368
	DAVID R. DIDUCH AND GILES R. SCUDERI	

Section 14   REVISION ARTHROPLASTY — 375

50	Component Removal	377
	PAUL N. SMITH AND CECIL H. RORABECK	
51	Three-Step Technique for Revision Total Knee Arthroplasty	384
	KELLY G. VINCE AND DANIEL A. OAKES	

Section 15   MANAGEMENT OF BONE LOSS IN REVISION ARTHROPLASTY — 391

52	General Concepts	393
	EMIL H. SCHEMITSCH AND THOMAS S. THORNHILL	
53	Classification of Bone Defects: Femur and Tibia	401
	GERARD A. ENGH	
54	Bone Defects: Tibial Modularity	409
	RUSSELL E. WINDSOR	
55	Bone Defects: Tibial Allograft	415
	BERNARD N. STULBERG	
56	Bone Defects: Femoral Allograft	424
	DOUGLAS A. DENNIS	

Section 16   FIXATION TECHNIQUES IN REVISION KNEE ARTHROPLASTY — 433

57	Cemented Revision Knee Arthroplasty	435
	WILLIAM J. MALONEY	
58	Cementless Fixation	440
	LEO A. WHITESIDE	
59	Press-Fit Stem Fixation	451
	WAYNE G. PAPROSKY, TODD D. SEKUNDIAK, AND JOHN KRONICK	

Section 17   INFECTION — 463

60	Single-Stage Revision of Infected Total Knee Replacement	465
	GARETH SCOTT AND MICHAEL A.R. FREEMAN	
61	Two-Stage Reimplantation	471
	GILES R. SCUDERI AND HENRY D. CLARKE	
62	Evolution and Design Rationale of the *PROSTALAC* Knee System in the Management of the Infected Total Knee Prosthesis	473
	BASSAM A. MASRI, CHRISTOPHER P. BEAUCHAMP, AND CLIVE P. DUNCAN	
63	Alternative Procedures for the Management of an Infected Total Knee	491
	AARON G. ROSENBERG AND RICHARD A. BERGER	

Section 18   EXTENSOR MECHANISM DYSFUNCTION — 503

64	Patellar Fracture	505
	MARK A. GREENFIELD, GEOFFREY H. WESTRICH, AND STEVEN B. HAAS	
65	Acute and Chronic Rupture of the Quadriceps Tendon Treated with Direct Repair	514
	ROBERT E. BOOTH AND FRANK P. FEMINO	

66	Reconstruction of the Extensor Mechanism with an Allograft Following Total Knee Arthroplasty ROBERT E. BOOTH AND FRANK P. FEMINO	516
67	Management of Patella Tendon Disruptions in Total Knee Arthroplasty GILES R. SCUDERI AND BRIAN C. DE MUTH	519
68	Revision of Loose Patellar Components ADOLPH V. LOMBARDI, JR., THOMAS H. MALLORY, AND STEPHEN M. HERRINGTON	524
69	Revision of Metal-Backed Patellar Components PAUL F. LACHIEWICZ	533
70	Patellar Dislocation PAUL F. LACHIEWICZ	539

Section 19	MANAGEMENT OF PERIPROSTHETIC FRACTURES	543
71	Femoral Periprosthetic Fractures: Nonoperative Treatment MICHAEL C. MORAN	545
72	Femoral Periprosthetic Fractures: Rush Rods JEFFREY R. GINTHER AND MERRILL A. RITTER	553
73	Femoral Periprosthetic Fractures: Retrograde Intramedullary Nail LAWRENCE A. SCHAPER AND DAVID SELIGSON	558
74	Femoral Periprosthetic Fractures: Blade Plates Fixation LAURENCE D. HIGGINS AND MARK P. FIGGIE	563
75	Revision of Periprosthetic Femur Fractures ROBERT E. BOOTH AND DAVID G. NAZARIAN	573
76	Classification of Periprosthetic Tibial Fractures ARLEN D. HANSSEN, MICHAEL J. STUART, AND NANCY A. FELIX	576
77	Tibial Periprosthetic Fractures: Nonoperative Treatment PHILIP M. FARIS	584
78	Tibial Periprosthetic Fractures: Open Reduction Internal Fixation WILLIAM L. HEALY	587
79	Revision Arthroplasty for Tibial Periprosthetic Fractures WAYNE G. PAPROSKY, TODD D. SEKUNDIAK, AND JOHN KRONICK	592

Section 20	SPECIAL SITUATIONS	599
80	Total Knee Arthroplasty Following High Tibial Osteotomy CHARLES L. NELSON AND RUSSELL E. WINDSOR	601
81	Total Knee Arthroplasty after Supracondylar Femoral Osteotomy GILES R. SCUDERI, JOHN N. INSALL, AND ALBERTO BOLANOS	610
82	Total Knee Replacement after Maquet Osteotomy DOUGLAS PADGETT	613
83	Total Knee Arthroplasty after Patellectomy FRANKIE M. GRIFFIN AND MICHAEL A. KELLY	621
84	Total Knee Arthroplasty for Patients with Prior Knee Arthrodesis PAUL A. LOTKE AND ELIZABETH A. COOK	627
85	The Effect of Extra-Articular Deformity on the Tibial Component DAVID S. HUNGERFORD	632

86	Total Knee Replacement with Associated Extra-Articular Angular Deformity of the Femur	635
	JOHN W. MANN III, GILES R. SCUDERI, AND JOHN N. INSALL	
87	The Effect of Extra-Articular Deformity on the Femoral Component	640
	DAVID S. HUNGERFORD	
88	Total Knee Replacement with Associated Extra-Articular Angular Deformity of the Tibia	645
	JOHN W. MANN III, GILES R. SCUDERI, AND JOHN N. INSALL	

Section 21   POSTOPERATIVE MANAGEMENT 649

89	Rehabilitation	651
	ROBERT S. GOTLIN AND ELIZABETH A. BECKER	
90	Postoperative Pain Management	680
	NIGEL E. SHARROCK	
91	The Stiff Knee	687
	VAN P. STAMOS AND JAMES V. BONO	
92	Deep Vein Thrombosis (DVT) and Total Knee Arthroplasty	694
	GILBERT B. CUSHNER, FRED D. CUSHNER, AND MICHAEL A. CUSHNER	

Glossary of Implants 705

Index 737

Contributors

PAOLO AGLIETTI, M.D.
Professor of Orthopaedics
Director, First Orthopaedic Clinic
University of Florence
Florence, Italy

JOSÉ ALICEA, M.D.
Assistant Clinical Professor
Department of Orthopaedics
Texas Tech Health Sciences Center
El Paso, TX, USA

THOMAS J. ALLARDYCE, M.D.
The Insall Scott Kelly Institute
Beth Israel Medical Center
New York, NY, USA

JONATHAN M. ARCHER, M.D.
The Insall Scott Kelly Institute
Beth Israel Medical Center
New York, NY, USA

C. LOWRY BARNES, M.D.
The Brigham and Women's Hospital
New England Baptist Hospital
Boston, MA, USA

CHRISTOPHER P. BEAUCHAMP, M.D.
Department of Orthopaedics
Vancouver Hospital and Health Science Center
Vancouver, British Columbia, Canada

ELIZABETH A. BECKER
Department of Physical Medicine and Rehabilitation
Beth Israel Medical Center
New York, NY, USA

MICHAEL W. BECKER, M.D.
Orthopaedic Associates of Portland
Portland, ME, USA

RICHARD A. BERGER, M.D.
Arthritis and Orthopaedic Institute
Rush Medical College
Rush Presbyterian – St. Luke's Medical Center
Chicago, IL, USA

ALBERTO BOLANOS, M.D.
Department of Orthopaedics
Beth Israel Medical Center
New York, NY, USA

JAMES V. BONO, M.D.
Department of Orthopaedics
New England Baptist Hospital
Boston, MA, USA

ROBERT E. BOOTH, JR., M.D.
Chief of Orthopaedics
Pennsylvania Hospital
Philadelphia, PA, USA

KENNETH W. BRAMLETT, M.D.
Alabama Sports Medicine and Orthopaedic Center
Birmingham, AL, USA

FREDERICK F. BUECHEL, M.D.
Clinical Professor of Orthopaedic Surgery
Chief, Total Joint Reconstructive and Arthritis
  Surgery Services
Department of Orthopaedics
UMDNJ – New Jersey Medical School
South Orange, NJ, USA

ROBERTO BUZZI, M.D.
Department of Orthopaedics
First Orthopaedic Clinic
University of Florence
Florence, Italy

JOHN J. CALLAGHAN, M.D.
Professor, Department of Orthopaedics
University of Iowa College of Medicine
Iowa City, IA, USA

HENRY D. CLARKE, M.D.
Attending Orthopaedic Surgeon
The Insall Scott Kelly Institute
Beth Israel Medical Center
New York, NY, USA

ELIZABETH A. COOK, M.D.
Department of Orthopaedics
University of Pennsylvania Hospital
Philadelphia, PA, USA

LAWRENCE S. CROSSETT, M.D.
Division of Adult Reconstruction
Department of Orthopaedic Surgery
University of Pittsburgh Medical Center
Pittsburgh, PA, USA

FRED D. CUSHNER, M.D.
Director, The Insall Scott Kelly Institute
Beth Israel Medical Center
New York, NY, USA
Assistant Clinical Professor of Orthopedic Surgery
Albert Einstein College of Medicine
Bronx, NY, USA

GILBERT B. CUSHNER, M.D.
Assistant Clinical Professor
The George Washington University
Washington, DC, USA

MICHAEL A. CUSHNER, M.D.
Attending Orthopaedic Surgeon
The Insall Scott Kelly Institute
Beth Israel Medical Center
New York, NY, USA

BRIAN C. DEMUTH, M.D.
The Insall Scott Kelly Institute
Beth Israel Medical Center
New York, NY, USA

DOUGLAS A. DENNIS, M.D.
Professor, Department of Orthopaedic Surgery
Colorado School of Mines
Division of Engineering
University of Colorado Health Science Center
Denver, CO, USA

DAVID R. DIDUCH, M.D.
Assistant Professor of Orthopaedic Surgery
Department of Orthopaedics
University of Virginia Health Sciences Center
Charlottesville, VA, USA

LAWRENCE D. DORR, M.D.
Director, The Bone and Joint Institute
Good Samaritan Hospital
Los Angeles, CA, USA

CLIVE P. DUNCAN, M.D.
Department of Orthopaedics
Vancouver Hospital and Health Science Center
Vancouver, British Columbia, Canada

GERARD A. ENGH, M.D.
Associate Clinical Professor
University of Maryland Medical School
Baltimore, MD, USA
President
Anderson Orthopedic Institute
Alexandria, VA, USA

PHILIP M. FARIS, M.D.
Department of Orthopedics
Kendrick Memorial Hospital
Mooresville, IN, USA

NANCY A. FELIX, M.D.
Department of Orthopaedics
Mayo Clinic
Rochester, MN, USA

FRANK P. FEMINO, M.D.
Department of Orthopaedics
Pennsylvania Hospital
Philadelphia, PA, USA

MARK D. FIGGIE, M.D.
The Hospital for Special Surgery
New York, NY, USA

MICHAEL A. R. FREEMAN, M.D.
Professor, School of Engineering
Southampton University
Hampshire, UK
Honorary Consultant Orthopaedic Surgeon
The Barts and the London NHS Trust
London, UK

KEVIN L. GARVIN, M.D.
Department of Orthopaedics
University of Nebraska Medical Center
Omaha, NE, USA

JEFFREY R. GINTHER, M.D.
Clinical Assistant Professor
Department of Orthopaedics
Uniformed Services University of the Health Sciences
Kendrick Memorial Hospital
Mooresville, IN, USA

VICTOR M. GOLDBERG, M.D.
Charles H. Herndon Professor
Chairman, Department of Orthopaedic Surgery
University Hospital of Cleveland
Case Western Reserve University
Cleveland, OH, USA

SERGIO GOMEZ, C.S.T.
The Insall Scott Kelly Institute
Beth Israel Medical Center
New York, NY, USA

ROBERT S. GOTLIN, D.O.
Assistant Chairman
Physician-in-Charge; Orthopaedic, Sports,
  Spine Rehabilitation
Department of Physical Medicine and Rehabilitation
Beth Israel Medical Center
New York, NY, USA

MARK A. GREENFIELD, M.D.
The Hospital for Special Surgery
New York, NY, USA

FRANKIE M. GRIFFIN, M.D.
The Insall Scott Kelly Institute
Beth Israel Medical Center
New York, NY, USA

STEVEN B. HAAS, M.D.
The Hospital for Special Surgery
New York, NY, USA

WILLIAM N. HALLER III, M.D.
University of Alabama at Birmingham
Birmingham, AL, USA

ARLEN D. HANSSEN, M.D.
Associate Professor of Orthopaedic Surgery
Mayo Medical School
Rochester, MN, USA

STEVEN F. HARWIN, M.D.
Associate Clinical Professor of Orthopaedic Surgery
Albert Einstein College of Medicine
Bronx, NY, USA
Chief, Adult Reconstructive Surgery
Department of Orthopaedic Surgery
Beth Israel Medical Center
New York, NY, USA

WILLIAM L. HEALY, M.D.
Chairman, Department of Orthopaedic Surgery
Lahey Hitchcock Clinic
Burlington, MA, USA

STEPHEN M. HERRINGTON, B.S.M.E.
Research Coordinator
Joint Implant Surgeons, Inc.
Columbus, OH, USA

LAURENCE D. HIGGINS, M.D.
The Hospital for Special Surgery
New York, NY, USA

AARON A. HOFMANN, M.D.
Professor, Department of Orthopaedics
University of Utah
Salt Lake City, UT, USA

DAVID S. HUNGERFORD, M.D.
Professor of Orthopaedic Surgery
Department of Orthopaedic Surgery
Johns Hopkins University School of Medicine
Baltimore, MD, USA

JOHN N. INSALL, M.D. (1930 – 2000)
Clinical Professor of Orthopaedic Surgery
Albert Einstein College of Medicine
Bronx, NY, USA
Director and Founder
The Insall Scott Kelly Institute
New York, NY, USA

NORMAN A. JOHANSON, M.D.
Associate Professor, Orthopaedic Surgery
Department of Orthopaedic Surgery
Temple University Hospital
Philadelphia, PA, USA

PETER A. KEBLISH, M.D.
Professor of Clinical Orthopaedics
Chief, Division of Orthopaedic Surgery
Department of Surgery
Pennsylvania State University College of Medicine
Allentown, PA, USA

MICHAEL A. KELLY, M.D.
Chief of Sports Medicine
Department of Orthopaedic Surgery
Beth Israel Medical Center
Director, The Insall Scott Kelly Institute
New York, NY, USA

MATTHEW J. KRAAY, M.D.
Department of Orthopaedic Surgery
University Hospital of Cleveland
Case Western Reserve University
Cleveland, OH, USA

KENNETH A. KRACKOW, M.D.
Department of Orthopaedic Surgery
The Buffalo General Hospital
Buffalo, NY, USA

WILLIAM D. KRAUSS, D.O.
Alabama Sports Medicine and Orthopaedic Center
Birmingham, AL, USA

JOHN KRONICK, M.D.
Central DuPage Hospital
Winfield, IL, USA

P. JOHN KUMAR, M.D.
The Bone and Joint Institute
Good Samaritan Hospital
Los Angeles, CA, USA

PAUL F. LACHIEWICZ, M.D.
Professor, Department of Orthopaedics
University of North Carolina
Chapel Hill, NC, USA

RICHARD S. LASKIN, M.D.
The Hospital for Special Surgery
New York, NY, USA

ADOLPH V. LOMBARDI JR., M.D., F.A.C.S.
Clinical Assistant Professor
Department of Orthopaedic Surgery
Ohio State University Hospitals
Columbus, OH, USA

PAUL A. LOTKE, M.D.
Professor, Department of Orthopaedics
University of Pennsylvania Hospital
Philadelphia, PA, USA

THOMAS H. MALLORY, M.D.
Chairman, Grant Orthopaedic Institute
Clinical Assistant Professor of Orthopaedic Surgery
Grant Medical Center
The Ohio State University Hospital
Columbus, OH, USA

WILLIAM J. MALONEY, M.D.
Professor of Orthopaedic Surgery
Washington University School of Medicine
Chief, Orthopaedic Surgery
Barnes-Jewish Hospital
St. Louis, MO, USA

JOHN W. MANN III, M.D.
Department of Medical Education
Carilion Roanoke Memorial Hospital
Roanoke, VA, USA

WILLIAM MARTIN, M.D.
Department of Orthopaedic Surgery
Mayo Clinic
Scottsdale, AZ, USA

BASSAM A. MASRI, M.D.
Department of Orthopaedics
Vancouver Hospital and Health Science Center
Vancouver, British Columbia, Canada

KEVIN R. MATH, M.D.
Department of Radiology
Beth Israel Medical Center
New York, NY, USA

MICHAEL C. MORAN, M.D.
Parkview Orthopaedic Group
Evergreen, IL, USA

LISA NASON, M.D.
Department of Orthopaedic Surgery
Beth Israel Medical Center
New York, NY, USA

Contributors

DAVID G. NAZARIAN, M.D.
Department of Orthopaedic Surgery
Pennsylvania Hospital
Philadelphia, PA, USA

CHARLES L. NELSON, M.D.
The Hospital for Special Surgery
New York, NY, USA

DANIEL A. OAKES, M.D.
Department of Orthopaedics
University of Louisville
Louisville, KY, USA

WILLIAM O'CONNOR, M.D.
The Hospital for Special Surgery
New York, NY, USA

DOUGLAS PADGETT, M.D.
The Hospital for Special Surgery
New York, NY, USA

MARK W. PAGNANO, M.D.
Assistant Professor of Orthopaedic Surgery
Mayo School of Medicine
Rochester, MN, USA

WAYNE G. PAPROSKY, M.D.
Department of Adult Joint Reconstruction
Rusk-Presbyterian-St. Lukes Medical Center
Chicago, IL, USA

HENRIK PEDERSEN, M.D.
The Insall Scott Kelly Institute
New York, NY, USA

PASCAL POILVACHE, M.D.
Assistant Professor
Department of Orthopaedic Surgery
Catholic University of Louvain
Saint-Luc University Hospital
Brussels, Belgium

CHITRANJAN S. RANAWAT, M.D.
Chairman, Department of Orthopaedic Surgery
Lenox Hill Hospital
New York, NY, USA

JAMES ALAN RAND, M.D.
Department of Orthopaedic Surgery
Mayo Clinic
Scottsdale, AZ, USA

MERRILL A. RITTER, M.D.
Professor of Orthopaedic Surgery
Indiana University Medical School
Surgeon-in-Chief for Hip & Knee Surgery
Department of Orthopaedics
Kendrick Memorial Hospital
Mooresville, IN, USA

JOSÉ A. RODRIGUEZ, M.D.
Department of Orthopaedic Surgery
Lenox Hill Hospital
New York, NY, USA

CECIL H. RORABECK, M.D., F.R.C.S.C.
Professor and Chairman
Department of Orthopaedic Surgery
University of Western Ontario
London, Ontario, Canada

AARON G. ROSENBERG, M.D.
Professor of Orthopaedic Surgery
Arthritis and Orthopaedic Institute
Rush Medical College
Rush Presbyterian – St. Luke's Medical Center
Chicago, IL, USA

HARRY RUBASH, M.D.
Professor and Chief
Department of Orthopaedic Surgery
Massachusetts General Hospital
Boston, MA, USA

LAWRENCE A. SCHAPER, M.D.
Assistant Clinical Professor
Department of Orthopaedics
University of Louisville
Louisville, KY, USA

ROBERT SCHEIDER, M.D.
The Hospital for Special Surgery
New York, NY, USA

EMIL H. SCHEMITSCH, M.D.
Department of Orthopaedic Surgery
The Brigham and Women's Hospital
Boston, MA, USA

DAVID F. SCOTT, M.D.
Department of Orthopaedics
University of Utah
Salt Lake City, UT, USA

GARETH SCOTT, M.D.
School of Engineering
Southampton University
Hampshire, UK

RICHARD D. SCOTT, M.D.
Professor of Orthopaedic Surgery
Harvard Medical School
Senior Surgeon
Department of Orthopaedic Surgery
The Brigham and Women's Hospital
Boston, MA, USA

W. NORMAN SCOTT, M.D.
Chairman, Department of Orthopaedics
Beth Israel Medical Center
New York, NY, USA
Director, The Insall Scott Kelly Institute
Clinical Professor of Orthopaedic Surgery
Albert Einstein College of Medicine
Bronx, NY, USA

GILES R. SCUDERI, M.D.
Chief, Section of Adult Knee Reconstruction
Department of Orthopaedics
Beth Israel Medical Center
Director, The Insall Scott Kelly Institute
New York, NY, USA
Assistant Clinical Professor of Orthopaedic Surgery
Albert Einstein College of Medicine
Bronx, NY, USA

THOMAS P. SCULCO, M.D.
Director of Orthopaedic Surgery
Chief, Surgical Arthritis Service
The Hospital for Special Surgery
New York, NY, USA

TODD D. SEKUNDIAK M.D.
Section of Orthopaedics
University of Manitoba
Winnipeg, Manitoba, Canada

DAVID SELIGSON, M.D.
Professor and Vice Chairman
Department of Orthopaedics
University of Louisville
Louisville, KY, USA

NIGEL E. SHARROCK, M.D, CH.B.
Attending Anesthesiologist
The Hospital for Special Surgery
New York, NY, USA

R.G. SIMON, M.D.
Department of Orthopaedics
University of Pennsylvania Hospital
Philadelphia, PA, USA

PAUL N. SMITH, M.D.
Department of Orthopaedic Surgery
University of Western Ontario
London, Ontario, Canada

VAN P. STAMOS, M.D.
Department of Orthopaedics
New England Baptist Hospital
Boston, MA, USA

STEVEN H. STERN, M.D.
Assistant Clinical Professor of Orthopaedics
Northwestern University
Chicago, IL, USA

JAMES B. STIEHL, M.D.
Clinical Associate Professor
Director, Midwest Orthopaedic Biomechanical
  Laboratory
Columbia Musculoskeletal Institute
Milwaukee, WI, USA

MICHAEL J. STUART, M.D.
Associate Professor
Department of Orthopaedic Surgery
Mayo Clinic
Rochester, MN, USA

BERNARD N. STULBERG, M.D.
Department of Orthopaedics
Lutheran Hospital
St. Vincent's Charity Hospital
Hillcrest Hospital
Cleveland, OH, USA

THOMAS S. THORNHILL, M.D.
Chairman, Department of Orthopaedics
The Brigham and Women's Hospital
Boston, MA, USA

ALFRED J. TRIA, M.D.
Clinical Professor of Orthopaedic Surgery
Robert Wood Johnson Medical School
Orthopaedic Center of New Jersey
Somerset, NJ, USA

KELLY G. VINCE, M.D.
Associate Professor
Department of Orthopaedics
University of Louisville
Louisville, KY, USA

PETER WALKER, PH.D.
Professor and Director of Biomedical Engineering
The Cooper Union for the Advancement of Science
   and Art
New York, NY, USA

GEOFFREY H. WESTRICH, M.D.
The Hospital for Special Surgery
New York, NY, USA

LEO A. WHITESIDE, M.D.
Director, Biomechanical Research Laboratory
Missouri Bone and Joint Center
Barnes-Jewish West County Hospital
St. Louis, MO, USA

RUSSELL E. WINDSOR, M.D.
The Hospital for Special Surgery
New York, NY, USA

DAVID J. YASGUR, M.D.
Katonah Medical Group
Katonah, NY, USA

SECTION 1
Preoperative Planning

CHAPTER 1
Indications and Patient Selection

Steven F. Harwin

INTRODUCTION: HISTORICAL AND AGE CONSIDERATIONS

Total knee arthroplasty has become a highly successful joint reconstruction procedure. Surgical outcomes, patient satisfaction, and implant survival have improved steadily since its inception and the operation has become widely accepted to afford relief of pain, restoration of range of motion and function.[1-9] In earlier years of total knee arthroplasty, the operation was offered usually to an older age group whose activity level was relatively sedentary.[10,11] It has now been shown that total knee arthroplasty is effective and durable in the younger, more active patient,[12-17] as well as in the elderly population.

Although arthroplasty has been shown to be successful in the younger population, ideally the more suitable patient will be more than 60 years of age so that an uncomplicated arthroplasty would more than likely last for the rest of the patient's life. Survivorship for cemented total knee arthroplasty ranges between 91% and 99% at 10 years[1,5] and between 91% and 96% at 15 years.[1,6] Patients are now living longer and remaining physically active well into their eighth, ninth, and even tenth decades. We have all been made aware of the importance and benefits of daily physical activity as it relates to cardiovascular and mental health. Disabling arthritis of the knee can prevent participation in these activities and can preclude patients from enjoying their leisure time and retirement years. Education of family practitioners and internists has also resulted in patients being referred at earlier stages, rather than as a "last resort." Patients are making decisions to have joint arthroplasty based on the quality of their life coupled with improved surgical and anesthetic techniques.

INDICATIONS: SYMPTOMATOLOGY AND DISEASE PROCESS

The prime indications for total knee arthroplasty (TKA) still are severe pain and functional disability. Relative indications include deformity, instability, and loss of motion. Diagnoses associated with the above problems and for which TKA has been successfully performed include osteoarthritis, rheumatoid arthritis, inflammatory arthritis, post-traumatic arthritis, osteonecrosis, arthritis associated with polio, Parkinson's disease, hemophilia, and other disabling disorders including those associated with tumors and fractures.[1-9,11,20,21,24-29] In special situations, TKA may be performed to salvage a knee with neuropathic arthropathy[30] or even to restore motion to a previously arthrodesed knee.[31] These indications, however, remain controversial and should be considered relative contraindications. Although total knee arthroplasty has been successfully performed in the face of extensor mechanism insufficiency by using complex allograft reconstructions,[31] this indication also remains controversial and no long-term studies are as yet reported.

CONTRAINDICATIONS

Patients with prior infection of the knee joint or its adjacent metaphyseal regions of the femur or tibia may be considered for TKA if sufficient time has elapsed and the disease process is arrested and "cured."[33] Certainly the risk of recurrence of the infection process must be considered. Recent, or active sepsis remains an absolute contraindication to TKA. Workup to exclude either local or systemic active infection must be carried out prior to consideration of arthroplasty. If any doubt exists about the possibility of acute inflammation, two-stage arthroplasty should be considered. In this situation, the initial stage consists of joint debridement and osteotomy of the distal femur and proximal tibia. An antibiotic impregnated spacer is inserted. Frozen sections are taken at the time of surgery to rule out any acute inflammation and cultures are sent to Pathology. If final cultures are negative, then second stage implant arthroplasty can be considered.

Other absolute contraindications to TKA include inadequate soft tissue coverage of the knee joint with or without associated poor vascularity. In some cases, joint salvage may be obtained by the use of soft tissue expanders.[34] Coverage with rotational or muscle pedicle flaps can also be considered to provide soft tissue coverage.[35] Those patients with poor limb perfusion and severe peripheral vascular disease are also not candidates for joint arthroplasty.

BENEFITS, RISKS, ALTERNATIVES, CAVEATS, AND INFORMED CONSENT

All patients considering total joint arthroplasty must be aware of the benefits, risks, and alternatives to the proposed procedure. The personal experience of the operating surgeon, longevity studies, and survivorship predictions of the implant used should be discussed. Particular mention should be made of the clinical history and performance record of the implant suggested. While often grouped into broad categories such as "cruciate retaining" or "posteriorly stabilized" implants, not all implants in these categories perform alike. It is important for surgeons to share their experience with a particular implant in order to give their patients a reasonable expectation of what result can typically be expected. The recuperative and rehabilitation process should be explained to the patient as well as the normal postoperative course and milestones. Discussion of the so-called "critical pathways" helps to improve the patient's understanding of their treatment. No amount of careful surgery will satisfy a patient who has unrealistic expectations or psychological impairment. Patients who can derive secondary gain either financially or emotionally from continued disability should be screened very carefully including an evaluation by a mental health specialist if necessary.[36]

Patients should be told of the reasonable expectation for correction of deformity and the predicted range of motion they can expect based upon the etiology of their condition, the deformity present, and the preoperative range of motion.

Patients should also be advised of known predictors of adverse outcomes. Patients with rheumatoid arthritis, diabetes, and those with multiple prior joint operations, severe deformities, and limited range of motion can be expected to have a higher incidence of complications, infection, and stiffness.[33,37,38] Patients who are obese are often told to put off joint arthroplasty, but statistically they do not seem to have any significant adverse outcomes.[39] It has been my experience that it is virtually impossible for a patient who is obese to lose any appreciable weight with severely arthritic knees because of the limitations it places on them in terms of exercising to supplement a dietary weight loss program.

Specific surgical complications referable to the total knee arthroplasty include failure or re-operation due to infection, wear, loosening, instability, fracture, implant breakage, dislocation, wound healing difficulties, or stiffness requiring manipulation. Also included should be more rare occurrences such as neurovascular compromise or reflex sympathetic dystrophy. Patients should be counseled about the need for prophylactic antibiotic protection to ensure that the joint does not become secondarily infected from subsequent intercurrent infections.

Medical complications including anesthesia complications, cardiovascular compromise, deep vein thrombosis, pulmonary embolus, urinary tract dysfunction, and blood-related issues should be discussed. The issue of autologous blood donation and the use of blood recovery drains should be addressed. Preoperative evaluation by a family doctor, internist, and/or cardiologist is essential.

If the patient has bilateral disease, the issue of performing both arthroplasties either sequentially or simultaneously should be discussed. Although an increase in the incidence of fat emboli has been reported,[40] others report no increase in intraoperative or perioperative complications.[41] The use of intramedullary instrumentation on both the femur and the tibia has been implicated in significant changes in the hematologic and hemodynamic values after arthroplasty.[42] In my own practice, bilateral simultaneous knee arthroplasty has been successfully accomplished on a routine basis. However, great care is taken to over drill the entry holes into the femur and tibia and the medullary contents are decompressed with suction. Fluted rods are used routinely. Bilateral knee arthroplasties should be considered when deformity is severe (especially flexion) and when not performing the arthroplasty on the other side would compromise the unilateral result.

Full disclosure should be given to the patient about the entire process including preoperative preparation, hospitalization, and recovery. In the current climate of shortened hospitalization and reduced length of stay, patients must know when they can expect to be discharged and early Social Service intervention is recommended. At the Beth Israel Medical Center, a presurgical class describing the entire process is mandatory for all patients undergoing joint arthroplasty. We have found a high degree of patient approval and a shorter length of stay after instituting this program.

Even though it may seem intuitively obvious, it must also be pointed out that the mere presence of gonarthrosis of the knee joint is not in and of itself an indication to proceed with total knee arthroplasty surgery. Alternatives such as medical management, rehabilitation therapy, and lifestyle alteration should be considered and discussed. Steroid injection in the elderly or infirm patient offers a temporizing palliative treatment that is variable in its length of relief. Surgical options such as arthroscopic joint debridement and tibial or femoral osteotomy should also be discussed if appropriate. These procedures must be excluded as choices before proceeding with TKA. Even though arthrodesis of the knee has traditionally been offered as a primary treatment option for gonarthrosis of the knee,[43] this is rarely offered or accepted by the patient.

EXAMINATION AND PATIENT ASSESSMENT

Regarding the patient's presenting complaints, it is worthwhile to take a lesson from our "sister" medical speciality of Radiology. Radiologists traditionally approach the reading of a radiograph by specifically ignoring, initially, the primary area of concern. Put another way, the radiologist will look at the corners and periphery of the radiograph before concentrating on its center. In this way, the likelihood of missing an associated lesion is diminished. We, as orthopedic surgeons, can do well to follow this example both radiographically and clinically. Even though almost all patients presenting for TKA will complain of pain, limp, deformity, swelling, and decreased range of motion related to the knee, it is important for us to rule out other causes that may contribute to, or even be uncovered as, the primary cause of this particular patient's disability. Conditions related to the spine, hip, and vascular systems must be addressed and ruled out as significant contributors. The time-honored teaching of examining the joint above and the joint below the one of concern certainly applies here. It is not uncommon for patients to have concomitant ipsilateral hip pathology or spinal disease. Although it may not change what we need to do for the knee, it behooves us to have this information *before* knee surgery and to assess its individual contribution to the patient's presenting complaints. The mere confirmation of arthritis of the knee based on clinical exam and radiographs may still lead us badly astray unless the above principles are followed.

GENERAL MEDICAL HISTORY

Obtaining a full medical history is essential not only to help in the planning of surgery, but also in the anticipation of the patient's postoperative care. Patients who are chronically ill or debilitated often present in poor nutritional health. These patients often have low albumin levels, which can cause difficulty with wound healing.[44,45] We must try to elicit a history of any infectious process, either systemic or cutaneous. Conditions such as diabetes mellitus, gout, rheumatoid arthritis, peptic ulcers, bleeding disorders, deep venous thrombosis, pulmonary embolus, peripheral vascular disease, skin ulcerations, and psoriasis can all affect the patient's outcome.[26,27,29,33,37] Patients with rheumatoid arthritis do have an increased incidence of complications, but it is unclear whether it is due to the disease process itself or due to the fact that many of these patients have taken or are taking steroids at the time of their surgery.

Additionally, a history of vascular insufficiency or bypass surgery of the extremity may preclude surgery itself or the use of a tourniquet during the procedure. Patients with a history of stroke or polio may exhibit circumstances such as instability or deformity that require a more constrained type of implant.[25] Patients with occult neuropathia, which is unrecognized, can also be at risk for complications or subsequent failure.[30]

Also essential is to note any prior difficulties with anesthesia. Patients with conditions such as rheumatoid arthritis or ankylosing spondylitis may require a formal anesthesia consultation prior to surgery in order to ensure the ability to insert an epidural catheter or to accomplish spinal anesthesia. In addition, patients with these conditions often have involvement of the mandible, which, in rare circumstances, may preclude the insertion of an endotracheal tube. Cervical instability must be ruled out with appropriate examination and radiographs in order to allow for uneventful intubation if this type of anesthesia is contemplated.

Eliciting a history of old fractures, rickets, renal osteodystrophy, femoral or tibial osteotomy, and other similar conditions is important because it may contribute to an associated extra-articular deformity that may need to be taken into account at the time of knee arthroplasty. A history of an ipsilateral total hip arthroplasty or an obliterated medullary canal may preclude the use of intramedullary instrumentation.

The patient's social history, including the family situation, is of great importance in terms of postoperative care and rehabilitation. Also, of importance, is whether or not the knee condition is work related, or related to any sort of accident in which litigation is pending. Patients who present with a history of many operations, but a paucity of radiographic and clinical findings, may have underlying psychological difficulties (such as Munchausen syndrome), which may require workup or evaluation prior to performing total knee arthroplasty.[36]

GENERAL PHYSICAL EXAMINATION

The busy orthopedic surgeon will commonly perform only a "regional" examination of the joint about which the patient is complaining. When the joint is the knee, a brief but satisfactory examination of the spine, hip, ankle, and foot is appropriate and necessary to rule out any associated disorders.

The patient's gait is observed and the type is recorded: normal, antalgic, varus/valgus attitude, with or without thrust, with or without a gluteal (Trendelenburg) component to it. Inspection is made for adaptive changes in the foot and ankle, such as a plano-valgus deformity commonly seen in rheumatoid arthritis. The skin of the extremity is scanned for prior incisions, old infections, skin grafts, poor or atrophied subcutaneous tissue, stasis changes, varicosities, chronic cellulitis, or any active infection or ulcer especially in the foot or toes. Pulses, skin temperature, proprioception, and vibratory senses are noted. The thigh and calf is inspected and any atrophy is noted. Even though this may be common in knee pathology, it may also be indicative of hip pathology, long-standing disuse, or spinal or neuromuscular disease. It may also be indicative of a prior surgery that the patient may not remember, especially if they are quite elderly. Incisions may have faded and can easily be missed if not searched for.

Alignment of both lower extremities is observed for obvious extra-articular deformities. Particular attention should be given to the patient mounting and dismounting the examination table, which can simulate stair climbing. In addition, the patient should be observed arising from and sitting down in a chair in the examining room.

THE KNEE EXAM

The appearance of the knee must be thoroughly examined. Any loss of the normal parapatellar contours or those of the distal thigh and proximal tibia must be noted. Swelling can be due to chronic long-standing deformity with gonarthrosis as well as from an effusion or chronic synovial thickening. Posteriorly, it is not uncommon to observe a prominent popliteal cyst. Patients often ask whether or not knee arthroplasty will take away the swelling that they have had. They must be counseled that swelling can persist for up to 6 to 12 months postoperatively and adaptive changes in their limb could account for permanent swelling compared to a "normal" knee.

Old incisions may not be readily observed. The patient must be asked about prior surgery and careful attention must be given in order to find them. Old short or long medial and lateral parapatellar incisions are not uncommon and, if faded, can be missed with disastrous consequences if a slough occurs.

Active and passive range of motion is recorded as well as the supine and standing leg alignment and deformity. Fixed and flexible deformities are noted as well as excessive laxity and hyperextension. Crepitation felt and heard during these maneuvers is noted.

Range of motion is best documented using a goniometer. Visual estimates are often inaccurate. Because the most important predictor of postoperative range of motion is that of the preoperative range of motion, the importance of this step cannot be overemphasized.

Stability of the knee is then assessed. The medial and lateral ligament complexes are tested in as much extension as possible and then in approximately 30 degrees of flexion. Exact quantification of instability is difficult. It may be characterized as mild, moderate, or severe and can be expressed in units of either millimeters or degrees of displacement: mild (0–5), moderate (5–10), or severe (>10). The softness or firmness of the endpoint should be noted. Lachman's test and anterior drawer sign are also noted as well as the presence or absence of a posterior sag. Although anterior cruciate ligament insufficiency is not uncommon, complete absence or insufficiency of the posterior cruciate ligament is rare except in post-traumatic cases or those with neuromuscular disease. When using the Knee Society rating, varus/valgus and medial-lateral instability is recorded as less than 5 degrees, 6 to 9 degrees, and 10 to 14 degrees, or greater. Anteroposterior stability is graded as less than 5 mm, 5 to 10 mm, or greater than 10 mm.

Large angular deformities with associated fixed flexion suggest significant ligament shortening on the concave side with concomitant stretching or lengthening on the convex side along with a contracture of the posterior cruciate ligament. Valgus deformities greater than 20 degrees may require extensive release with potential injury to the peroneal nerve or vascular structures. Therefore, the function of the peroneal nerve and the distal pulses must be checked thoroughly preoperatively.

It is important to note that what may feel like "ligamentous laxity" may indeed be secondary to a bony defect rather than from stretching of the ligament. This is commonly seen following lateral tibial plateau fractures.

The extensor mechanism is specifically examined for tone, strength, and competency. The patella is thoroughly inspected. The mobility of the patella, or lack thereof, is important to note. A patella that is virtually immobile may indicate difficulties in exposure and range of motion. A laterally displaced or dislocated patella alerts the surgeon to possible tracking problems, which can be addressed in preparation for the surgery by using, for example, less of a valgus cut on the femur.

Any effusion or synovial thickening is noted. Joint line or bursal tenderness is likewise noted. The posterior structures are examined and, if present, the size of the popliteal cyst is noted.

RADIOGRAPHS

After taking a history and performing a physical examination, a determination is made about the type of radiographs required. For total knee arthroplasty, at the

Beth Israel Medical Center, our standard protocol includes a standing anteroposterior view of both knees in extension, a standing posteroanterior view of both knees in 45 degrees of flexion, a lateral view, and a Merchant patellar view at 30° of flexion. Standing lateral radiographs are taken only in special circumstances. Often complete collapse of a joint compartment can only be appreciated on the standing P-A flexed knee views. It is not uncommon for a patient to present to the office for arthroscopic surgery of a "mildly" arthritic knee based upon supine non-weight-bearing radiographs. Once standing radiographs are taken, complete collapse of the joint space can be demonstrated and this patient could be better served by a joint arthroplasty.

A long (52-inch) radiograph of the hips, knees, and ankles on a single cassette will rule out extra-articular deformity and allow for calculation of the appropriate mechanical and femoral axes. It is not uncommon to see a prior total hip arthroplasty, an especially tight medullary canal, or an obstructed canal from prior fracture or prior surgery.

Radiographs should be taken at a standardized distance to allow for preoperative templating using standard total knee system templates. Most total knee systems use templates that take into account from 10% to 20% magnification.

PREPARATION FOR SURGERY

Combining the knowledge gained from our history, physical examination, and radiographic analysis we will be able to plan properly for all eventualities in the operating room. We must have available a full range of implants to address all technical problems from the simplest primary case to the most complex revision and to allow for changeover to any one of these implants depending on the intraoperative need. For example, we must have both intramedullary and extramedullary alignment guides available to compensate for extra-articular deformities and/or medullary compromise. In addition, a fully constrained implant should be available with the ability to add on modular augmentations to allow for deficient ligaments and bone stock.

PATIENT SELF-ASSESSMENT

In view of the importance now placed on "outcomes" as opposed to "results," the surgeon should consider having the patient complete a validated self-assessment evaluation for pain and function according to a standardized system. These instruments include the WOMAC and the SF-36 Form. The traditional "results-oriented" instruments such as the Knee Society rating and the Hospital for Special Surgery rating should be considered as well.

In summary, in order to achieve satisfactory outcomes for both the patient and surgeon, reconstructive surgery must be properly planned with regard and insight into the potential complications caused by medical, neurological, vascular, soft tissue, or emotional problems.

References

1. Scuderi GR, Insall JN, Windsor RE, Moran MC. Survivorship of cemented knee replacements. *J Bone Joint Surg Br.* 1989; 71B:798–803.
2. Ritter MA, Campbell E, Faris PM, Keating EM. Long term survival analysis of posterior cruciate condylar total knee arthroplasty: a ten year evaluation. *Journal of Arthroplasty.* 1989; 4:293–296.
3. Cobb AC, Ewald FC, Wright J, Sledge CB. The kinematic knee: survivorship analysis of 1943 knees. *J Bone Joint Surg.* 1990; 72B:532.
4. Stern SH, Insall JN. Posteriorly stabilized results after follow-up of nine years. *J Bone Joint Surg.* August 1992; 74A:980–986.
5. Ranawat CS, Flynn WF Jr, Saddler S, Hansraj KK, Maynard MJ. Long term results of the total condylar knee arthroplasty: a fifteen year survivorship study. *Clin Orthop.* 1993; 286:94–102.
6. Ritter MA, Herbst SA, Keating EM, Faris PM, Meding JB. Long term survival analysis of a posterior cruciate retaining total condylar knee arthroplasty. *Clin Orthop.* 1994; 309:136–145.
7. Malkani AL, Rand JA, Bryan RS, Wallrichs SL. Total knee arthroplasty with the kinematic condylar prosthesis. *J Bone Joint Surg.* March 1995; 77A; 423–431.
8. Emmerson KP, Moran CJ, Pinder IM. Survivorship analysis of the kinematic stabilizer total knee replacement: a 10 to 14 year follow-up. *J Bone Joint Surg.* May 1996; 78B(3): 441–445.
9. Weir DJ, Moran CG, Pinder IM. Kinematic condylar total knee arthroplasty: fourteen year survivorship analysis of 208 consecutive cases. *J Bone Joint Surg.* 1996; 78B(6):907–911.
10. Insall JN, Binazzi R, Soudry M, Mestriner LA. Total knee arthroplasty. *Clin Orthop.* 1985; 192:13–22.
11. Rand JA, Ilstrup DM. Survivorship analysis of total knee arthroplasty. Cumulative rates of survival of 9200 total knee arthroplasties. *J Bone Joint Surg.* March 1991; 73-A:397–409.
12. Diduch DR, Insall JN, Scott WN, Scuderi GR, Font-Rodrigues D. Total knee replacement in young, active patients. *J Bone Joint Surg.* April 1997; 79A:571–582.
13. Ewald F, Christie MJ. Results of cemented total knee replacement in young patients. *Orthop Trans.* 1987; 11:442.
14. Hungerford DS, Krackow KA, Kenna RV. Cementless total knee replacement in patients 50 years old and under. *Orthop Clin North Am.* 1989; 20:131–145.
15. Stern SH, Bowen MK, Insall JN, Scuderi GR. Cemented total knee arthroplasty for gonarthrosis in patients 55 years old or younger. *Clin Orthop.* 1990; 260:124–129.

16. Stuart MJ, Rand JA. Total knee arthroplasty in the young adult. *Orthop Trans.* 1987; 11:441–442.
17. Stulberg SD. Bi/tri-compartmental degenerative knee disease in the young patient. *Orthopedics.* 1995; 18:899–901.
18. L'Insalata JL, Stern SH, Insall JN. Total knee arthroplasty in elderly patients: comparison of tibial component designs. *J Arthro.* 1992; 7(3):261–266.
19. Colizza WA, Insall JN, Scuderi GR. The posterior stabilized total knee prosthesis. Assessment of polyethylene damage and osteolysis after a ten-year minimum follow-up. *J Bone Joint Surg.* November 1995; 77A:1713–1720.
20. Ewald FC, Jacobs MA, Miegel RE, Walker PS, Poss R, Sledge CB. Kinematic total knee replacement. *J Bone Joint Surg.* September 1984; 66-A:1032–1040.
21. Goldberg VM, Figgie MP, Figgie HE III, Heiple KG, Sobel M. Use of a total condylar knee prosthesis for treatment of osteoarthritis and rheumatoid arthritis. Long term results. *J Bone Joint Surg.* July 1988; 70-A:802–811.
22. Insall JN, Kelly M. The total condylar prosthesis. *Clin Orthop.* 1986; 205:43–48.
23. Insall JN, Hood RW, Flawn LB, Sullivan DJ. The total condylar knee prosthesis in gonarthrosis. A five to nine year follow-up of the first one hundred consecutive replacements. *J Bone Joint Surg.* June 1983; 65-A:619–628.
24. Horowitz SM, Lane JM, Otis JC. Prosthetic arthroplasty of the knee after resection of a sarcoma in the proximal end of the tibia. *J Bone Joint Surg.* 1991; 73A(2):286–293.
25. Patterson BM, Insall JN. Surgical management of patients with poliomyelitis. *J Arthro.* 1992 (suppl 2):419–426.
26. Stern SH, Insall JN, Windsor RE, et al. Total knee arthroplasty in patients with psoriasis. *Clin Orthop.* 1989; (24):108–110.
27. Vince KG, Insall JN, Bannerman CE. Total knee arthroplasty in patients with Parkinson's disease. *J Bone Joint Surg Br.* 1989; 1(1):51–54.
28. Bell KM, Johnstone AJ, Court-Brown CM, et al. Primary knee arthroplasty for distal femoral fractures in elderly patients. *J Bone Joint Surg.* 1992; 74B(3):400–402.
29. Figgie MP, Goldberg VM, Figgie HE, et al. Total knee arthroplasty for the treatment of chronic hemophilic arthropathy. *Clin Orthop.* 1989 (248):98.
30. Soudry M, Binazzi R, Johanson NA, et al. Total knee arthroplasty in Charcot and Charcot-like joints. *Clin Orthop.* 1986; 208:199–204.
31. Aglietti P, Windsor RE, Buzzi R, et al. Arthroplasty for the stiff or ankylosed knee. *J Arthro.* 1989; 4(1):1–5.
32. Harwin SF, Stein AJ, Stern RE. Extensor mechanism allograft with revision total knee arthroplasty complications in orthopedics. 11/93 8(4):79–82.
33. Jerry GJ, Rand JA, Ilstrup D. Old sepsis prior to total knee arthroplasty. *Clin Orthop.* 1988; (23):135.
34. Craig SM. Soft tissue considerations in the failed total knee arthroplasty. In: Scott WN, ed. *The Knee.* St. Louis, Mo: Mosby; 1994:1279–1295.
35. Gerwin M, Rothaus KO, Windsor RE, et al. Gastrocnemius muscle flap coverage of exposed or infected knee prosthesis. *Clin Orthop.* 1993; (286):64–70.
36. Sharma L, Sinacore J, Daugherty C, et al. Prognostic factors for functional outcome of total knee replacement: a prospective study. *J Gerontol.* 1996; 51(4):152–157.
37. England SP, Stern SH, Insall JN, et al. Total knee arthroplasty in diabetes mellitus. *Clin Orthop.* 1990; (260):130–134.
38. Parsley BS, Engle GA, Dwyer KA. Preoperative flexion. Does it influence postoperative flexion after total knee arthroplasty. *Clin Orthop.* 1992; (275):204–210.
39. Stern SH, Insall JN. Total knee arthroplasty in obese patients. *J Bone Joint Surg.* 1990; 72(9):1400–1404.
40. Dorr LD, Merkel C, Mellman MF, et al. Fat emboli in total knee arthroplasty: predictive factors for neurologic manifestations. *Clin Orthop.* 1989; 248:112–118.
41. Jankiewicz JJ, Sculco TP, Ranawat CS, et al. One stage versus two stage bilateral total knee arthroplasty. *Clin Orthop.* 1994; 309:94–101.
42. Stern SH, Sharrock N, Kahn R, et al. Hematologic and circulatory changes associated with total knee arthroplasty surgical instrumentation. *Clin Orthop.* 1994; 299;179–189.
43. Frymoyer J, Hoaglund F. The role of arthrodesis in reconstruction of the knee. *Clin Orthop.* 1974; (101):82.
44. Dickhaut SC, DeLee JC, Page CP. Nutritional status: predicting wound healing after amputation. *J Bone Joint Surg.* 1984; 661A:71–75.
45. Ecker MM, Lotke P. Postoperative care of the total knee patient. *Orthop Clin North Am.* 1989; (20):55–62.

CHAPTER 2
Preoperative Radiographic Assessment

Kevin R. Math and Giles R. Scuderi

Preoperative assessment of the knee prior to total knee arthroplasty primarily involves conventional radiographs; advanced imaging modalities such as MRI, CT, and nuclear imaging play an ancillary role in imaging these patients, and are sometimes helpful in clarifying equivocal plain film findings or for specific pathological conditions such as osteonecrosis.

STANDARD RADIOGRAPHIC VIEWS

AP View

For the evaluation of arthritic knees, the AP view is routinely performed with the patient standing (weight bearing) (Fig. 2.1). The radiographic joint space reflects the thickness of the articular cartilage, and the weight-bearing study provides a more accurate estimate of the presence and degree of cartilage thinning than a non-weight-bearing study[1] (Fig. 2.2). The X-ray beam is directed in an anteroposterior direction; angling the beam 5 to 7 degrees cephalad provides optimal visualization of the joint space. According to the classic paper by Ahlback,[2] the joint space on the weight-bearing AP film should be >3 mm or within 50% of the joint space of the contralateral knee.

The knee is normally in 7 degrees of valgus alignment on an AP view, and the lateral joint space is wider than the medial joint space. The articular surfaces of the medial and lateral joint compartments, and the presence of associated osteophytes and subchondral bony changes at the femoro-tibial joint are assessed to best advantage on this view.

Lateral View

This view is obtained on the radiography table with the patient lying on the imaged side (Fig. 2.3). By convention, the knee is flexed 30 degrees with the lateral aspect of the knee against the X-ray film cassette. The X-ray beam is directed at a 90-degree angle to the film; some advocate cephalad angulation of 5 degrees to best superimpose the femoral condyles. Patellar height is optimally assessed on the lateral view, and the suprapatellar region should be evaluated for the presence of a joint effusion and/or intra-articular loose bodies.

Regarding patellar height, several methods of assessment have been described; however, the Insall-Salvati method remains the most widely used[3,4] (Fig. 2.4). In their series, Insall and Salvati found that the average ratio of the length of the patellar tendon (LT) divided by the greatest diagonal length of the patella (LP) should equal 1.02 ± 0.2. In patella alta, the patella is relatively high in position (LT/LP > 1.2), and in patella baja the patella is relatively low (LT/LP < 0.8). The patellofemoral joint can be visualized on the lateral view; however, the alignment and articular surfaces at this joint are best evaluated on a tangential axial (Merchant) view.

Merchant View

The Merchant view[5] is the most widely used tangential axial view of the patella. The patient lies in the supine position on the radiography table, and the knees are flexed 45 degrees, resting on a firm surface (Fig. 2.5). Technically adequate reproducible Merchant images are best obtained using a homemade or commercially available Merchant apparatus (Mountain View, California); the degree of flexion on this apparatus can be fixed at 45 degrees or can be adjustable. The film cassette rests on the patient's shins and the beam is directed at an angle 30 degrees from the vertical, exposing both knees simultaneously.

This view provides the most optimal assessment of patellofemoral alignment, joint space, and articular surfaces. The axial tangential view is preferred for evalua-

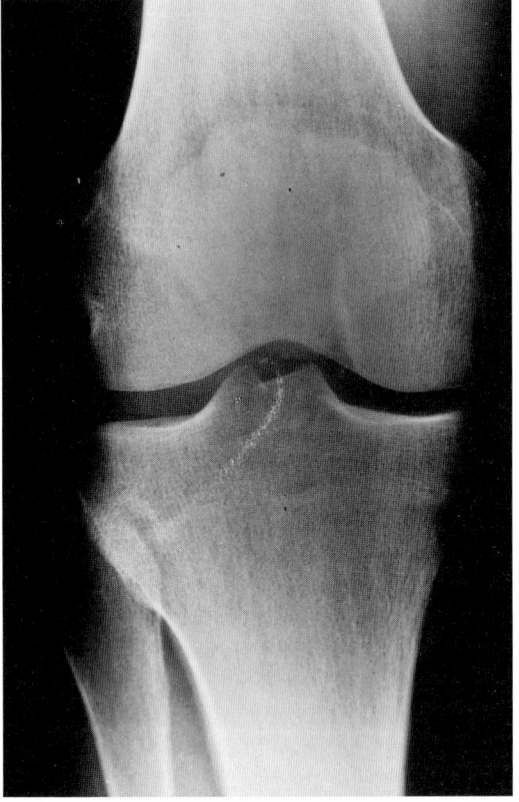

Figure 2.1. AP Knee: The lateral joint compartment is normally slightly wider than the medial compartment.

tion of patellofemoral osteoarthritis.[6] Several other tangential axial techniques have been described, including the Settegast, Hughston, and Laurin methods.[4]

SUPPLEMENTAL RADIOGRAPHIC VIEWS

Tunnel (Intercondylar Fossa) View

Also known as the "notch" view, this view is obtained with the knee flexed 45 degrees and the X-ray beam directed posteroanterior (Fig. 2.6).[7,8] The patient is placed in the prone position on the radiography table and the beam is directed obliquely 45 degrees to the horizontal. This view is ideal for imaging the posterior aspect of the intercondylar notch, and therefore is highly useful when evaluating younger patients with suspected osteochondritis dissecans or intra-articular loose bodies (Fig. 2.7). Also, osteophytes projecting into the intercondylar notch from the inner aspect of the femoral condyles can be seen to better advantage on the tunnel view than on the standard AP view.

Semiflexed Weight-Bearing AP View (Modified Tunnel)

This view can be helpful in detecting joint-space narrowing (cartilage thinning) that may be absent or underestimated on the standard AP view, obtained with

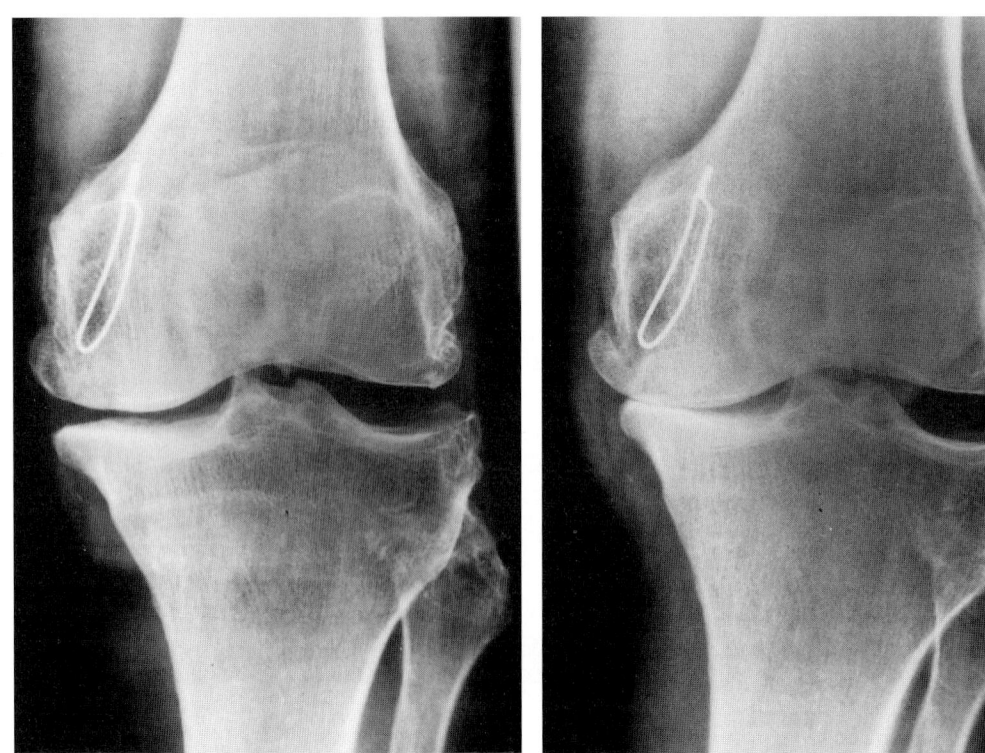

Figure 2.2. (A) AP Knee Supine View and (B) AP Knee Weight-Bearing View: The marked medial compartment joint-space narrowing is greater on the weight-bearing view, more accurately reflecting the severity of degenerative joint disease.

2. Preoperative Radiographic Assessment

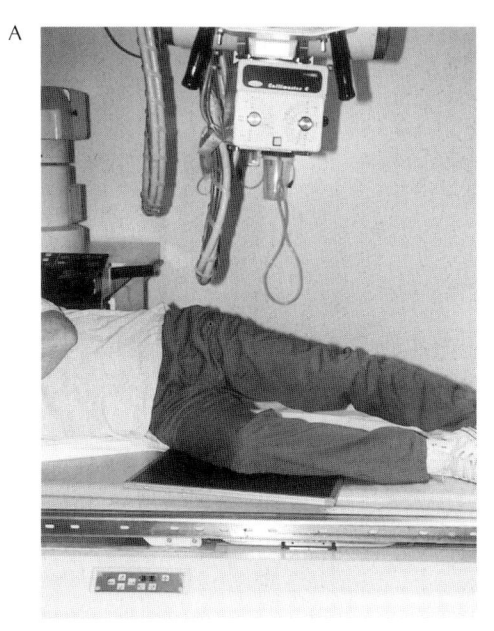

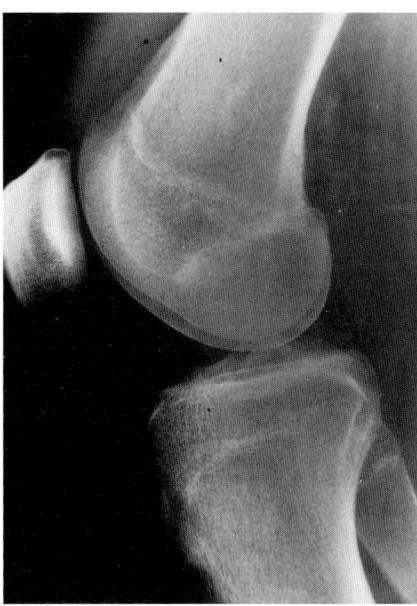

Figure 2.3. Lateral View: (A) The patient lies on the imaged side with the film underlying the lateral aspect of the knee. (B) The femoral condyles should be superimposed on a technically adequate true lateral view.

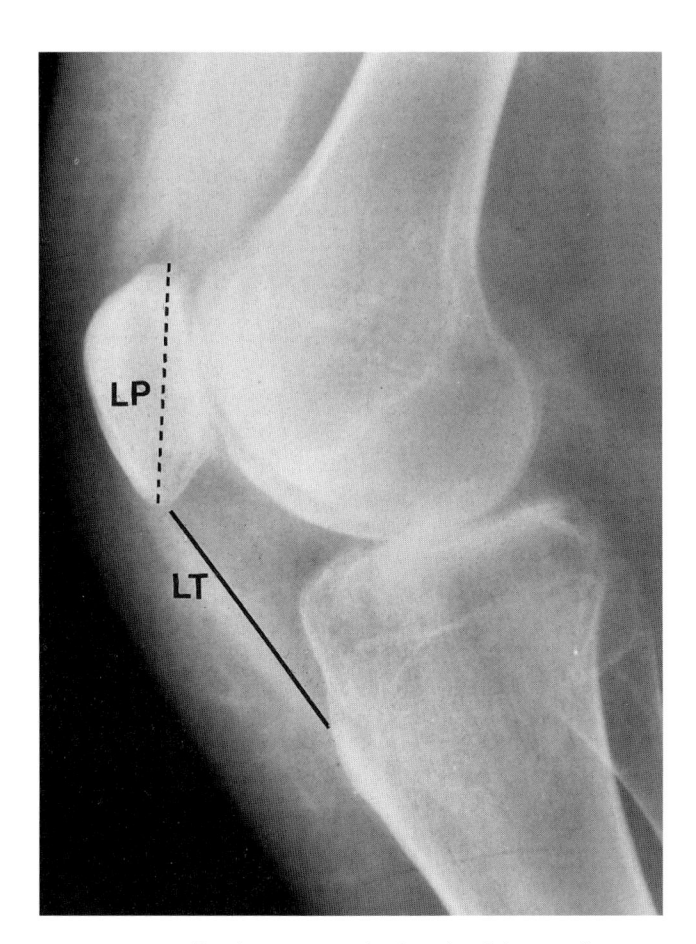

Figure 2.4. Insall-Salvati Ratio: The length of the patellar tendon (LT) and greatest diagonal length of the patella (LP) should be almost equal.

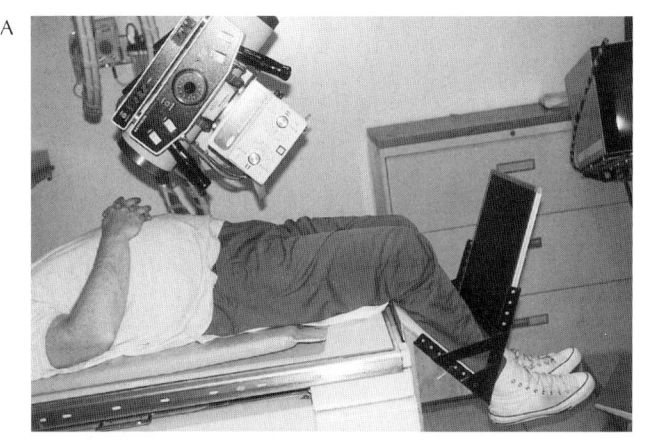

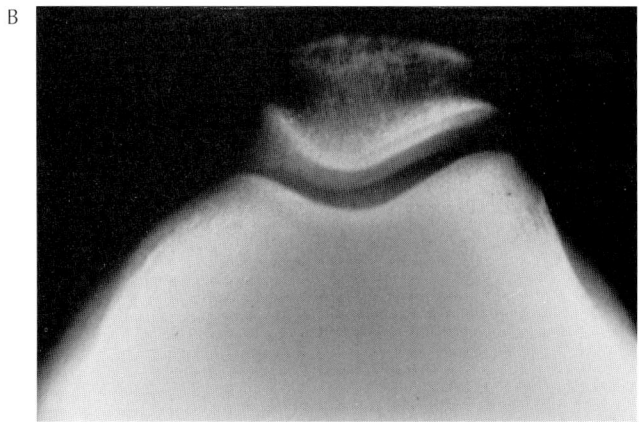

Figure 2.5. Merchant View: (A) The lower legs rest on an angled platform, and the film cassette is placed on the anterior shins. Note the tube angled inferiorly, tangent to the patellofemoral joints. (B) The medial facet of the patella is usually shorter and more steeply angled than the lateral facet.

AP.[9] The rationale for these views is based on the fact that when the knee is semiflexed, the posterior weight-bearing surfaces at the femoro-tibial joint are brought into apposition; those patients with more extensive cartilage thinning posteriorly will exhibit a greater degree of joint-space narrowing on this view (Fig. 2.9). Indeed up to 22% of patients with joint-space narrowing on the semiflexed view will have a normal appearing joint space on the standard AP image.[10] This view is most helpful when arthritic clinical symptoms are disproportionate to the degree of joint-space narrowing on the AP weight-bearing view, and is done routinely at some centers.

Standing 52-Inch Cassette ("Three Joint View")

A standing AP view of the lower extremities (including the hips and ankles) is helpful preoperatively for assessing the overall alignment (mechanical axis) of the lower extremity (Fig. 2.10). The 52-inch cassette allows accurate depiction of the degree of varus or valgus alignment at both knees, the relative leg length, and assesses for the presence of important extra-articular deformities, as may be seen in patients with prior trauma or Paget's disease. This view also provides limited assessment of the integrity of the hip and ankle joints, and allows detection of occasional incidentally discovered lesions in the femur or tibia.

DEGENERATIVE JOINT DISEASE

Degenerative joint disease (DJD) of the knee is the most common condition necessitating total knee arthroplasty. Radiographic findings of DJD are usually clearly evident at the time of presentation and include cartilage loss (joint-space narrowing), subchondral sclerosis and cyst formation, and osteophyte formation[2] (Fig. 2.11). The joint compartments are involved with the following frequency: medial > patellofemoral > lateral.

Conventional radiographs, while usually adequate for preoperative assessment of advanced arthritic knees may underestimate the severity and extent of DJD. Plain film findings of DJD occur late and often do not correlate with the patient's symptoms.[13,14] Furthermore, plain films fail to reveal the symptomatic synovitis and other soft tissue changes that may result in symptoms without significant bony changes.[13] This represents an important diagnostic limitation of plain films for those patients who require prompt medical treatment and clinical follow-up.

The radionuclide bone scan can be helpful for showing the typical increased uptake present at arthritic joints, especially when conventional radiographs are

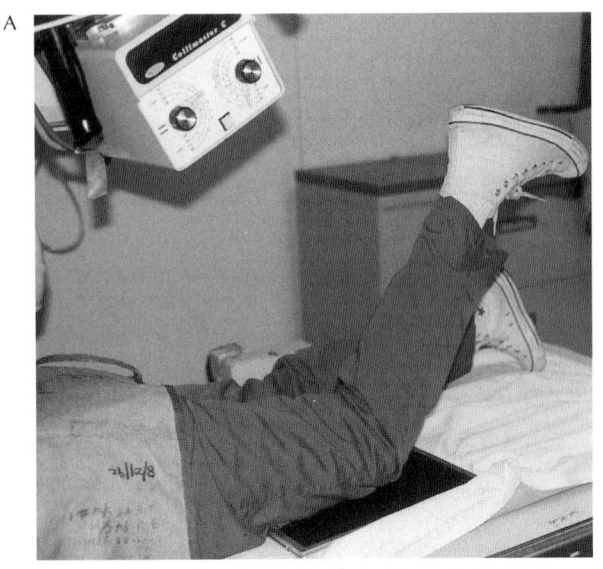

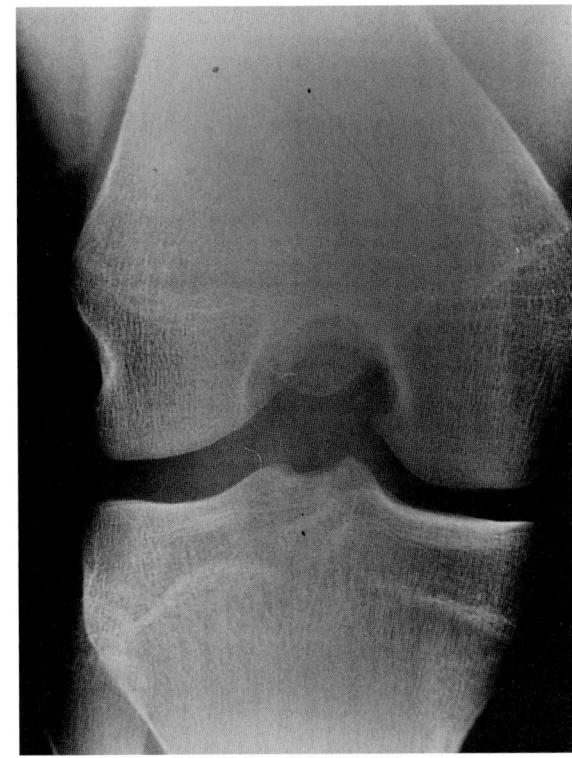

Figure 2.6. Tunnel View: (A) The knee is flexed 45 degrees and the tube is angled tangent to the joint line. (B) The intercondylar notch is optimally seen on this view. The lower patella is superimposed over the superior aspect of the notch.

the knee fully extended.[9–12] The knee is flexed approximately 45 degrees in the standing position, and the X-ray beam passes from anterior to posterior[10,12] (Fig. 2.8). One can also perform this view with the knee flexed up to 30 degrees in an attempt to bring the tibial plateau parallel to the floor and the beam passing PA rather than

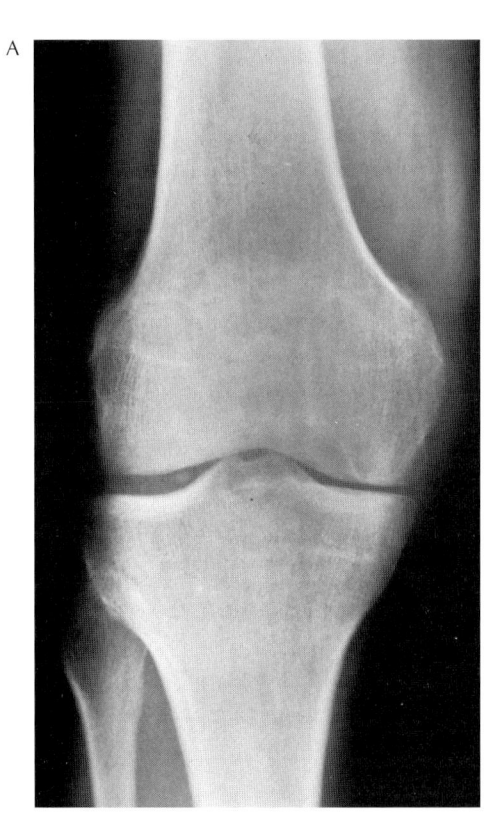

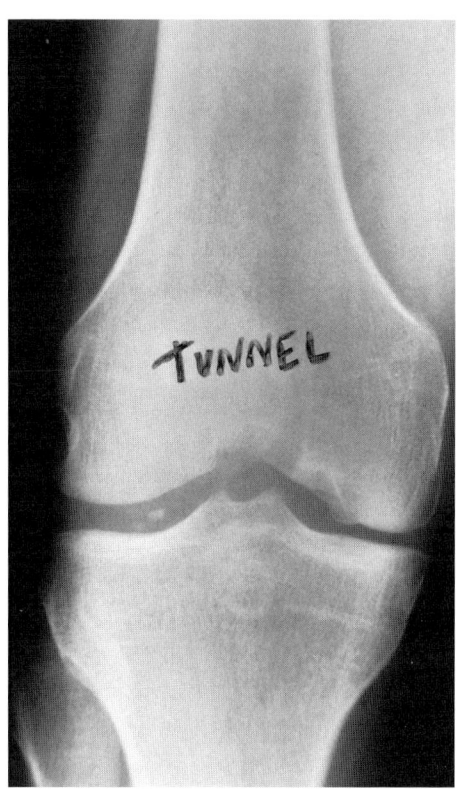

Figure 2.7. Osteochondritis Dissecans: (A) AP View: A calcified loose body overlies the lateral joint compartment. (B) Tunnel View: The donor site for this loose body is seen as an osteochondral defect at the lateral aspect of the medial femoral condyle. This is the characteristic location for osteochondritis dissecans.

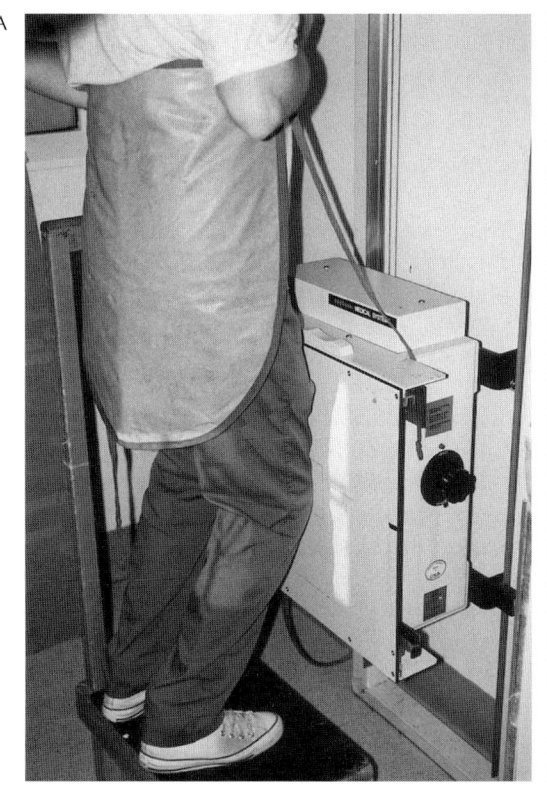

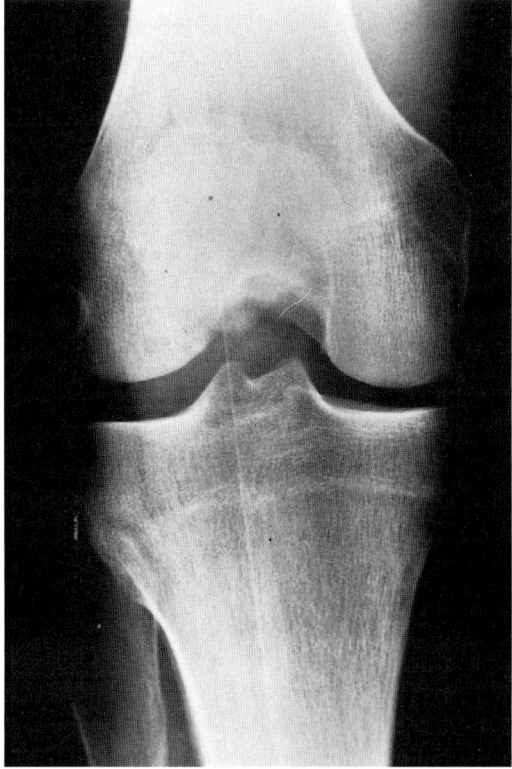

Figure 2.8. Semiflexed AP View: (A) The patient is in a shallow squatting position, with the patella resting on the film cassette holder. The lead shield should always be utilized for radiation protection. (B) The medial and lateral joint spaces should be equivalent on the semiflexed and standard AP films if the thickness of articular cartilage is uniform.

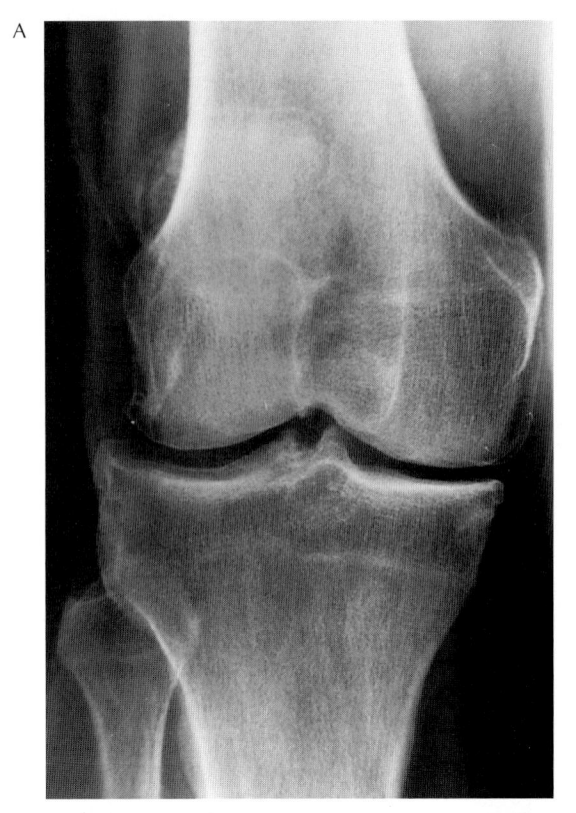

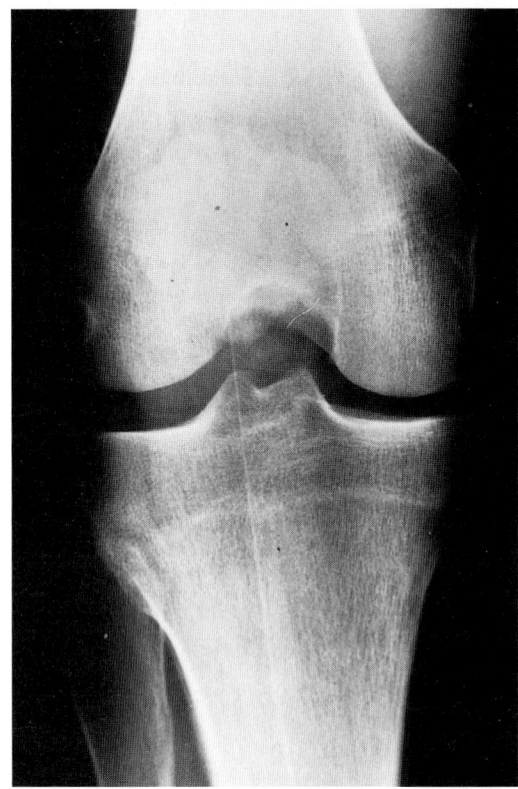

Figure 2.9. DJD Lateral Compartment: Value of Semiflexed AP View: (A) Standing AP view: Mild-moderate lateral compartment narrowing. (B) Semiflexed AP: Severe lateral compartment narrowing. These findings correlate with more severe thinning of cartilage at the posterior weight-bearing surfaces.

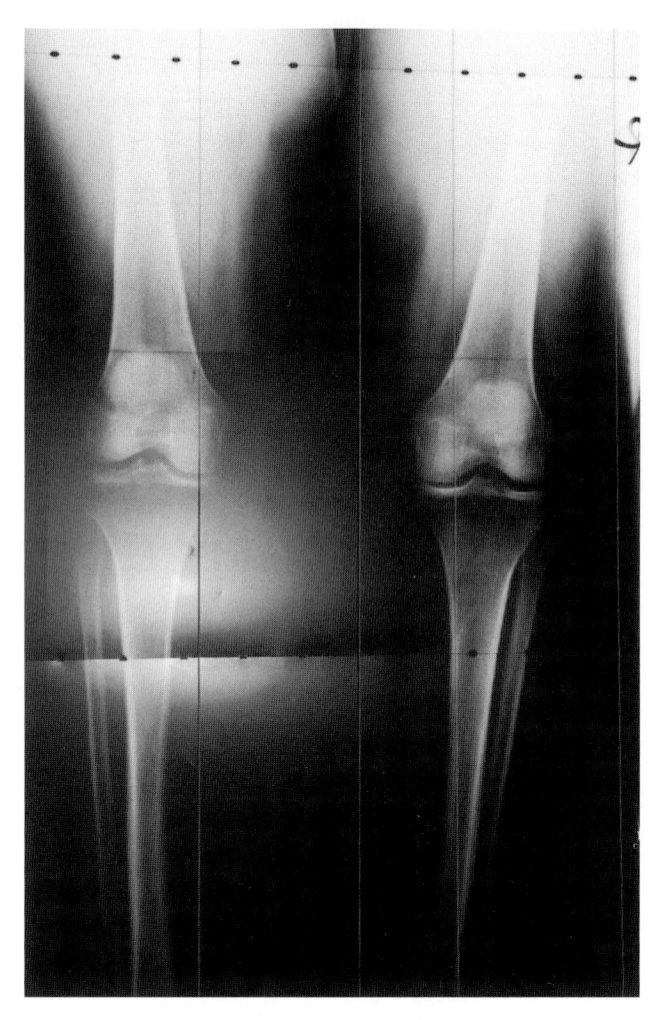

Figure 2.10. Standing AP Weight-Bearing View: Long Cassette: This film gives an overall assessment of alignment of the lower extremities. The cassette is long enough to extend from hips (not pictured) to ankles.

nearly normal. MR imaging, by virtue of its ability to directly image articular cartilage, synovial tissue, and subtle bone and marrow alterations, is more sensitive than conventional radiography at detecting early osteoarthritic changes and gives a more accurate assessment of the extent of disease and number of joint compartments involved[15,16] (Fig. 2.12). MR can be used as a supplemental modality for assessing those patients with suspected early clinically symptomatic DJD and nearly normal appearing radiographs.[17] It may also have a role in quantitatively monitoring progression and therapeutic response of arthritic disease.[18] Furthermore, MR allows detection of additional intra-articular abnormalities such as meniscal or cruciate ligament pathology. MR is ideal for assessment of the stability of osteochondral fragments in osteochondritis dissecans or osteochondral fracture; fluid extension beneath the osteochondral le-

2. Preoperative Radiographic Assessment

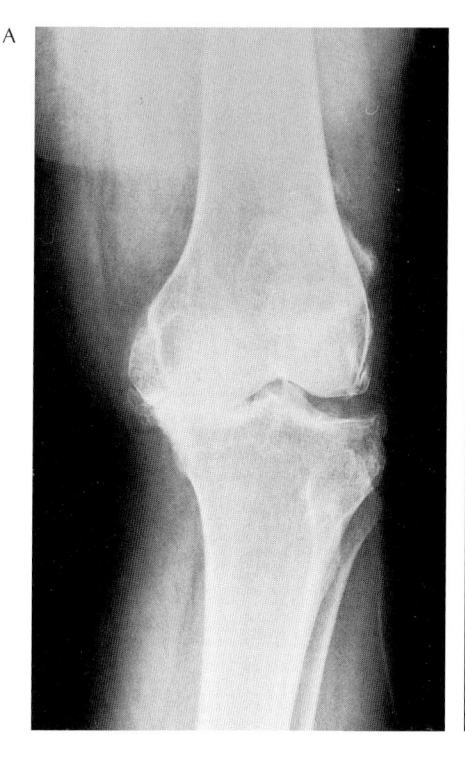

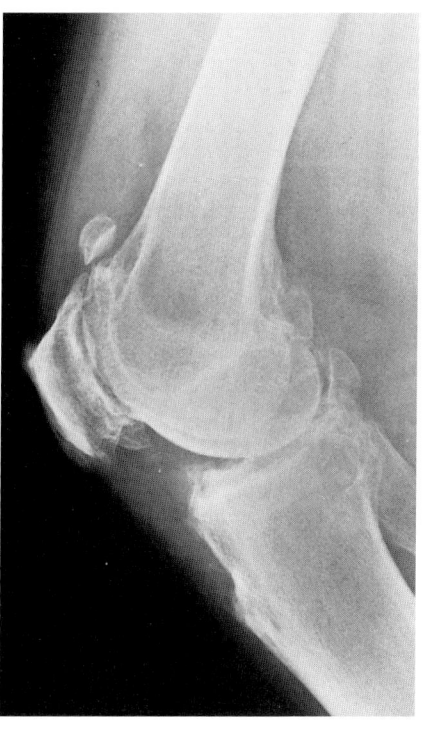

Figure 2.11. DJD—Medial and Patellofemoral Compartments: (A) AP View: Characteristic findings of DJD are seen, including severe joint-space narrowing, osteophytes and subchondral sclerosis. There is resultant genu varus. (B) Lateral View: Similar findings are present at the patellofemoral joint. There is a calcified loose body in the suprapatellar bursa as well as a joint effusion.

sion and/or subchondral cystic changes underlying the lesion correlate with a loose fragment (Fig. 2.13).

CT is of limited usefulness for preoperative evaluation; it is most helpful in complicated cases in which there is prior trauma and deformity requiring custom prosthetic components. Also, CT is helpful in cases of suspected chronic infection, for delineating the presence of a bony sequestrum. Computer-reformatted 2-dimensional and 3-dimensional images can be generated; however, these are more aesthetic than they are clinically useful (Fig. 2.14).

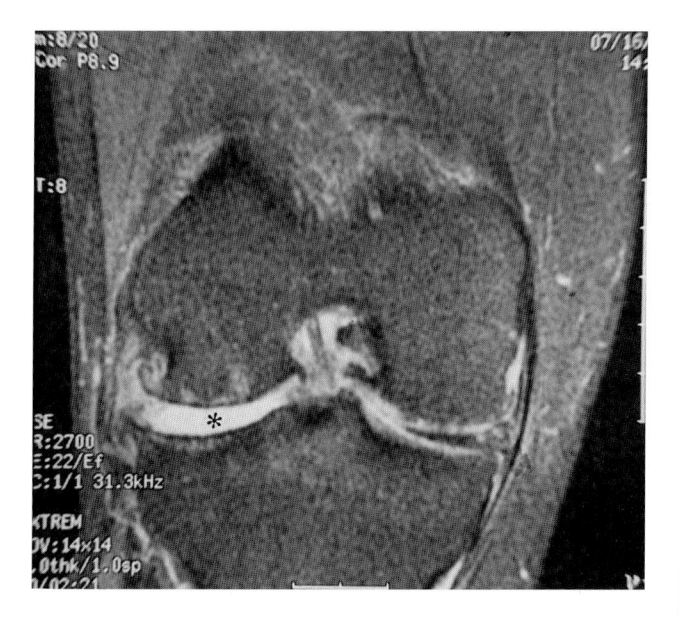

Figure 2.12. DJD—Magnetic Resonance Imaging: Coronal fat-suppressed proton density image: There is advanced thinning of articular cartilage at the lateral compartment with absence (degeneration) of the meniscus. There is joint fluid at the lateral compartment (asterisk) outlining the subchondral bone with mild cystic changes on the femoral and tibial sides. The joint space is maintained, causing the degenerative changes to be less apparent on conventional radiographs.

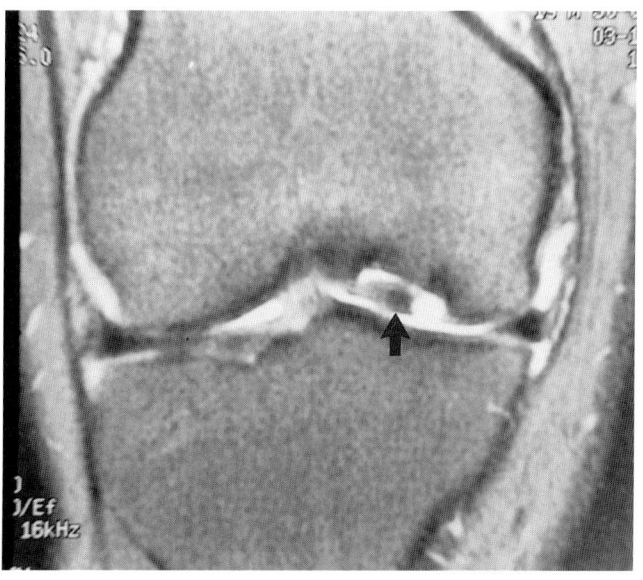

Figure 2.13. Osteochondritis Dissecans—Loose Fragment: Coronal fat-suppressed proton density image: There is a loose in situ osteochondral fragment at the medial femoral condyle (arrow). The fragment is surrounded by bright fluid, indicating that it is unstable.

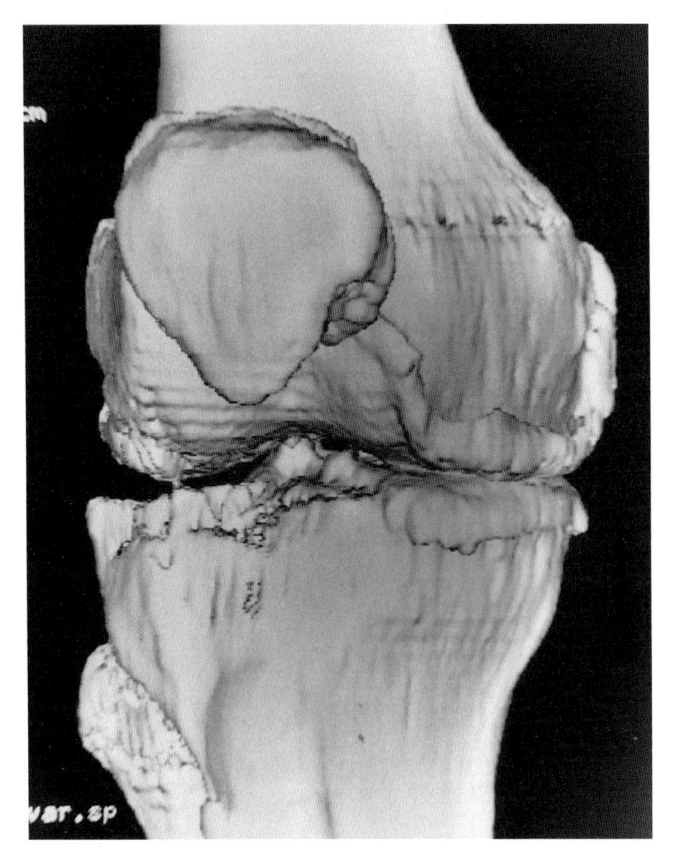

Figure 2.14. DJD—3-Dimensional CT: 3-Dimensional reformatted image of the knee shows advanced medial compartment disease, with a ridge of osteophytes at the margins of the tibial plateau and femoral condyle.

OSTEONECROSIS

Spontaneous osteonecrosis (SONC) has a classical clinical presentation of sudden onset severe knee pain and is most common in elderly women. Unfortunately, radiographic abnormalities are often absent or subtle at the time of presentation, and more advanced imaging modalities are often necessary for confirmation (Fig. 2.15). Plain film findings of osteonecrosis include sclerosis at the weight-bearing surface of the medial femoral condyle and often subchondral lucency. These findings are usually manifested several months following the onset of symptoms, and usually progress to flattening (collapse) of the articular surface (Fig. 2.16). The findings of SONC on the radionuclide bone scan (RNBS) of increased uptake at the abnormal femoral condyle on all three phases of a triple-phase bone scan have been shown to be sensitive for its detection and helpful for prognosis.[19,20]

Current MR technology allows comparable, if not greater, sensitivity[21,22] than the bone scan, and can also reveal important anatomic information. MRI can clearly demonstrate the narrow edema and subchondral crescentic signal abnormality present in this condition, and can also assess the integrity of the overlying articular cartilage. Furthermore, inasmuch as the size of an osteonecrotic lesion is of high prognostic value,[23] MR excels at depicting the precise size, location and extent of the abnormality,[24] features not afforded by the limited spatial resolution of nuclear imaging. MR can also detect concomitant intra-articular pathology such as

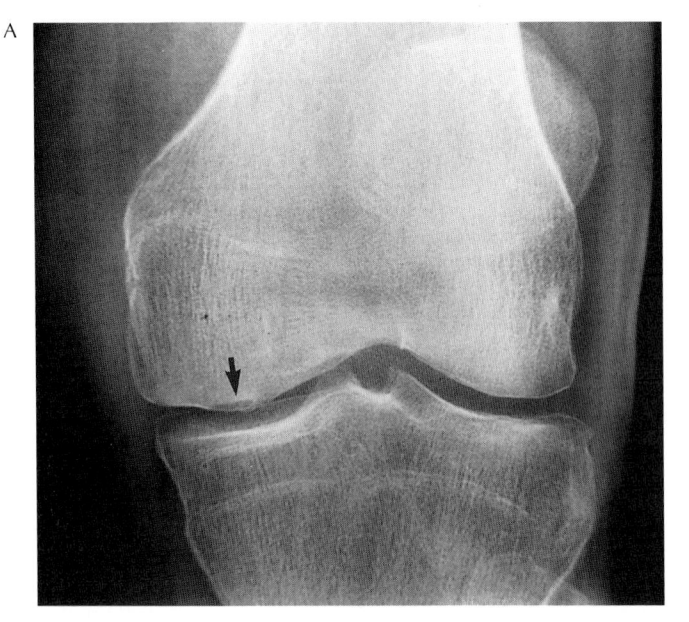

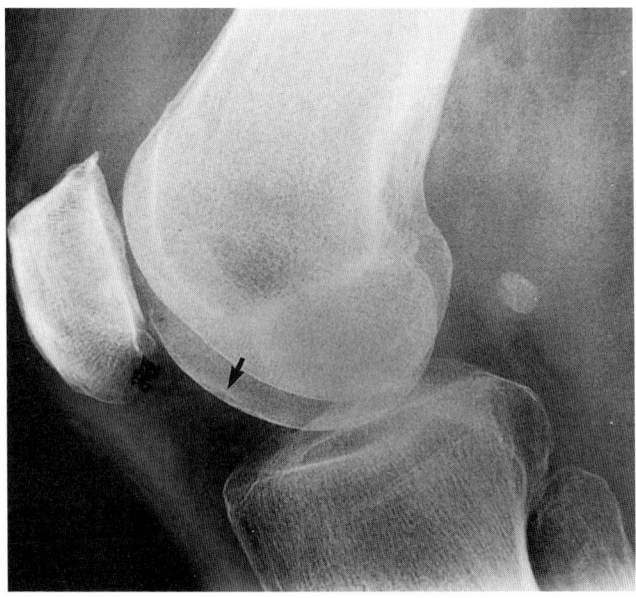

Figure 2.15. Early Osteonecrosis: (A) AP and (B) lateral views of the knee obtained in this 65-year-old man with sudden onset severe medial knee pain. A very subtle curvilinear lucency is seen at the weight-bearing surface of the medial femoral condyle (arrow), suspicious for osteonecrosis. (C) Coronal and (D) sagittal fat-suppressed MR images performed the same day, more clearly show the focal crescentic signal abnormality in the subchondral bone with significant bone marrow edema (bright signal in "D"). These findings are characteristic of spontaneous osteonecrosis.

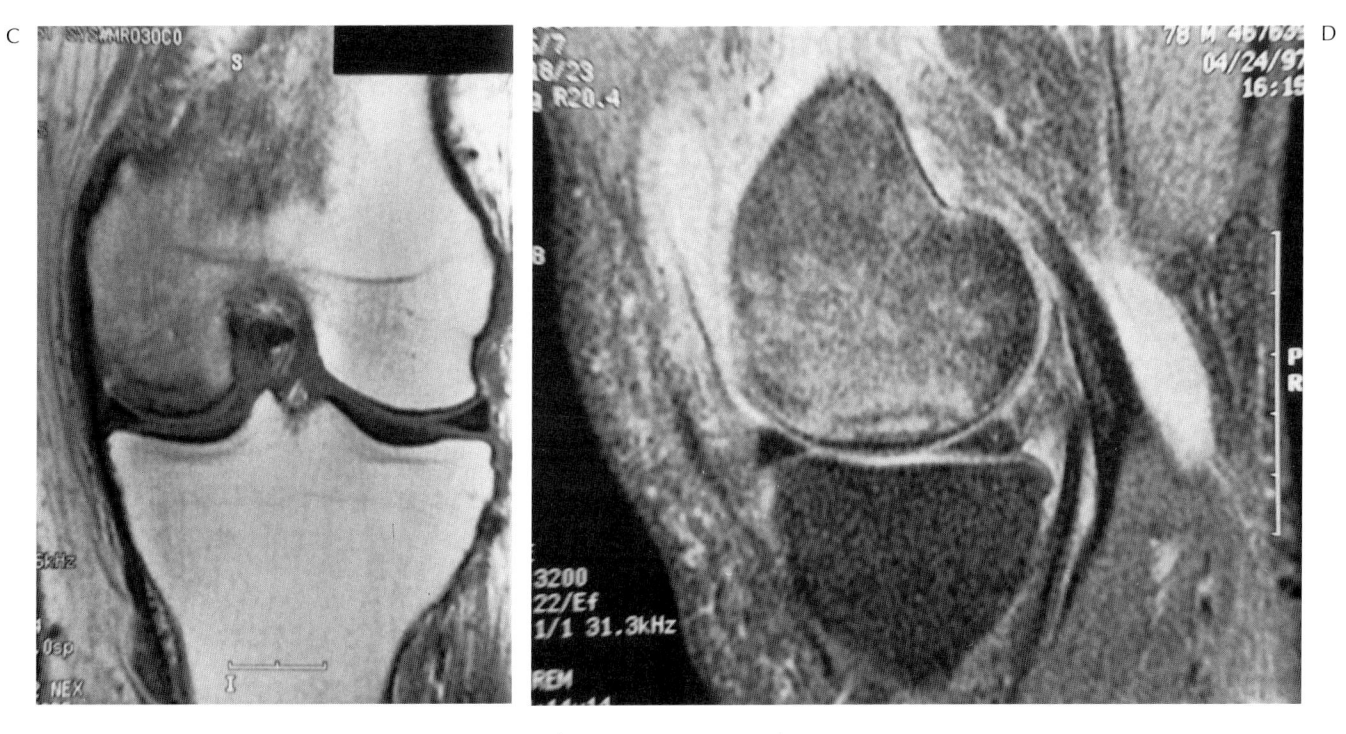

Figure 2.15. (continued).

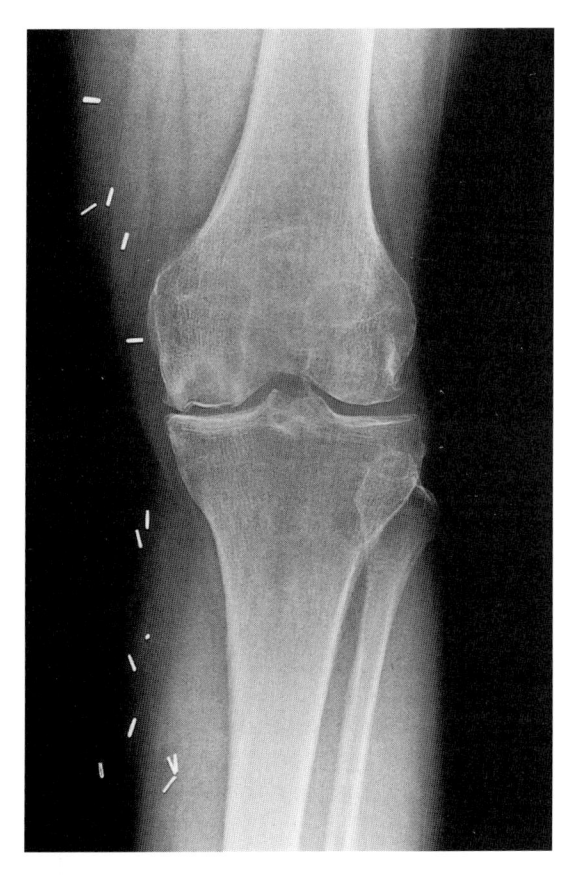

Figure 2.16. Advanced Osteonecrosis: AP view of the knee shows focal flattening of the weight-bearing articular surface of the medial femoral condyle, with underlying lucency and sclerosis, indicating osteonecrosis. There are moderate medial compartment degenerative changes.

meniscal tears. In view of the high specificity, sensitivity, and anatomic resolution of MR imaging, the authors suggest performing MR as the imaging modality of choice following equivocal or normal radiographs.

CONCLUSION

Prior to total knee arthroplasty, standard AP, lateral, and tangential axial views are usually sufficient for evaluation and surgical planning of most patients with significant arthritis. Supplemental views such as semiflexed standing and tunnel views can be helpful for detecting joint-space narrowing that is not evident on routine images. Advanced imaging modalities such as nuclear and magnetic resonance imaging can be useful for specific clinical indications such as diagnosis and prognostication of osteonecrosis and assessment of clinically significant arthritis in the face of nearly normal radiographs.

References

1. Leach RE, Gregg T, Siber FJ. Weight bearing radiography in osteoarthritis of the knee. *Radiology.* 1970; 97:265–268.
2. Ahlback S. Osteoarthritis of the knee: a radiographic investigation. *Acta Radiol Suppl.* (Stockh) 1968; 277:7–72.
3. Insall JN, Salvati E. Patella position in the normal knee joint. *Radiology.* 1971; 101:101–104.
4. Math KR, Ghelman B, Potter HG. Imaging of the patellofemoral joint. In: Scuderi GR, ed. *The patella.* New York: Springer Verlag, 1995.
5. Merchant AC, Mercer RL, Jacobsen RH, et al. Roenteno-

graphic analysis of patellofemoral congruence. *J Bone Joint Surg Am.* 1974; 56A:1391–1396.
6. Jones AC, Ledingham J, McAlindon T, et al. Radiographic assessment of patellofemoral osteoarthritis. *Ann Rheum Dis.* 1993; 52:655–658.
7. Camp JD, Coventry MB. The use of special views in roentgenography of the knee joint. *US Nav Med Bull.* 1944; 44:56–58.
8. Holmsblad E. Postero-anterior x-ray of the knee in flexion. *JAMA.* 1937; 109:1196–1197.
9. Messiah SS, Fowler PJ, Munro T. Anteroposterior radiographs of the osteoarthritic knee. *J Bone Joint Surg.* 1990; B72:639–674.
10. Buckland-Wright JC, Macfarlane DG, Jasani MK, Lynch JA. Quantitative microfocal radiographic assessment of osteoarthritis of the knee from weight bearing tunnel and semiflexed standing views. *J Rheumatol.* 1994; 21:1734–1741.
11. Resnick D, Vint V. The "tunnel" view in assessment of cartilage loss in osteoarthritis of the knee. *Radiology.* 1970; 97: 265–268.
12. Sartoris DJ, Resnick D. Plain film radiography: routine and specialized techniques and projections. In: Resnick D, Niwayama G, eds. *Diagnosis of Bone and Joint Disorders.* 2nd ed. Philadelphia: Saunders, 1988: 2–54.
13. Sabiston CP, Adams ME, Li DKB. Magnetic resonance imaging of osteoarthritis: correlation with gross pathology using an experimental model. *J Orthop Res.* 1987; 5164–5172.
14. Gresham GE, Rathey UK. Osteoarthritis in knees of aged persons: relationship between roentgenographic and clinical manifestations. *JAMA.* 1975; 233:168–170.
15. Chan WP, Lang P, Stevens MP, et al. Osteoarthritis of the knee: comparison of radiography, CT, and MR Imaging to assess extent and severity. *AJR.* 1991; 157:799–806.
16. Martel W, Adler RS, Chan K, et al. Overview: new methods in imaging osteoarthritis. *J Rheumatol.* 1991; 18:(suppl 27):32–37.
17. Li KC, Higgs J, Aisen AM, et al. MRI in osteoarthritis of the hip: gradations of severity. *Magn Resonance Imaging.* 1988; 6:229–236.
18. Peterfy CG, Majumdar S, Lang P, et al. MR imaging of the arthritic knee: improved discrimination of cartilage, synovium and effusion with pulsed saturation transfer and fat-suppressed T1-weighted sequences. *Radiology.* 1994; 191:413–419.
19. Greyson ND, Lotem MM, Gross AE, et al. Radionuclide evaluation of spontaneous femoral osteonecrosis. *Radiology.* 1982; 142:729–735.
20. Al-Rowaih A, Wingstrand H, Lindstrand A, et al. Three-phase scintimetry in osteonecrosis of the knee. *Acta Orthop Scand.* 1990; 61:120–127.
21. Healy WL. Osteonecrosis of the knee detected only by MRI. *Orthopedics.* 1991; 14:703–704.
22. Thomas RH, Resnick D, Alazraki NP, et al. Compartmental evaluation of osteoarthritis of the knee: comparative study of available imaging modalities. *Radiology.* 1975; 116:585–594.
23. Aglietti P, Insall JN, Buzz R, et al. Idiopathic osteonecrosis of the knee: aetiology, prognosis and treatment. *J Bone Joint Surg Br.* 1983; 65:588–597.
24. Bjorkengren AG, Al-Rowaih, Lindstrand A, et al. Spontaneous osteonecrosis of the knee: value of MR imaging in determining prognosis. *AJR.* 1990; 154:331–336.

CHAPTER 3
Cost Considerations: An Historical Perspective

Steven Stern

INTRODUCTION

Modern medicine has made significant strides over the last several decades. During this period emphasis has been on optimizing clinical outcomes, especially in "high-tech" procedures. In this regard, neither orthopedics nor knee arthroplasty has been an exception. Advances in instrumentation, design, and surgical technique have resulted in knee arthroplasty becoming one of the most common operative procedures performed by orthopedic surgeons. The procedure has become both predictable and durable. However, over this time period, there has been little emphasis placed on the cost issues associated with total knee arthroplasty.

In fact, it has been only recently that an emphasis has been placed on costs associated with medical care. Throughout the 1980s the cost of medicine rose exponentially and easily outpaced the rate of inflation[1] (Fig. 3.1). This exponential rise in health-care expenditures resulted in a new understanding and inspection of the cost associated with medical care. In addition, third-party payers began to employ various methods to control these expenditures (DRGs, preoperative certification, utilization review).

The pressure to control medical costs has affected almost all aspects of medical care. However, it has had a disproportionate impact on knee (and hip) arthroplasty procedures. This is because knee arthroplasty is a high-volume, relatively predictable procedure. Furthermore, the surgery is performed in a patient population in which Medicare is the predominant third-party payer.[2] Consequently, there has been a relatively recent emphasis on optimizing and analyzing the costs associated with total knee arthroplasty.[3,4] The pressure to manage costs has been felt by hospital administrators, insurance companies, physicians, and implant manufacturers. This new paradigm challenges the surgeon and institution to maintain high-quality care, while carefully monitoring the cost and effectiveness of each component of knee replacement surgery.

HISTORICAL ISSUES

One of the first efforts in controlling cost was undertaken by the federal government as part of the Medicare program. This occurred with passage of the Tax Equity and Fiscal Responsibility Act of 1982 (TEFRA) and Social Security Amendments of 1983. These statutes instituted diagnosis-related groups (DRGs) as a system of hospital reimbursement for hospital care rendered to Medicare recipients.[5] Prior to the institution of DRGs, hospitals were reimbursed under a traditional retrospective fee-for-service plan. Under fee for service, hospital reimbursement was tied to services rendered, with increased costs passed along to the third-party payers. This system encouraged hospitals and physicians to increase utilization, because reimbursement was almost always assured for these increased services. Thus, the greater the length of stay, the greater the reimbursement; the more expensive the supply (or implant), the greater the hospital markup and the greater the revenue. Under this system, hospitals had little incentive to reduce cost. In fact the opposite was true, increased utilization resulted in an improved revenue stream for the facility. It was against this backdrop that DRGs were instituted in an attempt to control costs and encourage efficiency.

The DRG system was a prospective payment system (PPS), by which hospitals were reimbursed a flat or capitated amount fixed in advance at an illness-specific rate.[5] The specific fixed payment for a particular DRG varied between hospitals based on certain parameters (i.e., geographic hospital location, resident education responsibilities). However, each individual hospital's reimbursement was fixed at a set amount for all Medicare patients with similar diagnoses (there

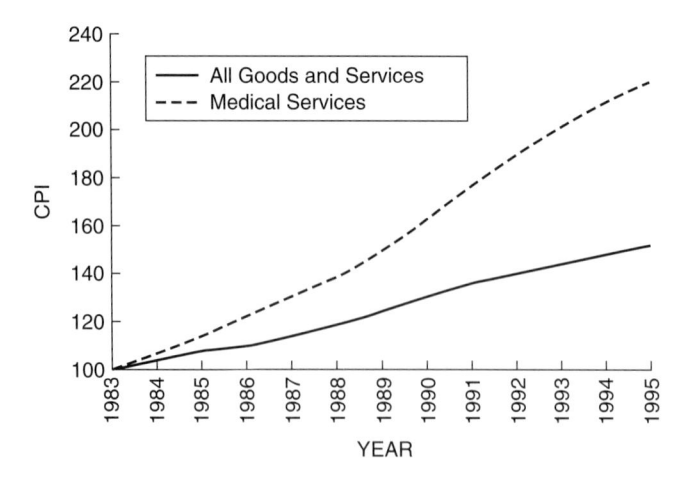

Figure 3.1. Consumer price index (CPI) for all goods and services (solid line) as compared with index for medical services (dashed line).[1]

was an adjustment for patients with significant co-morbidities). Thus, hospitals were no longer able to pass increased costs or their inefficiencies onto Medicare. Rather, the hospital became fully "at risk" for the difference between their average cost and the DRG payment.[5]

As a result of these changes, hospitals became increasingly concerned about cost issues, especially in areas with a high percentage of Medicare patients. Because over 60 percent of patients undergoing knee arthroplasty are Medicare recipients,[2] a significant portion of a hospital's revenue from this procedure came from these fixed DRG Medicare payments. Thus, knee arthroplasty became an area for particular scrutiny for hospital administrators.[3,4,6,7]

In addition to the institution of DRGs by Medicare, other third-party payers have recently instituted their own methods of controlling cost. These have taken varied forms, but tend to fall under the banner of "managed care." This emphasis on controlling cost has increased dramatically over the last several years, and now involves almost all third-party payers including private insurance, HMOs, and Medicaid.

ANALYSIS OF COST

Hospital Costs

The recent emphasis on expenditures associated with total knee replacements has resulted in several studies on this topic. Because different institutions use different accounting methodology, and stratify components of cost differently, it is difficult to perform exact comparisons of data between institutions. However, there are certain constants that become apparent when analyzing the available data. Thus, it is worthwhile to examine the published information on expenses associated with total knee arthroplasty.

The Lahey Clinic

One of the first widely reported studies on costs associated with total knee arthroplasty was done at the Lahey Clinic in Massachusetts.[6] In a published article, Healy and Finn reviewed the costs associated with knee replacements. The authors used a "top-down" type of methodology. This involved converting charge data to costs with the use of cost-to-charge ratios for each hospital service center. The authors pointed out that the ratios are hospital specific and represent government-mandated industry standards.

Healy and Finn reported that the average actual hospital costs for a knee arthroplasty procedure increased 17% from $10,122 in 1983 to $11,826 in 1991. However, when analyzing their data in inflation-controlled dollars, they actually found a 15% reduction in costs during this time period ($10,163 in 1983 reduced to $8,682 in 1991) (Table 3.1).

Table 3.1. Hospital expenditures associated with total knee arthroplasty. Data represents studies from the Lahey Clinic,[6] Northwestern Memorial Hospital,[7] and Hermann Hospital.[8] The costs are all in actual dollars

Costs	Lahey Clinic 1983	Lahey Clinic 1991	Northwestern Hospital 1992	Northwestern Hospital 1993	Northwestern Hospital 1994	Hermann Hospital 1991–1992
Operating/recovery room	$1,382	$2,532	$7,273	$5,021	$5,709	$2,601
Prosthesis	$1,359	$2,960	$2,369	$2,621	$2,984	$3,691
Hospital room/nursing	$4,804	$3,711	$4,006	$3,436	$3,148	$2,857
Other	$2,578	$2,623	$3,260	$3,059	$3,359	$3,412
Total	$10,122	$11,826	$16,908	$14,137	$15,200	$12,561
Variable costs			$8,294	$7,509	$8,821	
Fixed costs			$8,614	$6,628	$6,379	
Total			$16,908	$14,137	$15,200	
Length of stay (days)			8.7	6.9	6.1	7.9

3. Cost Considerations

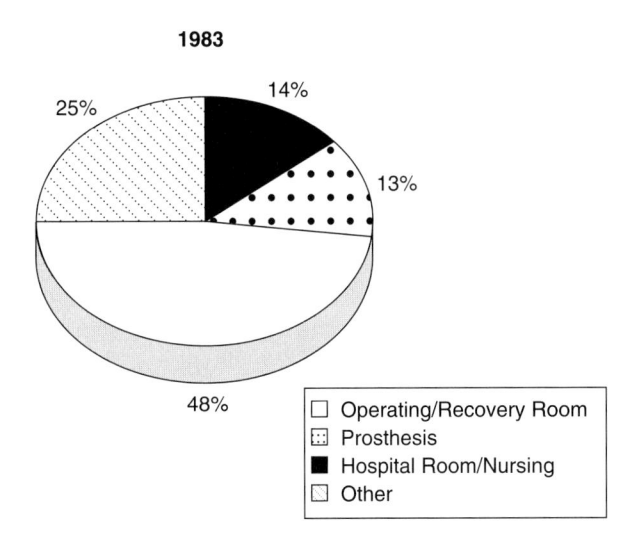

Figure 3.2. Allocation of costs for total knee arthroplasty at the Lahey Clinic in 1983.[6]

(1983 pie chart: Operating/Recovery Room 48%, Prosthesis 13%, Hospital Room/Nursing 14%, Other 25%)

The authors also stratified the costs associated with the knee replacements to various cost centers. These can be seen in detail in Figures 3.2 and 3.3. Notably, the costs for the hospital room decreased from 48% ($4,804) of total hospital costs in 1983 to 32% ($3,711) in 1991. This represented a decrease of 23% in actual dollars, and 46% in inflation-controlled dollars.

Conversely, the cost of the actual knee prosthesis increased from 13% of total costs in 1983 to 25% in 1991. The average cost of the prosthesis increased from $1,359 in 1983 to $2,960 in 1991 at their institution (Figs. 3.2 and 3.3). This represented a 118% increase in actual dollars, and a 59% increase in inflation-adjusted dollars.

Healy and Finn noted that the hospital cost of knee arthroplasty between 1983 and 1991 was controlled by utilization review. They felt this effectively reduced the volume of services and the supply costs associated with the operation at their institution. However, the individual unit cost of supplies, and specifically the cost of the prosthesis was not controlled. They recommended that the hospitals and surgeons work together to control the actual cost of the prostheses in the future.

Northwestern Memorial Hospital

A study of expenditures associated with total knee replacement surgeries was performed at Northwestern Memorial Hospital (NMH).[7] This is a large academic medical center located in downtown Chicago, Illinois. In this study, hospital costs associated with 15 index knee arthroplasty procedures from fiscal years 1992, 1993, and 1994 were analyzed.

During this time period, a major emphasis was made at the hospital to optimize the perioperative activities associated with knee arthroplasty. These changes included institution of an accelerated rehabilitation protocol and specific clinical pathways. These changes were instituted to both optimize the clinical results of surgery and to decrease the average length of stay (ALOS). The efforts were successful because ALOS for knee arthroplasty procedures decreased 30% (8.7 days to 6.1 days) (Table 3.1).

During this same time period, expenditures for total knee arthroplasty decreased only 10% ($16,908 to $15,200) in real dollars (Table 3.1) and 13% ($17,415 to $15,200) in inflation-controlled 1994 dollars. The cost associated with total knee arthroplasty over this time period were also stratified into the various components of costs for each year (Fig. 3.4). There were minimal changes in the cost distribution over the years studied. For all of the years studied, the majority of costs (approximately 56%) occurred during the patient's initial

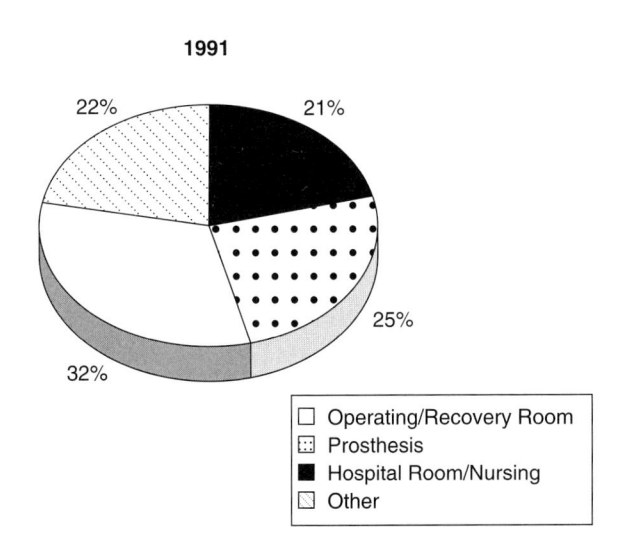

Figure 3.3. Allocation of costs for total knee arthroplasty at the Lahey Clinic in 1991.[6]

(1991 pie chart: Operating/Recovery Room 32%, Prosthesis 25%, Hospital Room/Nursing 21%, Other 22%)

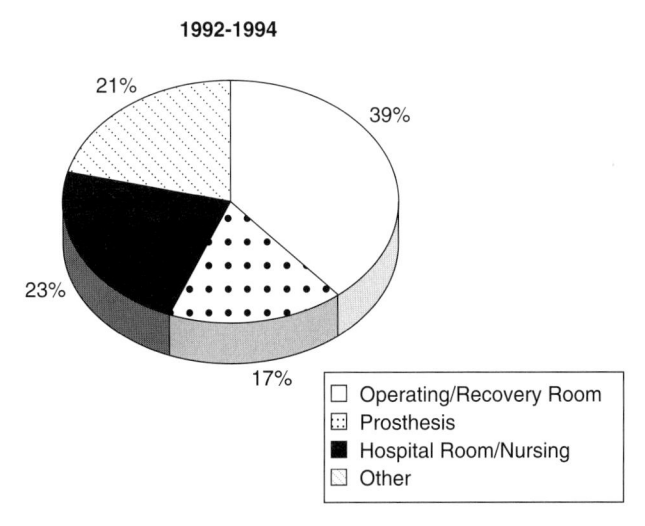

Figure 3.4. Allocation of costs for total knee arthroplasty at Northwestern Memorial Hospital for the years 1992 through 1994.[7]

(1992–1994 pie chart: Operating/Recovery Room 39%, Prosthesis 17%, Hospital Room/Nursing 23%, Other 21%)

hours in the operating and recovery rooms (operating room cost plus prosthesis cost).

The three largest cost items as a percentage of total cost for knee arthroplasty were the operating room (approximately 39%), implant cost (approximately 17%), and nursing cost (approximately 23%). The authors noted that despite a 30% reduction in ALOS, total costs fell only 10% during this time period. By using inflation-controlled dollars, the percentage decrease was slightly better (13% decrease), though still modest as compared with the drop in ALOS. They offered several explanations for this result.

First, they pointed out that at Northwestern Memorial Hospital, as at the Lahey Clinic,[6] by the early 1990s a significant portion of total hospital cost occurred during the actual operation (Figs. 3.5 and 3.4). Thus, attempts at NMH to reduce ALOS focused on the component of cost that occurred after the patient had left the operating room. The efforts were thereby focused at a point in time at which the majority of costs associated with the procedure had already been expended. The authors pointed out that reducing ALOS only effects the approximate 40% (or less) of expenses that are associated with the postoperative care.

Additionally, the largest individual component of cost was the prosthetic cost. During the period of the study, implant selection at NMH had been left solely to the discretion of the operating surgeon. There had been no attempt to influence implant selection, nor had any form of competitive bidding or volume price discounting been placed in effect. Thus, implant price was solely dictated by the price structure set by the prosthetic manufacturer.

The data in this study also stratified expenditures into fixed and variable costs (Fig. 3.5). Overall variable costs in real dollars totaled $8,208 (53%) and fixed costs $7,207 (47%) for total knee arthroplasty from 1992 to 1994. The variable costs actually increased ($527 increase) from 1992 to 1994. Even utilizing inflation-controlled dollars, analysis of variable costs revealed a continued rise of $278 over this time period.

Therefore, essentially all of the cost reductions achieved were in the fixed component of costs allocated to each patient. Variable costs remained unchanged or increased slightly. This is, in part, because the majority of costs associated with the hospital's daily room charge is classified as fixed. Because it is unclear if there was any change in the hospital's overall fixed cost structure, it is unclear to what degree, if any, the hospital actually realized savings from these perceived fixed cost reductions. The issue regarding the effect of ALOS reductions and fixed costs is discussed further in the ALOS section.

Hermann Hospital

Further work on cost issues associated with knee arthroplasty has also been done at Hermann Hospital in Houston, Texas.[8] Meyers and associates reported on expenditures associated with 37 primary total knee arthroplasty procedures performed between 1991 and 1992 at their institution. This report, like the one from Northwestern,[7] calculated the cost of the procedure directly from their institution's hospital-based cost accounting system. This is as opposed to the estimated hospital-specific, cost-to-charge ratios used in the Lahey Clinic study.[6] The patients from Hermann Hospital had an average length of stay of 7.9 days (s.d. 2.6 days). Their average total cost was $12,561 (s.d. $2,596) (Table 3.1). As in the other studies, the main components of cost were the operating room and surgical supplies (28%), the prosthesis (29%), and the hospital room (23%). Total costs correlated with length of stay, but they had no correlation with patient gender or age.

Similar to the other reports, the authors of this study found that the prosthetic cost represented the single most costly component of a knee arthroplasty procedure. They, like the Northwestern authors, pointed out that both the operating room and hospital room charges have a high component of fixed costs associated with them. Thus, they felt that it would be difficult for a hospital to reduce costs associated with these items without closing down operating rooms or hospital beds. Therefore they suggested that "reductions in the cost of the implant should be the most effective mechanism for cost savings."[8]

Posthospitalization (Rehabilitation) Costs

Posthospitalization costs associated with total knee arthroplasty have not been examined in the same manner as inpatient costs. There are a myriad of reasons for this. First, costs associated with posthospital treatment

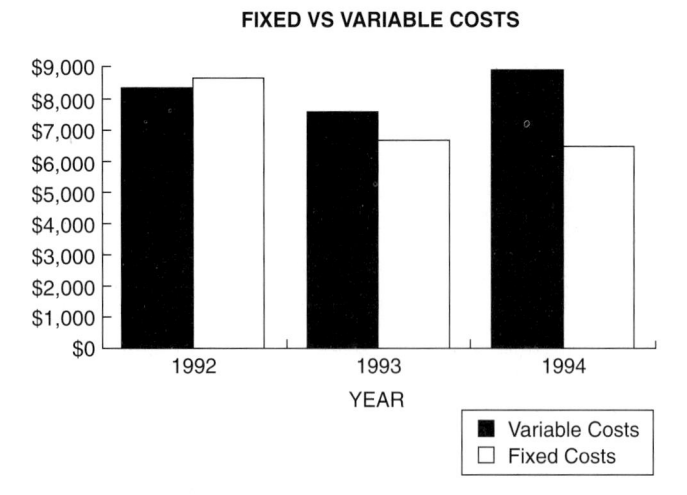

Figure 3.5. Fixed and variable costs in real dollars for total knee arthroplasty at Northwestern Memorial Hospital for the years 1992 through 1994.[7]

are even more difficult to obtain than those connected with the inpatient setting. Hospital inpatient costs can be tracked and analyzed via a hospital's inpatient accounting system. However, post hospitalization costs are much more diffuse. They consist of expenditures at extended care facilities and outpatient laboratories, as well as costs associated with home and outpatient nursing and physical therapy. Patients may have components of their postoperative care in more than one setting and reimbursement for these services may be covered by more than one third-party payer or even personally by the patient.

In addition, the Medicare DRG for joint arthroplasty includes only the inpatient hospital stay. Accordingly, this is the area that has come under the most scrutiny and analysis in cost optimization. In fact, many institutions have established posthospitalization units (i.e., skilled nursing facilities, step-down units, rehabilitation hospitals) as mechanisms to minimize hospital length of stay, while still allowing patients to remain in an inpatient setting. This practice has led to concern, and has been characterized by some as a cost-shifting, as opposed to a legitimate method of controlling costs.[6]

Prehospitalization Costs

Preoperative costs associated with knee arthroplasty have also not been well characterized. Thus, it is difficult to make definitive statements about the cost magnitude of this component of care. However, the author believes that in many cases expenditures in this area are significant. Specifically, these expenses include preoperative labs, medical "clearance," and autologous blood donations.

Professional Fees

Another area that has been largely ignored in most cost analysis of total knee arthroplasty is the professional cost component. These expenses are largely those associated with the surgeon, anesthesiologist, physiatrist (if any), and any other medical or surgical physician involved in the patient's care. Once again these expenses are not included in the hospital's capitated DRG reimbursement, so the tendency has been not to include them in most analyses.[6,7,8] The most significant professional expense would most likely be the surgeon's charge.

Surgeon fees for this procedure are largely controlled by Medicare, secondary to the large number of patients undergoing total knee replacement who have Medicare as their primary insurance coverage.[2] For 1997, the Medicare allowable charge for participating physicians performing a primary total knee arthroplasty in Chicago is ($2,155), which is only slightly lower than the maximum allowable charge for nonparticipating physicians ($2,355). The corresponding allowed charges for revision total knee surgery in which all components are revised is $2,493 for participating surgeons, as compared with $2,723 for nonparticipators.[9]

COST CONTAINMENT

ALOS Issues

Initial efforts to control costs began in a knowledge "vacuum." At first, neither hospital administrators nor surgeons had a good understanding of the true costs associated with knee arthroplasty, nor did they understand what percentage each individual component of care was of the total cost of care. Cost issues were not addressed at major orthopedic meetings, nor were they included in leading textbooks on knee replacement surgery.[10] It was against this backdrop that administrators and physicians began their attempts to optimize expenditures, and the length of stay (rightly or wrongly) is where most institutions began.

This initial emphasis resulted in the elimination of preoperative inpatient days, and early concentration on discharge planning. In addition, attempts were made to shift rehabilitation activities and costs out of the hospital inpatient setting. In the aggregate, all of these things successfully resulted in a decreased inpatient length of stay throughout the United States for patients undergoing knee arthroplasty. Average length of stay (ALOS) in the United States for knee arthroplasty procedures fell from approximately 13 days in 1985 to 8 days in 1993.[2]

However, there is a limit to savings that can be achieved with ALOS reductions alone. ALOS declines cannot continue indefinitely, because patients need to spend a reasonable amount of time hospitalized in the acute care setting. In fact, some authors feel that many institutions are approaching the plateau in terms of further ALOS reductions.[8]

ALOS reductions have eliminated the least expensive inpatient days (those prior to the day of surgery and those at the end of a patient's hospital stay). Many costly tests and procedures that were traditionally performed at the end of a patient's hospital stay, tended not to be eliminated, but rather simply transferred to an earlier day in the hospitalization.

In addition, as was pointed out in both the study at Northwestern Memorial Hospital[7] and the study at Hermann hospital,[8] decreased ALOS predominantly affects the fixed component of cost. The hospital's overall fixed costs are not necessarily reduced. This is because a hospital's total fixed costs (rent, insurance, utilities, and administrative expenses) may not change with small reductions in ALOS. Thus, cost savings in the fixed component of cost can be illusory and do not necessarily occur. Rather decreased ALOS yields a situation in which the total overall fixed costs allocated to inpatient days has to be apportioned over a smaller number of inpatient days.

It must be stressed that ALOS reductions can have a dramatic and positive effect on hospital expenditures. This occurs when the volume of inpatient days allows hospital administrators to initiate cost-saving measures such as closing inpatient nursing units or decreasing staffing levels. These global actions, which significantly reduce a hospital's overall fixed cost structure, can result in profound savings.

Alternatively, ALOS reductions will allow certain hospitals to increase surgical volume and hence revenue. This would occur at institutions that are turning patients away due to a lack of available beds. Although theoretically possible, at this time this scenario does not seem to be a common occurrence in the United States. Conversely, hospitals with chronic excess capacity may well benefit from concerted efforts to decrease this excessive capacity (decreasing their fixed cost structure), rather than focusing solely on decreasing ALOS.

Prosthetic Issues

As opposed to reductions in fixed costs, savings from declines in variable costs, especially supply and implant cost, represent an immediate direct cost savings. Because implants represent the largest single cost item in knee arthroplasty, and because they represent a totally variable expense, they deserve special scrutiny. Any reduction in the implant cost represents a real cash savings to the hospital. These cost savings will directly and immediately effect the hospital's net profit (or loss), as well as its cash flow. Particularly in an age of capitated reimbursement, implant cost reductions represent an area of possible profound impact, by which every dollar saved results in an increased dollar of profitability. Consequently, a variety of methods have been employed by hospitals and implant manufacturers to reduce prosthetic costs associated with joint arthroplasty in the United States. Many of the methods listed here were originally suggested by Healy and Finn in their 1994 paper.[6]

However, it must be stressed that in many instances, there is a trade-off that comes with decreasing implant costs. Specifically, many hospitals have grown accustomed to the level of service provided by the implant company's local representative. At many institutions, this takes a myriad of forms including helping with implant inventory, being available to bring in emergency supplies, checking instrument trays, and assisting in the teaching of hospital personnel. These functions heretofore borne by the implant vendor have tended to increase the implant price. As part of expecting cost reductions from vendors, hospitals must be ready to assume increased responsibility for some of these functions and services. Those hospitals most able to efficiently take on this increased responsibility will be in the best position to appropriately reap the greatest price reductions from the implant manufacturers.

Awareness

The first step at most institutions in controlling expenses, in general, and prosthetic costs, in particular, is increasing awareness of the issues associated with implant cost.[4,11] At the start of this decade there was a dearth of information available to hospital administrators and physicians on cost issues associated with total knee arthroplasty. At many institutions the accounting system had to be upgraded, so that the hospital could accurately track the true costs of this and other procedures.

However, there does appear to be a "sentinel" type effect. Thus, the simple step of gathering and analyzing data, along with making the appropriate personnel cognizant of actual costs, tends to, in and of itself, begin the process of cost reduction. This occurs because physicians, administrators, and vendors begin to feel a subtle, but definite, pressure to consider and reduce the costs associated with knee arthroplasty procedures. The benefits of increased levels of awareness have been documented by some authors as an important early step in cost reduction strategies.[4]

Volume Discounting

Volume discounting or bulk purchasing is a well-known method of cost cutting when purchasing almost anything. Accordingly, a seller will normally be willing to negotiate a lower unit price if the purchaser is willing to buy in bulk. This is as true for knee prostheses, as it is for other commodities. Thus, if a hospital, or a consortium of hospitals, can contract for bulk purchases of knee implants, they should be able to buy them at more favorable rates. Hospitals can achieve this goal in several ways. First, some hospitals have surgeons with large enough surgical volumes to simply approach the implant vendor. At other institutions, surgeons and administrators need to work together to discover if it is possible for there to be some degree of consensus among the professional staff in regards to prosthetic selection. If this can be achieved, the hospital may be able to purchase in quantity, and thereby to reduce its prosthetic unit cost.

Additionally, the institution of bulk purchasing tends to increase standardization within the operating room. Increased standardization can improve operating room efficiency because personnel have less prosthetic knee systems to master. This is especially true for knee arthroplasty procedures, because most systems are extremely instrument intensive. Consequently, allowing operating room staff to become familiar and expert with a specific set or sets of instrumentation can improve efficiency and morale. This improved efficiency can also help to reduce expenditures.

Competitive Bidding

Competitive bidding can be used as an adjunct to volume discounting in reducing prosthetic cost. It is an especially effective technique at institutions that are already doing a large number of surgeries. These high-volume institutions are in the best position when requesting competitive bids from implant vendors. This is because prosthetic knee manufacturers know that a successful bid at a high-volume institution can result in a significant number of implant sales. Thus, vendors tend to be more amenable to decreased profit margins on a per unit basis if they can compensate with increased sales volume at a busy joint replacement hospital.

It is imperative when attempting to institute any cost reduction strategy, but especially one involving competitive bidding, that there is cooperation between the hospital's administrative and professional staffs. If implant vendors know that individual surgeons are not willing to modify their implant selections, they will have little incentive to optimize price. Conversely, if vendors are aware that noncompetitive prices will result in limited implant sales, they will have a strong motivation to offer competitive prices to an institution. Thus, it is important that surgeons are both involved in, and "buy in" to the process used by an individual hospital to optimize cost.[4,6,7,11,12] Above all, physicians must be comfortable with any decisions made on implant selection. Physicians must appropriately act in their role as the patient's advocate. They also remain the individuals with the most expertise with the actual implantation and function of the knee components. Consequently, it is crucial that the surgeon is satisfied with any design being used.

It should be noted that competitive bidding does not mean that an institution necessarily agrees to purchase implants from whichever prosthetic manufacturer offers the lowest price. Institutions can appropriately solicit bids from manufacturers and then evaluate them in any way they desire. Thus, a vendor's bid can be evaluated in the context of the product offered, the service provided, the instrument quality, the preferences of the institution's surgeons, in addition to the price of the implant. Accordingly, institutions in bidding situations do not necessarily accept proposals offering the lowest implant price.

Because of the reproducibility of primary procedures (and the relative lack thereof in revision surgeries), volume discounting and competitive bidding are more commonly and easily employed for the prostheses routinely utilized in index procedures. It is harder to achieve consensus and unanimity for revision operations.

"Ceiling" Price

Another method of controlling implant costs that has been implemented at some institutions is the establishment of a "ceiling" or maximum price. In this strategy, the hospital defines a maximum price that it will be willing to pay for knee arthroplasty components. If this technique is to be effective, it is once again imperative to have appropriate interaction and input from both hospital administrators and physicians. The ceiling price must be a reasonable one. In addition, it is necessary to accurately define which components and technology are applicable to any specific "ceiling" price. Utilization of this procurement approach for total knee arthroplasty usually requires the breakdown of components into categories (i.e., porous components, cemented components with metal-backed tibia, and cemented components with all-polyethylene tibia). This is to ensure that the appropriate implant technology applies to the corresponding appropriate ceiling price.

The advantage of this strategy is that it may leave more room for individual surgeon preference. Conversely, depending on the level of the "ceiling" price, this method may not optimize the price to the same extent as competitive bidding, nor will it necessarily increase knee prosthesis standardization.

Other Techniques

It should be emphasized that cost control is not limited to prosthetic cost alone. Attention should be paid to all aspects of the total knee replacement procedure. Similar efforts to optimize the costs associated with other supplies can be carried out in an analogous manner to what has been discussed for the prosthesis. Efforts in these areas can also prove beneficial in reducing costs and increasing efficiency for total knee arthroplasty procedures.

Another strategy that can prove advantageous in reducing expenditures, as well as improving operating room efficacy, is cultivating surgeon standardization. If surgeons at an institution can maximize their operative similarities, it is easier for operating room personnel to efficiently service all of them. Preparing for the operation becomes easier and more straightforward. Surgical instruments and trays become easier to maintain. Of course, standardization must be carried out in a manner that allows for appropriate individual surgeon variation, so that patient care is not compromised.

Finally, individual parts of the total knee arthroplasty procedure will come under increased scrutiny in the coming years. Each portion of the procedure will need to be analyzed for its individual cost-effectiveness and efficacy. Certain segments of the operative and postoperative care may eventually be safely modified or even deleted. These changes may allow for both decreased

Table 3.2. American College of Rheumatology (ACR) functional classification.[18] Utility values assigned to each ACR class[19]

ACR Class	Description	Utility
I	Complete ability to carry on all usual duties without handicap	1.0
II	Adequate for normal activities despite handicap of discomfort of limited motion in the knee	0.8
III	Limited only to little or none of duties of usual occupation or self-care	0.5
IV	Incapacitated, largely or wholly bedridden or confined to wheelchair; little or no self-care	0.3

cost and improved outcomes. Already recent studies have suggested modifications in certain aspects of the procedure, including utilization of the CPM machine,[13,14] surgical drain,[14] and autologous blood.[15]

COST-EFFECTIVENESS ANALYSIS

Cost-effectiveness analysis (CEA) is a technique used to evaluate the health outcomes and costs associated with different health interventions. Advocates of this methodology believe that it can assist in showing the relative values of alternative interventions for improving health.[16] It may be especially important in an era when the health-care sector will have to live within increased budgetary restraint.

Total knee arthroplasty (like total hip arthroplasty) is an example of a health intervention that could come under increased scrutiny. This is because knee arthroplasty is a high-volume, elective procedure with a growing demand. It is perceived as expensive and is performed largely in a geriatric population. Despite this, there are few studies utilizing cost-effectiveness analysis to assess the long-term results of knee arthroplasty.

Gottlob and colleagues,[17] recently presented a study examining the long-term cost-effectiveness of total knee arthroplasty compared to nonoperative management for the treatment of severe knee osteoarthritis. Outcome states on each tree were based on function as defined by the American College of Rheumatology[18] (Table 3.2). The authors used commonly available data from the literature, government life tables, and their institution to drive the model. The model allowed for the calculation of life expectancy, total time spent in each functional class and total health-care costs over the remaining life of the patient. A utility value was assigned to each ACR class using a computer-based, continuous risk assessment protocol.[19]

The authors modeled as their base case a 70-year-old female with osteoarthritis. In addition they modeled as their best case (one that would tend to be biased toward surgical intervention) a 60-year-old female. Finally, they modeled for their worst case (one biased toward nonoperative treatment) an 85-year-old male.

The results of their study are listed in Table 3.3. For the base case patient, the operative strategy provided 11.71, 2.93, .29, and .08 years spent in ACR classes I through IV, respectively. This is in contrast to the nonoperative treatment that provided 11.03 and 4.08 years in ACR classes III and IV. In total, knee replacement procedures provided 9 QALY (Quality Adjusted Life Years) at a lifetime cost of $26,103. This is in contrast with the nonoperative treatment that provided 4.41 QALY at a cost of $77,119. Thus, the marginal cost-effectiveness ratio for total knee arthroplasty for the base-case patient was negative $11,112 per QALY. The negative figure indicates that knee arthroplasty was a cost-saving (cost beneficial) procedure for a 70-year-old female with osteoarthritis. That is, the procedure was both more ef-

Table 3.3. Years spent in each ACR class for the base-case patient scenario. Marginal CE ratio for base-case, best-case, and worst-case models. Note that negative numbers mean that the strategy is cost saving as compared with nonoperative treatment. Future costs and QALY were discounted at 5% per year

	Nonoperative treatment	TKR base case	TKR best case	TKR worst case
		70-yr-old female	60-yr-old female	85-yr-old male
Years in Class I	—	11.71		
Years in Class II	—	2.91		
Years in Class III	11.03	0.29		
Years in Class IV	4.08	0.08		
QALY (@ 5%)	4.41	9		
Lifetime cost (5%)	$77,119	$26,103		
Marginal CE Ratio ($/QALY)		($11,112)	($15,305)	$34,163

fective and less expensive than the nonoperative strategy. This is a result similar to what was obtained in a parallel study on total hip arthroplasty.[19]

The model for the best-case scenario revealed knee arthroplasty to be even more beneficial with cost savings of $15,305 per QALY for a 60-year-old female.

The worst-case scenario revealed a positive ratio of $34,163 per QALY for an 85-year-old male patient. Thus, in this instance there is a cost of $34,163 for every additional QALY obtained with the operative procedure. Even this pessimistic estimate is favorably cost-effective when compared to other commonly used interventions such as renal dialysis, screening mammography, and coronary artery bypass.

References

1. Bureau of Labor Statistics. Consumer price index for all urban consumers. Department of Labor, United States. WWW site: (http://stats.bls.gov); 1996.
2. Medenhall S. 1993 hip and knee implant review. *Ortho Network News.* 1994; 5:1–3.
3. Hand R. Hospitals review ortho process to trim costs. *Hospitals.* 1992; 66:54–56.
4. Zuckerman JD, Kummer FJ, Frankel VH. The effectiveness of a hospital-based strategy to reduce the cost of total joint implants. *J Bone Joint Surg.* June 1994; 76A(6):807–811.
5. Smith HL, Fottler MD. The path to prospective payment systems. Prospective rate setting based on DRGs. Prospective payment; managing for operational effectiveness. Rockville, Md: Aspen Publications; 1985: 1–18.
6. Healy WL, Finn D. The hospital cost and the cost of the implant for total knee arthroplasty. A comparison between 1983 and 1991 for one hospital. *J Bone Joint Surg.* June 1994; 76A(6):801–806.
7. Stern SH, Singer LB, Weissman SE. Analysis of hospital cost in total knee arthroplasty. Does length of stay matter? *Clin Orthop.* December 1995; (321):36–44.
8. Meyers SJ, Reuben JD, Cox DD, Watson M. Inpatient cost of primary total joint arthroplasty. *Journal of Arthroplasty.* 1996; 11(3):281–285.
9. Medicare Physician Fee Schedule 1997, Illinois Locality 16.
10. Insall JN, ed. *Surgery of the Knee.* New York: Churchill Livingstone; 1984: 41–54.
11. Levine DB, Cole BJ, Rodeo SA. Cost awareness and cost containment at the Hospital for Special Surgery. *Clin Orthop.* February 1995; (311):117–124.
12. American Academy of Orthopaedic Surgeons. Containing the cost of orthopaedic implants. Rosemont, Ill: The American Academy of Orthopaedic Surgeons, May 1992.
13. Jordan LR, Siegel JL, Olivo JL. Early flexion routine. An alternative method of continuous passive motion. *Clin Orthop.* June 1995; (315):231–233.
14. Ververeli PA, Sutton DC, Hearn SL, Booth RE Jr, Hozack WJ, Rothman RR. Continuous passive motion after total knee arthroplasty. Analysis of cost and benefits. *Clin Orthop.* December 1995; (321):208–215.
14. Ritter MA, Keating EM, Faris PM. Closed wound drainage in total hip or total knee replacement. A prospective, randomized study. *J Bone Joint Surg.* January 1994; 76A(1):35–38.
15. Birkmeyer JD, Goodnough LT, AuBuchon JP, Noordsij PG, Littenberg B. The cost-effectiveness of preoperative autologous blood donation for total hip and knee replacement. *Transfusion.* July 1993; 33(7):544–551.
16. Russell LB, Gold MR, Siegel JE, Daniels N, Weinstein MC. The role of cost-effectiveness analysis in health and medicine. *JAMA.* October 9, 1996; 276(14)1172–1177.
17. Gottlob CA, Pelissier JM, Wixson RL, Stern SH, Chang RW. Long-term cost effectiveness of total knee arthroplasty for the treatment of osteoarthritis. *Orthopaedic Transactions.* 1996; 20(1):32–33.
18. Steinbrocker O, Traeger CH, Batterman RC. Therapeutic criteria in rheumatoid arthritis. *JAMA.* 1949; 140:659–668.
19. Chang RW, Pellisier JM, Hazen GB. A cost-effectiveness analysis of total hip arthroplasty for osteoarthritis of the hip. *JAMA.* March 20, 1996; 275(11):858–865.

SECTION 2
Clinical Evaluation

CHAPTER 4
Knee Scores in Total Knee Arthroplasty

José Alicea

HISTORICAL PERSPECTIVE

The development of the modern total knee arthroplasty can be dated back to the 1960s. The polycentric knee designed by Frank H. Gunston introduced the use of two cemented polyethylene tibial components articulating on two cemented femoral components. In addition, specialized instrumentation was used to insert the prosthesis. The introduction of a reliable fixation agent, together with a metal on polyethylene articulation, led to a furious development of designs in knee arthroplasties.

With the introduction of a multitude of different prostheses with varying degrees of tibiofemoral conformity and different philosophies with regard to the sacrifice of the anterior and posterior cruciate ligaments, different methods of evaluating total knee arthroplasty performance were developed by investigators. Over time, investigators standardized reporting methods by selecting those they found most useful. The Hospital for Special Surgery Knee Scores[7,9–11] and the Knee Society Score[8] are scales most commonly used in the medical literature to report total knee arthroplasty results.

Over the last several years, there has been an effort to develop additional ways to measure the results of medical therapeutics. Some of this methodology, commonly known as outcome studies, was developed to evaluate the results of a particular treatment through the patient's opinion. Outcome studies in total joint arthroplasty are composed of two basic measurements: a health status questionnaire and a pain and function questionnaire. The health status questionnaire attempts to measure the patient's quality of life. The Western Ontario and MacMallister Osteoarthritis Index or WOMAC[2–5] score is currently being used by the Patient Outcome Research Team at the University of Indiana in their evaluation of total knee arthroplasty.

TOTAL KNEE REPLACEMENT SCORES

The two most commonly used scores for reporting the results of knee arthroplasty in the medical literature are the Hospital for Special Surgery Knee Score (HSS Knee Score) and the Knee Society Score (KSS). The Knee Society Score can be thought of as a derivation of the HSS Knee Score because it incorporates most aspects of the HSS Knee Score and it was created at a later date. The HSS Knee Score and the KSS are evaluations performed by an observer (usually a health-care professional) through an interview and physical exam.

The Hospital for Special Knee Surgery

The Hospital for Special Surgery Knee Score (Fig. 4.1) was introduced in the late 1970s. As physicians and investigators at the Hospital for Special Surgery reported their results with different types of prosthesis, they modified their rating scales until they finally agreed to the data collected by the HSS Knee Score.

The HSS Knee Score is based on a total of 100 points. The score is divided into seven categories, which include pain, function, range of motion, muscle strength, flexion deformity, instability, and subtractions. The knee is initially given a score of 0, and additions or subtractions are made according to specific criteria. The higher the score, the better the outcome. Approximately 50% of the score is based on a patient interview and the remaining on physical exam.

Pain

Thirty points are used to describe the amount of pain during ambulating and rest. The patient is asked to describe his or her level of pain as either "none," "mild," "moderate," or "severe" during walking and at rest. A response of "no pain" is awarded 15 points, "mild pain" is awarded 10 points, and "moderate pain is awarded 5 points, and "severe" pain receives 0 points.

THE HOSPITAL FOR SPECIAL SURGERY
KNEE SERVICE

Knee Rating Sheet

Name_____ HSS #_____ Preoperative date _____

	Score	LEFT						RIGHT					
		pre	6 mo	1 yr	2 yr	3 yr	4 yr	pre	6 mo	1 yr	2 yr	3 yr	4 yr
PAIN (30 points)													
Walking: none	15												
mild	10												
moderate	5												
severe	0												
At rest: none	15												
mild	10												
moderate	5												
severe	0												
FUNCTION (22 points)													
Walk:													
walking & standing unlimited	12												
5–10 blocks, standing >30 min	10												
1–5 blocks, standing 15–30 min	8												
walk ,1 block	4												
cannot walk	0												
Stairs: normal	5												
with support	2												
Transfer: normal	5												
with support	2												
ROM (18 points)													
each 8° = 1 point													
MUSCLE STRENGTH (10 points)													
cannot break quadriceps	10												
can break quadriceps	8												
can move through arc of motion	4												
cannot move through arc of motion	0												
FLEXION DEFORMITY (10 points)													
none	10												
5°–10°	8												
10°–10°	5												
>20°	0												
INSTABILITY (10 points)													
none	10												
0°–5°	8												
6°–15°	5												
>15°	0												
TOTAL													
SUBTRACTIONS:													
one cane	1												
one crutch	2												
two crutches	3												
extension lag of 5°	2												
10°	3												
15°	5												
Deformity (5° = 1 point)													
varus													
valgus													
TOTAL SUBTRACTIONS													
KNEE SCORE													

Figure 4.1. The Hospital for Special Surgery knee rating system.

Function

Twenty-two points are used to quantify the knee's function. The observer asks the patient how far she/he can walk before having to stop. The distance is measured in terms of city blocks. Twelve points are awarded if the patient is able to walk and ambulate indefinitely, 10 points for being able to walk 5 to 10 blocks and stand for more than 30 minutes, 8 points for being able to walk 1 to 5 blocks and stand 15 to 30 minutes, 4 points for walking less than 1 block, and 0 points for not being able to walk at all.

The remaining 10 points in the function evaluation are used to determine the patient's ability to transfer, and to go up and down stairs. If the patient is able to rise from a chair without assistance or pushing off the arms of the chair, the knee is awarded 5 points. If the patient needs minimal assistance, the knee is awarded 2 points. If the patient is able to go up and down stairs independently, without holding the railing, the knee is awarded 5 points; if she or he needs to hold on to the railing or needs minimal assistance, the knee is awarded 2 points. If the patient needs significant assistance to transfer, or to go up and down stairs, the knee is awarded 0 points.

Range of Motion

Eighteen points are used to evaluate range of motion. The scale is based on a maximum range of motion of 144 degrees. One point is awarded for each 8 degrees of motion. To determine the value for this category, the health-care professional measures the range of motion of the knee. That value is then divided by eight to arrive at the final score. A patient must gain a full 8 degrees of motion before a point can be awarded. For example, if a patient's range of motion is from −5 to 120, the total range of motion is 115 degrees. The value of 115 is then divided by 8, reaching a final score of 14 points.

Muscle Strength

Ten points are used to measure quadriceps muscle strength. It is easier for the examiner to measure this category with the patient sitting. The examiner asks the patient to extend her or his leg to the maximum point and then proceeds to try to break the quadriceps muscle contracture by pushing down on the leg. If the examiner cannot break the quadriceps contracture, 10 points are awarded. If the quadriceps contracture can be broken, 8 points are awarded. If the patient cannot extend the knee against gravity, but can lie on her or his side and move her or his knee through its arc of motion, 4 points are awarded. If the patient cannot move the knee through the arc of motion, 0 points are awarded.

Flexion Contractures

Ten points are used to measure flexion contractures. No flexion contracture carries a value of 10 points, a 5 to 10 degree flexion contracture carries a value of 8 points, a 11 to 20 degree flexion carries a value of 5, and more than a 20 degree contracture carries a value of 0.

Instability

Ten points are used to determine knee instability in the varus–valgus plane. The examiner applies a varus and valgus stress to a knee positioned at maximum extension and at 90 degrees of flexion. The examiner may place a goniometer in front of the knee to estimate the degree of instability. No instability carries a value of 10 points. A 0 to 5 degree instability to varus–valgus stress carries a value of 8 points. A 6 to 15 degree instability carries a value of 5 points. More than 15 degrees of instability carries a value of 0.

Subtractions

After adding the values of the previous six categories, the pre-total score is completed. This score is subject to subtractions. Subtractions are divided into three parts: the need of the patient to use ambulatory aides; the degree of extensor lag associated with the knee; and the amount of deformity from the normal anatomic axis of 7 degrees of valgus. If the patient ambulates with a cane, 1 point is deducted. If the patient ambulates with a crutch, 2 points are deducted. If two crutches are used, 3 points are deducted. An extension lag of 5 degrees carries a 2-point deduction, of 10 degrees carries a 3-point deduction, and of 15 degrees carries a 5-point deduction.

For every 5 degrees of deviation from the normal anatomic axis of 7 degrees in either valgus or varus direction, 1 point is subtracted. This value can be obtained by measuring the alignment of the knee in maximum extension with a goniometer. Values in varus are considered negative numbers. The obtained angle is then subtracted from 7 and this value is divided by 5. The absolute value of the calculation is used. For example, if a patient has a varus alignment of 3, the calculation of $(7 - -3)/5$ is performed to arrive at a value of 2. Two points would be the applied deduction in this example.

The Hospital for Special Surgery Knee Score offers a categorical description of the final score. Scores between 100 and 85 points are considered excellent results, scores between 84 and 70 points are considered good results. Scores between 69 and 60 points are considered fair, and scores less than 60 are considered poor results.

The Knee Society Score

Founded in 1983, the Knee Society is a private society of renowned physicians and scientists with special interest in total knee replacements. In 1989, the Knee Society introduced a new rating score for total knee arthroplasty. It attempts to address some of the shortcomings of the Hospital for Special Surgery Knee Score. The Knee Society Score (Fig. 4.2) added an instability evaluation in the anteroposterior plane and a classification system for patients with associated medical conditions. The KSS

	SCORE	LEFT						RIGHT					
		pre	1 yr	2 yr	3 yr	4 yr	5 yr	pre	1 yr	2 yr	3 yr	4 yr	5 yr
PAIN None	50												
Mild or Occ	45												
Stairs only	40												
Walking & stairs	30												
Moderate Occ	20												
Cont	10												
Severe	0												
ROM: (5° = 1 point)	25												
STABILITY (medt mov any pos)													
A/P < 5	10												
5–10 mm	5												
>10 mm	0												
M/L < 5°	15												
6–9°	10												
10–14°	5												
15°	0												
TOTAL =													
Deductions (Minus)													
FLEXION CONTRACTURE													
None	0												
5–10°	2												
11–15°	5												
16–20°	10												
>20°	15												
EXTENSION LAG None	0												
<10°	5												
10–20°	10												
>20°	15												
ALIGNMENT 5–10° (None)	0												
0–4° (3 pt each deg)													
11–15° (3 pt each deg)													
Other	20												
Total Deductions =													
KNEE SCORE =													
(If total is a minus)													
(score is zero)													
FUNCTION													
WALKING: Unlimited	50												
>10 blocks	40												
5 to 10 blocks	30												
<5 blocks	20												
Housebound	10												
Unable	0												
STAIRS Norm up & down	50												
Norm up: down rail	40												
Up & down rail	30												
Up rail: unable down	15												
Unable	0												
TOTAL =													
Deductions (Minus)													
Cane	5												
Two Canes	10												
Crutches/Walker	20												
Total Deductions =													
FUNCTION SCORE =													

NAME _____ OPERATIVE TIME _____

Patient Category: A. Unilateral or bilateral (opposite knee successfully replaced)
                 B. Unilateral − other knee symptomatic
                 C. Multiple arthritis or medical infirmity

Figure 4.2. The Knee Society rating sheet for pain and function.

also applies different point values to the criteria. The Knee Society Score is divided into three sections. It consists of the Knee Score (100 points), the Knee Function Score (100 points), and a patient classification system. The classification system assigns patients to three categories depending on their associated medical conditions. Both point scores are initially valued at zero, and points are awarded or deducted according to different criteria.

The Knee Score

The Knee Score of the Knee Society Score evaluates pain relief, range of motion and stability in the anteroposterior plane and mediolateral plane. It also offers deductions for flexion contractures, extension lag, and malalignment. Like its predecessors, the Hospital for Special Surgery Score, the Knee Score is based on the interview and physical exam of the patient as conducted by a health-care professional.

Pain

Fifty points are used to evaluate pain. The interviewer asks the patient if she/he has "mild," "moderate," or "severe" pain. Subcategories include whether the pain is "occasional" or "continuous," or whether the pain occurs only during stair climbing and walking. Based on the patient's answer, the interviewer selects the most appropriate score. If the patient has no pain, the knee is awarded 50 points. If the patient has "mild" or "occasional" pain, the knee is awarded 45 points. If the patient has "mild" or "occasional" pain during stair climbing, the knee is awarded 40 points. If the patient has "mild" or "occasional" pain during walking and stair climbing, the knee is awarded 30 points. If the pain is described as "moderate" and only occurring "occasionally," the knee is awarded 20 points. If the pain is described as "moderate" and "continuous," the knee is awarded 10 points. If the patient is described as "severe," no points are awarded.

Range of Motion

Twenty-five points are awarded for range of motion. One point is awarded for every 5 degrees of motion. Rare range of motions of more than 125 degrees can only receive 25 points.

Stability

Stability is measured in the anteroposterior plane and mediolateral plane. The stability on the anteroposterior plane is measured by the maximum degree of translation of the tibia on the femur in any position. The object of this measurement is to address the stability function of the posterior cruciate ligament or its mechanical substitute. This criteria is more easily tested with the patient sitting on an examining table, allowing the examiner to place a posterior force on the tibia in different positions. A perceived motion of less than 5 mm awards 10 points. If the motion is between 5 mm and 10 mm, the knee is awarded 5 points. If the knee translates more than one centimeter, it receives no points.

Stability in the mediolateral plane is evaluated in degrees. The stability on the mediolateral plane is measured by the maximum degree of alignment change to varus/valgus stress. The examiner may place a goniometer in front of the knee to estimate the degree of instability. If the knee opens less than 5 degrees, it is awarded 15 points. If the knee opens between 6 and 9 degrees, it gets awarded 10 points. Mediolateral instability between 10 and 14 degrees gets awarded 5 points. Any mediolateral instability of more than 15 degrees is awarded no points.

Deductions

Deductions are taken for flexion contractures, extension lag, and malalignment. Flexion contractures of less than 5 degrees receive no deductions. Contractures between 5 and 10 degrees receive a 2-point deduction. Contractures between 11 and 15 degrees receive a 5-point deduction. Flexion contractures between 16 and 20 degrees receive a 10-point deduction. Contractures over 20 degrees receive a 15-point deduction.

If the knee does not exhibit an extension lag, no points are deducted. If the extended lag is less than 10 degrees, 5 points are deducted. If the lag is between 10 and 20 degrees, 10 points are deducted. Extension lags over 20 degrees receive a 15-point deduction.

Alignment of the knee between 5 and 10 degrees of valgus receives no deduction. If the knee is malaligned between 0 and 4 degrees of valgus, the alignment value is subtracted from 5 and then multiplied by 3 points to calculate the correct deduction. For example, if a knee has a valgus alignment of 2 degrees, the number 2 would be subtracted from 5 and the result, 3, would then be multiplied by 3 to arrive at a final deduction of 9 points. The same procedure is used at the other end of the scale. If the knee has a valgus alignment between 11 and 15 degrees, the number 10 is subtracted from the alignment value and the result is multiplied by 3 points to calculate the correct deduction. Knees that are placed in varus, or in more than 16 degrees of valgus receive a deduction of 20 points.

Knee Function Score

The Knee Function Score of the Knee Society Score is based on an interview between the health-care professional and the patient. The score is divided in two sections that measure the ability to walk and the ability to go up and down stairs. The ability to walk is measured in city blocks.

Walking

If the patient is able to walk an unlimited amount of blocks, the knee gets awarded 50 points. For distances more than 10 blocks, but not unlimited, 40 points are awarded. Being able to walk between 5 to 10 blocks receives 30 points, less than 5 blocks receives 20 points, household ambulators receive 10 points, and patients unable to ambulate receive no points.

Stair Climbing
If the patient is able to go up and down stairs without assistance, the knee gets awarded 50 points. If the patient needs to hold on to the rail going down the stairs, but can climb normally, the knee gets awarded 40 points. If the patient is able to climb the stairs, but is not able to go down, the knee gets awarded 15 points. If the patient cannot go up and down stairs, no points are awarded.

Deductions
Deductions for function are based on the use of ambulatory aids during walking. Five points are deducted if the patient uses a cane, 10 if the patient uses two canes. If the patient uses crutches or a walker, 20 points are deducted.

Categorical Score

Recognizing that the outcome of a knee replacement is dependent on many variables, the Knee Society devised a categorical score to try to distinguish patients with other disabilities. The patient is assigned to three different categories depending on her or his functional impairment with relation to medical infirmity or other joints in their body.

Category A
Patients are assigned to this category if they have a unilateral total knee replacement or a bilateral replacement in which the knee not being measured has been successfully replaced. This category would also apply to asymptomatic total hip arthroplasties.

Category B
Patients are assigned to this category if they have a unilateral total knee replacement and their contralateral knee is symptomatic.

Category C
Patients are assigned to this category if they have multiple arthritic sites or have a significant medical infirmity compromising their function.

The Western Ontario and MacMallister Osteoarthritis Index (WOMAC Score)

Originally designed to test the effectiveness of nonsteroidal anti-inflammatory agents in the treatment of osteoarthritis, the WOMAC Score was chosen by the Patient Outcome Research Team at the University of Indiana to study total knee arthroplasty. It is based on a questionnaire completed by the patient without the help or intervention of the health-care provider. It has proven to be an effective and reproducible vehicle in medical research.

The WOMAC questionnaire score is based on 96 points. It consists of 24 questions—5 evaluate pain, 2 evaluate stiffness, and 17 evaluate function. The patient answers each question with the choices of "none," "mild," "moderate," "severe," or "extreme." Each one of these answers has a box underneath it in the printed questionnaire. The patient marks the box that best describes her or his answer. The answer "none" carries a value of 0 points, "mild" carries a value of 1 point, "moderate" carries the value to 2 points, "severe" carries the value of 3 points, and "extreme" carries the value of 4 points. In contrast to the HSS Knee Score and Knee Society Score, a high final score in the WOMAC questionnaire represents a poor result. The questions asked are as follows:

Section A (Pain)
How much pain do you have?
 Walking on a flat surface
 Going up or down stairs
 At night while in bed
 Sitting or lying
 Standing upright

Section B (Stiffness)
How severe is your stiffness after first wakening in the morning?
How severe is your stiffness after sitting, lying, or resting later in the day?

Section C (Function)
What degree of difficulty to you have with...
 Descending stairs?
 Ascending stairs?
 Rising from sitting?
 Standing?
 Bending to floor?
 Walking on flat?
 Getting in/out of car?
 Going shopping?
 Putting on socks/stockings?
 Rising from bed?
 Taking off socks/stockings?
 Lying in bed?
 Getting in/out of bath?
 Sitting?
 Getting on/off toilet?
 Heavy domestic duties?
 Light domestic duties?

Comparison between Outcome Measures

The HSS Knee Score, Knee Society Score, and WOMAC Score are the outcome measures most often used in total knee arthroplasty evaluations. The HSS Knee Score and the Knee Society Score are interview based and dependent on a physical examination. The two main weaknesses of these scores are that they are subject to examiner bias and that the physical examination parameters can carry a significant amount of inter-observer discrepancies.[6] However, they provide more detailed information about the physical dynamics of the prosthesis than the WOMAC Score. As a result, the KSS and the HSS Score are powerful tools for comparing specific dynamics of a knee replacement.

Although the HSS Knee Score and the Knee Society Score are different in organization and technique to the WOMAC Score, the three scales have been proven to correlate well with each other in their measurement of total knee replacement outcomes.[1]

Uses of Total Knee Replacement Scores

Until recently, most total knee replacement scores were being used by investigators to report on their results of total knee arthroplasties. Investigators evaluated the preoperative function of their patients prior to total knee arthroplasty, and compared them to postoperative scores at different postoperative times. In this manner, patient variables (co-morbidities) could be evaluated, as well as different types of prosthesis.

Over the last decade there has been increased pressure to decrease the cost of medical treatments. As a result, it has become increasingly important to evaluate the outcomes of different medical treatments. Outcome studies evaluate the change in the patient's quality of life, as well as the therapeutic result. In 1989, the Agency for Health Policy and Research decided to fund several Patient Outcome Research teams to study different medical therapeutics. This type of research has two objectives: to document the value of specific therapy relative to its cost, and to determine its impact on the patient's quality of life. If this type of research is successful, the results may be used to ration or direct medical care into more "effective" therapeutic means by the government and eventually third-party payers. Many providers are concerned that this data may eventually be used to judge the ability to deliver health care.

This has led many total joint physicians who previously had limited interest in objective measures of the results of their total knee arthroplasties to reevaluate their position. Due to concerns about the role of third-party payers in deciding health-care providers, practitioners are starting to gather more outcome data. Unfortunately, at this time no one score is used to determine these "effective" means. There are different commercial products that collect a multitude of information including some of the scores discussed in this chapter, financial data on the cost of the prosthesis, length of stay, and other parameters. Most of these products are computer database software that provide a variety of reports. Physicians can use these reports to study their own data and become more competitive. Some programs allow the practitioners to join a national data bank and compare their data to others in the country.

Most of these programs have been designed by physicians in conjunction with orthopedic companies; companies that have an interest in assuring that physicians use their products to stay competitive. Some companies collect and analyze the data free of charge for physicians who use their products. Other companies sell the software and allow physicians to use the data and reports as they want. Unfortunately, this adds cost to the business operations because data collection and analysis may require a separate dedicated computer system. Eventually, if outcome data are required of all practitioners, business software packages will most likely incorporate outcome data subroutines into their products.

References

1. Alicea JA, Insall JN, Scuderi GR. Comparative analysis of outcome scores in total knee arthroplasty. Presented at AAOS, Orlando, 1995.
2. Bellamy N. Pain assessment in osteoarthritis: experience with the WOMAC osteoarthritis index. *Semin Arthritis Rheum.* 1989; 18:14–17.
3. Bellamy N, Buchanan WW, Goldsmith CH, Campbell J, Stitt LW. Validation study of WOMAC: a health status instrument for measuring clinically important patient relevant outcomes to antirheumatic drug therapy in patients with osteoarthritis of the hip or knee. *J Rheumatol.* 1988; 15:1833–1840.
4. Bellamy N, Goldsmith CH, Buchanan WW, Campbell J, Duku E. Prior score availability: observations using the WOMAC osteoarthritis index [letter] [see comments]. *Br J Rheumatol.* 1991; 30:150–151.
5. Ballamy N, Kean WF, Buchanan WW, Gerecz-Simon E, Campbell J. Double blind randomized controlled trial of sodium meclofenamate (Meclomen) and diclofenac sodium (Voltaren): post validation reapplication of the WOMAC Osteoarthritis Index. *J Rheumatol.* 1992; 19:153–159.
6. Cartwright J, Oronoz J, Stevens W, Alicea JA. Reproducibility and reliability of the Knee Society Score. Presented at Society of Military Orthopaedic Surgeons, Vail, Colorado, 1996.
7. Insall J, Scott WN, Ranawat CS. The total condylar knee prosthesis: a report of two hundred and twenty cases. *J Bone Joint Surg Am.* 1979; 61(2):173–180.
8. Insall JN, Dorr LD, Scott RD, Scott WN. Rationale of the

knee society clinical rating system. *Clin Orthop*. 1989; 248: 13–14.

9. Insall JN, Hood RW, Flawn LB, Sullivan DJ. The total condylar knee prosthesis in gonarthrosis. A five- to nine-year follow-up of the first one hundred consecutive replacements. *J Bone Joint Surg Am* 1983; 65(5): 619–628.

10. Insall JN, Lachiewicz PF, Burstein AH. The posterior stabilized condylar prosthesis: a modification of the total condylar design: two- to four-year clinical experience. *J Bone Joint Surg Am*. 1982; 64(9):1317–1323.

11. Insall JN, Ranawat CS, Aglietti P, Shine J. A comparison of four models of total knee-replacement prostheses. *J Bone Joint Surg Am*. 1976; 58(6):754–765.

CHAPTER 5
Outcomes Data Collection

Norman A. Johanson

OUTCOME OR RESULT: WHAT'S THE DIFFERENCE?

Although the term *outcome* as it relates to surgical treatment may in some cases be synonymous with what has traditionally been called a result, the outcome of a procedure may be a much more multifaceted and complex issue, primarily because of the variety of disciplines that have focused on the cost and the effectiveness of medical care. The surgeon has traditionally been centrally located in the assessment and documentation of surgical results. The indications for performing various orthopedic procedures, and their results have typically been graded according to a set of prescribed data elements derived from the surgeon's impressions of the patient's symptoms and functional status, a physical examination, and the pertinent laboratory or radiographic studies. The relative importance of each of these elements may vary depending on who is performing the evaluation. For example, the patient may place the highest value on pain relief and functional improvement.[1] The surgeon may be interested in several additional features derived from the physical examination such as range of motion, limp, and leg lengths. Radiographic findings, which are not necessarily important to the patient, are very important to the surgeon because of their diagnostic value, their direct relationship to the technical features of surgery (alignment and fixation), and their prognostic value.

Disciplines such as health services research have approached outcomes from a more global perspective. Local, regional, or national rates of performance of various procedures have been analyzed to better understand how surgery is utilized and what the effect is on large populations.[2–9] Outcome measures for studies of this type are usually derived from telephone surveys, questionnaires, and large administrative databases; the objective is to demonstrate the effectiveness of a particular surgical procedure as it is used by many surgeons in different settings on populations that differ in demographics and in comorbidity. In contrast, traditional studies have primarily addressed the efficacy of a procedure, when applied under the well-defined indications and performed using the reproducible technique of one or relatively few particular surgeons.

Government health agencies also view outcome from a global perspective gleaned from administrative databases that contain information on volume and intensity of services.[10,11] Outcome data on morbidity, mortality, and rehospitalization are used as proxy measures for the actual clinical result. Economic outcomes are a high priority among the various payers for health care, especially among private insurers because of their immediate accountability to shareholders and the financial risks to corporate viability inherent to a highly competitive marketplace.[12,13]

In summary, there are many approaches to surgical outcomes taken by a diversity of disciplines that may not be directly involved with patient care. A variety of incentives drive the process. Although the outcome that primarily determines the value of a surgical procedure should be strongly related to the actual clinical result measured in a single patient or a population, the lack of reliable clinical data and the constant pressure for cost containment have placed clinical outcomes in a secondary role. Modern approaches to the assessment of clinical outcomes offer the technology and scientific credibility necessary for reengineering hospital and office information systems.[14] Success in adapting these advances promises to improve the environment for clinical outcome measurement, monitoring, and management that is patient-centered and scientifically valid. This process should help in more rigorously defining and improving quality of care.[15–19]

OUTCOMES ASSESSMENT IN TOTAL KNEE REPLACEMENT

The focus of clinical outcomes assessment in orthopedics in general, and in total joint replacement in particular, has been and should be centered around the patient. Recent research has demonstrated that the scoring systems that have traditionally been used to evaluate the results of total hip replacement have focused on the essential issues most important to the patients who undergo the procedure. Pain, difficulty walking, and difficulty on stairs are important complaints for over 90% of patients considering total hip replacement.[1] These issues are addressed by most of the commonly used hip or knee scores.[20,21] The weighting that each item receives for scoring purposes varies among the scores, reflecting disagreement between surgeons about an item's relative importance in demonstrating an indication or a desirable outcome of surgery. Therefore, the challenge of today is not to identify new items that need to be evaluated, but to work toward establishing uniformity in assessment and documentation. The future of outcomes assessment in total joint replacement depends on how the orthopedic community responds to the following questions: (1) Why use any uniform system to measure and document outcomes at all? (2) What is the current methodological approach to outcomes assessment? (3) What particular outcome assessment instruments should be used?

WHY MEASURE AND DOCUMENT OUTCOMES AT ALL?

Expense, Hassle, and Complexity

For the busy clinician, the fundamental issue raised by any new potentially labor-intensive office-based procedure is, "Why get involved in this in the first place?" Pioneering efforts in this sort of data collection have traditionally been at well-funded, academically oriented institutions that have placed a high priority on publication of results. Actually collecting data has been time consuming, expensive, and disruptive to the office routine. However, in today's health-care environment, reliable and accurate information systems containing outcome-based data is important from more than a strictly academic perspective. In fact, the financial viability of an office, a practice, or a health-care organization may be at stake.[22] Fortunately, developments in computer technology promise to bring powerful and affordable labor-saving equipment such as touch screens and scanners into the office and produce a more efficient transfer of data from the patient to a multipurpose database.[14]

Disruption of Patient Flow

Increasing volume in the office and in the operating room has become increasingly more difficult for busy surgeons to balance. Coordinating the assessment of follow-up patients at the appropriate intervals while continuing to provide enough new patient visits may be a stressful challenge for office staff. Modern outcomes assessment has provided some solutions, and will continue to promote efficiencies realized by those who become involved. The addition of validated questionnaires that will be further discussed next, and software functions that automatically alert staff and print mailing labels at the appropriate time intervals promise to streamline the follow-up process. "Ticklers" such as these have the added potential of alerting the surgeon to any lost patients who may be having problems.

Data Overload

Concerns may also arise about the volume of data being collected. Is it really necessary to collect so much? How will this benefit the patient in exchange for the added cost to the surgeon and his or her staff? The first efforts by the American Academy of Orthopaedic Surgeons (AAOS) to collect outcomes data centrally in a pilot project in 1995 were noteworthy for the additional workload for patients and office staff. It is likely, however, that this process will be streamlined. Ultimately, fewer data elements will need to be collected than those that were originally advocated. Reductions in the so-called respondent burden (number of questions that the patient has to answer) have already been made, and there are more to come. The problem is that it remains unclear about which elements will be eliminated. For example, the SF-36, a 36-question general health status instrument that has been popularized in the orthopedic community, has been recently reduced to 12 questions in the SF-12.[23-24] Several of the questions that were eliminated related to physical functioning, and it is yet unclear how successfully this change will demonstrate the changes effected by many orthopedic procedures, particularly total joint replacement. Therefore, it seems safer at this time to continue to collect all data elements of the SF-36 until an adequate comparison between the two instruments can be made in orthopedic patients. The most important factor is that a common data set of essential elements be developed at a national level and that item reduction proceed according to a methodologically sound process.

Medicolegal Risk and Confidentiality

There are many concerns that significant medicolegal problems will arise from such comprehensive data collection, and computerization in a system either designed to become or to have a significant interface with medical records of the office, clinic, or hospital.[25] Issues such as patient confidentiality and medical malpractice exposure must be monitored and managed if outcomes assessment is to be successful on a large scale. Patient confidentiality in the computerized environment is currently the subject of intensive interest and investigation. Electronic encryption systems are being developed that promise to offer the patient the desired level of security during data transmission. The medicolegal issue is yet to be tested extensively, but the risk of having comprehensive data hurting the surgeon should be compared with the theoretical benefits of having the patient actively participate in the preoperative and postoperative assessment process by way of a questionnaire.

WHAT IS THE CURRENT APPROACH TO ORTHOPEDIC OUTCOMES ASSESSMENT?

Essential Data Elements

Over the past five years, several groups representing specialty societies and the general membership of the AAOS have identified essential data sets that constitute the framework of a modular system for office-based orthopedic outcomes assessment.[23] This process has resulted in the release in 1996 of several instruments designed to be used for outcomes measurement in the upper extremities, lower extremities, spine, and in pediatric patients. Except for the pediatrics instrument, which possesses unique characteristics, the instruments share identical elements that describe the following: (1) patient demographics (age, gender, race, education, marital status, living arrangements, employment, disability status, compensation status), (2) comorbidity, (3) patient's expectations (symptom reduction, functional gain, sleep improvement, return to work and recreational activities), (4) patient's satisfaction with current symptoms, and (5) general health status. Disease-specific symptoms and related functional questions are included in core instruments that relate to the region of interest such as the upper or lower extremity, or in specialty-related modules that address issues such as sports knee injuries, or hip and knee arthritis.

How Should Outcomes Data Be Collected?

Instruments used to collect outcomes data are similar to laboratory instruments that have been traditionally thought of as sources of "hard" data.[26] The hardness or softness of any data is determined by a few important characteristics that need to be tested before using the instrument in practice. This testing process is referred to as validation, and it involves three basic steps: (1) reproducibility or reliability, (2) validity, and (3) responsiveness.

The reproducibility of an instrument is a very important feature because it represents the "background noise" generated by differing responses by the same stable patient when tested within a few days.[27–30] The better the reproducibility, the lower the noise. As noise increases with poor reproducibility, real clinical change becomes harder to detect, either in an individual or in a population. Consequently, more patients need to be measured in order to detect significant differences between two procedures, or to conclusively state that no difference exists.[30,31]

The validity of an instrument relates to its ability to measure or demonstrate the concept that it purports to be measuring.[27–30] Face validity involves seeking a consensus among experts that the issues addressed and the response categories are appropriate for the condition or procedure being studied. Criterion validity utilizes an acknowledged "gold standard" for comparison with selected items dealing with a single concept. For example, a question (or questions) that assesses the patient's walking distance can be validated by comparing the patient's own assessment of capability to the actual performance during a timed walking distance test. When tested in a series of patients, the finding of a correlation between self-assessment and actual performance would tend to provide validity to the instrument's claims to assess walking ability.[30]

The responsiveness of an instrument is its ability to demonstrate the appropriate change (improvement or deterioration) when the patient actually changes, in distinction to its stability, which is a measure of an instrument showing no change when the patient's clinical status is stable. The ideal instrument will demonstrate stability or reproducibility in a stable patient, and will be sensitive enough to change appropriately when the patient's status either improves or deteriorates. The magnitude of change that is sought in a given treatment (clinically important difference) and the reproducibility of the instrument are essential determinants of the number of patients that need to be followed in comparing two or more treatments in a clinical trial.[30,31] A poorly reproducible instrument that does not show much change with a particular treatment will require more patients to provide adequate power for conclusions regarding relative effectiveness of those procedures.

The interrelatedness of the three cardinal features of instrument validation can be best appreciated when considering how the instruments will be focused. For clinical use, the data elements must be of interest to the clinician (face validity). In addition, the instrument change affected by treatment should match the judgment of a skilled clinician regarding the quality of the result (responsiveness). These features must be combined with the scientific rigor of an instrument that does not change when the patient's clinical status is stable (reproducibility). It should be noted that even though knee scores have been widely accepted by the orthopedic community, there are none that have comprehensively passed through all three stages of the validation process.[21,27,28] The publication of a knee score is not the equivalent of validation. On the other hand, it is likely that the difficulties associated with validation of traditional physician-administered knee scores can be explained by the method of administration rather than the content of the questions.

The potential for bias in the evaluation of a postoperative result has been well documented. Lieberman has reported significant differences between questionnaire-based responses from patients' and physicians' evaluations following total hip replacement.[32] The physician's evaluation was consistently more favorable than the patient's, and the difference increased in patients with inferior surgical results. The possible causes of the observed discrepancy were different expectations and definitions of the quality of outcome. The physician's communication style and his or her relationship with the patient may also have an impact on the evaluation of a surgical result. McGrory found differences between physician and patient evaluation of walking distance and limp following total hip replacement, but noted many more differences when the outcome of total knee replacement was studied.[33] After total knee replacement, the surgeon's evaluation was always better than the patient's in the categories of pain, walking distance, stairs, transfer, range of motion, and strength. When excellent, good, fair, and poor categories were used to classify the outcomes among 200 one hip and knee arthroplasties, 70 (35%) patients would be recategorized when comparing the surgeon's with the patient's own evaluation. Fifty of the 70 (71%) patients were placed in an inferior category by a patient-based questionnaire compared to a surgeon-generated hip or knee score. The question regarding which evaluation, a patient-administered questionnaire or the surgeon's assessment, is more accurate and reliable awaits further study. However, in light of the validation issues mentioned earlier, the questionnaire is likely to become the standard approach. A trained, unbiased observer who administers an instrument may provide the same or better reliability as a self-administered questionnaire, but the cost of such a process would be prohibitively high in most cases. On the other hand, patients who have difficulty filling out questionnaires because of problems such as illiteracy or poor comprehension may need special assistance.

WHICH OUTCOME ASSESSMENT INSTRUMENTS SHOULD BE USED?

Disease-Specific Instruments

In the 1970s Kettlekamp and Thompson advocated the development of a uniform knee rating system according to the following criteria: (1) important measurable characteristics of the knee should be used, (2) the arbitrary assignment of point values should be avoided, (3) the actual clinical result should be related to the total point value derived by the scoring system, (4) the clinical variables should be easily quantified, and (5) the system should be simple to use.[34] Traditional knee scores have typically involved the clinician's evaluation of knee symptoms, the assessment of associated functional impairment, and important physical findings such as knee deformity, stability, and range of motion. An example is the Hospital for Special Surgery (HSS) Knee Score, which has gained wide acceptance.[35] The HSS Knee Score was found by Drake to be used to rate the outcome of primary total knee arthroplasty in 66% of 210 studies published in the English language literature from 1972 to 1992.[21] It was among the earliest of the scoring systems to be developed, and the other 33 systems cited by Drake were relatively recent additions. Subsequent scores have included minor variations, but the primary data elements dealing with pain, walking, function, range of motion, and deformity have emerged as a consensus. In an effort to consolidate the important data elements into a uniform approach to evaluating the outcome of total knee arthroplasty, the Knee Society developed the two-part Knee Society Clinical Rating System.[36] By consensus the knee score that included the assessment of pain severity and physical examination (range of motion, stability, and deformity) were separated from the function score (walking, stairs, and support). The rationale for this was that the function of an aging individual deteriorates without necessarily being affected by the actual condition of the knee. Therefore, a single global score may not adequately reflect the true outcome of knee surgery. Consequently, the knee and function scores were represented by separate 100-point scales. Deductions from each scale were based on the degree of deformity (knee score) and the amount of support used for walking (function score).

Questionnaire Adaptations of Knee Scores

Because follow-up evaluations may be difficult to perform in person, the various knee scores have been adapted to a questionnaire format. In such a questionnaire, the patient is queried regarding symptoms and functional activities using standardized questions with four to six graded response categories from which to choose. Because there can be no clinician-performed physical examination, the score can be truncated, leaving out those elements that require a physical exam and reducing the possible maximum point score.[33] In lieu of a physical exam proxy questions may be developed for the translation of such functional issues as difficulty with stairs to muscle strength. Rather than directly measuring range of knee motion, asking the patient to mark a diagrammatic representation may give some sense about the actual range. McGrory adapted the HSS Knee Score to a questionnaire format and eliminated the sections relating to flexion contracture and instability, truncating the maximum score to 80.[33] Range of motion, however, was retained, and determined from the patient's response to a diagram depicting the knee in various positions from 0 to 120 degrees. Muscle strength was determined by the patient's assessment of his or her own ability to climb stairs, the support required, and the presence or absence of a limp.

Crosslinks from Validated Instruments

An alternative approach to generating traditional knee scores from questionnaire data is to utilize a scientifically validated questionnaire and construct crosslinks from the response categories of the questionnaire to the appropriate symptom or functional level specified in the traditional scoring system. Questionnaires that have been validated have a higher probability of providing reliable data and scores that will generate statistically significant differences among appropriate patient populations for reasons listed earlier. For example, the WOMAC (Western Ontario and McMaster University Osteoarthritis Index) questionnaire for hip and knee arthritis is a published and validated scale that contains most of the data elements for constructing crosslinks to traditional knee scores.[37] The WOMAC includes 5 questions about pain, 2 regarding stiffness, and 17 functional questions. To generate a knee score, some supplementary questions would be required that deal with walking distance, walking support, muscle strength, and range of motion. The WOMAC has been accepted by the AAOS Committee on Outcome Studies as the Arthritis Module for lower extremity data collection.[23]

General Health Status Instruments

General health status instruments are useful for evaluating the health of patients with a variety of medical conditions. Unlike disease-specific measures, they facilitate the comparison of treatments across disease boundaries. The SF-36 was developed during the Medical Outcomes Study, an observational study conducted between 1986 and 1990 on adult patients in Boston, Chicago, and Los Angeles.[24] Over a 2-year period, 2546 patients were surveyed at 6-month intervals. The short form is a 36-item questionnaire that measures three major health attributes and eight health concepts. Each health concept is scored on a scale of 0 (worst) to 100 (best). There is no global score calculated. Functional status as an attribute takes into account the concepts of physical function, social function, and role limitations caused by either physical or emotional problems. Well-being encompasses mental health, energy or fatigue, and pain. The attribute of overall health includes the patients' perceptions of their current health, expectations of the future, and the changes in their health over the past year. The results of total joint replacement correlate best with the postoperative improvements in the physical Functioning and Pain scales.[38-40] Recently the SF-36 has been reduced to the SF-12, eliminating all but 2 of the original 10 physical function questions. The impact of this change on the sensitivity of the instrument to the effects of total joint replacement has not been reported.

The Arthritis Impact Measurement Scales (AIMS) is a 45-item questionnaire that was developed for use in rheumatoid arthritis, but has also been used to evaluate patients with degenerative arthritis.[30,41-43] There are nine scales that are scored from 0 (best health) to 10 (worst health). In addition to the nine specific scales, a global rating utilizing a visual analog scale has been used. The scales can be combined to form an overall 100-point scale (0 = best, 100 = worst). The results of total joint replacement correlate best with the pain, mobility, physical activity, and global evaluation scales.[30]

CONCLUSION

The orthopedic community has been a leader in outcomes assessment for nearly 100 years since E.A. Codman instituted his "End Result System" at the turn of the century.[44] Throughout the twentieth century there have been various attempts to uniformly categorize musculoskeletal symptoms and functional impairments that make up the indications and outcomes of medical and surgical treatments. The current approach to outcomes assessment is not a significant departure from this tradition, but is simply a continuation of the same effort, with the addition of scientifically valid measurement instruments; and convenient, affordable computer technology. The new information should assist clinicians in making their practice more cost-effective, a clear mandate in today's health-care environment. At the same time, a clearer definition of quality and efficiency of care should begin to emerge as the data is shared on a local, state, and national level. The utilization of common data elements in the evaluation of outcomes following total knee replacement has been advocated for several years, but the method of data collection has been such that the reliability of the data has been an important mitigating factor in assembling a large national or international database. Patient-administered questionnaires have emerged as a reliable way to document a patient's preoperative and postoperative status. If a consensus is reached on the use of questionnaire-based data elements, this would open the way for the establishment of large databases that will be able to educate clinicians about issues of quality improvement, and protect quality itself from being dominated by the tyrannical forces of cost containment.

References

1. Wright JG, Rudicel S, Feinstein AR. Ask patients what they want: evaluation of individual complaints before total hip replacement. *J Bone Joint Surg.* 1994; 76-B:229–234.
2. Chassin MR, Brook RH, Park RE, Keesey J, Fink A, Kosecoff J, Kahn K, Merrick N, Solomon DH. Variations in the use of medical and surgical services by the medicare population. *N Engl J Med.* 1986; 314:285–290.
3. Friedman B, Elixhauser A. Increased use of an expensive, elective procedure: total hip replacements in the 1980's. *Med Care.* 1993; 31(7):581–596.
4. Keller RB, Soule DN, Wennberg JE, Hanley DF. Dealing with geographic variations in the use of hospitals. *J Bone Joint Surg.* 1990; 72-A:1286–1293.
5. Keller RB, Rudicel SA, Liang MH. Outcomes research in orthopaedics. *J Bone Joint Surg.* 1993; 75-A:1562–1574.
6. Madhok R, Lewallen DG, Wallrichs SL, Ilstrup DM, Kurland RL, Melton LJ. Trends in the utilization of primary total hip arthroplasty, 1969 through 1990: a population-based study in Olmsted County, Minnesota. *Mayo Clin Proc.* 1993; 68:11–18.
7. Melton LJ, Stauffer RN, Chao EYS, Ilstrup DM. Rates of total hip arthroplasty: a population-based study. *N Engl J Med.* 1982; 307:1242–1245.
8. Peterson M, Hollenberg J, Szatrowski T, Johanson NA, Mancuso CA, Charlson ME. Geographic variations in the rates of elective total hip and knee arthroplasties among Medicare beneficiaries in the United States. *J Bone Joint Surg.* 1992; 74-A:1530–1539.
9. Wennberg J, Gittelsohn A. Variations in medical care among small areas. *Sci Amer.* 1982; 246(4):120–134.
10. Melfi C, Holleman E, Arthur D, Katz B. Selecting a patient characteristics index for the prediction of medical outcomes using administrative claims data. *J Clin Epidemiol.* 1995; 48(7):917–926.
11. Mitchell JB, Bubolz T, Paul JE, Pashos CL, Escarce JJ, Muhlbaier LH, Weisman JM, Young WW, Epstein RS, Javitt JC. Using Medicare claims for outcomes research. *Med Care.* 1994; 32(7):JS38–JS51.
12. Emanuel EJ, Brett AS. Managed competition and the patient-physician relationship. *N Engl J Med.* 1993; 329(12): 879–882.
13. Inglehart JK. Physicians and the growth of managed care. *N Engl J Med.* 1994; 331(17):1167–1171.
14. Wallace S. The computerized patient record. *Byte.* 1994; May:67–75.
15. Angell M, Kassirer JP. Quality and the medical marketplace—following elephants. *N Engl J Med.* 1996; 335:883–885.
16. Blumenthal M. Quality of health care: part 1. Quality of care—what is it? *N Engl J Med.* 1996; 335:891–893.
17. Brook RH, McGlynn EA, Cleary PD. Quality of health care: part 2. Measuring quality of care. *N Engl J Med.* 1996; 335: 966–969.
18. Chassin MR. Quality of care: time to act. *JAMA.* 1991; 266(24):3472–3473.
19. Inglehart JK. The national committee for quality assurance. *N Engl J Med.* 1996; 335:995–999.
20. Bryant MJ, Kernohan WG, Nixon JR, Mollan RAB. A statistical analysis of hip scores. *J Bone Joint Surg.* 1993; 75-B:705–709.
21. Drake BG, Callahan CM, Dittus RS, Wright JG. Global rating systems used in assessing knee arthroplasty outcomes. *J Arthroplasty.* 1994; 9(4):409–417.
22. Relman AS. Shattuck Lecture—The health care industry: Where is it taking us? *N Engl J Med.* 1991; 854–859.
23. American Academy of Orthopaedic Surgeons, Council of Musculoskeletal Specialty Societies. Lower Limb, Upper Limb, Spine, and Pediatrics Outcomes Data Collection Packages, Version 1.0, February, 1996.
24. Ware JE, Sherbourne CD. The MOS 36-item short-form health survey (SF-36). *Med Care.* 1992; 30:473.
25. Woodward B. The computer-based patient record and confidentiality. *N Engl J Med.* 1995; 333(21):1419–1422.
26. Fries JF. Toward an understanding of patient outcome measurement. *Arth Rheum.* 1983; 26(6):697–704.
27. Bellamy N, Campbell J. Hip and knee rating scales for total joint arthroplasty: a critical but constructive review. Part 1. *J Orth Rheum.* 1989; 3:3–21.
28. Bellamy N, Campbell J. Hip and knee rating scales for total joint arthroplasty: a critical but constructive review. Part 2. *J Orth Rheum.* 1989; 2:63–76.
29. Charlson M, Johanson N, Williams P. Scaling, staging and scoring. In: Troidl H, Spitzer W, and McPeek B, et al., eds. Principles and practice of research: strategies for surgical investigators. New York: Springer-Verlag, 1991:192–200.
30. Johanson NA, Charlson M, Sztrowski T, Ranawat CS. A self-administered hip-rating questionnaire for the assessment of outcome after total hip replacement. *J Bone Joint Surg.* 1992; 75-A:1619–1626.
31. Guyatt G, Walter S, Norman G. Measuring change over time: assessing the usefulness of evaluative instruments. *J Chronic Dis.* 1987; 40:171–178.
32. Lieberman JR, Dorey F, Shekelle P, Schumacher L, Thomas B, Kilgus DJ, Finerman GA. Differences between patients' and physicians' evaluations of outcome after total hip arthroplasty. *J Bone Joint Surg.* 1996; 78-A:835–838.
33. McGrory BJ, Morrey BF, Rand JA, Ilstrup DM. Correlation of patient questionnaire responses and physician history in grading clinical outcome following hip and knee arthroplasty: a prospective study of 201 joint arthroplasties. *J Arthroplasty* 1996; 11(1):47–57.
34. Kettlekamp DB, Thompson C. Development of a knee scoring scale. *Clin Orthop.* 1975; 107:93.
35. Insall JN, Ranawat CS, Aglietti P, Shine J. A comparison of four models of total knee replacement. *J Bone Joint Surg.* 1976; 58-A:754.
36. Insall JN, Dorr LD, Scott RD, Scott WN. Rationale of the Knee Society clinical rating system. *Clin Orthop.* 1989; 248: 13.
37. Bellamy N, Buchanan WW, Goldsmith CH, Campbell J, Stitt LW. Validation study of WOMAC: a health status instrument for measuring clinically important patient relevant outcomes to antirheumatic drug therapy in patients with osteoarthritis of the hip or knee. *J Rheumatol.* 1988; 15:1833–1840.
38. McGuigan FX, Hozack WJ, Moriarty L, Eng K, Rothman

RH. Predicting quality-of-life outcomes following total joint arthroplasty: limitations of the SF-36 health status questionnaire. *J Arthroplasty*. 1995; 10(6):742–747.
39. Rissanen P, Aro S, Slatis P, Sintonen H, Paavolainen P. Health and quality of life before and after hip or knee arthroplasty. *J Arthroplasty*. 1995; 10(2):169–175.
40. Ritter MA, Albohm MJ, Keating EM, Faris PM, Meding JB. Comparative outcomes of total joint arthroplasty. *J Arthroplasty*. 1995; 10(6):737–741.
41. Dawson J, Fitzpatrick R, Carr A, Murray D. Questionnaire on the perceptions of patients about total hip replacement. *J Bone Joint Surg*. 1996; 78-B:185–190.
42. Liang MH, Larson MG, Cullen KE, Schwartz JA. Comparative measurement of efficiency and sensitivity of five health status instruments for arthritis research. *Arthrit and Rheumat*. 1985; 28:542–547.
43. Liang MH, Fossel AH, Larson MG. Comparisons of five health status instruments for orthopaedic evaluation. *Med Care*. 1990; 28:632.
44. Codman EA. *The Shoulder*. Boston, Mass, 1934: v–xl.

SECTION 3
Prosthetic Design

CHAPTER 6
PCL-Sparing Total Knee Arthroplasty

Paul N. Smith and Cecil H. Rorabeck

THE CASE FOR RETENTION OF THE POSTERIOR CRUCIATE LIGAMENT IN TOTAL KNEE ARTHROPLASTY

The posterior cruciate ligament is known to be present in the vast majority of knees undergoing total joint arthroplasty.[1] The arguments for and against retention of the posterior cruciate ligament have been joined over (1) range of motion, (2) the phenomenon of femoral rollback, (3) stability, (4) correction of deformity, (5) gait analysis, (6) stresses at the bone–prosthesis interface, (7) wear, and more recently, (8) proprioception.[2,3,4,5] We will consider these in turn to demonstrate the rationale for retention of the posterior cruciate ligament in total knee arthroplasty.

Range of Motion

It has been argued that the phenomenon of rollback of the femur on the tibia during flexion prevents the impingement of the femur on the posterior border of the tibia with flexion.[2] Therefore, range of motion should be higher in a knee that has normal posterior femorotibial contact in flexion. A second means of achieving posterior articulation of the femur with the tibia in the replaced knee in flexion was mooted by shifting the axis of motion permanently posteriorly[3] as in the Freeman-Samuelson knee. In this situation it is important to realize the importance of achieving full coverage of the tibial plateau by the tibial component, because incomplete coverage can predispose to component migration. Hence, one may be constrained in the position that one can place the tibial component, depending on the need to obtain full plateau coverage and by the geometry of the component. A more elegant solution is to allow rollback to occur and to use an appropriately designed tibial component to permit this motion.

The literature does not support an advantage in range of motion for posterior cruciate sacrifice over retention. A study by Becker and associates[6] in which 30 paired bilateral cruciate retaining and cruciate substituting total knee arthroplasties were evaluated found no clinical advantage of one type over another. Dorr and colleagues[7] analyzed 11 patients with paired bilateral cruciate retaining and cruciate sacrificing total knee arthroplasties and noted that the range of motion and knee scores were equal at 5 years for both sets of knees.

Femoral Rollback

Femoral rollback is defined as the posterior shift of the tibiofemoral contact areas. Kapandji[8] credits Weber in 1836 with performing an experiment in which they marked on the cartilage corresponding points of contact between the femoral and tibial condyles. They noted that the point of contact moved back during flexion and that the distance between the points of contact marked on the femoral condyle was double that marked on the tibial plateau, demonstrating a combination of rolling and sliding of the femoral condyle on the tibial plateau.

Lindahl and Movin[9] in investigating the mechanics of extension of the knee found that rollback of the femur on the tibia occurred; however, they did not differentiate between motion at the medial and lateral condyles. They found that the rollback occurred in the first 30 degrees of knee flexion and that thereafter rollback did not occur. Nisell[10] likewise found significant rollback of the tibiofemoral contact point of 40% of the plateau sagittal breadth. This study showed a rollback at flexion angles of greater than 30 degrees, but agreed that most of the rollback occurred in the first 30 degrees of flexion. Walker and Hajek[11] in 1972 investigated the load-bearing area in the cadaver knee and found the average contact areas for the lateral and medial condyles were 1.4 and 1.8 cm^2. These areas diminished as the angle of flexion increased and also moved well posteriorly on the tibia with flexion on both lateral and medial sides.

Goodfellow and O'Connor[12] demonstrated that the contact areas in the cadaveric knee are anterior in extension and posterior in flexion. They note that this phenomenon maximizes the power of the quadriceps to extend the knee and minimizes the compressive forces at the articular surfaces.

Kurosawa and associates[13] analyzed the relative motion of the medial and lateral condylar centers of motion in both cadaver and volunteer knees. Results in both groups were comparable, with the medial center moving forward by 4.5 mm to midflexion and then moving back 2.3 mm. The lateral center moved back progressively throughout flexion a total of 17 mm. This movement of centers occurred with a 20 degree external rotation of the tibia through knee flexion. This result is somewhat surprising; however, these authors note that the forward motion of the center of motion of the medial condyle does not necessarily reflect forward movement of the contact points.

Walker, Rovick, and Robertson[14] used a computer model generated by embedding, slicing, and digitizing the bone outlines and ligament coordinates. They used as their flexion-extension axis a line joining the centers of radii of the essentially circular posterior condyles. They found that for average knee motion the contact points on the lateral and medial sides moved posteriorly with flexion and that the rate of this posterior movement decreased with increasing angle of flexion. For the lateral plateau the initial contact point was near the midpoint in the anteroposterior axis and moved back 10 mm by 30 degrees, 14 mm by 45 degrees, and then remained constant. The contact point medially at full extension was 30% from the anterior edge of the plateau. It moved posteriorly and uniformly 13 mm up to 45 degrees flexion, after which it stayed constant.

Shapeero and colleagues[15] used an ultra-fast cine-CT technique to investigate the functional dynamics of 12 cadaver knee joints. They found that the lateral femoral condyle moved an average of 2.3 times farther on the tibial plateau than the medial condyle. The percentage of rolling movement of the lateral condyle was 46% versus the medial condyle at 21%. The overall gliding motion was 54% for the lateral condyle and 79% for the medial condyle. The average lateral condyle arc on the tibia was longer (average of 2.34 cm) than the medial condylar arc (average of 1.01 cm).

Thompson and colleagues[16] used MRI to assess the behavior of the meniscus during flexion-extension in cadaver knees. They found that both menisci translated posteriorly with knee flexion, the lateral virtually double the distance of the medial. In this article the authors publish elegant series of parasagittal images through the medial and lateral femoral condyles at varying angles of knee flexion. These images clearly show significant posterior translation of the femorotibial contact points on both medial and lateral plateaus with progressive knee flexion.

Freeman and Railton[3] state that the section of the anterior cruciate ligament and retention of the posterior cruciate ligament destroys the normal mechanism of femoral rollback and rollforward. The implication here is that the anterior cruciate ligament deficient knee will not display rollback. Schoemaker and associates[17] used a testing rig with 6 degrees of freedom to examine the motion of cadaveric knees with the anterior cruciate ligament intact, sectioned, and reconstructed. Normal rollback was seen in all these scenarios. The anterior cruciate deficient group not surprisingly exhibited additional anterior displacement throughout the flexion range. Therefore, the section of the anterior cruciate ligament does not stop normal rollback. Normal rollback will still occur with the addition of a further degree of freedom due to the loss of the restraint of the anterior cruciate. Rollback is therefore not solely dependent on an intact functioning anterior cruciate ligament. Whether or not rollback occurs in the knee without both an anterior or posterior cruciate ligament is not known.

The question of what occurs with respect to rollback in the prosthetically replaced knee is not yet clear. Kurosawa and associates[13] used radiographic evaluation to assess the motion of the replaced knee in 14 patients with kinematic 1 condylar prostheses. They found that the posterior translations of the center of motion of both the medial and lateral condyles averaged 2.2 mm through the arc of flexion. This was notably less than in the normal knees they assessed. They also noted that almost all the femoral axis points were over the central third of the tibial surface and concluded that the posterior cruciate in preventing excessive anterior movement of the femur on the tibia aided in this more central contact, thereby reducing eccentric loading on the components.

Soudry and colleagues[18] measured contact point location in 10 fresh knee specimens with prosthetic joints inserted and found that the contact point locations were similar for both the medial and lateral plateaus. They found that rollback occurred through the range of flexion and was of the order of approximately 5 mm for the flat and the dished plastic trays tested.

El Nahass and associates[19] used an electromagnetic device to track the motion of the knee in 25 normal volunteers and 25 total knee patients (Kinematic 2). Motion of the total knees was similar to that of the normal knees. For standing, sitting, and free-swing, the knee rotated internally by 5 to 10 degrees and the femur displaced posteriorly by 9 to 14 mm, through a flexion range from 0 to 90 degrees. This result would imply that rollback does occur in the replaced knee with posterior cruciate retention.

Stability

There is no question that the posterior cruciate ligament is the primary physiologic stabilizer of the knee to posterior displacement of the tibia on the femur and that this importance increases with increasing flexion. The posterior cruciate ligament also acts as a secondary stabilizer in mediolateral displacement, varus-valgus angulation, and axial rotation.[20,21,22] In the absence of the posterior cruciate forces that are normally supported by this ligament must be either taken up by secondary soft tissue restraining structures, or supported by the implant itself. These forces are not solely compressive but also shear and may predispose to either wear of the polyethylene component or to failure at the bone-prosthesis or bone-cement interface. The use of a physiological stabilizer rather than a prosthetic articulation to stabilize the knee arthroplasty removes a potential source of wear from the prosthetic construct. Soudry and colleagues[18] showed that retention of the posterior cruciate stabilized femorotibial contact points close to the center of the tibial plastic surface using a series of tibial plastic designs. When the posterior cruciate was sacrificed, they found that the contact points moved to the extreme anterior of the plastic, theoretically placing the anterior component under high compression and also the posterior component-bone interface under tension. Such assymetric loading predisposes to wear of the plastic and may predispose to mechanical failure of the component- or cement-bone interface.

Correction of Deformity

Ligament balancing is an integral part of the operation of total knee arthroplasty. Equalization of the flexion and extension gaps must be performed with any ligament releases that are required to achieve this objective. In the vast majority of cases appropriate ligament balancing can be performed without the need to sacrifice the posterior cruciate ligament.[23] Only in the rare case of extreme deformity, either varus or valgus greater than 20 degrees of the knee, is it necessary to sacrifice the posterior cruciate ligament to achieve soft tissue balancing. The process of ligament balancing in posterior cruciate ligament retention must include assessment of posterior cruciate ligament tension throughout the range of motion.[24] A posterior cruciate ligament that is too tight in flexion will restrict flexion range and produce inappropriate translation of the femur posteriorly on the tibia at the extreme of flexion. This phenomenon manifests as tilting or posterior hinging of the tibial trial insert during trial range of motion testing. If the posterior cruciate is judged to be too tight, subperiosteal recession of the ligament is performed from the posterior aspect of the proximal tibia to the point at which a full range of motion is obtained without component tilting. Ritter and colleagues[24] found that 30% of patients required this form of posterior cruciate ligament balancing and that this was performed without sacrificing posterior stability of the knee. In summary, the vast majority of total knee arthroplasties can be successfully performed with preservation of the posterior cruciate ligament as a functioning biological stabilizer of the prosthetic knee joint.

Gait Analysis

The mechanics of gait on level ground and in stair climbing have been addressed by Andriacchi and colleagues.[25] There is no question that gait is not normal following total knee arthroplasty. It is suggested that adaptive gait patterns caused by degenerative joint disease do not return to normal despite a successful arthroplasty. An interesting observation is that there is high symmetry in gait between the operated and unoperated sides in unilateral total knee arthroplasty.[26,27,28] The explanation for this is that the normal side adapts to the prosthetic gait to produce symmetry. In a subsequent study, Andriacchi's group analyzed five different total knee replacement designs with varying degrees of constraint.[29] They found that all groups had abnormalities of gait when compared to normal and all groups performed in a similar fashion in walking on level ground. They were, however, able to identify significant differences between groups in stair climbing, with patients with the least constrained cruciate retaining prosthesis having the closest to normal mechanics.

Dorr and associates[7] analyzed the gait of 11 patients with bilateral paired posterior cruciate sacrificing and cruciate retaining arthroplasties. They found the sacrificed cruciate is less efficient when walking on level ground and in climbing stairs. On level ground the increased flexion moment required more quadricep work, on stairs the soleus was more active to stabilize the tibia and due to the greater varus moment and forward trunk leaning the biceps femoris was more active. They also noted that the increased varus moment produced eccentric loading medially and theorized that this may predispose to early wear.

In summary, no study has demonstrated an advantage with respect to gait for the resection of the posterior cruciate ligament in total knee arthroplasty. On the contrary, advantage has been demonstrated for the retention of the posterior cruciate ligament in total knee arthroplasty in terms of objective gait assessment.

Stresses at the Bone-Prosthesis Interface and Wear

Total knee arthroplasties with high inherent conformity of the articular surfaces may transmit to the bone-cement-prosthesis interface stresses that in less conforming designs would be taken up by the surrounding soft tissues.[1,12,30] The posterior cruciate ligament acts to secondarily stabilize the knee against varus-valgus moments and aids to prevent lateral liftoff due to adduction moments at the knee. Excision of the PCL predisposes to eccentric loading of the tibial component and hence eccentric force transfer to the interfaces. El Nahass[19] examined knee motions in differing activities and found that a knee prosthesis should allow rotational freedom of −12 to 12 degrees and anteroposterior displacement of 13 mm, to minimize transfer of force via the componentry.

Soudry and Walker and colleagues[18] examined the effect of total joint design on tibiofemoral contact conditions. They found that a compromise situation existed by which, when the PCL was retained, shear and rocking force transmitted to the components was less than when the PCL was sacrificed. The trade-off was that with the posterior cruciate ligament retained the compressive forces transmitted to the components was greater than when the posterior cruciate was excised. However, this study noted that posterior cruciate retention produced contact points centrally on the tibial component versus more eccentrically for the posterior cruciate excision group.

Wear of the articulating polyethylene surface is a complex interaction between knee joint kinematics, component alignment, patient demands, thickness of the polyethylene, geometric design of the articulation, and polyethylene processing. There has been an assumption that the wear of the plastic insert increases with contact stress.[31] However, the picture is not so simple. Blunn and associates[32] created a wear model of a spherical femur on a flat tibial plateau that demonstrated that cyclic sliding and oscillating produced severe surface and subsurface cracking of the tibial insert and concluded that more conforming components would be less susceptible to wear as they limit sliding. Sathasivam and Walker[33] generated a computer model of optimization of the bearing surfaces in total knee arthroplasty and found that lowest contact stresses occurred with higher conformity and that it was most important to have high conformity in the coronal plane. They found that moderate conformity in the sagittal plane was required to allow sufficient laxity, avoiding excessive restraint. A similar modeling exercise was undertaken by Bartel and colleagues.[34] They found that contact stresses in tibial components were reduced most when the articulating surfaces were more conforming in the coronal plane and were much less sensitive to changes in geometry in the sagittal plane.

Retrieval studies have placed emphasis on a number of these points. Landy and Walker[35] analyzed 90 retrieved total knee arthroplasties, finding that abrasive (from cement or bone) and delamination wear were particularly pronounced. They noted that delamination was initiated by material defects and propagated due to high subsurface stresses. Collier and associates[36] examined 122 retrieved tibial inserts. They noted that the contact pressures in poorly conforming inserts were higher than the yield stress of the polyethylene and also that unconsolidated polymer powder was found in 44% of the inserts and correlated with severe wear of the articular surface. It is notable that the majority of these components were very thin, for example less than 6 mm, well below the currently recommended 8 mm.[34]

In summary, polyethylene wear is a problem due to a number of factors. Absolute conformity is not the answer as the stresses transferred to interfaces cause early failure at these interfaces. Neither is absolute nonconformity the answer as contact stresses in the polyethylene are manifestly too high, contributing to early wear of the insert. The ideal is a compromise with sufficient conformity to minimize wear (particularly with high conformity in the coronal plane and moderate conformity in the sagittal plane) and sufficient laxity to prevent interface overload. The well-balanced posterior cruciate retaining total knee arthroplasty with appropriate contour of insert meets this requirement. This issue has been recognized by Scott and Thornhill[37] who have recently reported on a series in which the posterior cruciate ligament was retained and appropriately balanced and the tibial insert was sagittally more conforming. They found range of motion to be identical with a matched group of patients in which a flat insert was used and noted that this practice achieved an attractive compromise between the schools of cruciate preservation and sacrifice, allowing theoretical improvement in polyethylene wear with higher conformity of bearing surfaces to be combined with the advantages of preservation of the posterior cruciate.

Early designs of the posterior cruciate-retaining total knee replacement were often flawed in technique and design. Particularly use of polyethylene, which we now know was too thin, flat nonconforming tibial inserts and insufficient attention to balance of both collateral structures and posterior cruciate ligament led to early wear and reports of failure.[38,39,40] There is no question that total knee replacement is a highly successful procedure with the vast majority of patients having successful results to 10 years and beyond. Long-term studies of modern forms of both posterior cruciate ligament-retaining and posterior cruciate ligament-sacrificing designs have shown equivalent survivorship of prostheses[41,42,43] with survivorship of around 95% at 10 years. Ritter and associates[44] have published their 10- to 18-year survival analysis of the posterior cruciate-retaining posterior cruciate condylar total knee replacement (Howmedica, Rutherford, NJ). Kaplan-Meier survival analysis revealed a 96.8% survival at 12 years. In 1993, Ranawat and colleagues[45] reported a 94% 15-year survival of 112 posterior cruciate ligament-sacrificed total condylar prostheses. Stern and Insall[43] examined 229 total knee arthroplasties using an all polyethylene posterior stabilized tibial component and found a survival rate of 94% at 13 years. Rand[46] evaluated a series of posterior cruciate-sparing arthroplasties and found a 96% survival at 10 years. Another posterior cruciate ligament-sparing design, the AGC knee system, has been recently shown to have at least equivalent survival figures to the total condylar knee in the Swedish Knee Arthroplasty Register.[47] The inevitable conclusion is that a well-performed total knee arthroplasty with either posterior cruciate retention or sacrifice have equivalent survival figures. Hence, because there is no demonstrated advantage to sacrifice of the posterior cruciate ligament in respect of long-term outcome, we recommend its retention.

Proprioception of the Knee

Proprioception of the knee has until recently received little attention with regard to total joint arthroplasty. A notable observation is the protective function for joints of proprioception, exemplified by neuropathies where proprioception is preserved but other sensation lost.[48] There is no question that the posterior cruciate ligament (PCL) has a proprioceptive role. Studies in animal models[49,50] and in human cadavers[51,52] and amputation specimens[53] have demonstrated mechanoreceptors in the posterior cruciate ligament. These mechanoreceptors powerfully influence gamma motor neurons so that even minor stretch of the posterior cruciate ligament can produce major changes in the muscle spindle afferents.[54]

Skinner and associates[55] assessed joint position sense of the knee in 29 subjects and found that proprioception deteriorated with increasing age. This finding was noted by Barrett and colleagues,[48] who also noted that proprioception improved following replacement of the osteoarthritic knee joint. Warren and associates[56] examined proprioception after total knee joint arthroplasty, in particular the role of prosthetic design on proprioception. They found that a PCL-retaining prosthesis conferred a statistically significant greater improvement in proprioception than a PCL-sacrificing design. They postulate that the more sensitive detection of joint position is due to the effective recreation of joint height, which occurs more readily in posterior cruciate-retaining prostheses.

To summarize, total knee replacement of the arthritic knee confers proprioceptive benefit, which is enhanced by retention of the posterior cruciate ligament.

Does the Posterior Cruciate Ligament Work after Total Knee Arthroplasty?

This question is predicated by the claim that for the posterior cruciate ligament to function normally following arthroplasty then normal joint line and contour must be restored. This is plainly a purist view that ignores the practical realities of joint replacement. The best approximation to normality is achieved using the correct sizing of components for a particular patient. No one is the same and hence we cannot expect normality. The assumption that the posterior cruciate ligament must function normally following arthroplasty is also unrealistic. One expects it to function; one does not expect it to function as in a normal knee. The fact that the posterior cruciate ligament does not function after joint replacement as it does in the normal knee has been demonstrated in several cadaver studies in which strain in the posterior cruciate ligament has been measured after prosthetic replacement.[57,58] These studies have shown that it is difficult to reproduce the precise normal strain in the PCL following joint replacement, a finding not at all surprising given the limitations of modularity and size ranges in total knee replacement systems. Notwithstanding, the posterior cruciate ligament appropriately retained and balanced is an excellent stabilizer of the prosthetic knee against posterior displacement of the tibia on the femur. In our current series of 442 posterior-cruciate-retaining total knee arthroplasties, at 3- to 8-year follow-up no knee had significant posterior instability and no knee was revised for problems with posterior instability. Further evidence of the functionality of the posterior cruciate ligament in posterior cruciate-retaining arthroplasty is in the work by Montgomery and associates,[59] who documented three patients who had late rupture of the posterior cruciate ligament after posterior cruciate-retaining arthroplasty. All three cases experienced severe posterior knee instability and were sufficiently symptomatic despite nonoperative therapy including physiotherapy and bracing that revision to a posterior stabilized system was deemed necessary. After revision stability was restored, symptoms resolved.

Summation

No benefit has been demonstrated in sacrifice of the posterior cruciate ligament in respect to knee range of motion or knee stability. Proprioception is inferior with posterior cruciate sacrifice. There is no evidence that posterior cruciate-sacrificing total knee arthroplasties are superior in gait performance to posterior cruciate-retaining; in fact, the reverse holds. There are also advantages in transmitting less stress to the component-bone interface and also the ease of maintaining the physiological joint line level. Long-term outcome studies also show no clear benefit to routine sacrifice of the posterior cruciate. It has been demonstrated that conforming inserts are compatible with posterior cruciate retention in total knee arthroplasty and thus concerns regarding wear of flat inserts are no longer germaine to the debate. Therefore, we support the routine retention of the posterior cruciate ligament in total knee replacement and recommend its routine sacrifice only in the rare case in which deformity is sufficiently severe.

TECHNIQUE OF POSTERIOR CRUCIATE LIGAMENT RETAINING KNEE ARTHROPLASTY

Preparation of the Patient

The patient is positioned supine on the operating table under appropriate anesthesia. A pneumatic tourniquet is applied to the upper thigh with care to ensure appropriate padding of the tourniquet site, and the tourniquet is applied sufficiently high on the thigh to allow free access to the proximal thigh for draping and to allow unrestricted access for proximal exposure of the knee. To assist with positioning of the limb we use a sandbag taped to the operating table to act as a foot rest when the knee is positioned in the flexed position. In addition a bolster or rest positioned at the level of the greater trochanter will prevent the patient's leg externally rotating at the hip when the knee is positioned in the flexed position. These measures simplify the issues of combined issues of leg positioning and retraction for the surgical assistant during the operation. Ideally, using these measures the leg should require no support in the flexed position, leaving the assistant's hands free for retraction and other purposes. Prior to skin preparation any previous skin incisions are clearly marked using an indelible marking pen to prevent any confusion regarding the appropriate line of incision once the limb is prepared and draped. The skin is prepared with a standard prep solution such as iodine. Draping is begun with placing of a stocking over the foot and ankle up to the level of the tourniquet. Care is taken to ensure that this stocking is not bulky because this may interfere with extramedullary cutting guides and that the malleoli are freely palpable. The draping proceeds with application of impervious draping material over the whole leg. A window is then made in the stocking material to expose the anterior knee, and an adhesive drape is then applied to occlude the skin. Following draping it is important to have the bony landmarks of the pelvis as well as the malleoli readily palpable in order to confirm alignment intraoperatively. A surgical marking pen is then used to mark the projected incision. The limb is exsanguinated using an Esmarch bandage and the tourniquet inflated to an appropriate pressure.

Exposure of the Knee

As a general rule a longitudinal straight anterior incision is preferred. Such an incision is extensile both proximally and distally and allows easy eversion of the patella following arthrotomy. Rarely, preexisting scars will dictate the line of approach, because there is a real risk of producing skin slough by creating "railway tracks" on the front of the patient's knee. The problem lies not so much in transverse scars as are often the result of prior high tibial osteotomy, but other more oblique, longitudinal, and paramidline scars that cannot be crossed or paralleled without concern for skin viability. Where there are parallel incisions, the most recent should be utilized, or if this is not known, the most lateral is preferred.

The incision is developed through subcutaneous fat and through the thin layer of deep fascia overlying the medial retinaculum. We prefer to perform a medial parapatellar arthrotomy, except in knees with a severe fixed valgus deformity. The arthrotomy is extended proximally in the substance of the quadriceps tendon, curves smoothly around the medial border of the patella and distally alongside the patellar tendon down to its insertion. Care is taken to preserve a tough border of tissue along the line of the arthrotomy to allow secure closure of the retinaculum at the completion of the operation. We do not routinely use modifications of this approach such as the lateral arthrotomy[60] or the subvastus approach;[61] however, recently we have used the vastus medialis splitting approach and have had no problems with this technique.

The medial proximal tibia is exposed by subperiosteal reflection of the soft tissues past the midline in the coronal plane in order to facilitate the external rotation of the tibia, which occurs during exposure of the tibial plateau. The patella is reflected laterally, with great care taken to protect the insertion of the patellar tendon in this maneuver. In cases of difficult exposure one can utilize either proximal releasing techniques such as the quadriceps snip[62] or turndown[63,64] or distally osteotomize the tibial tubercle.[65-67] Following patellar reflection, the knee is flexed, again taking care not to damage the patellar tendon insertion.

With the knee thus exposed, the joint is then debrided. Overhanging osteophytes are excised to reveal the true bony contours of the joint and to allow free access to the bone of cutting guides. Removal of osteophytes also aids in achieving balance of the soft tissues later in the procedure. If necessary a synovectomy can be performed at this stage. The anterior cruciate ligament is excized if present; however, the posterior cruciate is preserved. The infrapatellar fat pad may be either retracted, or, if this is not satisfactory, it can be excised as the situation demands. The goal at this point is to display the relevant bony anatomy unimpeded by either bony distortion or soft tissue interposition.

Cutting the Femur

Contemporary total knee replacement systems use intramedullary guide systems to assure correct alignment of cutting jigs. These intramedullary systems are preferable to extramedullary guiding systems because they are subject to less error and hence allow greater reproducibility of cuts.[68] The starting point for the initial drill is normally just medial to center above the insertion of the posterior cruciate ligament on the femur (Fig. 6.1). This point should always be checked by reference to preoperative radiographs to ensure that the correct starting point is chosen. This is marked with a punch and the initial drill introduced proximally into the femoral medullary canal. The drill is rotated to produce a widening of the hole to allow some venting of intramedullary fat to occur on introduction of intramedullary guide rod.

To prevent fat embolization a slotted or fluted intramedullary guide rod is used. We use a distal cut of 6 degrees to correspond with the normal anatomic valgus of the femur. With the cutting jig in place the intramedullary guide is inserted. Rotational alignment is then checked using the posterior femoral condyles as reference points. With rotation stabilized in the desired position, the distal femoral cutting block is pinned in place (Fig. 6.2).

The distal femoral cut should not be proximal to the fibers of the posterior cruciate ligament. After the distal femoral cut is performed, the femoral sizing jig is used to determine the appropriate size of femoral component, referencing from the anterior cortex of the femur (Fig. 6.3).

It is important to not oversize the femoral component and if in doubt one should go to the smaller size to avoid oversizing. An oversized femoral component will impair flexion range and place higher stress on the patellofemoral mechanism, also predisposing to patellar maltracking. An anterior referencing system is used to ensure the risk of notching the anterior femur is minimal. In addition, we use an anterior cut that has a built-in flexion of 4 degrees, which further protects against accidental notching of the anterior femur. Following this step, the anterior and posterior femoral cuts are completed.

Cutting the Tibia

The proximal tibia is exposed through subluxing the tibia anteriorly and externally rotating using a blunt retractor passed to the lateral side of the posterior cruciate ligament to maintain this position (Fig. 6.4). It is important to preserve the posterior cruciate ligament in this process, taking care to place the posterior retractor so damage does not occur. Further retractors can be passed medially and laterally to complete the exposure.

Again, modern arthroplasty systems will allow both intramedullary and extramedullary guide systems. It is our practice to routinely use extramedullary guides. We aim to resect sufficient tibial bone to allow for a *minimum* of 10 mm of polyethylene insert. The tibial cut is made at right angles to the long axis of the tibia in the coronal plane and incorporates approximately 3 degrees of posterior slope to mirror normal anatomy and to facilitate flexion of the prosthetic knee. We do not routinely retain a bone block anterior to the cruciate ligament but rather perform the tibial cut through the tibial plateau and then sharply dissect the remaining posterior cruciate ligament fibers from the cut fragment, taking care to preserve the continuity of the posterior cruciate ligament.

The appropriate tibial trial baseplate is selected to achieve complete coverage of the cut tibial surface without significant overhang of the tray, which may cause impingement on soft tissues in motion.

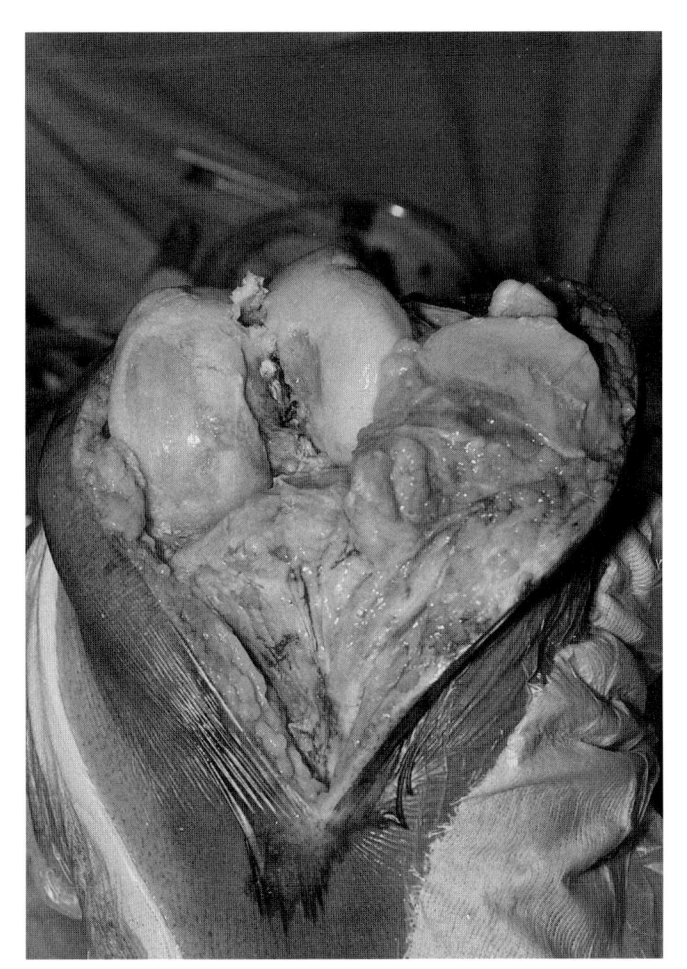

Figure 6.1. Position of the starting hole in the distal femur for the intramedullary guide rod. Note the position is just medial to center and anterior to the femoral origin of the posterior cruciate ligament.

Ligament Balancing

After the tibial cut has been made, ligament balancing is performed, ensuring equal flexion and extension gaps. Graduated blocks are utilized in this process and appropriate ligament releases are performed to achieve balance of the soft tissues with equal flexion and extension gaps (Fig. 6.5). Attfield and colleagues[69] have considered the effect of correct soft tissue balancing in both flexion and extension on knee joint proprioception. They found a significant improvement in proprioception in knees for which soft tissues had been balanced in both flexion and extension over those knees for which balance had been performed only in extension (Fig. 6.6).

Following this step the chamfer cuts on the distal femur are completed. At this stage it is important to check

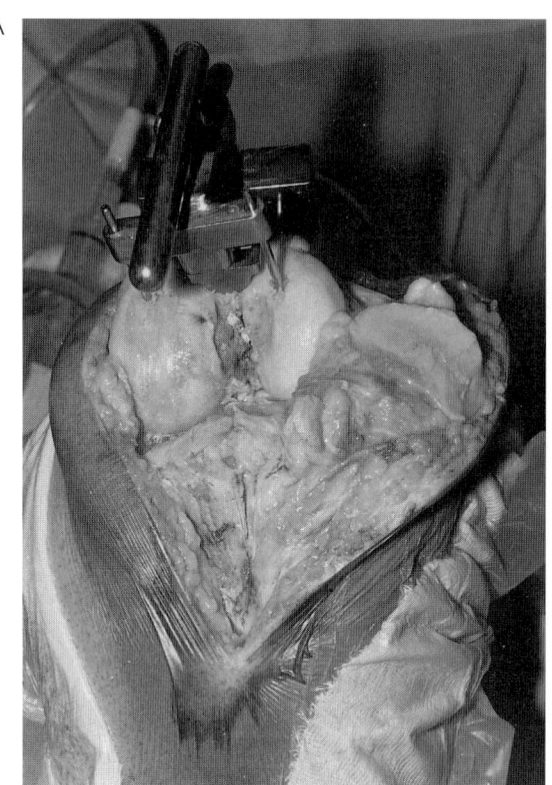

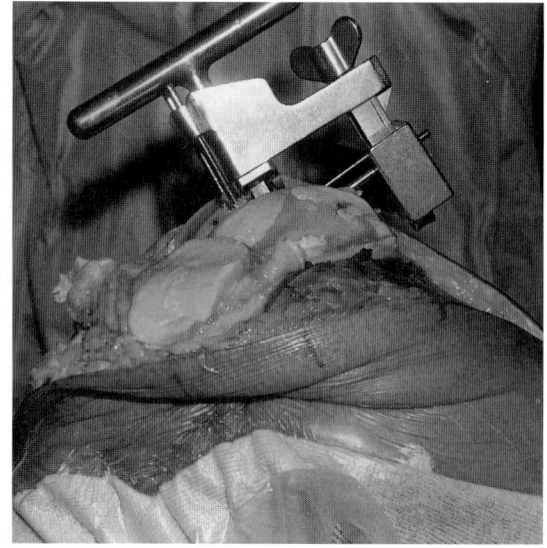

Figure 6.2. The distal femoral cutting block in position.

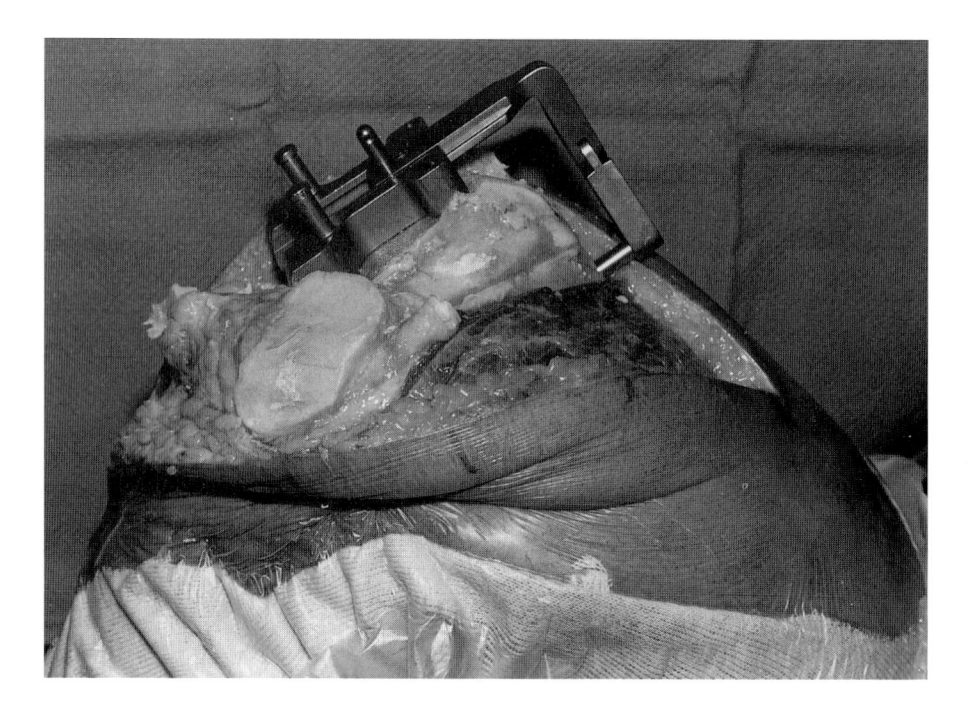

Figure 6.3. The distal cut has been performed and the sizing block applied using the anterior femoral cortex for referencing.

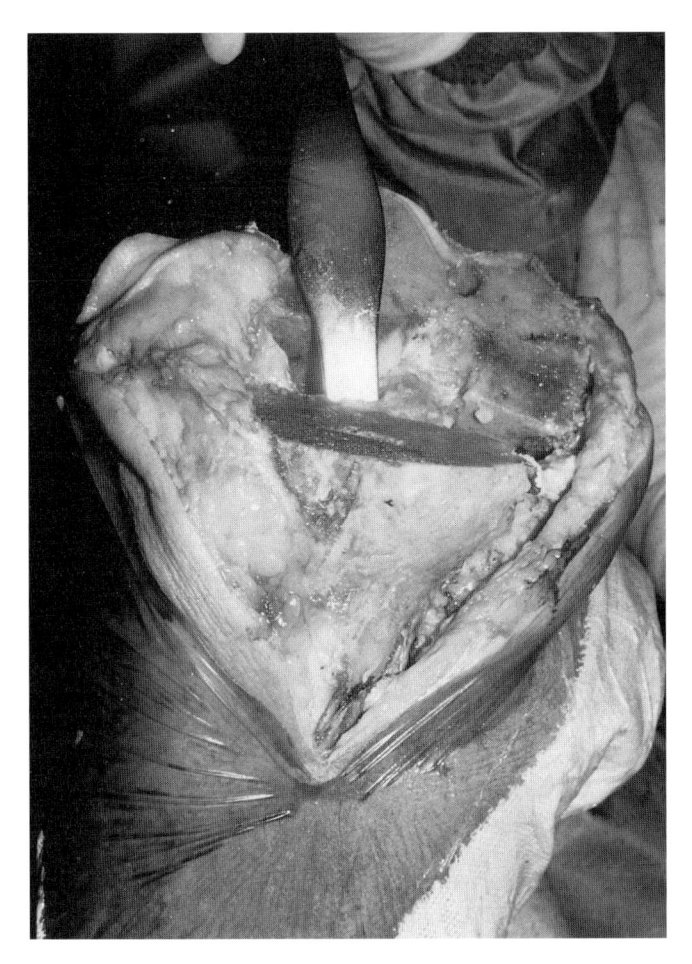

Figure 6.4. Complete exposure of the proximal tibia with posterior retractor placed lateral to the posterior cruciate ligament, which is shown well preserved after the tibial cut is performed.

for and to remove any posterior osteophytes from the femoral condyles because these can prevent full extension by tenting the posterior capsule and may also impinge on the tibial component during flexion.

After removal of these osteophytes the trial tibial and femoral components are inserted, using the graduated blocks to calculate the appropriate thickness of the tibial insert. The knee is then taken through a range of motion, first, to assess the tension of the posterior cruciate ligament, second, to enable rotational position of the tibial component to be checked, and third, to assess patellar tracking. The posterior cruciate ligament must be evaluated for tension through the range of knee motion. If the ligament is too tight, then flexion range will be reduced with anterior subluxation of the tibia on the femur as the knee flexes and stress concentration posteriorly on the polyethylene insert. The technique of balancing the posterior cruciate ligament has been previously described by Ritter and colleagues.[24] This technique takes advantage of the long insertion of the posterior cruciate ligament on the posterior proximal tibia. As the knee with trial components in situ is taken through a range of motion, the motion of the tibial component is observed. If during flexion of the knee anterior subluxation or superior tilting of the tibial tray or insert occur, the posterior cruciate ligament is judged to be too tight and the ligament is recessed by subperiosteal dissection from the proximal tibia. Release is continued in 2 to 3 mm increments until smooth component motion without either anterior subluxation or tilting is achieved.

The Patella

The patella is addressed once the femoral and tibial cuts have been completed and ligament balancing both collateral and posterior have been performed. The patella thickness is measured using a Vernier caliper. The aim is to resurface the patella, recreating the original thickness of the bone with the prosthesis. Excess removal of bone may compromise patellar viability or predispose to fracture, whereas inadequate bony resection will produce an "overstuffed" patella, which may impair flexion range and predispose to maltracking. To ensure correct patellar tracking it is important to medialize the patellar component to reduce the lateral vector acting on the patella, reducing the likelihood of maltracking.

Patellar tracking is once again checked with all trial components in situ. The patella should run centrally in its groove without tilt without using any restraint—the so-called "no-thumb" test. If the patella does not track well at this stage, it is worth checking the rotation of the tibial component because by slightly realigning this into more external rotation will produce a relative internal rotation of the tibial tubercle, thus reducing the lateral vector on the patella. Should the patella still not track well, a lateral retinacular release may be performed.

After the patella tracking has been optimized, the tibial baseplate rotation is confirmed and drill holes for stabilizing posts made in the final position of rotation.

Implantation of the Definitive Components

Once the definitive components have been chosen, the bone is prepared for component implantation. We implant the tibial component first, followed by the femoral component, and lastly the patellar button. The bone is cleaned of all debris using pulsatile lavage and carefully dried to produce an optimal surface for cementation. Cement is applied to the cut tibial surface using a cement gun to obtain maximum cement interdigitation. The tibial baseplate is then inserted and excess cement removed from about the component. The tibial polyethylene insert is then placed in position and locked in place using the locking pin and clip. The femur is then carefully brought over the newly cemented tibial com-

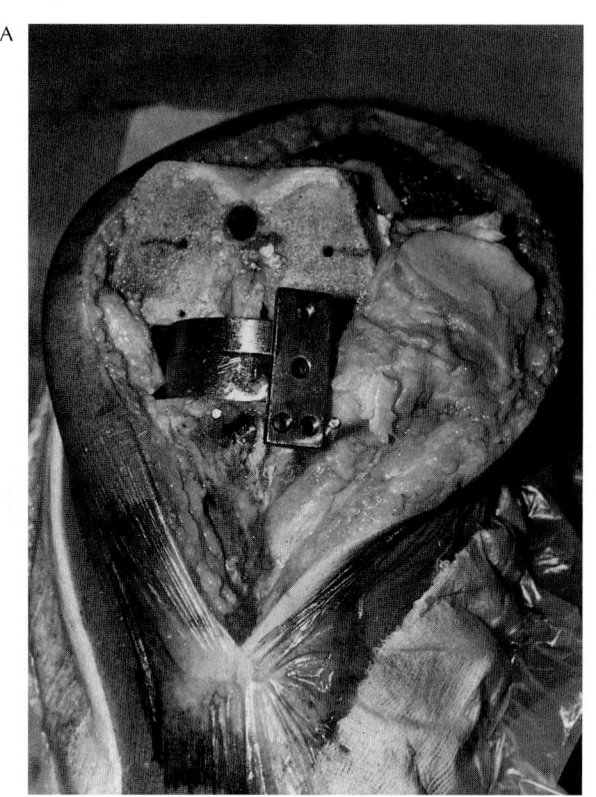

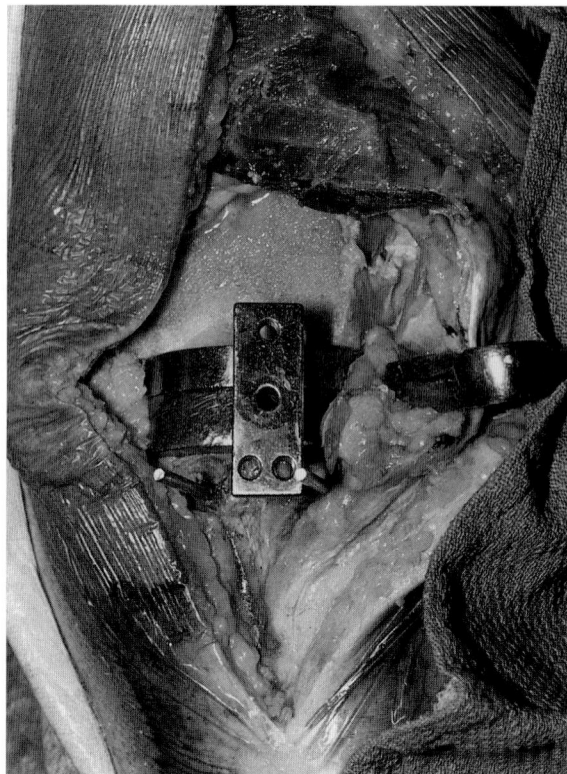

Figure 6.5. The femoral distal, anterior, and posterior cuts and the tibial cut have been performed allowing the balancing of flexion (A) and extension (B) gaps using the technique of graduated blocks.

ponent so as not to disturb the implant. The cement gun is used again to apply cement to the femur and further cement is applied to the femoral component that is then implanted using the femoral impactor. Excess cement is removed from about the component edges and the knee brought out to extension with the heel supported on a padded rest. The patellar button is then cemented in position and held steady with the patellar clamp until the cement is dry. Once the cement is dry, the knee is inspected for further cement, which needs to be removed and is done using narrow osteotomes. The joint is thoroughly cleaned of any debris and washed out using the pulsatile lavage. The knee is put through a final range of motion to ensure all components track well. A drain is inserted and the wound securely closed in layers.

Postoperatively

The patient is transferred to the bed and immediately placed on continuous passive motion (CPM) machine

Figure 6.6. The knee is flexed to 90 degrees with trial tibial components in situ showing central tracking of the femoral component on the tibial polyethylene insert without any evidence of anterior tibial subluxation or tilting of the tibial tray. This implies appropriate balance of the posterior cruciate ligament.

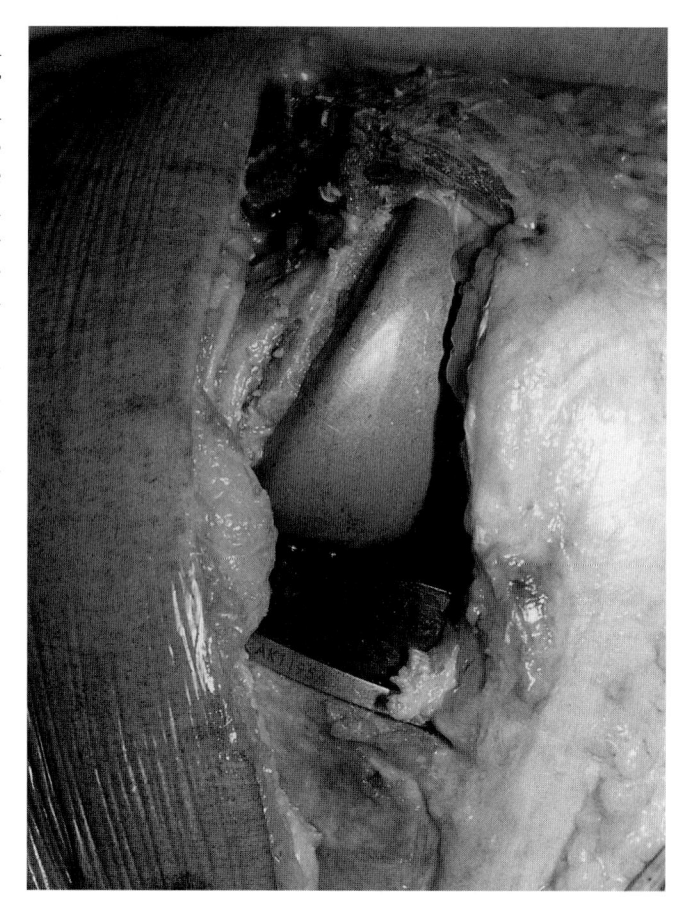

beginning in the range of 70 to 100 degrees and increasing steadily to 0–100 degrees by the first postoperative day. Central to this aggressive range of motion rehabilitation is adequate analgesia. All patients have patient-controlled analgesia morphine pumps and are given indomethacin in suppository form for the first 48 to 72 hours postsurgery. Patients are mobilized fully weight bearing as tolerated, using a walker under the supervision of a physiotherapist from the first postoperative day. Wound drains are removed by 24 hours and antibiotics are ceased at this time also. The goal is independent mobilization with the aim of achieving readiness for discharge to either home or rehabilitation facility by 5 days postsurgery. The patient should be able to flex the knee to 90 degrees or beyond by discharge from hospital. An aggressive range of motion program while an inpatient enables easy achievement of this goal for virtually all patients.

References

1. Scott RD, Volatile TB. 12 years experience with posterior cruciate retaining total knee arthroplasty. *Clin Orthop.* 1986; 205:100–107.
2. Andriacchi TP, Galante JO. Retention of the posterior cruciate in total knee arthroplasty. *J Arthroplasty.* 1988; 3(suppl):S13.
3. Freeman MAR, Railton GT. Should the posterior cruciate ligament be retained or resected in condylar nonmeniscal knee arthroplasty. *J Arthroplasty.* 1988; 3(suppl): S3.
4. Ritter MA, Li E. Total knee arthroplasty: the case for retention of the posterior cruciate ligament. *J Arthroplasty.* 1995; 10:560–564.
5. Moilenan T, Freeman MAR. Total knee arthroplasty: the case for resection of the posterior cruciate ligament. *J Arthroplasty* 1995; 10:564–568.
6. Becker MW, Insall JN, Faris PM. Bilateral total knee arthroplasty—one cruciate retaining and one cruciate substituting. *Clin Orthop.* 1991; 271:122–124.
7. Dorr LD, Ochsner JL, Gronley J, Perry J. Functional comparison of posterior cruciate retained versus cruciate sacrificed total knee arthroplasty. *Clin Orthop.* 1988; 236:36–43.
8. Kapandji IA. *The Physiology of the Joints, Vol 2, The Lower Limb.* 5th ed. Edinburgh: Churchill Livingstone, 1985.
9. Lindahl O, Movin A. The mechanics of extension of the knee joint. *Acta Orthop Scandinav.* 1967; 38:226–234.
10. Nisell R. Mechanics of the knee—a study of joint and muscle load with clinical applications. *Acta Orthop Scandinav.* 1985; 56(suppl):216.
11. Walker PS, Hajek JV. The load-bearing area in the knee joint. *J Biomechanics.* 1972; 5:581–589.
12. Goodfellow J, O'Connor J. The mechanics of the knee and prosthesis design. *JBJS.* 1978; 60B:358–369.
13. Kurosawa H, Walker PS, Abe S, Garg A, Hunter T. Geometry and motion of the knee for implant and orthotic design. *J Biomechanics.* 1985; 18:487–499.
14. Walker PS, Rovick JS, Robertson DD. The effects of knee brace hinge design and placement on joint mechanics. *J Biomechanics.* 1988; 21:965–974.
15. Shapeero LG, Dye SF, Lipton MJ, Gould RG, Galvin EG, Genant HK. Functional dynamics of the knee joint by ultrafast cine-CT. *Invest Radiol.* 1988; 23:118–123.
16. Thompson WO, Thaete LF, Fu FH, Dye SF. Tibial meniscal dynamics using three dimensional reconstrucion of magnetic reconstrucion images. *Am J Sports Med.* 1991; 19:210–216.
17. Schoemaker SC, Adams D, Daniel DM, Woo SL. Quadriceps/anterior cruciate graft interaction. *Clin Orthop.* 1993; 294:379–390.
18. Soudry M, Walker PS, Reilly DT, Kurosawa H, Sledge CB. The effect of total knee replacement design on femoraltibial contact conditions. *J Arthroplasty.* 1986; 1:35–44.
19. El Nahass B, Madson MM, Walker PS. Motion of the knee after condylar resurfacing—an in-vivo study. *J Biomechanics.* 1991; 24:1107–1117.
20. Markolf KL, Mensch JS, Amstutz HC. Stiffness and laxity of the knee—the contributions of the supporting structures. *JBJS.* 1976; 58A:583–594.
21. Piziali RL, Seering WP, Nagel DA, Schurman DJ. The function of the primary ligaments of the knee in anterior-posterior and medial-lateral motions. *J Biomechanics.* 1980; 13:777–784.
22. Seering WP, Piziali RL, Nagel DA, Schurman DJ. The function of the primary ligaments of the knee in varus-valgus and axial rotation. *J Biomechanics.* 1980; 13: 785–794.
23. Faris PM, Herbst SA, Ritter MA, Keating EM. The effect of preoperative knee deformity on the initial results of cruciate retaining total knee arthroplasty. *J Arthroplasty.* 1992; 7:527–530.
24. Ritter MA, Faris PM, Keating EM. Posterior cruciate ligament balancing during total knee arthroplasty. *J Arthroplasty.* 1988; 3:323–326.
25. Andriacchi TP, Andersson GBJ, Fermier RW, Stern D, Galante JO. A study of lower limb mechanics during stair climbing. *JBJS.* 1980; 64A:749–757.
26. Berman AT, Zarro VJ, Bosacco SJ, Israelite C. Quantitative gait analysis after unilateral or bilateral total knee replacement. *JBJS.* 1987; 69A:1340.
27. Rittman N, Kettelkamp DB, Pryor P, Schwartzkopf GL, Hillberry B. Analysis of knee motion walking for four types of total knee replacement. *Clin Orthop.* 1981; 155:111–117.
28. Kelman GJ, Biden EN, Wyatt MP, Ritter MA, Colwell CW. Gait laboratory analysis of a posterior cruciate sparing total knee arthroplasty in stair ascent and descent. *Clin Orthop.* 1989; 248:21–26.
30. Werner F, Foster D, Murray DG. The influence of design on the transmission of torque across knee prostheses. *JBJS.* 1978; 60A:342–348.
31. Rostoker W, Galante JO. Contact pressure dependence of wear rates of ultra high molecular weight polyethylene. *J Biomed Mater Res.* 1979; 13:957–964.
32. Blunn GW, Walker PS, Joshi A, Hardinge K. The dominance of cyclic sliding in producing wear in total knee replacements. *Clin Orthop.* 1991; 273:253–260.
33. Sathasivam S, Walker PS. Optimisation of the bearing surface geometry of total knees. *J Biomechanics.* 1994; 27:255–264.
34. Bartel DL, Bicknell VL, Wright TM. The effect of conformity, thickness and material on stresses in ultra high mol-

ecular weight components for total joint replacement. *JBJS.* 1986; 68A:1041–1051.
35. Landy MM, Walker PS. Wear of ultra high molecular weight polyethylene components of 90 retrieved knee prostheses. *J Arthroplasty.* 1988; 3:S73–S85.
36. Collier JP, Mayor MB, McNamara JL, Surprenant VA, Jensen RT. Analysis of the failure of 122 polyethylene inserts from uncemented tibial knee inserts. *Clin Orthop.* 1991; 273:232–242.
37. Scott RD, Thornhill TS. Posterior cruciate supplementing total knee replacement using conforming inserts and cruciate recession. *Clin Orthop.* 1994; 309:146–149.
38. Swany MR, Scott RD. Posterior polyethylene wear in posterior cruciate ligament retaining total knee arthroplasty. *J Arthroplasty.* 1992; 8:439–446.
39. Lewis P, Rorabeck CH, Bourne RB, Devane P. Posteromedial tibial polyethylene failure in total knee replacements. *Clin Orthop.* 1994; 299:11–17.
40. Feng EL, Stulberg SD, Wixson RL. Progressive subluxation and polyethylene wear in total knee replacements with flat articular surfaces. *Clin Orthop.* 1994; 299:60–71.
41. Ritter MA, Campbell E, Faris PM, Keating EM. Long term survival analysis of the posterior cruciate condylar total knee arthroplasty. *J Arthroplasty.* 1989; 4:293–296.
42. Vince KG, Insall JN, Kelly MA. The total condylar prosthesis. 10–12 yr results of a cemented knee replacement. *JBJS.* 1989; 71B:793–797.
43. Stern SH, Insall JN. Posterior stabilised prosthesis: results after follow up of nine to twelve years. *JBJS.* 1992; 74A:980–986.
44. Ritter MA, Herbst SA, Keating EM, Faris PM, Meding JB. Long term survivorship analysis of a posterior cruciate retaining total condylar total knee arthroplasty. *Clin Orthop.* 1994; 309:136–145.
45. Ranawat CS, Flynn WF, Sadder S, Hansraj KK, Maynard MJ. Long term results of the total condylar knee arthroplasty: a 15 yr survivorship study. *Clin Orthop.* 1993; 286:94–102.
46. Rand JA. Comparison of metal-backed and all polyethylene tibial components in cruciate condylar total knee arthroplasty. *J Arthroplasty.* 1993; 8:307–313.
47. Knutson K, Lewold S, Robertsson O, Lidgren L. The Swedish Knee arthroplasty register—a nationwide study of 30,003 knees 1976–1992. *Acta Orth Scand.* 1994; 65:375–386.
48. Barrett DS, Cobb AG, Bentley G. Joint proprioception in normal, osteoarthritic and replaced knees. *JBJS.* 1991; 73B:53–56.
49. Yahia LH, Newman NM, St Georges M. Innervation of the canine cruciate ligaments. A neurohistological study. *Anat Histol Embryol.* 1992; 21:1–8.
50. Marinozzi G, Ferrante F, Gaudio E, Ricci A, Amenta F. Intrinsic innervation of the rat knee joint articular capsule and ligaments. *Acta Anat Basel.* 1991; 141:8–14.
51. Katonis PG, Assimakopoulos AP, Agapitos MV, Exarchou E. Mechanoreceptors in the posterior cruciate ligament. Histological study on cadavers. *Acta Orthop Scand.* 1991; 62:276–278.
52. Johansson H, Sjolander P, Sojka P. A sensory role for the cruciate ligaments. *Clin Orthop.* 1991; 268:161–178.
53. Schultz RA, Miller DC, Kerr CS, Micheli L. Mechanoreceptors in human cruciate ligaments. *JBJS.* 1984; 66A:1072–1076.
54. Sojka P, Johansson H, Sjolander P, Lorentzon R, Djupsjobacka M. Fusimotor neurones can be reflexly influenced by activity in receptor afferents from the posterior cruciate ligament. *Brain Res.* 1989; 483:177–183.
55. Skinner HB, Barrack RL, Cook SD. Age related decline in proprioception. *Clin Orthop.* 1984; 184:208–211.
56. Warren PJ, Olanlukun TK, Cobb AG, Bentley G. Proprioception after knee arthroplasty—the influence of prosthetic design. *Clin Orthop.* 1993; 297:182–187.
57. Mahoney OM, Noble PC, Rhoads DD, Alexander JW, Tullos HS. Posterior cruciate function following total knee arthroplasty. *J Arthroplasty.* 1994; 9:569–578.
58. Incavo SJ, Johnson CC, Beynnon BD, Howe JG. Posterior cruciate ligament strain biomechanics in total knee arthroplasty. *Clin Orthop.* 1994; 309:88–93.
59. Montgomery RL, Goodman SB, Csongradi J. Late rupture of the posterior cruciate ligament after total knee replacement. *Iowa Orthop J.* 1993; 13:167–170.
60. Keblish PA. Valgus deformity in total knee replacement—the lateral approach. *Orthop Trans.* 1985; 9:28–29.
61. Hoffman AA, Plaster RL, Murdock LE. Subvastus (southern) approach for primary total knee arthroplasty. *Clin Orthop.* 1991; 209:70–.
62. Garvin KL, Scuderi G, Insall JN. Evolution of the quadriceps Snip. *Clin Orthop.* 1995; 321:131–137.
63. Coonse K, Adams JD. A new operative approach to the knee joint. *Surg Gynaecol Obstet.* 1943; 77:344–347.
64. Trousdale RT, Hanssen AD, Rand JA, Cahalan TD. V-Y quadricepsplasty in total knee arthroplasty. *Clin Orthop.* 1993; 286:48–55.
65. Whiteside LA, Ohl MD. Tibial tubercle osteotomy for exposure of the difficult total knee arthroplasty. *Clin Orthop.* 1990; 260:6–9.
66. Dolin MG. Osteotomy of the tibial tubercle in total knee replacement. A technical note. *JBJS.* 1983; 65A:704–706.
67. Wolff AM, Hungerford DS, Krakow, KA, Jacobs MS. Osteotomy of the tibial tubercle during total knee replacement. *JBJS.* 1989; 71A:848–852.
68. Tillet ED, Engh GA, Peterson TA. A comparative study of extramedullary and intramedullary alignment systems in total knee arthroplasty. *Clin Orthop.* 1988; 230:176–184.
69. Attfield SF, Wilton TJ, Pratt DJ, Sambatakakis A. Soft tissue balance and recovery of proprioception after total knee arthroplasty. *JBJS.* 1996; 78B:540–545.

CHAPTER 7
Posterior Cruciate-Sacrificing Total Knee Arthroplasty

P. John Kumar and Lawrence D. Dorr

INTRODUCTION

Posterior cruciate-sacrificing total knee arthroplasty was popularized in the 1970s at the Hospital for Special Surgery. It was there that Walker, Ranawat, and Insall designed the Total Condylar Knee (Howmedica, Rutherford, NJ). This prosthesis relied on resection of the posterior cruciate ligament.[5,7,12,13,22,24] Stability was imparted by a congruent prosthesis articulation, soft tissue balance, and proper axial limb alignment. This was one of the first designs that permitted resurfacing of the patella. Instrumentation provided standardized cuts of the femur and tibia. Adequate cementing technique gave predictable fixation. Today, in spite of many changes in the 1980s, total knee arthroplasty is the most predictable total joint arthroplasty.

INDICATIONS FOR SURGERY

At this time we perform total knee arthroplasty in patients with debilitating pain or functional loss from osteoarthritis, avascular necrosis, or inflammatory arthritis such as rheumatoid arthritis, systemic lupus erythematosus, or ankylosing spondylitis. We feel that a correctly performed total knee arthroplasty may be either cruciate retaining or cruciate sacrificing.[1,5,6,7,13,22,24,25,28] Currently we do not perform cruciate-sacrificing arthroplasty without also substituting for the posterior cruciate. A posterior cruciate-sacrificing arthroplasty can be performed without a posterior substituting design if the principles of total knee arthroplasty are maintained and a conforming polyethylene insert design is utilized. This design of knee also provides protection for those cruciate-retaining knees in which the PCL inadvertently is cut at surgery or ruptures postoperatively. The PCL should be sacrificed in cases of moderate to severe deformity such as flexion contracture >20 degrees or angulation >20 degrees in which the soft tissue releases necessary compromise the cruciate length or intrinsic stability.

CONTRAINDICATIONS

A relative contraindication for sacrifice of the PCL without substitution is patellectomy because both the anterior and posterior soft tissue constraints for the knee are then absent. However, with PCL substitution this contraindication is not present. With an absent or severely attenuated medial collateral ligament, or in those few situations in which soft tissue balancing cannot be obtained and the flexion space is greater than the extension space, a constrained implant such as Total Condylar III (Johnson and Johnson, Braintree, Mass) is required. This is most common with valgus deformities.

PRINCIPLES OF SURGERY

Total knee replacement with sacrifice of the PCL requires a close match of the flexion and extension spaces. Spacer blocks help in confirming this equality of gaps. Most current instrumentation employs measured resection techniques so that release of the PCL may increase the flexion space by as much as 4 mm.[19] With sacrifice of the PCL, less tibial bone should be resected than is common when using a cruciate-retaining design. Dorr suggested that no more than 5 to 6 mm bone be removed from the medial tibial condyle to permit maintenance of strong bone[9,20] and to also prevent an excessive flexion space. With trials in place and the posterior drawer sign tested at 90 degrees, the front of the tibial trial must remain 1 cm anterior to the front of the femoral component or the knee will not have the stability for the patient to walk downstairs in a reciprocal fashion. If the tibial component subluxes under the femoral component, then dislocation of the knee could occur. The eminence of the posterior stabilized (PS) knees helps prevent femoral-tibial dislocation although this can still occur if the flexion gap is too large. Currently no designs are used that promote sacrifice of the PCL without substitution.

One complaint of PCL-sacrificing knees was a lack of flexion motion. The total condylar knee was expected to achieve 90 degrees of flexion. In fact, in our experience this was true when the tibia was cut in the anteroposterior plane at 90 degrees. However, when we cut the tibia 5 degrees posteriorly the flexion motion increased to 115 degrees. Furthermore, the Insall-Burstein PS knee (Zimmer, Warsaw, Ind) designed a 7-degree posterior slope into the tibial plastic and achieved a 120-degree flexion motion. Therefore, the restricted motion with the total condylar knee was not secondary to sacrifice of the PCL, but to the absence of posterior slope.

Patella complications with the total condylar knee design have been rarely reported. Three factors account for this: first, the knee did not roll back (and in fact had anterior slide) so the extensor mechanism was seldomly too tight. Second, restriction of flexion was considered an advantage for the patella. Third, the tibial component was aligned with the tibial tubercle, which reduces the Q angle of the patella ligament.

DESIGN OF COMPONENTS

Long-term results with the total condylar knee and the Insall-Burstein knee, which have high conformity between the components, have shown excellent long-term durability and wear characteristics.[5,7,12,17,22,24] Nonconforming designs lead to high-point contact stresses and increasing shear forces on the polyethylene causing accelerated polyethylene wear with osteolysis and failure.[14,21] We use the Apollo knee design (Intermedics Orthopedics, Austin, Tex), which has round femoral condyles in both the sagittal and coronal planes. The tibial insert is "dished" to permit good congruence with resultant high-contact areas and low-contact stresses.[10] The tibial contact point is located 3 mm posterior to the coronal center. The tibial design does *not* promote "rollback." Ideally, the femur rotates at the same contact point during flexion and extension. This decreases sliding, which helps to preserve the polyethylene.

The design of the Apollo knee was evaluated by radiographs in a study of 50 patients with range of motion from at least 0 to 90 degrees after surgery.[10] The average flexion in these patients was 115 degrees. The center of rotation of the knee was in the 3 mm posterior to the coronal midline position and the contact point of the femur in flexion or extension varied by only ±0.7 mm. Clearly, this design limits the amount of shear force that is transmitted to the polyethylene and helps to prevent catastrophic wear. The high conformity between the polyethylene insert and the femoral component is similar to, but significantly improved from, the total condylar design, which has no reports of clinically problematic wear. The Apollo PS knee improves patella tracking when compared to traditional PS designs because of the anterior tibial post position. The Apollo prosthesis has an all polyethylene patellar button. At this time, we feel that metal-backed patellar components should be avoided because of many reports of failure.[3,4,17]

SURGICAL TECHNIQUE

Today, only inadvertently would we sacrifice the PCL and not substitute for it. This can occur by cutting it with a saw during preparation of the tibia or by excessive release during recession of the PCL. Because the Apollo knee has congruent surfaces, we can tolerate PCL loss *provided* the tibial component is stable in flexion. Stable in flexion means that the tibial component (and the tibial bone) remain one fingerbreadth (at least 1 cm) anterior to the femoral component (Figs. 7.1 and 7.2). However, if the tibial component can be pushed under the femur, then two options are available. One option is to use a thicker polyethylene in flexion to achieve stability. This usually means the knee is now tight in extension and the femur must be cut again. The second option is to convert to a posterior-stabilized design.

With the Apollo knee conversion to a PS is simple because the articulation surfaces are nearly the same for both the cruciate-retaining and posterior-stabilized knees. Therefore soft tissue balance will be the same except for the flexion gap. The femur intercondylar bone block is removed with the appropriate jig and the same tibial trial height previously stable in extension is placed. Because of the tibial eminence, stability is almost always now also satisfactory in flexion. In flexion of 90 degrees, contrary to a cruciate-retaining knee, the tibial *bone* can be pushed 1 cm under the tibial trial (Fig. 7.3). To do this test, the tibial trial should not have a peg into the tibia. This laxity in flexion is too much if the tibial bone displaces more than 2 cm or, if using a pegged tibial trial, the trial tilts forward on the bone with flexion. The appropriate laxity in flexion promotes easier flexion with this PCL-sacrificed knee.

Mediolateral soft tissue balance is not affected if the PCL is sacrificed. Therefore, no alterations in soft tissue balance technique are necessary. With PCL sacrifice the threat of postoperative instability is anteroposterior and this is controlled by equal flexion or extension spaces as determined by blocks or use of trials as described ear-

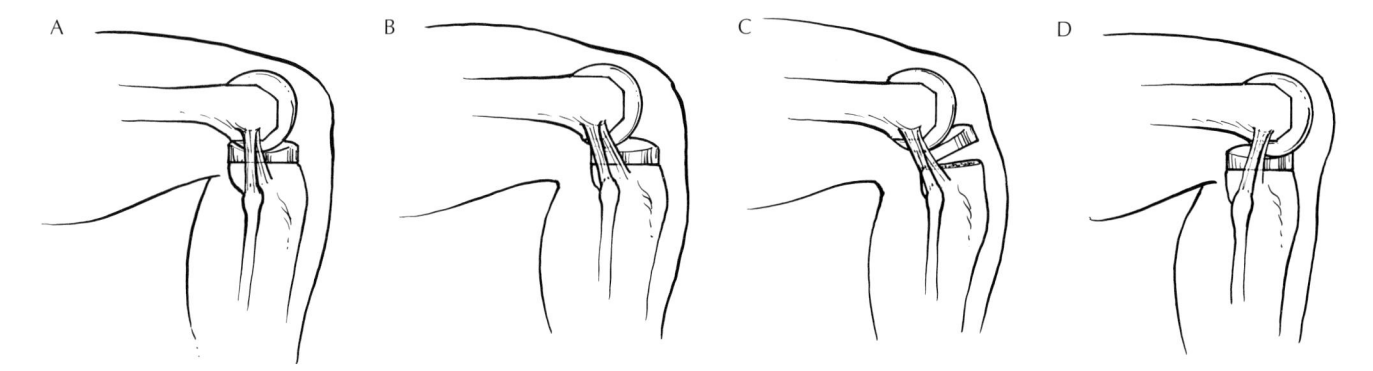

Figure 7.1. This figure illustrates component positions in flexion when the component is balanced, tight or loose. (A) This illustrates the desired amount of flexion stability. The femoral component sits in the center of the tibial tray and the tibia is anterior to the femur. (B) This represents the situation in which the flexion space is too tight. At 90 degrees of flexion the femoral component will sit on the posterior aspect of the tibial component rather than in the center. (C) This is a second example of a flexion space that is too tight. The tibial component "lifts off" the anterior tibial bone at 90 degrees of flexion. (D) This depicts the situation in which the flexion space is loose. The femoral component will sit on the anterior part of the tibial component rather than in the center.

lier. To ensure that the flexion space is correctly prepared, we always insert a lamina spreader at 90 degrees of flexion and remove loose bodies, osteophytes, and tight soft tissue from the medial and lateral compartments. This technique improves flexion and pain relief.

One reason PCL-sacrificed knees such as the total condylar had so few patellar problems was because the femur was centered on the tibia in flexion or often slid *anteriorly.* This position allows the patella ligament to track vertically between the patella and the tibial tubercle. This principle should be maintained when cruciate-retaining or cruciate-sacrificing knee designs are used so as to optimize patella tracking. This is the reason for recession of the PCL—to prevent rollback of the femur and keep the femur centered on the tibia. This principle is also the reason the tibial eminence post on the Apollo PS knee is positioned anteriorly so that rollback is avoided and the patella ligament tracks vertically.

Patella tracking with current trochlear designs with

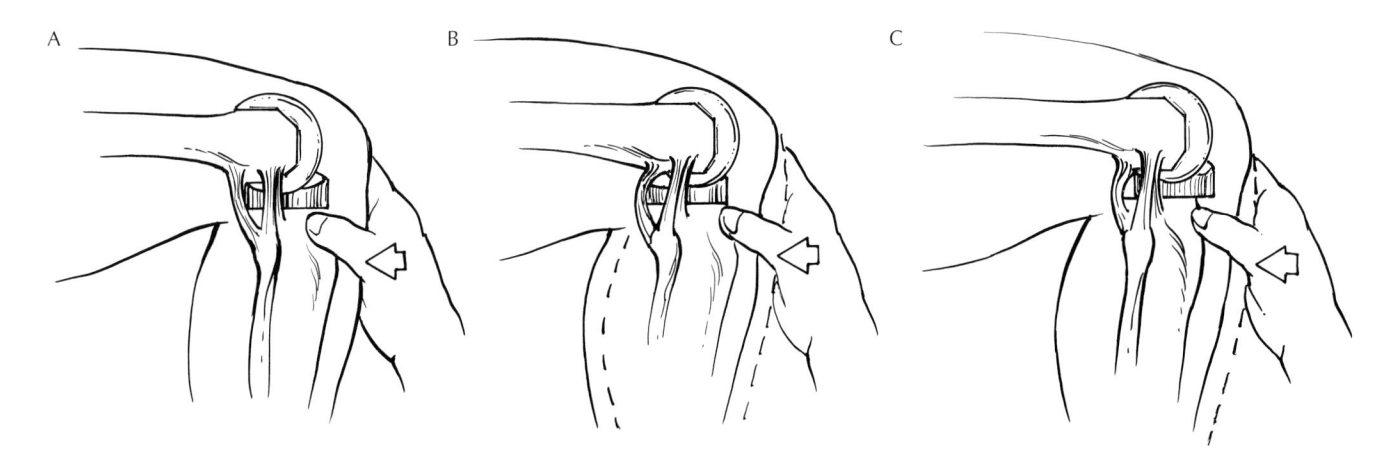

Figure 7.2. This sequence depicts assessment of the flexion stability of cruciate-retaining implants. All of these assessments are made with trials without a keel. (A) This figure represents desired stability with flexion and an applied posterior drawer. The femur should sit in the center of the tibial tray and no posterior subluxation of the tibial component under the femur or of the tibia under the pegless trial should occur. (B) This figure demonstrates a loose flexion space with an applied posterior drawer. The tibial component slides posteriorly underneath the femoral component with a pegged trial. (C) A loose flexion space with a pegless trial allows the tibial bone to sublux under the tibial implant. Neither of these situations are acceptable with cruciate-retaining total knee arthroplasty. With this instability, conversion to a posterior-stabilized implant is recommended.

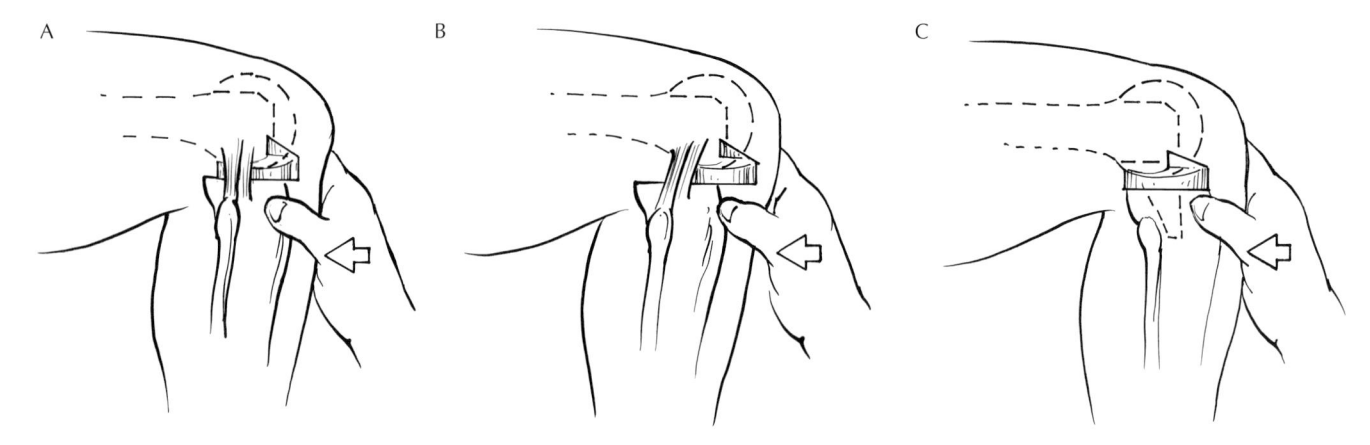

Figure 7.3. This sequence represents assessment of the flexion stability with posterior-stabilized implants with an applied posterior drawer with trials. (A) The femoral component sits in the center of the tibial component and the high eminence prevents the posterior drawer of the trial underneath the femur. The tibial bone should sublux posteriorly 1 cm underneath the pegless trial. This allows for improved flexion. (B) Flexion space instability is present when the tibia subluxes 3 to 4 cm underneath the pegless trials with the posterior drawer. In this situation, when the actual implants are used, the potential for posterior dislocation is high. (C) Flexion stability is correct with the actual implants when no tilt of the tibia occurs around the central peg and no dislocation occurs with varus and valgus stress combined with rotation.

deep grooves must be closely observed in the *first 30 degrees*. In a normal knee patella tilt in the first 30 degrees is medial so that if the patella tilts laterally in this first 30 degrees a lateral release must be bone. We do this release by an oblique incision from the tibial bone (this origin is most important) to the superior pole of the patella (Fig. 7.4). This release protects the lateral geniculate artery, which courses 3 mm superior to the superior pole of the patella.

We cement all three components using the same cement mix. This requires experienced operative personnel and experience with the technique. The bony surfaces are carefully pulse-lavaged and dried. Methylene blue is used to mark the holes for the pegs in the patella. We use Simplex cement (Howmedica, Rutherford, NJ), which is "set" in our operating room at 12 to 14 minutes. The patella is cemented at 2 minutes after mixing and at 3 to 4 minutes the tibial component is cemented by manually pressurizing cement into the condylar bone and the stem hole. Cement is also placed on the keel. Excessive cement is removed and the femoral trial placed and the knee is brought to extension to compress the tibial component and to pressurize the cement. This maneuver extrudes more cement from around the tibia, which requires removal of this extruded cement. Cement is applied to femoral bone, except the posterior condylar cuts, and manually pressurized. Cement is placed on the metal posterior condyles of the femoral component. After the femur is implanted, the knee again is brought to extension for compression and any extruded cement removed. All excess cement should be removed and no cement should be left in the posterior compartment of the knee. When the cement has fully polymerized, closure is commenced. The tourniquet is deflated to obtain hemostasis with electrocautery prior to closure of the wound.

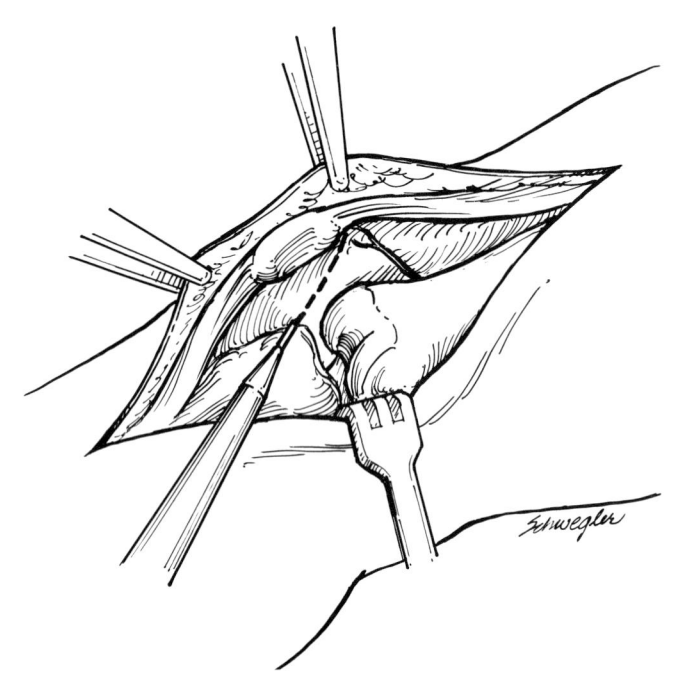

Figure 7.4. This illustrates the oblique lateral release. The incision is made from the inside out, starting from the tibial bone and coursing obliquely to the superior pole of the patella. This prevents injury to the lateral geniculate artery.

We place one suture at the superior corner of the patella and flex the knee completely. If the suture does not break and the patella does not tilt, then the extensor mechanism is not excessively tight. We place 2 to 3 sutures cephalad and caudad to this single suture in full flexion and the remainder of the closure is completed with the knee in extension. After this wound closure is obtained, dressings are applied and postoperative rehabilitation should be performed according to the surgeon's desired protocol. We do not use a continuous passive motion (CPM) machine, but use a drop and dangle routine.[16] This routine is often combined with the use of a "skateboard" for passive motion. The drop and dangle routine and the use of a skateboard necessitate training by the physical therapist. In this protocol, the patient's pain is adequately controlled with analgesics, and a program of passive and active assisted flexion is performed at bedside. Initially, the patient sits at the edge of the bed and the foot is held firmly fixed to the ground. This is done by the therapist. The therapist then encourages the patient to slowly slide forward on the bed so that the knee is held in a position of flexion. This is done until 90 degrees of flexion is obtained or maximum flexion is tolerated by the patient. The leg is then held in this position for approximately 20 minutes twice a day. This drop and dangle routine is augmented with the use of a skateboard, in which the patient will sit at the side of the bed with the foot fixed firmly to a skateboard and then will gradually be passively flexed and actively flexed and extend the knee on the skateboard. We have been able to eliminate the use of continuous passive motion in routine total knee arthroplasty with this protocol.

CONCLUSIONS

Posterior-sacrificing total knee arthroplasty certainly has an excellent track record. Total knee arthroplasty performed under this technique has shown excellent long-term results and very little has changed with this technique over the last 20 years. Proper performance of this technique requires meticulous attention to detail, particularly balancing the flexion and extension gaps, and the use of conforming polyethylene. The main limitations of this technique were restricted flexion caused by the lack of posterior slope with the original technique, and instability in flexion, especially going downstairs. Currently we would recommend substitution for the PCL, if one performs posterior cruciate-sacrificing arthroplasty. In total knee arthroplasty with a cruciate-retaining design in which the posterior cruciate is inadvertently resected, conversion does not need to be performed if the flexion and extension gaps are adequately balanced, the knee is stable, and the articulation surface is conforming.

References

1. Barnes LC, Sledge C. Total knee arthroplasty with posterior cruciate ligament retention design. In: Insall J, Windsor R, Scott WN, et al., eds. *Surgery of the Knee.* 2nd ed. New York: Churchill Livingstone; 1993: 815–827.
2. Bartell D, Bicknell NS, Ithaca A, Wright TM. The effect of conformity, thickness and material on stresses in ultra high molecular weight components for total joint replacement. *J Bone Joint Surg.* 1986; 68A:1041–1051.
3. Bayley JC, Scott RD, Ewald FC, Holmes GB. Metal-backed patellar component failure following total knee replacement. *J Bone Joint Surg.* 1988; 70-A:668–674.
4. Bayley JC, Scott RD. Function observation on metal-backed patellar component failure. *Clin Orthop.* 1988; 236:82–87.
5. Brugioni DJ, Andriacchi TP, Galante JO: A functional and radiographic analysis of the total condylar knee arthroplasty. *J Arthroplasty.* 1990; 5:173–180.
6. Colizza WA, Insall JN, Scuderi GR. The posterior stabilized total knee prosthesis. *J Bone Joint Surg.* 1995; 77A:1713–1720.
7. Donaldson WF III, Sculco TP, Insall JN, Ranawat CS. Total condylar III knee prosthesis. *Clin Orthop.* 1988; 226:21–28.
8. Dorr LD. Technique of correction of varus deformity. *Techiques Orthop.* 1988; 3:77–85.
9. Dorr LD, Boiardo R. Technical considerations in total knee arthroplasty. *Clin Orthop.* 1996; 205:5–11.
10. Dorr LD, Little G, McPherson E. *Cemented Total Knee Replacement, Current Concepts in Primary and Revision Total Knee Arthroplasty.* Philadelphia: Lippencott Raven Publishers; 1996; 91–98.
11. Firestone TP, Krackow KA, Davis JD, Teeny SM, Hungerford DS. The management of fixed flexion contractures during total knee arthroplasty. *Clin Orthop.* 1992; 284:221–227.
12. Hohl WM, Crawfurd E Zelicof SB, Ewald F. The total condular III prosthesis in complex knee reconstruction. *Clin Orthop.* 1991; 273:91–97.
13. Hood RW, Vanni M, Insall J. The correction of knee alignment in 225 consecutive total condylar knee replacements. *Clin Orthop.* 1981; 160:94–105.
14. Kilguss DJ, Funahashi TT, Campbell PA. Massive femoral osteolysis and early disintegration of a polyethylene-bearing surface of a total knee replacement. *J Bone Joint Surg.* 1992; 74A:770.
15. Krackow KA, Jones MM, Teendy SM, Hungerford DS. Primary total knee arthroplasty in patients with fixed valgus deformity. *Clin Orthop.* 1991; 273:9–18.
16. Kumar PJ, McPherson EJ, Dorr LD, Wan Z, Baldwin K. Rehabilitation after total knee arthroplasty. *Clin Orthop.* 1996; 331:93–101.
17. Lombardi AV, Engh GA, Volz RG, Albrigo JL, Brainard BJ. Fracture/disassociations of the polyethylene in metal-back patellar components in total knee arthroplasty. *J Bone Joint Surg.* 1988; 70A:675–679.

18. Merritt J, Conaty P, Dorr LD. The effect of soft tissue releases on results of total knee replacement, total arthroplasty of the knee. Proceedings of the Knee Society, 1985–1986. Rockville, MD: Aspen Publications; 1987.
19. Oschner JL, Johnson WD. Flexion and extension gap measurements in total knee arthroplasty after sacrifice of the posterior cruciate ligament. *J of Southern Orthopedic Assoc.* 1994; 3(4):290–294.
20. Passick JM, Dorr LD. Primary total knee arthroplasty for the 1990's. *Techniques Orthop.* 1990; 5:57–66.
21. Peters PC, Engh G, Dwyer KA, Vinh TN. Osteolysis after total knee arthroplasty without cement. *J Bone Joint Surg.* 1992; 74A:864.
22. Ranawat C, Flynn W Jr, Saddler S, Hansraj K, Maynard MJ. Long term results of the total condylar knee arthroplasty. *Clin Orthop.* 1993; 286:94–102.
23. Rhoads D, Noble P, Reuben J, Mahoney O, Tullose H. The effect of femoral component position and patellar tracking after total knee arthroplasty. *Clin Orthop.* 1990; 260: 43–51.
24. Shoemaker SC, Markolf K, Finerman G. In vitro stability of the implanted total condylar prosthesis. *J Bone Joint Surg.* 1992; 64A:1201–1213.
25. Stern SH, Insall J. *Total Knee Arthroplasty with Posterior Cruciate Ligament Substitution Design, Surgery of the Knee.* 2nd ed. Insall J, Windsor R, Scott WN, et al., eds. New York: Churchill Livingstone; 1993; 980–986.
26. Stern SH, Moecklel BH, Insall JN. Total knee arthroplasty in valgus knees. *Clin Orthop.* 1991; 273:5–8.
27. Teeny SM, Krackow KA, Hungerford DS, Jones M. Primary total knee arthroplasty in patients with severe varus deformity. *Clin Orthop.* 1991; 273:19–31.
28. Vince KG, Insall J, Kelly M. The total condylar prosthesis. *J Bone Joint Surg. Br.* 1989; 71B:793–803.
29. Walker PS. *Total Condylar Knee in Its Evolution, Total Condylar Knee Arthroplasty, Techniques, Results and Complications.* Ranwat C, ed. New York: Springer-Verlag, 7–16.

CHAPTER 8
The Insall-Burstein® Posterior Stabilized Condylar Knee Prosthesis

Thomas J. Allardyce, Giles R. Scuderi, and John N. Insall

HISTORY OF DEVELOPMENT

The posterior-stabilized condylar knee prosthesis is one of the many successful condylar prostheses developed at the Hospital for Special Surgery.[1] It was introduced as a modification of the total condylar knee prosthesis, which, with its unmatched durability, has been called the "gold standard" for total knee arthroplasty longevity[2] (Fig. 8.1). Despite clinical survivorship exceeding 94% at 15 years, shortcomings with the total condylar knee exposed the weaknesses of the prosthesis and provided the impetus for design change. In 1978, the posterior-stabilized condylar knee prosthesis was first implanted at the Hospital for Special Surgery. The most recent clinical survivorship studies prove that its durability has surpassed that of the total condylar knee prosthesis.[3] The posterior-stabilized condylar knee prosthesis has since undergone many subtle design changes, with each modification incorporating the merits and eliminating the weaknesses of the preceding design.

Although the total condylar prosthesis, which was introduced in 1974, is considered to be the predecessor of the posterior-stabilized condylar knee prosthesis, the total condylar knee prosthesis and the posterior-stabilized condylar knee prosthesis are separate types of arthroplasties. The total condylar knee prosthesis is a "posterior cruciate ligament-sacrificing" prosthesis, which allows for a larger proximal tibial cancellous surface area for tibial component fixation.[4] The posterior-stabilized condylar knee prosthesis is similar to the total condylar knee prosthesis in that both technically require excision of both cruciate ligaments for prosthesis implantation; however, the posterior-stabilized condylar knee prosthesis is radically different. It is a "posterior cruciate ligament-substituting" prosthesis, which has a tibial and femoral component articulation, that allows for femoral rollback during knee flexion. This "posterior cruciate ligament-substituting" mechanism makes the posterior-stabilized condylar knee prosthesis both clinically and mechanically a better prosthesis choice for patients requiring a total knee arthroplasty. The Insall-Burstein I was the original posterior-stabilized condylar prosthesis developed at the Hospital for Special Surgery and was the successor of the total condylar prosthesis (Fig. 8.2). It was introduced as a modification of the total condylar prosthesis to specifically improve joint stability, range of motion, and ability to climb stairs. These goals were to be achieved with the use of a "posterior cruciate ligament-substituting mechanism." A transverse cam on the femoral component articulating with a central polyethylene post on the tibial component combined with a change in the center of curvature of the femoral condyles allowed for femoral rollback during flexion to improve motion and knee stability. In the original reports on the performance of the posterior-stabilized condylar prosthesis, these goals were indeed achieved.[5] It was thought that the design change that incorporated more component constraint would lead to either more lucencies around the components or early loss of fixation. These negative effects were not seen in the early reports nor in the long-term follow-up. The horizontal shear force associated with the cam and post mechanism actually contributed minimally to the resultant vector force acting on the tibial component in flexion, most of which is pure axial compression (Fig. 8.4). It was felt that the posterior-stabilized condylar prosthesis design with the posterior femoral rollback would tend to decrease quadriceps forces for any given extension moment that would lead to a lower incidence of patellar complications. However, it became evident that patellar complications were increasing with this new design. There were 10 patellar fractures out the original 118 total knee arthroplasties performed with the posterior-stabilized condylar knee prosthesis. Most of

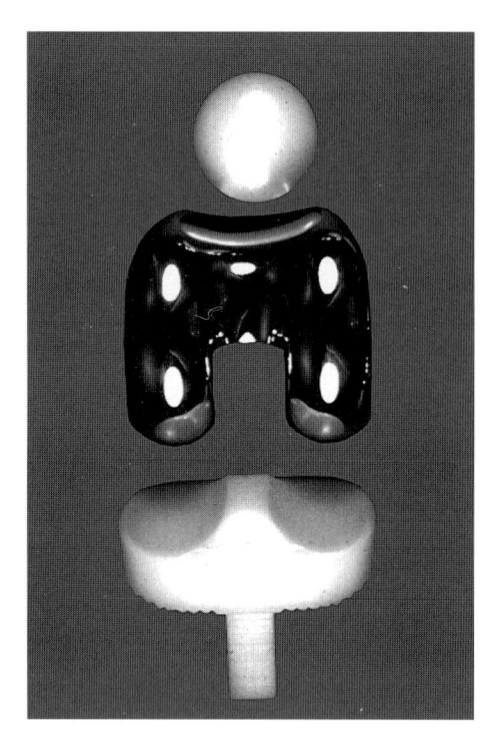

Figure 8.1. Total condylar prosthesis

these fractures occurred with the larger patellar buttons and nearly all were associated with excellent knee function when treated nonoperatively.[5] These fractures have since been attributed to overstuffing of the patellofemoral joint and to the increased motion realized by the new design rather than to the femoral rollback mechanism of the femoral cam and tibial post.

There was another troublesome clinical occurrence with the patellofemoral articulation in the new design. Fibrous tissue tended to accumulate in the quadriceps tendon just above the patellar button. This fibrous tissue frequently became lodged between the leading edge of the femoral intercondylar box and the patellar button when the knee extended from a flexed position. This phenomenon has been well described in the original report on the posterior-stabilized condylar prosthesis.[5] This condition, treatment, and the outcome have since been well described and has been coined the "patellar clunk" syndrome.[6] Different degrees of quadriceps tendon irritation have been described with the original posterior-stabilized condylar knee design.[7] As a result, modifications to the original prosthesis have been made. In 1982, the leading edge of the femoral box at the distal end of the trochlear groove was cambered to prevent this quadriceps irritation.[7] In 1983, the trochlear groove was deepened to inhance the patellofemoral tracking.[8] Although this change was minor, it did reduce the incidence of patellofemoral symptoms in patients with the posterior-stabilized condylar knee prosthesis. In a series of patients reported by Aglietti,[7] the incidence of patellar impingement symptoms was reduced from 25% to 15% after the modifications to the patellofemoral articulations of the posterior-stabilized condylar knee prosthesis were made.

A major change to the posterior-stabilized condylar knee prosthesis came about in November 1980,[8] when a posterior-stabilized prosthesis with a metal-backed tibial component was first implanted at the Hospital for Special Surgery. It was determined that in the revision setting, the primary mode of failure had been the loosening of the tibial component due to poor cancellous osseous support of the tibial tray.[9] Frequently the best cancellous bone is missing in the proximal tibia after a failed primary total knee arthroplasty. Therefore, the tibial tray should be indirectly supported by the cortical shell of the tibia, because its stiffness increases distally and the cancellous bone stiffness decreases correspondingly.[10] As a result, metal backing was introduced into the tibial component to evenly distribute proximal tibial loads

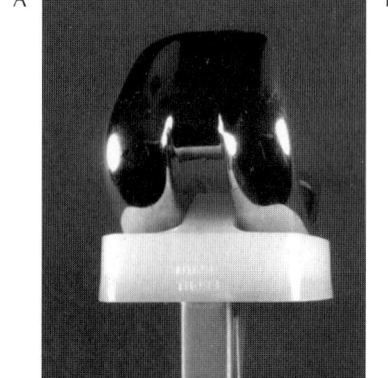

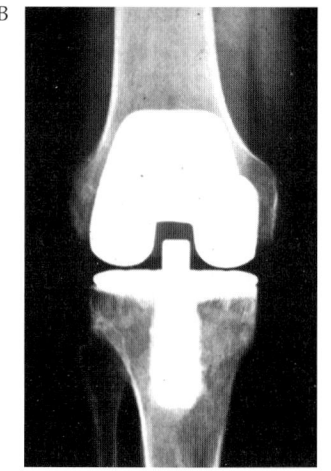

Figure 8.2. The (A) Install Burstein I prosthesis and (B) antero-posterior radiographic appearance.

to the tibial cortical shell rather than the proximal cancellous bed. Even in primary total knee arthroplasty with an all-polyethylene tibial component, the most frequent cause of failure is tibial loosening.[11] In one of the original series of total condylar knees with an all polyethylene tibia, Hood reported that two of the three failures that occurred were due to aseptic tibial component loosening.[12] In Stern's 9- to 12-year follow-up study posterior-stabilized condylar knee prosthesis with an all-polyethylene tibial component,[13] there were twice as many aseptic failures on the tibial side as compared to the femoral side. Additionally, fewer radiographic lucencies have been reported around metal-backed tibial components compared to all-polyethylene tibial components. In Colizza's 10-year follow-up of posterior-stabilized condylar knee prosthesis with a metal-backed tibial component,[14] nonprogressive lucencies were reported in only 10% of cases. Contrast this with the 49% incidence of radiolucencies in Stern's 9- to 12-year follow-up of posterior-stabilized condylar knees with an all-polyethylene tibial component. Unequivocally the introduction of metal backing into the tibial component reduced the incidence of radiolucencies around the prosthesis and aseptic loosening of the tibial component. In October 1981, the last posterior-stabilized condylar knee prosthesis with an all-polyethylene tibial component was implanted at the Hospital for Special Surgery.

Other significant changes were made to the original posterior-stabilized condylar knee prosthesis, all with the intention of improving upon the original design. In September 1988, the Insall-Burstein II was introduced.[15] Modularity of components and more component sizes were the key issues with the new prosthesis. Stems and wedges became available to enhance component fixation, and constrained condylar components became available to enhance stability. Other changes were incorporated, including deepening of the trochlear groove to facilitate patellar tracking. The radii of curvature of the femoral condyles and the tibial articular surfaces in the coronal plane were increased to enhance mediolateral rotation. The tibial polyethylene insert was also significantly changed to enhance knee flexion by shortening the tibial post by 2 mm and translating it posteriorly 2 mm.[15]

One of the initial goals of the Insall-Burstein I posterior-stabilized condylar knee prosthesis was to improve upon the stability of the total condylar prosthesis in the anteroposterior direction. The original Insall-Burstein II tibial post made the articulation more susceptible to dislocation by shortening the tibial post. Galinat[16] reported the first two cases of dislocation of the Insall-Burstein posterior-stabilized condylar prosthesis, both occurring in patients with a preoperative valgus deformity. Lombardi,[15] in a review of over 3000 Insall-Burstein posterior-stabilized condylar prosthesis between 1981 and 1991, identified 15 cases of posterior tibial dislocation. There was a statistically significant higher incidence of Insall-Burstein II dislocations versus Insall-Burstein I dislocations. This was attributed to the shortening and posterior translation of the tibial post with the Insall-Burstein II. In January 1990, the Insall-Burstein II tibial polyethylene insert was modified by beveling the anterior margin of the polyethylene to decrease patellar button impingement. The tibial post was also lengthened by 2 mm and translated anteriorly by 2 mm (Fig. 8.5). This Insall-Burstein II modified version is known as the "2+2" design, and it remains as the present posterior-stabilized condylar knee tibial insert. With this design, the cruciate-substituting mechanism of the femoral cam and the tibial post engages at about 75 degrees of knee flexion. This articulation causes femoral rollback during flexion, but it does tend to "ride up" the tibial post with increased knee flexion. This is thought to predispose the prosthesis to dislocate with increasing amounts of flexion. In Lombardi's series of posterior-stabilized condylar knees,[15] a statistically higher average range of motion was documented in those patients who had dislocated compared to those who had not dislocated. Extensor mechanism complications have also been implicated in total knee arthroplasty instability. Sharkey[17] reported that all patients with a posterior-stabilized condylar knee prosthesis who had dislocated and who had a complete clinical and radiographic review had a history of a valgus deformity and a lateral patellar retinacular release. Most importantly all patients who had dislocated had some form of extensor mechanism disruption with either a patellar dislocation, patellar tendon rupture, or fracture. Since this data was collected on patients operated on between 1985 and 1989, most of these patients probably had Insall-Burstein I prostheses, as opposed to Lombardi's series of knee dislocations for which most of the prostheses were the original Insall-Burstein II designs. Therefore, surgical, anatomic, and prosthetic design factors all contribute to instability with the posterior-stabilized condylar knee prosthesis.

Knee instability in both the primary total knee arthroplasty and the revision knee was a major consideration in the development of the constrained condylar knee prosthesis (Fig. 8.3). The constrained condylar knee, a more constrained version of the posterior-stabilized condylar knee prosthesis, was developed in 1987 to provide more constraint in both flexion and extension.[8,18] It descended from an earlier design developed at the Hospital for Special Surgery, known as the total condylar III prosthesis (Fig. 8.4). The major difference between the constrained condylar knee and the total condylar III prosthesis is stem fixation of the femoral and tibial components. The femoral and tibial stems in

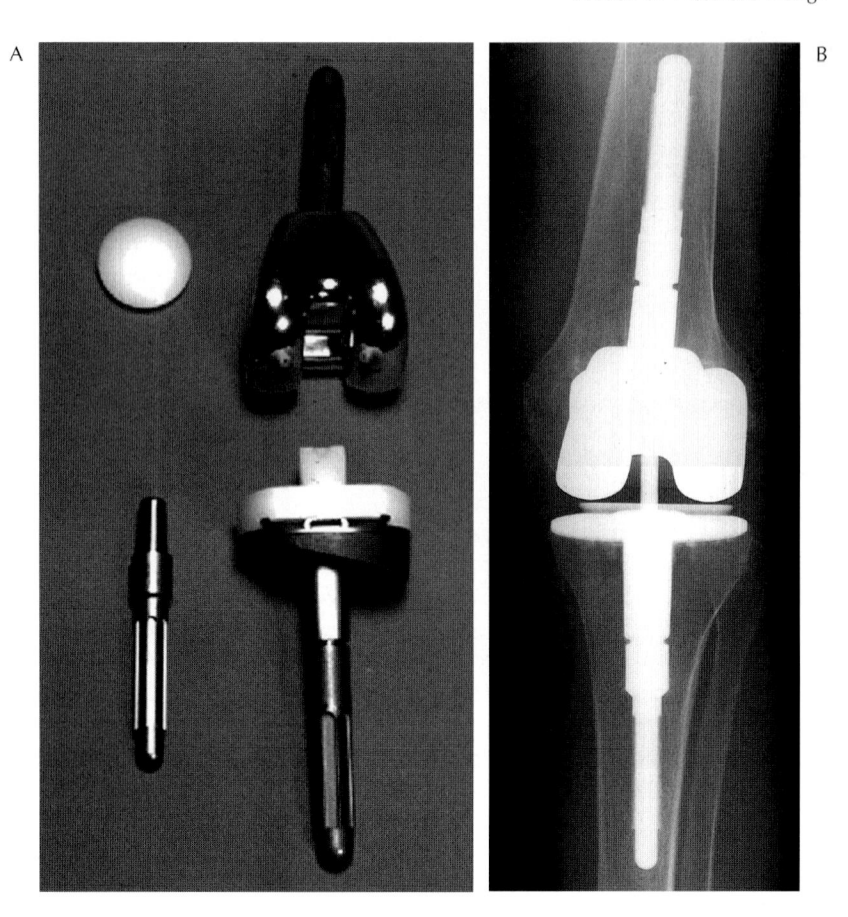

Figure 8.3. Constrained condylar knee prosthesis

the constrained condylar knee prosthesis are completely modular and do not require cement fixation. The total condylar III prosthesis stems are nonmodular and were designed for supplemental cement fixation. The femoral intercondylar box and tibial post articulation are identical in the two prostheses.

The constrained condylar knee prosthesis, in addition to increasing articulation constraint, also enhances component fixation in the presence of bone deficiency in both primary and revision total knee arthroplasty with the use of stems, wedges, and augments. The constrained condylar knee femoral component has the same femoral condyle design as the posterior-stabilized condylar knee prosthesis but it incorporates a deeper intercondylar box to accommodate a higher tibial intercondylar post. The constrained condylar knee femoral intercondylar box and tibial post articulation allow for 0 to 120 degrees of knee flexion, 5 degrees of internal and external rotation, and 3 degrees of varus and valgus freedom in full extension.[18] The higher tibial post prevents knee dislocation in flexion by creating a longer "jumping distance" for the femoral cam. The increased constraint with the tibial and femoral components in the constrained condylar knee system has made it an attractive surgical treatment choice in the revision knee, but it has also been used in the primary setting.[18] Good early results have been reported, but it remains to be seen whether the increased constraint of the constrained condylar knee articulation will lead to early loosening and prosthetic failure in the primary total knee arthroplasty.

SHORT-TERM RESULTS

Like most other total knee arthroplasty designs, the early clinical results with the posterior-stabilized condylar prosthesis were uniformly excellent. The 2- to 4-year experience in the first 118 patients who had a posterior-stabilized condylar prosthesis implanted showed 96% good and excellent results according to the Hospital for Special Surgery Knee Scoring System.[5] Groh[19] has reported similar results with the posterior-stabilized condylar knee. In a review of 137 posterior-stabilized total knee arthroplasty with an average follow-up of 29 months, there were 98% good and excellent results with few major complications. However, other designs have shown similar promising early results, only to have design flaws exposed with long-term follow-up.[20]

The posterior-stabilized condylar knee was specifically designed as a modification of the total condylar prosthesis to improve stair-climbing ability and range

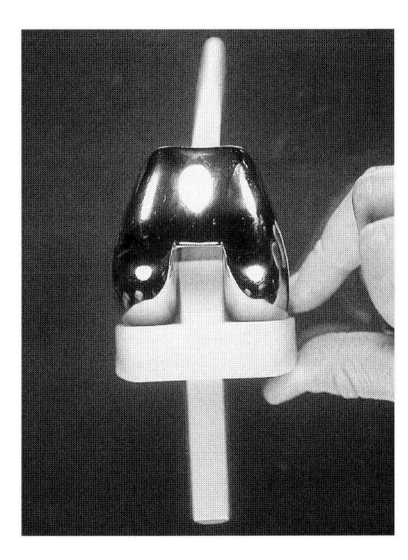

Figure 8.4. Total condylar III prosthesis

of motion and to prevent posterior tibial subluxation. These goals were certainly achieved with the new "cruciate-substituting" design. Insall reported a significant improvement in the range of motion in the posterior-stabilized condylar knee group compared to the total condylar prosthesis group.[5] Fewer than one-quarter of the patients with the total condylar prosthesis could climb stairs reciprocally compared to 97% of patients with the posterior-stabilized condylar prosthesis. These favorable early results with the posterior-stabilized condylar knee were seen in patients who were not good candidates for the total condylar prosthesis implant. Direct clinical comparison of the total condylar prosthesis and the posterior-stabilized condylar prosthesis patient groups is difficult in these retrospective analyses because of the biases in patient selection. The posterior-stabilized condylar prosthesis was initially implanted in patients who had either severe deformity or persistent instability with the total condylar prosthesis with intact collateral ligaments. These were patients who either required more extensive soft tissue release or in patients with rheumatoid arthritis where the flexion gap is frequently looser than the extension gap.[4]

The motion obtained in patients with the posterior-stabilized condylar prosthesis improved from 95 degrees to 115 degrees, whereas those patients with the total condylar prosthesis had only 90 degrees of motion postoperatively. This difference in motion was statistically significant. Maloney and Schurman[21] questioned the increased motion that was realized with the "cruciate-substituting" mechanism of the posterior-stabilized condylar knee design. In their series of 104 arthroplasties including the posterior-stabilized condylar knee and total condylar knee, the maximum flexion achieved was similar in both groups. The posterior-stabilized group actually achieved more flexion but the preoperative motion was greater in this group. The maximum flexion gained with surgery actually occurred in the total condylar group, which supports the widely held theory that postoperative motion is best predicted by preoperative motion and stiffer knees paradoxically gain more motion with surgery.

The increased motion and increased stability with the new "cruciate-substituting" design certainly enhanced knee function by allowing a greater percentage of patients to reciprocally negotiate stairs. In the early series, the motion came at considerable cost to the overall performance of the knee extensor mechanism. It was felt at the outset that the new design with the "femoral rollback" during flexion would effectively lengthen the moment arm of the extensor mechanism and therefore decrease the quadriceps and patellar forces for any given extension moment. This, in turn, was supposed to lead to fewer patellar and extensor mechanism complications, but the early results prove this to be incorrect. In the short-term follow-up with the posterior-stabilized condylar knee,[5] there was an 11% incidence of major patellar and extensor mechanism complications, including 10 patellar fractures. The early results reported with the total condylar prosthesis including the total condylar II prosthesis and the total condylar III prosthesis revealed only a 0.8% incidence of major patellar complications.[22] This included only one patellar fracture. Insall[22] felt that the increased incidence of patellar fractures with the posterior-stabilized condylar knee was not caused by the cruciate-substituting mechanism of the femoral cam and tibial post but rather to the increased motion realized with the new design. Aglietti[7] also felt that the extensor mechanism complications, including impingement types of symptoms, were not related to the femoral rollback but rather to the femoral component design itself. Because many of the early patellar fractures occurred in patients with larger patellar buttons, it became apparent that the patellofemoral joint should not be "overstuffed" with the posterior-stabilized condylar knee prosthesis. Daluga[23] has shown that an increase in the overall anterior to posterior dimensions of the knee by more than 12% was a critically independent variable that correlated with the need for knee manipulation after arthroplasty. Other variables have been demonstrated to correlate well with motion, and therefore, function of the knee. Figgie[24] has shown in a series of 116 posterior-stabilized condylar knees that the best functional knee results were associated with neutral or posterior tibial component position with respect to the center line of the tibia, elevation of the joint line by no more than 8 mm and patellar height between 10 and 30 mm above the joint line. Patellar height has also been shown to be directly related to the incidence of impingement symptoms, including the "patellar clunk," with the original Insall-Burstein I posterior-stabilized condylar knee.[7,24] Meticulous surgical technique needs to be followed with the posterior-stabilized condylar knee in that the joint line is normally elevated and the patellar height is lowered an average of 12 mm with the standard bone resection and component insertion.[24]

One concern with the development of the "cruciate-substituting" mechanism of the tibial post and femoral cam was that it would increase the horizontal shear forces across the tibial component, which may predispose to early tibial component loosening. This was certainly a potential problem because of the already high incidence of radiolucencies at the bone-cement interface around the all-polyethylene tibial component in the total condylar knee.[2] Vector force analysis of the posterior-stabilized condylar knee tibial post and femoral cam mechanism shows that the majority of forces across the tibial component are not shear but are compressive forces. Short-term follow-up of the total condylar prosthesis and the posterior-stabilized condylar knee show a nearly identical incidence of tibial component radiolucencies. The vast majority of lucencies are observed around the tibial tray, with tibial keel lucencies occurring only rarely. The all-polyethylene tibial component makes radiographic analysis of bone-cement interfaces more accurate and precise, which makes clinical comparison between the all-polyethylene tibial component of the total condylar prosthesis and the posterior-stabilized condylar knee more meaningful. The 5-year radiographic follow-up of the total condylar knee revealed a 36% incidence of nonprogressive bone-cement radiolucencies around the tibial component, most of which occurred around the tibial tray. There was only a 0.8% incidence of tibial component loosening with the total condylar knee (3 of 354). The 2- to 4-year follow-up of the posterior-stabilized condylar knee[5] with an all-polyethylene tibial component revealed a very similar 32% incidence of nonprogressive radiolucencies around the tibial component and an identical 0.8% incidence (1 of 118) of tibial component loosening. Radiographic evaluation of femoral bone-cement lucencies is more difficult and imprecise due to component rotation, which tends to obscure bone-cement interfaces. Femoral loosening with both the total condylar prosthesis and posterior-stabilized condylar knee, however, is very uncommon.[2,5,11,19]

The posterior-stabilized condylar knee has clearly been associated with more patellofemoral complications than either the cruciate-sacrificing or the cruciate-retaining knees.[2,20,25] Theories have been proposed and supported with retrospective clinical data; however, the reason is probably multifactorial.[5,6,7,8,24] Despite the unforgiving patellofemoral mechanism, it still remains the prosthesis of choice for patients who have had a previous patellectomy.[25,26] Martin reported better overall clinical results in posterior-stabilized arthroplasties compared to total condylar arthroplasties in patients with a history of a prior patellectomy.[25] The best results correlated with the amount of time that had elapsed between the patellectomy and the total knee arthroplasty. Paletta and Laskin[26] reported similar results. They found better pain and function scores in their cohort of posterior-stabilized arthroplasties compared to posterior cruciate ligament-retaining arthroplasties. In their series, better pain relief was observed in patients who had a patellectomy for a diagnosis of a fractured patella. Less predictable results occurred in patients with a history of patellectomy for chondromalacia and osteoarthrosis.

The design of the cruciate-substituting mechanism of the femoral cam and tibial post in the posterior-stabilized condylar knee offers several advantages in the patellectomized patient. Posterior tibial subluxation and knee recurvatum are prevented with the posterior-stabilized condylar knee. The predictable rollback in the posterior-stabilized condylar knee compared to cruciate-retaining designs[27] also functionally lengthens the extensor mechanism moment arm resulting in increased torque for a given quadriceps contraction. Extensor lags have been reported in up to 32% of patellectomized patients undergoing total knee arthroplasty and pain relief is not as predictable as in primary total knee replacement. For these reasons, total knee arthroplasty with the posterior-stabilized condylar knee in the patellectomized patient should still be considered a salvage operation.

LONG-TERM RESULTS

One method of determining the long-term outcome of a prosthesis is survivorship analysis.[28,29,30] This provides a tool to predict the probability of implant success and also an estimate of time to failure. Survivorship analysis is based on the assumption that the clinical outcomes are the same for those patients who are followed for short and long periods of time and for those who are lost to follow-up. This may be one of the flaws in survivorship analysis in that it provides the best-case scenario because the vast majority of total knee arthroplasty procedures are successful. Another important point in survivorship analysis is the definition of end points, which usually include loosening, revision surgery, or planned revision surgery. Therefore, survivorship analysis usually gives the probability of not having a total knee arthroplasty failure without giving any information about the quality of the result. The total condylar knee prosthesis has the longest available follow-up, however, the posterior-stabilized condylar knee is associated with fewer failures in comparative survivorship studies.

In a series of posterior-stabilized condylar knees using an all-polyethylene tibial component, Stern[13] reported 94% clinical survival at 13 years. Good and excellent results were reported in 87% of patients using the HSS knee score, but 49% of the patients had radiolucencies around the tibial component. Even though there was only a 0.4% failure rate per year, most of the failures (9 of 14) were due to aseptic loosening and 6 of the 9 aseptic failures were due to tibial component loosening. In a recent study of the posterior-stabilized condylar knees using a metal-backed tibial component, 96.4% clinical survivorship at 11 years was reported.[14] These statistics are very similar to those reported by Stern,[13] however, with the introduction of metal-backing to the tibial component, there was only a 10% incidence of nonprogressive radiolucencies around the tibial component. Additionally, none of the 159 knees that were followed were revised for aseptic tibial loosening.

Osteolysis secondary to polyethylene damage and wear debris is a known cause of total knee arthroplasty failure. However, in the long-term follow-up study of the posterior-stabilized condylar knee with a metal-backed tibial component, Colizza[14] has shown specifically that this knee design is not prone to polyethylene wear with only 8 cases of slight polyethylene wear in a series of 101 knees. There was also no clinical evidence of knee joint reaction (synovitis or swelling) to wear debris in those 8 cases and only 3 cases of progressive radiolucencies were observed, none of which showed clinical evidence of loosening.

Several papers have looked specifically at the survivorship analysis of total knee arthroplasty, but only a few have follow-up equal to or greater than 15 years.[3,30,31,32] These papers include either the total condylar knee or the posterior-stabilized condylar knee with either a metal-backed or an all-polyethylene tibial component. Even at 21 years, the estimated clinical survivorship with the total condylar knee is greater than 90%.[3] More impressively, the failure rates with the total condylar knee successor, the posterior-stabilized condylar knee with a metal-backed tibial component, were cut in half and a greater than 98% survival has been reported at 16 years.[3]

The excellent long-term results associated with the posterior-stabilized condylar knee prosthesis have surpassed that of the "gold standard" of total knee arthroplasty, the total condylar prosthesis. These impressive statistics are reflective of thoughtful patient selection and preoperative planning, meticulous surgical technique and appropriate postoperative patient management. Good and excellent outcomes cannot be guaranteed even with the use of the posterior-stabilized condylar knee prosthesis, however, the best chance at a good result starts with the appropriate prosthesis selection. The Insall-Burstein posterior-stabilized condylar knee prosthesis has become the prosthesis of choice with its unmatched survivorship and is now the benchmark by which all other prostheses will be compared.[33]

References

1. Insall J, Ranawat C, Aglietti P, Shine J. A comparison of four models of total knee replacement prostheses. *J Bone Joint Surg.* 1976; 58-A:754–765.
2. Ranawat C, Flynn W, Saddler S, Hansraj K, Maynard M. Long-term results of the total condylar knee arthroplasty. A 15-year survivorship study. *Clin Orthop.* 1993; 286:96–102.
3. Font-Rodriguez D, Scuderi G, Insall J. Unpublished data.
4. Insall J, Ranawat C, Scott W, Walker P. Total condylar knee replacement. Preliminary report. *Clin Orthop.* 1976; 120:149–154.
5. Insall J, Lachiewicz P, Burstein A. The posterior stabilized condylar prosthesis: a modification of the total condylar design. Two to four year clinical experience. *J Bone Joint Surg.* 1982; 64-A:1317–1323.
6. Hozack W, Rothman R, Booth R, Balderston R. The patellar clunk syndrome. A complication of posterior stabilized total knee arthroplasty. *Clin Orthop.* 1989; 241:203–208.
7. Aglietti P, Buzzi R, Gaudenzi A. Patellofemoral functional results and complications with the posterior stabilized total condylar knee prosthesis. *J Arthroplasty.* 1988; 3:17–25.
8. Scuderi G, Insall J. Total knee arthroplasty. Current clinical perspectives. *Clin Orthop.* 1992; 276:26–32.
9. Bartel D, Burstein A, Santavicca E, Insall J. Performance of the tibial component in total knee replacement. Conventional and revision designs. *J Bone Joint Surg.* 1982; 64-A:1026–1033.
10. Harada Y, Wevers H, Cooke T. Distribution of bone strength in the proximal tibia. *J Arthroplasty.* 1988; 3:167–175.
11. Windsor R, Scuderi G, Moran M, Insall J. Mechanisms of failure of the femoral and tibial components in total knee arthroplasty. *Clin Orthop.* 1989; 248:15–20.
12. Hood R, Vanni M, Insall J. The correction of knee alignment in 225 consecutive total condylar knee replacements. *Clin Orthop.* 1981; 160:94–105.
13. Stern S, Insall J. Posterior stabilized prosthesis. Results after follow-up of nine to twelve years. *J Bone Joint Surg.* 1992; 74-A:980–986.
14. Colizza W, Insall J, Scuderi G. The posterior stabilized total knee prosthesis: assessment of polyethylene damage and osteolysis after a ten-year-minimum follow-up. *J Bone Joint Surg.* 1995; 77-A:1716–1720.
15. Lombardi A, Mallory T, Vaughn B, Krugel R, Honkala T, Sorscher M, Kolczun M. Dislocation following primary posterior stabilized total knee arthroplasty. *J Arthroplasty.* 1993; 8:633–639.
16. Galinat B, Vernace J, Booth R, Rothman R. Dislocation of the posterior stabilized total knee arthroplasty. A report of two cases. *J Arthroplasty.* 1988; 3:363–367.
17. Sharkey P, Hozack W, Booth R, Balderston R, Rothman R. Posterior dislocation of total knee arthroplasty. *Clin Orthop.* 1992; 278:128–133.

18. Bullek D, Scuderi G, Insall J. The constrained condylar knee prosthesis. An alternative for the valgus knee in the elderly. In: Insall J, Scott W, Scuderi G, eds. *Current Concepts in Primary and Revision Total Knee Arthroplasty.* Philadelphia: Lippincott Raven Publishers, 1996:85–89.
19. Groh G, Parker J, Elliott J, Pearl A. Results of total knee arthroplasty using the posterior stabilized condylar prosthesis. A report of 137 consecutive cases. *Clin Orthop.* 1991; 269:58–62.
20. Hungerford DS, Kenna RV. Preliminary experience with a total knee prosthesis with porous coating used without cement. *Clin Orthop.* June 1983; 176:95–107.
21. Maloney W, Schurman D. The effects of implant design on range of motion after total knee arthroplasty. Total condylar versus posterior stabilized total condylar designs. *Clin Orthop.* 1992; 278:147–152.
22. Insall J, Tria A, Scott W. The total condylar knee prosthesis. The first five years. *Clin Orthop.* 1979; 145:68–77.
23. Daluga D, Lombardi A, Mallory T, Vaughn B. Knee manipulation following total knee arthroplasty. Analysis of prognostic variables. *J Arthroplasty.* 1991; 6:119–128.
24. Figgie H, Goldberg V, Heiple K, Moller H, Gordon N. The influence of tibial-patellofemoral location on function of the knee in patients with the posterior stabilized condylar knee prosthesis. *J Bone Joint Surg.* 1986; 68-A:1035–1040.
25. Martin S, Haas S, Insall J. Primary total knee arthroplasty after patellectomy. *J Bone Joint Surg.* 1995; 77-A:1323–1330.
26. Paletta G, Laskin R. Total knee arthroplasty after a previous patellectomy. *J Bone Joint Surg.* 1995; 77-A:1708–1712.
27. Stiehl J, Komistek R, Dennis D, Paxson R, Hoff W. Fluoroscopic analysis of kinematics after posterior cruciate retaining knee arthroplasty. *J Bone Joint Surg.* 1995; 77-B:884–889.
28. Malkani A, Rand J, Bryan R, Wallrich S. Total knee arthroplasty with the kinematic condylar prosthesis. A ten-year follow-up study. *J Bone Joint Surg.* 1995; 77-A:423–431.
29. Rinonapoli E, Mancini G, Azzara A, Aglietti P. Long-term results and survivorship analysis of 89 total condylar knee prostheses. *J Arthroplasty.* 1992; 7:241–246.
30. Scuderi G, Insall J, Windsor R, Moran M. Survivorship of cemented knee replacements. *J Bone Joint Surg.* 1989; 71-B:798–803.
31. Diduch D, Insall J, Scuderi G, Scott W, Font-Rodriguez D. Unpublished data.
32. Ranawat C, Insall J, Shine J. Duocondylar knee arthroplasty. Hospital for Special Surgery design. *Clin Orthop.* 1973; 94:2–3.
33. Allardyce T, Scuderi G, Insall J. Long-term results of cemented total knee replacement. *Bombay Hosp J.* 1996; 38:512–517.

CHAPTER 9
Constrained Prostheses

Kelly G. Vince

INTRODUCTION

Constrained knee arthroplasties, like life boats, are nice to have but not to use. The considerable forces on the knee (and an arthroplasty) are more reliably and durably dissipated by the ligaments around the joint. Living and elastic soft tissues are far more suited to the task than nonresilient, mechanical devices. Mechanically constrained knee prostheses, despite the advantage of easily stabilizing even the difficult knee reconstruction, are more susceptible to loosening, breakage, and wear than conventional resurfacing prostheses.

BACKGROUND AND DESIGNS

Constrained implants include linked and nonlinked designs. The former are synonymous with hinges, from the original Walldius[1–6] to the more recent kinematic rotating hinge[7] (Fig. 9.1). Nonlinked constrained devices, such as the Total Condylar III,[8–10] were first introduced in the 1970s. The additional stability or constraint came from a tall central post on the tibial component that rested between the two femoral condyles. These implants resist varus and valgus forces, decreasing as well, the risk of posterior dislocation of the tibia (Fig. 9.2).

Hinged devices were some of the earliest knee replacements available, having been introduced in the early 1950s. The detailed history of these implants is instructive.[11] Most were implanted in exceedingly small numbers. Work on hinged knee prostheses spanned three decades, until the entire concept was largely abandoned.

The literature on hinged arthroplasties teaches several important lessons:

1. Short-term results must be viewed critically. Most hinges did reasonably well over the first 2 years. Later, it seemed everyone wanted to forget about them.
2. There is always a need for follow-up literature from institutions and individuals who were not involved in the original design. Despite glowing reports from the developers of the GUEPAR device,[12–14] it was independent surgeons who identified problems with the implants.[15,16]
3. Misguided work may persist for many years before a bad concept is abandoned. Hinges were introduced in 1953, and there followed at least three decades of active development and implantation.

Hinges were gradually abandoned. Hui and Fitzgerald reported a 23% incidence of major complications in 77 hinged arthroplasties, concluding that "whenever possible, a moderately constrained replacement arthroplasty should be considered."[17] Eventually, hinges were reserved for revision surgery. Bargar and colleagues found that the GUEPAR and Herbert prostheses they had used in difficult reconstructions ultimately failed in large numbers and did not solve the problems of the revision patient.[18] "There is *no* indication for hinge prosthesis in revision surgery," wrote Insall and Dethmers in 1982.[19] This is sound advice, with general consensus. There are a very few surgeons, in a very few circumstances, who would argue that a linked implant is necessary or appropriate.

CURRENT MODELS

Nonlinked constrained knee prostheses, though mechanically more sound, are also used infrequently. Numerous styles are available from a variety of manufacturers, all based to a greater or lesser extent on the original total condylar III. Although this type of constrained implant has fared surprisingly well in clinical studies, they are still susceptible to breakage[20] and recurrent instability as a result of cold flow (Fig. 9.3). The spectrum of designs has been described well and in detail by Lombardi.[21]

Hinged prostheses are still available. Most are rotationally unconstrained, often allowing amounts of rotation, that clearly exceed the physiologic performance or requirements of the knee. A knee prosthesis may be con-

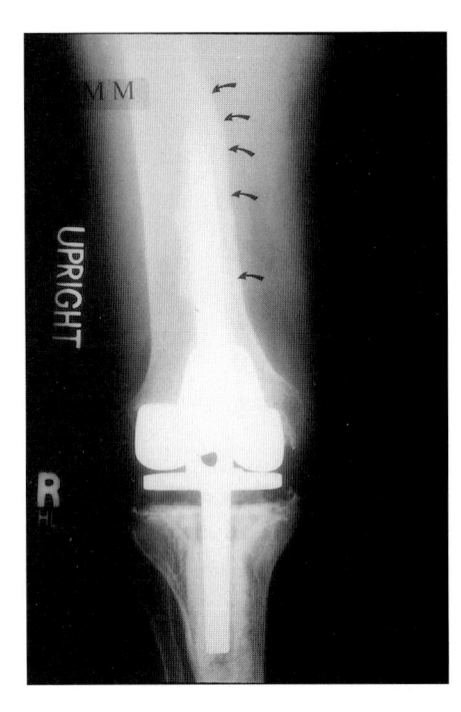

Figure 9.1. Kinematic Rotating Hinge Knee Prosthesis. Despite the rotational freedom permitted by the design, this implant was removed because of painful loosening. Radiograph shows radiolucent lines.

strained in numerous directions (Table 9.1). Some types of constraint are employed frequently, to a greater or lesser degree in the majority of condylar type resurfacing arthroplasties. Medial lateral translation, for example, is inhibited by a central, usually polyethylene eminence in even the most unconstrained replacements. The need for this was recognized early and has

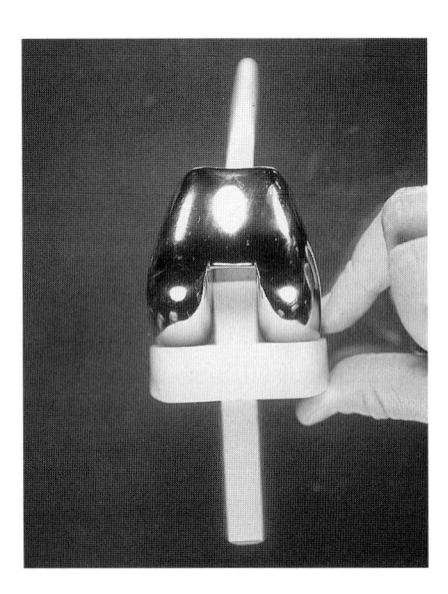

Figure 9.2. Constrained condylar type implant. The mechanism of a prominent tibial spine, housed tightly in a box, between the two femoral condyles confers stability to varus and valgus forces in the absence of solid collateral ligaments.

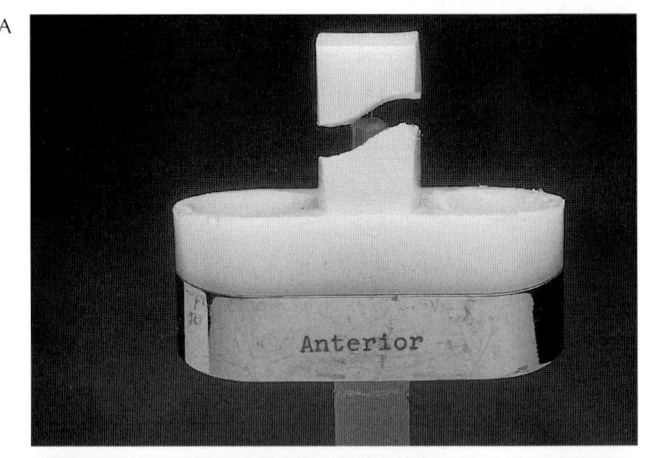

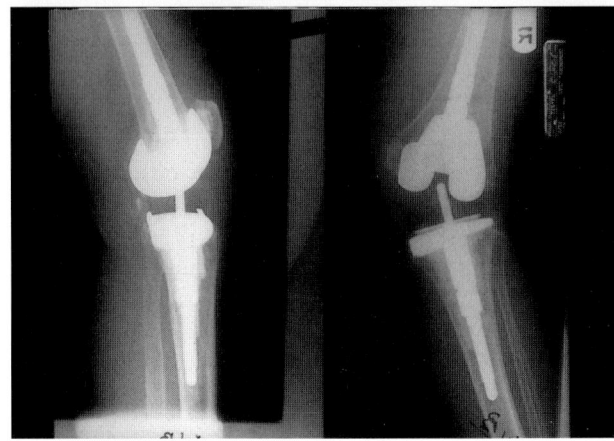

Figure 9.3. (A) Broken TC III tibial spine resulting in clinical instability. (B) Recurrent instability in a constrained condylar knee arthroplasty secondary to malalignment of the knee, overload of the prosthesis and cold flow of the tibial spine.

been incorporated into designs for over two decades.[22] Except for the flattest articular geometries, now obsolete due to concerns over accelerated polyethylene wear due to "point loading," there is usually some "dishing" of the articular surface from the front to the back that resists anteroposterior translation. Cruciate-retaining devices rely more heavily on the posterior cruciate ligament for this mode of stability and posterior-stabilized implants have a spine and cam mechanism that prevent posterior tibial subluxation in the flexed position. Most of these resurfacing implants have excellent long-term results without suffering loosening as an effect of constraint.

Accordingly, when we assess constraint, neither the conformity of the articular geometry nor simple mechanisms like the posterior-stabilized spine and cam mechanism are likely to be the source of trouble.

Constraint to varus or valgus stresses is problematic, however. There is general agreement that this constraint can lead to loosening. The more "play" in the constraint (i.e., the less constrained) the less likelihood there is of loosening, but probably the greater risk of instability

Table 9.1. Modes of constraint in knee arthroplasty prostheses

Direction	Type of motion	Problem?
Anteroposterior	Translation	No
Mediolateral	Translation	No
Varus-valgus	Arc	Yes
Rotation	Arc	No
Flexion extension stop	Arc	Definitely

and breakage of the device.[23] Both the constrained condylar type of implants and the hinges provide this type of constraint.

Rotational freedom, mentioned earlier, has been included in several linked designs with the argument that this will protect against loosening. True, very tight constraint to rotation of the tibia on the femur is unphysiologic and will likely expose the device to undue stresses with normal activities. Generally speaking, it would be difficult to argue, based on the published series of implants or laboratory testing that rotational constraint alone is a significant cause of arthroplasty failure by loosening. This is specifically supported by the observation that total condylar III type designs, as reported by several independent institutions, have performed well, perhaps surprisingly well, given a relatively high degree of rotational constraint.[24] By contrast, rotating hinges have done far less well, despite complete rotational freedom.[7] What is the most significant mechanical difference between these two constrained devices—one linked and the other unlinked? One rotationally unconstrained, the other with some constraint to rotation?

The hyperextension stop is the qualitative difference between constrained condylar implants and rotating hinges. And, the author suggests, it is the most damaging mode of constraint. With every step of the gait cycle the hyperextension stop may engage. The moment arm of the knee and the mechanical forces are large. Retrieved hinges usually have polyethylene bumpers (that engage during hyperextension), with severe wear or breakage. Constrained condylar type devices, by contrast, require soft tissue stability from posterior structures to prevent hyperextension. If the soft tissue structures are available posteriorly, yet the surgeon depends on an implant to limit hyperextension, a price will be paid unnecessarily for stability.

Other situations, such as limb salvage for tumor reconstruction, may create a situation in which virtually all stabilizing structures have been resected and only the implant can stabilize the joint.[25] Clearly these are particularly difficult and fortunately infrequent circumstances.

It can be argued then that the most damaging mode of constraint may well be the hyperextension stop. Constraint should be avoided when possible, and when required, the minimum amount necessary should be employed. Devices with a hyperextension stop should be avoided whenever possible.

INDICATIONS

Even the best-constrained designs are required infrequently. They should be avoided, when possible, in favor of good soft tissue technique. The two most common situations that arise where constraint may be indicated are:

1. The flexion gap that is much larger than the extension gap and cannot be equalized
2. Varus-valgus instability due to collateral ligament incompetence

Consider the first situation in which the flexion and extension gaps *cannot* be equalized by the selection of appropriate component sizes and sound soft tissue surgery. A relatively common scenario in difficult revisions and in correction of severe fixed flexion contractures during primary surgery is the flexion gap that gapes widely and is tremendously bigger than the extension gap. The surgeon must ensure, in revision arthroplasty that the size of femoral component, specifically its anteroposterior dimension has been chosen with an attempt to stabilize the knee in flexion (refer to Chapter 55 in this text on revision TKR technique) and not simply to fit whatever bone happens to be left after the failed components are removed. If standard components that are undersized are implanted, there will be a risk of posterior tibial dislocation. This risk will be heightened if the patient has also had a patellectomy, because the patella, by augmenting the mechanical effect of the extensor mechanism, is a buttress to posterior dislocation of the tibia. There may be a need for some constraint in this situation. A posterior-stabilized implant suffices, if the discrepancy is well under a centimeter, but a constrained condylar type device will be required for greater disparity in the gaps. Before opting for a linked implant in this situation the surgeon may consider adjunctive soft tissue reconstruction. Additionally, in this situation, if the extensor mechanism is tightened with a distal advancement of the vastus medialis, the risk of dislocation will decrease, although flexion may also be reduced. Additionally, there has been limited application of ligament advancement techniques, in this case anterior advancement of the femoral attachment of the medial collateral ligament to selectively tighten the flexion gap. This technique, combined with a constrained implant, will keep the central tibial spine between the femoral condyles, which prohibits posterior dislocation.[26]

The difficult primary knee arthroplasty may also pose problems of matching flexion and extension gaps. This occurs most commonly in the correction of a profound fixed flexion contracture. Elevation or transection of the posterior capsule often leads to greater increases in the flexion space than the extension space. This usually can be remedied with a constrained device, though rarely a linked device.

Conversely, the flexion extension gap mismatch may also occur when the extension gap exceeds the dimensions of the flexion gap. This would be a very dangerous problem to try and solve with any kind of constraint. The linked device or hinge can only salvage this situation with the use of a hyperextension stop. This applies damaging forces to the joint that will lead to rapid failure. If indeed this type of implant is used and the knee remains shortened, an incapacitating extensor lag is also likely to ensue. The true cause of this mismatch should be appreciated and corrected. In most cases it is the loss of distal femoral bone that leads to an excessively large extension gap. Small amounts can be reconstituted with distal femoral augments on modular femoral components. Larger defects will require structural femoral allografts. This type of mismatch cannot be corrected with constraint alone. Reconstruction of bone is necessary to restore collateral ligament and posterior capsular soft tissue tension. In the rare case in which an overly large extension gap and the concomitant recurvatum deformity result from neurovascular causes, arthroplasty may be impossible and arthrodesis is indicated.

Constraint is commonly employed when there has been some degree of plastic failure in the collateral ligaments, most importantly on the medial side. Consider for a moment the relative importance of the two collateral ligaments. A knee arthroplasty must be aligned with a valgus tibial femoral angle. This is sometimes described as a neutral or slightly valgus mechanical axis, referring to the line drawn from the center of the femoral head, through the knee, and then to the ankle. With this alignment, there is generally tension on the medial collateral ligament with each step, and so the ligament functions as a tension band. The patient may tolerate some laxity in the lateral stabilizers reasonably well. This lesson was demonstrated with the first techniques for correction of valgus deformity by complete transection to release the structure on the lateral side.[27] These knees remained stable when reconstructed, if they had been aligned in valgus. This technique has been superseded by more elegant and less severe lateral releases, because of occasional posterior (not varus) instability. Accordingly, many knee arthroplasty patients function well with a healthy and strong medial collateral ligament and compromised lateral structures if the appropriate valgus alignment has been achieved.

This is not true for the knee without a good or balanced medial collateral ligament. Such a knee will be unstable with standing and walking. Constraint is usually required for severe deficiencies of the medial side, but must never be considered as an alternate or substitute for the conventional techniques of ligament release.

Constraint should only be considered in the knee with valgus instability after the lateral structures have been released. Once surgical releases are complete on the lateral side (as an attempt to lengthen the lateral side equal to the length of the stretched medial ligaments),[28] then the knee should be stabilized with thicker polyethylene inserts on the tibia. The best indication that the medial collateral ligament is unsatisfactory will be the observation that medial instability persists even after progressively thicker inserts have begun to create a flexion contracture. After all, the medial collateral ligament is abnormally long due to years of valgus deformity, and even though the lateral side has been released and lengthened, the posterior structures remain intact. The posterior structures define the limit to which thicker polyethylene can be expected to help.

Whether a constrained condylar, as opposed to a hinge, can be employed in the functional absence of a medial collateral ligament is debated. Some surgeons argue that a constrained implant cannot hope to stabilize this type of knee. The author would favor ligament advancements or even the use of prosthetic materials for ligament reconstruction over a linked constrained device. We might argue further that the role of all varus-valgus constraint is to *temporarily* support the knee, until some soft tissue healing has occurred. The analogy to fracture fixation devices applies; unless the fracture heals, the fixation device is doomed to break. Corollary to knee arthroplasty is that unless some collateral-stabilizing soft tissue heals, no amount of mechanical constraint can continue to stabilize the arthroplasty.

TECHNIQUE

The surgical technique for each constrained device will differ by manufacturer and according to the instruments that are used. There are, however, some principles that are useful for implantation of a constrained device.

All constrained devices will require enhanced fixation, usually in the form of medullary stem extensions. There is currently no data to recommend uncemented fixation of the constrained implant.

Intramedullary stem extensions may be used with one of five basic strategies:

1. Large diameter, tightly fitting "press fit stems"[2] (Fig. 9.4)
2. Small diameter, intermediate length stems—"dangling stems"
3. Very long, narrow diameter "three-point fixation" stems
4. Fully cemented stems of intermediate diameter and usually intermediate length
5. Curved or offset stems that accommodate the asymmetry of the femur and tibia, achieving superior fit without compromising component position (Fig. 9.4).

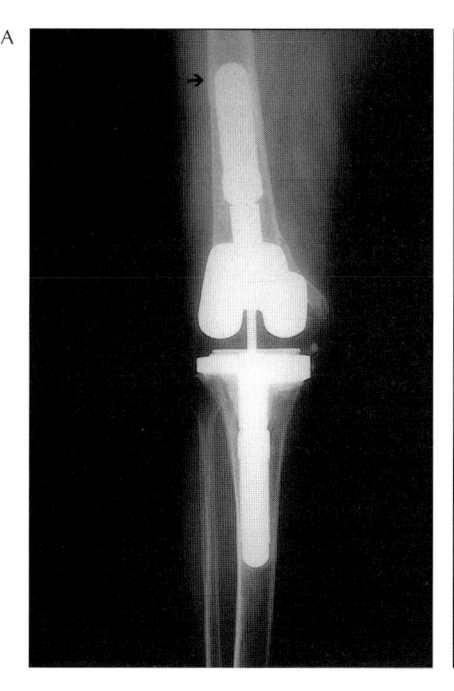

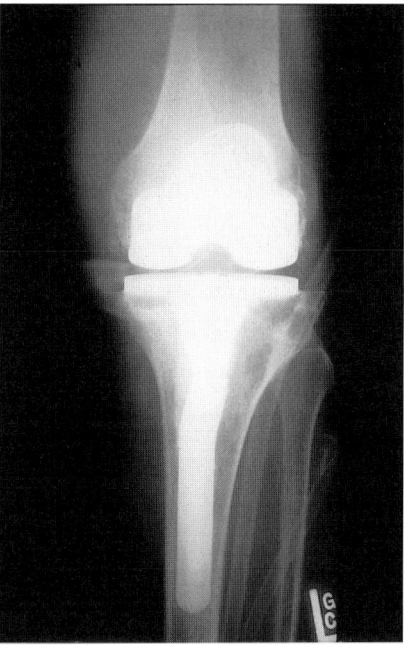

Figure 9.4. Strategies for stem use to augment fixation in total knee arthroplasty: (A) large diameter, tightly fitting "press fit stems," (B) curved or offset stems that accommodate the asymmetry of the femur and tibia, achieving superior fit without compromising component position.

Most intramedullary stems for knee arthroplasty have been relatively crude and nonanatomic designs. Unlike hip arthroplasty femoral stems, which have been scrutinized intensely to develop geometries that yield superior fit in the proximal femoral canal, most knee prosthesis stems have been straight and cylindrical. The designs have serious implication for surgical technique.

Because of the destruction that was associated with fully cemented hinges in the past, surgeons became reluctant to cement knee arthroplasty stems. Removal of the fully cemented stem is difficult. Extrication of all methacrylate in the event of infection is even more problematic. Enhanced fixation then, without cement, required a wide stem. Modularity enables the surgeon to select the necessary width to engage the medullary canal. However, problems emerge as the stem begins to determine component position. Wherever a large diameter stem sits in the tibia or femur, is where the component will lie.

Since the early 1980s, there has been general consensus that varus position leads to loosening of knee replacements.[29] However, with the exception of patellar tracking and appearance, valgus has not been considered problematic. Due to the asymmetry of the tibia, large diameter stems invariably sit in 3 to 4 degrees of valgus relative to the long axis of the shaft of the tibia. When combined with the 5 to 7 degrees of valgus cast into most stemmed femoral components and compounded by potential femoral component position in additional valgus, some revision knee arthroplasties have ended up in 10 and more degrees of valgus. Although this was not associated with loosening of condylar type replacements, the mechanics of constrained implants differ distinctly. Revision knee arthroplasty in patients with poor-quality bone using constrained components and uncemented canal filling stem extensions has led to failures in some cases.[30]

The so-called "dangling stem" would appear not to augment fixation, because it is not wedged into the tibia. The cross section of the tibial medullary canal is triangular however, and the appearance of a conventional radiograph may not reveal to what extent the longer, more narrow stem is, in fact, wedged into the canal. The great advantage of not filling the canal maximally is that alignment is not subservient to fit of the stem or the geometry of the medullary canal. Alignment is of greater importance.

The very long, but narrow diameter medullary stem extension has been described in revision arthroplasties, using unconstrained and sometimes uncemented replacements.[31] Very little has been written on the use of these stems with constrained devices. The advantage of this strategy is that modularity is not required. The narrow diameter stems can be cast as a single unit with the component with the expectation that the narrow diameter will fit any canal. The fixation advantage derives from the three-point contact that occurs down the canal.

Cemented stems nonetheless have some appeal. Fixation is immediate and rigid without compromising the alignment of the arthroplasty. The results with this approach have been excellent[32] but the difficulty of removal, if it is ever required, remains the great drawback. Fortunately, the technologies that have been developed for removal of implants and cement in revision hip surgery lend themselves well to the equally difficult task in the knee.

SUMMARY

The constrained knee prosthesis must be regarded as an occasionally necessary evil. Some difficult primary and revision knee surgeries must be reconstructed in the absence of dependable ligamentous structures. When the flexion gap sags open and the knee is well balanced in extension, or when the medial collateral ligament in particular is not functional, some additional maneuver will be required to stabilize the joint. Constraint, preferably nonlinked, whether alone or combined with ligamentous reconstruction is often the answer.

Constrained prostheses differ qualitatively and quantitatively. The immediate qualitative difference lies between the linked (hinged) and unlinked prosthesis. The hinges undoubtedly fail at a more rapid rate than constrained condylar designs. The argument is made here that this is due in large part to the extension stop inherent in the design. Constraint should never be regarded as a substitute for classic techniques of ligament releases to correct deformity and stabilize the knee. Hinges should not be used where a constrained condylar type device will suffice. Newer, infrequently used techniques for ligament reconstruction may enable the surgeon to stabilize the difficult knee without recourse to a hinge and perhaps without a constrained condylar device either.

References

1. Freeman PA. Walldius arthroplasty: a review of 80 cases. *Clin Orthop*. 1973; 94:85–91.
2. Bain AM. Replacement of the knee joint with the Walldius prosthesis using cement fixation. *Clin Orthop*. 1973; 94:65–71.
3. Jackson JP, Elson RA. Evaluation of the Walldius and other prostheses for knee arthroplasty. *Clin Orthop*. 1973; 94: 104–114.
4. Haberman ET, Deutsch SD, Rovere GD. Knee arthroplasty with the use of the Walldius total knee prosthesis. *Clin Orthop*. 1973; 94:72–84.
5. Jones GB. Total knee replacement—the Walldius hinge. *Clin Orthop*. 1973; 94:50–57.
6. Walldius B. Arthroplasty of the knee using an acrylic prosthesis. *Acta Orthop Scan*. 1953; 23:121.
7. Rand JA, Chao EY, Stauffer RN. Kinematic rotating-hinge total knee arthroplasty. *J Bone Joint Surg*. 1987; 69A:489–497.
8. Rosenberg AG, Verner JJ, Galante JO. Clinical results of total knee revision using the total condylar III prosthesis. *Clin Orthop*. 1991; 273:83–90.
9. Hohl WM, Crawford E, Zelicof SB, Ewald FC. The total condylar III prosthesis in complex knee reconstructions. *Clin Orthop*. 1991; 273:91–97.
10. Lachiewicz PF, Falatyn SP. Clinical and radiographic results of the total condylar III and constrained condylar total knee arthroplasty. *J Arthroplasty,* 1996; 11:916–922.
11. Vince K. The evolution of knee arthroplasty design in surgery of the knee. In: Scott WN, ed. *The Knee*. St. Louis: Mosby, 1994: 1045–1078.
12. Deburge A, GUEPAR. GUEPAR hinge prosthesis: complications and results with two years' follow-up. *Clin Orthop*. 1976; 120:47–53.
13. Deburge A, Aubriot JH, Jenet JP, GUPAR. Current status of a hinge prosthesis. (GUEPEAR). *Clin Orthop*. 1979; 145: 91–93.
14. Accardo NJ, Noiles DG, Pena R, Noiles NJ Jr. Noiles total knee replacement procedure. *Orthopedics*. 1979; 2:37–45.
15. Jones EC, Insall J, Inglis AE, Ranawat CS. GUEPAR knee arthroplasty results and late complications. *Clin Orthop*. 1979; 140:145–152.
16. Shindell R, Neumann R, Connolly JF, Jardon OM. Evaluation of the Noiles hinged knee prosthesis. *JBJS*. 1986; 68A: 579–585.
17. Hui FC, Fitzgerald RH Jr. Hinged total knee arthroplasty. *JBJS*. 1980; 62A:513–519.
18. Bargar WL, Cracchiolo A 3d, Amstutz HC. Results with the constrained total knee prosthesis in treating severely disabled patients and patients with failed total knee replacements. *J Bone Joint Surg*. 1980; 62A:504–512.
19. Insall JN, Dethmers DA. Revision of total knee arthroplasty. *Clin Orthop*. 1982; 170:123–130.
20. MacPherson E, Vince K. Case report of broken TC III.
21. Lombardi A. Constrained knee arthroplasty. In: Fu F, Harner C, Vince K, eds. *Knee Surgery, Vol II*. Baltimore: Williams and Wilkins 1994: 1331–1350.
22. Ewald FC, Scott RD, Thomas WH, et al. The importance of intercondylar stability in knee arthroplasty. *J Bone Joint Surg*. 1975; 57A:1033.
23. Scott C, Heiner J, Worzala FJ, Vanderby R. Condylar failure of the Lacey rotating-hinge total knee. *J Arthroplasty*. February 1996; 11(2):214–216.
24. Rosenberg AG, Verner JJ, Galante JO. Clinical results of total knee revision using the total condylar III prosthesis. *Clin Orthop*. 1991; 273:83–90.
25. Choong PF, Sim FH, Pritchard DJ, Rock MG, Chao EY. Megaprostheses after resection of distal femoral tumors. A rotating hinge design in 30 patients followed for 2–7 years. *Acta Orthop Scand*. August 1996; 67(4):345–351.
26. Vince K, Berkowitz R, Spitzer A. Ligament reconstruction in the difficult primary and revision total knee arthroplasty. Presented at the Annual Meeting of the Knee Society. San Francisco, Calif. January 1997.
27. Insall JN. Total knee replacement. In: Insall JN, ed. *Surgery of the Knee*. New York: Churchill Livingstone, 1984: 587–696.
28. Vince K. Leg length discrepancy in total knee arthroplasty. *Techniques in Orthopedics*.
29. Vince K, Insall JN, Kelly MA. The total condylar prosthesis: 10- to 12-year results of a cemented knee replacement. *J Bone Joint Surg*. 1989; 71B:793–797.
30. Vince K, Long W. Revision knee arthroplasty: The limits of press fit medullary fixation. *Clin Orthop*. 1995; 317: 172–177.
31. Bertin K, Freeman MA, Samuelson KM, Ratcliffe SS, Todd RC. Stemmed revision arthroplasty for aseptic loosening of total knee replacement. *JBJS*. 1985; 67:242–248.
32. Murray PB, Rand JA, Hanssen AD. Cemented long-stem revision total knee arthroplasty. *Clin Orthop*. December 1994; (309):116–123.

CHAPTER 10
Meniscal-Bearing Total Knee Arthroplasty

Frederick F. Buechel

INTRODUCTION

Human knee joint replacements have been developed with specific bioengineering requirements to provide near-normal kinematics, maintain fixation, and minimize wear. A mechanical solution to the bearing overload problem that causes excessive wear has been to use more congruent meniscal-bearing surfaces[1,2,3,4] to lower the contact stresses below 10 MPa,[5] which is reported as the maximum permissible compressive stress limit of ultrahigh-molecular-weight (UHMW) polyethylene. Lowering contact stresses to within the reported medical load limit of 5 MPa[6] while allowing kinematically acceptable motion provides a meniscal-bearing surface that is resistant to fatigue wear and demonstrates normal abrasive wear behavior over a 10-year period as seen in both simulator and retrieval studies.[2,7,8,9,10] (Figs. 10.1 and 10.2).

The first complete systems approach to total knee replacement using meniscal bearings was developed at the New Jersey Medical School in 1977 and first reported in 1986.[1] Unicompartmental, bicompartmental, and tricompartmental disease were managed with a variety of primary and revision components that allowed retention of both cruciates, the posterior cruciate ligament (PCL) only, or no cruciate ligaments. Additionally, the first metal-backed, rotating-bearing patella replacement was developed in 1977 to provide mobility with congruence in patellofemoral articulation. This New Jersey Low-Contact-Stress (LCS) total knee system (DePuy, Warsaw, Ind), initially used with cement in 1977, was expanded to noncemented use in 1981 with the availability of sintered-bead porous coating[11] and remains the only knee system in the United States to have undergone formal Food and Drug Administration (FDA)-Investigational Device Exemption (IDE) clinical trials in both cemented and cementless applications before being released for general clinical use[12,13,14,15] (Fig. 10.3).

SURGICAL TECHNIQUE
Preparation

Preoperatively, obtain a standing AP X ray of both femora and tibia centered on the knee joint. On the X ray, draw a line through the center of each femoral canal to the center of the knee joint (anatomic axis). Draw a line through the center of each femoral head to the center of the knee joint (mechanical axis). The angle between these two lines is the "valgus angle" (Fig. 10.4). Measure the valgus angle of both knees. The normal angle varies from 3 to 8 degrees and should be individualized for each patient in the distal femoral resection. It is recommended by this author that the following valgus angles be used based on the patient's height:

Height < 5'11"	5 degrees
Height from 5'11" to 6'1"	4 degrees
Height > 6'1"	3 degrees

Incision and Exposure

With the knee slightly flexed, make a straight midline incision from 8 cm above the patella, over the patella, and ending at the tibial tubercle (Fig. 10.5a). With neutral alignment or a varus deformity, make a median parapatellar incision through the retinaculum, capsule, and synovium (Fig. 10.5b). If significant valgus deformity exists, a lateral parapatellar deep incision as part of a lateral release may be preferred (Fig. 10.5c).[16,17]

Following a median parapatellar incision, reflect the patella laterally to expose the entire tibiofemoral joint

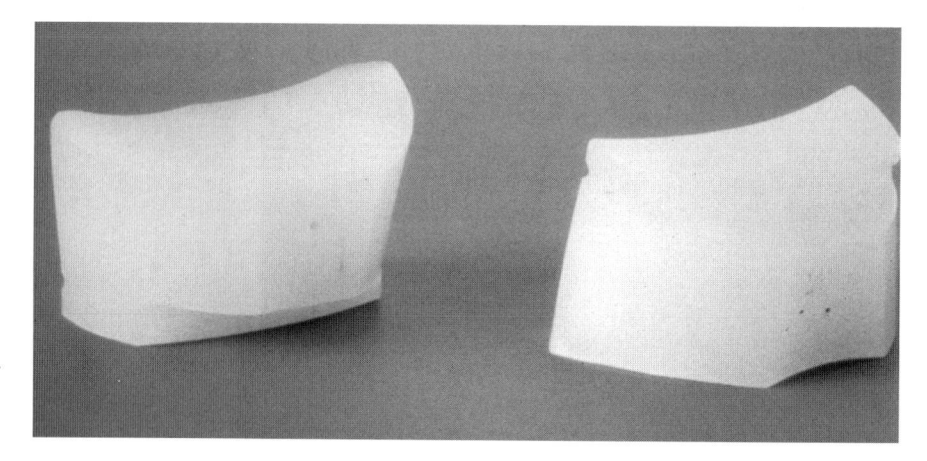

Figure 10.1. Meniscal-bearing simulator specimen after 10 million cycles under loads of 2,200 NS.

(Fig. 10.6). Should tension prevent adequate lateral displacement of the patella, detach the medial one-fourth to one-third of the patellar tendon from the tibial tubercle. To further mobilize the extensor mechanism, continue the sharp incision of the medial portion of the quadriceps tendon proximally or, while proximal, perform a "quadriceps snip"[18] across the quadriceps tendon at a 45-degree angle.

Following a lateral parapatellar incision in the valgus knee, incise the anterior compartment fascia longitudinally one centimeter from the tibial tubercle. Elevate the tibial tubercle with an osteoperiosteal flap if necessary or use a reverse "quadriceps snip." Reflect the patella and periosteal attachments medially.[16,17]

Excise hypertrophic synovium and a portion of the infrapatellar fat pad to allow access to the medial, lateral, and intercondylar spaces. Excise redundant synovium to prevent possible impingement or postoperative overgrowth. Evaluate the condition of the cruciate ligaments to determine the appropriate tibial component to use.[19]

Ligament Balancing

Remove femoral and tibial osteophytes, especially any deep to the collateral ligaments. Lateral soft tissue release and, occasionally, osteotomy and removal of the fibular head[16] will enable correction of valgus contracture (Fig. 10.7a). Medial sleeve release may be necessary for a fixed varus deformity[20] (Fig. 10.7b). An extensive medial tibial subperiosteal sleeve may be necessary in severe varus angulation.

Nine basic steps are then performed using precision instruments to gain a perpendicular tibial component orientation in the frontal plane, anatomically sloped posteriorly in the lateral plane; balanced flexion-extension gaps; and reasonable mechanical axis positioning. These steps are as shown in Figure 10.8.

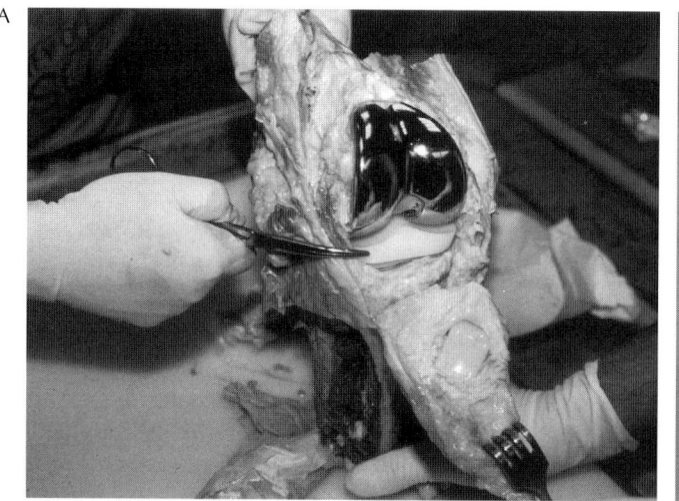

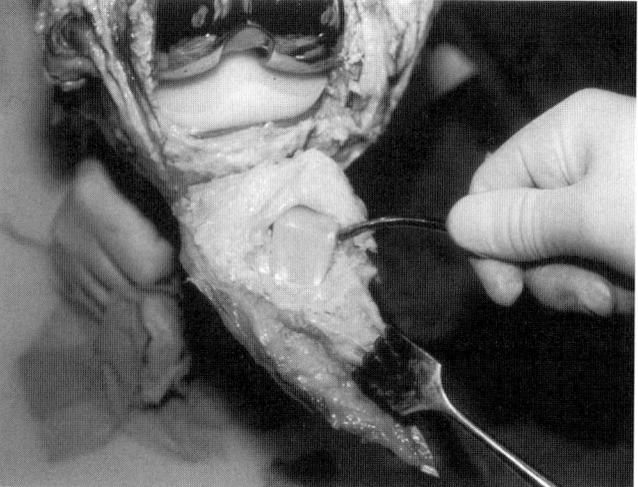

Figure 10.2. (A) Ten-year postmortem retrieval of an asymptomatic rotating platform prosthesis demonstrating continued rotation of the tibial bearing. (B) The same retrieval specimen demonstrating continued axial rotation of the rotating patella bearing.

LCS™ Total Knee System

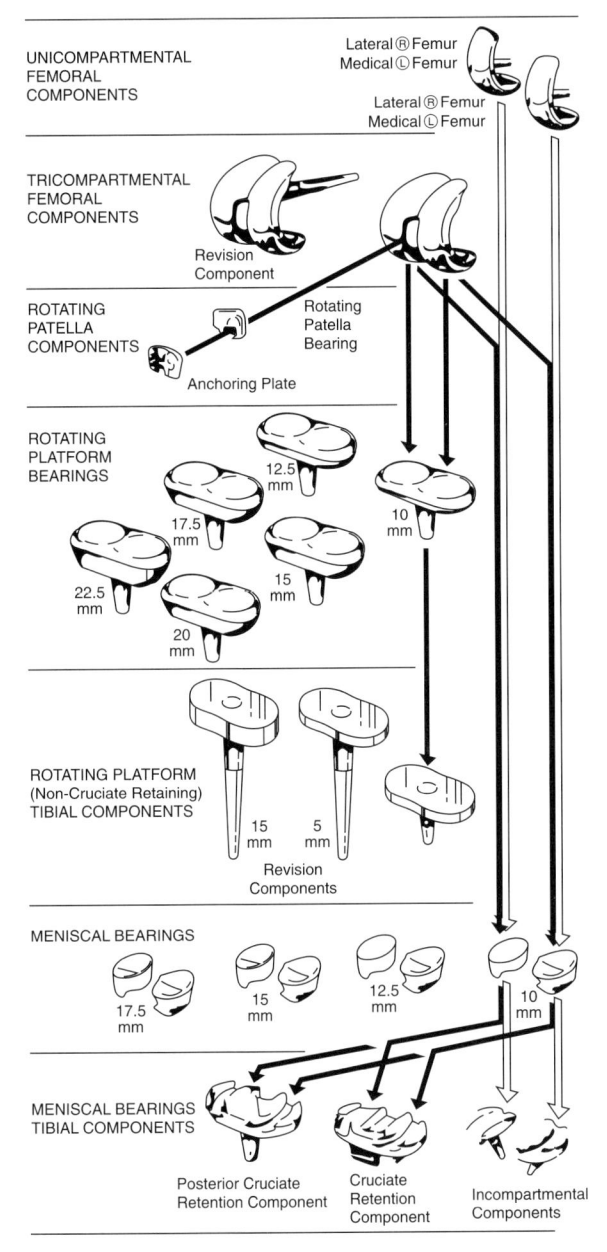

Figure 10.3. New Jersey LCS knee replacement system components.

Implantation

After a satisfactory trial reduction of all components, remove the trials and implant the final components in the following order.

1. Tibial tray
2. Tibial bearings
3. Femoral component
4. Patellar component

The bicruciate-retaining, posterior cruciate-retaining, and cruciate-sacrificing components are seen on Figure 10.9.

The patella is reduced into its anatomical position and checked for congruent tracking in the femoral groove using "thumb pressure" to maintain contact. If thumb pressure fails to maintain full-bearing contact, perform a sequential lateral release until full contact; then unrestricted motion is appreciated with all components (Fig. 10.10).

Closure

The tourniquet is released and the deep retinacular tissues are closed with #1 absorbable suture with the knee in greater than 100° of flexion. Subcutaneous tissue is approximated with 2-0 absorbable suture in extension and the skin is closed in flexion with staples. The use of a drain is optional.[21]

POSTOPERATIVE REHABILITATION

The patient is allowed progressive ambulation with weight bearing to tolerance on the first postoperative

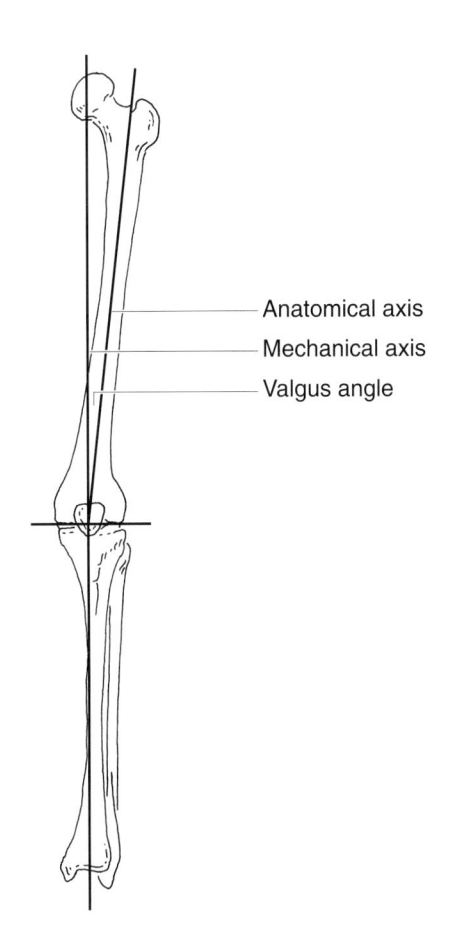

Figure 10.4. Frontal plane axis of the knee.

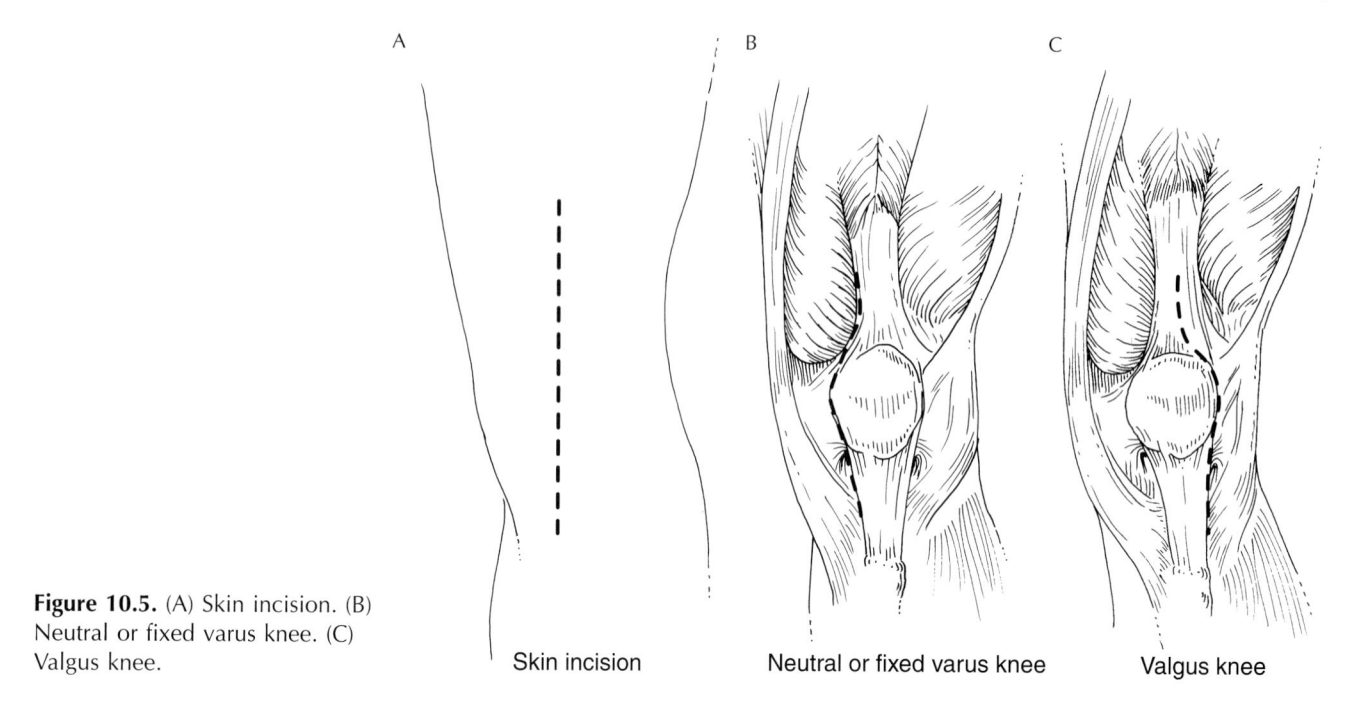

Figure 10.5. (A) Skin incision. (B) Neutral or fixed varus knee. (C) Valgus knee.

day regardless of cemented or cementless fixation. Active-assistive and gravity-assistive range of motion of the knee are also begun on the first postoperative day in conjunction with isometric quad sets of 50 to 100 per day with a 5-second hold for each contraction. Unassisted gait and a ROM of 0–120° is usually achieved in 6 to 12 weeks in primary knee replacements using this program.

SURVIVORSHIP ANALYSIS OF CEMENTED AND CEMENTLESS MENISCAL-BEARING KNEE REPLACEMENTS

Survivorship of at least 90% at the 10-year interval, using as an end point revision of any component for any reason, has been recommended as a standard for primary TKR.[22] Any knee replacement that does not

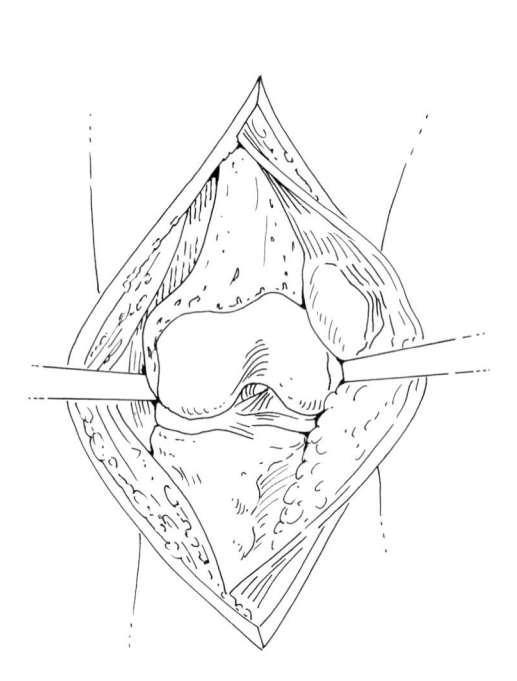

Figure 10.6. Deep exposure of the knee.

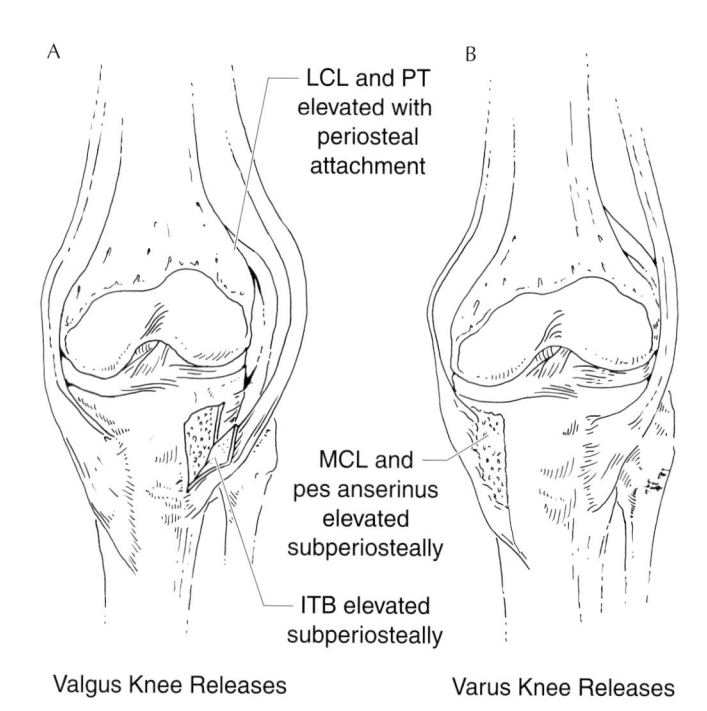

Figure 10.7. (A) Valgus knee releases. (B) Varus knee releases.

achieve this level of success should not be routinely used until design improvements can clearly demonstrate advantages over standard designs.

Meniscal-bearing knee replacements have demonstrated this high level of survivorship in several designs. The Oxford meniscal knee has been specifically indicated for medial, unicompartmental, noninflammatory arthritis, and in such conditions, when both cruciate ligaments are intact, has a reported 99.1% survivorship at 10 years when used with methyl methacrylate bone cement.[23] Cementless long-term use of the Oxford device has not been reported and its use in bicompartmental and lateral unicompartmental applications is not recommended because of loosening and dislocation problems.[24]

The cemented LCS unicompartmental meniscal knee replacement has a reported 91% survivorship at 10 years when used for either the medial or lateral compartments

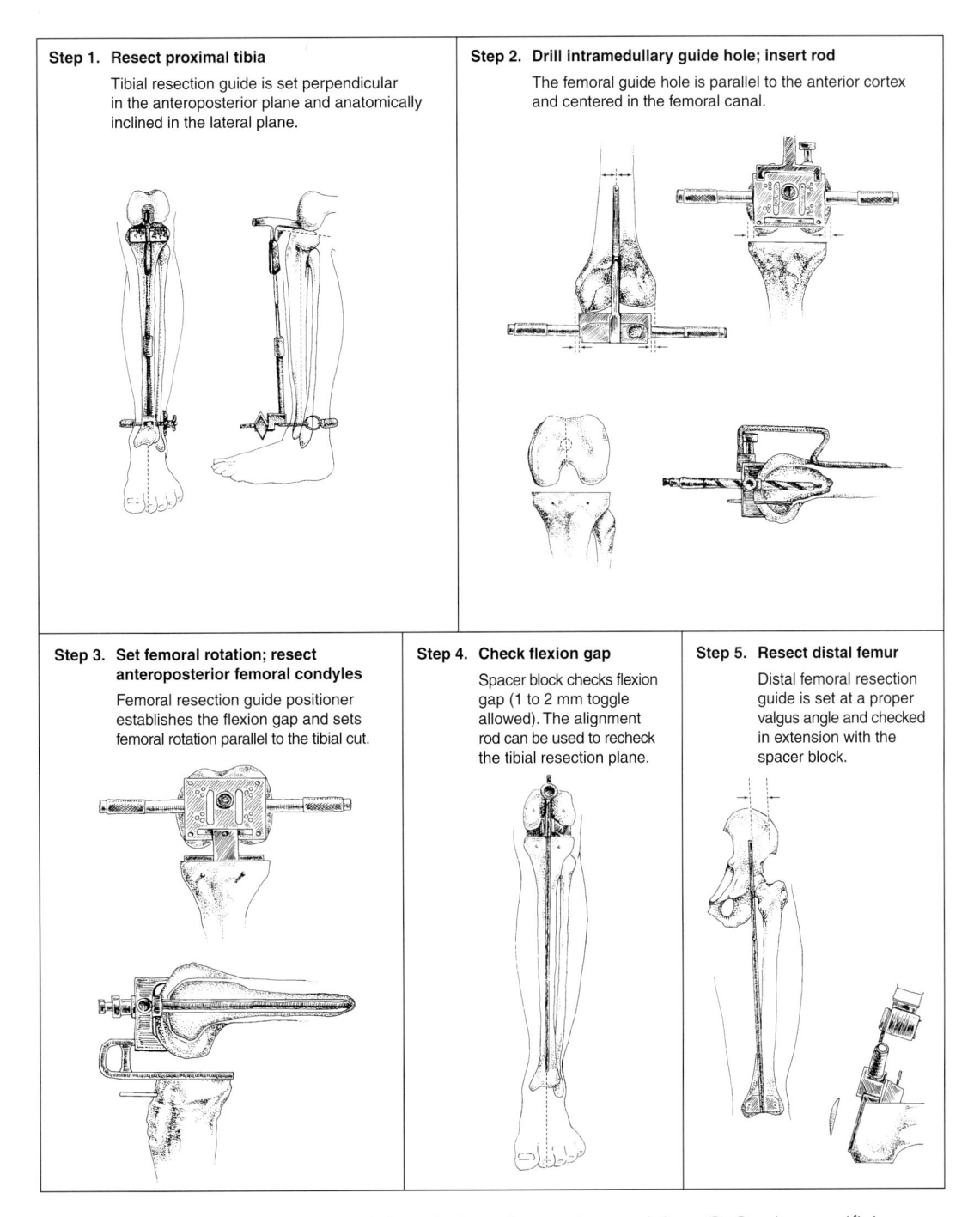

Step 1. Resect proximal tibia
Tibial resection guide is set perpendicular in the anteroposterior plane and anatomically inclined in the lateral plane.

Step 2. Drill intramedullary guide hole; insert rod
The femoral guide hole is parallel to the anterior cortex and centered in the femoral canal.

Step 3. Set femoral rotation; resect anteroposterior femoral condyles
Femoral resection guide positioner establishes the flexion gap and sets femoral rotation parallel to the tibial cut.

Step 4. Check flexion gap
Spacer block checks flexion gap (1 to 2 mm toggle allowed). The alignment rod can be used to recheck the tibial resection plane.

Step 5. Resect distal femur
Distal femoral resection guide is set at a proper valgus angle and checked in extension with the spacer block.

Figure 10.8. (A) Bicruciate retaining. (B) Posterior cruciate retaining. (C) Cruciate sacrificing

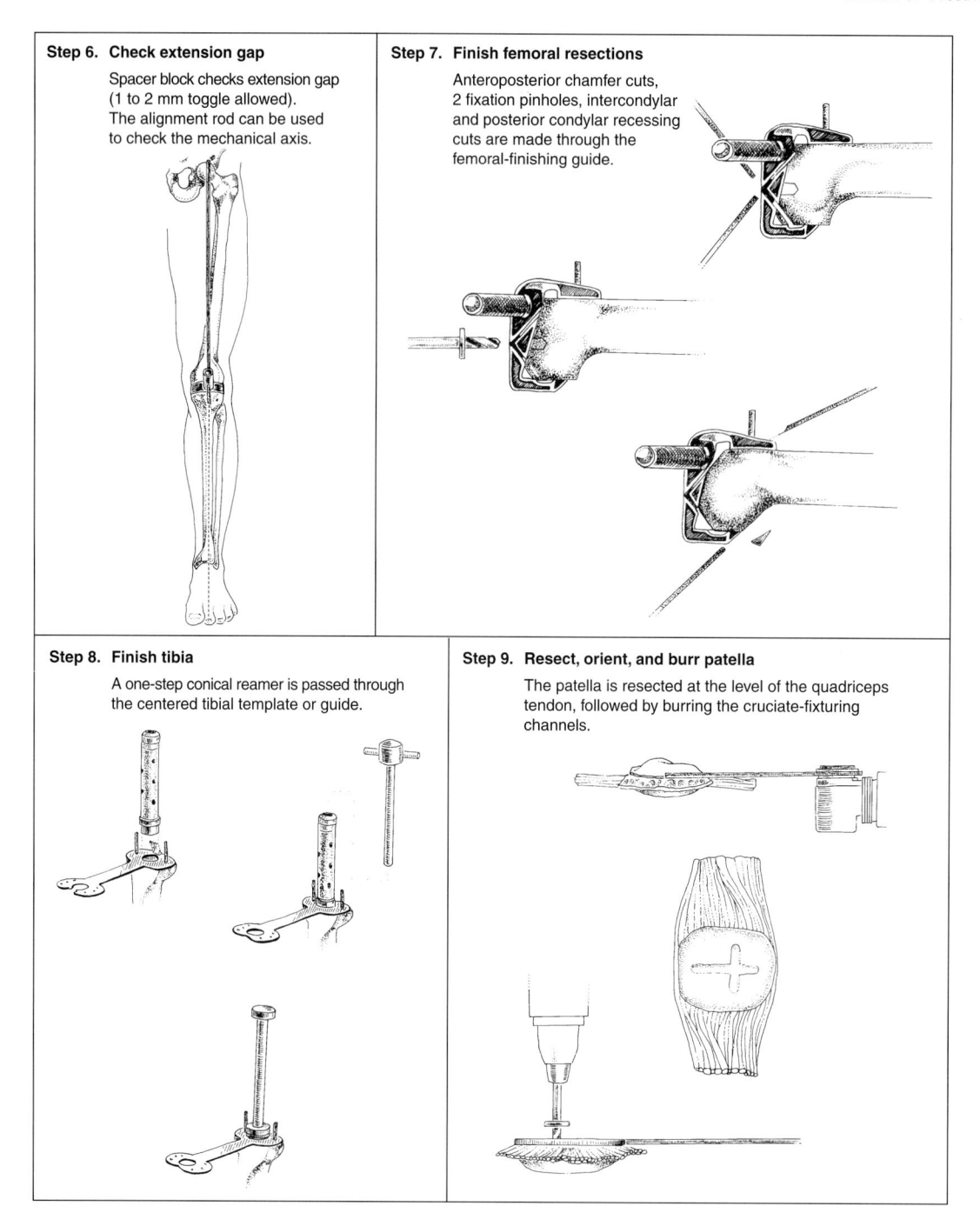

Step 6. Check extension gap
Spacer block checks extension gap (1 to 2 mm toggle allowed). The alignment rod can be used to check the mechanical axis.

Step 7. Finish femoral resections
Anteroposterior chamfer cuts, 2 fixation pinholes, intercondylar and posterior condylar recessing cuts are made through the femoral-finishing guide.

Step 8. Finish tibia
A one-step conical reamer is passed through the centered tibial template or guide.

Step 9. Resect, orient, and burr patella
The patella is resected at the level of the quadriceps tendon, followed by burring the cruciate-fixturing channels.

Figure 10.8. (continued).

in conjunction with intact cruciate ligaments in noninflammatory degenerative arthritis. The cementless LCS unicompartmental replacement has a reported 98% survivorship at 10 years when indicated for the same conditions as the cemented device. Inflammatory conditions such as rheumatoid arthritis, severe osteoporosis, and ACL deficiency are contraindications for LCS meniscal-bearing unicompartmental replacement and are a documented source of failure in such cases.[14]

The cemented LCS bicruciate-retaining meniscal-bearing TKR has a reported 90% survivorship at 10 years and the cementless device has a 95% survivorship at the same follow-up interval. Undersizing the tibial component in the cemented group and previous high tibial osteotomy or tibial plateau fracture in the cementless group are causes for failure and are now contraindicated for these devices. Additionally, it is not recommended to use the bicruciate device when the ACL has been dis-

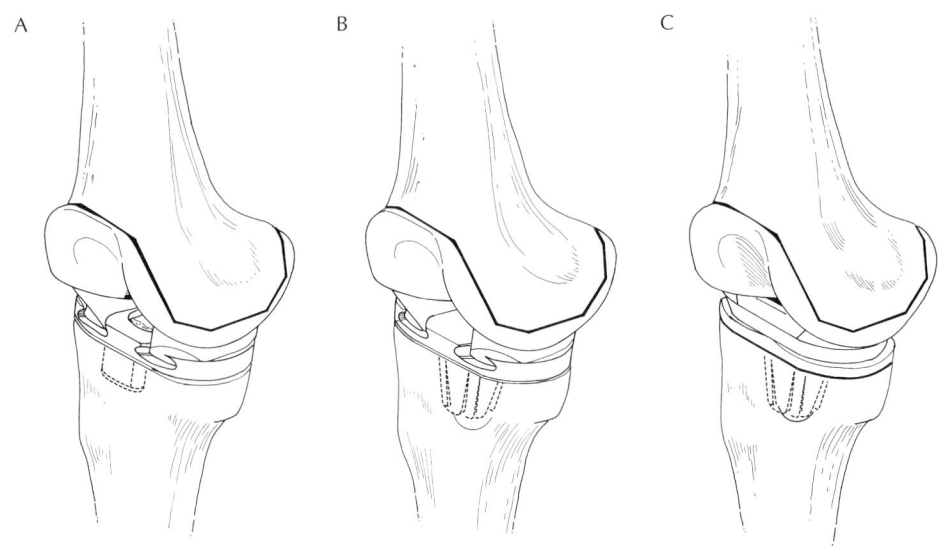

A	B	C
Bicruciate retaining	Posterior cruciate retaining	Cruciate sacrificing

Figure 10.9. Final knee components with unrestricted motion.

rupted or is deficient, but rather the centrally stabilized, PCL-retaining meniscal-bearing tibial component is preferred.

The cementless LCS PCL-retaining meniscal-bearing TKR has a 97% survivorship over the initial 10 years. It was released for clinical use in 1984 and remains the most popular meniscal-bearing knee replacement worldwide at the present time. Flexion instability,[25,26] rotational malalignment,[27] and late rupture of the PCL can compromise the long-term results with this device. It is important to be sure of PCL integrity, proper rotation of the tibial tray, and balanced flexion-extension gaps at surgery[28] for reproducible long-term results with this implant.

The cemented LCS rotating platform TKR used for cruciage ligament deficiency has a reported 97% survivorship at 16 years and the cementless device has a 98% survivorship at the 15-year interval. Flexion instability has been identified as unusual but the main problem with this device. The cemented and cementless survivorship of this implant represents a new standard for successful TKR to which future designs should be compared.

Cementless total knee fixation represents an advance over cemented fixation in that a temporary bone-cement interface is eliminated in favor of a permanent bone-prosthesis interface. Thus, it is reasonable to assume that a 10-year survivorship of a cementless device that improves upon a cemented device of the same design would be preferred as a means of long-term fixation. As such, the improved contact stresses of mobile bearings over fixed bearings would also be preferred, especially if long-term survivorship studies demonstrate such improvement. Such is the case, when one reviews the reported survivorship of a wide variety of fixed-bearing knee replacements used in cementless applications compared to the long-term survivorship of LCS cementless knee replacements (Fig. 10.11).

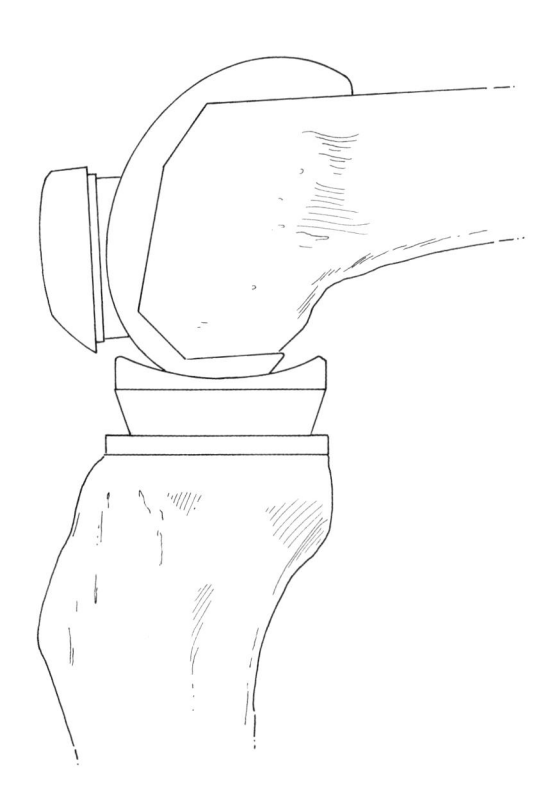

Figure 10.10. Survival estimates of cementless TKRs compared with the cemented total condylar knee.

The fact that wear resistance is also superior to fixed-bearing designs makes cementless mobile bearings the current implant choice for joint replacement of the knee in patients with active loading demands.

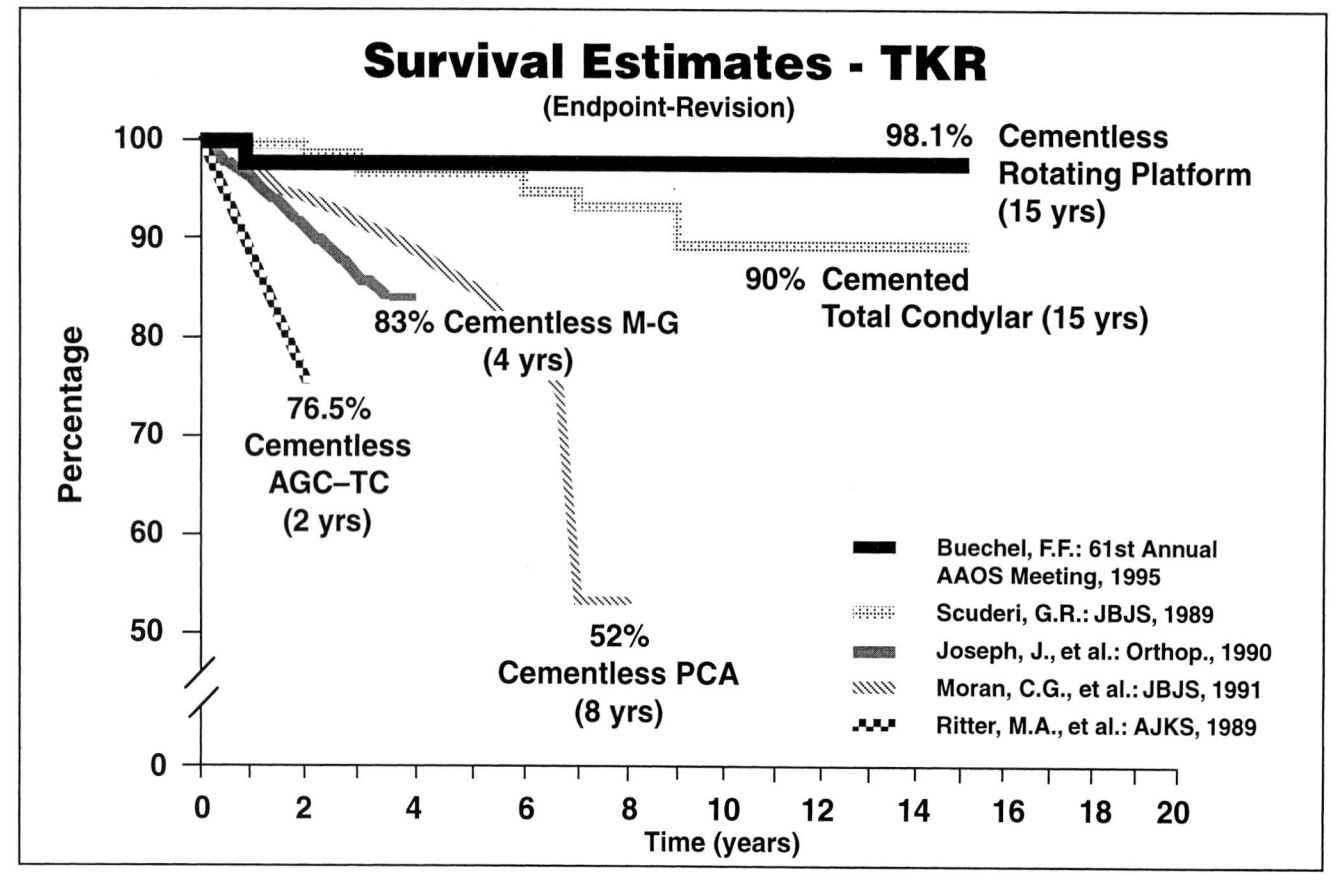

Figure 10.11. Survivorship of total knee replacement.

References

1. Buechel FF, Pappas MJ. The New Jersey low contact stress knee replacement system: biomechanical rationale and review of the first 123 cemented cases. *Arch Orthop Trauma Surg.* 1986; 105:197–204.
2. Goodfellow J, O'Conner J. The mechanics of the knee and prosthesis design. *J Bone Joint Surg BR.* 1978; 60:358–369.
3. Huson A, Spoor CW, Verbout AJ. A model of the human knee derived from kinematic principles and its relevance for endoprosthesis design. *Acta Morphol Ned Scand.* 1989; 270:45.
4. Schlepckow P. Three dimensional kinematics of total knee replacement systems. *Arch Orthop Trauma Surg.* 1992; 3:204–209.
5. Hostalen GUR. Hoechst aktiengellschaft. Frankfurt, Germany, 1982: 22.
6. Buechel FF, Pappas MJ, Makris G. Evaluation of contact stress in metal-backed patellar replacements: a predictor of survivorship. *Clin Orthop.* 1991; 273:190–197.
7. Buechel FF, Pappas MJ. New Jersey LCS knee replacement system: biomechanical rationale and comparison of cemented and noncemented results (a two to five year follow-up). *Contemp Orthop.* 1987; 14:52–60.
8. Buechel FF, Pappas MJ. New Jersey LCS knee replacement system: 10 year evaluation of meniscal bearings. *Orthop Clin North Am.* 1989; 20:147–177.
9. Coll BF, Jacquot P. Surface modification of medical implants and surgical devices using TiN layers. *Surface Coating Technol.* 1988; 36:867–878.
10. O'Connor J, Goodfellow J, Biden E. Designing the human knee. In: Stokes IAF, ed. *Mechanical Factors and the Skeleton*; London: John Libbey, 1981.
11. Pilliar RM, et al. Radiographic and morphologic studies of load-bearing porous-surfaced structured implants. *Clin Orthop.* 1981; 156:249–257.
12. Buechel FF, Pappas MJ. New Jersey integrated total knee replacement system: biomechanical analysis and clinical evaluation of 918 cases. FDA Panel Presentation, Silver Spring, Md. July 11, 1984.
13. Buechel FF, et al. New Jersey LCS posterior cruciate retaining total knee replacement: clinical, radiographic, statistical, and survivorship analyses of 395 cementless cases performed by 13 surgeons. Food and Drug Administration Panel Presentation. Rockville, Md. June 1, 1990.
14. Buechel FF, et al. New Jersey LCS unicompartmental knee replacement: clinical, radiographic, statistical and survivorship analyses of 106 cementless cases performed by 7 surgeons. Food and Drug Administration Panel Presentation. Rockville, Md. August 16, 1991.

15. Buechel FF, Sorrels B, Pappas MJ. New Jersey rotating platform total knee replacement: clinical, radiographic, statistical, and survivorship analyses of 346 cases performed by 16 surgeons. Food and Drug Administration Panel Presentation. Gaithersburg, Md. November 22, 1991.
16. Buechel FF. A sequential three-step lateral release for correcting fixed valgus knee deformities during total knee arthroplasty. *Clin Orthop*. 1990; 260:170–175.
17. Keblish PA. The lateral approach to the valgus knee surgical technique and analysis of 53 cases with over two-year follow-up evaluation. *Clin Orthop*. 1991; 271:52–62.
18. Garvin KL, Scuderi G, Insall JN. Evolution of the quadriceps snip. *Clin Orthop*. 1995; 321:131–137.
19. Keblish PA, Pappas MJ. Rationale and selection of prosthetic types in mobile bearing total knee arthroplasty (scientific exhibit). Presented at the 59th Annual American Academy of Orthopaedic Surgeons. Washington, DC, February 20–25, 1992.
20. Install, JN. Surgical approaches to the knee. In: Insall JN, ed. *Surgery of the Knee*. New York: Churchilll Livingstone; 1984; 4–54.
21. Ritter M, Keating M, Faris P. Closed wound drainage in total hip or total knee replacement. A prospective randomized study. *J Bone Joint Surg Am*. 1994; 35–38.
22. Buechel FF, Pappas MJ, Greenwald AS. Use of survivorship and contact stress analyses to predict the long term efficacy of new generation joint replacement designs: a model for FDA device evaluation. *Orthop Rev*. 1991; 20:50–55.
23. Carr AJ, Keyes G, Miller RK. Medial unicompartmental arthroplasty: a survival study of the Oxford Meniscal Knee. Presented at the Ninth Combined Meeting of the Orthopaedic Association of the English-Speaking World (poster exhibit). Toronto. June 21–26, 1992.
24. Goodfellow J, O'Conner J. Clinical results of the Oxford Knee surface arthroplasty of the tibio-femoral joint with a meniscal bearing prosthesis. *Clin Orthop*. 1986; 205: 21–42.
25. Bert JM. Dislocation/subluxation of meniscal bearing elements after New Jersey low-contact stress total knee arthroplasty. *Clin Orthop*. 1990; 254:211–215.
26. Buechel FF. Dislocation/subluxation of the LCS knee replacement (letter). *Clin Orthop*. 1991; 264:309.
27. Weaver JK, Derkash RS, Greenwald AS. Difficulties with bearing dislocation and breakage using a movable bearing total knee replacement system. *Clin Orthop*. 1993; 290:244–252.
28. Buechel FF. New Jersey LCS API surgical procedure. Warsaw, Ind. 1989, DePuy Division of Boehringer Mannhelm Corp.

CHAPTER 11
Meniscal-Bearing Knee—Principles, Technique, and Preliminary Results

Paolo Aglietti, John N. Insall, Roberto Buzzi, and Peter Walker

INTRODUCTION

Many mobile-bearing knees have been used since the late seventies. The most widely known include the Oxford (Biomet, USA), the LCS (De Puy), the Rotaglide (Corin), the T.A.C.K. (Link), and the S.A.L. (Protek). The concept of a meniscal-bearing knee appears attractive because it mimics the normal anatomy. With an adequate prosthetic design, the developers of these prostheses intend to achieve better joint kinematics and reduced polyethylene wear. Good mid- to long-term results have been published with the Oxford[1] and LCS knee.[2] The results obtained with these implants therefore represent the base line of comparison for other mobile-bearing knees being introduced.

In 1992 a new design was developed and called the MBK prosthesis (meniscal-bearing knee, Zimmer, Warsaw, Ind, USA). The concept underlying the design of this prosthesis is to have complete congruency between the femoral component and the polyethylene insert at all degrees of flexion while allowing rotation between polyethylene and the tibial tray. The prosthesis was first implanted in October 1993. This chapter includes a description of the principles, technique, and preliminary results that were obtained with this implant.

PRINCIPLES

Rotation around the tibial axis occurs at the knee during most activities including walking. It has been calculated in walking volunteers[3] that 5 degrees of internal tibial rotation take place during the stance phase and 10° of external rotation occur during the swing phase. It is an accepted principle that some freedom of rotation in the knee is required in everyday activities and certainly in sports. Rotation is decreased by weight bearing and at least 10 to 12 degrees of rotational freedom are required by modern total knee designs.[4]

During physiologic motion of the knee femoral rollback occurs in flexion. This is more evident in the lateral compartment.[5,6] This fact causes a simultaneous internal tibial rotation in flexion, which occurs around a center located in the medial compartment. At the same time a few millimeters of anteroposterior motion take place, again more pronounced laterally. The interpretation of these events is not universally accepted. Some authors believe that the rollback phenomenon is mostly apparent and due to the shape of the femur. According to them a good kinematics can be reestablished simply by placing the axis of flexion permanently in a posterior position rather than by imposing a femoral rollback with the posterior cruciate ligament (PCL).[7]

Classic femoral anatomy describes a decreasing radius for the posterior condyles,[8] but recent studies[9,10] have shown a constant posterior condylar radius in the order of magnitude of 21 to 23 mm for the medial femoral condyle.

Wear is a long-term problem that may become apparent only years after implantation. It involves three mechanisms, adhesive and abrasive wear (superficial wear), and fatigue (delamination or deep wear). The latter modality is predominant in knee prostheses, whereas the first two predominate in hip replacements. Wear is also a multifactorial problem. Some factors are under industry control, whereas others are under surgeon control. The manufacturers control the quality of the polyethylene, including fusion defects, molecular weight, and the sterilization method. Oxidative degradation, the formation of cross-linking, and in general the stiffness of polyethylene influence wear resistance. The surgeon chooses the thickness of the polyethylene and above all the prosthetic design. The most important design factors in this respect are the conformity of the prosthetic surfaces and the contact stresses that are generated in the bearing area. Polyethylene wear in knee prostheses is related to the sliding motion between femur and polyethylene and to high contact stresses.[11] Contact stresses increase significantly when the ratio between the radii of the prosthetic surfaces becomes larger.[12] An increasing potential for polyethylene damage occurs with increasing contact stresses. Ten MPa or even better 5 MPa is considered the safe limit. For a load of 4000 N, equivalent to 5 times body weight, a contact surface of at least 400 sqmm is required to stay within the 10 MPa limit.

Wear, bearing surfaces, and PCL function are interrelated. A flat design with low conformity requires an intact PCL for stability. This increases the risks of wear[13] due to a sliding mechanism if the PCL is lax or due to increased compression forces if the PCL is too tight. Experience with PCL-preserving knees has shown that tension in the PCL is frequently abnormal, either excessive or insufficient. PCL strain was measured at surgery before and after implantation of a total knee prosthesis.[14] Out of 10 knees the PCL was found lax in 6, tight in 3, and with normal tension in only 1.

Proprioception as measured by threshold of motion or reproduction of position was found no different for PCL-saving or PCL-substituting designs.[15,16] PCL receptors were studied in osteoarthritic knees and in a control group with a gold chloride staining and an isomorphometric computerized method in 40 to 80 transverse sections.[17] The neural component area was found significantly larger in normal knees, confirming the finding of others.[18]

Gait analysis studies[19] showed the same flexion up and down the stairs with the PCL-preserving and the PCL-substituting types, contradicting the findings of previous studies.[20] Fluoroscopic analysis of PCL-retaining knee arthroplasties with a flat tibial component[21] showed abnormal kinematics with erratic or even paradoxical motion of the femorotibial contact point. The femorotibial contact point was noted to be posterior with the knee near full extension, possibly due to the flat tibial design and to the absence of the anterior cruciate ligament (ACL). An in vivo determination of condylar liftoff using an inverse perspective technique with fluoroscopy[22] showed lateral liftoff again possibly due to the absence of the ACL.

For the reasons mentioned earlier PCL preservation with a flat tibial component design without a functioning ACL does not restore a normal kinematics and increases the risks of wear. The risk of wear is particularly increased with a flat tibial design in which there is a higher potential for lateral translocation, instability, and edge loading if the prosthesis is malaligned.

We believe that in order to use a more conforming curved design, which decreases contact stresses and wear, a reasonable solution is PCL recession or release to adjust its tension. PCL release can be performed in various degrees. Removal of the tibial spine and the posterior condylar osteophytes already allows for some release. A more formal release can be performed by selectively cutting the anterior fibers off the femur or subperiosteally elevating the tibial insertion.

PROSTHETIC DESIGN

The MBK prosthesis has complete femorotibial conformity throughout motion owing to the fixed radius of the posterior femoral condyles (Fig. 11.1). The radius ratio is 1 to 1 in both the sagittal and frontal planes. Axial rotation takes place between the tibial tray and the polyethylene insert, around a medial center of rotation for a total of about 25 degrees. Some anteroposterior motion (3–4 mm) is also possible between the polyethylene insert and tibial tray. The PCL is preserved but may be released.

The femoral component has separate femoropatellar and femorotibial surfaces. The femorotibial surfaces (the posterior femoral condyles) are separated from the patellar flange by two condylo-trochlear grooves (Fig. 11.2). The femoral condyles have a constant radius of curvature. Its magnitude changes with the prosthetic size (Fig. 11.3). The patellar sulcus is deep and pro-

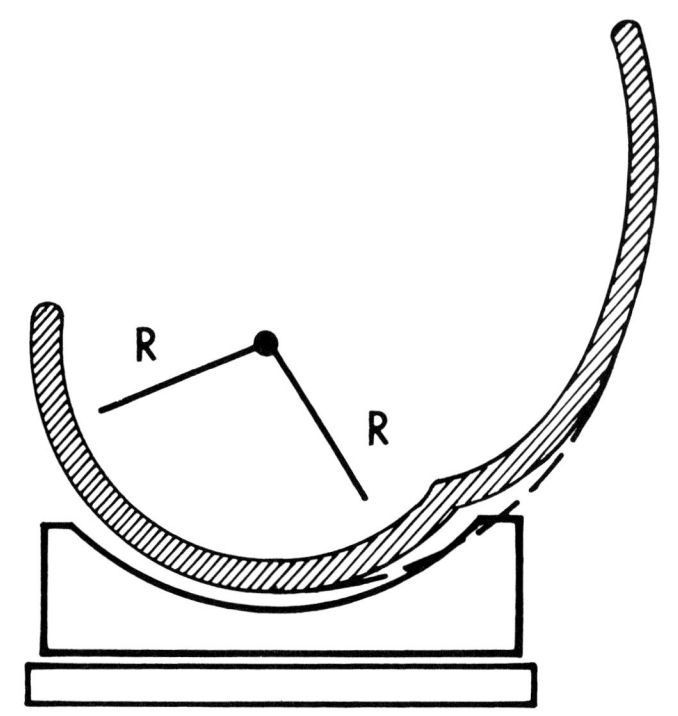

Figure 11.1. Schematic drawing of the prosthetic design in the sagittal plane. The radius of the posterior condyles (R) is constant and complete femorotibial congruity is present in the whole arc of flexion. The dotted line represents the outline of the patellar sulcus.

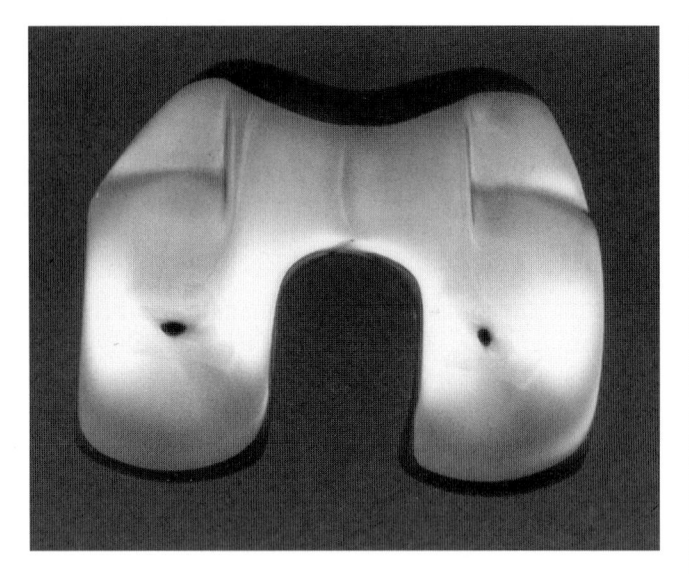

Figure 11.2. Left MBK femoral component as seen from the distal aspect. The femoral condyles are separated from the patellar flange by two condylo-trochlear grooves. The patellar groove extends distally and merges with the central aspect of the condyles.

longed distally. It is slightly displaced laterally to improve patellar tracking (Fig. 11.4). There are right and left femoral components. The profile of the patellar component is in between the "dome" and the "sombrero" designs in order to maintain a linear contact area in the arc of motion.

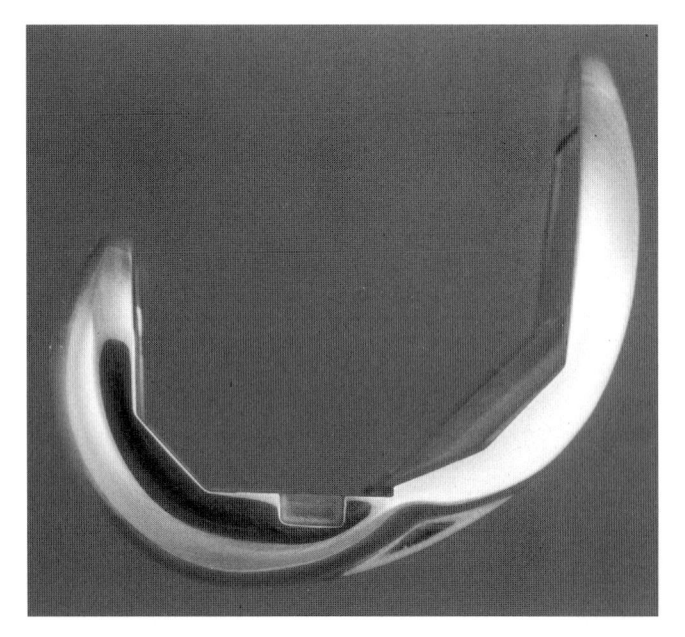

Figure 11.3. The MBK femoral component as visualized from the side. The constant radius of the posterior femoral condyles is evident, together with the condylo-trochlear groove and the profile of the patellofemoral surface.

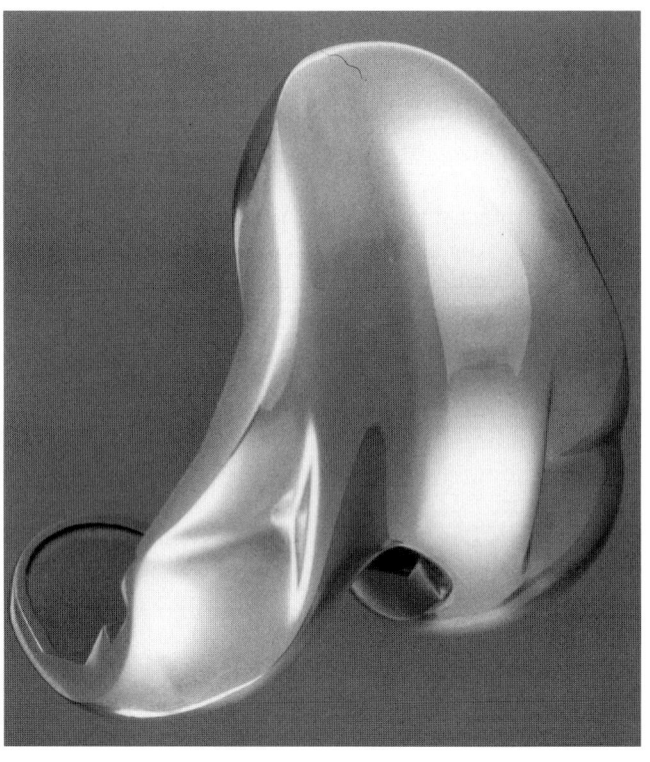

Figure 11.4. Anterior aspect of the MBK femoral component. The patella sulcus is deep and prolonged distally to merge with the condyles.

The tibial component has a metal tray and a single mobile polyethylene insert. The guiding mechanism is in the form of a mushroom placed on the tibial tray, which fits into a slot of the undersurface of the polyethylene. The polyethylene insert can be loaded from the top to enhance insertion or change of the insert at surgery. The tibial tray has an anterior stop to prevent anterior subluxation of the plastic insert (Fig. 11.5). The polyethylene insert can rotate externally by 8 degrees and internally by 17 degrees. The upper surface of the polyethylene insert has two cupped surfaces for articulation with the femoral condyles and a prominent intercondylar "saddle" eminence to prevent translocation (Fig. 11.6). The prosthetic design allows 12 degrees of hyperextension. This is necessary because the tibial component is implanted with 5 to 7 degrees of posterior tilt and the femoral component with 3 degrees of flexion.

Contact areas of various prostheses have been evaluated using either Fuji films or computer-assisted methods[23,24] (Blamey J, personal comunication, Swindon, UK, 1995). It has been found that the average fixed-bearing prosthesis has only about 100 sqmm, per condyle, the LCS has approximately 200 sqmm, the Rotaglide 400 sqmm, the Oxford almost 600 sqmm, and the MBK 535 sqmm (size E). Therefore for the MBK pros-

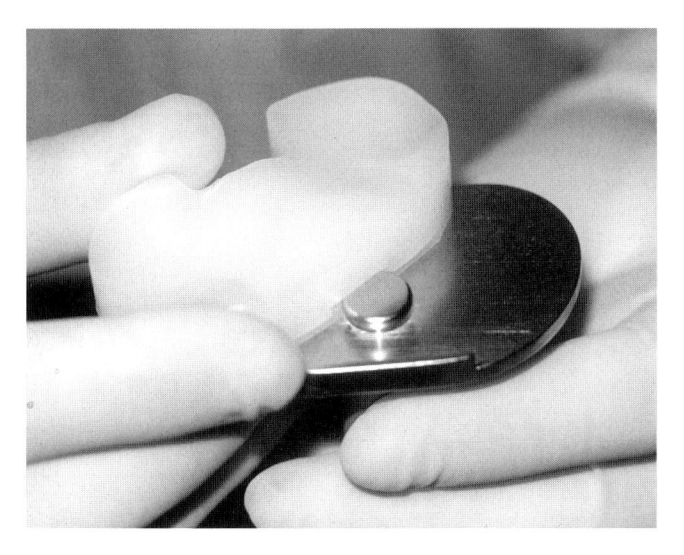

Figure 11.5. The MBK tibial tray and polyethylene insert. The tibial tray has a guiding mechanism formed by a mushroom that fits into a slot of the undersurface of the polyethylene insert. An anterior stop is present in the front of the tibial tray. The polyethylene insert rotates around a medial center of rotation.

thesis at a given load of 4000 N if contact occurs symmetrically in both condyles contact stresses should be 3.6 MPa. If contact occurs in only one condyle, contact stresses should be no more than 7.0 MPa. Experimental studies in a knee simulator (Walker, personal comunication, 1995) have shown only little scratches in the upper and lower surface of the plastic up to 10 million cycles equivalent to 10 years of life. In vivo fluoroscopic studies (Barrett D, personal comunication, 1996) have shown meniscal motion with a near normal kinematic pattern.

SURGICAL TECHNIQUE

The surgical approach involves a straight longitudinal skin incision with anteromedial arthrotomy and lateral eversion of the patella. Adequate medial and lateral releases are performed for correction of angular deformities. The operation includes the following steps: distal femoral cut, anterior and posterior femoral cuts with adjustment of rotational alignment, tibial cut, insertion of the trial components, possible PCL release, and finally patellar resurfacing.

The distal femoral cut is performed using an intramedullary aligned instrument with an extramedullary check. The distal 8 to 10 mm of bone are removed from the normal condyle, and an alignment of 6 degrees of valgus in relationship to the anatomical axis is obtained. The distal femoral cut has 3 degrees of flexion in relationship to the distal femoral axis. This is useful to avoid notching of the anterior cortex of the femur, particularly in the cases in which the anteroposterior dimensions of the femur are in-between sizes and the lower size is implanted.

The preparation of the distal femur continues with exposure of the epicondyles, which are useful landmarks for adjusting the rotational position of the femoral component.[25] We try to achieve a few[3] degrees of external rotation in relationship to the posterior condylar line. There are varius methods of achieving a good rotatory position. The traditional method involves referencing from the posterior condylar line. Using this method there are difficulties in knees with posterior condylar erosion or dysplasia. In valgus deformities erosion of the posterior aspect of the lateral condyle may lead to a relative internal rotation of the femoral component. Erosion of the posterior aspect of the medial condyle may lead to an excessive external rotation of the femoral component. The second method of adjusting femoral component rotation involves creating the tibial cut first, tensing the ligaments in flexion and resecting the posterior condyles parallel to the tibial cut (parallel flexion gap method). Laminar spreaders or other specialized devices may be used to tense the ligaments in flexion. The third method requires the drawing of the trochlear anteroposterior line (Whiteside's line). This has been found particularly useful in the valgus knee. Finally the method we prefer requires identification of the epicondyles.[26] It has been found that by referencing off the epicondylar line we obtain an automatic external rotation of a few degrees (average 3.6 degrees, range 1 to 7 degrees) in relationship to the posterior condyles. The degree of external rotation varies according to the deformity and averages 3 degrees in the varus knee and 4.5 degrees in the valgus. This method has the advantage that the

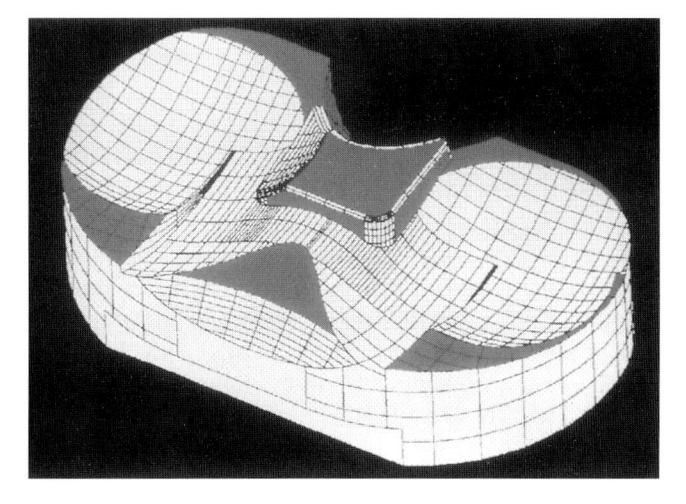

Figure 11.6. The design of the tibial polyethylene insert with the two articulating surfaces separated by a raised intercondylar eminence to prevent instability and translocation (courtesy of Zimmer Inc.).

epicondyles represent the collateral ligament insertion and the axis of flexion. The epicondylar line is always perpendicular to the tibial axis at all degrees of flexion.[27]

The epycondyles are exposed at surgery by reflecting the synovium and dividing the lateral patellofemoral ligament. The lateral epicondyle is more easely identified because it is well pointed. On the medial side there are more difficulties because the epicondyle is larger and fan-shaped. The epicondylar line is drawn on the resected distal femur using methylene blue and a slotted instrument is aligned along the line itself. A saw is used to produce a slot perpendicular to the epicondylar line in the center of the resected surface of the distal femur. This does not damage the PCL. The anteroposterior cutting block of the appropriate size is engaged into the slot. The cutting block is displaced in an anteroposterior direction using the anterior femoral cortex and the posterior condyles as a reference. Probes are fitted on the block to aid in this purpose. The anterior probe should touch the anterior femoral cortex on its lateral and more prominent aspect. The posterior probe should indicate an average resection of 10 mm from the posterior condyles. Because a few degrees of external femoral rotation are desired, resection of the posterior condyles is usually more than 10 mm medially and less than 10 mm laterally.

The proximal tibial cut is accomplished using an extramedullary guide. This guide references off the malleoli distally. The alignment of the cut is perpendicular to the tibial axis in the frontal plane and with a 5- to 7-degree posterior slope, according to individual variations. We try to remove 8 to 10 mm of bone from the normal tibial plateau. At this point flexion and extension gaps have been established and they are sized with spacers. At the same time mediolateral stability and overall limb alignment are evaluated.

The PCL is protected while performing femoral and tibial bone cuts. In particular during the proximal tibial cut an osteotome may be inserted in front of the posterior spine to protect the PCL insertion. Alternatively, the surgeon may choose to cut across the proximal tibia and therefore automatically obtain at this stage a partial release of the PCL. After insertion of the trial components (Fig. 11.7) the knee is taken through range of motion while assessing the tension in the PCL. Tension in the PCL is seldom correct, more frequently with the MBK it is excessive, causing limitation of flexion, excessive rollback, and/or an anterior liftoff of the plastic insert. The liftoff is more evident if the patella is everted, and therefore it should be assessed with the patella dislocated. In the case of excessive tension, the PCL is released. This can be done off the femur, by selectively cutting the anterior fibers, or from the tibia, by releasing the insertion either with the knife or with a periosteal elevator. We prefer the release from the tibial side because it leaves the PCL attached to the posterior capsule so that it may later heal to the back of the tibia.

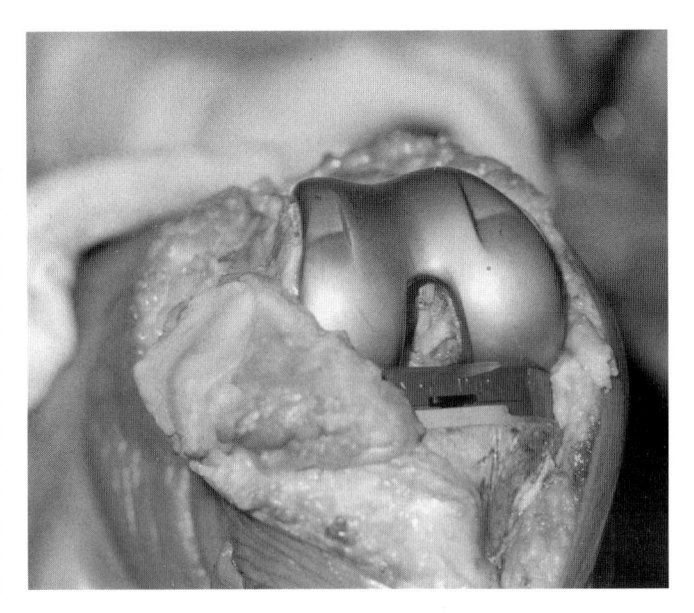

Figure 11.7. The trial components of the MBK prosthesis at surgery.

PRELIMINARY RESULTS

Two series of cases have been operated with implantation of the MBK prosthesis. The first series includes 23 patients operated from 1993 to 1994. The second series includes 22 cases operated in 1995. The Mark I prosthesis was implanted in the first series while the Mark II prosthesis was implanted in the second. The average age of the 45 patients was 65.4 years (range 56 to 83 years). There were 7 males and 38 females. The diagnosis was osteoarthritis in 42, rheumatoid arthritis in 2, and osteonecrosis in 1 patient. The condition of the PCL at the end of surgery was as follows: in 22 cases (49%) the PCL was intact, in 18 (40%) it was released, and in 5 (11%) it was attenuated. A lateral retinacular release was performed in 14 cases (31%).

We were able to follow 44 patients with at least 1 year of follow-up. One patient had died from unrelated reasons. The knee score according to the Knee Society rating system[28] increased from an average of 40 preoperatively to 89 points at follow-up. There were 28 (64%) excellent results, 10 (23%) good, 5 (11%) fair, and 1 (2%) poor. The Knee Society functional score improved from an average of 55 points preoperatively to 86 points at follow-up. There were 26 (59%) excellent, 12 (27%) good, 5 (11%) fair, and 1 (2%) poor result. The 1 to 10 visual analogue scale for subjective satisfaction revealed that 39 (89%) patients scored 8 or more and no patients were below 5. The 1 to 10 visual analogue scale for pain revealed the same figures. The average postoperative flexion was 110 degrees with a range of 90 to 130 degrees. Extension loss was present in 3 knees postoperatively. It measured 5 degrees in 2 knees and 8 degrees in 1. Walking was unlimited in 29 (66%) patients and over 10 blocks in 10 (23%). Twenty-one (48%) patients could manage stairs normally, 9 (20%) could walk down stairs holding on to the rail, and 13 (30%) could walk up and down stairs with the rail.

Radiographic analysis (Fig. 11.8) of the angle between the mechanical axes of the femur and tibia in long-standing films showed that 34 (77%) cases were within 2 degrees from the neutral, 6 (14%) knees were 3 to 5 degrees of varus, 1 (2%) knee was in 7 degrees of varus, 2 (4.5%) knees were in 3 to 5 degrees of valgus and 1 (2%) knee in 6 degrees of valgus. Tibial radiolucent lines were studied according to the Knee Society evaluation system.[29] Radiolucent lines were present in zone 1 in 18 (41%) cases, in zone 2 in 11 (25%) cases, and in zone 4 in 1 (2%) knee. The thickness of the radiolucency was 1 mm in all the cases except 1 in which it was 2 mm. Patella symptoms were absent in 42 (95%) cases. In 2 (4.5%) knees there was a moderate patellofemoral crepitation.

According to the Knee Society rating system, there were 5 fair and 1 poor result. The reasons for the 5 fair were as follows: 3 patients complained of knee pain, 1 patient had hip pain, and 1 had objective mediolateral instability. There was 1 poor result, which was due to varus alignment of the limb (7 degrees of varus) in an otherwise asymptomatic knee.

One knee of the Mark I series complained of some instability while approaching extension. The phenomenon was attributable to anterior tibial subluxation because the prosthesis did not allow sufficient hyperextension. It should be pointed out that implantation of the tibial component with 7 degrees of posterior slope and of the femoral component with 3 degrees of flexion already requires a prosthesis that allows 10 degrees of hyperextension. Some more hyperextension is required if the knee goes into recurvatum. This problem was corrected in the Mark II prosthesis by moving anteriorly and proximally the condylo-trochlear groove of the femoral component. A further modification has been recently introduced, the Mark III prosthesis. In this model the height of the intercondylar eminence has been raised to prevent translocation of the components and the patellar groove has been displaced laterally to improve patellar tracking.

COMMENTS

Posterior cruciate ligament substitution has been in our experience a valuable option in the field of total knee replacement. With the Insall-Burstein posterior-stabilized total knee replacement most deformities can be corrected, the mild as well the severe ones. It has proved valuable in the treatment of stiff knees, in knees with severe flexion contractures, patellar dislocation, insufficient PCL, and in most of the revisions. The Insall-Burstein knee replacement has been used for many years with minor design modifications from the original form. Good long-term results have been reported by the originators[30,31] as well as by others.[32,33] Therefore, we feel that a posterior stabilized knee will maintain its place in the field of total knee replacement as a generic knee to be used by most surgeons in most of the cases, with a standard technique and reliable results. However, there is a place for a "high-tech" knee to be used by specialized surgeons in younger patients with increased demands. This implant should allow improved performance with reduced polyethylene wear. The results are initial but promising and require a longer-term evaluation. The MBK appears based on sound principles and offers the advantages of full conformity throughout flexion and the possibility of keeping the PCL and releasing it.

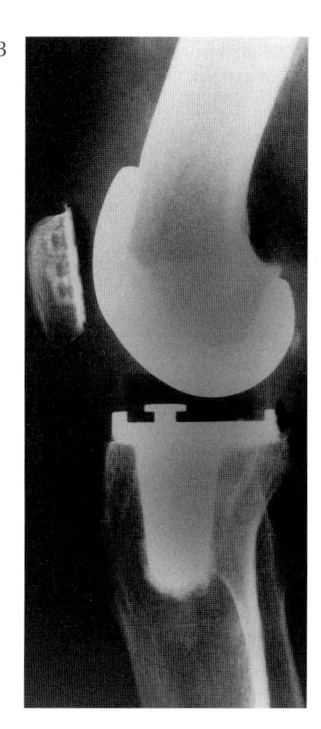

Figure 11.8. (A) Anteroposterior and (B) lateral radiographs of the MBK prosthesis. In the lateral radiograph the guiding mechanism of the polyethylene insert, in the form of a mushroom, is visualized.

References

1. Goodfellow JW, O'Connor J. Clinical results of the Oxford knee. *Clin Orthop*. 1986; 205:21–42.
2. Buechel FF, Pappas MJ. Long-term survivorship analysis

of cruciate-sparing versus cruciate-sacrificing knee prostheses using meniscal bearings. *Clin Orthop*. 1990; 260:162–169.
3. Lafortune MA, Cavanagh PR, Sommer MS, Kalenak A. Three dimensional kinematics of the human knee during walking. *J Biomech*. 1992; 25(4):347–357.
4. Nahass BE, Madson MM, Walker PS. Motion of the knee after total condylar resurfacing. An in vivo study. *J Biomech*. 1991; 24(12):1107–1117.
5. Barnes CL, Sledge CB. Total knee arthroplasty with posterior cruciate ligament retention designs. In: Insall JN, ed. *Surgery of the Knee*. New York: Churchill-Livingstone; 1993: 815–827.
6. Thompson WO, Thaete FL, Fu FH, Dye SF. Tibial meniscal dynamics using three-dimensional reconstruction of magnetic resonance images. *Am J Sports Med*, 1991; 19(3):210–216.
7. Freeman MAR, Railton GT. Should the posterior cruciate ligament be retained or resected in condylar nonmeniscal knee arthroplasty? *J Arthroplasty*. 1988; (suppl):3–12.
8. Kapandj IA. Profilo dei condili e delle glenoidi. In: Kapandji IA, ed. *Fisiologia articolare*. Roma: Editrice Demi; 1974; II:88–89.
9. Elias SG, Freeman MAR, Gokcay EI. A correlative study of the geometry and anatomy of the distal femur. *Clin Orthop*. 1990; 260:98–103.
10. Hollister AM, Jatana S, Singh AK, Sullivan WW, Lupichuck H. The axes of rotation of the knee. *Clin Orthop*. 1993; 290:259–268.
11. Walker PS. Design of total knee arthroplasty. In: Insall JN, ed. *Surgery of the Knee*, 2nd ed. New York: Churchill-Livingstone; 1993:723–738.
12. Andriacchi TP, Natarajan RN. Conformity and polyethylene damage in total knee replacement. Zimmer, technical paper, 1996.
13. Engh GA, Dwyer KA, Hanes CK. Polyethylene wear of metal backed tibial components in total and unicompartmental knee prostheses. *J Bone Joint Surg*. 1992; 74B:9–17.
14. Lotke PA, Corces A, Williams JL, Hirsch HS. Strain characteristics of the posterior cruciate ligament after total knee arthroplasty. *Am J Knee Surg*. 1993; 6(3):104–107.
15. Cash RM, Gonzales M, Garst J, Barmada R. Proprioception thresholds in PCL retaining versus substituting total knee arthroplasty. Presented at the scientific meeting of the Knee Society, Atlanta, February 1996.
16. Barrack RL, Simmons S, Lephart S, Rubash H, Pifer GW. Proprioception following unicondylar versus total knee arthroplasty. Presented at the scientific meeting of the Knee Society, Atlanta, February 1996.
17. Franchi A, Zaccherotti G, Aglietti P. Neural system of the human posterior cruciate ligament in osteoarthritis. *J Arthroplasty*. 1995; 10(5):679–682.
18. Alexiades M, Scuderi G, Vigorita V, Scott N. A histologic study of the posterior cruciate ligament in the arthritic knee. *Am J Knee Surg*. 1989; 2:153–157.
19. Wilson J, Insall JN. Functional gait analysis of the Insall-Burstein posterior stabilized knee prosthesis. Presented at the AAOS, Atlanta, 1992.
20. Andriacchi TP, Galante JO, Fermier RW. The influence of total knee replacement design on walking and stair climbing. *J Bone Joint Surg Am*. 1982; 64:1328–1335.
21. Sthiel JB, Komistek RD, Dennis DA, Paxon RD. Fluoroscopic analysis of kinematiks after posterior cruciate retaining knee arthroplasty. *J Bone Joint Surg*. 1995; 77B:884–889.
22. Dennis DA, Komistek RD, Hoff W, Gabriel SM. In vivo knee kinematik derived using an inverse perspective technique. Presented at the scientific meeting of the Knee Society, Atlanta, February 1996.
23. Greenwald SA, Heim CS, Postak PD, Plaxton N. Factors influencing the longevity of UHMWPE tibial components. Scientific exhibit, AAOS, Atlanta, February 1996.
24. Polyzoides JA. The rotaglide knee. Presented at the interim meeting of the Knee Society, Boston, September 1995.
25. Berger R, Rubash H, Seel M, Thompson W, Crossett L. Determining the rotational alignment of the femoral component in total knee arthroplasty using the epicondylar axis. *Clin Orthop*. 1993; 286:40–47.
26. Poilvache P, Insall JN, Scuderi GR, Font-Rodriguez DE. Rotational landmarks and sizing of the distal femur in total knee arthroplasty. Presented at the scientific meeting of the Knee Society, Atlanta, February 1996.
27. Yoshioka Y, Siu D. The anatomy and functional axes of the femur. *J Bone Joint Surg Am*. 1987; 69:873–888.
28. Insall JN, Dorr LD, Scott RD, Scott NW. Rationale of the Knee Society rating system. *Clin Orthop*. 1989; 248:13–14.
29. Ewald FC. The Knee Society total knee arthroplasty roentgenographic evaluation and scoring system. *Clin Orthop*. 1989; 248:9–12.
30. Stern SH, Insall JN. Posterior stabilized prosthesis. Results after follow-up of nine to twelve years. *J Bone Joint Surg Am*. 1992; 74A:980–986.
31. Colizza WA, Insall JN, Scuderi GR. The posterior stabilized total knee prosthesis. Assessment of polyethylene damage and osteolysis after a ten-year minimum follow-up. *J Bone Joint Surg Am*. 1995; 77A:1713–1720.
32. Aglietti P, Buzzi R, Segoni F, Zaccherotti G. Insall-Burstein posterior-stabilized knee prosthesis in rheumatoid arthritis. *J Arthroplasty* 1995; 10(2):217–225.
33. Aglietti P, Buzzi R, De Felice R. The Insall-Burstein total knee replacement in osteoarthritis. A ten year minimum follow-up. *J Arthroplasty*. Submitted for publication, 1996.

CHAPTER 12
Constrained Total Knee Designs for Revision Arthroplasty

James Rand and William Martin

INTRODUCTION

Revisions of total knee arthroplasty (TKA) in patients with extensive bone loss or ligamentous instability have frequently been performed using constrained prostheses.[7–9,13–17,20] Early hinge designs did not reproduce normal knee kinematics. Early hinge prostheses had a high frequency of aseptic loosening and patellar instability.[2,5–7] When early hinge designs were utilized for revision, the results were satisfactory in only 48% of the cases.[5] When utilized for revisions, survival probabilities among newer implants are better for the less-constrained prostheses (such as the anametric, total condylar, cruciate condylar, and kinematic condylar) than for the more-constrained prostheses (total condylar II, total condylar III, kinematic stabilizer, and kinematic rotating hinge prosthesis).[5]

Since early fixed hinges, progress has been made in both prosthesis design and in surgical technique. Several studies have reported varying degrees of success with the use of constrained prosthesis for revision.[4,6–8,10,11,13,15–17,20] The results of revision TKA using constrained devices depend upon a number of different factors and include the reasons for failure, the number of previous implants, the extent of bone loss, and the quality of the soft tissues. The aim of this chapter is to discuss the design, indications, results, and complications of constrained total knee prostheses for revision.

IMPLANT DESIGNS

There are six possible degrees of freedom at the knee, three rotational and three linear. The less inherently stable the knee being treated, the more degrees of freedom need to be controlled by the prosthesis. Levens identified a transverse rotation of at least 8 degrees that occurred during gait.[1,18]

Early total knee implant designs used single axis hinges that did not allow for the normal rotational motion of the knee. In addition, single axis hinges do not allow for the changing instant center of rotation of the normal knee. The failure of the early hinge prostheses to mimic normal knee kinematics placed increased loads on the bone-cement interface leading to a high incidence of loosening. Abnormal motion, impingement on flexion, and distraction of the femur were identified on motion studies of hinge prostheses in vivo. The abnormal forces and high frictional forces contributed to wear of the bearing surfaces with metal fracture and creation of wear debris.[18]

The problems with the early hinge designs led to a new generation of constrained prostheses in an attempt to improve the results over the single axis early hinge designs. The total condylar III prosthesis provides a deepened femoral intercondylar recess into which an elongated polyethylene peg articulates—providing varus-valgus and anteroposterior stability (Figs. 12.1A–D). Extended femoral and tibial stems transfer the loads away from the condylar bone prosthesis interface.

Newer hinge prostheses allow flexion-extension, distraction, and some degrees of rotation. The kinematic rotating hinge prosthesis (Howmedica, Rutherford, NJ) is a constrained hinge that allows axial rotation and distraction between the inner tibial bearing and the outer sleeve[7] (Figs. 12.2A–D). The Noiles knee prosthesis was introduced in the late 1970s as a modified constrained hinged prosthesis. The Noiles has an uncemented tibial stem, set within a cemented sleeve, and reported to allow a 20-degree arc of both medial and lateral rotation in flexion as well as reduced tensile loading[3,6] (Figs. 12.3A–B).

In the revision knee arthroplasty the quality of bone is often inferior and deficient. Because of the poor bone stock, the tibial and femoral surfaces are inadequate be-

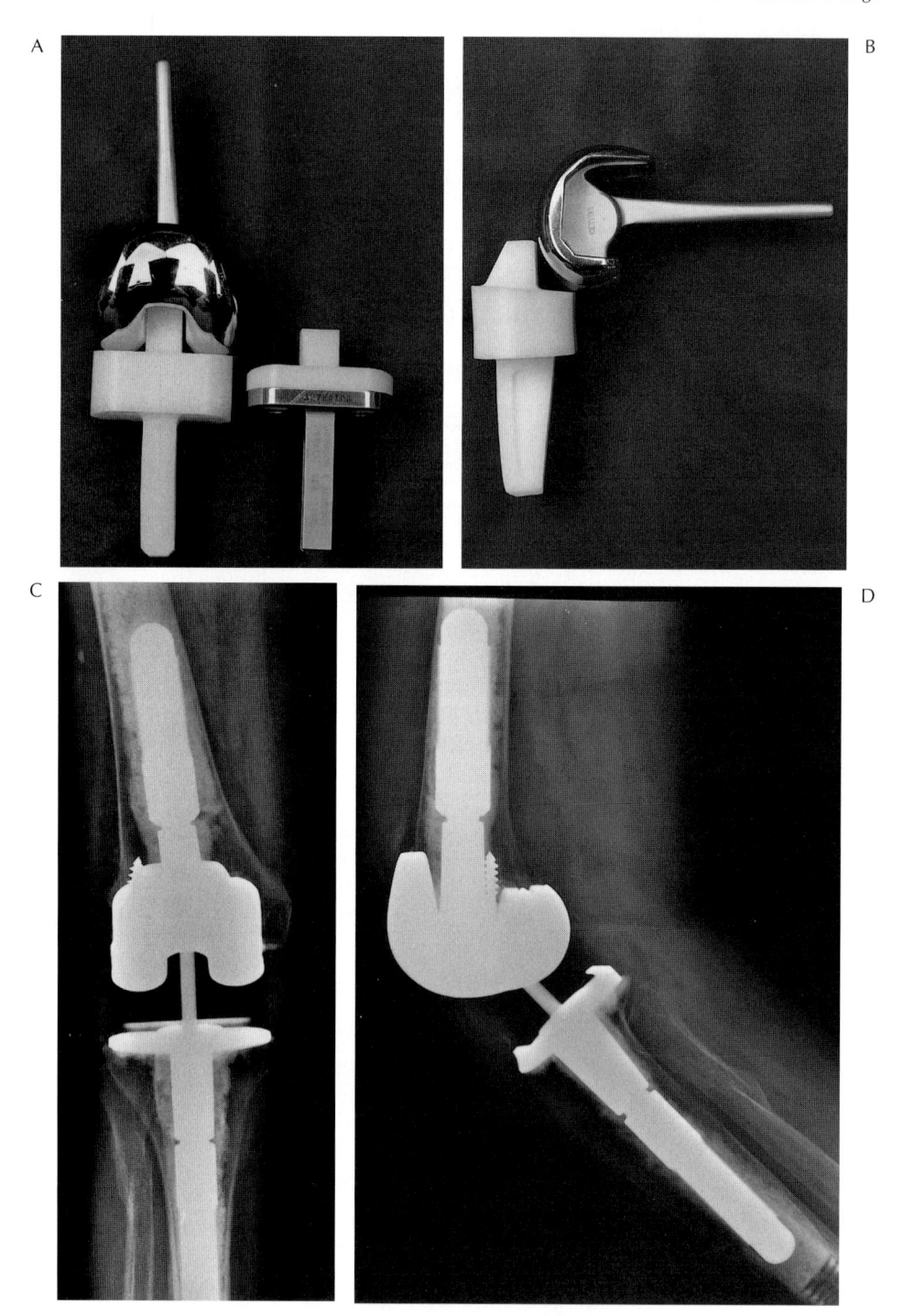

Figure 12.1. (A) Anteroposterior and (B) lateral photograph and (C) anteroposterior and (D) lateral radiograph of total condylar III prosthesis.

cause the main load-bearing surfaces for implant fixation and the loads must be transferred to the intramedullary area of the tibia and femur via stems. Custom implants have been utilized to assist in situations in which there is marked bone loss and/or instability.[12] Custom implants are limited by their cost, inflexibility for unanticipated anatomy at the time of surgery, and by the length of time that it takes to manufacture the implant. Custom implants have been largely replaced by modular designs. Modular total knee systems allow for varying length of stems. In addition, modular implants allow for distal and/or posterior femoral wedge augmentation for asymmetric bone loss. Augmentation blocks or wedges may also be added to the undersurface of the tibia for similar reasons (Figs. 12.4A–C).

The type of intra-articular constraint desired may also be varied with modular total knee systems depending upon the clinical setting. A posterior-stabilized or

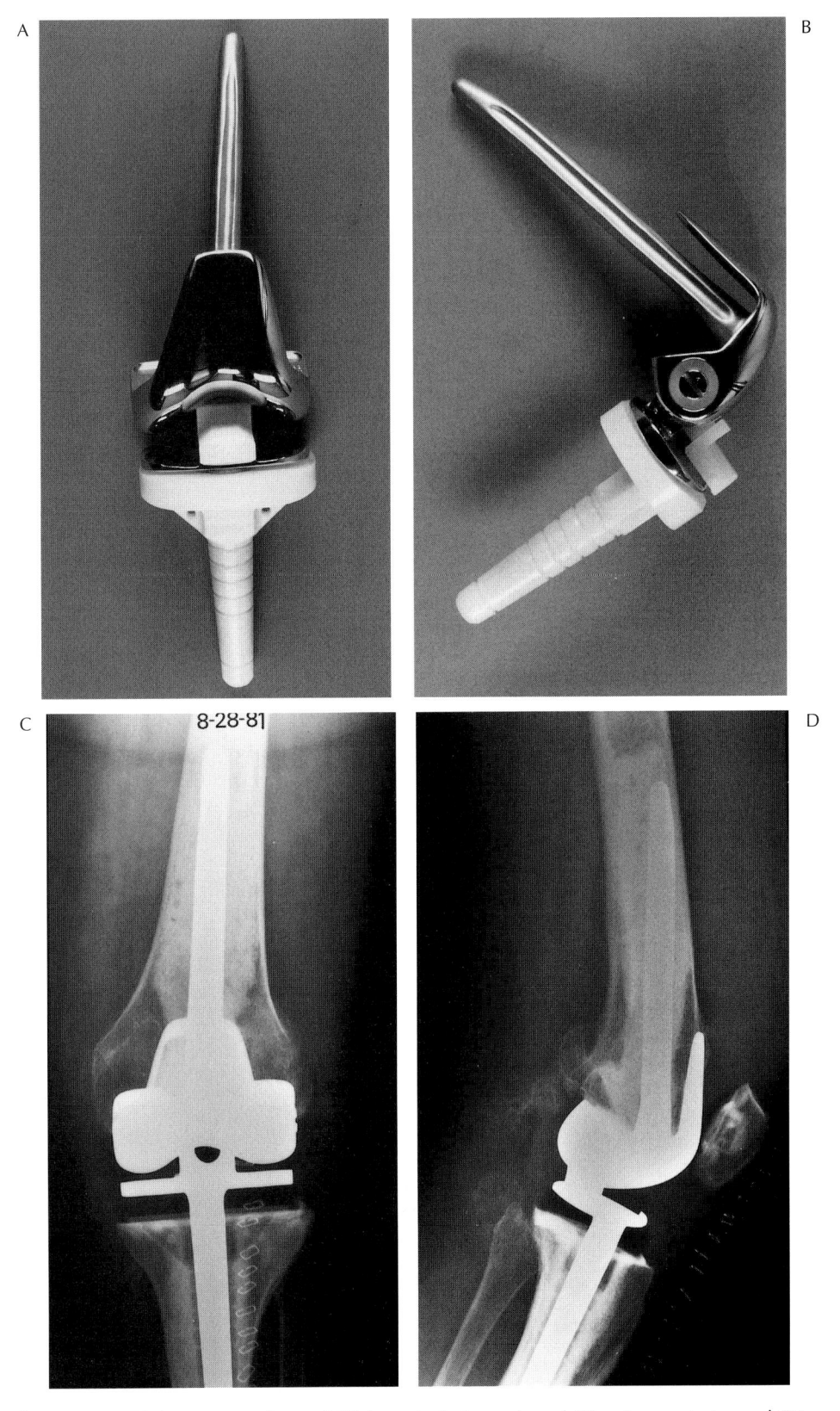

12. Constrained Total Knee Designs for Revision Arthroplasty

Figure 12.2. (A) Anteroposterior and (B) lateral photograph and (C) anteroposterior and (D) lateral radiograph of kinematic rotating hinge prosthesis.

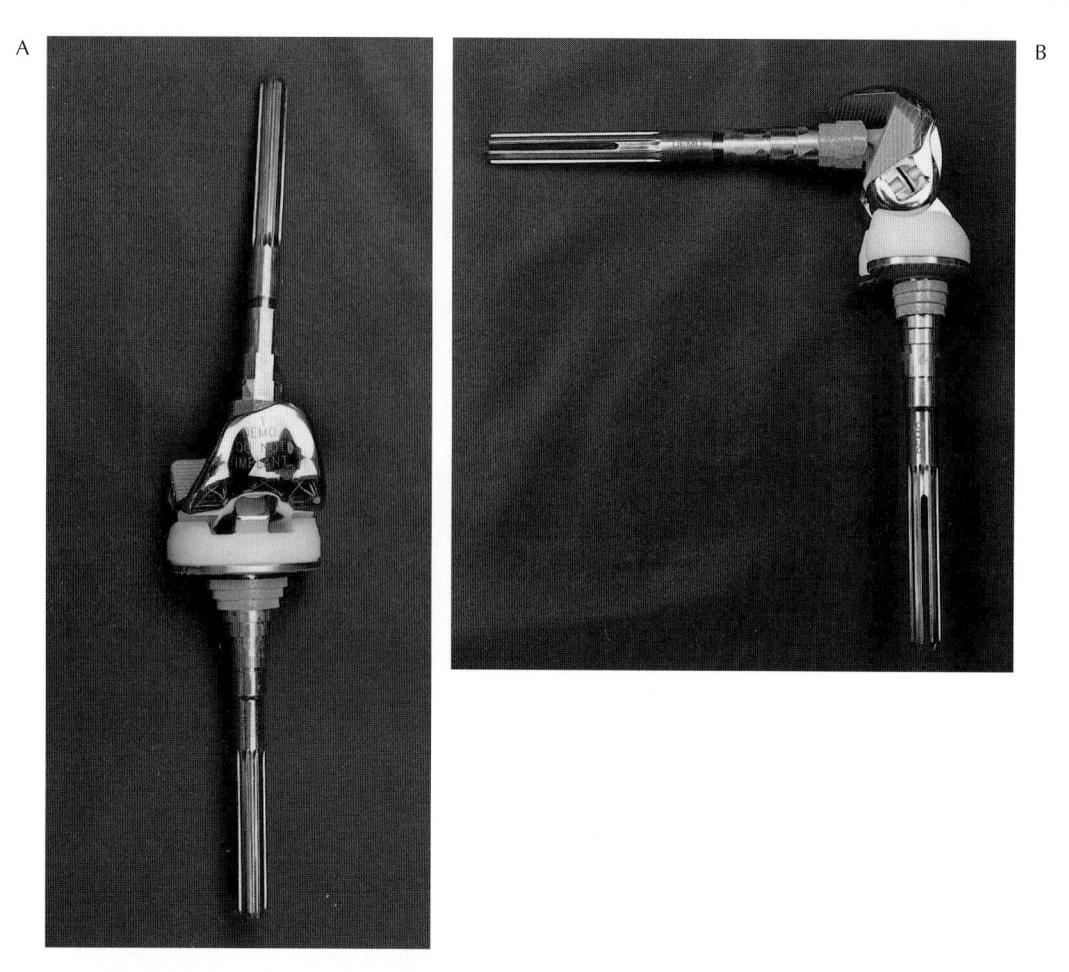

Figure 12.3. (A) Anteroposterior and (B) lateral photograph of Noiles rotating hinge prosthesis.

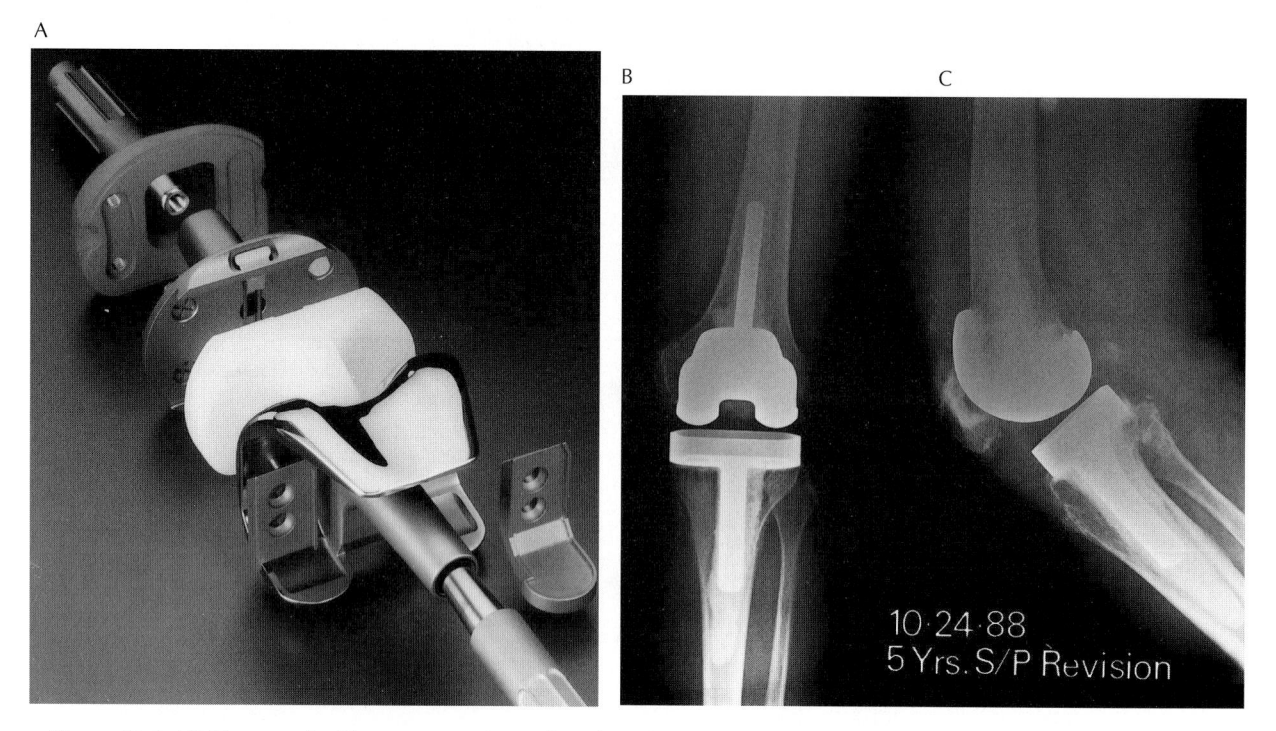

Figure 12.4. (A) Photograph, (B) anteroposterior and (C) lateral radiograph of constrained condylar total knee prosthesis.

12. Constrained Total Knee Designs for Revision Arthroplasty

Figure 12.5. (A) Anteroposterior radiograph of nonunion of supracondylar femur fracture in an 85-year-old woman. (B) Anteroposterior and (C) lateral radiographs following custom kinematic rotating hinge total knee. (D) Anteroposterior and (E) lateral radiographs at 5 years following revision.

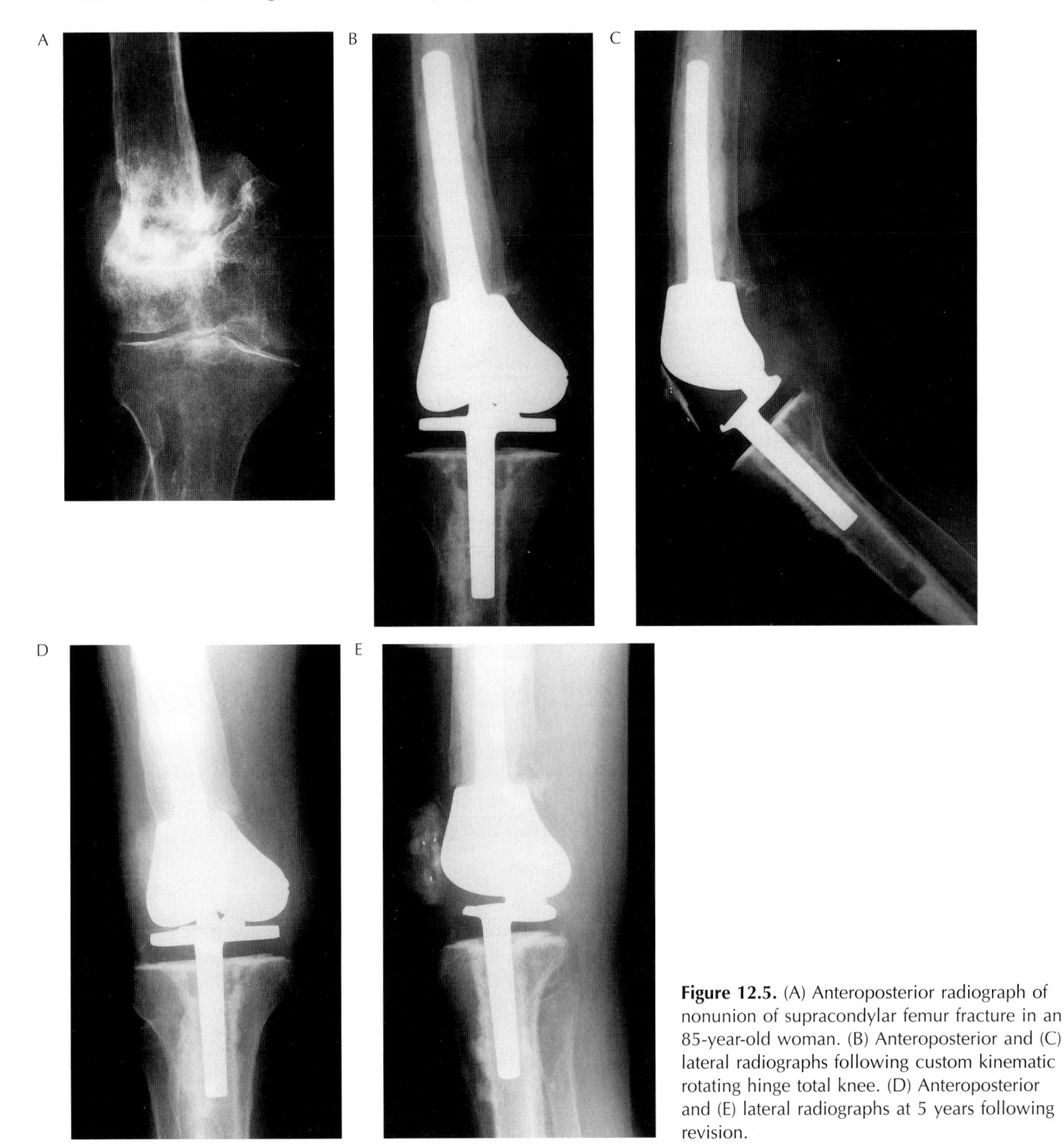

cruciate-retaining tibial polyethylene implant may be used, or, in situations in which instability is greater, a more constrained tibial polyethylene component may be used that provides a thick intercondylar peg similar to the total condylar III design.

INDICATIONS

Constrained total knee prostheses have been selected for a wide variety of reasons. The most common reasons for use of a constrained prosthesis are ligamentous instability,[4,6,7,10,11,13,15–17,20] bone loss,[4,7,11,15] deformity,[6,10,16] revision of a prior failed TKA,[6,10,13,16] septic or aseptic loosening,[11,17,20] or supracondylar femur fracture[15,20] (Figs. 12.5A–E). Additional indications for use of a constrained prosthesis are cases of unstable revision in which a resurfacing arthroplasty will not suffice,[10] anticipated heavy use of the knee,[6] implant malposition,[15] inadvertent transection of the medial collateral ligament during standard total knee arthroplasty,[13] extreme imbalance in the flexion-extension gaps,[20] recurrent dislocation of previous posterior-stabilized constrained knee arthroplasty,[20] and exposure obtained by the so-called "femoral peel."[8,20] The authors limit the use of constrained designs to knees with a deficient collateral ligament, supracondylar femur fracture with extensive bone loss in an elderly patient, or cases with large soft tissue imbalance after appropriate ligament releases.

RESULTS

The results of revision TKA using constrained devices are variable and affected by prosthesis design, surgical technique, and length of follow-up. Most studies have demonstrated inferior results to primary knee replacement procedures. It is important, however, to view these results in light of the evolving technical aspects of revision total knee replacement and the improvements in implants used for these revision procedures.

Hinge Prostheses for Revision

The largest and most recent series for revision TKA using constrained prosthesis, to date, is reported by Lombardi.[20] Using the Hospital for Special Surgery rating system, they studied 113 rotating hinge revision TKAs. The mean follow-up was 6 years. Eighteen knees (16%) were rated excellent, 58 knees (51%) were rated good, 26 knees (23%) were rated fair, and 11 knees (10%) were rated poor.

Rand and associates[7] reported the results of 23 kinematic rotating hinge total knee arthroplasties used for revision at the Mayo Clinic. Using the Hospital for Special Surgery scoring system, at a mean of 50 months, of the revision knees 9 (39%) were rated excellent, 7 (30%) good, 3 (13%) fair, 2 (9%) poor, and 2 were unavailable for follow-up.

Shaw and colleagues[11] reported the results of revision using the kinematic rotating hinge prosthesis using the Brigham and Women's Hospital and Harvard Medical School knee rating system. Mean follow-up was 50 months; 22% had excellent results, 40% had good results, 13% had fair results, and more than 10% had poor results. Shindell and associates reported on 18 Noiles hinged prostheses of which 4 were revisions.[6] All 4 revisions failed at a mean of 31 months. Femoral component subsidence occurred in 17 of 18 knees.

Total Condylar III Prostheses for Revision

Lombardi,[20] using the Hospital for Special Surgery rating system, reported 66 revision TKAs using a posterior-stabilized constrained prosthesis. The posterior-stabilized constrained prosthesis had a mean follow-up of 14 months; 19 knees (30%) were rated excellent, 36 knees (53%) were rated good, 6 knees (9%) were rated fair, and 5 knees (8%) were rated poor.

Donaldson and colleagues[10] studied 31 knees in 25 patients using the total condylar III knee prosthesis. There were 17 primary arthroplasties and 14 revisions with an average follow-up period of 3.8 years. Using the Hospital for Special Surgery knee-rating score for the revision arthroplasties, 2 (14%) were rated as excellent, 5 (36%) were rated as good, 1 (7%) was rated as fair, and 1 (7%) was rated as poor. There were 5 (36%) failures.

Kavolus and associates[13] studied the total condylar III knee prosthesis in elderly patients. Sixteen knee arthroplasties were performed in 14 patients with 11 of the 16 being revisions. Mean follow-up was 4.5 years. In this age group, 15 of 16 implants had a good or excellent Hospital for Special Surgery knee score.

Rand and colleagues[15] reported revision TKA using the total condylar III prosthesis in 21 knees in 19 patients. At 4-year follow-up using the Hospital for Special Surgery knee score, 25% were excellent, 25% were good, 25% were fair, and 25% were poor. The results were not influenced by the number of prior revisions or the prior prosthesis type.

Rosenberg and associates[17] also reported the clinical results of total knee revision using the total condylar III prosthesis. At mean follow-up of 45 months, 11 patients (30%) were graded excellent, 14 patients (39%) good, 6 (17%) fair, 4 (11%) poor, and there was one failure.

Hohl reported the results of the total condylar III prosthesis in complex knee reconstruction at a mean of 6.1 years for 29 revised TKAs.[16] Using the Knee Society scoring system, 71% of the patients had good or excellent results.

Kim reported the results of fourteen hinge prostheses that were revised to a total condylar III design.[8] The patients were followed for 4 years. The Hospital for Special Surgery Knee Score improved from 58 to 81.

The results of Lombardi and Hohl are similar to those reported by Rand, Donaldson, Shaw, Kavolus, and Rosenberg, which demonstrate 50 to 92% of the patients with good or excellent results following revision TKA using constrained devices (Table 12.1).

Table 12.1. Results of revision total knee arthroplasty using constrained devices

Author	Number	Follow-Up	Excellent	Good	Fair	Poor	Failures
Rand et al.[7]*	38 Knees (21 revised)	4.2 years	9 (43%)	7 (33%)	3 (14%)	2 (9%)	0
Donaldson et al.[10]*	31 Knees (14 revised)	3.8 years	2 (14%)	5 (36%)	1 (7%)	1 (7%)	5 (36%)
Kavolus et al.[13]*	16 Knees (11 revised)	4.2 years	5 (45%)	5 (45%)	1 (9%)	0	0
Rand et al.[15]*	21 Knees	4.0 years	5 (24%)	5 (24%)	5 (24%)	4 (19%)	1 (5%)
Hohl et al.[16]**	35 Knees (29 revised)	6.1 years	18 (51%)	7 (20%)	2 (6%)	5 (14%)	3 (9%)
Rosenberg et al.[17]**	36 Knees	3.75 years	11 (30%)	14 (39%)	6 (17%)	4 (11%)	1 (3%)
Lombardi et al.[20]*	113 Knees	2.1 years	18 (16%)	58 (51%)	26 (23%)	11 (10%)	0

(*) Hospital for Special Surgery Score
(**) Knee Society Score

COMPLICATIONS

Stuart and associates[19] discussed various reasons for reoperation after knee revision surgery that included implant loosening, sepsis, extensor mechanism problems, fractures of bone or prosthetic components, wear debris, and limited range of motion. The most common complications following revision TKA using constrained devices involve problems with the patella. Walker[4] in a series of 22 knees (21 revisions) noted one patellar subluxation and one patellar dislocation. Rand[7] in a series of 38 knees (23 revisions) noted patellar instability in 9, patellar implant loosening in 2, patellar fractures in 2, and patellar tendon ruptures in 2 knees. Shaw[11] noted in a series of 38 knees (18 revisions) that 36% of the revisions had perioperative patellar subluxation. Many other authors have elucidated problems with the extensor mechanism following revision TKA using constrained prostheses.[10,13-17,20]

Inglis and colleagues[14] noted that a major complication and cause of failure of revision total knee arthroplasty was fracture of the femur at the level of the tip of the intramedullary stem. This was due to the close proximity of the tip to the lateral cortex. This complication occurred in 38% of the first revisions and in 31% of the second revisions, comprising more than half the failures.

Donaldson and associates[10] noted failures included three prostheses removed for deep infections. Additional failures included aseptic loosening in two knees. Hohl and colleagues[16] noted three failures (8.6%); two failures were from infection and one from implant loosening.

Rosenberg and associates[17] noted four hemarthroses, four patients with chronic and symptomatic patellar subluxation, one superficial wound infection, one symptomatic deep vein thrombosis, one pulmonary embolism, one cerebrovascular accident, and one late neuroma. Two knee manipulations were required to gain flexion, one of which suffered a femoral fracture at manipulation that healed after cast brace treatment. One metal-backed patella was revised for excessive wear.

Rand[16] noted that complications consisted of two atraumatic patellar fractures, one patellar tendon rupture, one transient skin ischemia, one superficial infection, one deep infection, and one nonunion of a preexisting supracondylar femur fracture. Two of the extensor mechanism complications adversely affected the results with two poor and only one good knee score. The one transient skin ischemia resolved with cessation of knee motion, and the patient had an excellent knee score. The one deep infection required an above-knee amputation for control of sepsis. The patient who had revision using a cemented long-stem femoral component for a preexisting supracondylar femur fracture developed nonunion at the fracture site and had a poor knee score.

Other complications following revision TKA using constrained devices include breakage, loosening, superficial infection, deep infections, arthrofibrosis, femur and/or tibial shaft fractures, peroneal nerve palsies, shortening, nonunion, and screw disengagements (Table 12.2).

CONCLUSIONS

The need of constraint is relatively infrequent in primary versus revision total knee arthroplasty. Indications include deficient collateral ligaments, inadequate soft tissue balancing that cannot be salvaged, and marked metaphyseal bone loss (i.e, supracondylar femur or proximal tibia). The results of revision arthroplasty in this difficult group of patients will be satisfactory in 50% with a complication rate of 30 to 50%. Our preference is to use the least amount of constraint for revision.

Table 12.2. Complications of revision total knee arthroplasty using constrained devices

Author	Number	Patellar	Tibial	Femoral	Loosening	Sup. Infection	Deep Infection	Breakage	Arthro-fibrosis	Wound	Bleeding	Nerve Palsies	Other
Walker et al.[4]	21 revisions	1 subluxation; 1 dislocation	1 avulsion of tubercle; 1 shaft perforation	2 shaft perforations									
Rand et al.[7]	23 revisions	9 instabilities 2 loosening; 2 tendon rupture; 2 fracture		2 fractures	3 with aseptic leading to revision (2/3)	6	8	8					
Donaldson et al.[10]	14 revisions	1 fracture			2 with aseptic loosening					1 knee manipulation	5 wound complications	2 intra-articular bleeding		
Shaw et al.[11]	18 revisions	36% revisions with subluxation	1 fracture			3						1 peroneal nerve palsy	
Kavolus et al.[13]	11 revisions	2 dislocations					8						1 shortening > 60 mm; 1 removal of cement debris
Inglis et al.[14]	40 revisions	1 ligament rupture	1 fracture				1			1 transient skin ischemia			1 non-union of a pre-existing supracondylar fracture
Rand[15]	21 Knees	2 fractures; 1 tendon rupture	2 fractures	14 fractures		1	2		3 knee manipulations	1 wound slough; 1 decubitus ulcer		2 peroneal nerve palsies	1 tibial post dislocation
Hohl et al.[16]	29 revisions	1 subluxation			2 aseptic loosening	1	1		2 knee manipulations		4 hematomas		1 DVT; 1 PE; 1 late neuroma
Rosenberg et al.[17]	36 Knees	4 subluxations; 1 metal backed revised for excessive wear		1 fracture									
Lombardi et al.[20]	113 Knees	1 subluxation; 2 fractures			6 femoral component loosening secondary to allograft failure	2	4		5 knee manipulations				2 femoral-tibial dislocations; 2 screw disengagements

References

1. Levens AS, Berkeley CE, Inman VT, and Blosser JA. Transverse rotation of the segments of the lower extremity in locomotion. *J Bone Joint Surg.* 1948; 30A:859–872.
2. Nogi J, Caldwell JW, Kavzlanich JJ, Thompson RC Jr. Load testing of geometric and polycentric total knee replacement. *Clin Orthop.* 1976; 114:235–242.
3. Accardo NJ, Noiles DG, Pena R, Accardo NJ Jr. Noiles total knee replacement procedure. *Orthopedics.* 1979; 2:37–45.
4. Walker PS, Emerson R, Potter T, Scott R, Thomas WH, Turner RH. The kinematic rotating hinge: biomechanics and clinical application. *Orthop Clin of North Am.* 1982; 13(1):187–199.
5. Rand JA, Peterson LFA, Bryan RS, Ilstrup DM. Revision total knee arthroplasty. Instructional Course Lectures XXXV: 1986: 305–318.
6. Shindell R, Neumann R, Connolly JF, Jardon OM. Evaluation of the Noiles hinged knee prosthesis. *J Bone Joint Surg.* 1986; 68A(4):579–585.
7. Rand JA, Chao YS, Stauffer RN. Kinematic rotating-hinge total knee arthroplasty. *J Bone Joint Surg.* 1987; 69A(4):489–497.
8. Kim YH. Salvage of failed hinge knee arthroplasty with a total condylar III type prosthesis. *Clin Orthop.* 1987; 221:272–277.
9. Sculco TP. Total condylar III prosthesis in ligament instability. *Orthop Clin of North Am.* 1989; 20(2):221–226.
10. Donaldson WF, Sculco TP, Insall JN, Ranawat CS. Total condylar III knee prosthesis—long-term follow-up study. *Clin Orthop.* 1988; 226:21–28.
11. Shaw JA, Balcom W, Greer RB. Total knee arthroplasty using the kinematic rotating hinge prosthesis. *Orthopedics.* 1989; 12(5):647–654.
12. Goldberg VM, ed. *Controversies of Total Knee Arthroplasty.* New York: Raven Press, 1991.
13. Kavolus CH, Faris PM, Ritter MA, Keating EM. The total condylar III knee prosthesis in elderly patients. *J of Arthroplasty.* 1991; 6(1):39–43.
14. Inglis AE, Walker PS. Revision of failed knee replacements using fixed-axis hinges. *J Bone Joint Surg.* 1991; 73B(5):757–761.
15. Rand JA. Revision total knee arthroplasty using the total condylar III prosthesis. *J of Arthroplasty.* 1991; 6(3):279–284.
16. Hohl WM, Crawfurd E, Zelicof SB, Ewald FC. The total condylar III prosthesis in complex knee reconstruction. *Clin Orthop.* 1991; 273:91–97.
17. Rosenberg AG, Verner JJ, Galante JO. Clinical results of total knee revision using the total condylar III prosthesis. *Clin Orthop.* 1991; 273:83–90.
18. Morgan CL, Rand JA. Results of total knee arthroplasty using older constrained implant designs. In: Rand JA, ed. *Total Knee Arthroplasty.* New York: Raven Press; 1993:177–191.
19. Stuart MJ, Larson JE, Morrey F. Reoperation after condylar revision total knee arthroplasty. *Clin Orthop.* 1993; 286:168–173.
20. Lombardi AV Jr, Mallory TH, Eberle RW, Adams JB. Results of revision total knee arthroplasty using constrained prostheses. *Seminars in Arthroplasty,* in press, 1996.

CHAPTER 13
Unicondylar Replacement

C. Lowry Barnes and Richard D. Scott

Despite almost two decades of controversy, the status of unicompartmental knee replacement remains uncertain.[16,36] In the early 1970s several authors reported early poor results in unicompartmental knee arthroplasty, with the exception of lateral compartment replacement.[9,10,17] With refined surgical technique and instrumentation, more encouraging results have been reported.

Marmor reported 70% of his patients with satisfactory results at 10 years when treated with medial compartment replacement.[21] Failures were attributed to improper patient selection and technical problems. Others reported good results in 3- to 5-year follow-up studies.[1,30] Eight- to twelve-year follow-up of a series of 100 unicompartmental knee replacements demonstrated survivorship of the components in 90% of the patients at 9 years, 85% at 10 years, and 82% at 11 years.[28] The early results using metal-backed tibial components were encouraging,[15] but these have since become somewhat discouraging because of early failure of the 6 mm tibial components.[22,35]

The concept of unicompartmental knee replacement is attractive as an alternative to tibial osteotomy or tricompartmental replacement in selected osteoarthritic patients with unicompartmental disease confirmed at arthrotomy.[15,16,34] Compared to osteotomy, there is a higher initial success rate and fewer early complications with unicompartmental arthroplasty.[5,8,30] Patients with bilateral disease can have both knees operated during the same anesthetic with full recovery within three months of surgery following unicompartmental replacement. Patients who undergo bilateral osteotomies often have their surgeries spaced from 3 to 6 months apart, and as much as a year may be required to achieve full recovery from the time of the initial procedure.[16]

Unlike standard tricompartmental arthroplasty, unicompartmental replacement has the advantage of preserving both cruciate ligaments, which may yield a knee with near-normal kinematics.[16,36] Attrition of the anterior cruciate ligament, however, may occur following unicompartmental replacement. This may lead to femoraltibial subluxation and development of arthritis in the unresurfaced compartment.[33] A study of 42 patients with a tricompartmental arthroplasty on one side and a unicompartmental arthroplasty on the other side showed that a majority of the patients preferred the unicompartmental side because it felt more like their normal knee.[18] Patients with unicompartmental replacement, as compared to tricompartmental replacement, may also have a better range of motion and ambulatory function.[26]

A theoretic advantage of unicompartmental knee replacement, as compared to tricompartmental knee replacement, is that revision surgery should be easier in the unicompartmentally replaced knee because of the maintenance of bone stock.[13] However, two reviews of revision of unicompartmental arthroplasty patient have not supported this theoretic advantage.[2,23] Augmentation with special components or bone graft was often necessary due to bone deficiency, and the results were no better than revisions of standard total knee replacement procedures. A more recent report, however, shows that modern techniques using surface replacements on the femoral and tibial sides have made the procedure as conservative in practice as it is in theory.[19]

Two studies have compared results following revision of unicompartmental replacement or tibial osteotomy. Gill and associates demonstrated that either can be predictably revised to a tricompartmental replacement. The unicompartmental group, however, required more major osseous reconstruction.[7] Jackson and colleagues also reported significant manageable bone loss following unicompartmental failure. However, they also report an increased complication rate (30%) in patients who had revision of failed tibial osteotomy to total knee replacement.[12]

PATIENT SELECTION

Osteotomy remains the procedure of choice in young, heavy, active patients with unicompartmental osteoarthritis. Poor range of motion and pain at rest are relative contraindications to osteotomy.

For many years, the ideal candidate for unicompartmental replacement was the osteoarthritic patient with a physiologic age older than 60 and a sedentary lifestyle.[16] With survivorship studies of tricompartmental arthroplasty superior to unicompartmental arthroplasty after the first decade, the selection process must be reconsidered. Patients in their sixties and seventies would seem to have a greater chance of living out their life without a revision if they undergo a tricompartmental procedure.

Unicompartmental replacement now assumes a role in two groups of patients. One is the middle-aged osteoarthritic patient (especially female) as their "first arthroplasty." Advantages include a very reliable initial result, anatomic realignment (versus osteotomy with potentially cosmetically objectional clinical valgus), retention of both cruciates for higher performance, and easy salvage.

The second group of patients is the osteoarthritic octogenarian as their "first and last" arthroplasty. Advantages include faster surgery, faster recovery, less blood loss, less deep vein thrombosis, less energy consumption, and a less expensive prosthesis. An unpublished series of 42 octogenarians from our clinic shows that at 5 to 10 years after surgery, the prosthesis survived the patient in all but one case.

In assessing patient candidacy, the disease process should not have an inflammatory component, which may be indicated by an effusion or significant pain at rest. The patient should have greater than 90 degrees of flexion and should have a flexion contracture of less than 15 degrees. Relative contraindications to unicompartmental replacement include subluxation and an anatomic alignment greater than 10 degrees of varus or 12 degrees of valgus. Occasionally, interpositional unicompartmental arthroplasty with metallic inserts may be indicated when an osteotomy is not appropriate and the patient is too heavy, too young, or too active for total knee replacement.[6,29]

The ultimate decision between a tricompartmental replacement and a unicompartmental replacement must be made at the time of arthrotomy.[30] Although the patient may be an ideal candidate for unicompartmental arthroplasty by clinical examination and radiography, contraindications to the procedure may be discovered at the time of arthrotomy. An absent anterior cruciate ligament is a contraindication to unicompartmental replacement because subluxation can occur and lead to early arthritic change in the opposite compartment. The patellofemoral joints and the other femoral-tibial compartment must also be thoroughly examined for any arthritic involvement. Mild areas of grade I chondromalacia in the opposite compartment are acceptable, but eburnated bone is a contraindication. Synovial proliferation or chondrocalcinosis at the time of arthrotomy suggests an inflammatory component to the knee arthritis, and unicompartmental replacement should not be performed.

SURGICAL PROCEDURE

A longitudinal skin incision is made just medial to the midline of the patella. A medial parapatellar arthrotomy is then performed to allow eversion of the patella and adequate exposure. Although this arthrotomy can be used for both medial and lateral replacement, some surgeons favor a lateral approach for valgus knees.[14] This would provide excellent exposure of the lateral compartment but may make bicondylar replacement more difficult, if deemed necessary following arthrotomy.

For medial compartment arthroplasty, the coronary ligament is incised at the anterior horn of the medial meniscus and a periosteal sleeve is elevated from the anteromedial aspect of the tibia. The lateral dissection is performed within the fat pad anterior to the coronary ligament, avoiding detachment of the anterior horn of the lateral meniscus. Similarly, during lateral compartment replacement, the medial aspect of the coronary ligament is protected and an anterolateral periosteal sleeve is raised from the lateral aspect of the tibial plateau to Gerdy's tubercle.

Following adequate exposure, the patellofemoral, medial, and lateral compartments are thoroughly inspected to determine the number of compartments that should be replaced as noted previously, unicompartmental replacement is contraindicated if there is inflammatory synovitis or if crystalline deposits are noted. The anterior cruciate ligament should be intact and functional. The cartilage in the opposite and patellofemoral compartments should also appear healthy. Although grade I or II chondromalacia in the patellofemoral compartment is not a contraindication to unicompartmental arthroplasty, eburnated bone on the patella or trochlea probably mandates tricompartmental replacement.

Peripheral osteophytes are usually present at the medial aspect of the femoral condyle and on the medial aspect of the tibial plateau in an osteoarthritic varus knee with isolated medial compartment arthritis. They often prevent passive correction of the varus deformity because of relative shortening of the capsule and medial collateral ligament as they pass over these osteophytes. Their removal will usually allow passive correction of the varus deformity.[30] If a more significant medial release is required to obtain proper alignment, this probably implies a more severe varus deformity, which should be treated with bicompartmental or tricompartmental replacement.

Patients who have medial compartment arthritis may also develop intercondylar "kissing osteophytes" because the lateral tibial spine impinges on the medial aspect of the lateral femoral condyle. If not removed, these osteophytes will impinge, producing pain with weight-bearing. Bicompartmental or tricompartmental arthroplasty may be necessary if the area of impingement is large (Fig. 13.1).

As lateral compartment osteoarthritis progresses, lateral subluxation of the tibia on the femur usually does not occur until the deformity is so severe that unicompartmental arthroplasty is not appropriate. The medial collateral ligament and medial capsule gradually elongate as the valgus increases. With significant medial laxity, the knee can no longer be stabilized by unicompartmental arthroplasty. This situation usually requires bi- or tricompartmental arthroplasty and a lateral release.

Proper sizing of the components is important, and the femoral component should reproduce the anteroposterior dimension of the native femoral condyle. The larger component should be used in borderline cases because this would provide better capping of the subchondral bone of the condyle. This will help resist loosening and subsidence. The posterior condyle must be resected to at least the thickness of the femoral implant. It is better to resect too much of the posterior condyle rather than too little, because tightness in flexion must be avoided. The femoral component should not protrude anteriorly, or it may disrupt patellar tracking (Fig. 13.2). The femoral component should, however, extend far enough anteriorly to fully cover the weight-bearing surface that is in contact with the tibia in full extension.

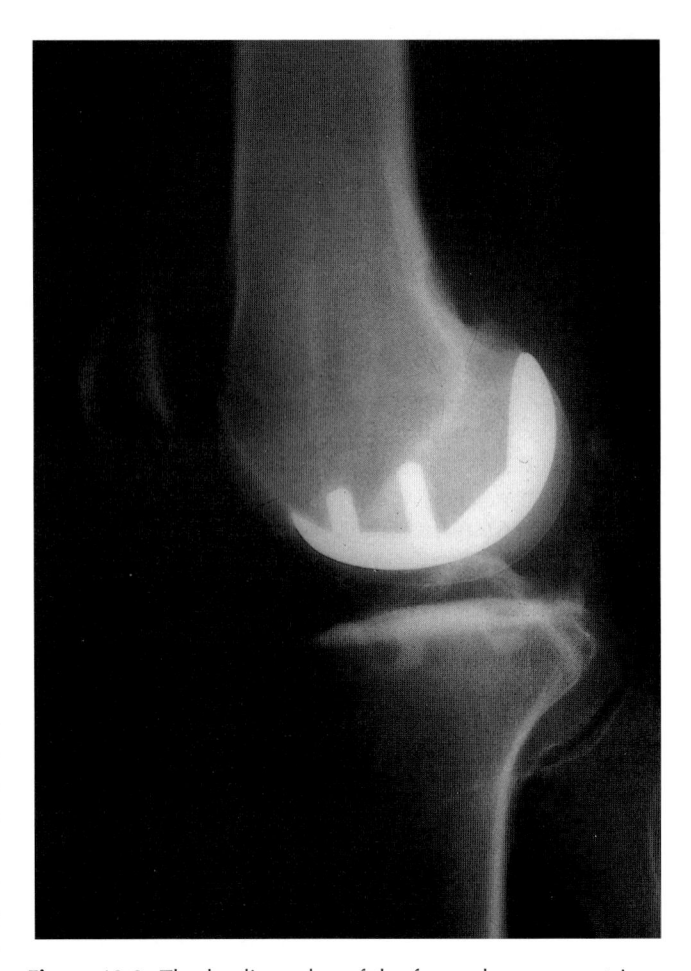

Figure 13.2. The leading edge of the femoral component is recessed to avoid patellar impingement during flexion.

The tibial component should be thick enough to restore the tibial plateau to its original height. Appropriate medial peripheral osteophyte resection should allow for correction of the varus deformity without requiring thicker tibial components. Following medial unicompartmental replacement, the medial joint space should open 1 to 2 mm with application of a valgus stress in full extension. Similarly, the lateral joint space should open 1 or 2 mm with the application of varus stress in full extension following isolated lateral replacement. Components placed too tightly could cause the tibia to subluxate toward the opposite compartment, producing excessive pressure and increased wear.

IMPLANT DESIGN

Twenty years of experience has led to a better understanding of the ideal design features for unicompart-

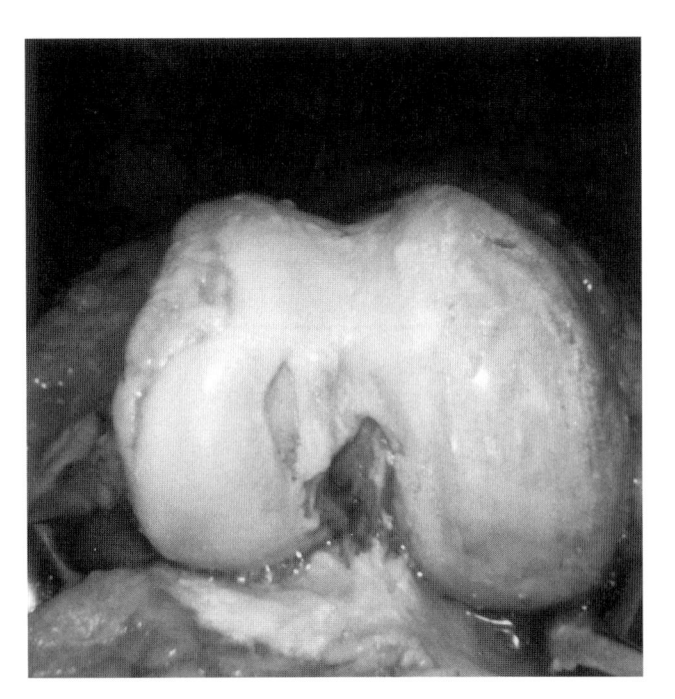

Figure 13.1. Secondary erosion of the medial aspect of the lateral femoral condyle due to lateral subluxation of the tibia.

mental replacement. Many of the early femoral components subsided into the condylar bone of the femur because they were too narrow in the medial to lateral dimension. The ideal component should, therefore, be wide enough to maximally cap the resurfaced condyle so that it will adequately distribute the weight-bearing forces. Therefore, there should be multiple sizes of femoral components available. The fixation pegs must not invade the femoral condyle too deeply because of the possibility of significant bone loss in the revision situation. Two relatively small fixation lugs to control rotation appear to be sufficient. The resected posterior condyle of the femur must be completely capped with the posterior condylar portion of the component to allow full range of motion without impingement.

Although in theory it would be preferable to resurface the subchondral bone of the femur without making a distal resection, more tibial bone stock would have to be sacrificed to accommodate the components. An appropriate compromise is to resect up to 4 mm of distal femoral condyle, which retains subchondral bone for fixation of the prosthesis and conserves enough distal femur to allow easier conversion to a standard total knee replacement. This allows for preservation of 4 mm of tibial bone stock, which also should make revision surgery easier.

Backing of the tibial component with metal remains controversial. Although initially thought to deliver more uniform weight-bearing forces across the tibia, early failures have been noted due to the thin polyethylene.[22,35] Failures resulting from polyethylene wear have been seen mainly in the 6 mm thick, metal-backed, tibial component. Failure occurred most frequently in the designs with a sharp angle between the metal base and the polyethylene at the periphery, creating an area in which the polyethylene was only 2 mm thick. This is not significantly different from problems seen with metal-backed patellar components.[3,20] Because of these problems, there may be a trend back to all polyethylene tibial components in unicompartmental replacements.

Retrievals of worn unicompartmental tibial components have yielded important information regarding wear patterns and their implication on prosthetic design. It appears that the wear pattern of the prosthetic components tends to reproduce the preoperative wear pattern of the osteoarthritic knee[22] (Fig. 13.3). As noted

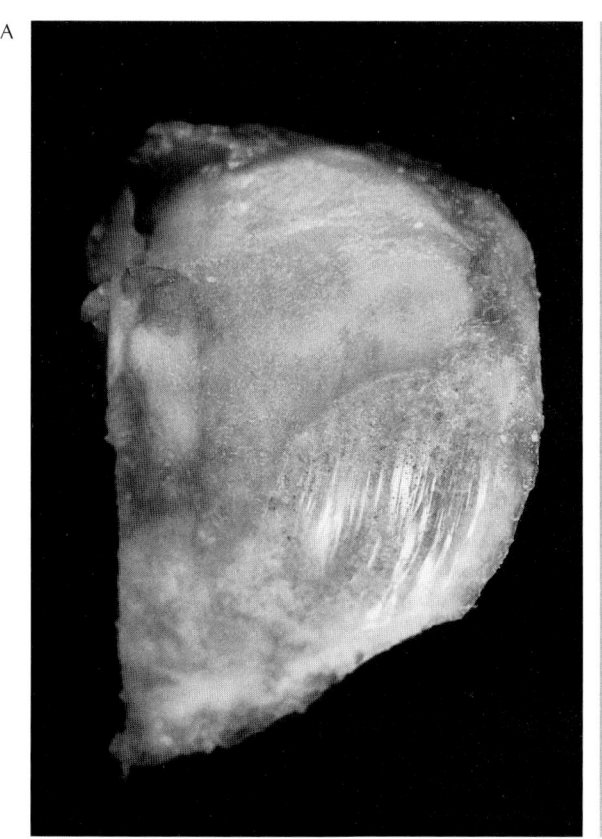

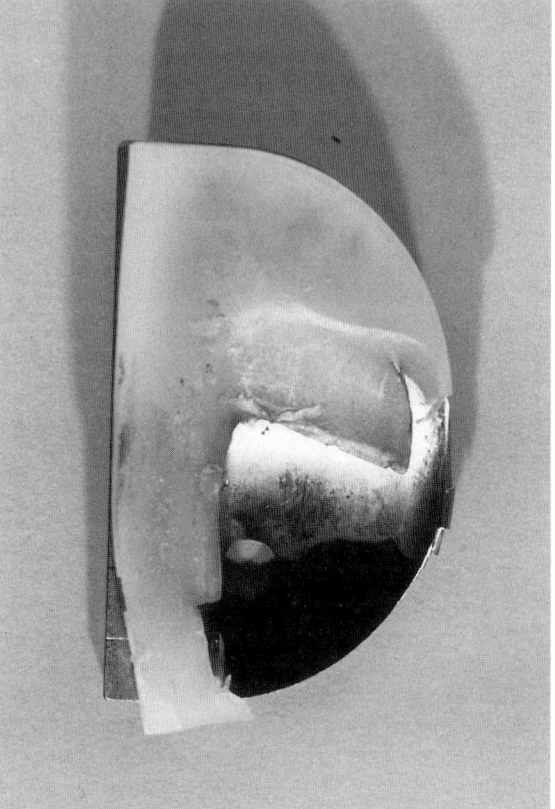

Figure 13.3. The wear pattern of the unicompartmental arthroplasty reproduces the wear pattern of the osteoarthritic knee. Typically this occurs anteriorly and peripherally.

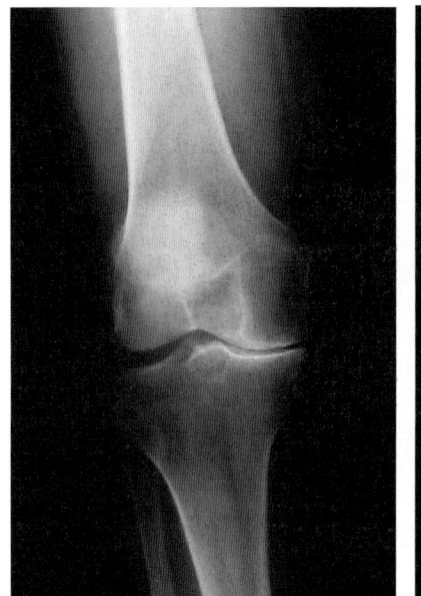

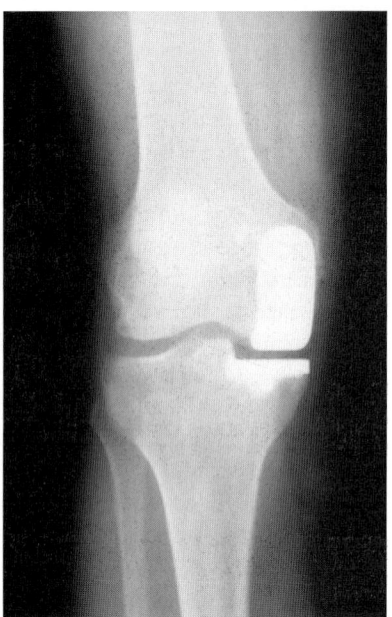

Figure 13.4. (A) Preoperation roentgenogram of an ideal candidate for unicompartmental arthroplasty. (B) Postoperative roentgenogram showing conservative bone resection and restoration of normal anatomic alignment.

by White and associates, this tends to be anterior and peripheral on the medial tibial plateau in a varus knee.[37] Tibial components, therefore, are best designed to be asymmetrical in shape to maximally cap this portion of the tibial, and they must have an adequate thickness of polyethylene in this area.

REHABILITATION

Postoperative rehabilitation following cemented unicompartmental knee replacement is similar to that in standard total knee replacement. However, rehabilitation goals are often met sooner because patients usually have less pain and swelling.

Use of a continuous passive motion machine is initiated in the recovery room with the machine initially set at 30 to 40 degrees following a general anesthetic or at 70 to 90 degrees following a long-acting spinal or an epidural anesthetic. The continuous passive motion machine is then advanced 10 to 20 degrees per day, as tolerated by the patient, until 90 degrees of flexion is achieved and maintained. A knee immobilizer is applied at night to prevent the development of a flexion contracture.

Mobilization is begun quickly, and the patient continues to use a knee immobilizer when walking until straight leg raises can be easily performed. Weightbearing is protected with a walker or crutches until 6 weeks following surgery, after which patients can use a cane outdoors and can walk without support for short distances indoors. The cane is usually discontinued 3 months following surgery.

SUMMARY

Despite two decades of experience, the role of unicompartmental arthroplasty remains controversial and uncertain. It has been suggested as the appropriate operation in 6% of patients with gonarthrosis.[32] Unicompartmental replacement appears to offer an attractive alternative to osteotomy or tricompartmental arthroplasty in selected patients with unicompartmental arthritis (Fig. 13.4). Compared to osteotomy, there is a higher initial success rate and fewer complications. Compared to tricompartmental arthroplasty, there tends to be a better quality result with a faster recovery and improved function. The procedure can be conservative regarding preservation of both cruciate ligaments and bone stock in the opposite compartment and patellofemoral joint. With appropriate patient selection, prosthetic design, and operative techniques, unicompartmental knee arthroplasty should assume its proper role in our armamentarium, functioning as the initial conservative arthroplasty in qualified patients. It may, however, also be appropriate in the very elderly patient with a life expectancy of less than 10 years. Osteotomy should still be utilized as a conservative procedure in the young, heavy, active individual, especially males.

References

1. Bae KK, Guhl JF, Keane SP. Unicompartmental knee arthroplasty for single compartment disease. *Clin Orthop.* 1983; 176:233–238.
2. Barrett WP, Scott RD. Revision of failed unicondylar arthroplasty. *J Bone Joint Surg.* 1987; 69A:1328–1335.
3. Bayley JC, Scott RD, Ewald FC, Holmes GB. Failure of the

metal-backed patellar component after total knee replacement. *J Bone Joint Surg.* 1988; 70A:668–674.
4. Bernasek TL, Rand JA, Bryan RS. Unicompartmental porous coated anatomic total knee arthroplasty. *Clin Orthop.* 1988; 236:52–59.
5. Broughton NS, Newman JH, Bailey RA. Unicompartmental replacement and high tibial osteotomy for osteoarthritis for the knee. *J Bone Joint Surg.* 1986; 68B:447–452.
6. Emerson RH, Potter T. The use of the metallic McKeever hemiarthroplasty for unicompartmental arthritis. *J Bone Joint Surg.* 1985; 67A:208–212.
7. Gill T, Schemitsch EH, Brick GW, Thornhill TS. Revision total knee arthroplasty after failed unicompartmental knee arthroplasty or high tibial osteotomy. *Clin Orthop.* 1995; 321:10–18.
8. Inglis G. Unicompartmental arthroplasty of the knee. *J Bone Joint Surg.* 1984; 66B:682–684.
9. Insall J, Aglietti P. A five to seven-year follow-up of unicondylar arthroplasty. *J Bone Joint Surg.* 1980; 62A:1329–1337.
10. Insall JN, Walker PS. Unicondylar knee replacement. *Clin Orthop.* 1976; 120:83–85.
11. Ivarsson I, Gillquist J. Rehabilitation after high tibial osteotomy and unicompartmental arthroplasty. *Clin Orthop.* 1991; 266:139–144.
12. Jackson M, Sarangi PP, Newman JH. Revision total knee arthroplasty. Comparison of outcome following primary proximal tibial osteotomy or unicompartmental osteotomy. *J Arthroplasty.* 1994; 9:539–542.
13. Jones WH, Bryan KS, Peterson LR, Ilstrup DM. Unicompartmental knee arthroplasty using polycentric and geometric hemicomponents. *J Bone Joint Surg.* 1981; 63A: 946–954.
14. Keblish PS, Valgus deformity in total knee replacement. The lateral retinacular approach. *Orthop Trans.* 1985; 9:28–29.
15. Kozinn CS, Marx C, Scott RD. Unicompartmental knee arthroplasty. *J Arthroplasty.* 1989; 4:S1–S10.
16. Kozinn SC, Scott. Current concepts review, unicompartmental knee arthroplasty. *J Bone Joint Surg.* 1989; 71A:145–150.
17. Laskin RS. Unicompartmental tibiofemoral resurfacing arthroplasty. *J Bone Joint Surg.* 1978; 60A:182–185.
18. Laurencin CT, Zelicof ST, Scott RD, Ewald FC. Unicompartmental versus total knee arthroplasty in the same patient. A comparative study. *Clin Orthop.* 1991; 273:151–156.
19. Levine WN, Ozuna RM, Scott RD, Thornhill TS. Conversion of failed modern unicompartmental arthroplasty to total knee arthroplasty. *J Arthroplasty.* 1996; 11(7):797–801.
20. Lombardi AV Jr, Engh GA, Volz RG, et al. Fracture/dissociation of the polyethylene in metal-backed patellar components in total knee arthroplasty. *J Bone Joint Surg.* 1988; 70A:675–679.
21. Marmor L. Unicompartmental knee arthroplasty. Ten to thirteen year follow-up study. *Clin Orthop.* 1987; 226:14–20.
22. McCallum JD, Scott RD. Duplication of medial erosion in unicompartmental knee arthroplasties. *J Bone Joint Surg.* 1995; 77-B:726–728.
23. Padgett DE, Stern SH, Insall JN. Revision total knee arthroplasty for failed unicompartmental replacement. *J Bone Joint Surg.* 191:73A:186–190.
24. Ranawat CS, Oheneba RB. Survivorship analysis and results of total condylar knee arthroplasty. *Clin Orthop.* 1988; 226:6–13.
25. Rand JA, Ilstrup DM. Survivorship analysis of total knee arthroplasty. Cumulative rates and survival of 9200 total knee arthroplasties. *J Bone Joint Surg.* 1991; 73A:397–409.
26. Rougraff BT, Heck DA, Gibson AE. A comparison of tricompartmental and unicompartmental arthroplasty for the treatment of gonarthrosis. *Clin Orthop.* 1991; 273:157–164.
27. Scott RD. Robert Brigham unicondylar knee surgical techniques. *Orthop.* 1990; 5:15.
28. Scott RD, Cobb AG, McQueary FG, Thornhill TS. Unicompartment knee arthroplasty, eight to twelve year follow-up with survivorship analysis. *Clin Orthop.* 1991; 271:96–100.
29. Scott RD, Joyce MJ, Ewald FC, Thomas WH. McKeever metallic hemiarthroplasty of the knee in unicompartmental degenerative arthritis. *J Bone Joint Surg.* 1985; 67A:203–207.
30. Scott RD, Santore R. Unicondylar unicompartmental replacement for osteoarthritis of the knee. *J Bone Joint Surg.* 1981; 63A:536–544.
31. Scuderi GR, Insall JN, Windsor RE, Moran MC. Survivorship of cemented knee replacement. *J Bone Joint Surg.* 1989; 71B:798–803.
32. Stern SH, Becker MW, Insall JN. Unicondylar knee arthroplasty. An evaluation of selection criteria. *Clin Orthop.* 1993; 286:143–148.
33. Swank M, Stulberg SD, Jiganti J, Machairas S. The natural history of unicompartmental arthroplasty. An eight year follow-up study with survivorship analysis. *Clin Orthop.* 1993; 286:130–142.
34. Thornhill TS. Unicompartmental knee arthroplasty. *Clin Orthop.* 1986; 205:121–131.
35. Thornhill TS, Clark AE, McManus J, Bergman T, Scott RD. Metal-backed unicompartmental knee replacement. Presented at 58th Annual Meeting of the American Academy of Orthopedic Surgeons, Anaheim, California, March 11, 1991.
36. Thornhill TS, Scott RD. Unicompartmental total knee arthroplasty. *Clin Orthop.* NA. 1989; 20:245–256.
37. White SH, Ludkowski PF, Goodfellow JW. Anteromedial osteoarthritis of the knee. *J Bone Joint Surg.* 1991; 73B:582–586.

SECTION 4
Surgical Approaches

CHAPTER 14
Medial Parapatellar Arthrotomy

Steven H. Stern

INTRODUCTION

All operative procedures begin with exposure of the relevant anatomy. It is imperative that this visualization of the appropriate structures is excellent in order to optimize the surgical outcome. Thus adequate exposure must be attained, while at the same time, minimizing risks to neurovascular structures and muscle tissue, promoting soft tissue healing and maximizing postoperative function.

In this regard, knee arthroplasty is no different from other operative procedures. However, there are several unique aspects of knee replacement surgery that place an extra burden on the implant surgeon. First, the knee is a relatively superficial joint with a limited soft tissue envelope. In addition, postsurgical outcome is related both to the healing of this soft tissue envelope, as well as maximizing knee motion. Thus, the soft tissues within this envelope are routinely stressed early on in the postoperative period, when attempts are made to regain knee motion. Therefore, exposure must minimize skin and soft tissue tension in an attempt to reduce any skin problem, especially skin necrosis, which is a definite concern in knee surgery.[1–5]

In general, anterior surgical approaches are the basic method of achieving exposure in knee arthroplasty. The superficial nature of the joint aids the surgeon in dissecting directly down to the applicable anatomy. Patellar eversion allows easy visualization of all three knee compartments. The neurovascular bundle is located posteriorly, thus injury to these structures is minimized with an anterior approach. The basic variations in the anterior surgical approaches involve modification of the plane of muscle dissection, with each method possibly resulting in different degrees of visualization and postsurgical clinical function.

The basic tenets of surgical exposure should be kept in mind. Generally, extensile exposures are preferred. This allows for dissection to be extended, as needed, either proximally or distally. One long incision is preferable to several shorter incisions. However, it is widely accepted that prior transverse incisions can be successfully crossed perpendicularly by a new longitudinal incision.[1–3,5,6] If at all possible, prior longitudinal incisions should be incorporated into current skin incisions and parallel vertical incisions avoided. However, on occasion, prior vertical incisions are in areas that make inclusion of them in a current longitudinal exposure unrealistic. If this is the case, then the second vertical incision should be made in a manner as to leave as wide a soft tissue bridge between the two wounds as practically possible.

ANTERIOR APPROACH FOR KNEE ARTHROPLASTY

The anterior approach is the basic workhorse of exposure in knee surgery. It is extensile, allowing easy access to both distal femur and proximal tibia. The technique can be used for fractures, arthroplasty, arthrodeses, and extensor mechanism procedures. Multiple procedures can be performed through the same incision with excellent visualization of both medial and lateral structures and minimal neurovascular injury. The specifics of exposure in total knee arthroplasty follow.

Preparation

The first step in any surgical procedure is the induction of satisfactory anesthesia. Suitable exposure can be achieved for knee arthroplasty surgery with either general, epidural, or spinal anesthesia. However, it is important that a complete motor block is maintained throughout the procedure. This is necessary in order to minimize the risk of patellar tendon avulsion secondary to a forceful intraoperative quadriceps contraction.

After the induction of successful anesthesia, the patient is positioned on the operative table with all pressure points carefully padded. A pneumatic tourniquet is applied to the upper thigh. It is imperative that the tourniquet is as proximal as possible in order to minimize interference with the operative field.

The lower extremity is then prepped and draped for surgery according to the particular hospital's protocol and surgeon's preference. Adhesive drapes can be used to seal off the foot and groin area. The lower extremity is elevated and exsanguinated with an Esmarch bandage. The pneumatic tourniquet is then routinely inflated to 350 mm Hg.

In certain cases of severe lower extremity peripheral vascular disease or after lower extremity vascular bypass procedures, it may be worthwhile to consider minimizing or eliminating tourniquet use. Knee arthroplasty surgery can be accomplished in these instances. However, increased attention must be paid to achieving hemostasis and minimizing bleeding. Visualization, although compromised from the increased bleeding, is normally still adequate for successful knee arthroplasty.

Skin and Superficial Dissection

The actual positioning of the skin incision varies among different surgeons. In most instances, this variation is simply a matter of personal preference. However, in certain circumstances, the actual location of the skin cut represents an integral part of the surgical procedure. Skin incisions can be directly straight in the midline, or curved slightly either medially or laterally (Fig. 14.1). Some authors believe that a slightly curved medial parapatellar incision offers a theoretical benefit for wound healing.[4] However, large curves necessitate increased undermining of skin, which others feel is undesirable.[3,5] In general, lateral skin incisions associated with medial arthrotomies are rarely performed because of the increased undermining they require.

The most common incision at our institution (if the knee does not have any prior scars) is a straight midline one. The incision is positioned over the medial one-third of the patellar and carried distally 1 cm medial to the tibial tubercle. The proximal pole of the incision extends about 8 cm superior to the top of the patellar and concludes about 2 cm distal to the patellar tendon's insertion on the tibial tubercle.

Any prior scars or incisions must be taken into account at the commencement of the exposure. In general, prior well-healed arthroscopic portals and transverse skin incisions can be ignored, and new vertical incisions made with impunity. Care should be taken to position the new exposure so that it is perpendicular to the old scars. However, prior vertical medial arthrotomy incisions, if at all possible, are best incorporated into any new skin approach. This tends to position the incision more medially than routinely desired and requires some skin undermining in order to perform the retinacular

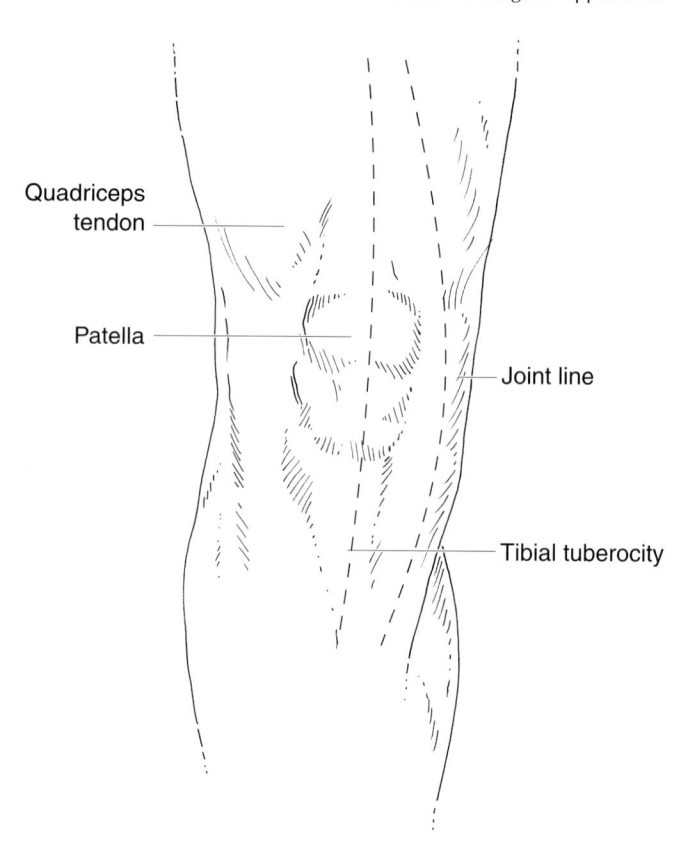

Figure 14.1. Skin incisions that can be utilized for the anterior approach to the knee.

arthrotomy. However, in these instances, it is normally felt that accepting some undermining and the attendant risks is preferable to creating an avascular area between two vertical incisions.

A more difficult problem is encountered in knees in which a prior lateral skin incision is present. In many cases, these are too far lateral to be incorporated into a new skin incision and still allow a medial retinacular arthrotomy. In these instances, it is usually necessary to make a second longitudinal incision that does not incorporate the prior lateral scar. When this method is necessary, the newer incision should be positioned as far medial as practically possible, so that as large a skin bridge as possible is created between the two incisions.

After the initial incision is made, dissection is normally carried directly down to the extensor mechanism. A bovie electrocautery is used to coagulate any bleeding or potential bleeding vessels. Large varicosities are tied with appropriate suture, though ligature ties are not routinely needed. Care should be taken at all times to minimize both trauma to the soft tissue, as well as undermining of skin. Dissection is carried directly down to the extensor mechanism, so that the quadriceps tendon, patella, and patellar tendon are all easily visualized. After adequate exposure of the extensor mecha-

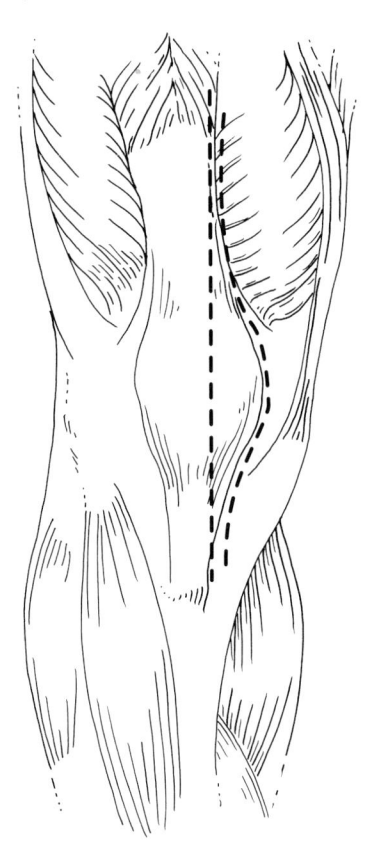

Figure 14.2. Various options for the retinacular capsular incision in knee arthroplasty. These include the midline and medial parapatellar incisions.

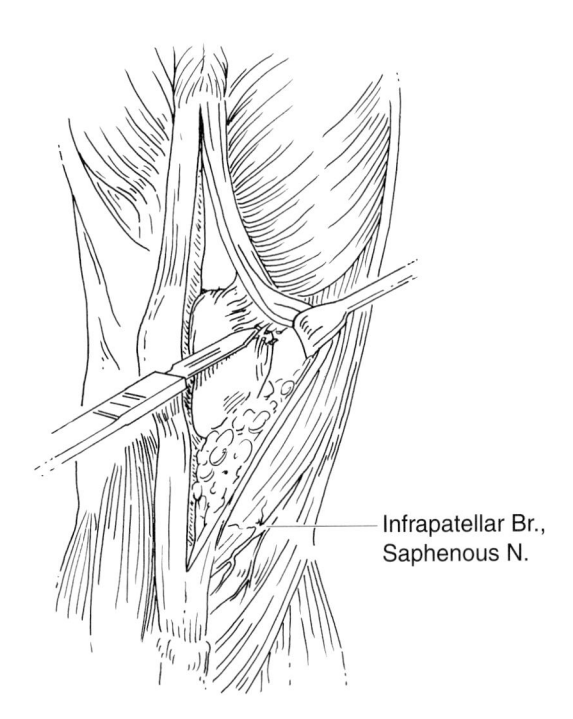

Figure 14.3. The quadriceps expansion is sharply dissected from the medial aspect of the patella in a subperiosteal manner.

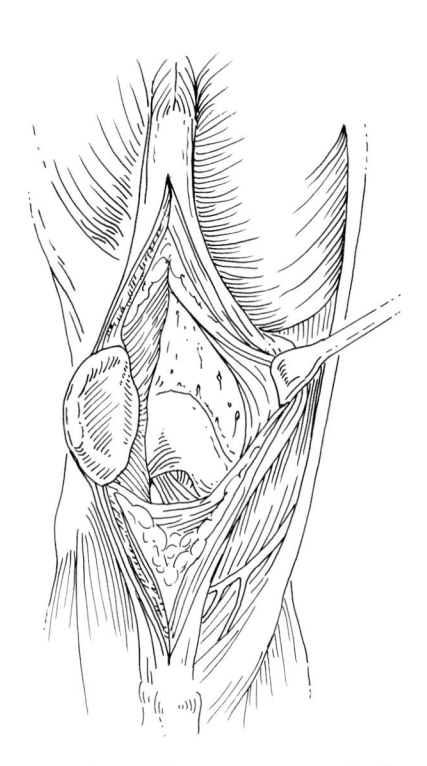

Infrapatellar Br., Saphenous N.

Figure 14.4. After the quadriceps expansion is dissected from the patella, the extensor mechanism is retracted laterally.

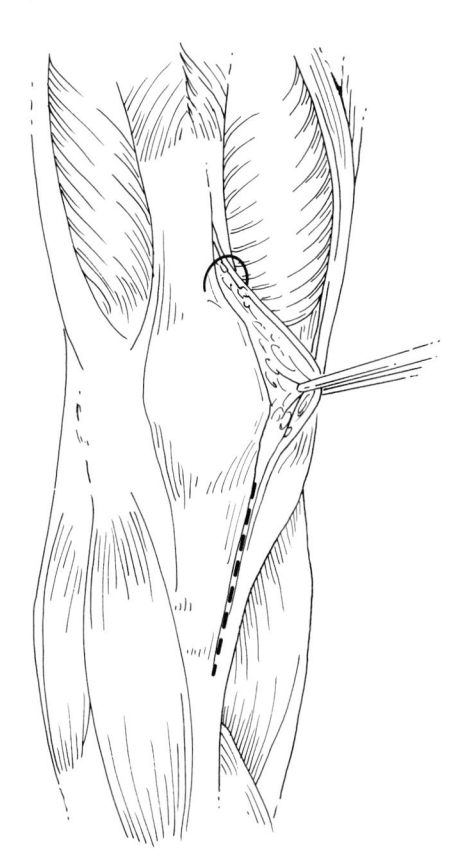

Figure 14.5. Placement of the initial retinacular suture during closure to minimize postoperative patella baja complications.

nism is achieved, attention can be turned to performing a medial arthrotomy.

Arthrotomy

At this point in the surgical procedure, attention can be turned to the retinacular arthrotomy. Adequate exposure through the skin and soft tissue should have yielded excellent visualization of the extensor mechanism. Most surgeons expose the inner aspects of the knee joint via a medial retinacular arthrotomy. This technique allows the patella to be everted and retracted laterally. The medial retinacular incision can either be curvilinear or straight (Fig. 14.2).

The curvilinear (or parapatellar arthrotomy) is arguably the most common method of achieving exposure in knee arthroplasty surgery.[1,7,8] In this technique, the retinacular incision extends along the medial aspect of the quadriceps tendon. At the level of the patella, the retinacular incision is carried medial to the patella through the anteromedial knee capsule. Distally, the incision curves back to the medial aspect of the patellar tendon and continues distally along its medial margin. Using this technique, the surgeon leaves a thick cuff of soft tissue on the medial aspect of the patella for repair during closure.

Other surgeons advocate a straight medial retinacular exposure.[3,9] In this technique the goal is to make a straight retinacular incision. This routinely necessitates carrying the exposure directly over the patella bone. At the level of the patella the quadriceps expansion is sharply dissected from the medial aspect of the patella in a subperiosteal manner (Figs. 14.3 and 14.4). This is in contrast to the curvilinear technique in which the incision is purposefully medial to the patellar bone. The distal limb of the incision extends onto the anterior tibial cortex in a similar manner to the curvilinear technique.

Insall condemns routine use of a curved retinacular incision, feeling it disrupts the insertion of the vastus medialis into the patella.[2,3] He feels that repair of the extensor mechanism with this approach is not as strong as with a straight midline retinacular incision. Theoretically, the straight arthrotomy minimizes disruption of the vastus medialis' attachment to the patella, thereby ensuring a straight pull of the extensor mechanism.

At this point in the procedure the knee is flexed and the patella everted. Care should be taken to minimize tension on the extensor mechanism. A bent Hohman retractor (bent at 90 degrees) can be placed over the lateral aspect of the tibial plateau and used to retract the extensor mechanism laterally and aid in exposure.

The knee arthroplasty can then be carried out in the standard fashion, depending on the alignment of the knee and the types of components to be implanted.

Closure

Care must be taken in closure of a knee, because healing of the soft tissue is crucial to achieving a successful result. Unfortunately, even in the best of circumstances, there always remains a risk of problems with the soft tissue and wound healing. Closure of the knee joint is routinely accomplished with the use of synthetic sutures (absorbable or nonabsorbable) meticulously placed in an interrupted fashion. Careful positioning of the sutures can be done in an attempt to minimize patellar baha, which is known to be associated with knee procedures.[10] The initial sutures can be placed in an oblique fashion to counteract the natural tendency of the patella to drift into a baha location[5] (Fig. 14.5). Subsequent interrupted synthetic sutures can then be placed in a sequential manner. The subcutaneous tissues are copiously irrigated, and then closed with the use of interrupted sutures in a meticulous layered fashion. The skin can be approximated in a number of ways depending on the individual surgeon's preference.

References

1. Boiardo RA, Dorr LD. Surgical approaches for total knee replacement arthroplasty. *Contemporary Orthopaedics* 1986; 12:60.
2. Insall JN. Surgical approaches to the knee. In: Insall JN, ed. *Surgery of the Knee.* New York: Churchill Livingstone; 1984: 41–54.
3. Insall JN. Surgical approaches. In: Insall JN, Windsor RE, Scott WN, Kelly MA, Aglietti P, eds. *Surgery of the Knee.* New York: Churchill Livingstone; 1993: 135–148.
4. Johnson DP, Houghton TA, Radford P. Anterior midline or medial parapatellar incision for arthroplasty of the knee. A comparative study. *J Bone Joint Surg.* 1986; 68B:812.
5. Stern SH. Surgical exposures in total knee arthroplasty. In: Fu F, Harner CD, Vince KG, eds. *Knee Surgery.* Baltimore: Williams & Wilkins; 1994: 1289–1302.
6. Vince KG. Revision arthroplasty technique. In: Heckman J, ed. *Instructional Course Lectures.* Rosemont, Il: American Academy of Orthopaedic Surgeons; 1993: 325–339.
7. Hoppenfeld S, DeBoer P. *Surgical Exposures in Orthopaedics: The Anatomic Approach.* 2nd ed. Philadelphia: J.B. Lippincott Company, 1994.
8. Krakow KA. *The Technique of Total Knee Arthroplasty.* St. Louis, MO: C.V. Mosby; 1990: 168–197.
9. Insall JN. A midline approach to the knee. *J Bone Joint Surg.* 1971; 53A:1584.
10. Scuderi GR, Windsor RE, Insall JN. Observations on Patellar Height after Proximal Tibial Osteotomy. *J Bone Joint Surg.* 1989; 71(2):245–248.

CHAPTER 15
Subvastus Approach

Kelly G. Vince

The subvastus surgical approach is appealing. Some surgeons hail it as a tremendous advance over other, more conventional surgical approaches to the knee.[1] It is more "anatomic" than the medial parapatellar arthrotomy, but the functional advantages have not been measurable in all studies.[2] The subvastus surgical approach is really a matter of surgeon preference, an issue more of style than substantive advantage.

Not all knees can be exposed easily with the subvastus approach. The obese, stiff, or muscular knee is more amenable to standard arthrotomies. It has been said that badly deformed knees are poor candidates for this approach. The author would disagree. The bad valgus knee is usually quite supple with a patella that everts easily. The bad varus knee will yield to any approach more readily if a medial release is incorporated into the approach so that the tibia can be externally rotated, repositioning the tubercle laterally, making it easier to evert the patella. The subvastus approach, though feasible for revision surgery, is not the best choice.

The steps described in this chapter describe a personal adaptation of the technique.[3] These are neither the only published description nor the only possible. Much of this technique inevitably borrows from other surgeons. The subvastus arthrotomy is applicable to many types of arthroplasty surgery with the exception of a lateral compartment unicompartmental replacement. If a medial unicompartmental replacement is planned, then the lateral meniscus should not be detached anteriorly as is described in Figure 15.17. The steps are executed so that a minimum number of instrument changes are required. In short, everything should be accomplished that can be, before time is expended asking for new instruments.

Dissection against bone that will dull knife blades should be the least step before the scalpel is laid down for different instruments. The steps described next can be completed in 3 to 5 minutes.

1. Cutaneous landmarks (Fig. 15.1). It is useful to identify the patella and the tibial tubercle to guide the skin incision. A poorly placed incision may stretch and compromise the skin. It will hamper exposure of the joint for the duration of the surgery.

2. Incision (Fig. 15.2). With fingers on the tubercle, incise the skin from a point proximal and lateral to the knee, over the patella ending about a centimeter medial to the tibial tubercle. It is wise to keep the incision off the tubercle for two reasons: (1) Healing is compromised over prominent subcutaneous bones, such as the olecranon in the elbow, and (2) incisions directly over the tubercle inevitably lie directly over and jeopardize the patellar tendon, essential to the arthroplasty.

The incision originates laterally to create a smaller lateral skin and subcutaneous flap that facilitates eversion of the patella. When the incision lies straight down the center of the knee, the lateral skin flap may well be stretched when the patella is everted. This is particularly true in the obese patient in whom it may lead to skin necrosis.

3. The medial skin flap (Fig. 15.3). Although there is generally reluctance to create any flap in the exposure of the knee for arthroplasty surgery, the medial side tolerates this well. The medial flap is neither stretched nor everted. This flap is dissected with a scalpel or scissors, establishing a plane that keeps the light fascial layer with the skin flap because it is a source of circulation to the skin.

4. Lifting up the vastus medialis (Fig. 15.4). The deeper layer of this dissection is more safely developed with a finger, given the contents of the subsartorial (Hunter's canal) at this level. When the medial border of the vastus medialis is palpable, the finger should be driven forcefully against the medial femur and under the muscle. The muscle edge can be lifted up, revealing the relatively thin capsule and synovium on the medial part of the suprapatellar pouch. This sets the stage for the arthrotomy itself. With a little care, there will be two well-defined edges of capsule that are available for a synovial closure at the completion of the arthroplasty. (The arthrotomy is "L shaped" as indicated by the dotted line.)

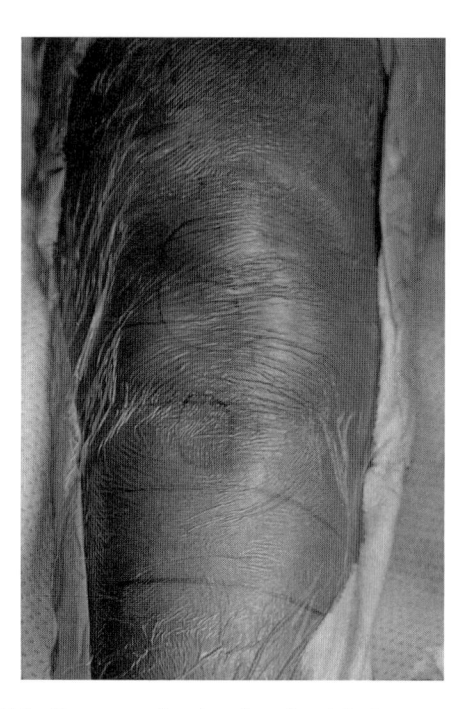

Figure 15.1. Cutaneous landmarks of a right knee, prepped for arthroplasty. (The top of the photo is proximal.) The distal portion of the incision should not lie on the tibial tubercle (small circle), but rather, just medial to it. Orient the proximal incision laterally as it crosses the patella (large circle) to facilitate eversion of the flap. The transverse lines on the skin facilitate approximation of the skin edges at the time of closure.

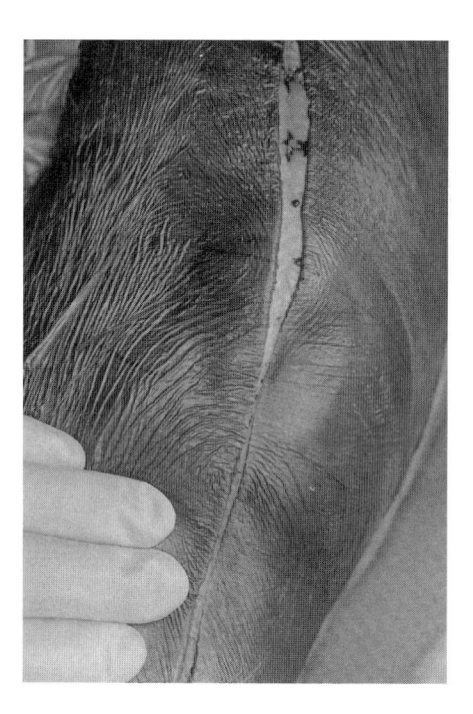

Figure 15.2. Incision. Fingers of the hand without the scalpel (here the left hand) protect the tubercle.

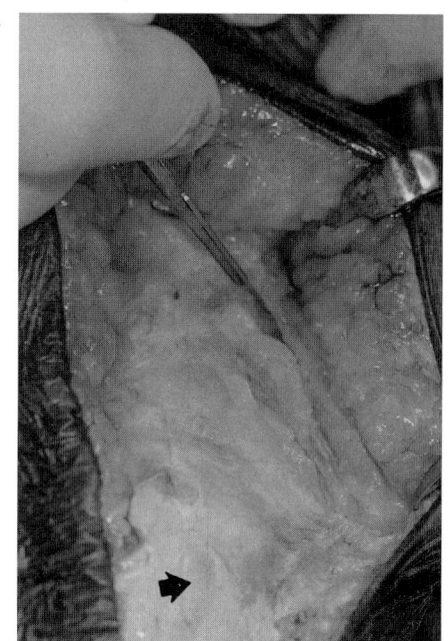

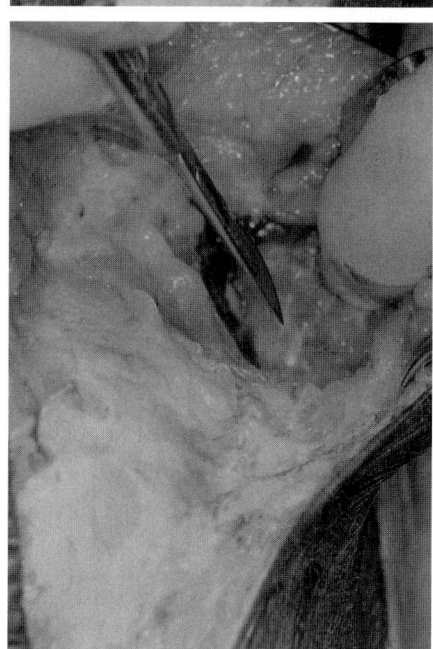

Figure 15.3. The medial skin flap, located here under a Langenbeck retractor, can be developed with a scalpel or scissors. The former is quicker and obviates the need to change instruments. (The pre-patellar bursa is apparent in the left lower quadrant of the figure at the arrow, and the quadriceps tendon is on the upper left quadrant.)

5. The medial limb of the arthrotomy (Fig. 15.5). The arthrotomy will be L shaped. An incision made from posterior to anterior through the capsule, across the medial femoral condyle, and up to the edge of the patella will release synovial fluid.

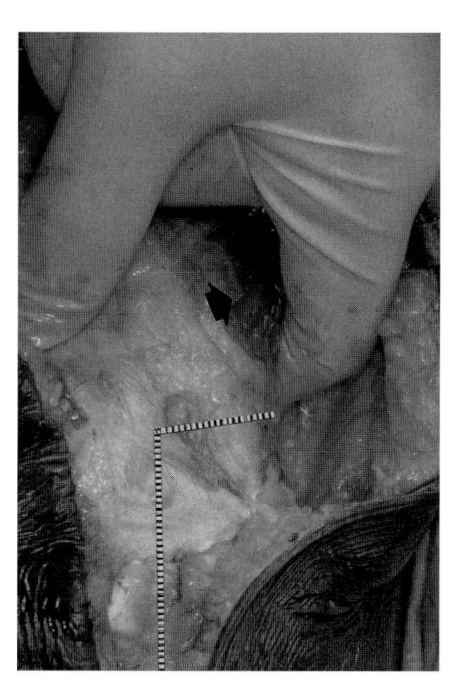

Figure 15.4. It is safer to plunge into the adductor canal with a fingertip rather than a sharp instrument. The fibers of the vastus medialis (arrow) can be seen between the thumb and forefinger in this figure. Lifting the muscle places the suprapatellar pouch under tension and facilitates creating the arthrotomy, which will be "L shaped" as indicated by the line.

6. Preserving the capsule for later closure (Fig. 15.6). If the index (second) finger is then inserted into the suprapatellar pouch through this arthrotomy and the third finger is placed on the other side of the capsule (outside and above the knee joint) superiorly, an edge of capsule will be grasped between the fingers. This will later be retrievable for the capsular closure.

7. Dividing the capsule of suprapatellar pouch (Fig. 15.7). The capsule should be cut across to the midline of the femur, with a scalpel, just under the dorsum of the fingers. Unless this part of the arthrotomy is performed, it will not be possible to evert the patella.

8. The lower limb of the arthrotomy (Fig. 15.8). The lower or vertical limb of the L-shaped arthrotomy begins at the anterior end of the transverse incision. The lower incision proceeds along the medial border of the patella, within a centimeter of the medial border of the patellar tendon and down onto the anterior tibia. Drive the knife blade hard into the bone of the anterior tibia (shown in Fig. 15.8) and respect this well-defined line. Too often, surgeons elevate the medial capsule with a series of parallel knife strokes that create multiple ribbons of soft tissue that cannot be used in the closure. If the knee has a varus deformity that will require a for-

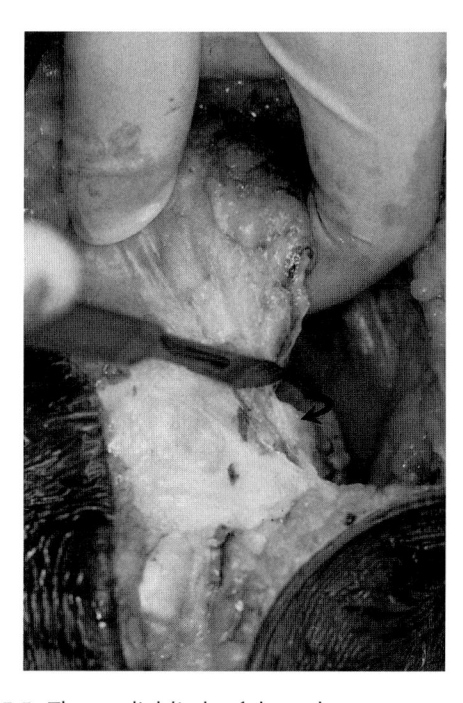

Figure 15.5. The medial limb of the arthrotomy crosses the medial femoral condyle (curved arrow) and runs to the medial edge of the patella.

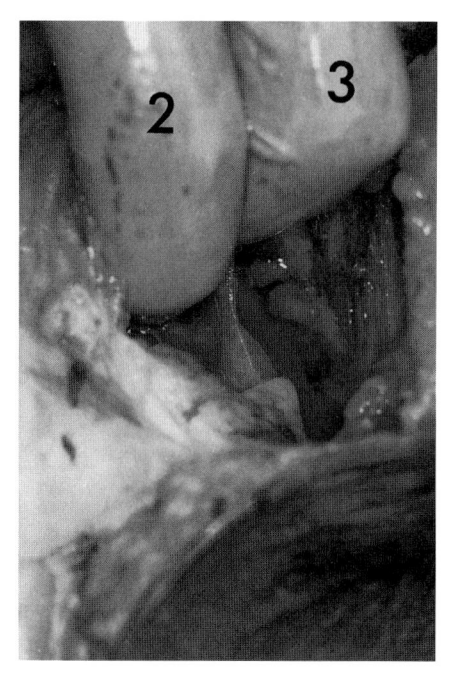

Figure 15.6. The suprapatellar pouch can be preserved for a better, synovial closure at the completion of the surgery. By placing the index (second) finger into the suprapatellar pouch (numeral 2), and the third finger (numeral 3) above the pouch, an edge of tissue is preserved between the two digits, ready for closure. Otherwise, this somewhat flimsy tissue is difficult to find and re-approximate at the time of closure.

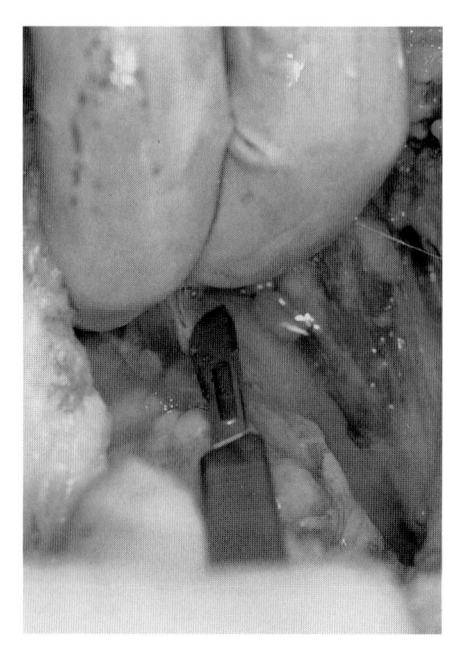

Figure 15.7. The suprapatellar pouch is divided with a scalpel, across to the midline or the patella will not evert easily.

mal medial release, this tissue will be tight to close at best and at worse, uncloseable.

9. Elevating the medial capsule from the tibia (Fig. 15.9). Start to elevate the medial capsule at its superior and lateral tip, using sharp dissection to develop a tri-

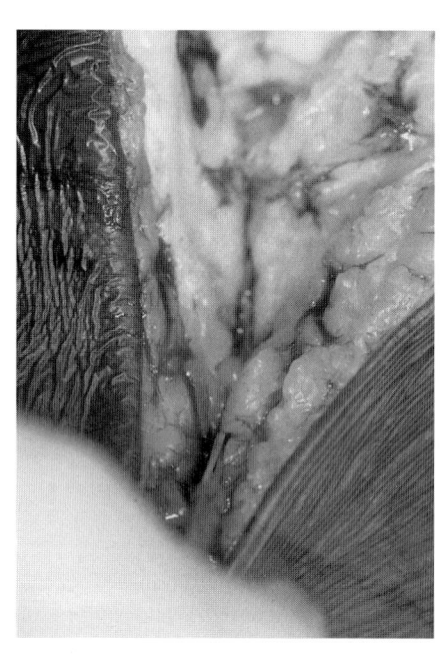

Figure 15.8. The distal limb of the arthrotomy is created at right angles to the horizontal limb on the medial side of the patella tendon. The knife should be driven hard through the periosteum over the anterior tibia and all the soft tissue elevated as a single sleeve. This provides for later closure.

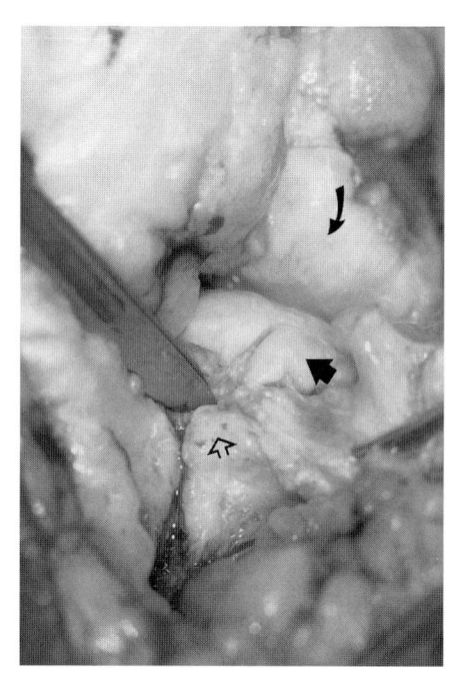

Figure 15.9. The medial femoral condyle (curved arrow) and anterior tibia with osteophytes (solid dark arrow) are apparent here. Start to elevate the medial capsular tissue (open arrow) with a sharp dissection at the apex of its attachment. Some tension will be required on the flap with forceps.

angular flap. The goal is to create a solid, intact flap of periosteum that will be available to close. Before taking the time to change instruments, use the scalpel under the patellar tendon, as shown in Figure 15.10. The blade will have dulled somewhat with the incision along the tibia, but it remains sharp enough for the flimsy fat pad.

10. Separate the patellar tendon from the anterior tibia (Fig. 15.10). Several maneuvers facilitate eversion of the patella, which must be accomplished without threatening the integrity of the extensor mechanism. Lift the patella straight up off the anterior femur with two flexed fingers, without pulling the extensor mechanism off to the lateral side. With the knee fully extended it will be easy to separate the fat pad from the anterior tibia. Introduce the scalpel blade against the anterior tibia, immediately proximal to the junction of the tendon and the tubercle, with the sharp edge directed proximally. Penetrate to the lateral border of the patellar tendon. Sweep the blade proximally, away from the attachment of the patellar tendon. With the patellar tendon free to twist, the patella will evert more easily.

11. Elevate the medial capsule (Fig. 15.11). A key elevator efficiently raises a smooth flap of medial capsule. If used with a small mallet, discrete amounts of force can be directed to the tissue, without the risk of forcing, slipping, and plunging. The medial collateral ligament, situated farther around the corner of the tibia is really

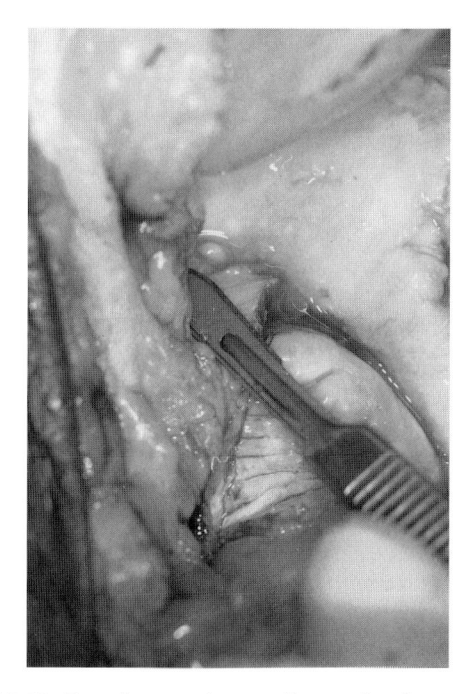

Figure 15.10. Free the anterior patellar tendon from the anterior tibia and fat pad. Cut up and away from the tubercle to avoid damage to the extensor mechanism. See where the initial sharp dissection of the apex of the medial tissue has left a series of parallel knife marks. We want a smoother separation of periosteum from bone for the rest of this dissection.

a consolidation of the medial capsule layers, which at this location are neither as thick nor as strong as the "ligament" itself.

Remember at this stage that the fibers to be elevated are oriented vertically, free proximally, and attached distally. Orient the elevator accordingly, so that it becomes a wedge, driven between the soft periosteum and the bone.

12. Remove the medial osteophytes (Fig. 15.12). With a triangle of tissue freed from the tibia, reorient the elevator, pointing proximally, with its sharp edge under the osteophytes, if present, on the edge of the tibia. Sharp mallet blows break them off, freeing the medial soft tissues nicely. Continue this more medially, at least to the mid-coronal line. Irrespective of the deformity of the knee, elevate the most proximal attachment of the deep medial collateral ligament from the tibia. When exposing a varus knee, for which a medial release is anticipated, by all means continue this elevation around the posteromedial corner, detaching the semimembranosus insertion. This medial release enables you to externally rotate the tibia at the moment of flexion and patellar eversion. External rotation places the tubercle more laterally and facilitates exposure. (Spare the attachment of the per anserinus, except in the most severe varus deformities.)

13 and 14. Tricks for the difficult exposure. What if the patella will not evert easily and safely? Above all

Figure 15.11. A smoother elevation of the bulk of the medial capsule, and in the varus knee, of the deep medial collateral ligament can be accomplished with a periosteal elevator and a small mallet. (The arrow indicates the medial tibia.)

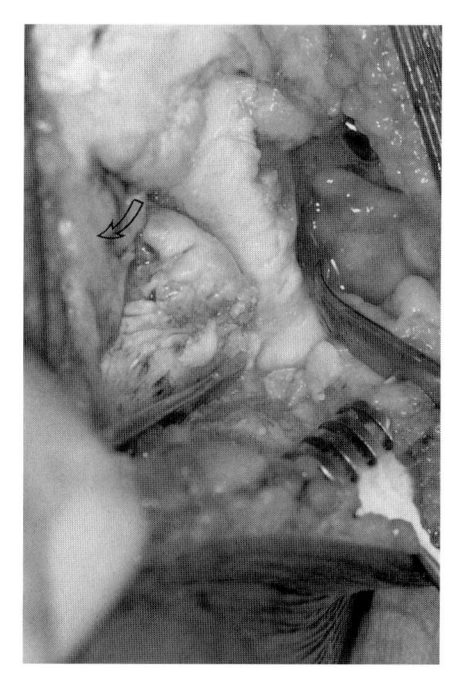

Figure 15.12. Once the medial capsule has been elevated, there may be osteophytes present. These can be knocked off of the proximal tibia by sharp blows to the elevator that is oriented proximally. (The arrow indicates the patellar tendon.)

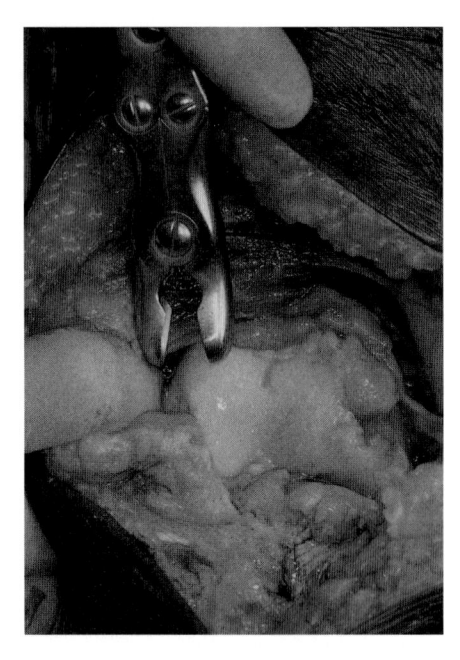

Figure 15.13. If the patella is difficult to evert, consider using a rongeur to remove osteophytes and some of the articular cartilage of the lateral femoral condyle.

else, be patient. At times, it is difficult to hold the patella everted even with the knee in full extension. With a large rongeur, nibble the cartilage and small amounts of bone off of the anterior aspect of the lateral femoral condyle, precisely where the patella rests against the femur (Fig. 15.13). By decreasing the prominence of the lateral condyle and eliminating the slippery cartilage, the patella will evert more easily, and rest firmly on the exposed cancellous bone (Fig. 15.14).

If the knee is still difficult to evert, push a thumb proximally at the far posterior edge of the vastus medialis between the muscle and the subcutaneous layer. This will be directly in the vicinity of the major vessels and nerves. Check also that the transverse arthrotomy in the superior part of the suprapatellar pouch extends far enough to the lateral side, so that the entire extensor mechanism can twist and sublux laterally. Now, the patella should evert in full extension, but it may slip back as you try to flex the knee. Keep the patella everted with the thumb of one hand and place the other hand on the foot. You may need an assistant to place a hand behind the knee and gently induce flexion, while you maintain the patella eversion and while you firmly externally rotate the foot to drive the tubercle laterally.

If the patella still flips back out of the everted position, make a mental note not to try this surgical approach again on a patient who is as muscular, obese, or tight as this patient. The other maneuvers that are available now effectively negate most of the advantages of this approach.

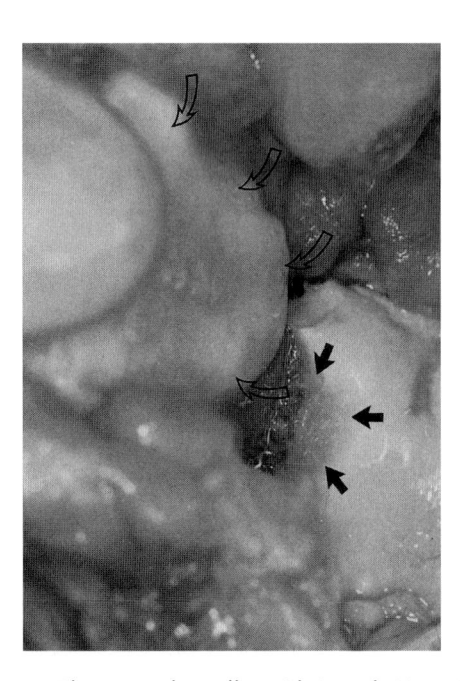

Figure 15.14. The everted patella, with its arthritic articular surface held under the surgeon's thumb on the left of this photo (white curved arrows), will lodge on the lateral femoral condyle where osteophytes and residual cartilage have been removed with the rongeur (solid dark arrows).

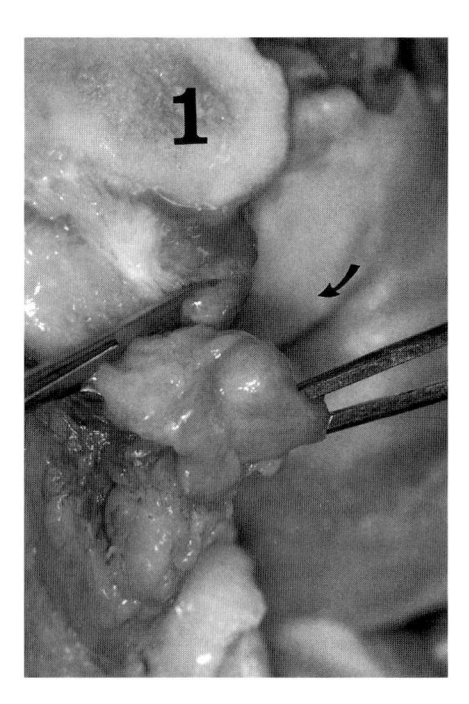

Figure 15.15. Four final steps with scalpel and forceps are performed with the knee flexed and the patella everted laterally. The first step is to reduce the size of the patellar fat pad. (Patella is at "1.") With some of the fat pad out of the way, it is easier to see the posterior femoral condyle (femoral condyle at curved arrow), which helps to ensure correct rotational position of the femoral component.

A complete lateral patellar retinacular release may be useful, enabling the patella to evert more easily. An extension of the arthrotomy through the tendon of the vastus medialis, superior to the patella can be performed. This converts the subvastus approach largely to a medial parapatellar arthrotomy with the disadvantage of an extra flap created under the medial soft tissues. The author has been reluctant to extend the incision any farther than this, converting it into a quadriceps snip or patellar turndown. The ultimate maneuver for a difficult exposure would be a tibial tubercle osteotomy, tedious but preferable to damaging the extensor mechanism.

15 (Fig. 15.15). Four final steps with scalpel and forceps. First the patellar fast pad. Once the knee has been safely flexed, pick up the scalpel and forceps once more. Four small steps now avail the knee completely for arthroplasty.

First, debride the patellar fat pad sufficiently so that the posterior lateral condyle can be seen fully. This is important to ensure correct rotational positioning of the femoral component.

16 (Fig. 15.16). The anterior cruciate ligament. Divide the anterior cruciate ligament, which enables the tibia to translate forward, revealing the tibial surface more completely.

17 (Fig. 15.17). The lateral meniscus. Separate the anterior attachment of the lateral meniscus so that it can reflect to the lateral side when a retractor is in-

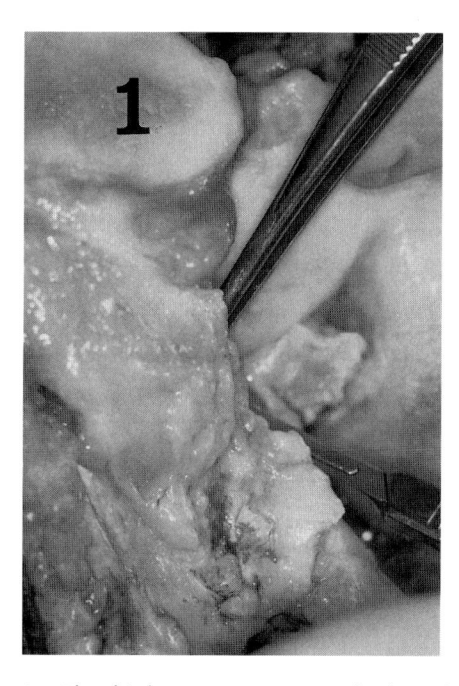

Figure 15.17. The third step is to separate the lateral meniscus from its anterior attachment. (The patella is seen at the figure "1," but the lateral meniscus itself is obscured behind the fat pad in this photo.) This facilitates eversion of the patella. The entire meniscus can be better and more completely removed at a later step in the procedure.

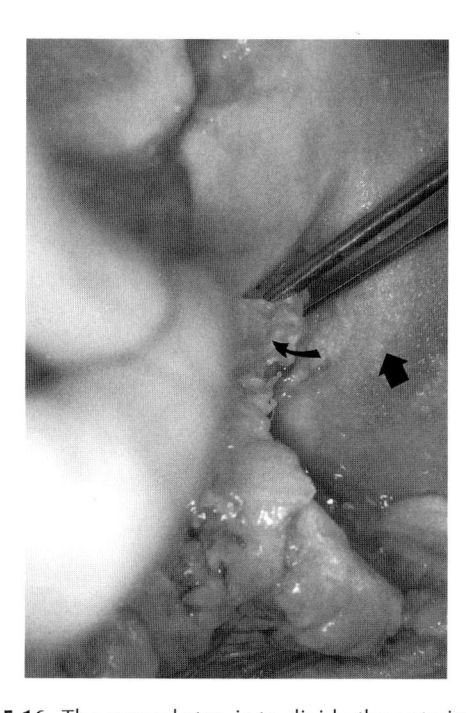

Figure 15.16. The second step is to divide the anterior cruciate ligament (curved arrow), which enables the tibia to translate forward, revealing the tibial plateau more completely. (The solid arrow indicates an arthritic medial femoral condyle.)

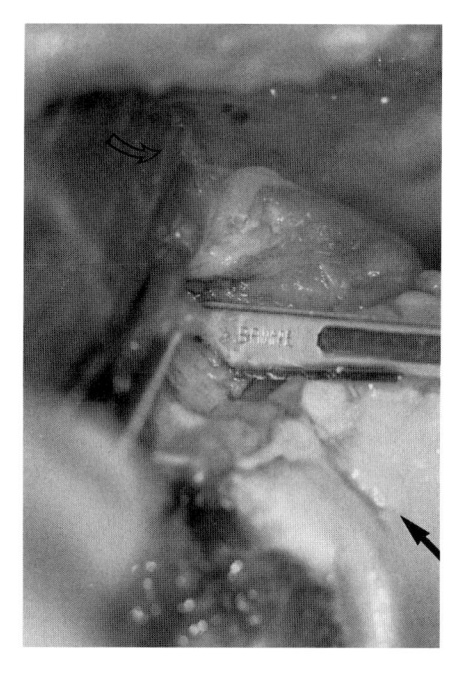

Figure 15.18. The fourth step exposes the anterior femur by cutting down through all soft tissue in the supracondylar area over the anterior femur. (The dark arrow indicates anterior femoral trochlear groove; border of everted vastus medialis is apparent at open arrow.) Elevate a triangle of soft tissue on either side of this incision. Better visualization prevents notching of the femur in this area, enhances rotational positioning, and avoids a prominent position of the femoral component.

serted under the extensor mechanism. It will become easier to resect the entire meniscus later, when it becomes more accessible.

18. The anterior femur (Fig. 15.18). Expose the anterior femur so that instruments and trial components can be placed accurately. Good visualization avoids *supracondylar* notches, unappealing flexed, internally rotated, and prominent positions of the femoral component. Incise the fat and periosteum firmly, driving the knife onto the bone longitudinally down the anterior femur for about 3 cm above the articular surface. A triangle of tissue can be elevated on either side of this incision. Some surgeons, fearing adhesion of the quadriceps tendon to the exposed bone, may resist this step or prefer to close the elevated flap over the bone. This fear is unfounded in an arthroplasty that mechanically permits adequate flexion.

References

1. Hofman AA, Plaster RL, Murdock LE. Subvastus (Southern) approach for primary total knee arthroplasty. *Clin Orthop*. 1991; 269:70–77.
2. Ritter MA, Keating EM. Comparison of two anterior medial approaches to total knee arthroplasty. *Am J Knee Surgery*. 1990; 3:168–171.
3. Vince K. The subvastus surgical approach to the knee for arthroplasty surgery. In: Insall JN, Scott N, eds. *Insall Scott's VideoBook of Knee Surgery*. New York: J.B. Lippincott; 1992.

CHAPTER 16
Midvastus Approach

Gerard A. Engh

INTRODUCTION

The midvastus muscle-splitting approach to the knee is different from the medial parapatellar and the subvastus approaches in that it involves opening an interval in the midsubstance of the vastus medialis muscle (Fig. 16.1). The stabilizing contribution of an intact extensor mechanism above the patella is maintained by preserving the portion of the vastus medialis that inserts into the quadriceps tendon. Complete eversion and lateral displacement of the patella are not inhibited by the portion of the vastus medialis that attaches along the medial side of the patella. The extraosseous blood supply is not likely to be compromised with this surgical approach, because the supreme genicular artery is generally avoided.

INDICATIONS AND CONTRAINDICATIONS

The midvastus muscle-splitting approach is routinely used as our approach of choice for total knee arthroplasty in all patients who have at least 90 degrees of knee flexion and are undergoing elective total knee arthroplasty. Patients with less than 90 degrees of knee flexion should be approached through a midline or a medial parapatellar approach (Fig. 16.2). A quadriceps or rectus snip can then be performed to improve exposure. Excessive weight is not a contraindication to the midvastus approach. This approach also provides excellent surgical exposure in both varus and valgus knee deformities.

Revision surgery can also be performed through a midvastus surgical approach. Again, more than 90 degrees of knee flexion would eliminate the need for a quadriceps snip. An ideal patient for a midvastus approach in a revision would be a person with excellent knee flexion who underwent a primary knee arthroplasty through a midvastus approach. If exposure is compromised with a midvastus approach the incision is easily extended cephalad along the medial border of the quadriceps tendon. If necesssary, a quadriceps snip could then be performed.

SURGICAL TECHNIQUE

The midvastus muscle-splitting approach is performed through a standard anterior midline skin incision. This incision is best performed with the knee in flexion, which applies tension to the skin and retracts the skin margins as the incision is made. The incision is carried down directly through the adipose tissue and deep fascia lata. The fascia is opened downward over the aponeurosis of the vastus medialis along the medial border of the patella. The deep fascia is divided to the distal end of the tibial tubercle, where the periosteum is incised just medial to the patellar tendon insertion.

The muscle-splitting part of the approach is performed first. A subfascial layer is opened far enough to expose the vastus medialis and its insertion into the quadriceps tendon and the medial aspect of the patella. The superomedial border of the patella is identified with the knee in flexion and the vastus medialis is parallel to the muscle fibers. The full thickness of the muscle is opened over a distance of 4 to 5 cm ending at the superomedial corner of the patella (Fig. 16.1). With this incision, the capsule is entered above the patella. The quadriceps tendon is not incised. A well-defined muscular aponeurosis is noted on the deep but not on the superficial surface of the vastus medialis muscle. The extracapsular adipose tissue that fills the suprapatellar pouch often herniates between the muscle fibers.

Next the capsular portion of the approach is per-

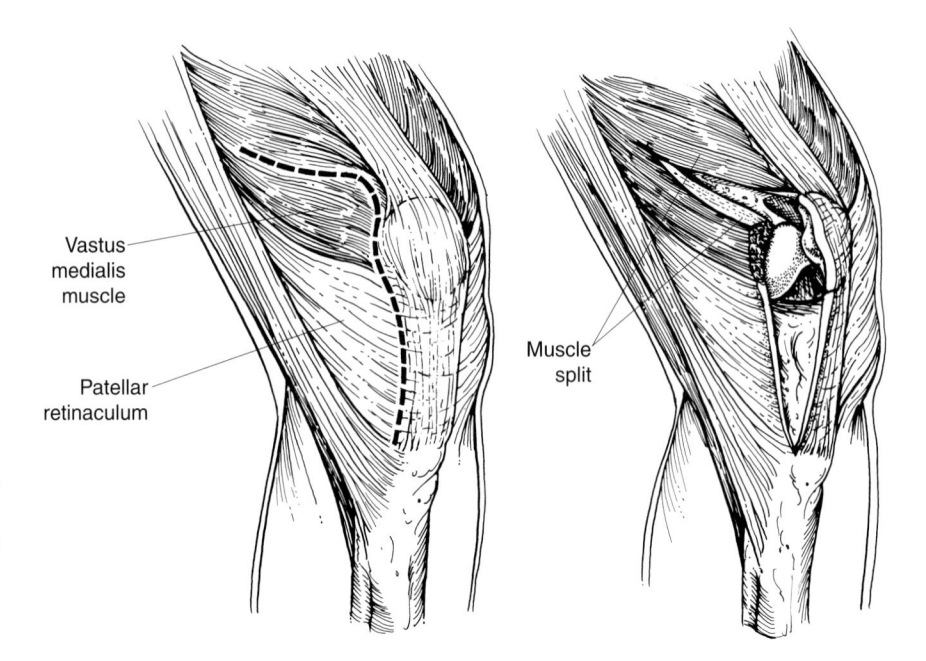

Figure 16.1. The midvastus muscle-splitting approach splits the vastus medialis parallel with its fibers. The muscle-splitting portion extends from the superomedial pole of the patella 4 to 5 cm into the muscle.

formed by carrying the capsular opening at the superomedial border of the patella distally, releasing the muscular insertion of the vastus medialis and the medial joint capsule from the medial side of the patella. A cuff of soft tissue attached to the patella is preserved for later capsular repair. The capsule and synovium of the knee are reflected medially to the coronal midline of the tibia and laterally to the medial border of the tibial tubercle. This is performed subperiosteally with a cautery or with sharp dissection, and should continue until the retropatellar bursa directly behind the superior aspect of the patellar tendon insertion is entered. A drop of clear yellow fluid is characteristically encountered when the bursa is entered. The most medial fibers of the patellar tendon may need to be released to adequately evert the patella and gain full exposure to the lateral tibial plateau. It is important not to release more than one-quarter of the patellar tendon from the tibial tubercle. This precaution will avoid jeopardizing the integrity of the tendon.

Capsular folds of the suprapatellar pouch are released to aid eversion of the patella. The surgeon completes exposure of the knee by everting the patella and dividing the lateral patellofemoral ligament. A portion

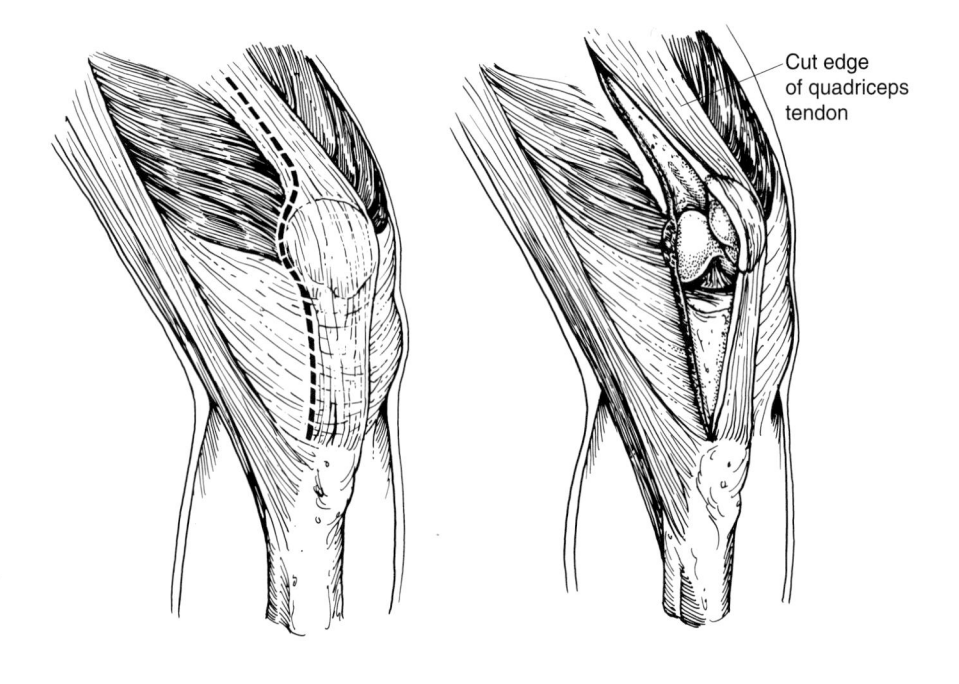

Figure 16.2. The medial parapatellar approach splits the medial aspect of the quadriceps tendon.

of the fat pad is excised and the joint capsule is reflected until the lateral tibial plateau is fully visible.

At wound closure, the muscle-splitting portion of the midvastus approach is not sutured with wound closure. The muscle approximates well after repair of the medial joint capsule and patellar retinaculum. The majority of the vastus medialis, including the entire portion of the muscle inserting into the quadriceps tendon, remains intact with this surgical approach. No portion of the quadriceps tendon should be entered if the midvastus approach is properly performed.

NEUROVASCULAR ANATOMY OF THE VASTUS MEDIALIS

In the words of Abbott and Carpenter, "The operating surgeon should be so familiar with the anatomy that he can plan his own approach, basing it upon the anatomical accessibility of the lesion. This fundamental knowledge of anatomy is most important in the surgery of bones and joints."[1] The point where the vastus medialis inserts into the superomedial border of the patella is a safe location for a muscle-splitting incision. The vastus medialis muscle is innervated by terminal branches of the saphenous nerve.[2] The saphenous nerve branches from the femoral nerve and courses deep in the vastus, close to its origin along the medial intermuscular septum. The midvastus approach splits the muscle fibers near the insertion of the vastus into the extensor mechanism, well away from the terminal branches of the saphenous nerve. We performed Cybex muscle strength testing on a comparative group of patients operated on through midvastus or medial parapatellar surgical approaches. At the six-week follow-up interval, there was no significant difference in quadriceps muscle strength between the two groups although the midvastus group was slightly stronger.[3]

The medial superior genicular artery is distal to the region of the vastus medialis where the midvastus incision splits the muscle. The medial superior genicular artery branches from the popliteal artery. It courses from the back of the knee deep to the tendon of the adductor magnus and divides into two branches. One of these branches supplies the vastus medialis, before anastomosing with the highest genicular artery medial to the patella.[2] Terminal small branches of these genicular branches are occasionally encountered in the muscle-splitting part of a midvastus surgical approach.

The highest genicular (descending genicular) artery arises from the femoral artery and divides into saphenous and musculoarticular branches. The musculoarticular branch descends in the substance of the vastus medialis to the medial side of the knee, where it anastomoses with the medial superior genicular artery and anterior recurrent tibial artery. A branch crosses above the patellar surface, forming an anastomotic arch with the lateral superior genicular artery, supplying branches to the knee joint.[2] This branch is routinely divided with a quadriceps tendon-splitting incision, but is proximal to the muscle-splitting part of a midvastus approach.[1,4]

EVOLUTION OF THE MIDVASTUS APPROACH

Medial parapatellar and midline surgical approaches have been advocated for total knee arthroplasty because of familiarity, simplicity, and the excellent exposure achieved for bone preparation and component placement.[1] The excellent surgical exposure achieved is due in part to the destabilizing effect of detaching the medial side of the quadriceps tendon from the patella. Obese patients and those with limited knee flexion may require the additional release of medial fibers of the patellar tendon where the fibers insert into the tibial tubercle. Patients with severely restricted knee motion may require further relaxation of the extensor mechanism by transversely dividing the quadriceps tendon near its proximal origin to the rectus femoris muscle ("quadriceps snip"). This further destabilizes the patellofemoral articulation.

Before 1991, a medial parapatellar approach was our standard approach for knee arthroplasty. The quadriceps tendon was routinely divided in its medial one-third by staying a constant distance from the vastus medialis insertion. Exposure was excellent, but patellar maltracking frequently required a lateral retinacular release. Patellofemoral instability was further increased if we failed to recognize the junction between rectus and vastus as the muscles insert into the quadriceps tendon. The fibers of the rectus femoris muscle insert more distally on the medial side of the quadriceps tendon. If the incision inadvertently follows the rectus rather than the vastus musculotendonous junction, the quadriceps tendon is partially divided at its proximal end, akin to a quadriceps or rectus snip.

Recovery of quadriceps muscle control was another problem we often encountered with the medial parapatellar approach. Many patients with a standard parapatellar approach required three or four days to regain enough quadriceps strength to perform an independent straight leg raise. Our theory was that the incision into the quadriceps mechanism was responsible for this problem. A quicker recovery of quadriceps function that occurred when we subsequently used a subvastus or midvastus muscle-splitting approach confirmed this hypothesis.

We performed a prospective clinical study comparing the subvastus surgical approach to a standard medial parapatellar approach in 1991.[5] With the subvastus approach, an improvement in postoperative quadriceps function and reduction of pain was apparent.[5,6] In addition, we noted a marked reduction in the need for lateral retinacular releases. However, surgical exposure for performing a total knee arthroplasty, as reported by others, was compromised in patients with (1) limited preoperative flexion, (2) excessive weight over 200 pounds, (3) revision total knee arthroplasty, (4) a previous major arthrotomy, or (5) a prior high tibial osteotomy.[5]

We abandoned the subvastus approach because of the unpredictability of achieving satisfactory surgical exposure for TKA. Our standard approach became a modification of the medial parapatellar approach. Rather than splitting the quadriceps tendon, we detached the vastus medialis muscle along the medial border of the quadriceps tendon. This modification of a medial parapatellar approach provided a more rapid recovery of quadriceps strength when compared to a tendon-splitting incision. Patellofemoral stability improved and surgical exposure was excellent with this modification. However, surgical repair of muscle fibers to tendon was less secure and more difficult than repair of a split tendon.

The midvastus approach evolved as a means of achieving the excellent surgical exposure of conventional surgical approaches with the improvement in extensor mechanism function demonstrated with the subvastus approach and with our modified approach. Initially we opened the knee in extension for the muscle-splitting part of a midvastus exposure, but gradually found the surgical technique easier with the knee in the flexed position.

SURGICAL EXPERIENCE

We first investigated the midvastus muscle-splitting approach in a prospective randomized study from April 1992 to April 1993.[3] There were 61 midvastus cases and 57 modified medial parapatellar exposures (described earlier). Both approaches gave excellent surgical exposure for primary total knee replacement surgery.[3] Patients rapidly recovered quadriceps function and had relatively minimal pain. Occasionally a patient developed fluid in the prepatellar bursa, but aspiration was not necessary because this fluid collection rapidly resolved. Aggressive use of a continuous passive motion device may have been responsible for the prepatellar fluid collection in such cases.

The midvastus approach, which was easier to perform, required less tissue dissection than did other approaches. Surgical closure did not require the tedious and precarious reattachment of muscle fibers to the quadriceps tendon. In addition operative time was minimized because of the simplified wound closure that did not involve repairing an incision along the quadriceps mechanism.

The midvastus muscle-splitting approach has not been previously described in standard texts or surgical approach manuals. This approach represents the culmination of efforts to achieve satisfactory exposure without compromising the stabilizing effects of an intact extensor mechanism. Since April 1993, all our primary knee arthroplasties have been performed through the midvastus approach, constituting over 500 total and unicompartmental knee replacements.

References

1. Abbott LC, Carpenter WF. Surgical approaches to the knee joint. *J Bone Joint Surg Am.* 1945; 27:277–310.
2. Gray H. *Anatomy of the Human Body.* Philadelphia: Lea & Febiger, 1959.
3. Engh GA, Holt BT, Parks NL. A midvastus muscle-splitting approach for total knee arthroplasty. *J Arthroplasty.* 1996; in press.
4. Insall JN. *Surgery of the Knee.* New York: Churchill Livingstone; 1984.
5. Knezevich S, Engh GA, Preidis FE, et al. Comparison of subvastus quadriceps-sparing and standard anterior quadriceps-splitting approaches in total and unicompartmental knee arthroplasty. *Orthop Trans.* 1992; 16:101.
6. Hofmann AA, Plaster RL, Murdock LE. Subvastus (Southern) approach for primary total knee arthroplasty. *Clin Orthop.* 1991; 269:70–77.

CHAPTER 17
The Trivector-Retaining Arthrotomy

Kenneth W. Bramlett, William N. Haller III,
and William D. Krauss

ABSTRACT

Patellofemoral complications occur in 5 to 30% of all total knee arthroplasty cases. Contemporary efforts to decrease this prevalence have focused on implant design, particularly the tracking of the patella in the patellofemoral groove. In addition, a lateral release is frequently recommended as a means of overcoming patellofemoral complications. However, the influence of the vector forces acting on the patella and the inadequacy of the standard parapatellar incision in preserving these vectors in their natural biomechanical function may require further explanation. Therefore, a reevaluation of the standard medial parapatellar exposure is offered and an arthrotomy retaining the major divisions of the trivector anatomy of the quadriceps tendon unit acting on the patella is provided. The trivector-retaining arthrotomy (TRA) technique provides extensile exposure for primary and revision TKA, while sparing the anatomic trivector arrangement of the vastus medialis, vastus intermedius, rectus femoris, and the vastus lateralis.

INTRODUCTION

Following total knee arthroplasty surgery, one of the most common noted complications is patellofemoral instability.[1–3] Patellofemoral complications occur in 5 to 30% of all total knee cases,[4] with the most common complications being subluxation,[1–3,5,6] component wear,[6] dislocations,[2,4,5] fractures,[3,5–9] and pain.[5,6] Numerous proposed causes of these complications include mechanical axis malalignment, inadequate soft tissue balancing, tibiofemoral component malrotation, and tilted patella implantation.[6,10] Grace and Rand[11] suggested the four most common causes of patella instability following TKA surgery were prosthetic design, quadriceps imbalance, surgical technique (most common), and trauma. Merkow and associates[4] supported this belief, suggesting that surgical technique, including inadequate soft tissue balancing and prosthetic malposition and malignment, was the most predominant cause. According to Moreland and colleagues, malalignment of the quadriceps muscle system is the most common cause of patella dislocation or subluxation. Several authors[2,4,12,13] have advocated the use of a lateral release for maltracking the patella and an extensive vastus medialis oblique (VMO) advancement and imbrication,[14] if the implantation alignment alone was ineffective.

The most commonly utilized incision to gain exposure during a TKA is the medial parapatellar arthrotomy (Fig. 17.1). The actual clinical application of the traditional medial parapatellar arthrotomy splits the quadriceps tendon in a variable manner. The standard parapatellar arthrotomy is a curvilinear incision beginning at the apex of the quadriceps tendon proper down its midline to the patella superior pole. It is then extended inferiorly around the radius of the patella along the medial border to its inferior pole and downward to the tibial tubercle (Fig. 17.1). Alternate applications extend the initial incision of the quadriceps tendon across the midline into the vastus lateralis musculotendinous insertion or even transversely if increased exposure is necessary. In each of these parapatellar variations, the transection of the quadriceps tendon across the midline diminishes the natural stabilizing forces acting on the patella, and in some cases, patella tracking is distorted.

A surgical option to the medial parapatellar arthrotomy is the trivector-retaining arthrotomy (TRA), which provides a standardized extensile exposure while maintaining and preserving the critical trivector-stabilizing forces of the vastus medialis, vastus intermedialis, and vastus lateralis on the patella. Early results of our use of this approach were first published by Fu in his text *Knee Surgery* in 1994.[15] The purpose of this chapter is to further explicate the trivector-retaining arthrotomy technique and to discuss the clinical outcome of this technique on primary, unicondylar, and revision total knee arthroplasty patients.

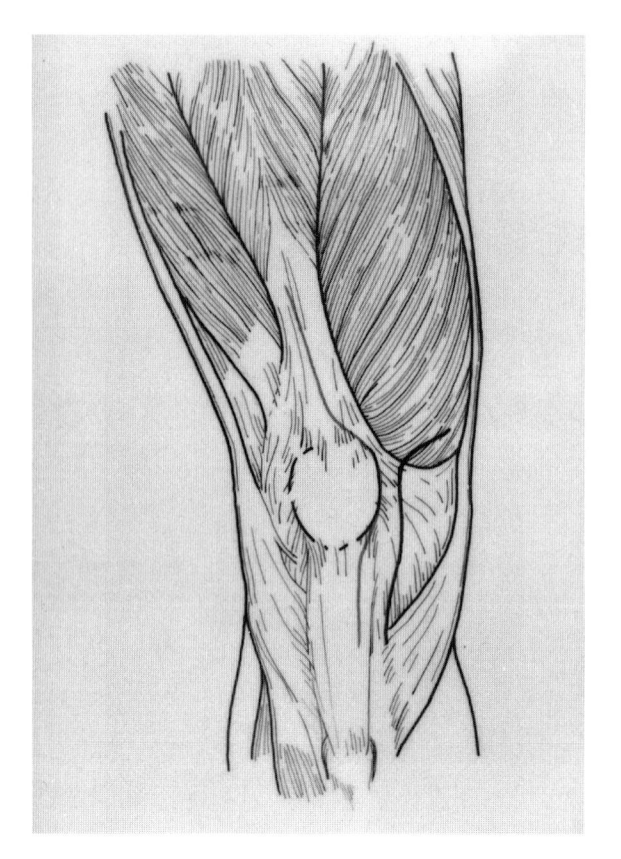

Figure 17.1. Common knee arthroplasty exposure techniques: (A) Red: medial parapatellar; (B) Blue: subvastus.

MATERIALS AND METHODS

Surgical Technique

The trivector-retaining arthrotomy (TRA) technique begins with a transection of the VMO fibers 1.5 to 2 cm medial to the medial border of the quadriceps tendon proper, three finger breadths above the superior pole of the patella (Fig. 17.2). The arthrotomy is extended directly inferiorly 1 cm medial to the patella border and 1 cm medial to the patella tendon to the level of the tibial tubercle (Figs. 17.2 and 17.3). The benefit of this arthrotomy is the reproducibility of the exposure despite previous surgeries or severe varus or valgus deformities.

In this series, a routine midline skin incision was performed for each of the total knee arthroplasty surgeries. The straight skin incision was made four finger breadths above and below the patella and extended through to the quadriceps and retinacular fascia. The well-defined triangular tendon insertion of the rectus femoris with the three separate vasti muscle groups was easily visualized, normally above the patella. The trivector-retaining arthrotomy was then made three finger breadths above the superior pole of the patella with the knee at 90 to 110 degrees of flexion if possible. A straight arthrotomy incision was performed 1.5 cm medial to the insertion of the vastus medialis into the quadriceps tendon proper. It was extended inferiorly in a straight line, passing 1 cm from the medial patellar border to the level of the tibial tubercle (Fig. 17.3). In revision cases, the same technique was also used despite expected fibrosis and anatomical distortion of the quadriceps tendon. A tourniquet was used in all cases, and it was released prior to closure to confirm hemostatic control.

The incision is most effectively closed to reproduce the normal anatomic configuration with the knee in 115 degrees of flexion. Our preference is to begin the arthrotomy closure using a 0-nylon inverted figure of eight sutures starting at the inferior pole of the patella. These sutures are placed in a proximal to distal direction for approximately 1 inch. At this point 0-absorbable running suture is then placed from the inferior pole of the patella to the most distal aspect of the incision and doubled back on itself. This assures a watertight closure of the inferior part of the incision. Finally the proximal two-thirds of the incision is closed with 0-nonabsorbable suture by reapproximating the undersurface fascia of the vastus medialis to the quadriceps tendon. The skin and subcutaneous tissue are closed in a routine manner.[16]

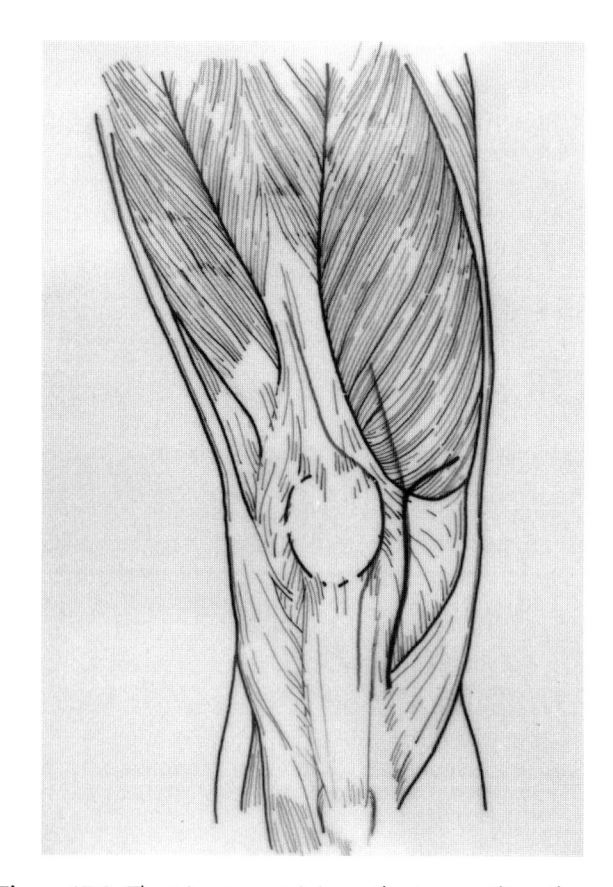

Figure 17.2. The trivector-retaining arthrotomy utilizes the optimal features of the (A) Red: standard parapatellar; (B) Blue: subvastus exposures allowing universal application; and (C) Brown: trivector exposure.

1) Flex knee 100 degrees.
2) Place Arthrotomy incision 3 finger breadths (approximately 3 cm) above patella; 1 finger breadth 1–2 cm medical to the Quad tendon border.
3) Extend incision above and below midline of patella approximately 8 cm, retaining a 1cm medical border to facilitate closure.
4) Closure is commonly performed at 100 degrees of flexion.

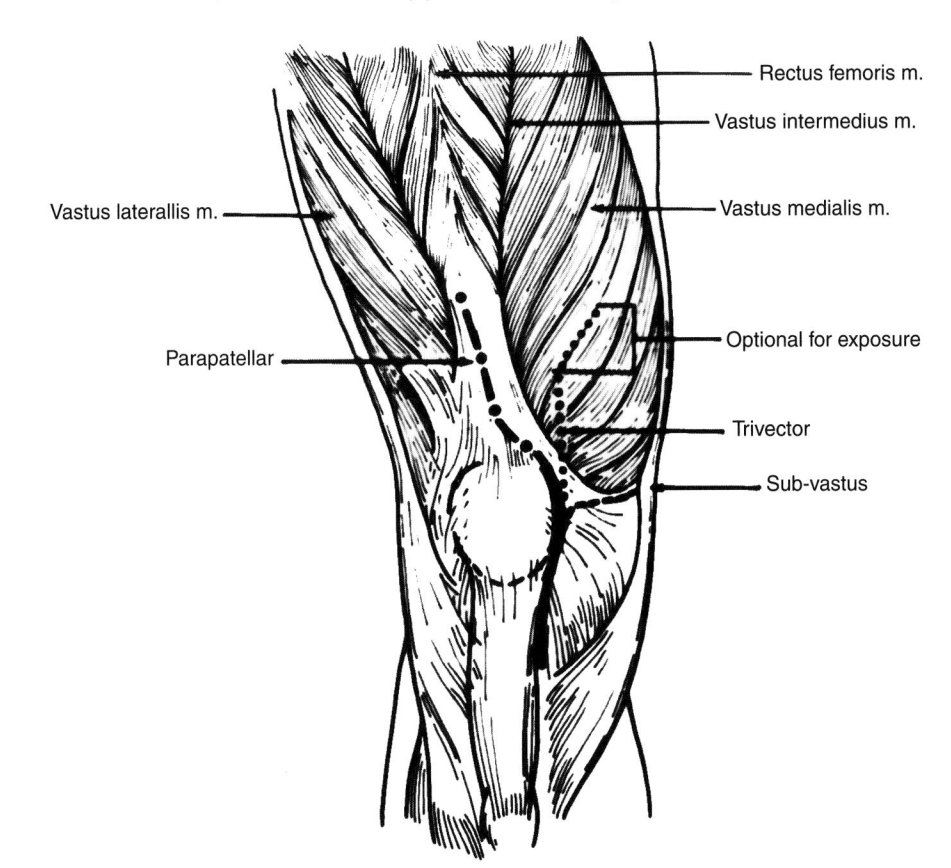

Figure 17.3. Surgical techniques for trivector arthrotomy exposure for knee surgery. Anatomic relationships reveal the benefit of a combined exposure with ease of possible extension if indicated.

Subjects

This surgical exposure technique was utilized on 234 consecutive total knee arthroplasties in a 33-month period from February 1991 to December 1993. The patient population consisted of 77 males and 157 females, and the mean age of the group was 68.5 (range 41 to 87). Of the 234 arthroplasties performed, 179 were primary arthroplasties, 23 revision arthroplasties, and 28 medial and 4 lateral unicondylar arthroplasties. The TRA technique was used during the initial exposure in each case. Five different implant designs were utilized on these patients based on templating, revision needs, ligament integrity, and physiological demands.

Once the TRA technique was executed, a complete synovectomy was performed, and patella eversion and posterior lateral exposure was possible. The subsequent ligamentous and bony procedures were completed and the prosthesis was implanted. Of the 234 patients, 224 received a hybrid fixation method and 10 were cementless.

Postoperative Management

Postoperatively, all patients began weight-bearing as tolerated (WBAT) ambulation activities on the first postoperative day. All patients received similar preoperative and postoperative treatment protocols based on ORTHOPC.A.C.E.™ practice management system. All patients were established on an independent rehabilitation program at the time of discharge. Each patient was reevaluated in the clinic at 10 to 14 days, 4 to 6 weeks, 3 months, 6 months, and one year following surgery and annually thereafter.

RESULTS

The average follow-up for these patients is 31.4 months. The ongoing follow-up for these patients ranges from approximately 1 to 4 years. The average hospital length of stay for the primary total knee group was 3.4 days, the revision total knee group was 3.6 days, and the unicondylar knee replacement group was 2.8 days. Three

Table 17.1. Summary of trivector knee arthroplasty results

Primary arthrotomy (n = 179)		Revision arthrotomy (n = 23)		Unicondylar arthrotomy (n = 32)	
Lateral Release	1	Lateral Release	4	Lateral Release	0
Tendon Rupture	0	Tendon Rupture	0	Tendon Rupture	0
Avulsion	0	Avulsion	1	Avulsion	0
Infection	1	Infection	0	Infection	0
Revision Patella	1	V-Y Quadraplasty	1	Revision	0
Subluxation Patella	1	Subluxation Patella	3	Subluxation Patella	0
Dislocation Patella	0	Dislocation Patella	0	Dislocation Patella	0
Patella Fracture	0	Patella Fracture	0	Patella Fracture	0
Reoperation	0	Reoperation	2	Reoperation	0

*Outcome follow-up on all procedure range from approximately 1 to 4 years.

patients (1.7%) who received a primary total knee and two (8.7%) who received a revision total knee were evaluated and found to require extended rehabilitation placement (ERP). None of the patients who received a unicondylar knee replacement required extended rehabilitation placement.

The complications due to the trivector-retaining arthrotomy technique are listed in Table 17.1. Clinical variance occurred in the revision group when one patella tendon avulsion occurred in a rheumatoid arthritic patient who had received prednisone therapy for 15 years. Three patients (13%) of the revision group exhibited 25 to 50% parital patellar subluxations; however, only one was symptomatic, and none have required surgery for patella instability. One patient who was referred required a V-Y advancement while undergoing a third revision. None of the patients in the primary, revision, or unicondylar replacement groups exhibited patellae dislocations, and none of the revision group required reoperation for patella instability.

Within the primary total knee group, there were no patellar tendon ruptures or avulsions, and only one patient exhibited symptomatic patella subluxation (0.1%). In the primary replacement group 2 of 179 (1.1%) received a lateral retinacular release. Three reoperations were required in this group, one for the repair of a synovial fistula and the other two following disruption of the posterior cruciate ligament resulting in posterior instability. These two cases were treated with one patient receiving a revision procedure to exchange the tibial polyethylene spacer with an anterior-lipped component, and in the other case, a posterior-stabilized knee was implanted.

Regarding the unicondylar group, one reoperation was required due to a traumatic fracture, but patella instability has not been observed or reported in any of the cases. There were no cases requiring a lateral retinacular release.

Overall in the three knee arthroplasty groups, one patient developed ischemia of the inferior skin flaps and required operation. Otherwise no vascular or nervous system complications have been reported. Two infections occurred in two primary cases who were diabetic patients, 9 months and 18 months postoperatively, and both have undergone revision procedures with no recurrence of infection. One patient developed a clinically proven deep venous thrombosis. One patient in the primary group required resurfacing of the nonresurfaced patella due to bone erosion and pain. No patient in the series has developed recurrent dynamic patella subluxation or patella dislocations. There have been no fractures, patella loosenings, prosthesis failures, or musculotendinous unit failures. None of the patients exhibited significant scarring of the medial quadriceps musculature, which restricted knee flexion or was a site for pain. Average range of motion for the primary group was 112 degrees, for the revision group 108 degrees, and for the unicondylar group 119 degrees.

With all of the above taken into account, the overall complication rate for patellofemoral disorders was less than 0.5%.

DISCUSSION

Advances in implant technology have aided in the continued success of total knee arthroplasty.[2] Several studies have documented 90% survival rate of prosthetic knee implants at 10 years following surgery;[17,18] however, the rate of extensor mechanism and/or patellofemoral joint complications have remained a concern.[4–6,10,11] Most patellofemoral joint dysfunction complications (70%) occur within the first eight weeks following prosthetic implantation.[1] This suggests that this complication occurs during the soft tissue challenge phase, and the surgeon and their technique are important.[1] Additionally, patellar complications following TKA appear directly related to a compromised residual medial vector force arising from the vastus medialis oblique due to the surgical technique or quadriceps (VMO) inhibition.[1]

In this series of 233 consecutive total knee arthroplasties using the trivector-retaining arthrotomy technique, the complication rate for patellofemoral disorders was less than 0.5% as compared to 5 to 30% seen historically with standard parapatellar arthrotomies.[19] In the primary total knee group (n = 179), one patient who did not receive patella resurfacing was identified with patellar erosion and received a patellar resurfacing due to abrasion and gradual subluxation of the patella one year postoperative. In the revision arthrotomy group (n = 23), three patients were diagnosed with a subluxing patella (13%), and one patient received a V-Y quadriplasty due to extreme extensor tendon rigidity (arthrofibrosis). No patients in the unicondylar knee replacement group experienced extensor mechanism problems or patellar instability. The higher rate of patellar complications in the revision patients can be attributable to arthrofibrosis and the loss of normal compliance of the knee retinaculum. Other investigators have also noted a similar higher occurrence rate in revision total knee arthroplasty.[20,21]

Additionally, utilizing this technique, none of the 234 patients developed excessive leg edema, retarded progression of range of motion or strength, and only one patient required treatment for the clinical development of deep venous thrombosis. The average hospital length of stay was 3.3 days for all patients included in the study with all medical and surgical conditions included. The implementation of this surgical exposure does not appear to cause an increase in joint effusion, postoperative blood loss, or postoperative pain. Physical therapy requirements were not different from our normal patient care regime, and to date, no patella fractures have occurred in any of the trivector-retaining arthrotomy arthroplasty patients.

The trivector-retaining arthrotomy (TRA) technique bears some similarity to the subvastus approach.[19] The medial subvastus arthrotomy utilizes a parapatellar tendon incision extending in a cephalad direction to the inferior fibers of the VMO. Then a medially directed oblique incision is made along the VMO fibers (Fig. 17.1). The medial subvastus arthrotomy technique is beneficial in that the dynamic stabilizers of the patella are not interrupted and intrinsic patella stability is retained. However, its limited use in large patients, short legs, and revision cases is considered a disadvantage of this technique. Additionally, it is difficult to use the subvastus approach in valgus patients requiring posterolateral exposure unless extended dissection is used.[19]

The TRA offers the advantages of the subvastus such as maintenance of intrinsic patellar stability without the limitations of exposure. In this study 23 revision arthroplasties and 4 lateral unicondylar arthroplasties were preformed using the TRA without a tubercle osteotomy. In revision cases and other cases in which the patella was difficult to evert, the synovium of the lateral gutter was thoroughly removed and the capsule along the anterior lateral rim of the tibia was dissected to free the lateral meniscus from the tibial plateau. These two procedures were all that were necessary in all but the most obese patients. In very obese patients, the patella was slid laterally into the gutter until all of the cuts were made, then it was everted.

One theoretical disadvantage of the TRA when compared to the subvastus approach is that the TRA, like the standard parapatellar approach, does sacrifice the medial superior geniculate artery. However, this has had few proven consequences with the TRA or traditional standard medial parapatellar approaches.

CONCLUSION

The trivector-retaining arthrotomy is easily reproducible and serves to provide the advantages of the standard parapatellar arthrotomy in regards to the knee joint extensile exposure, yet minimizes the specific disadvantages regarding extensor mechanism dysfunction and resultant vector force displacement, which leads to patellar complications. The TRA has reduced the need for lateral patellar retinacular releases and other procedures designed to reduce postoperative patellar instability. It appears this type of procedure has enhanced the patients' postoperative rehabilitation potential, and has aided in reducing the frequency of complications associated with patellofemoral motion in total knee arthroplasty, including primary, unicondylar, and revision cases.

References

1. Brick GW, Scott RD. The patellofemoral component of total knee arthroplasty. *Clin Orthop.* 1988; 231:163–178.
2. Murray DG. Total knee arthroplasty. *Clin Orthop.* 1985; 192:59–68.
3. Webster DA, Murray DG. Complications of variable axis total knee arthroplasty. *Clin Orthop.* 1985; 193:160–167.
4. Merkow RL, Soudry M, Insall JN. Patellar dislocation following total knee replacement. *J Bone Joint Surg.* 1985; 67A: 1321–1327.
5. Insall JN, Binazzi R, Soudry M, Mestriner LA. Total knee arthroplasty. *Clin Orthop.* 1985; 192:13–22.
6. Leblanc JM. Patellar complications in total knee arthroplasty. A literature review. *Orthop Rev.* 1989; 18(3):296–304.
7. Roffman M, Hirsh DM, Mendes DG. Fracture of the resur-

faced patella in total knee replacement. *Clin Orthop.* 1980; 148:112–116.
8. Scott RD, Turoff N, Ewald FC. Stress fracture of the patella following duopatellar total knee arthroplasty with patellar resurfacing. *Clin Orthop.* 1982; 170:147–151.
9. Terry GC. The anatomy of the extensor mechanism. *Clin Sports Med.* 1989; 8(2):163–177.
10. Doolittle KH, Turner RH. Patellofemoral problems following total knee arthroplasty. *Orthop Rev.* 1988; 17(7):696–702.
11. Grace JN, Rand JA. Patellar instability after total knee arthroplasty. *Clin Orthop.* 1988; 237:184–189.
12. Moreland JR, Thomas RJ, Freeman MAR. ICLH replacement of the knee. *Clin Orthop.* 1979; 145:47–59.
13. Cheal EJ, Hayes WC, Harry JD, Gerhart TN, Page D. Influence of component orientation on peg failure of patella surface replacements. *32nd Annu Orthop Res Soc.* New Orleans, February 17–20, 1986.
14. Huberti HH, Hayes WC. Patellofemoral contact pressures. The influence of Q angle and tendofemoral contact. *J Bone Joint Surg.* 1984; 66A:715–724.
15. Stern SH. Surgical exposure in total knee arthroplasty. In: Fu FH, Harner CD, Vince KG, eds. *Knee Surgery.* Vol. 2. Baltimore: Williams & Wilkins; 1994:1289–1302.
16. Bramlett KW. *The Trivector Arthrotomy Approach.* AAOS Instructional Videotape, June 1994.
17. Scuderi GR, Insall JN, Windsor RE, Moran MC. Survivorship of cemented knee replacements. *J Bone Joint Surg.* 1989; 71B(5):798–803.
18. Vince KG, Insall JN, Kelly MA. The total condylar prosthesis. 10- to 12-year results of a cemented knee replacement. *J Bone Joint Surg.* 1989; 71B(5):793–797.
19. Hofmann AA, Plaster RL, Murdock LE. Subvastus (Southern) approach for primary total knee arthroplasty. *Clin Orthop.* 1991; 269:70–77.
20. Figgie HE, Goldberg VM. Some success rates of revision total knee arthroplasty. *Orthop Rev.* 1988; 17(5): 464–466.
21. Goldberg VM, Figgie MP, Figgie HE, Sobel M. The results of revision total knee arthroplasty. *Clin Orthop.* 1988; 226:86–92.

CHAPTER 18
The Lateral Approach

Peter A. Keblish

INTRODUCTION

Fixed valgus deformity presents a major challenge in total knee arthroplasty (TKA), especially in moderate or severe cases (Fig. 18.1). The literature suggests that correction of fixed valgus deformities via the standard medial parapatellar approach leads to higher failure rates, primarily at the patellofemoral joint. In a prospective case-controlled study, Karachalios and associates[1] reported poorer clinical outcomes and significantly higher patellar subluxation or dislocation in patients with preoperative fixed valgus deformities. Merkow and colleagues[2] reported that of 12 cases presenting to the Hospital for Special Surgery with patellar dislocation following TKA, nine had preexisting valgus deformities. Because valgus deformity represents under 15% of TKA cases, this failure rate is extremely high. Personal clinical experience[3,4] (1974 to 1980) with 23 fixed valgus knees (greater than 15 degrees) utilizing the medial approach resulted in patellar maltracking in 8, peroneal neuropraxia in 3, and 3 deep skin sloughs. Stern and associates[5] stated that TKA is reliable in valgus deformity but represents a greater challenge than their varus counterparts, primarily because of greater difficulty in achieving ligamentous equilibrium. Many reports of patellar problems in TKA do not cite the preexisting deformities, but the consensus in the literature supports the relationship of increased patellar complications in (preoperative) fixed valgus deformities. A common factor in all reports is the medial surgical approach.

This chapter will (1) define the pathologic anatomy of the valgus knee, (2) analyze the reasons for increased patellar complications in valgus TKA, (3) define the technical problems and disadvantages of the medial approach in fixed valgus deformity, and (4) illustrate the technique specifics and advantages of the direct lateral approach in fixed valgus deformity.

PATHOLOGIC ANATOMY—VALGUS KNEE

Fixed valgus deformity is usually associated with external tibial rotation. The deformity is prevalent in females (9:1), and rheumatoid arthritis is an underlying disease in a higher number of cases as compared to the more common osteoarthritic knee. In severe cases (Fig. 18.2), the skin can be fragile with little underlying subcutaneous tissue, especially following the required releases and prosthetic insertion. Vascularity of the skin and subcutaneous tissue occurs through the larger superficial longitudinal vessels as well as the perforating flower spray capillary circulation. Therefore, excessive undermining, increased tension, or lack of a soft tissue layer between skin and prosthesis can lead to skin necrosis, a potentially devastating complication of TKA.

Extra-Articular Layer (Figs. 18.1 and 18.3)

The fascia lata extension envelops the quadriceps with attachment to the posterior aspect of the femur. The distal lateral confluence becomes the iliotibial (I-T) band with distinct insertion into Gerdy's tubercle and the lateral tibial plateau. Transverse and oblique fibers extend to the patellar mechanism. This distinct layer is referred to as the lateral retinaculum.[6] The fascia attaches to bone via Sharpey's fibers and into the myofascia of the anterior compartment of the calf.

The I-T band and the lateral retinaculum are, by definition, deforming factors in the fixed valgus knee. The I-T band attachment to the upper tibia produces a valgus moment with external rotation. The lateral retinaculum (oblique and transverse extensions) produces a lateral (subluxing) moment to the patellar mechanism. The lateral retinaculum is a distinct layer from the deeper capsular or fat pad and vastus lateralis attachments.

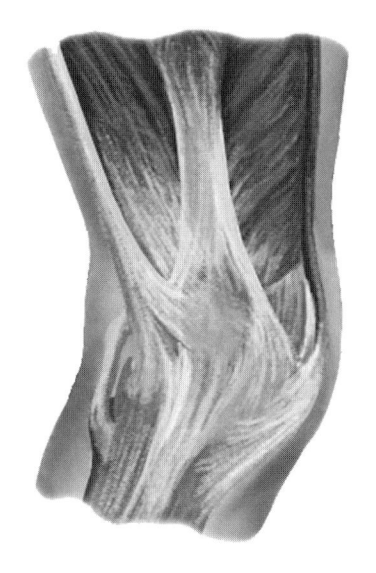

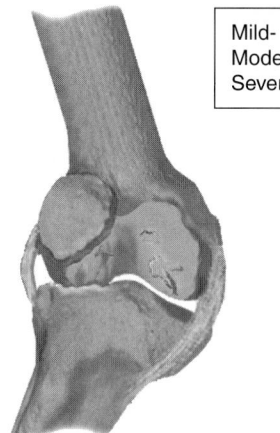

Figure 18.1. Fixed-valgus deformity.

Mild-   <15°
Moderate- 15-30°
Severe-   >30°

The extra-articular layer also includes the lateral hamstring (biceps femoris), the fabello-fibular ligament,[7,8] the lateral head of the gastrocnemius, and the popliteus muscle, which becomes an intra-articular tendon insertion. These structures may be contracted secondary to the long-standing valgus, especially in rheumatoid or inflammatory conditions with myofibrosis. Bony deformity (hereditary, acquired, or posttraumatic) further increases the contractures.

The lateral superficial layer differs from the (compliant) medial oblique retinaculum of the vastus medialis in that the lateral retinaculum is relatively noncompliant. This noncompliant lateral fascial extension to the patellar mechanism, coupled with contractures of the deeper layer, becomes a major determinant of the soft tissue deformity in the valgus knee.

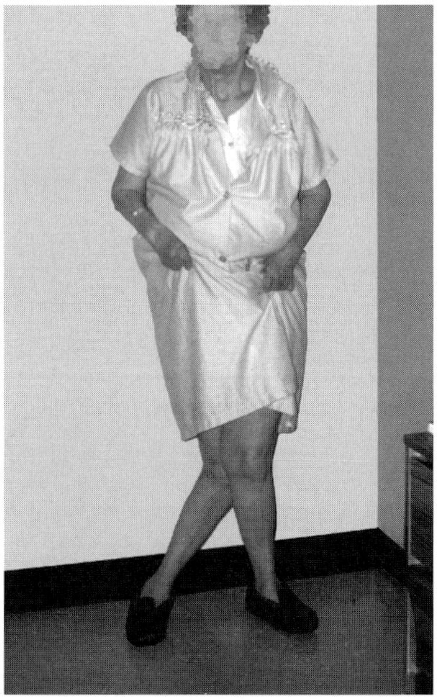

Intra-Articular (Deep Layer—Fig. 18.3)

The popliteus tendon, lateral collateral ligament (LCL), fabello-fibular ligament, arcuate ligament and capsule form the posterolateral complex.[7-9] Anteriorly, the vastus lateralis inserts at the proximal patellar facet. The tendon of the vastus lateralis is usually of substantial thickness and joins the lateral aspect of the central quadriceps (rectus tendon). These structures are covered by a capsular and/or synovial layer in the joint. The muscles, by definition, have an extra-articular origin. The LCL differs from the medial collateral ligament (MCL) in that the distal insertion is at the fibular head, not the upper tibia—a determinant of increased anteroposterior tibial translation on the lateral side. The MCL sleeve may be stretched or elongated and, at times, may require surgical advancement.

The deep anterior and posterior lateral soft tissue layers are contracted to different degrees, depending on factors such as the underlying pathology, longevity of the deformity, bony pathology, and others. Management of this deep layer in valgus TKA represents the key to

Figure 18.2. Patient with clinical valgus. Elderly female with severe rheumatoid arthritis and compromised soft tissue envelope.

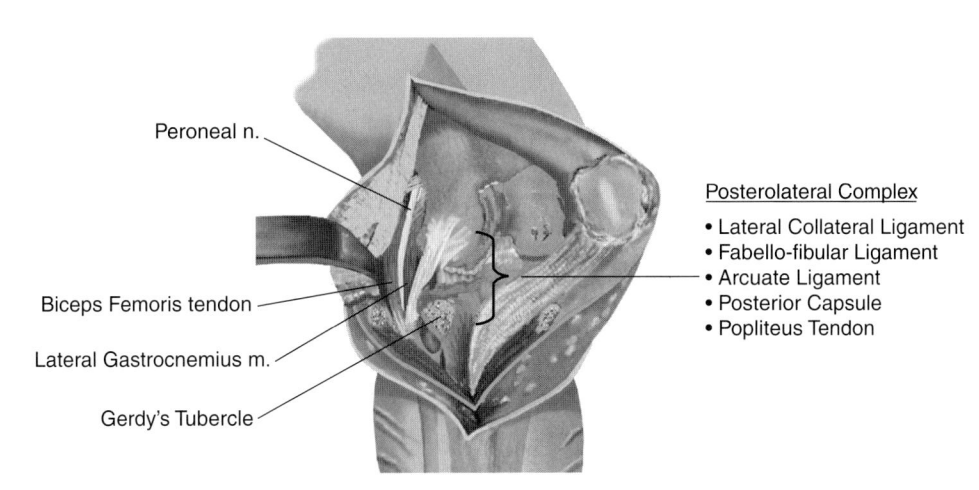

Figure 18.3. Deep posterolateral corner of the valgus knee. The I-T band is shown released from the upper tibia for illustration purposes.

correction of the tibial rotation and centralization of the patella following prosthetic insertion.

Bone Deformities (Developmental) (Figs. 18.1 and 18.2)

Femur—The lateral femoral condyle is smaller and eroded secondary to arthritic changes. Peripheral osteophytes and intercondylar notch stenosis are common. The anatomic femoral axis is significantly increased.

Tibia—The tibia is externally rotated, and the tibial tubercle is positioned laterally. The lateral plateau has varying degrees of central bone resorption and peripheral osteophyte encroachment.

Patella—The patella is often subluxed laterally. The lateral facet is frequently deformed (flattened or concave), with large traction osteophytes secondary to lateral overpull. Patella alta, with an expanded suprapatellar pouch, is common. The suprapatellar soft tissue is hypertrophied.

Bone deformities secondary to the lateral femoral condyle or tibial plateau fractures may contribute to or accentuate preexisting valgus. If the deformity is minor and/or correctable and limited to the lateral compartment, supracondylar varus osteotomy or lateral unicompartment replacement is an option to TKA. In either case, the direct lateral approach enhances exposure and provides other advantages that will be discussed in the technique section.

MEDIAL APPROACH

The standard medial parapatellar approach is the most commonly utilized procedure for all total knees.[9–12] The subvastus and, more recently, the midvastus[13] variations have been described. There is a general consensus that sequential releases should be performed from the femoral side prior to instrumentation in fixed valgus.[14–17] Releases include the posterolateral complex, the posterior cruciate ligament (PCL), and the I-T band. In extremely severe deformities, lengthening of the lateral hamstring and/or lateral gastrocnemius, with or without resection of the fibular head, can be performed. A second posterolateral incision may be required. However, inside-out releases are the norm, without consideration of joint seal.

The medial approach in valgus TKA fails to address the pathologic anatomy rationally and biomechanically. Patellar maltracking is more common, and there is increased potential for inaccurate flexion-extension gap balancing and less than optimum femorotibial stability. Technical disadvantages of the approach include: (1) it is indirect; (2) it increases external rotation of the tibia; (3) access to the posterolateral corner is more difficult; (4) an extensive lateral release is still required; (5) joint seal and prosthetic soft tissue coverage is difficult, if not impossible; (6) vascularity to the quadriceps patella tendon (QPT) mechanism and lateral skin (beneath the extensive lateral release) is decreased;[18] (7) it does not allow for correction of the external rotation contracture of the tibia; and (8) it may encourage overreleasing of deep soft tissues.

LATERAL APPROACH—RATIONALE

The lateral approach in valgus deformity, by contrast, addresses the pathologic anatomy in a rational and sequential manner.[3,4,19–21] The approach (1) is direct, (2) accomplishes the extensive "lateral release" with the exposure; (3) decreases skin undermining; (4) internally rotates the tibia with improved access to the pathologic posterolateral corner; (5) allows for better titration of sequential releases based on flexion-extension gap balance requirements; (6) preserves vascularity because the medial side is untouched;[18] (7) allows for planned soft tissue gap and prosthetic coverage; (8) centralizes the QPT mechanism, which optimizes patella tracking; (9) improves femorotibial alignment stability; and (10) rehabilitation is unimpeded because the medial quadriceps remains intact.

The approach from skin incision to soft tissue closure will be described and illustrated in detail in the next section. The six major steps are:

Step I.   I-T Band Release or Lengthening
Step II.   Lateral Arthrotomy—Coronal Plane Z-plasty
Step III. Patella Dislocation—Joint Exposure
Step IV.   Tibial Sleeve Release—Osteoperiosteal
Step V.   Femoral Sleeve Release—Osteoperiosteal
Step VI.   Soft Tissue (Prosthetic Joint) Closure

SURGICAL TECHNIQUE

The surgical technique of the direct lateral approach differs substantially from the standard medial parapatellar approach. The surgeon is less familiar with the lateral side of the knee; orientation is reversed, and a more careful handling of the soft tissues is required. The recommended skin incision in the virgin knee follows the Q-angle and is slightly lateral to the patella, lateral border of the patellar tendon, and the tibial tubercle (Fig. 18.4). Long incisions are preferred, especially in large knees. It is important to avoid unnecessary undermining. In previously operated knees, the existing incision should be incorporated and extended proximally and distally. If multiple incisions are present, select the most direct or the latest operated tract.

STEP I: I-T BAND RELEASE OR LENGTHENING (FIG. 18.5)

The I-T band is frequently a deforming force. Proximal and/or distal releases are required for correction of deformities over 15 degrees. Performing the release proximally (1) decreases the "bow string" effect of the I-T band, (2) allows for some initial correction, (3) prevents proximal migration of the distal tibial sleeve (following release) in severe deformities, (4) allows for anatomical reattachment of the distal sleeve, and (5) decreases potential for peroneal nerve compression.

Proximal I-T band exposure is gained by freeing and retracting the vastus lateralis from the fascial envelope to expose the posterior femur. The broad fascial band is released from the femoral attachment and stripped proximally and distally to the condylar attachments. Dissection is initiated with a hemostat and completed with a finger or blunt instrument. Following exposure and longitudinal stripping from the femur, a varus moment is placed at the knee joint, bow-stringing the I-T band. The "pie crust" lengthening, as used in percutaneous Achilles tendon lengthening, is preferred because it allows the fascia to remain in continuity. However, transverse, Z-plasty, or V-Y techniques can also be utilized.[10,14] The lengthening is performed from inside-out, taking care not to undermine the subcutaneous layer. The peroneal nerve can be exposed as needed in severe cases.

Initial correction of 10 to 15 degrees can be accomplished by this lengthening technique. The proximal relaxation allows for more precise or titrated release at the joint level. In moderate cases, sleeve releases of the tibia and/or femur may not be required if the intra-articular pathology is primarily bone loss. If the deformity is mild or totally correctable under anesthesia, Step I can be eliminated.

STEP II: LATERAL ARTHROTOMY—CORONAL Z-PLASTY (FIGS. 18.6 AND 18.7)

Lateral Retinoacular Incision (Fig. 18.6)

The lateral arthrotomy incision separates the superficial from the deep layers via a coronal plane Z-plasty technique. The proximal, middle, and distal segments require different anatomic dissection techniques. The superficial or first layer incision extends proximally from

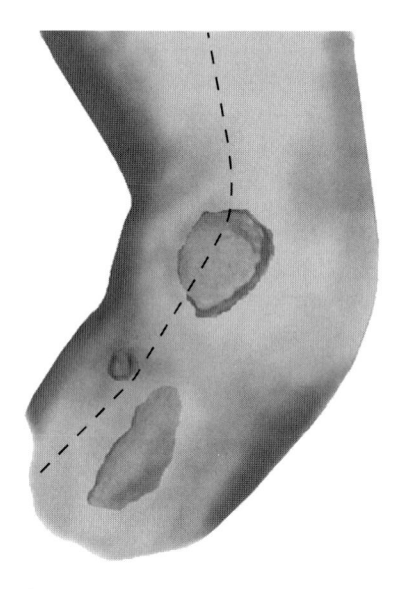

Figure 18.4. Skin incision is placed laterally to decrease undermining.

18. The Lateral Approach

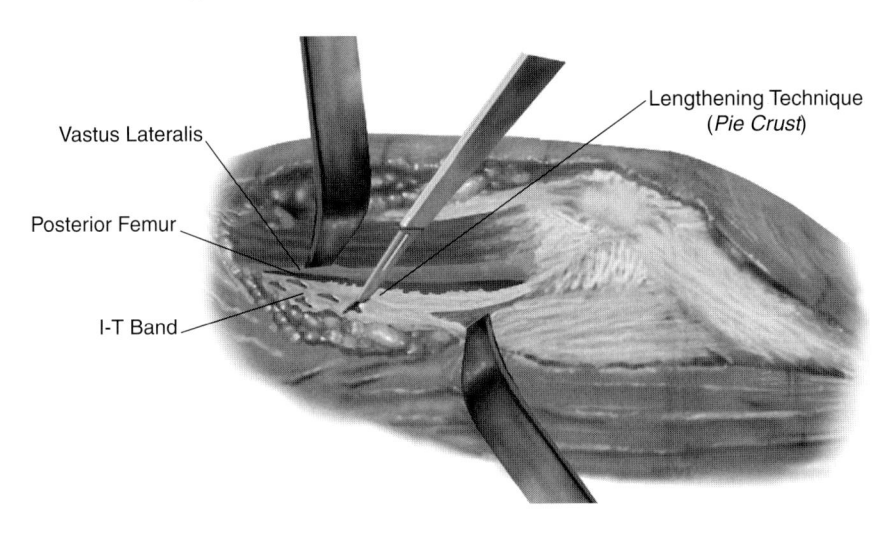

Figure 18.5. Step I: I-T Band Release/Lengthening. The I-T band is released longitudinally from the posterior femoral attachments. A varus stress is applied to the knee joint as the multiple puncture (pie crust) lengthening of the I-T band is performed.

the lateral border of the rectus femoris to, but not through, the musculotendinous junction of the vastus lateralis (V-L); in the midsegment, it proceeds laterally 2 to 4 cm from the patella border, and distally through the anteromedial aspect of Gerdy's tubercle and the anterior compartment fascia.

Proximally, the incision extends from superficial lateral to deep medial, entering the suprapatellar pouch at an estimated 45-degree angle. The laminations of the central quadriceps tendon allow for a natural plane dissection to the proximal or musculotendinous junction of the V-L. The V-L tendon inserts at the proximal lateral patella. The tendon is substantially thick (6 to 10 mm), which allows for a relaxation (coronal plane Z-plasty) approach. The incision continues from the musculotendinous junction superficially, through 50% of the tendon, ending at the patella. Finger tension from the undersurface of the patella and V-L tendon allows for a controlled (sharp knife) coronal plane dissection (Fig. 18.7). The deep (50%) fibers are detached from the patella rim, maintaining the lateral sleeve. Plicae bands are sectioned medially in order to enhance the soft tissue gap closure. The distal aspect of the V-L insertion blends into the lateral capsular attachment and becomes more compliant after the proximal dissection has been completed.

The midsegment dissection extends from 2 to 4 cm lateral to the patellar border through the lateral retinaculum without penetrating the capsule. The natural retinaculum capsular plane allows for an anatomical

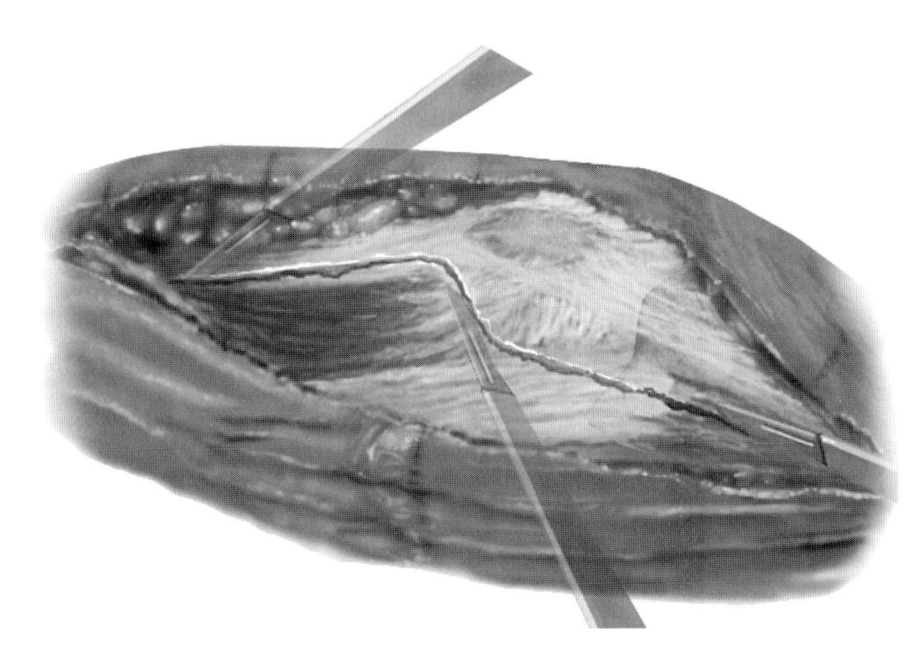

Figure 18.6. Step II: Lateral Retinacular Incision (Superficial). The course of the lateral parapatellar incision extends laterally to the patella by 2 to 4 cm and into the anterior aspect of Gerdy's tubercle.

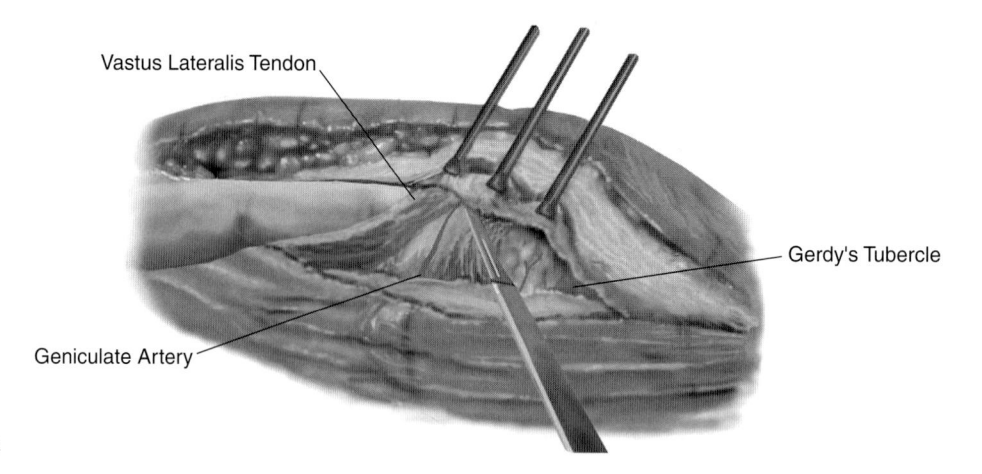

Figure 18.7. Step II: Lateral Arthrotomy (Deep Layer). The superficial layer is separated from the deep layer with a coronal plane Z-plasty.

separation of the capsule to the lateral patellar rim. The capsule is protected or separated with a wide osteotome or careful sharp knife dissection and is detached from the patellar rim. The fat pad blends into the lateral capsule at this point.

The fat pad is incised obliquely to include the lateral meniscus, preserving approximately 70% of the fat pad with the meniscus and 30% with the patellar tendon (Fig. 18.8). Lateral fat pad mobilization and preservation can vary according to soft tissue defects and surgeon preference. The lateral inferior geniculate artery provides excellent vascularization. The fat pad incision can be made prior to or as the patella is being everted. The advantage of incising with patella eversion is that soft tissue tension is increased and a more definite incision path is defined. The lateral fat pad-meniscal sleeve can be mobilized and expanded for soft tissue closure in very severe cases.[4]

The distal extension of the retinacular incision splits the medial aspect of Gerdy's tubercle and continues distally into the anterior compartment fascia. Osteoperiosteal elevation (using a sharp osteotome) beginning at mid-Gerdy's to, but not including, the tibial tubercle protects the patellar tendon attachment (Fig. 18.8). Including the medial fibers of the anterior tibial muscle maintains continuity of the sleeve and allows for safer dislocation of the patellar mechanism. The medial sleeve broadens the effective width of the patellar tendon attachment by 2 to 3 cm; it protects the insertion of the patellar tendon and enhances the internal rotation moment of the tibia. Care must be taken to control (cauterize) or avoid the recurrent branch of the anterior tib-

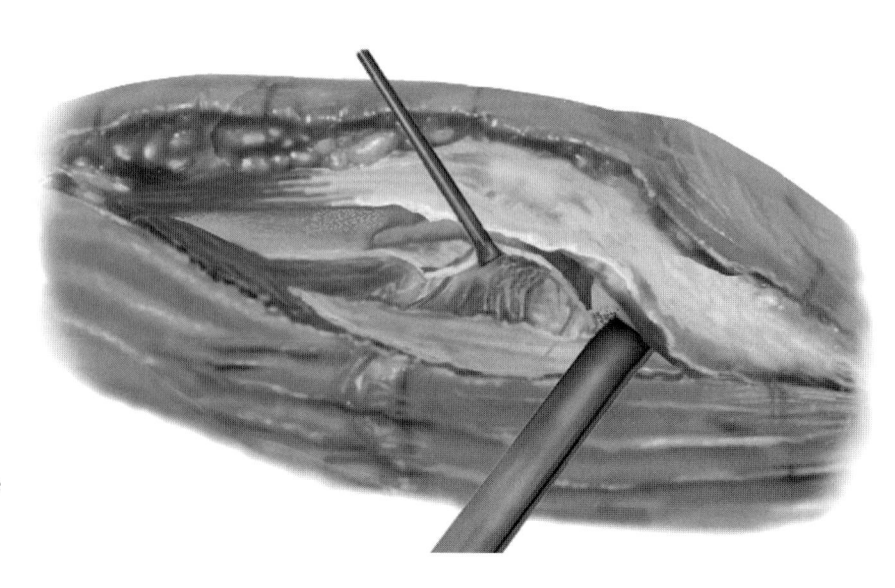

Figure 18.8. Step II: Gerdy's Tubercle Elevation. Osteoperiosteal sleeve release from mid-Gerdy's tubercle to, but not including, the tibial tubercle.

ial artery. The patella is now prepared for translocation and/or eversion.

The lateral approach preserves the surgical option of formal tibial tubercle osteotomy, preferred by some surgeons and reported in the literature[16,17,22] via the medial approach. Performing the osteotomy from lateral to medial (with the extended sleeve) is more anatomical and maintains other benefits of the direct lateral approach. Personal experience has shown that formal tubercle osteotomy is rarely required if the osteoperiosteal technique is mastered. A proximal soft tissue incision, including a lateral to medial rectus snip, is helpful to enhance exposure and is preferred over formal tibial tubercle osteotomy.

STEP III: PATELLA DISLOCATION—JOINT EXPOSURE (FIG. 18.9)

Following the expanded lateral exposure and Gerdy's tubercle elevation, the patella is dislocated to the medial side as the knee is flexed with a varus stress. If the patella dislocates easily, proceed with the next step. If there is soft tissue resistance to dislocation proximally, the incision should be extended, with or without a rectus snip (lateral to medial). If there is bony resistance, pre-cuts of 5 to 10 mm of the much larger distal and posterior medial condyle and tibial spine are recommended. The pre-cut maneuver decompresses the medial side and allows ease of translocation and/or eversion of the QPT mechanism. The lateral extension of the patellar tendon (to Gerdy's tubercle) protects the insertion at the tibial tubercle by dissipating the stress to the anterior compartment sleeve.

The medial-posterior corner is the most difficult exposure with the lateral approach. Soft tissue elevation from the upper medial tibial plateau is best accomplished with electrocautery. The medial meniscal rim is preserved. A Homan-type retractor placed through or inside the meniscal rim and behind the posterior medial tibial plateau levers the tibia forward. The cruciate attachments and capsule may be released from the posterior femur at this time or following tibial sleeve release (Step IV). When exposure is completed, the tibia rotates internally, and the pathologic posterolateral corner translates forward—a major advantage of the approach.

STEP IV: TIBIAL SLEEVE RELEASE—OSTEOPERIOSTEAL (FIG. 18.10)

The tibial sleeve can be released prior to and/or following patella dislocation. The recommended sequence begins with the knee in extension (prior to patella dislocation) and is completed in flexion (following formal joint exposure). Sleeve release of the upper tibia begins at the midportion of Gerdy's tubercle. Subperiosteal elevation with a sharp osteotome begins anteriorly and extends around the posterior corner to the insertion of the PCL (which is released). The technique maintains the continuity of the fascial sleeve from the I-T band proximally to the anterior compartment fascia distally. Peripheral osteophytes and loose bodies are removed. Capsular release from the femur should be completed at this time.

In extreme cases, the dissection is extended to the proximal fibula, which can be resected from inside to the outer cortex. This technique preserves the attachments of the LCL and biceps femoris and decompresses the peroneal nerve as it passes around the upper fibula.

Direct visualization, with the tibia internally rotated, ensures that safe, sequential or titrated releases are per-

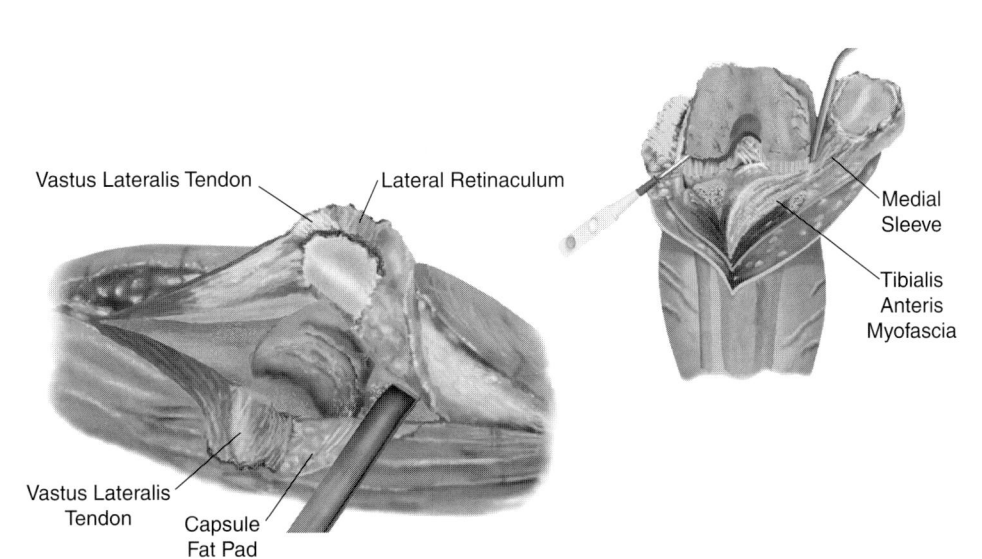

Figure 18.9. Step III: Patella Dislocation—Joint Exposure. Exposure can be enhanced with pre-cuts of the larger posteromedial condyle and/or tibial spine.

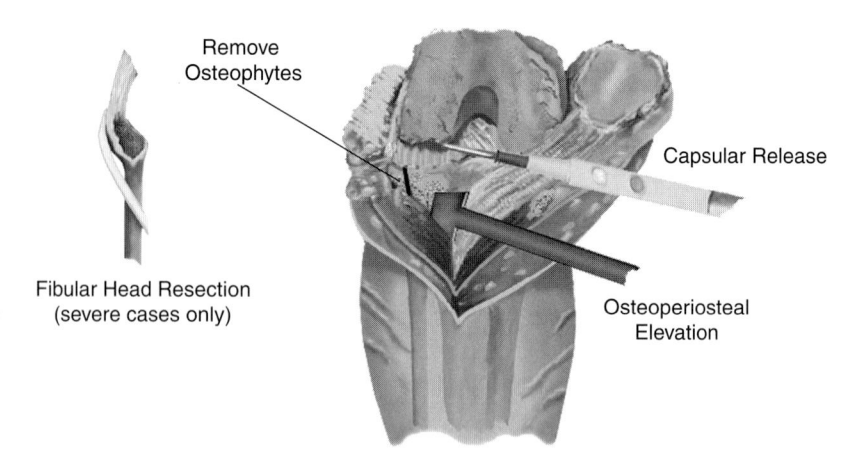

Figure 18.10. Step IV: Tibial Sleeve Release or Capsular Release. Osteoperiosteal release from mid-Gerdy's tubercle to the posterolateral tibia. In extreme cases, the proximal fibula can be resected to decompress the peroneal nerve (inset).

formed. The knee should be extended and flexed following tibial sleeve release to evaluate correction (Fig. 18.11). Use of lamina spreaders aids in assessment. If there is an obvious need for femoral sleeve release, proceed to the next step. If gaps have been corrected to a reasonable mechanical axis, proceed to bone resections and fine-tune with trial components.

STEP V: FEMORAL SLEEVE RELEASE—OSTEOPERIOSTEAL (FIG. 18.12)

The femoral attachment of the popliteus, LCL, and posterolateral capsular attachments must be released in severe and some moderate deformities. Technically, a subperiosteal release with a sharp osteotome is preferred. The osteotome is placed beneath the periosteum of the popliteus insertion and continues proximally. The LCL and posterior capsular complex structures are included. In moderate deformities, selected or titrated releases are preferable and best performed at the time of flexion-extension gap evaluation (spacer blocks or tensors) and/or at the time of trial reduction (Figs. 18.11, 18.13, and 18.14). Preservation of posterolateral stability is the goal. In extreme contractures, the lateral head of the gastrocnemius and the lateral hamstring are released or lengthened. Flexion-extension gap spaces should be checked as the releases progress. Fine-tuning at the time of spacer-tensor instrumentation or at trial reduction allows for more accurate balancing of the femoral sleeve.

INSTRUMENTATION—BONE RESECTIONS (FIGS. 18.13 AND 18.14)

The philosophy of surgical technique or rationale varies with surgeon and instrument systems. Two basic approaches, with variations, include (1) soft tissue first-tibia resection and (2) femoral resection first-soft tissue

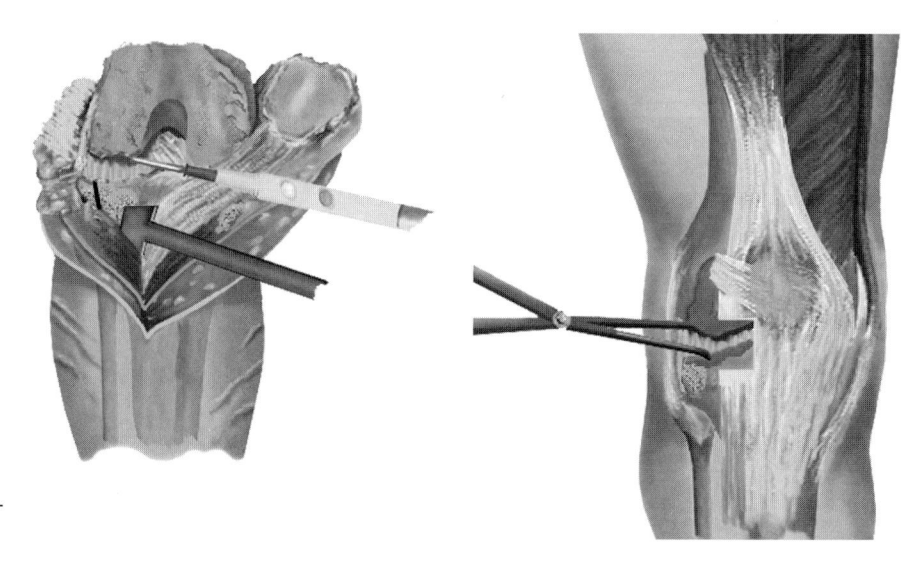

Figure 18.11. Flexion-Extension Gap Evaluation. Use of lamina spreaders aids in release and evaluation of mechanical axis.

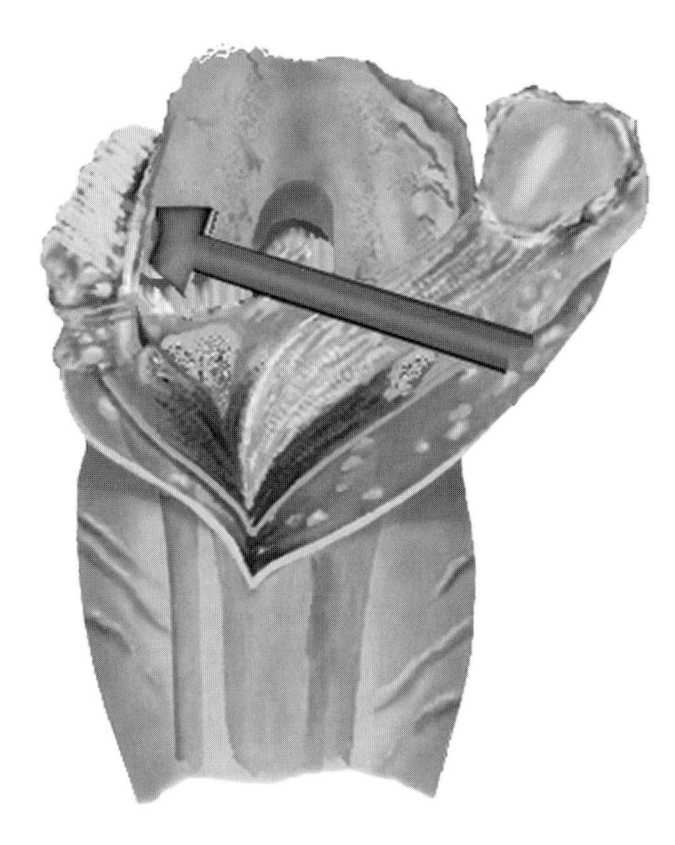

Figure 18.12. Step V: Femoral Sleeve Release. Osteoperiosteal release begins under the popliteus insertion and extends proximally as illustrated.

release. Regardless of approach, initial soft tissue steps, as described, must be completed in order to expose the distal femur and/or the proximal tibia. With the direct lateral approach, resection of the upper tibia is somewhat more difficult as the broadened patellar tendon and internal tibial rotation alter the anatomic landmarks. Good exposure and proper rotational orientation of the tibial resection guides are mandatory for accurate upper tibial resection. Attention to the exposure techniques will help to avoid instrumentation or resection errors.

The recommended resection of the proximal tibia is perpendicular to the mechanical (anatomical) axis with a 7- to 10-degree posterior inclination. Proper rotational orientation (proximal tibia to ankle or foot), therefore, is critical because curvatures in one plane can affect angulation in another plane. Failure to correct the external tibial rotation may influence the plane of resection. The medial approach in valgus TKA increases external rotation of the tibia, whereas the direct lateral approach internally rotates the tibia, allowing for better assessment of anatomical landmarks, depth, and plane of resection.

The depth of tibial resection follows normal guidelines. The lesser involved medial plateau should dictate the depth of resection. Minimal lateral resection is the norm. Grafting (or shimming) of the lateral tibial plateau is preferable (within reason) to deeper resections because the depth of resection will affect flexion gap stability, joint line, and patella position.

The femoral resection may be influenced by the distorted anatomy. The prominent medial and pathologic lateral compartment may skew the instrumentation (intra- or extramedullary). Minimal to no resection of the lateral distal and posterior femoral condyle is the norm in severe deformity.

Rotational resections are based on various landmarks with different instrument systems.[15,16,23,24] Systems based on the posterior femoral condyles produce an internally positioned femoral component, much exaggerated in the valgus knee. Systems based on the transepicondylar axis[25] or the tibial axis (and flexion ten-

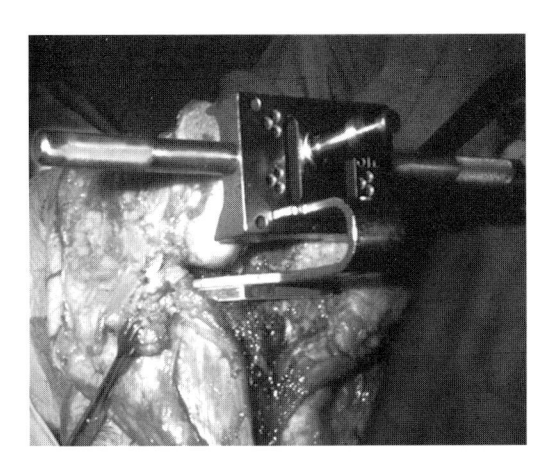

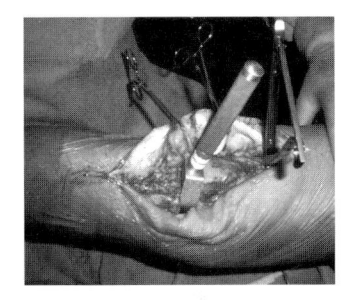

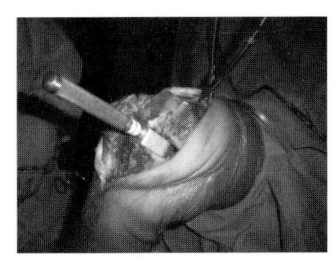

Figure 18.13. Instrumentation (Fine-Tuning). Instrumentation with flexion gap or femoral positioner allows for fine-tuning of soft tissue balancing. Flexion and extension gaps are checked with appropriate spacer blocks.

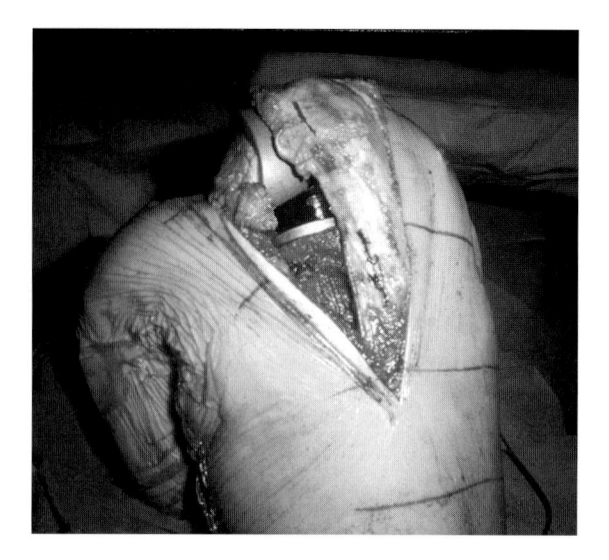

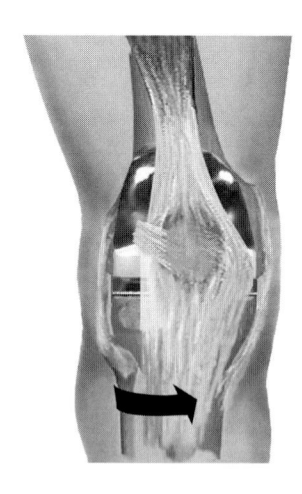

Figure 18.14. Trial Reduction. Intraoperative example of trial reduction with LCS rotating platform prosthesis. Note the correction of tibial rotation and natural patella tracking.

sion)[3,19,24] more accurately position the femur for the rotational (coronal plane) resection and a balanced flexion gap. Patellar tracking is critically dependent on proper femoral rotation alignment, in addition to soft tissue balancing and a proper (anatomic) femoral prosthetic component.

The distal femoral resection plane recommended is 4 to 5 degrees valgus, and the depth of resection is based on extension gap requirements (instrument systems dependent). The goal is to mate the extension gap to a stable flexion gap. Fine-tuning is accomplished with spacers (Fig. 18.13) or at the time of trial reduction (Fig. 18.14). Trial reduction allows for assessment of stability and mobility at the femorotibial and patellofemoral joints. Note the natural patella tracking, tibial tubercle position, and stable flexion at 130 degrees in the clinical case following LCS rotating platform insertion (Fig. 18.14). External tibial rotation has been corrected, and the (untouched) medial forces now balance the soft tissues through the flexion-extension arc of motion.

The direct lateral approach best prepares and exposes the distal femur and proximal tibia for the critical axial and rotational cuts. The advantages cited will decrease the potential for malresections and will allow for better assessment of stability in all planes (varus-valgus, rotation, anteroposterior, patellofemoral). The need for medial ligament advancement is eliminated as the soft tissues realign with correction of mechanical axis.

STEP VI: SOFT TISSUE (PROSTHETIC JOINT) CLOSURE (FIG. 18.15)

Soft tissue closure is completed with the knee flexed. The expanded lateral soft tissue sleeve (coronal Z-plasty) is positioned to the medial sleeve. Towel clips or

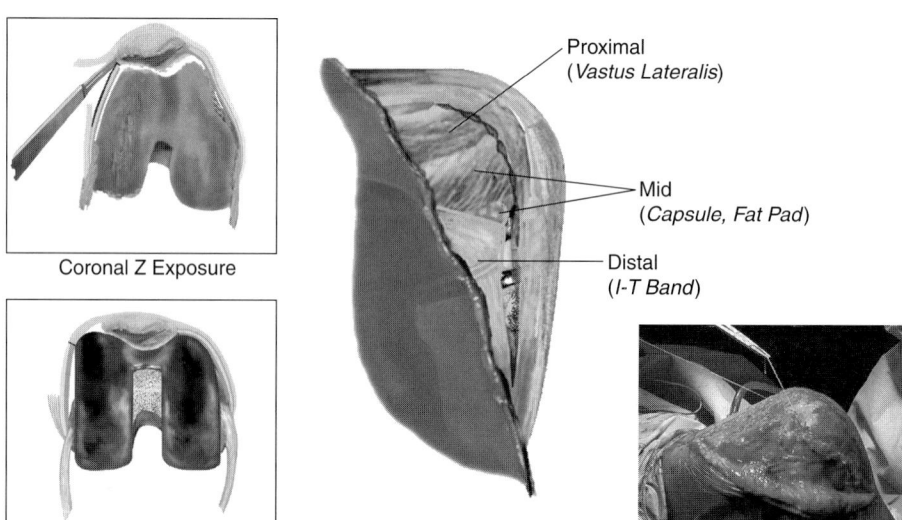

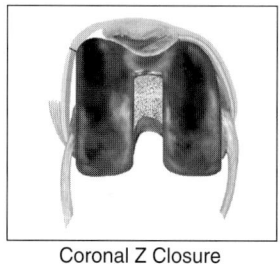

Figure 18.15. Step VI: Soft Tissue (Prosthetic Joint) Closure. Closure in flexion. The expanded soft tissue sleeve seals the prosthetic joint. The I-Y band is reattached anatomically to Gerdy's tubercle or medial sleeve.

stay sutures are utilized, and the knee is extended and flexed through the maximum range. Distal to proximal closure is recommended.

Distally, anatomic reattachment of the I-T band and posterolateral sleeve to Gerdy's tubercle and the medial sleeve stabilizes the posterolateral corner. In the midsegment, the capsule is sutured to the lateral border of the retinaculum. Proximally, the vastus lateralis tendon is reattached in the expanded (coronal plane Z-plasty) position with the knee in maximal flexion. The knee is ranged to a full flexion position (140 to 150 degrees), and soft tissue compliance and integrity of the joint seal are checked. Appropriate adjustments or reinforcing sutures can be implemented at this time. The preoperative noncompliant-deforming lateral soft tissue structures are now more compliant and allow for coverage of the prosthetic joint.

DISCUSSION

Management of soft tissues has become recognized as a key ingredient in TKA outcome. Femorotibial stability and extensor mechanism alignment are influenced by many factors including preoperative deformity, prosthetic instrumentation or design, and surgical approach. Fixed valgus deformity presents a different and more difficult challenge to the operating surgeon. The surgical approach should be designed and executed to correct the soft tissue contractures for balanced bony resections.

The medial approach is the recommended surgical approach in all standard textbooks relating to TKA, including correction of fixed valgus deformity.[9–11,26,27] Technique points stressed are sequential release of extra- and intra-articular soft tissue contractures from the femoral side. Insall[10] stressed the importance of proximal I-T band release. Ranawat[14] and others[1,15–17] stress the need for an extensive lateral retinacular release (with coagulation of the lateral geniculate vessels), proximal release of the I-T band, and cautery release of the posterolateral (arcuate) complex from the femur in valgus deformities over 15 degrees (moderate) and over 30 degrees (severe). Release or lengthening of the lateral gastrocnemius and lateral hamstring is recommended if the above steps are not adequate. Hungerford and associates[16] categorized fixed-valgus deformity into two types based on medial soft tissue integrity. Type I includes intact medial stabilizers, and Type II has attenuated medial stabilizers. Type II (severe) deformities are treated with medial soft tissue advancement, a step most surgeons prefer to avoid. If flexion-extension or mediolateral balancing is unsatisfactory, they recommend use of a more stable prosthesis.

The direct lateral approach best addresses the technical challenges of fixed valgus and provides the surgeon with a surgical option to the standard medial approach. Cameron and colleagues[28] discussed the lateral approach in TKA as an option but did not describe specifics of the technique. Buechel[21] described a sequential three-step lateral release via the lateral approach, a slight variation of the technique described herein. This author's initial clinical experience and technical steps[3] were described in 1985[4] with early follow-up results reported in 1991.[3]

The technical steps described have been refined from the original description and are available for viewing on videotext.[20] Significant changes include (1) soft tissue expansion using a coronal plane Z-plasty, rather than expanding the fat pad to provide soft tissue gap coverage; (2) osteoperiosteal elevation from mid-Gerdy's tubercle rather than adjacent to the tibial tubercle, protecting the patellar tendon insertion; and (3) more extensive osteoperiosteal elevation from mid-Gerdy's tubercle to the posterior tibia, improving the tibial external rotation contracture prior to release from the femoral side, which may not be required.

These refinements in technique have improved the understanding of the anatomical correction and have

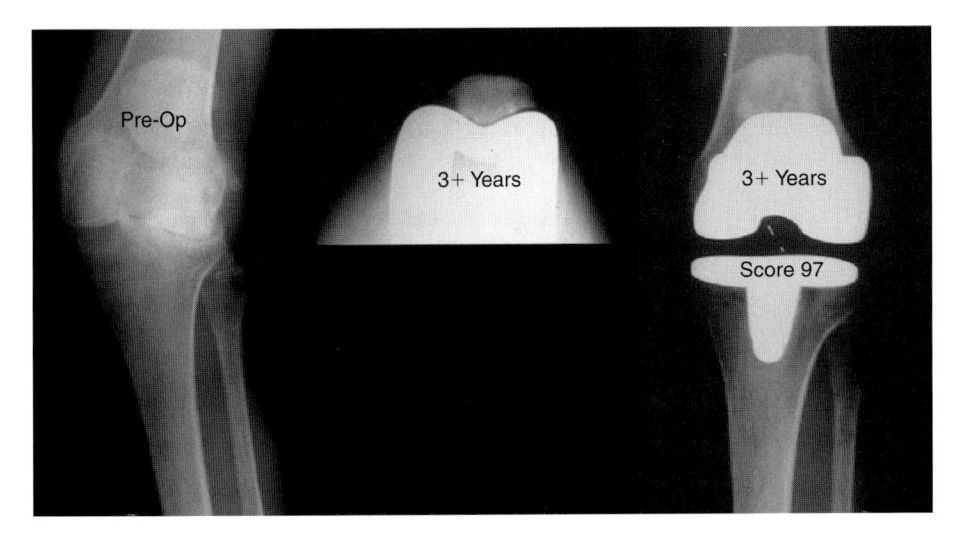

Figure 18.16. X-ray example of severe valgus correction in a 63-year-old white female. Patellofemoral tracking and femoro-tibial stability are excellent at 3 years.

decreased the learning curve for the approach. The approach requires an appreciation of the lateral soft tissue structures of the knee and is more technically demanding. Patellar eversion and orientation are reversed, and instrumentation and tibial exposure (posteromedial) are somewhat more difficult. However, clinical results[3,21] of the direct lateral approach in valgus TKA have eliminated patellar maltracking and have improved alignment stability—the basic goals of TKA (Fig. 18.16).

SUMMARY/CONCLUSIONS

The soft tissue challenge in valgus TKA is to achieve balance and prosthetic coverage with relatively noncompliant tissue. The bone alignment challenge is to restore the mechanical and rotational axis, allowing the femorotibial and patellofemoral articulations to function in a stable manner through a maximum flexion-extension arc of motion. The lateral approach allows direct access to the deformities and optimal assessment and correction of the soft tissue and bone deformities that are more challenging in the valgus knee.

References

1. Karachalios T, Sarangi PP, Newman JH. Severe varus and valgus deformities treated by total knee arthroplasty. *J Bone Joint Surg.* 1994; 76B:938–942.
2. Merkow TL, Soudry M, Insall JN. Patellar dislocation following total knee replacement. *J Bone Joint Surg.* 1985; 67A:1321–1327.
3. Keblish PA. The lateral approach to the valgus knee: surgical technique and analysis of 53 cases with over two-year follow-up evaluation. *Clin Orthop.* 1991; 271:52–62.
4. Keblish PA. Valgus deformity in TKR: the lateral retinacular approach. *Orthop Trans.* 1985; 9:28–29.
5. Stern SH, Moeckel BH, Insall JN. Total knee arthroplasty in valgus knees. *Clin Orthop.* 1991; 273:5–8.
6. Fulkerson JP, Gossling HR. Anatomy of the knee joint lateral retinaculum. *Clin Orthop.* 1981;153:188–196.
7. Kapandji IA. *The Physiology of the Joints: Annotated Diagrams of the Mechanics of the Human Joints.* 2nd ed. Edinburgh, Scotland: Churchill Livingstone; 1970.
8. Kaplan EB. The fabello fibular and short lateral ligaments of the knee joint. *J Bone Joint Surg.* 1961; 43:169–179.
9. Scott WN. *The Knee. Vol II.* St. Louis: CV Mosby; 1994.
10. Insall JN. *Surgery of the Knee.* New York: Churchill Livingstone; 1984: 587–696.
11. Krackow KA, ed. *The Technique of Total Knee Arthroplasty.* St. Louis: CV Mosby; 1990.
12. Morrey BF, ed. *Joint Replacement Arthroplasty.* New York: Churchill Livingstone; 1991.
13. Engh GA, Parks NL, Ammeen DJ. The influence of surgical approach on lateral retinacular releases in TKA. Presented at The Knee Society and AAHKS. Atlanta, GA; February 1996.
14. Ranawat CS. Total-condylar knee arthroplasty for valgus and combined valgus-flexion deformity of the knee. *Techniques in Orthopaedics.* 1988; 3:67–76.
15. Krackow KA, Jones MM, Teeny SM, et al. Primary total knee arthroplasty in patients with fixed valgus deformity. *Clin Orthop.* 1991; 273:9–18.
16. Hungerford DS, Krackow K, Kenna R. *Management of Fixed Deformity in TKA: A Comprehensive Approach.* Baltimore: Churchill Livingstone; 1984: 41–54.
17. Whiteside LA. Correction of ligament and bone defects in total arthroplasty of the severely valgus knee. *Clin Orthop.* 1993; 288:234–245.
18. Scapinelli R. Blood supply of the human patella. *J Bone Joint Surg.* 1967; 49B:563.
19. Buechel FF, Pappas MJ. New Jersey low contact stress knee replacement system ten-year evaluation of meniscal bearings. *Orthop Clin North Am.* 1989; 2:147–177.
20. Insall JN, Scott WN, Keblish PA, et al. Total knee arthroplasty exposures and soft tissue balancing. In: Insall JN, Scott WN, eds. *VideoBook of Knee Surgery.* Philadelphia: JB Lippincott; 1994.
21. Buechel FF. A sequential three-step lateral release for correcting fixed valgus knee deformities during total knee arthroplasty. *Clin Orthop.* 1990; 260:170–175.
22. Wolff AM, Hungerford DS, Krackow KA, et al. Osteotomy of the tibial tubercle during total knee replacement. A report of twenty-six cases. *J Bone Joint Surg.* 1989; 71A:848–852.
23. Callaghan JJ, Dennis DA, Paprosky WG, et al., eds. *Orthopaedic Knowledge Update: Hip and Knee Reconstruction.* Rosemont, IL: American Academy of Orthopaedic Surgeons, 1995.
24. Keblish PA, Varma AK, Greenwald AS. Patella resurfacing or retention in total knee arthroplasty: a prospective study of patients with bilateral replacements. *J Bone Joint Surg.* 1994; 76B:930–937.
25. Cooke TD, Scudamore RA, Bryant JT, et al. A quantitative approach to radiography of the lower limb. *J Bone Joint Surg.* 1991; 73-B:715–723.
26. Laskin RS, ed. *Total Knee Replacement.* London, UK: Springer-Verlag; 1991: 41–74.
27. Rand JA, ed. *Total Knee Arthroplasty.* New York: Raven Press; 1993.
28. Cameron HU, Fedorkow DM. The patella in total knee arthroplasty. *Clin Orthop.* 1982; 165:197–199.

CHAPTER 19
Quadriceps Snip

Kevin L. Garvin

Adequate exposure is one of the most common difficulties encountered in revision knee arthroplasty. The quadriceps snip offers a unique alternative and evolved from more traditional surgical approaches. For many years, the approach initially described by Coonse and Adams[1] in 1943 was utilized (Fig. 19.1). In 1983 this approach was modified by Insall[2,3] to allow extensive exposure but preserve the blood supply to the turned down segment, and maintain the integrity of the vastus medialis (Fig. 19.2). This modification, also known as the patellar turndown, was used by Insall until 1988 as a standard approach for treatment of the stiff, ankylosed, or revised knee when exposure was difficult. It was at this time that Insall serendipitously noted that the proximal portion of the quadriceps had been transected in an oblique fashion. The surgeons were impressed with the additional exposure provided. At the completion of the observed surgical procedure, the tendon was repaired in a standard fashion. The patient's postoperative course was uneventful, and motion was not impaired, emphasizing the innocuous nature of the quadriceps incision. Since that time, the procedure, now known as the quadriceps snip, has been refined and has provided an alternative to the patellar turndown. This chapter will describe the quadriceps snip surgical technique, report the results in a group of patients, and outline the main advantages of the procedure.

SURGICAL TECHNIQUE

The initial aspect of the surgical technique is the selection of the skin incision. A standard anterior midline or paramedian incision is preferred. When feasible, prior incisions are included or incorporated in the incision. Narrow skin bridges must be avoided so skin necrosis does not occur.

The deep incision is a standard slightly medial incision through the extensor mechanism that begins at the tendinous portion of the proximal quadriceps. As the incision continues distally, the vastus medialis is left in continuity over the patella. The distal incision is completed 1 cm medial to the tibial tubercle that helps to prevent avulsion of the tendon during exposure. If the exposure is unsatisfactory, the quadriceps snip should be performed. The quadriceps snip portion of the exposure is an incision through the proximal aspect of the tendon from a proximal and lateral position directed distally and medially until it intersects the other portion of the quadriceps incision (Fig. 19.3). The quadriceps snip allows the patella to be mobilized in a distal and lateral fashion (Fig. 19.4). Excision of peripatellar tissue, capsule, and hypertrophic scar is helpful to mobilize the patella (Fig. 19.5). Occasionally, a lateral retinacular release is performed to allow the patella to be everted or subluxed laterally. The lateral superior and inferior geniculate vessels are identified and preserved when possible. The lateral inferior geniculate is normally cauterized when the lateral meniscus is excised. The limited dissection of the quadriceps snip may theoretically preserve the collateral vessels about the patella from the lateral geniculate that would be sacrificed during a more extensive lateral release for exposure.

If after the quadriceps snip and lateral release the exposure is still unsatisfactory, then a quadriceps turndown may be performed. In the author's experience, the quadriceps turndown procedure has not been necessary where exposure was provided using the quadriceps snip (Figs. 19.6 and 19.7).

PATIENT SELECTION

Patients undergoing knee replacement or revision knee surgery who have sepsis of the knee or limited motion are candidates for the quadriceps snip procedure. When the technique was first described, it was not clear if patients would have difficulty achieving active knee extension or develop other problems because of the technique. As more experience was gained, the innocuous

Figure 19.1. The original techniques as described by Coonse and Adams. In (A) the quadriceps incision for the turndown is marked and in (B) the quadriceps has been reflected distally.

Figure 19.2. The modified Coonse-Adams patellar turndown. In (A) the standard incision is shown. In (B) the segment has been reflected distally and laterally.

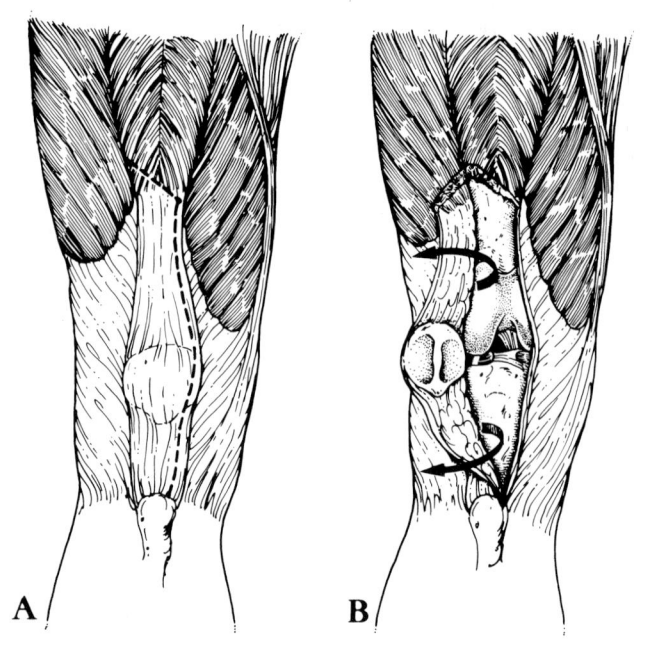

Figure 19.3. The quadriceps snip is shown in (A). In (B) the tissues have been mobilized for exposure of the knee.

nature of the quadriceps snip became clear, lessening the concern about intraoperative and postoperative complications.

A group of 16 patients were reported in 1995.[8] Ten of the patients had a revision (2 septic, 8 aseptic), and 6 had primary knee replacement. The patients were followed postoperatively for an average of 30 months (range: 2 to 4 years) after the procedure. Information on the patient's quadriceps function was obtained at the follow-up. In addition to this, and a standard Hospital for Special Surgery knee score, patients' quadriceps were also evaluated using the Cybex 6000 (Lumex, Ronkonkoman, NY). Ten patients were tested 3 months after surgery and 11 were tested one year after surgery when peak torque and work were recorded at speeds of 60 and 180 degrees/second. The quadricep and hamstring strength and endurance of both legs were tested with the Cybex with three repetitions and the results averaged for each patient (Table 19.1).

SURGICAL OUTCOME

The result of primary and revision knee replacement should not be compromised in any way because of the quadriceps snip technique. More importantly, the increased exposure, and minimal complications we observed, may allow the surgeon and patient to have an optimal result. Of the 16 patients in this investigation,

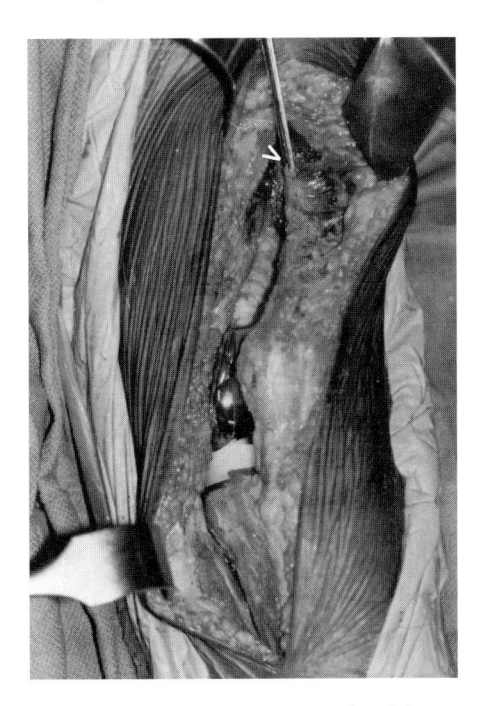

Figure 19.4. The intraoperative photograph of the quadriceps snip (arrow) and medial parapatellar approach.

10 were rated as excellent and 6 as good, using the Hospital for Special Surgery knee score. Furthermore, 4 of these patients were able to return to their presurgical work and their activity level was not limited. One patient could walk up to 10 blocks, and 9 patients could walk 1 to 5 blocks, while 2 patients could only walk short distances (less than 1 block) after surgery. All of these patients' knee scores improved at least one grade and their activity level improved.

Knee range of motion improved in 14 of the 16 patients by an average of 38 degrees (range: 5 to 85 degrees). Five of the patients did have a postoperative knee flexion contracture that averaged 5 degrees, but none of these had a contracture greater than 10 degrees. The results of Cybex testing of the knees, which included peak torque and work, showed no significant difference between the quadriceps snip knee and the opposite knee, which had undergone total knee replacement. The difference in the peak torque, which was statistically significant when the knee with the quadriceps snip was compared to the opposite knee that had not been operated ($p < 0.04$, $p < 0.034$), although the difference in work was not significant.

DISCUSSION

Surgical technique in total knee arthroplasty depends on adequate exposure of the area to properly inspect reference points about the knee for alignment and component placement. Furthermore, exposure is essential when preparing the bone to accept placement of the prosthesis. In 1943, Coonse and Adams reported a new approach to the knee that provided good exposure of the knee with less trauma to the structures of the knee joint.[1] It was simple to perform, but an associated risk was devascularization of the patella and the attached proximal tongue of the quadriceps tendon.

In 1983, Insall modified the Coonse-Adams approach to exposure of the knee.[2,3] His approach, also known as the patellar turndown, provided good exposure with the added benefits of maintaining the integrity of the vastus medialis, and preserving the inferior lateral geniculate artery to the turned down segment. This remains a standard approach and one of the most popular and often used techniques by knee surgeons for similar problems. The exposure allowed by these techniques is excellent, but both require postoperative immobilization of the knee in extension for up to three weeks. A resultant extension lag may prolong the postoperative recovery of the patient and, in some cases, persist for several months.

An alternative to the procedures described is tibial tubercle osteotomy. This was first described by Dolin[4] in 1983, and has since been reported on by other authors. Wolf and associates[5] reported on 24 patients who had 26 tibial tubercle osteotomies in conjunction with total knee replacements. In five of the knees an extension lag averaging 24 degrees occurred. An extension

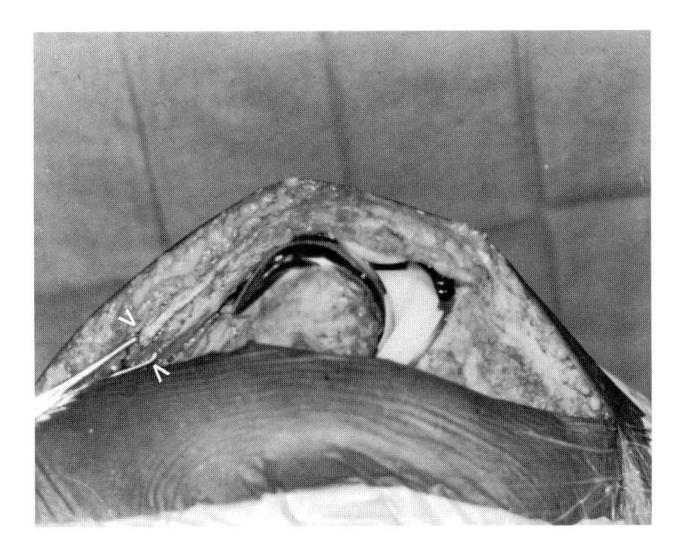

Figure 19.5. The intraoperative photograph demonstrates patellar tracking during total knee replacement, which can be accomplished by placing longitudinal traction on the quadriceps.

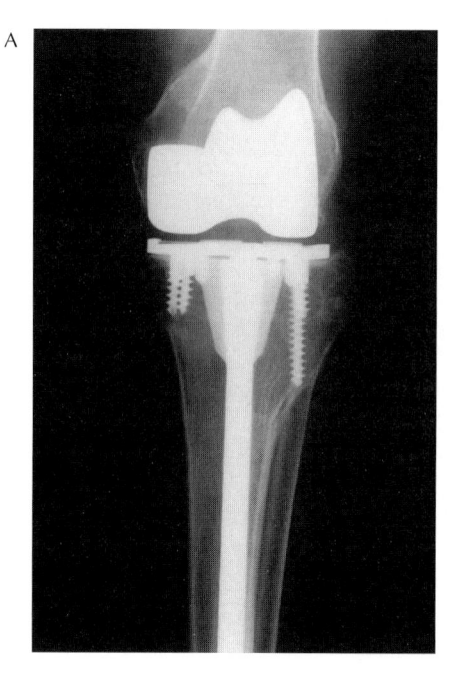

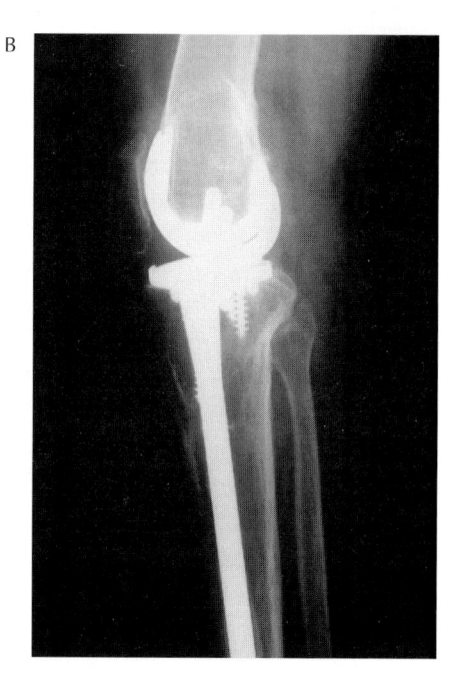

Figure 19.6. The X-rays are of a 62-year-old female who, 10 years prior to this evaluation, sustained a femur fracture above a total knee arthroplasty during manipulation for stiffness.

lag occurred only in knees that had disruption of the extensor mechanism. Whiteside and Ohl made modifications to the procedure, and in 1990 reported on 71 patients who had the procedure to expose the joint for total knee arthroplasty.[6] In follow-up none of the tibial tubercles fractured or pulled loose. In one case the tibial tubercle migrated proximally 1 cm, causing mild patella alta, but did not result in extension lag. No extension lag was found in this series and mean flexion contracture was 2.5 degrees.

The quadriceps snip is a safe, simple alternative that does not require special equipment or instrumentation. It is technically much easier to do and the patient's postoperative physical therapy routine does not have to be altered. Furthermore, if it becomes necessary that more exposure be obtained, the quadriceps snip can be converted to a V-Y quadricepsplasty to provide this exposure.[7] At the time of this writing, it has not been necessary to convert the quadriceps snip to a V-Y quadricepsplasty or turndown.

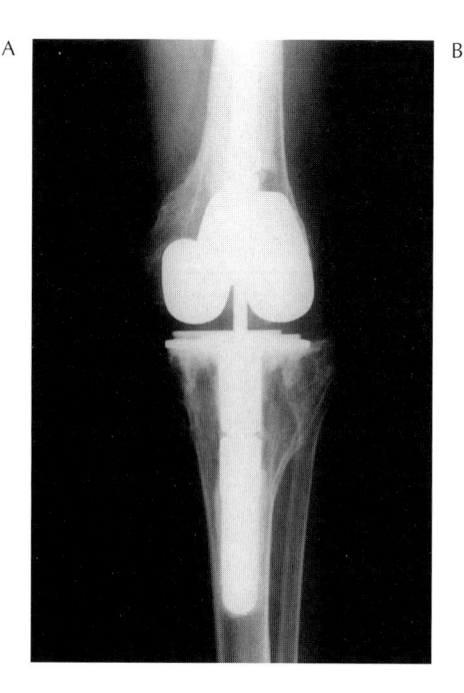

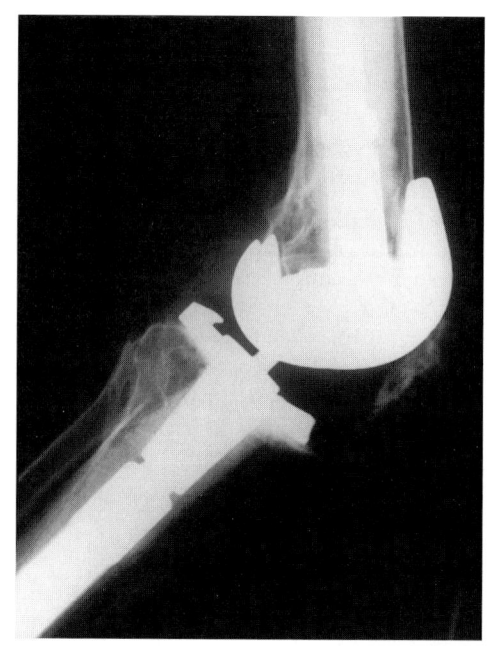

Figure 19.7. The X-rays are at the 1-year follow-up of the patient. At that time, the patient had no complaints, was able to negotiate stairs, and walk unlimited distances. Range of motion showed full extension and flexion to 80 degrees.

Table 19.1 Results with the quadriceps snip

Case	Age/Gender	Preoperative Diagnosis	Procedure	Length of Follow-up	Range of Motion Preoperative	Range of Motion Postoperative	Knee Score Preoperative	Knee Score Postoperative
1.	67/F	Rheumatoid Arthritis	L Total Knee Revision	35 months	−45 to 60	0 to 70	33	80
2.	68/M	Infected L Total Knee Arthroplasty	R Reimplantation	24 months	−20 to 70	0 to 90	41	91
3.	66/M	Mechanically Failed L Total Knee Arthroplasty	L Revision	24 months	−10 to 112	−5 to 115	46	97
4.	73/M	Mechanically Failed L Total Knee Arthroplasty	L Revision	24 months	−10 to 95	−5 to 120	57	83
5.	59/M	Arthrofibrosed after Total Knee Arthroplasty	L Revision	24 months	−25 to 80	−10 to 112	59	93
6.	50/F	Mechanically Failed R Total Knee Arthroplasty	R Revision	24 months	fixed 30	0 to 115	9	88
7.	66/F	Infected R Total Knee Arthroplasty	R Reimplantation	30 months	−20 to 80	−10 to 92	32	88
8.	73/M	Mechanically Failed L Total Knee Arthroplasty	L Revision	31 months	0 to 115	0 to 90	57	76
9.	67/M	Mechanically Failed L Total Knee Arthroplasty	L Revision	48 months	−30 to −60	0 to 100	7	81
10.	68/M	Mechanically Failed L Total Knee Arthroplasty with Instability	R Revision	24 months	0 to 100	0 to 100	57	78
11.	68/M	Mechanically Failed L Total Knee Arthroplasty	L Revision	24 months	0 to 90	0 to 120	56	90
12.	66/M	Post-Traumatic Arthritis with Arthrofibrosis	L Total Knee Revision	24 months	−20 to 40	0 to 70	55	92
13.	68/M	Status Post High Tibial Osteotomy—Osteoarthritis	L Total Knee Revision	24 months	0 to 90	0 to 105	55	93
14.	65/F	Psoriatic Arthritis	L Total Knee Revision	24 months	−5 to 75	−5 to 80	57	89
15.	58/M	Status Post High Tibial Osteotomy	L Total Knee Revision	24 months	−10 to 90	0 to 110	49	94
16.	63/M	Post Traumatic Arthritis with Arthrofibrosis	R Total Knee Revision	24 months	−30 to 45	0 to 60	51	84

SUMMARY

The evolution of the surgical technique was a fortuitous observation by a master surgeon with a keen sense of awareness. What some may have thought was a complication has developed into a procedure that in our experience does no harm, and greatly improves the surgical exposure in knee surgery for the stiff, ankylosed joint, and revision knee surgery.

References

1. Coonse K, Adams JD. A new operative approach to the knee joint. *Surg Gynecol Obstet.* 1943; 77:344–347.
2. Insall JN. Chapter 3. Surgical approaches to the knee. In: Insall JN, ed. *Surgery of the Knee.* New York: Churchill Livingstone; 1984: 41–54.
3. Insall JN. Miscellaneous Items: arthrodesis, the stiff knee, synovectomy, and popliteal cysts. In: Insall JN, ed. *Surgery of the Knee.* New York: Churchill Livingstone; 1984: 733–737.

4. Dolin MG. Osteotomy of the tibial tubercle in total knee replacement. A technical note. *J Bone Joint Surg.* 1983; 65A: 704–706.
5. Wolff AM, Hungerford DS, Krackow KA, Jacobs MS. Osteotomy of the tibial tubercle during total knee replacement. *J Bone Joint Surg.* 1989; 71A:848–852.
6. Whiteside LA, Ohl MD. Tibial tubercle osteotomy for exposure of the difficult total knee arthroplasty. *Clin Orthop.* 1990; 260:6–9.
7. Trousdale RT, Hanssen AD, Rand JA, Cahalan TD. V-Y quadricepsplasty in total knee arthroplasty. *Clin Orthop.* 1993; 286:48–55.
8. Garvin KL, Scuderi GS, Insall JN. Evolution of the quadriceps snip. *Clin Orthop.* 1995; 321:131–137.

CHAPTER 20
V-Y Quadricepsplasty

John J. Callaghan and Russell E. Windsor

When performing a total knee arthroplasty in a stiff knee, several special considerations are warranted. The goal of the surgeon in these circumstances is to gain adequate exposure to the knee so as to allow release of the contracted tissues without avulsion of the patella tendon from the tibial tubercle. Patella tendon avulsion is one of the most disabling complications following total knee replacement and reconstruction for this problem does not always provide satisfying functional results.[2] An additional problem with the stiff knee is the contracted quadriceps tendon that prevents adequate flexion (to 90 plus degrees).

Several approaches have been utilized at the time of surgery to address these problems associated with performing total knee arthroplasty in the stiff knee. Options in these situations include tibial tubercle osteotomy, quadriceps snip, and V-Y quadricepsplasty (Fig. 20.1). The potential benefit of V-Y quadricepsplasty over tibial tubercle osteotomy and quadriceps snip procedures is the ability to lengthen the quadriceps tendon, in addition to gaining knee joint exposure, while preserving patella tendon-tibial tubercle continuity.

Coonse and Adams initially described the quadriceps turndown in 1943 as an alternative surgical approach to the knee joint.[3] Their quadriceps incision was an inverted V with the distal limbs extending symmetrically (medially and laterally) inferior to the patella (Fig. 20.2A). This incision was modified by John Insall in 1983 to theoretically preserve the inferior lateral genicular artery and to avoid violation of the vastus medialis.[1] The modification involved the use of a medial parapatellar quadriceps incision (standardly used for total knee arthroplasty) with the addition of an inverted V. The apex of the V is at the top of the medial parapatellar incision and the lateral limb extends across the quadriceps mechanism distally 2 to 4 cm lateral to the superior pole of the patella (Fig. 20.2B). The surgeons at the Mayo Clinic have modified this procedure by starting the lateral limb of the quadriceps incision approximately 1 cm above the superior pole of the patella (Fig. 20.2C).[6]

OPERATIVE PROCEDURE

A midline skin incision is made unless previous parapatellar incisions are present. A modified medial parapatellar arthrotomy is performed after visualizing the proximal origin of the quadriceps tendon. When the extensor mechanism is contracted several maneuvers are performed before quadricepsplasty in an attempt to increase the mobility and to allow eversion of the patella. The lateral and medial gutters around the femoral condyles are freed of any scar tissue. Subperiosteal medial release from the proximal tibia is performed all the way posterior to allow external rotation of the tibia as well as anterior translation. If the patella cannot be everted without undue tension and if further lateral retinacular release and quadriceps snip will not allow adequate exposure or extensor mechanism reconstruction (usually cases with less than 60 degrees of flexion and less than 30 to 40 degrees of total motion), a quadriceps turndown is performed. The medial limb of the inverted V has already been performed with the medial arthrotomy. The lateral limb is performed using a sharp knife to cut across the quadriceps tendon from proximal medial to inferior lateral ending 1 cm lateral to the middle of the patella (in the superior inferior direction). After performing the turndown, the medial proximal tibia is exposed in a subperiosteal manner and an entire femoral peel with subperiosteal release of all femoral attachments (medial, lateral, and posterior including the heads of the gastrocnemius muscles) can be performed. When reattaching the turndown at the end of the procedure we recommend flexing the knee to 90 degrees and reapproximating the tendon with abundant number two nonabsorbable suture. This provides the appropriate V-Y lengthening of the tendon. The illustration and photographs in Figures 20.3A–K demonstrate the specifics of the procedure.

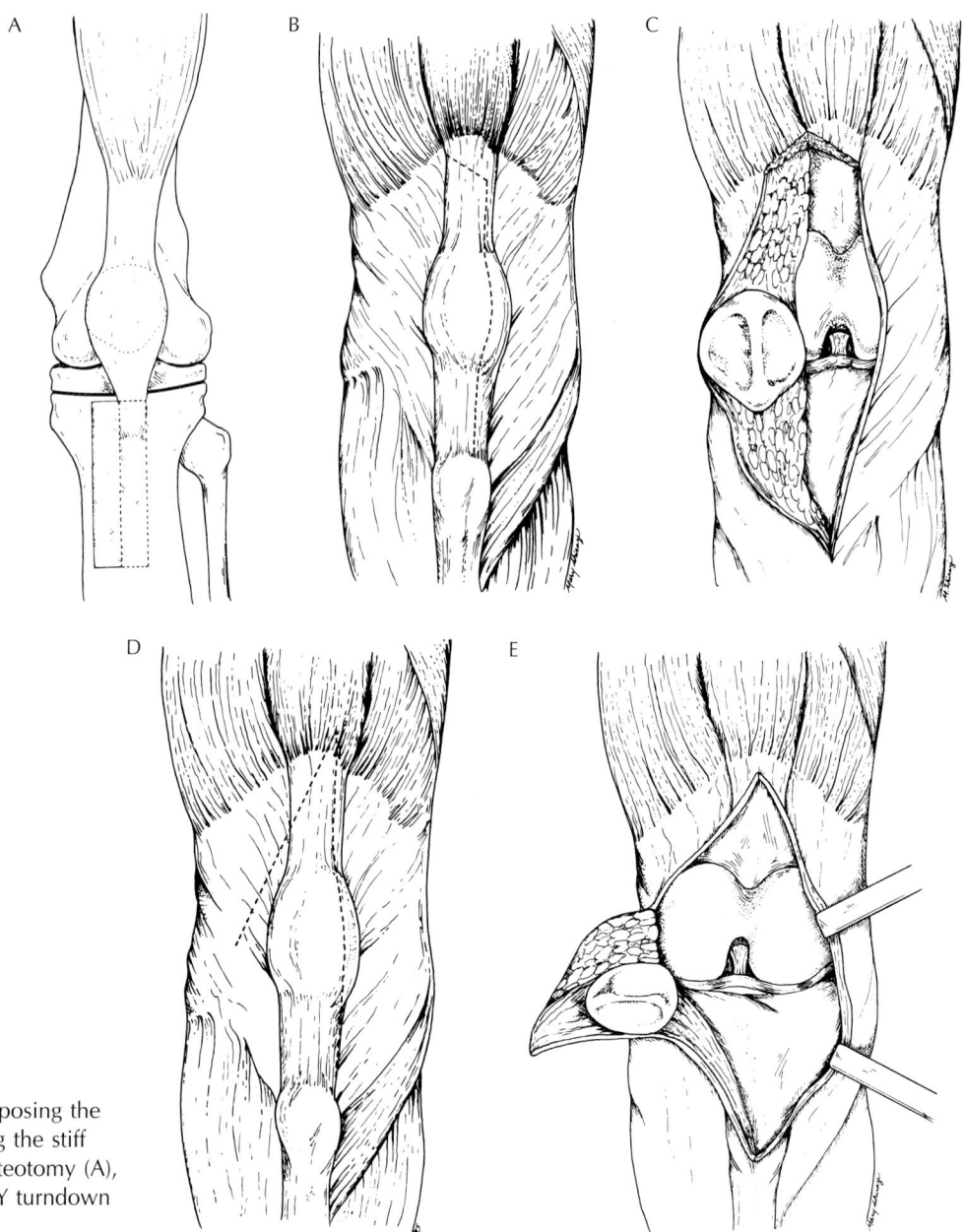

Figure 20.1. Techniques for exposing the stiff knee: Options for exposing the stiff knee include tibial tubercle osteotomy (A), quadriceps snip (B, C), and V-Y turndown quadricepsplasty (D, E).

POSTOPERATIVE REHABILITATION

Initially when the V-Y turndown was utilized for exposure of the stiff knee during total knee arthroplasty, the patients' knees were kept in extension in splints for two weeks. Presently we allow 30 degrees of active flexion with passive extension in the first week. The patients are kept touch weight-bearing and in an immobilizer when not working on active flexion and passive extension. This helps to prevent an extensor lag. After one week, active flexion is advanced 10 degrees a day up to the degree at which flexion was obtained at the time of intraoperative repair. Attempt at further flexion and active extension is not begun until 6 or 7 weeks postop to allow soft tissue healing.

RESULTS OF V-Y QUADRICEPSPLASTY IN TOTAL KNEE ARTHROPLASTY

Scott and Siliski reported using a V-Y quadricepsplasty in 7 total knee arthroplasty procedures. The average increase in flexion was 49 degrees. The average extension lag was 8 degrees.[5] Aglietti and colleagues reported on 26 stiff knees.[1] Flexion improved from an average of 60 degrees before surgery to 85 degrees at the time of follow-up. Flexion contracture was reduced from 28 degrees to 7 degrees, and the total arc of motion significantly increased from 32 to 78 degrees. V-Y quadricepsplasty was used in 11 cases. Trousdale and associates[6] evaluated 16 knees at the Mayo Clinic where a V-Y quadricepsplasty was used to perform to-

20. V-Y Quadricepsplasty

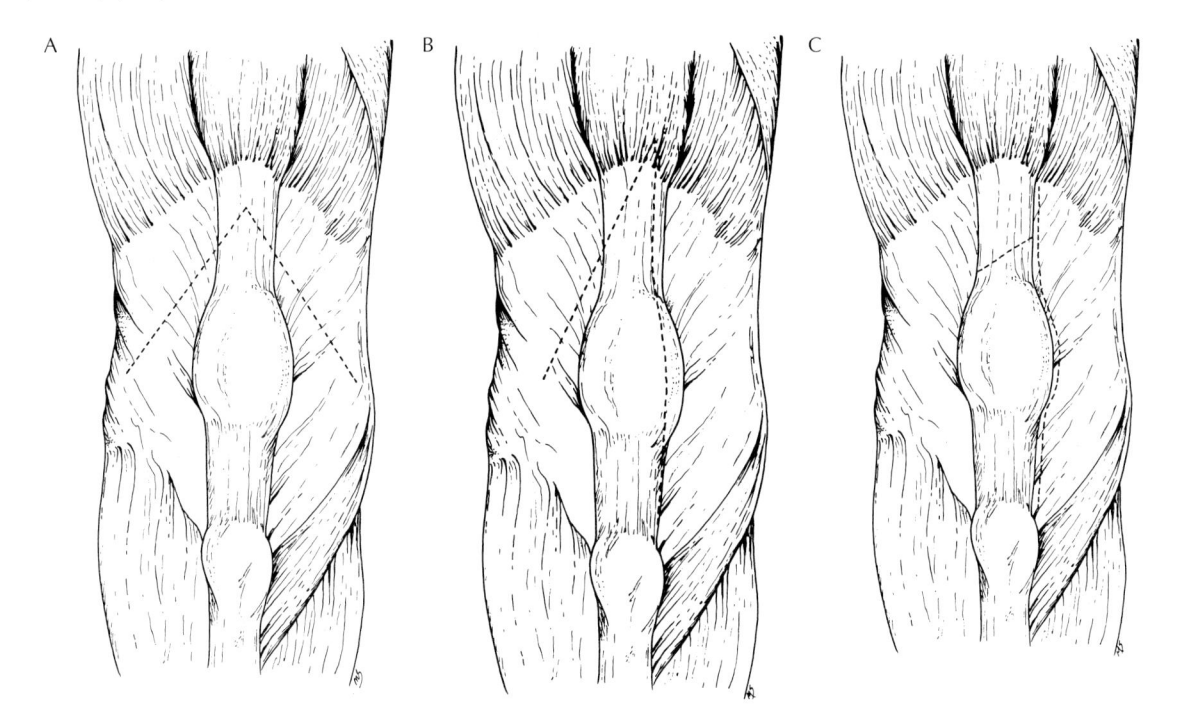

Figure 20.2. Evolution of V-Y quadricepsplasty: Coonse-Adams (A) initially described the quadricepsplasty. Insall (B) modified the approach using a medial parapatellar incision as the medial limb of the incision and Mayo Clinic surgeons (C) further modified the incision using a short lateral limb.

tal knee arthroplasty in stiff knees. Average active range of motion at the time of follow-up was from 4 to 85 degrees. On Cybex-II testing, the extensor mechanisms in knees with V-Y quadricepsplasties were slightly weaker than contralateral knees.

CONCLUSIONS

The V-Y quadricepsplasty has been used less frequently for exposure of the stiff knee when performing total knee arthroplasty since the quadriceps snip was devel-

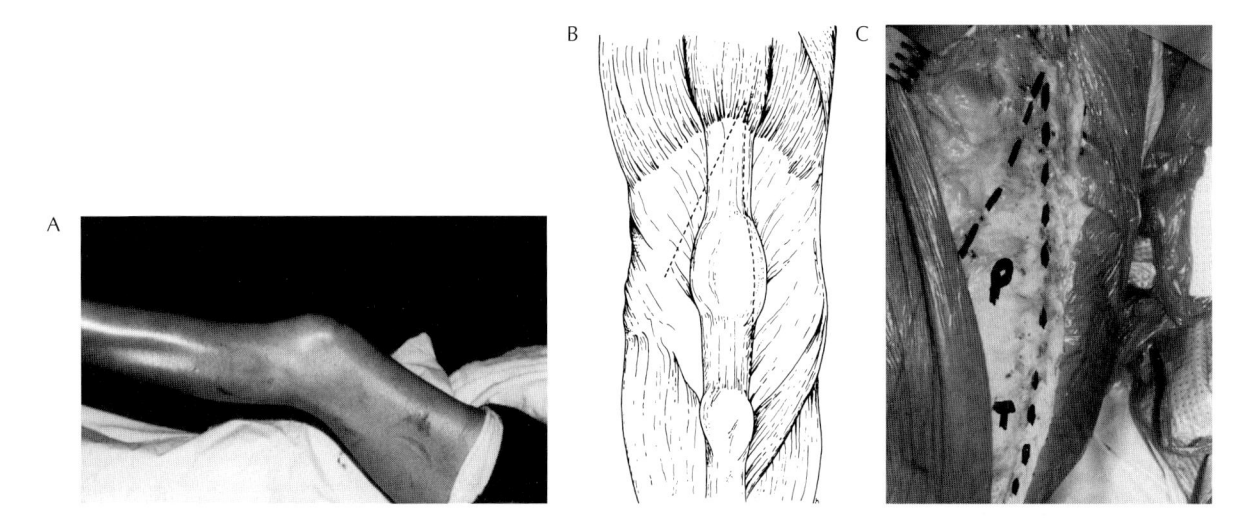

Figure 20.3. Technique of V-Y quadricepsplasty: A typical case (A) for which quadricepsplasty is indicated. Patient could flex knee from 30 to 65 degrees; (B) illustrates the incision in the quadriceps mechanism and (C) is an actual case with P marking the patella and T the tibial tubercle; (D) illustrates the initial turndown and (E) the medial tibial subperiosteal exposure; (F) is a revision case for which the quadriceps tendon has been turned down; (G) illustrates the femoral peel and (H) is a case example; (I) demonstrates the exposure available to insert components when the quadricepsplasty has been utilized; (J) demonstrates the closure of the quadriceps tendon that provides lengthening of the extensor mechanism; (K) demonstrates the 90-degree flexed position where the extensor mechanism is reapproximated.

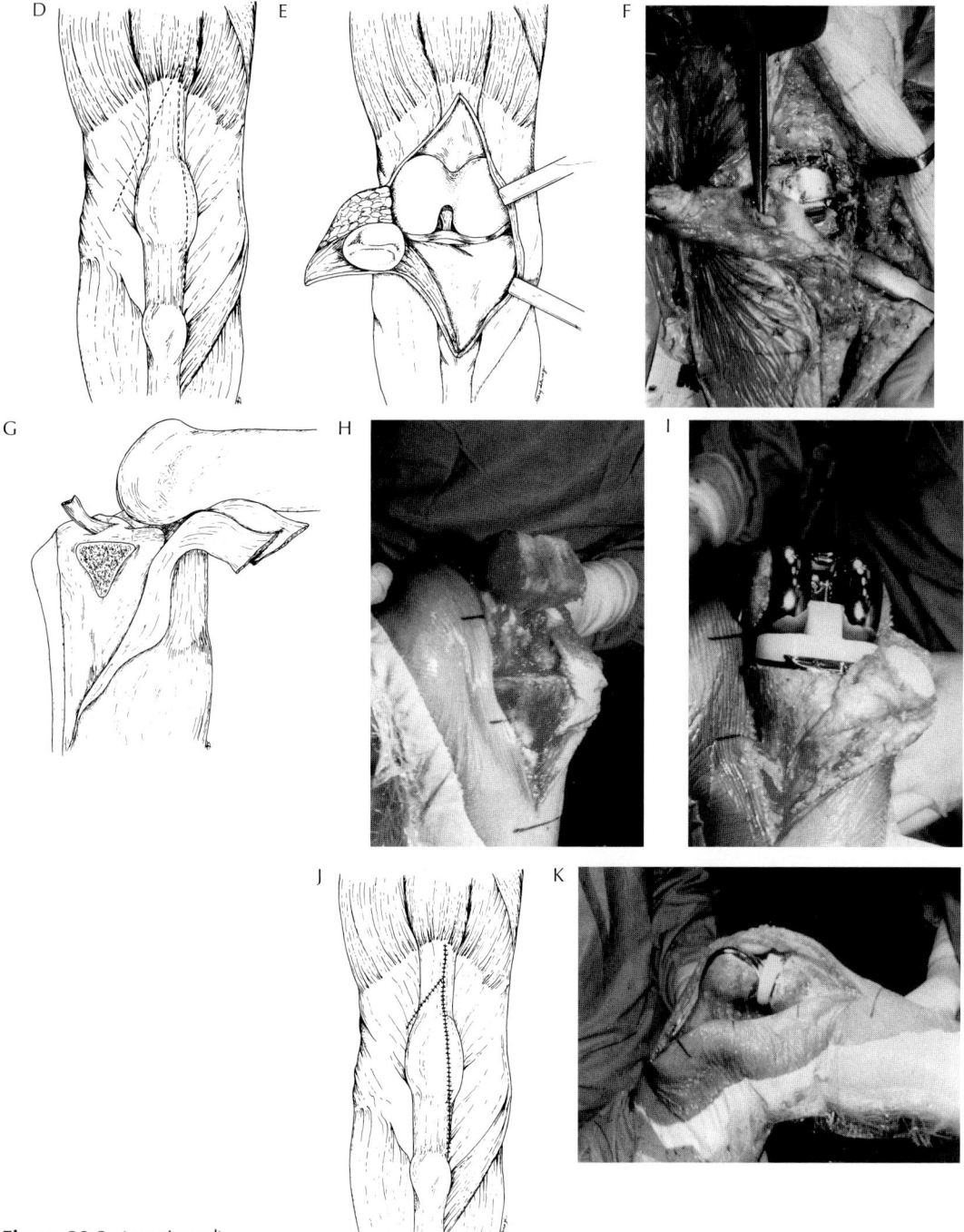

Figure 20.3. (continued).

oped.[4] It still should be considered in the knee with significant flexion contractures (35 to 45 degrees) and limited flexion (65 to 75 degrees). It remains the one procedure that enables elongation of the quadriceps mechanism without disturbing the tibial tubercle.

References

1. Aglietti P, Windsor R, Buzzi R, Insall J. Arthroplasty for the stiff or ankylosed knee. *J Arthroplasty*. 1989; 4:1–5.
2. Cadambi A, Engh G. Use of a semitendinosus tendon autogenous graft for rupture of the patella ligament after total knee arthroplasty: a report of seven cases. *J Bone Joint Surg*. August 1992; 74-A:974–979.
3. Coonse K, Adams J. A new operative approach to the knee joint. *Surg Gynecol Obstet*. 1943; 77:344.
4. Garvin K, Scuderi T, Insall J. Evolution of the quadriceps snip. *Clin Orthop*. 1995; 321:131–137.
5. Scott R, Siliski J. The use of a modified V-Y quadricepsplasty during total knee replacement to gain exposure and improve flexion in the ankylosed knee. *Orthopaedics*. 1985; 8:45.
6. Trousdale R, Hanssen A, Rand J, Cahalan T. V-Y quadricepsplasty in total knee arthroplasty. *Clin Orthop*. 1993; 286:48–55.
7. Windsor R, Insall J. Exposure in revision total knee arthroplasty. The femoral peel. *Techniques Orthop*. 1988; 3:1.

CHAPTER 21
Tibial Tubercle Osteotomy

Leo A. Whiteside

Exposure in difficult total knee replacement is often compromised by fibrosis in the quadriceps mechanism. Transection of the quadriceps tendon above the patella can aid exposure,[1-3] but if repeated entry into the knee is necessary, exposure through this route can compromise quadriceps function.[4] Reports of exposure using the quadriceps tendon approach during difficult total knee replacement generally mention a significant number of knees with moderate to severe quadriceps lag.[4] This suggests that transection of the quadriceps tendon weakens the muscle group, and may cause scarring and fibrosis. During active knee extension, tensile forces are higher in the quadriceps tendon than in the patellar tendon,[5] so release below the patella would seem less likely to fail.

Previous studies of tibial tubercle osteotomy with total knee arthroplasty have reported varying success.[6-8] In 1984 an osteotomy technique was devised to expose knees with dense fibrous adhesions and quadriceps contracture. This technique was reported initially in 1990,[9] and has been used exclusively for exposure of the knee since 1984.

SURGICAL PROCEDURE

The standard surgical approach to total knee replacement generally is used in the first attempt to expose the knee, but full exposure in difficult cases requires an extension of the standard approach. Osteotomy of the tibial tubercle is especially effective when extensive exposure to the lateral half of the knee is required and when a vastus medialis splitting or a subvastus approach has been made. This procedure offers the most extensive exposure to the knee in patients with severe quadriceps contracture, and it is especially useful in patients with fibrous ankylosis and with takedown of knee fusion.

A flap approximately 4 cm long, measured from the top of the tibial tubercle, is elevated through a medial osteotomy that is carried transversely under the tubercle through the lateral cortex (Fig. 21.1). The initial saw cut is made distally at an oblique angle approximately 30 degrees above horizontal with the saw blade directed proximally. The saw also is used to osteotomize the proximal medial cortex. A curved half-inch osteotome is used to make the transverse proximal cut just above the attachment of the patellar tendon into the tubercle. This osteotome cut should be made at a 45-degree angle to create a notch in the tibial bone and a ledge on the tibial tubercle. The half-inch osteotome then is used to elevate the flap of bone 4 cm long, 2 cm wide, and 1 cm thick, and to cut through the lateral cortex of the tibia. The lateral attachments of the muscles and the periosteum are left intact (Fig. 21.2). The stress riser effect of the osteotomy is minimized by the oblique saw cut at the distal end of the osteotomized segment. The soft tissue attachments between the fat pad and anterior tibia must be severed, and a small amount of the anterolateral capsular attachment of the tibia must be released to allow the quadriceps mechanism to turn laterally. Where there is dense contracture of the quadriceps group, an extended incision proximally is necessary (Fig. 21.2). When intraosseous exposure of the proximal tibia is necessary, and a long stem is planned for the tibial component of the total knee arthroplasty, a longer tubercle osteotomy often is indicated. Care should be used that the stem of the tibial component extends well below the distal end of the osteotomy, especially in patients with decreased proprioception.

When the tubercle osteotomy is used for exposure of

Reprinted in part with permission from the American Academy of Orthopaedic Surgeons and from Lippincott-Raven Publishers. In: *Instructional Course Lectures Volume 46*, "Surgical Exposure in Revision Total Knee Arthroplasty" by Leo A. Whiteside; and In: "Exposure in difficult total knee arthroplasty using tibial tubercle osteotomy," *Clin Orthop* 321:32–35, 1995, by Leo A, Whiteside, MD.

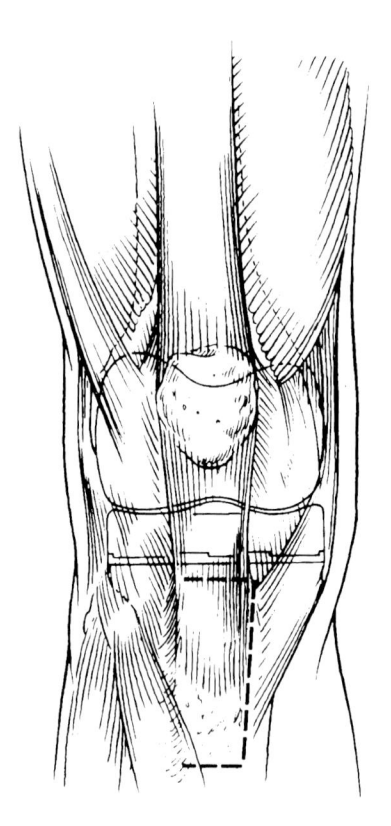

Figure 21.1. Outline of the tibial tubercle osteotomy. The distal portion of the osteotomy is made with a saw, and the medial, superior, and lateral portions are made with a curved osteotome. Lateral soft tissue attachments are left intact.

the knee, it is not necessary to transect the main rectus tendon. Instead, the proximal incision is allowed to follow the cleavage plane between the vastus medialis and vastus intermedius (Fig. 21.3). The nerve and blood supply to the vastus medialis enter from above and posteriorly, and spread throughout the muscle distally, but the plane between the vastus medialis and vastus intermedius is crossed by few motor nerve fibers and thus can be dissected without compromising healing or muscle function. Often the quadriceps mechanism is tightly adherent to the anterior aspect of the femur, and must be dissected carefully from the bone to allow the quadriceps to be turned laterally; however, it is not necessary to transect any of the lateral aspect of the quadriceps mechanism. The lateral soft tissue attachments to the tibial tubercle allow the bone flap to turn laterally while maintaining its blood supply. These fibers also maintain attachment of the bone fragment and prevent its proximal migration.

Careful reattachment of the tibial tubercle osteotomy will avoid fracture of the proximal pole of the osteotomized fragment. Because the lateral soft tissue hinge has been left intact, the lateral edge does not need to be fixed. However, the medial edge requires firm attachment to bone. When screws are used to reattach this segment, they must be placed through the central or medial aspect of the fragment to be effective. Drill holes in this area significantly weaken the bone fragment and often cause fractures. The proximal screw hole, placed in the soft cancellous bone of the tubercle, is especially vulnerable to fracture.[8] Severe extension lag can result if a fracture occurs through the proximal pole, and surgical repair is difficult. Fixation of the tibial tubercle with wires, however, is highly effective and is safe from fracture. The drill holes are placed along the lateral edge of the tibial tubercle and directed obliquely distally to penetrate the posteromedial edge of the tibial cortex. The wires are passed through these drill holes and twisted down. They pull obliquely downward across almost the entire width of the tibial tubercle and provide semirigid fixation.

CLINICAL RESULTS

One hundred thirty-six total knee replacements were exposed using the extended tibial tubercle osteotomy tech-

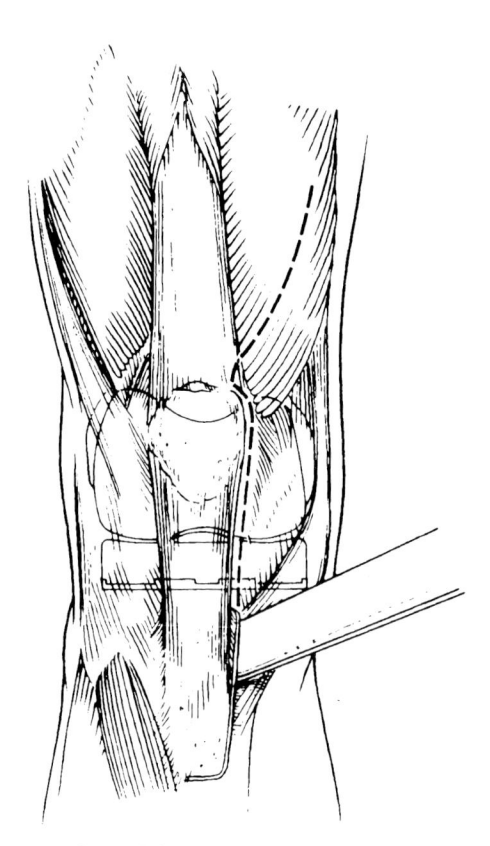

Figure 21.2. Outline of the incision used with tibial tubercle osteotomy exposure of the knee. The incision can be placed medially to the main quadriceps tendon, and can be allowed to extend proximally in line with the fibers of the vastus medialis. The osteotomy is made from the medial side to maintain the lateral soft tissue hinge.

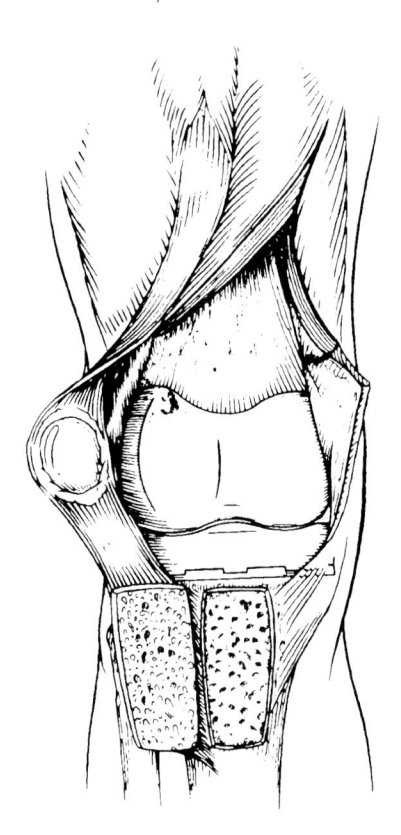

Figure 21.3. Exposure of the knee with tibial tubercle osteotomy. The interval between the vastus medialis and vastus medialis obliquus has been split in line with the muscle fibers. The lateral soft tissue attachments to the tibial tubercle are oriented longitudinally, so the bone fragment does not slip proximally.

nique from 1986 to 1994.[10] Twenty-six knees had primary total knee arthroplasty, 76 had first revision total knee arthroplasty, 10 had repeated revision total knee arthroplasty, 19 had infected total knee arthroplasty, and five had repeated revision for infected total knee arthroplasty. The patients ranged in age from 34 to 88 years. Sixty-one patients were men and 75 were women.

After the surgical procedure, patients were started on early mobilization, allowed leg raising as tolerated, and placed on the same rehabilitation program as the primary total knee replacement patients. This included full weight-bearing both in primary cases and in revision cases with good bone support.

At two years after surgery, the mean range of motion in these cases was 93.7 degrees (range, 15 to 140 degrees). Two knees had extension lag, but it was present in both cases before the surgery. The tibial tubercle in two knees had partial proximal avulsion fracture, but did not separate widely. Healing occurred in all cases, even in the infected ones in which repeated elevation of the tibial tubercle flap and quadriceps mechanism was done. Three wires were removed due to pain or because of late penetration of the skin.

Three tibial fractures occurred, two in a patient who had diabetic Charcot arthropathy and wear of the tibial components. Short stems were used during revision surgery to secure fixation of the tibial components. Early weight-bearing was allowed because of good proximal bone support. Three weeks after surgery the patient noted sudden collapse of her left knee while walking, followed by a similar collapsing phenomenon in the right knee. Radiographs revealed fracture of both tibias through the distal pole of the tibial tubercle osteotomy. These fractures failed to heal, and the tibial components were revised with long-stemmed implants. Subsequent healing occurred and the patient now is functioning well with full range of motion and no extension lag.

The third fracture occurred in a patient who had tibial tubercle osteotomy for open lysis of adhesions. Two weeks after the procedure, the patient had a manipulation under anesthesia, and a fracture occurred through the distal pole of the tibial tubercle osteotomy. This required casting, and the fracture healed with no significant displacement.

DISCUSSION

Loss of fixation of the tibial tubercle has not occurred in our series. The two cases of partial avulsion of the proximal tibial tubercle did not result in dysfunction of the quadriceps mechanism.

Wolff and associates reported a high rate of fixation failure with tibial tubercle osteotomy, but complications related to fixation in their series involved only those cases in which the tibial tubercle fragment was less than 3 cm long and was fixed with screws.[8] It is not clear if the lateral soft tissue attachments were left intact in those cases. The length of the tibial tubercle segment in our series was probably responsible for the absence of fracture and for the minimal problems with fixation. The intact lateral muscular attachments and lateral capsular structures maintained blood supply to the tibial tubercle and patellar tendon and probably contributed to rapid healing of the osteotomy. At first glance screw fixation might appear to be preferable to fixation with wires because the feeling of rigid fixation is easier to achieve with screws. However, screw holes in this fragile bone segment are likely to weaken it enough to precipitate catastrophic failure through the upper screw hole as was noted in Wolff's series.[8] By passing the wires through the lateral edge of the tibial tubercle and through the medial tibial cortex, the entire substance of the tibial tubercle is used to resist the wires as they are pulled through the bone. These drill holes along the lateral edge of the tubercle and tibial crest fragment do not appear to significantly weaken it. This wiring technique is especially helpful when a large tibial stem is used on the tibial component.

Although transecting the quadriceps tendon offers a means for effective exposure of the knee, it violates an already compromised soft tissue structure and could restrict knee flexion and produce extension lag. Denham and Bishop found that tensile loads often are much higher in the quadriceps mechanism above the patella than in the patellar tendon below.[5] The tendency to fail in tension should be lower with repairs distal to the patella, especially if strong wire fixation through robust bony structures are used to maintain the repair. With tibial tubercle osteotomy, one relies on heavy wire loops passed through bone to resist lower tensile load. When the quadriceps mechanism itself is transected and repaired, one must rely on sutures passed through soft tissue to hold a higher tensile load.

Occasionally transfer of the tibial tubercle is necessary to correct patellar maltracking, and rarely must the tibial tubercle be elevated to prevent impingement of the patella against the tibial polyethylene component in cases of patella infera. Exposing the difficult knee through the tibial tubercle offers a convenient means to deal with these difficult cases.

Extended tibial tubercle osteotomy weakens the upper tibia, and predisposes it to fracture in cases of unusually high stress. The three cases of fracture of the proximal tibia in this series resulted in significant clinical consequences, and these cases illustrate the importance of caution after using this approach to the knee. In the insensate knee or in cases in which manipulation is expected, tibial components with stems that bypass the osteotomized area of the tibia would be a prudent choice.

CONCLUSION

Exposure of the knee for total knee arthroplasty can be hindered by a variety of conditions that affect the quadriceps muscle and tendons, patella, patellar tendon, capsule, and ligaments of the knee. Most conditions are addressed directly by the arthroplasty, or are reversible by rehabilitative efforts after surgery. Because the rehabilitative potential of the quadriceps mechanism is difficult to predict, surgical approaches that transect the quadriceps tendon, or even lengthen it, may produce disappointing results long term. Tibial tubercle osteotomy is especially attractive for exposure of the knee because it does not add additional injury to the quadriceps muscle and tendons, and allows early vigorous rehabilitation.

ACKNOWLEDGMENT

The author appreciates the editorial assistance of Diane Morton, BA, in the preparation of this manuscript.

References

1. Coonse K, Adams JD. A new operative approach to the knee joint. *Surg Gynecol Obstet*. 1943; 77:344–347.
2. Scott RD, Siliski JM. The use of a modified V-Y quadricepsplasty during total knee replacement to gain exposure and improve flexion in the ankylosed knee. *Orthopedics*. 1985; 8:45–48.
3. Windsor RE, Insall JN. Exposure in revision total knee arthroplasty: the femoral peel. *Tech Orthop*. 1988; 3:1–4.
4. Trousdale RT, Hanssen AD, Rand JA, Cahalan TD. V-Y quadricepsplasty in total knee arthroplasty. *Clin Orthop*. 1993; 286:48–55.
5. Denham RA, Bishop RED. Mechanics of the knee and problems in reconstructive surgery. *J Bone Joint Surg*. 1978; 60B:345–352.
6. Dolin MG. Osteotomy of the tibial tubercle total knee replacement. A technical note. *J Bone Joint Surg*. 1983; 65A: 704–706.
7. Levy RN. Osteotomy of the tibial tubercle in total knee replacement (letter). *J Bone Joint Surg*. 1983; 65A:1207–1208.
8. Wolff AM, Hungerford DS, Krackow KA, Jacobs MA. Osteotomy of the tibial tubercle during total knee replacement. *J Bone Joint Surg*. 1989; 71A:848–852.
9. Whiteside LA, Ohl MD. Tibial tubercle osteotomy for exposure of the difficult total knee arthroplasty. *Clin Orthop*. 1990; 260:6–9.
10. Whiteside LA. Exposure in difficult total knee arthroplasty using tibial tubercle osteotomy. *Clin Orthop*. 1995; 321:32–35.

SECTION 5
Principles of Primary Total Knee Arthroplasty

CHAPTER 22
The Basic Principles

Giles R. Scuderi

In primary total knee arthroplasty, whether a posterior cruciate-retaining or posterior cruciate-substituting design is implanted, the clinical results are influenced by the surgical technique. Adherence to the basic principles of the surgical technique ensures a successful outcome.

The goal of primary total knee arthroplasty is to reestablish the normal mechanical axis with a stable prosthesis that is well fixed (Fig. 22.1). This is achieved by both the bone resection and the soft tissue balance. The femoral component should be aligned with 5 to 10 degrees valgus angulation in the coronal plane and 0 to 10 degrees of flexion in the sagittal plane. The tibia should be resected at 90 ± 2 degrees to the long axis of the tibia in the coronal plane. In the sagittal plane, the posterior slope is dictated by the prosthetic design, but it appears preferable to recreate the posterior slope of the natural tibia.

Regardless of prosthetic design there are three basic bone cuts in primary total knee arthroplasty: the proximal tibia, the distal femur, and the posterior femur (Fig. 22.2). Each one influences the arthroplasty in a different manner (Table 22.1). Usually the amount of bone resected corresponds to the thickness of the component being implanted. Resection of the proximal tibia influences both the flexion and extension gaps and is replaced by the tibial component. The more tibial bone resected, the thicker the tibial component. Resection of the distal femur selectively influences the extension gap. Usually the distal femur is resected 9 to 10 mm from the unaffected or normal side, which in the case of a varus knee is the lateral femoral condyle. This concept of removing as much bone as being replaced by the femoral component helps to reassure reestablishment of the joint line. Over-resection of the distal femur creates an extension gap that is larger than the flexion gap resulting in recurvatum, whereas under-resection creates a flexion contracture. Resection of the posterior femur selectively influences the flexion space. If the flexion gap is larger than the extension gap, then posterior flexion instability will occur. It is recommended that the amount of bone resected be replaced by the implant.

There is a fourth cut that seems to receive less attention. The anterior femoral resection influences both the flexion space and the patellofemoral joint. The amount of bone resected from the anterior femur is dependent upon sizing of the femur and position of the anteroposterior cutting guide. Under-resection of the anterior femur is caused by an inappropriately large femoral component or by anterior placement of the correct size component with excessive posterior resection. This leads to overstuffing of the patellofemoral joint, which may possibly lead to limited motion and patellofemoral dysfunction. Conversely, over-resection of the anterior condyles may result in notching of the distal femur.

The ligament releases, to correct fixed angular deformities, are discussed elsewhere in this text and should be reviewed, but the basic principles will be highlighted. For the fixed-varus deformity, the medial soft tissue release includes the deep medial collateral ligament, the posteriomedial corner (including the semitendinosus), and the superficial medial collateral ligament. Correction of a fixed-valgus deformity tends to be sequential with release of the posterolateral capsule, the iliotibial band, and the lateral collateral ligament. If possible, it is preferable to preserve the integrity of the popliteus tendon in order to maintain flexion stability. Whatever the fixed deformity, balancing of the tight contracted soft tissues is critical in reestablishing the normal mechanical axis of the knee.

Of prime importance is establishing equal flexion and extension gaps (Fig. 22.3). Anteroposterior stability depends on balanced flexion and extension gaps. These gaps are influenced by femoral component sizing, asymmetry of the flexion space, flexion contracture, and release of the posterior cruciate ligament. Each variable affects the knee in a different way. Failure to address these issues may result in posterior subluxation or dislocation, irrespective of prosthetic design. It is a misconception that proper soft tissue releases that restore

```
                    Fixation
                       ↑
Alignment   ←   Total Knee Arthroplasty   →   Stability
                       ↓
                   Kinematics
```

Figure 22.1. The goals of total knee arthroplasty.

Table 22.1. The basic principles of total knee arthroplasty

1. Restoration of the mechanical axis
2. Restoration of the joint line
3. Balance of the soft tissues
4. Equalize flexion and extension gaps
5. Restore patellofemoral alignment and mechanics

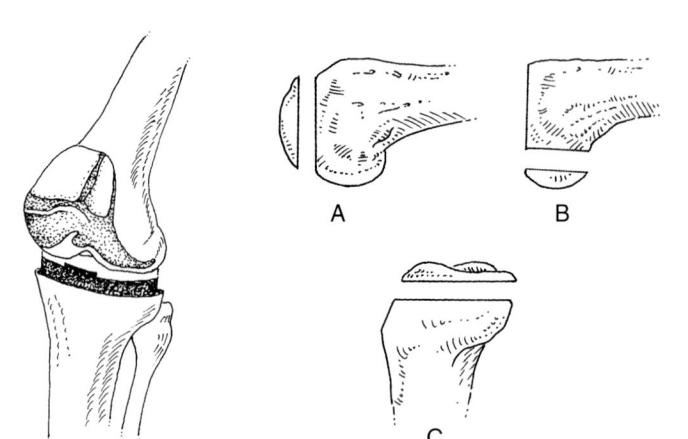

Figure 22.2. The three basic cuts in total knee arthroplasty include the distal femur (A), the posterior femur (B), and the proximal tibia (C). Correct positioning and spacing of these cuts will ensure a stable and well-aligned prosthesis.

the mechanical axis to neutral in extension will ensure stability in flexion. As each variable is reviewed, their influence will be better understood.

Matching the femoral component to the anteroposterior dimension of the femur has always been recommended. When the femur measures in-between sizes, it may be preferable to downsize the femoral component. In this situation, an anterior-referencing system will resect more bone from the posterior femur enlarging the flexion gap, whereas a posterior-referencing system will resect more bone from the anterior femur resulting in an anterior notch (Fig. 22.4). The ideal system should allow the additional bone resection to be divided between the anterior and posterior condyles. Slight flexion of the distal femoral resection avoids anterior notching and permits blending of the anterior femur. There may be situations in which upsizing of the femoral component is preferable, this is usually the case with a wide distal

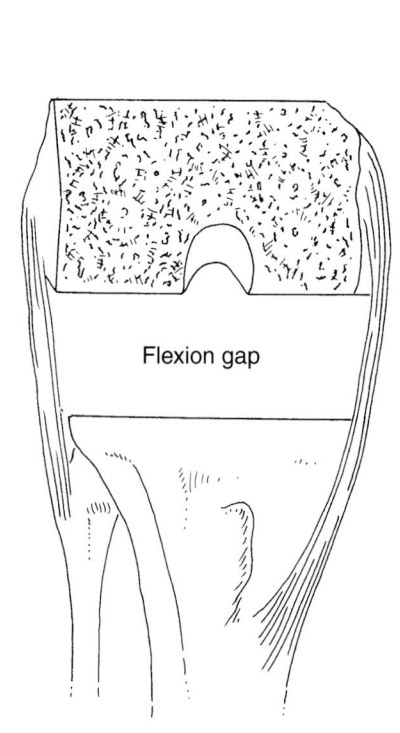

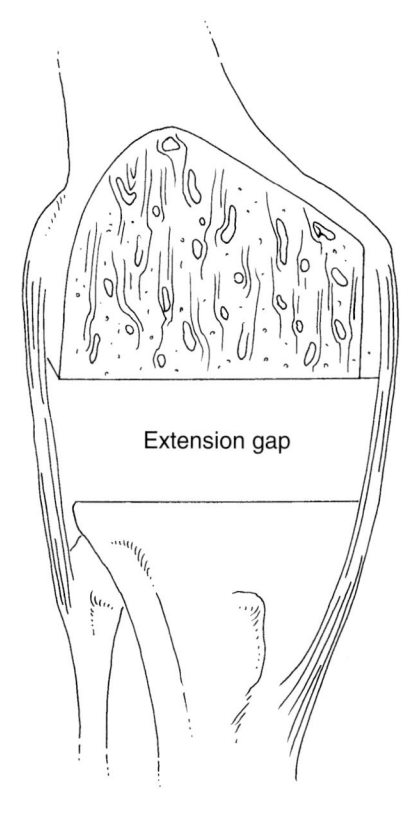

Figure 22.3. The flexion gap must equal the extension gap.

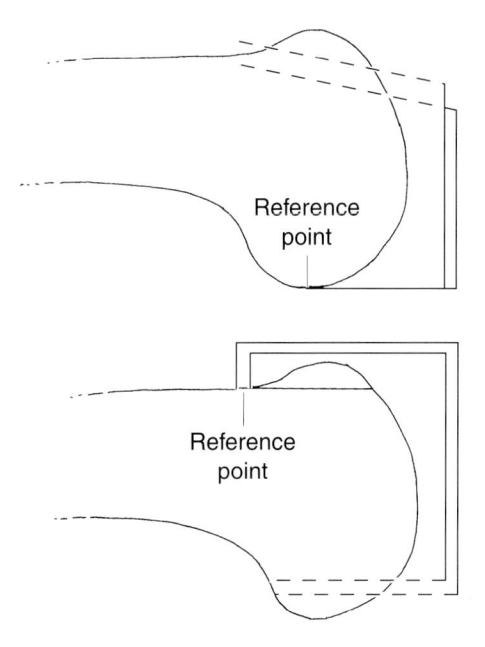

Figure 22.4. When sizing the femur the level of resection can be referenced from the posterior or anterior femur. The posterior reference point causes variation in the anterior resection when the femur measures in between sizes, while an anterior reference point causes variation in the posterior cuts.

femur whose anteroposterior measurement is within 1 to 2 mm of the next larger femoral component.

External rotation of the femoral component has always been advocated. Whether the rotation is set at a predetermined 3 degrees, referenced off the posterior condyles or set in line with the epicondylar axis, a certain amount of external rotation is desirable. The femoral epicondylar axis is a reliable and reproducible landmark for setting femoral component rotation. Following soft tissue balancing, setting the femoral component along the epicondylar axis creates a balanced rectangular space. In addition to its influence on patellar tracking, internal rotation of the femoral component must be avoided because this will cause asymmetry of the flexion space. This asymmetry results in a trapezoidal flexion space that would be tight on the medial side and loose on the lateral side.

Asymmetry of the flexion space can also be related to over-release of a valgus deformity. As discussed elsewhere in this text, there are several techniques described for correction of a fixed-valgus deformity. Although complete release of the lateral supporting structures will correct the axial alignment in extension, over-release will result in an asymmetry of the flexion space. The resultant trapezoidal space would be larger on the lateral side than on the medial side. Correction of the valgus deformity should be sequential, lengthening the lateral soft tissues and attempting to maintain flexion stability.

Following standard resection of the femur and tibia, a knee with a preoperative flexion contracture will probably have a flexion-extension space imbalance. The flexion space would be larger than the extension space. Although it might be appealing to use a thinner tibial polyethylene component, this would cause flexion instability. The correct management of this situation should be a posterior capsule release and resection of additional bone from the distal femur so that the extension space equals the flexion space.

Finally, correct preparation of the patella ensures improved performance of the extensor mechanism and reduces the incidence of complications. The preparation of the patella includes a measured resection that is parallel to the anterior cortex. The bone-patellar component composite should be as thick as the original patella. Even though lateralization of the femoral and tibial components are advocated, the patellar component should be medialized. The assessment of patella tracking is judged by the rule of "no thumbs." Further details of patellar preparation will be discussed in later chapters.

Adhering to these basic principles in both the simple and complex cases ensures a successful outcome.

CHAPTER 23
Draping Technique for Total Knee Arthroplasty

Sergio Gomez, David J. Yasgur, Giles R. Scuderi, and John N. Insall

INTRODUCTION

Preparation of the patient is an important initial step in total knee arthroplasty (TKA). We present a technique that has been utilized for the past 10 years and has been found to be very useful. The technique is easily applied from a unilateral TKA to a bilateral TKA with little modification, allowing the surgical team to proceed to the second knee without redraping. It also has the potential advantages of minimizing operating room time and anesthesia time, while maximizing sterility and cost-effectiveness.

TECHNIQUE

The patient's leg is shaved in the holding area prior to bringing the patient into the operating room (OR). Epidural anesthesia is then administered to help minimize the risk of postoperative deep venous thrombosis.[4] A urinary catheter is inserted and a pneumatic tourniquet is applied over cotton cast padding. The leg is then scrubbed circumferentially with an iodophor solution for 5 minutes. Prophylactic antibiotics are given within 30 minutes of making the skin incision, and are continued for 24 hours.

The procedure is done under vertical laminar flow, with an average of 100 air exchanges per hour. All of the surgeons, operative assistants, and scrub technicians within the laminar flow panels wear helmets that are equipped with a battery operated air filtration system. Sterile hoods are donned prior to sterile gowns and gloves, so that each individual's exhausted air leaves beneath the gowns. This is believed to reduce cross-contamination between patient and staff. Furthermore, laminar flow ORs with occlusive staff garments are proven to have significantly cleaner air than conventionally ventilated ORs,[2] and are generally recommended when available for total hip and knee arthroplasty.[1,3]

The legs are then elevated and painted with povidone iodine topical solution, beginning at the foot. A rolled cotton stockinette is placed over the foot, and the remainder of the leg is painted (Fig. 23.1A). The stockinette is then unrolled fully, to the level of the tourniquet, and gloves are then changed (Fig. 23.1B). The leg is kept elevated while a sterile field is established on the OR table. This consists of an impervious drape, followed by a folded half-sheet. The leg is then lowered onto the table.

A three-quarter sheet is then placed over the tourniquet, and is unfolded to cover the patient's body and the contralateral arm board. A second top sheet is then placed, consisting of another half-sheet, and is used to drape off the ipsilateral arm board. The top and bottom sheets are secured to the stockinette at the level of the tourniquet with nonpenetrating Kelly clamps (Fig. 23.2A). The leg is elevated and an operative extremity drape is applied and advanced as far proximally as possible (Fig. 23.2B). If a bilateral TKA were to be draped, the identical procedure would be done, except that a bilateral operative extremity drape would be applied. The extremity drape is applied reversed (i.e., "inside-out"), so that better adherence to incise drapes (applied next) will be achieved.

The leg is then sealed in impervious incise drapes, of which five are used in the draping of a unilateral TKA. The leg is elevated and a single incise drape is placed under the lower leg and foot (Fig. 23.3A). It is sealed tightly anteriorly and excess drape is cut away (Figs. 23.3B and 23.3C).

The operative field is then exposed by cutting a long elliptical hole in the stockinette. The knee is then dried of excess paint with a lap pad. The skin of the operative site is marked with transverse lines beginning four finger breadths (8 to 10 cm) above the patella to four fin-

23. Draping Technique for Total Knee Arthroplasty

then cut three times into four pieces (one-half, one-fourth, one-eighth, and one-eighth portions). The lower portion of the isolation drape is split and secured to the third incise drape with a one-fourth portion of a fourth incise drape (Fig. 23.7B). The electrocautery, suction tubing, and pulsatile lavage devices are then secured to the isolation drape on the contralateral side of the patient.

A pocket is then created between the end of the OR table and two Mayo stands. The leg is elevated and a three-quarter sheet is unfolded onto the foot of the OR table. Another half portion of the fourth incise drape is used to secure this sheet to the operative extremity drape, taking care to overlap the incise drape with the second incise drape previously placed onto the posterior aspect of the extremity (Fig. 23.8). The pocket is then created as this three-quarter sheet is unfolded onto the two Mayo stands (Figs. 23.9A and 23.9B). The edges of the sheet are each secured to the Mayo stands with one-fourth portions of the fourth incise drape (Figs. 23.9B and 23.9C). Finally, a fifth incise drape is used to cover the lower portion of the operative extremity drape, tak-

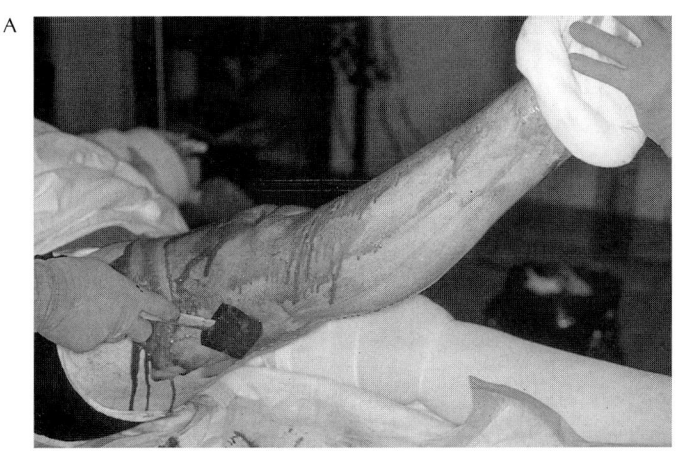

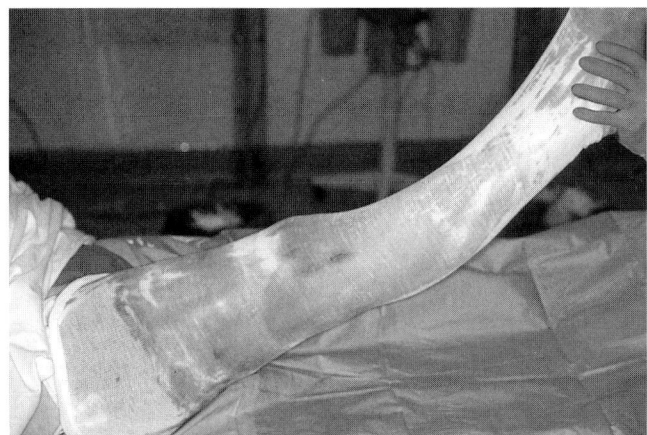

Figure 23.1. (A) and (B) Cotton stockinette applied from toes to tourniquet following preparation with Betadine scrub and paint from toes to tourniquet.

ger breadths below the patella, spaced 4 to 5 cm apart (Fig. 23.4). These markings will serve to help align the skin edges at the time of closure.

Next, the second and third incise drapes will be placed on the leg to form a sandwich of incise drape around the knee. The leg is elevated maximally with the knee extended and the second incise drape is applied to the posterior aspect of the leg, making sure to overlap both the first incise drape and the operative extremity drape (Figs. 23.5A and 23.5B). The third incise drape is then applied over the anterior surface of the knee, taking care to stretch the drape tightly over the skin (Figs. 23.6A and 23.6B). These last two incise drapes completely seal the extremity with a sandwich of tightly applied, impervious incise drape. Excess incise drape is then trimmed (Fig. 23.6C). A bilateral case would then require that the process be repeated for the other knee.

A plastic "shower curtain" isolation drape, similar to one used for hip fractures, is then used to seal off the laminar flow panels from the sterile field, and gloves are changed again (Fig. 23.7A). A fourth incise drape is

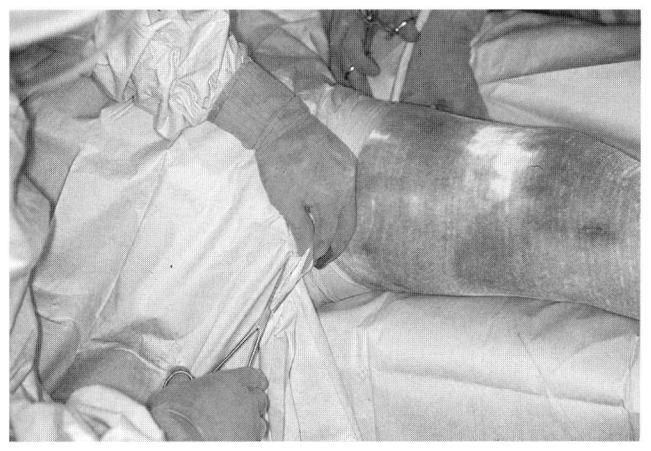

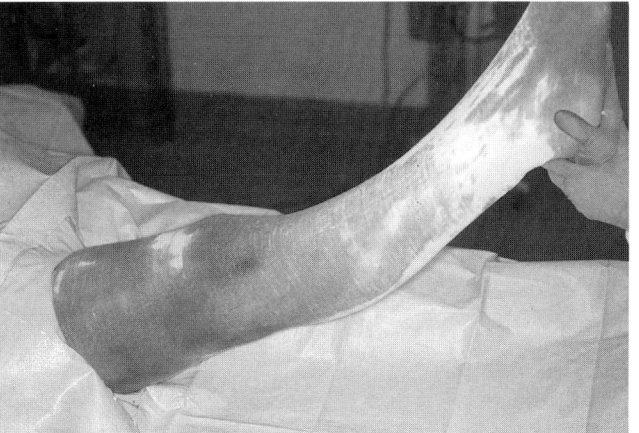

Figure 23.2. (A) Two bottom half sheets and two three-quarter top sheets applied and clamped to stockinette at the level of the tourniquet. (B) Reversed extremity drape applied.

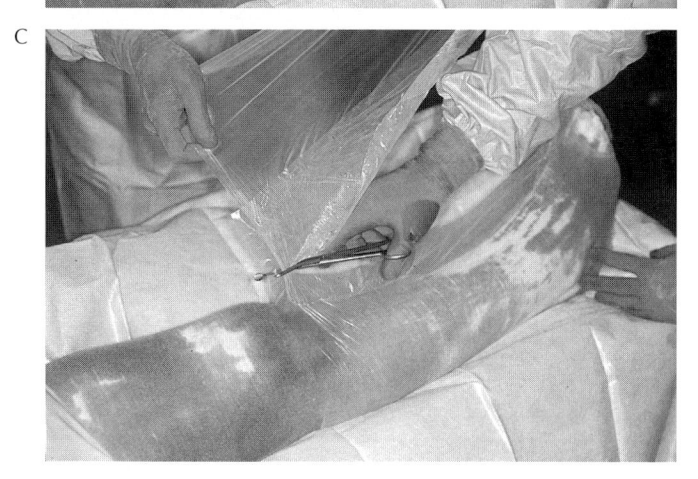

Figure 23.3. (A) The first incise drape applied to the posterior surface of lower leg, (B) sealed anteriorly, and (C) trimmed.

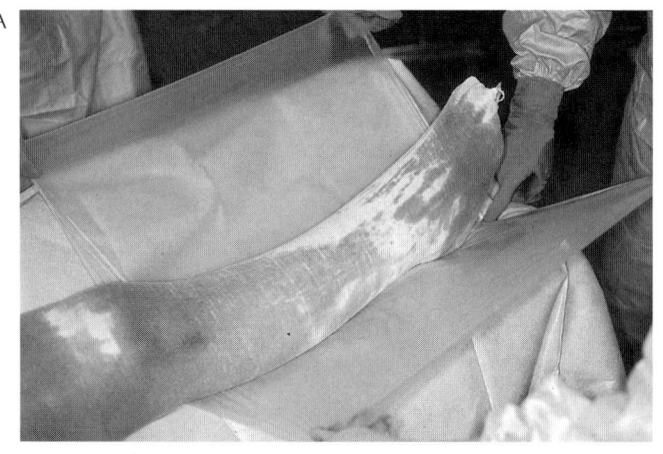

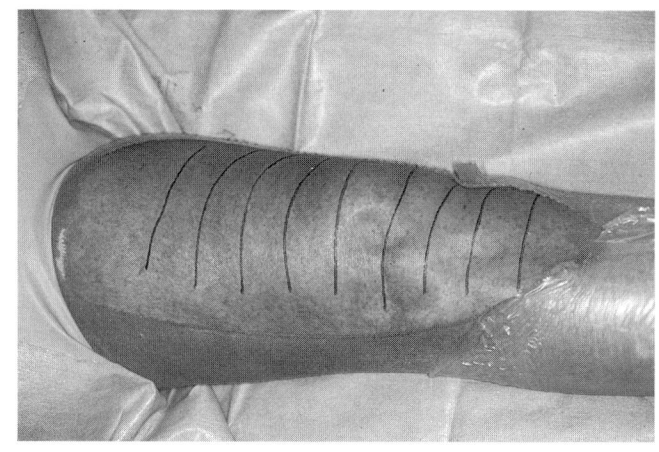

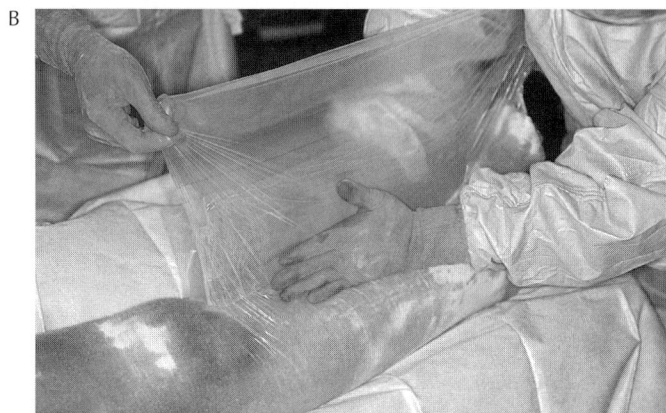

Figure 23.4. A hole is cut into the stockinette and the skin is marked transversely.

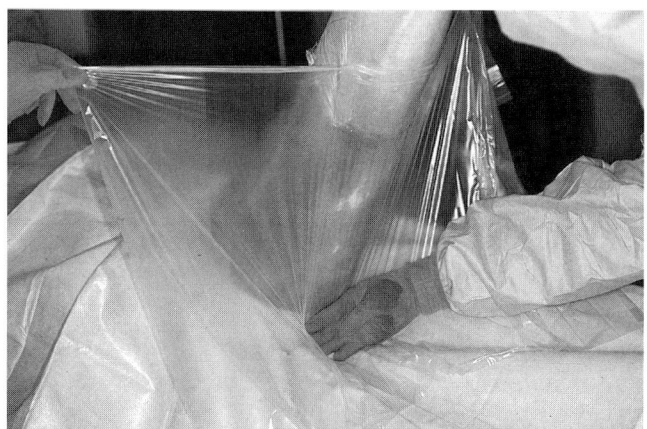

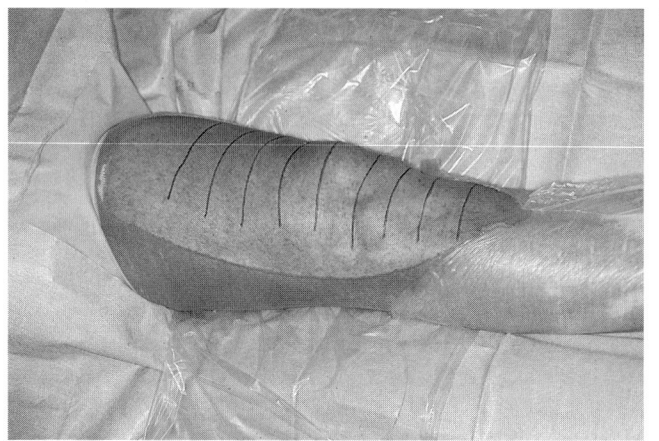

Figure 23.5. (A) and (B) The second incise drape is applied to the posterior surface of the thigh with the adhesive facing anteriorly, overlapping both the first incise drape and the extremity drape.

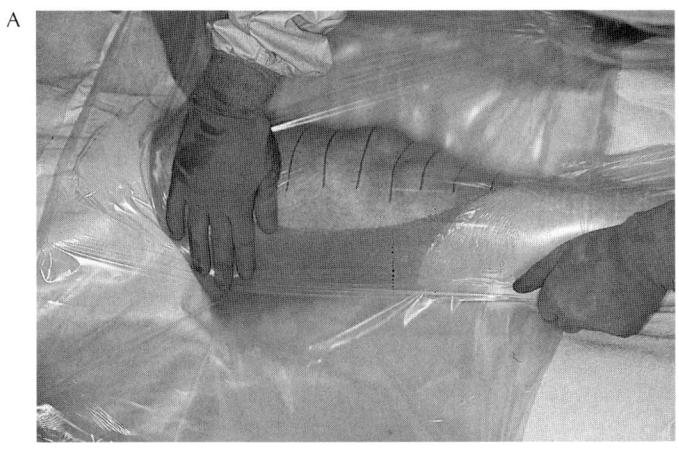

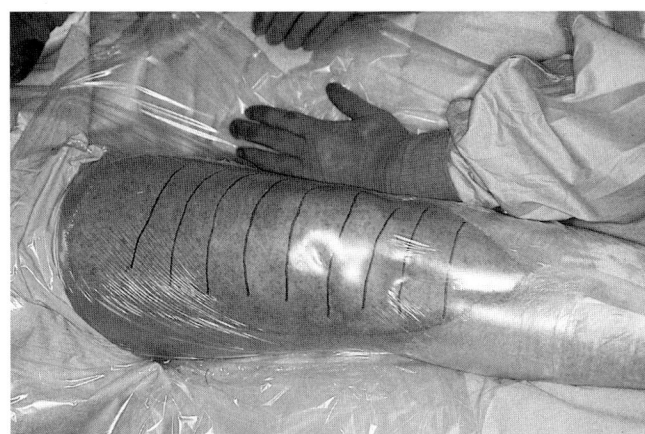

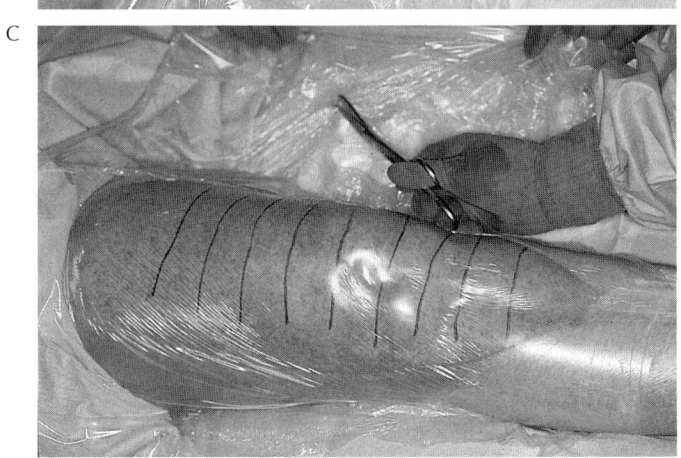

23. Draping Technique for Total Knee Arthroplasty

Figure 23.6. (A) and (B) The third incise drape is carefully applied anteriorly, overlapping both the first incise drape and the extremity drape. It is sealed first medially, then laterally, taking care to ensure that bubbles are eliminated and that the skin is not distorted during application. (C) Excess is trimmed.

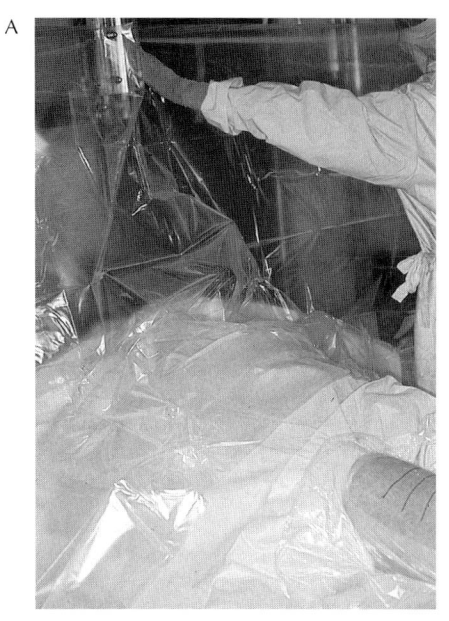

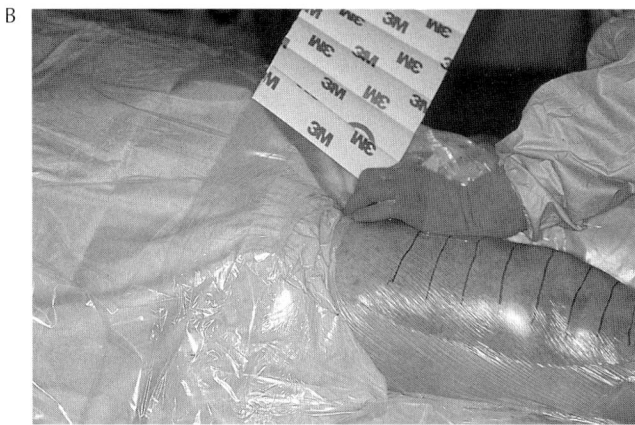

Figure 23.7. (A) The plastic isolation "shower curtain" drape seals off the sterile field from the laminar flow panels. (B) A portion of a fourth incise drape is used to seal the isolation drape with the third incise drape.

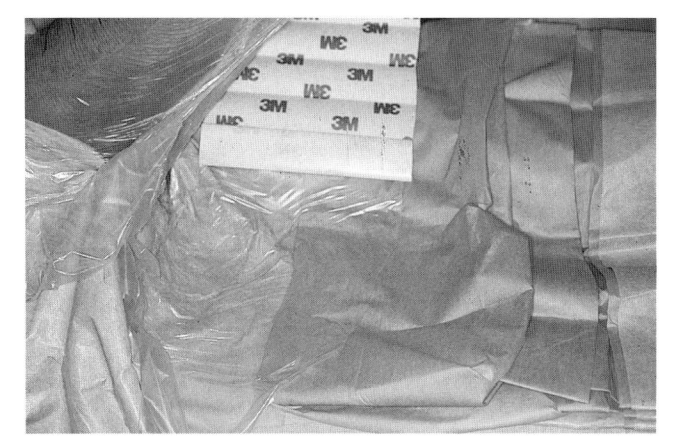

Figure 23.8. A pocket is created with another three-quarter drape secured to the foot of the table while the leg is elevated maximally. This is done with another portion of the fourth incise drape, making sure to overlap the second incise drape applied to the posterior thigh.

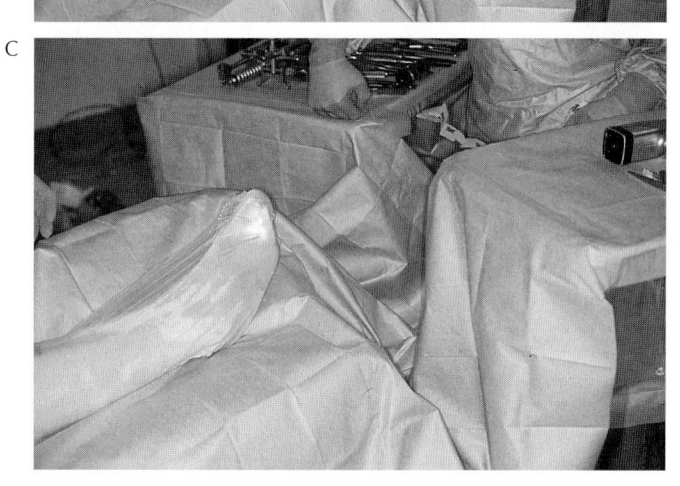

Section 5. Principles of Primary Total Knee Arthroplasty

Figure 23.9. (A), (B), and (C) The pocket is then formed at the foot of the table as the drape is secured to two Mayo stands. Portions of the fourth incise drape are used to secure the drapes.

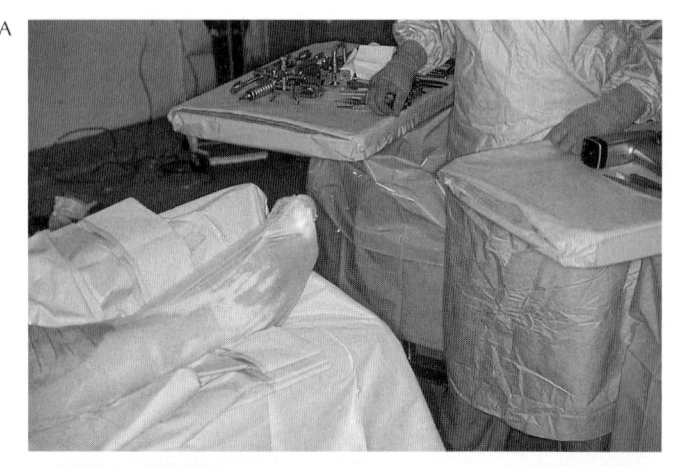

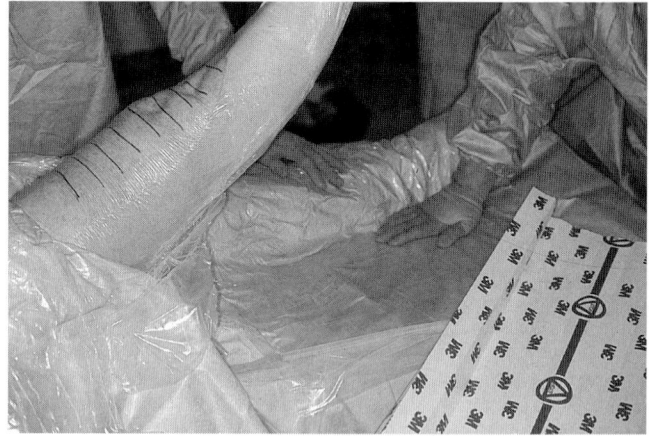

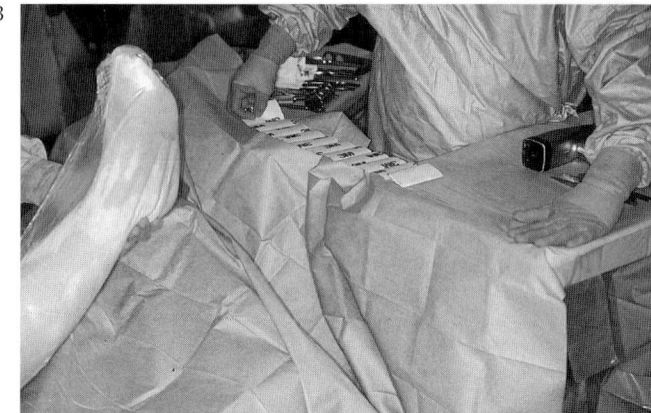

Figure 23.10. The fifth incise drape is then applied to the extremity drape at the foot of the table, being sure to overlap with the previously applied portion of the fourth incise drape.

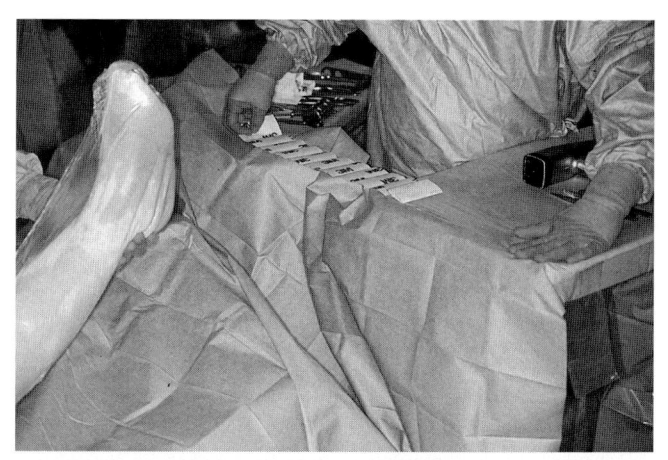

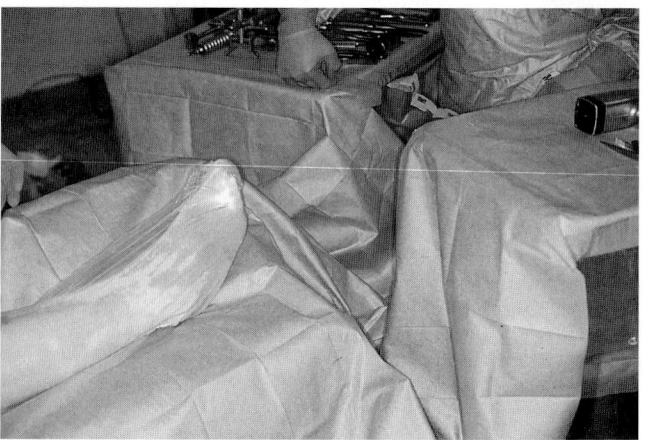

Figure 23.11. (A) and (B) The extremity is now ready for the surgery to begin. Note the instruments placed on the two Mayo stands (see text).

ing care to overlap it with previously applied incise drape (Fig. 23.10). The extremity is then ready to be exsanguinated and the skin incision made (Fig. 23.11A). Note the items placed onto the two Mayo stands to facilitate delivery of instruments, including scalpels, heavy tissue forceps, vascular forceps, Kocher clamps, periosteal elevators, curved and flat osteotomes, bent Hohmann retractors, right angle retractors, and a battery operated saw and drill (Fig. 23.11B).

CONCLUSIONS

We find this method of draping to be very useful and have had no cases of sepsis in the immediate postoperative period. Such a draping technique, coupled with laminar flow, occlusive exhaust suits, and appropriate antibiotics may actually save OR and anesthesia time, and may be more cost effective and safer for the patient because it may serve to reduce the risk of cross-contamination between patient and staff, thereby minimizing the risk of infection.

References

1. Aebi B, Gerber C, Ganz R. Prevention of infection in elective orthopedic interventions with special reference to alloplastic joint replacement. *Helv Chir Acta*. 1989; 56:387–397.
2. Ahl T, Dalen N, Jorbeck H, Hoburn J. Air contamination during hip and knee arthroplasties. Horizontal laminar flow randomized vs. conventional ventilation. *Acta Orthop Scand*. 1995; 66:17–20.
3. Schutzer SF, Harris WH. Deep-wound infection after total hip replacement under contemporary aseptic conditions. *JBJS*. 1988; 70A:724–727.
4. Sharrock NE, Haas SB, Hargett MJ, Urquhart B, Insall JN, Scuderi G. Effects of epidural anesthesia on the incidence of deep-vein thrombosis after total knee arthroplasty. *JBJS*. 1991; 73A:502–506.

SECTION 6
Instrumentation

CHAPTER 24
Total Knee Arthroplasty

Alfred J. Tria, Jr.

INTRODUCTION

In the early 1970s the total condylar knee arthroplasty was designed at the Hospital for Special Surgery and emphasized the concepts of ligament balance and knee alignment.[1] After the introduction of polymethylmethacrylate, there was a rapid increase in design work because the major obstacle of fixation was relieved. Although the knee implant designs continued to undergo refinement, instrumentation lagged significantly behind the design technology. This dichotomy occurred because the emphasis was given to the development of better anatomic and biomechanical prostheses that could take advantage of the new fixation and improve upon the early loosening and increase the range of motion. The technique for the implantation of the knee was not a central issue. Thus, instruments were designed after the prostheses had been developed and oftentimes were not even available for the initial surgical procedures.

In the 1980s the knee designs became more sophisticated and the concept of a cementless prosthesis was introduced.[2] The cementless components required more accurate bone cuts in order to increase the surface area of contact between the prosthesis and the bone. This placed a much greater demand upon the instrumentation and required a parallel technology to complete the prosthesis and the instruments as one unified system. It became evident that the results of the new implants were dependent both upon the design rationale of the prosthesis and the surgical technique. It was no longer acceptable to rely upon the "surgeon's eye" to establish proper positioning of the implant. Implant design and instrument design became equally important.

PRINCIPALS OF INSTRUMENTATION
Tibiofemoral Alignment

The overall alignment of the knee must be in 5 to 10 degrees of anatomic valgus. The alignment is determined by the position of both the femoral and tibial components in the coronal plane of the joint. There are two basic schools of thought concerning the position of the knee joint.[3,4] The most popular school references the *mechanical axis* of the lower leg. The tibial cut is made perpendicular to the tibial shaft and the femoral cut is made parallel to the mechanical axis of the femur (i.e., the line drawn from the femoral head through the middle of the tibia and through the middle of the ankle). The *anatomic alignment* references the mechanical axis of the lower leg but allows for the fact that the proximal tibial plateau is actually in a few degrees of varus. In this system the tibial cut is set anatomically (i.e., in 2 to 3 degrees of varus) and the femoral cut is made parallel to the mechanical axis with the addition of the 2 or 3 degrees. Hungerford and Krackow popularized this concept hoping to improve knee arthroplasty with greater anatomic precision (Fig. 24.1).

The Femoral Component

The preceding discussion has only considered the angular relationship of the femur and the tibia in the coronal plane. The instruments must align *each component* in the sagittal, coronal, and horizontal planes. The femoral component should include a valgus angle of 4 to 6 degrees, should be centered on the end of the femoral shaft with respect to the anteroposterior plane, should not be significantly flexed or extended, and should include external rotation of 3 to 4 degrees.

The femoral valgus angle can be referenced with respect to the femoral shaft. The anterior to posterior position and the external rotation can be verified with respect to the posterior condylar axis, the anterior cortex of the shaft of the femur, the intramedullary canal, the epicondyles, and the flexion gap. Each of the references has an individual variability. The posterior femoral condyles are easily defined. However, as the varus or valgus deformity of the knee increases the posterior aspect of the medial condyle (in varus) and the lateral condyle (in valgus) can become deficient. With this atrophy, the anterior to posterior thickness will be under-

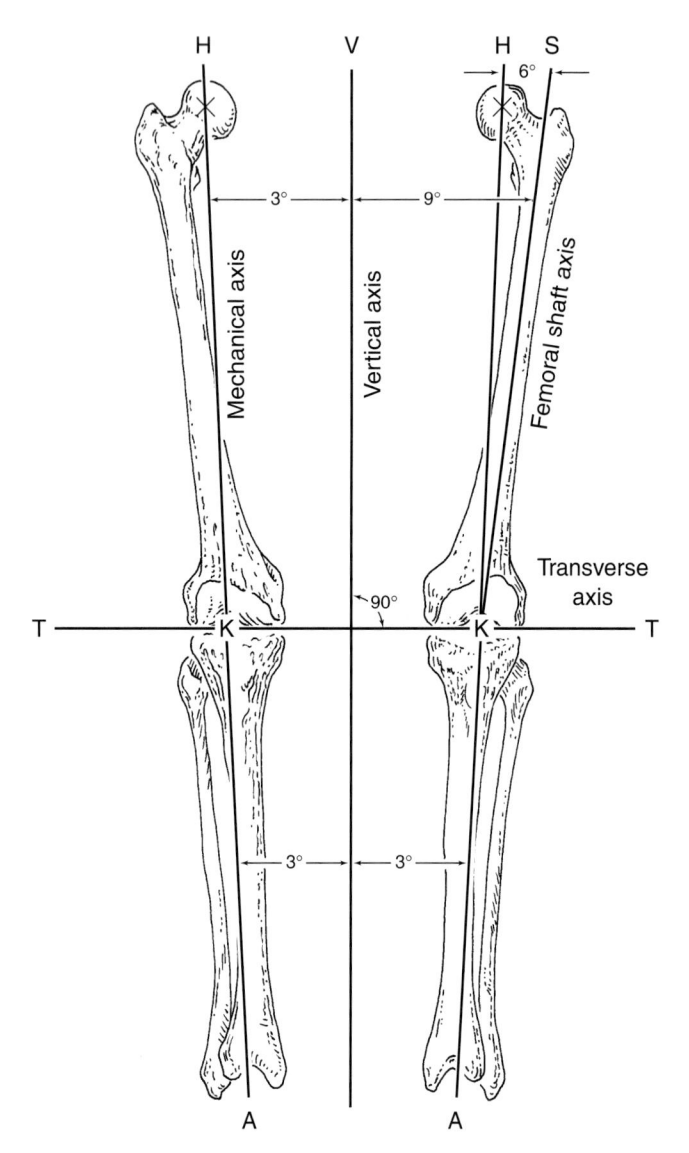

Figure 24.1. The figure on the left illustrates the mechanical axis of the knee. The figure on the right shows the femoral anatomic axis with the tibial reference line drawn to allow for the anatomic varus of the tibia of 3 degrees.

estimated and the femoral cuts will be internally rotated in the valgus deformity and externally rotated in the varus deformity if the posterior condylar axis is the primary reference (Fig. 24.2). The anterior cortex of the femur is readily available for referencing.[5] Because the lateral femoral condyle rises higher than the medial condyle in the femoral sulcus area, the surgeon must choose between the high lateral referencing or the low medial referencing. If the anterior cut is elevated, the forces in the patellofemoral joint will be increased because of the increased distance of the patella from the center of rotation of the knee. Anterior positioning of the femoral component will also increase the flexion space. If the cut is lowered on the anterior surface, there is the chance of femoral notching. A notch defect of 1 or 2 mm is probably not significant; however, deeper defects can be associated with supracondylar fracture. If all femoral cuts are referenced from the anterior cortex despite the size of the chosen component, the smaller component will increase the flexion gap, perhaps out of proportion to the extension gap, and may remove an undesirable amount of bone. The larger femoral component will decrease the flexion gap without a proportionate effect on the extension space (Fig. 24.3).

The intramedullary canal of the femur is a stable referencing point, especially in the revision case in which there can be significant bone deficits and loss of palpable bone landmarks. The canal helps with the anteroposterior position and with the valgus distal cut. The intramedullary referencing rod is most accurate if the length is increased to engage the isthmus of the femoral shaft. The accuracy can also be increased if the width of the intramedullary rod is increased to engage both the medial and lateral cortex of the femur. The intramedullary canal itself does not provide good rotational referencing.

The epicondyles are especially helpful with respect to rotational positioning; however, it is sometimes difficult to identify the exact center point, most especially of the medial epicondyle.[6,7] Rubash has reported some excellent anatomic studies comparing the epicondylar axis with the posterior condylar axis and he has shown that they do indeed correlate with each other.[8] The transepicondylar axis of the distal femur does represent a reproducible landmark. The epicondyles are identified and the component is rotated until it is parallel to the axis. This reference is based solely upon the femoral anatomy, much the same as the posterior condyles. The surgeon should not confuse the rotational positioning of the femoral component with the flexion-extension gap in reference to the tibial component. With this technique the balancing is considered as a completely separate issue. The flexion gap technique for femoral rotation is based upon the reference to the tibial cut with the *collateral ligaments balanced* in flexion. The knee is distracted in flexion after the tibial cut has been completed. The collateral ligaments are balanced equally and the posterior femoral cut is made parallel to the proximal tibial cut surface to create a rectangular space (the "gap" technique as described by Insall) (Fig. 24.4).[9] This technique assures ligament balance in flexion but if either collateral is abnormally tight or lax, the femoral rotation can be incorrect and interfere with patellar tracking.

The rotational alignment of the femoral component effects both the tracking of the patella and the balance of the collateral ligaments in flexion. The sulcus of the femoral component must articulate with the patella and maintain normal contact from extension to full flexion. Internal rotation of the femoral component will allow the patella to track laterally with respect to the femoral

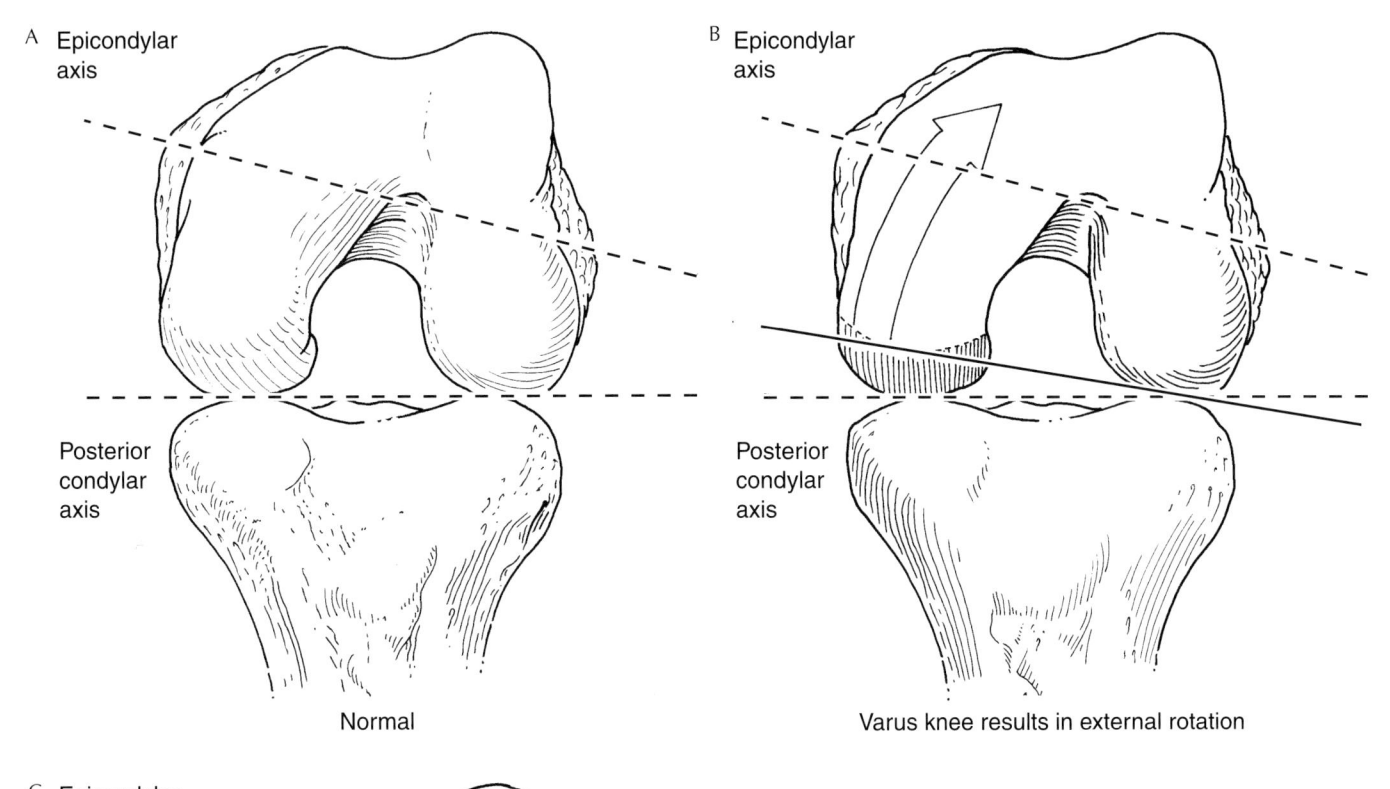

A Epicondylar axis

Posterior condylar axis

Normal

B Epicondylar axis

Posterior condylar axis

Varus knee results in external rotation

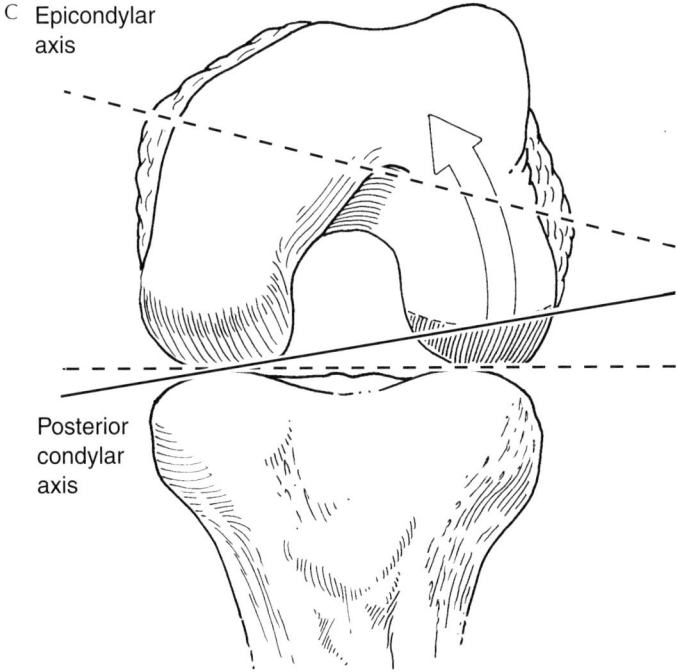

C Epicondylar axis

Posterior condylar axis

Valgus knee results in internal rotation

Figure 24.2. (A) The relationship of the posterior condylar axis and the epicondylar axis. (B) The varus knee presents with an atrophic medial femoral condyle, especially posteriorly. This can result in increased external rotation of the femoral component if the posterior condylar axis is used as the only reference point. (C) The valgus knee presents with an atrophic lateral femoral condyle, especially posteriorly. This can result in increased internal rotation of the femoral component if the posterior condylar axis is used as the only reference point.

sulcus. Internal rotation will also tighten the medial flexion space and open up the lateral flexion space gap. External rotation of the femoral component favors the tracking of the patella; however, if the external rotation is excessive, the patella can track medially and the flexion gap can become too large on the medial side and too small on the lateral.

The Tibial Component

The tibial component must also be considered as a separate entity similar to the femoral component. Most tibial cuts are perpendicular to the tibial shaft in the coronal plane unless the knee system incorporates an anatomic 3 or 4 degrees of varus. In the sagittal plane

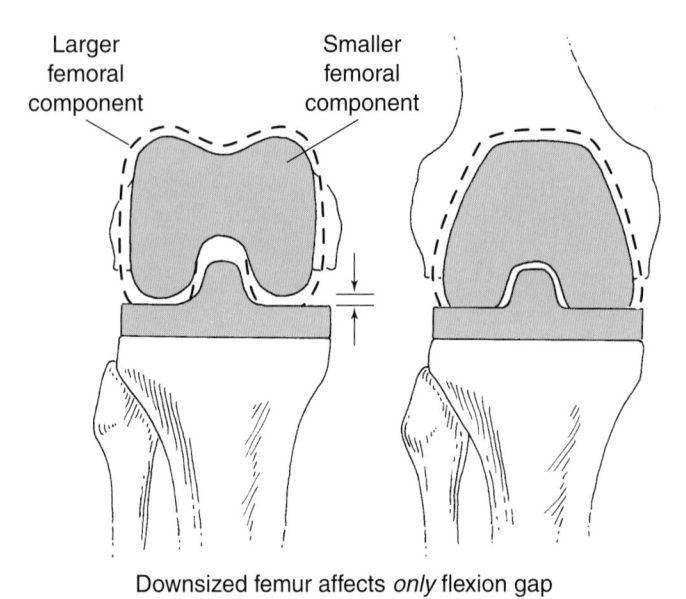

Figure 24.3. The flexion gap is affected by the size of the femoral component without significant effects on the extension space.

the tibial cut is usually perpendicular or includes a slight posterior angulation to help with the flexion range of motion improving the rollback of the femoral component on the tibial surface. Many knee systems include a slight posterior angulation in the polyethylene surface and cut the tibial plateau at a 90-degree angle. If the slope is built into the polyethylene, there must be some thinning of the polyethylene from the anterior to the posterior aspect of the surface. With the thinner inserts, it is possible to approach the critical thickness of 6 mm or less. Thus, some designs incorporate the slope in the tibial cut and then implant a polyethylene that is of uniform thickness from anterior to posterior and avoid the issue of changing polyethylene thickness.

The tibia must also be rotated in the horizontal plane with respect to the tibial tubercle.[6,7] The tibial rotation is slightly less complicated than the femoral (Fig. 24.4). The tibial tubercle is the major landmark for referencing. Most component systems center upon the tubercle unless there is a marked external or, less commonly, internal rotation of the tibial tuberosity. With abnormal tubercle anatomy, the tibial rotation is usually determined with respect to the femoral component in the flexed position and then referenced in extension to check the entire range of motion. It can become difficult to choose the proper position when the existing tubercle is markedly rotated. If the tibial tray is internally rotated, the patella will track with the patellar ligament and tend to shift laterally. If the tray is externally rotated, the patella will track more centrally but the tibiofemoral contact will not be anatomic and the rotational torque can lead to loosening or wear.

The Patellar Component

As the technology for knee arthroplasty improves, the last area of difficulty is the patellofemoral articulation. The patella must track centrally throughout the range of motion despite the individual position of the femoral and tibial components. Soft tissue procedures and/or tubercle osteotomies are sometimes required to center the patella on the femoral sulcus.[10,11] The thickness of the patella has become a point of concern and instruments can be helpful with this problem. Although the literature is scant at the present time, there is a tendency to favor decreasing the overall thickness of the resurfaced patella versus the original presenting thickness. Thinning the patella brings the component closer to the center of rotation of the knee and decreases the forces on the surface, hopefully decreasing wear and fracture. Most surgeons favor retaining a minimum of 10 mm of the original patellar bed. The patellar cut should be parallel to the anterior cortical surface and the thickness should be equal to or less than the original thickness. The patella can also be placed eccentrically on the cut bed. The author favors a central position; however, some groups recommend medial placement of the patella to favor better tracking on the femoral surface.

If the patellar component is facetted, the alignment becomes even more important. The patella may track centrally; yet, there may still be an element of torque if the facets are rotated out of position versus the femoral condyles. The problem of facet alignment can be somewhat corrected if the patella is a mobile-bearing surface

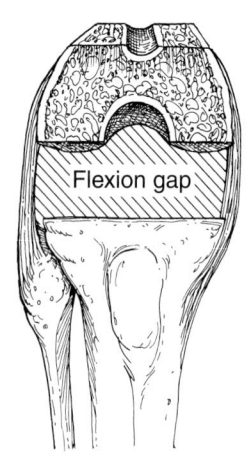

Figure 24.4. With the collateral ligaments balanced in flexion, the posterior femoral cut can be made parallel to the proximal tibia to create a rectangular space in flexion which must then be matched in extension.

that can rotate throughout the range of motion. The mobile-bearing designs require a metal baseplate and often will increase the overall thickness of the patella leading to increased forces and possible increased wear.

INSTRUMENTATION

Cutting Instruments

Early knee arthroplasty was performed with simple hand implements and without sophisticated cutting guides. With the introduction of power tools, the cuts became more reproducible and the surgeons demanded better guides. Cutting blocks were introduced and the sawblade rested upon the block for support and direction (Fig. 24.5). Cutting slots were then introduced to grasp the blade better and protect it from roaming across the guide block. The slots took the sawblade to the best accuracy that it could afford. Then, the concept of frames was introduced. The frame can be applied to the bone and the cutting blade is locked into a slot for the various cuts. The advantage of the frame is the single application with several cuts completed at the same step (Fig. 24.6). Multiple blocks and slots lead to multiple opportunities for the introduction of inaccuracies. The frame eliminates several steps and, thus, eliminates more of the chances for inaccurate cuts. The next logical step was to introduce rotary blades to be used with the frames. The rotary blade eliminates the wobble of the long oscillating blade, decreases the temperature of the cut bone surface, and controls the depth of the cut. At the present time the sawblade with the cutting slots still represents the gold standard in knee arthroplasty. The author favors the use of the frames with rotary blades and looks to the future for greater improvement of these devices.

Although lasers have gained a great deal in other specialties, open knee procedures do not favor the user of the laser. The electrocautery remains the primary device

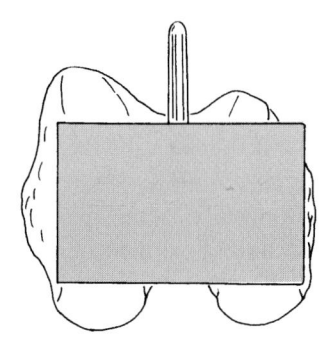

Figure 24.5. The femoral cutting block is pinned on the distal surface with proper rotation.

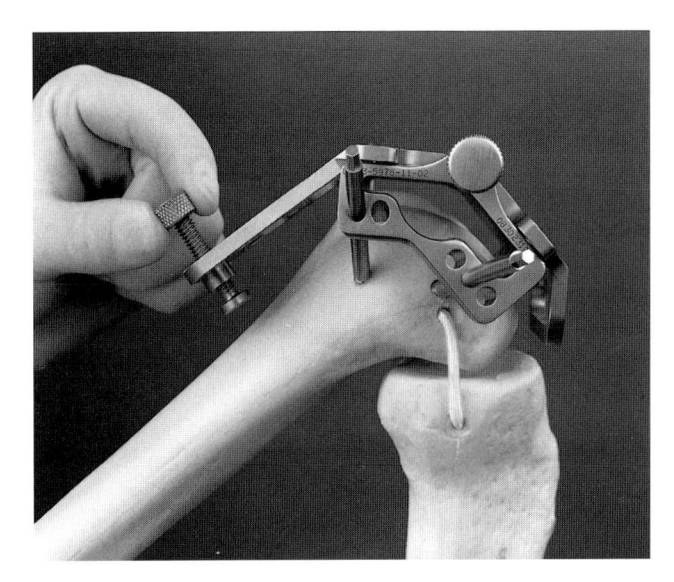

Figure 24.6. An external frame applied to the distal femur allows all of the subsequent cuts to be completed with a single reference point.

for hemostasis and the power tools cut the bone quite accurately and acceptably.

There have been some attempts to apply robotic arms to the knee surgery and this may become more popular in the future when the instruments become more accurate and lock the cutting devices into place about the bone. It is also difficult for the arm to use the standard bone landmarks that are presently used. When the landmarks become more accurate and reproducible, it may be more appropriate to visit this technology again.

Instrument Design

The designer's choice of anatomic references concerning alignment and balance of the knee arthroplasty components significantly affects the type of instrument that is subsequently designed. The discussion earlier outlines the multitude of parameters that are available for referencing each component.

During the arthroplasty, the surgeon must address the femur, the tibia, and the patella as separate entities and then as an integrated unit. Various systems begin on the femoral or the tibial side. With either approach, the considerations are the same but are addressed at different points during the surgical procedure. This chapter will begin with the tibial preparation and proceed to the femur and then to the patella.

Tibial Preparation

The instruments for the tibial preparation are based upon intramedullary or extramedullary referencing. Because the anterior prominence of the tibial shaft and the malleoli of the ankle joint are usually readily palpable, extramedullary rods for the tibia are very reliable. The tibial tubercle and the fibular head are usually available for referencing except in the worst revision cases. The initial tibial cut is usually perpendicular to the shaft with a slight posterior angulation according to the system that is being used. The tibial jigs attach to the anterior tibia in line with the tubercle and include either a capture slot to enclose the oscillating sawblade or a cutting block upon which the sawblade rests. Capture slots control the oscillating sawblade but tend to block the full view of the underlying bone. Cutting blocks allow more complete visualization of the bone surface but they also allow more sawblade deviation. The tibial cutting slots can accommodate angled cuts to prepare the plateau surface to accept a wedge attached to the tibial tray. Rotary blade power cutters are presently being considered to fashion the tibia and femur. These devices create significant bone debris and require capture slots that often obscure the bone surface from the operating surgeon.

Intramedullary tibial jigs are also available for this primary cut. The tibial shaft is often too narrow for the rod, or the shaft is curved, or the proximal tibial surface requires offset from the central canal, making intramedullary placement difficult or sometimes impossible. Simmons studied the accuracy of the intramedullary devices and reported neutral alignment in 83% of the varus knees and only 37% of the valgus knees.[12] The major source of the difficulty was the tibial bowing, which was present in 66% of the valgus knees. He recommended preoperative long films or cross checking with external alignment in the genu valgus deformity (Table 24.1). The literature indicates that either the extramedullary or the intramedullary instruments are equally accurate for the tibial cut; however, the intramedullary technique may not be possible in the setting of the valgus knee.

Femoral Preparation

The femoral preparation is the more difficult portion of the knee arthroplasty. The femoral shaft is less visible and palpable than the tibia because of the bulk of the thigh musculature, the proximal arterial tourniquet, and the commonly associated thigh obesity. The femoral head is not a palpable landmark and the anterior superior iliac spine is often difficult to identify beneath the surgical drapes. The femoral shaft has the natural anterior bow and may also include a varus bow. Multiple studies have been performed to evaluate the accuracy of either the extramedullary or the intramedullary alignment rods (Table 24.2).[13–22] At the present time the intramedullary rod systems appear to be more helpful and can be checked with extramedullary backup. In 1988, Tillett and Engh compared extramedullary and intramedullary alignment systems for the distal femoral cut and found no significant difference.[13] The femoral head was located for the extramedullary system using a radio opaque marker with roentgenographic verification in the operating room before the procedure was undertaken. The authors admitted that the roentgenogram required greater time and that the intramedullary system was more expedient. The same authors subsequently published a comparative experience using similar techniques for both the extramedullary and intramedullary alignment guides.[15] They reported 87.5% correct alignment with the intramedullary system and only 68.8% correct with the extramedullary. They explained the difference in their two papers by indicating that in the newer paper they used longer X-ray cassettes for greater measuring accuracy. Second, they reported greater variation with larger discrepancies in the extramedullary group.

If the intramedullary canal of the femur is particularly large, it is possible to ream the canal eccentrically and insert the reference rod into the canal in an incorrect varus or valgus position. Bertin reviewed these possibilities and showed that a lengthened rod with an increased diameter helped to prevent some of the discrepancies (Fig. 24.7).[23] Once the intramedullary rod is properly placed, the distal end of the femur can be resected with the appropriate valgus angulation to reestablish the biomechanical axis of the lower extremity. The exact choice of the angle can be made with preoperative full-length standing films or with intraoperatively placed markers that are roentgenographically positioned and checked. Despite the modifications of the intramedullary devices, extramedullary confirmation of the component position is still advised during

Table 24.1. The accuracy of the intramedullary and extramedullary tibial jigs varies in the reported literature

	Intramedullary	Extramedullary
Manning[17]	90%	—
Engh[15]	—	82%
Brys[18]	94%	85%
Dennis[20]	72%	88%
Laskin[21]	97%	—

Table 24.2. The published results of intramedullary and extramedullary femoral jigs clearly favor the intramedullary devices

	Intramedullary	Extramedullary
Manning[17]	90%	—
Engh[15]	87.5%	68.8%
Cates[19]	85.6%	72%
Siegel[22]	—	>2–3° (unacceptable)

24. Total Knee Arthroplasty

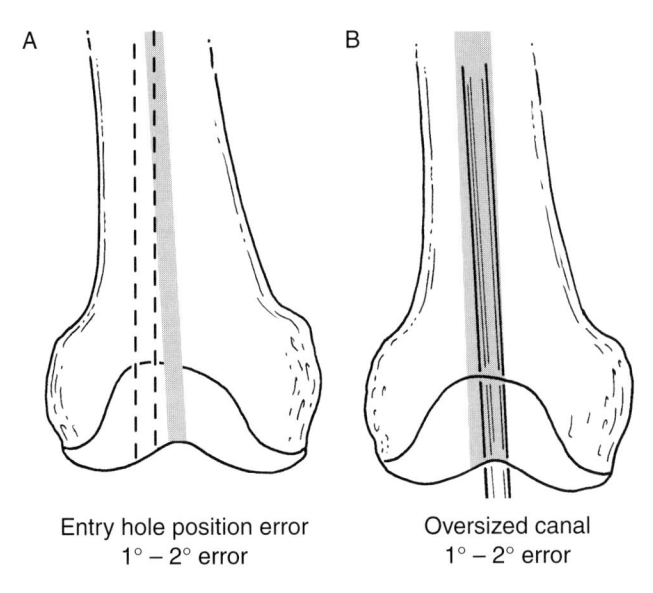

Figure 24.7. The femoral hole on the left is eccentric and will lead to increased valgus. The intramedullary rod on the right is centrally placed but can shift into varus or valgus if the rod is too short.

the operative procedure. The author does not rely upon full-length standing roentgenograms for the valgus alignment. In the varus knee, the intramedullary guide is positioned and 4 degrees of valgus is set in place. In the valgus knee we chose 2 to 3 degrees of valgus for the intramedullary guide. With these choices we have found that the femorotibial angle is 5 to 10 degrees on the postoperative roentgenograms. This somewhat arbitrary angle assignment allows us to perform the arthroplasty in a timely fashion and to avoid significant malalignment.

Keying from the intramedullary rod helps to prevent flexion or extension of the femoral component. The intramedullary reference permits direct visualization of the anterior and posterior cortices and allows the surgeon to choose the anterior to posterior placement of the femoral component that is the best solution for the relationship of the patellofemoral joint and the tibiofemoral flexion gap.

Although the intramedullary femoral guide does appear to solve most of the femoral problems, the surgeon is still left with the choice of the rotational position. Except in the most deformed cases, the epicondyles of the femur are readily palpable. The difficulty with the epicondyles has been the problem of establishing the exact center of each prominence. Insall has contributed significant insight into the anatomy with his new epicondylar instruments and Rubash has shown that the medial epicondyle has a central depression that can be clearly identified if the overlying synovium is thoroughly removed.[8] The central depression can also be confirmed with a circle of marker dots that are placed about the base of the medial epicondylar prominence and then connected across to identify the center of the circle. Krackow's textbook refers to the epicondyles for the rotational alignment.[24] Whitesides' article identifies the anteroposterior axis of the femoral sulcus and relates this to the epicondyles and the posterior condylar axis (Fig. 24.1).[25] Rubash's work shows the relationship of the posterior condylar axis and the epicondylar axis and confirms the correlation between the two.[8]

Patellar Preparation

Instruments for cutting the patellar surface are still at the early design level. There are many surgeons who believe that the patella can be best cut with the power saw and a well-trained eye. Even though experience is one of the most valuable instruments, cutting guides can only help to improve the accuracy. The patella is most commonly cut with an oscillating saw locked into a capture slot or with the sawblade resting on a cutting block. It is true that the blade can wobble on the top of a block and can also angle in the cutting slot, if the slot is not made tight enough. There are also cutting devices that encircle the patella and then use a rotating type blade to remove the posterior surface. The holding devices are somewhat bulky and it is also true that the cutting device obscures the patella while the reaming is completed. At the present time, there is no ideal solution and resurfacing of the patella must be completed as accurately as possible. The author uses a rotating type blade and confirms the position in the middle of the reaming so that any necessary correction can be made before the entire procedure is completed with an off angle cut (Fig. 24.8).

Balancing the Knee

After the tibia and the femur have been appropriately prepared, the flexion and extension gaps must be

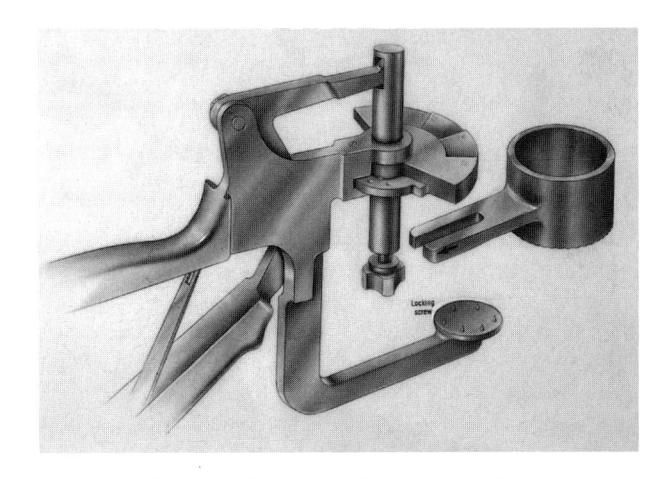

Figure 24.8. The patellar cutting guide.

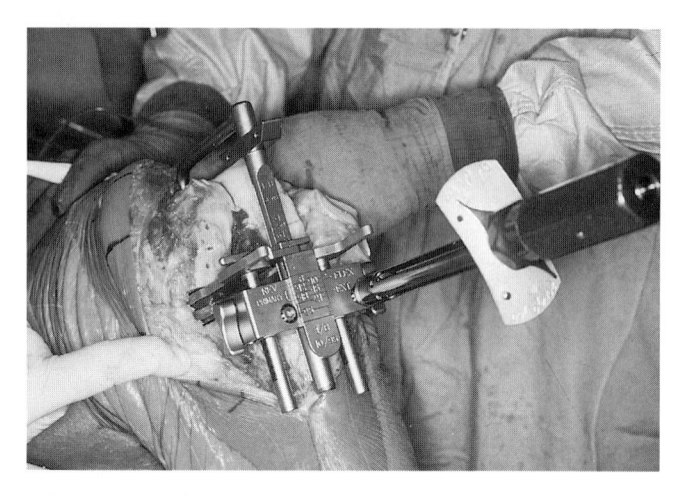

Figure 24.9. The tensor for flexion and extension balancing.

equaled. At the present time, this soft tissue balancing is completed at full extension and at 90 degrees of flexion. Most knee systems do not incorporate an instrument to perform or confirm the balancing. Tensing devices have been introduced that spread the tibia and femur and allow measurements of the gaps that are established with the ligaments balanced. In the past, the instruments have been bulky and have not added precision beyond hand tensioning. Dr. Robert Booth has developed a new tensor that establishes the soft tissue balance and predicts the size of the femoral component and the thickness of the tibial insert with a comparison from flexion to extension (Fig. 24.9). The author has had the opportunity to use the instrument with some early successes. If such a device can be refined, it may be possible to eliminate some of the guesswork that is involved in matching the flexion and extension spaces.

CONCLUSIONS

Instruments for total knee arthroplasty continue to be refined. Most systems develop the implants and the instruments at the same time with two different teams leading the investigations. There is no question that the more accurate the surgery performed, the better the result and longevity of the prosthesis.

At the present time, extramedullary tibial jigs, intramedullary femoral jigs, and patellar resurfacing with reference to the original thickness represent the standard. Instruments for the flexion and extension balancing are still in their infancy. The references and landmarks for the instruments will probably change over the next few years; however, the principle will remain the same.

References

1. Insall JN, Scott WN, Ranawat CS. The total condylar knee prosthesis: a report of two hundred and twenty cases. *J Bone Joint Surg.* 1979; 61(A):173–180.
2. Hungerford DS, Kenna RV. Preliminary experience with a porous coated total knee replacement used without cement. *Clin Orthop.* 1983; 176:95–107.
3. Moreland JR, Bassett LW, Hanker GJ. Radiographic analysis of the axial alignment of the lower extremity. *J Bone Joint Surg.* 1987; 69(A):745–749.
4. Krackow KA. *The Technique of Total Knee Arthroplasty.* St. Louis, Mo: The CV Mosby Company; 1990: Chap. 4, page 87.
5. Insall JN. *Surgery of the Knee.* 2nd ed. New York: Churchill Livingstone; 1993: Chap. 26, page 745.
6. Lotke PA, Ecker ML. Influence of positioning of prosthesis in total knee replacement. *J Bone Joint Surg.* 1977; 59(A): 77–79.
7. Jiang C-C, Insall JN. Effect of rotation on the axial alignment of the femur. *Clin Orthop.* 1989; 248:50–56.
8. Berger RA, Rubash HE, Seel MJ, Thompson WH, Crossett LA. Determining the rotational alignment of the femoral component in total knee arthroplasty using the epicondylar axis. *Clin Orthop.* 1993; 286:40–47.
9. Insall JN. *Surgery of the Knee.* 2nd ed. New York: Churchill Livingstone; 1993: Chap. 26, page 746.
10. Wolff AM, Hungerford MD, Krackow KA, Jacobs MA. Osteotomy of the tibial tubercle during total knee replacement. *J Bone Joint Surg.* 1989; 6:848–856.
11. Whiteside LA, Ohl M. Tibial tubercle osteotomy for exposure of the difficult total knee arthroplasty. *Clin Orthop.* 1990; 260:6–9.
12. Simmons ED, Sullivan JA, Rackemann S, Scott RD. The accuracy of tibial intramedullary alignment devices in total knee arthroplasty. *J Arthroplasty.* 1991; 6:45–50.
13. Tillett ED, Engh GA, Petersen T. A comparative study of extramedullary and intramedullary alignment systems in total knee arthroplasty. *Clin Orthop.* 1988; 230:176–181.
14. Petersen TL, Engh GA. Radiographic assessment of knee alignment after total knee arthroplasty. *J Arthroplasty.* 1988; 3:67–72.
15. Engh GA, Petersen TL. Comparative experience with intramedullary and extramedullary alignment in total knee arthroplasty. *J Arthroplasty.* 1990; 5:1–8.
16. Whiteside LA, Summers RG. Anatomical landmarks for an intramedullary alignment system for total knee replacement. *Orthop Trans.* 1983; 7:546–547.
17. Manning M, Elloy M, Johnson R. The accuracy of intramedullary alignment in total knee replacement. *J Bone Joint Surg.* 1988; 70(B):852–858.
18. Brys DA, Lombardi AV, Mallory TH, Vaughn BK. A comparison of intramedullary and extramedullary alignment systems for tibial component placement in TKA. *Clin Orthop.* 1991; 263:175–179.
19. Cates HE, Ritter MA, Keating EM, Faris PM. Intramedullary versus extramedullary femoral alignment systems in total knee replacement. *Clin Orthop.* 1993; 286: 32–39.

20. Dennis DA, Channer M, Susman MH, Stringer EA. Intramedullary versus extramedullary tibial alignment systems in total knee arthroplasty. *J Arthroplasty*. 1993; 8(1): 43–47.
21. Laskin RS, Turtel A. The use of an intramedullary tibial alignment guide in TKR arthroplasty. *The American J of Knee Surgery*. 1989; 2(3):123–130.
22. Siegel JL, Shall LM. Femoral instrumentation using the anterosuperior iliac spine as a landmark in total knee arthroplasty. An anatomic study. *J Arthroplasty*. 1991; 6(4):317–320.
23. Bertin CB. Intramedullary instrumentation for total knee arthroplasty. In: Goldberg VM, ed. *Controversies in Total Knee Arthroplasty*. New York: Raven Press, Ltd., 1991; Chap. 18.
24. Krackow KA. *The Technique of Total Knee Arthroplasty*. St. Louis, Mo: The CV Mosby Company; 1990: Chap. 5, page 137.
25. Whiteside LA, Arima J. The anteroposterior axis for femoral rotation alignment in valgus total knee arthroplasty. *Clin Orthop*. 1995; 321:168–172.

SECTION 7
Correction of Deformity

CHAPTER 25
Medial Release for Fixed-Varus Deformity

David J. Yasgur, Giles R. Scuderi, and John N. Insall

INTRODUCTION

Varus deformity of the knee is one of the most common deformities seen at the time of total knee arthroplasty. When a fixed deformity is present, the pathoanatomy usually involves erosion of medial tibial bone stock with medial tibial osteophyte formation, and contractures of the medial collateral ligament (MCL), posteromedial capsule, pes anserinus, and semimembranosus muscle (Fig. 25.1). Elongation of the lateral collateral ligament is a late event. A flexion contracture may coexist, which is manifested by contractures of both posterior capsule and posterior cruciate ligament.

Success and longevity of total knee arthroplasty is predicated in part on achieving proper limb alignment of 5 to 10 degrees of valgus.[1] The limb should be corrected to this ideal alignment without regard to the contralateral alignment, because a varus deformity often exists bilaterally. Furthermore, the ideal alignment of the femoral component is 7 ± 2 degrees of valgus angulation, whereas that of the tibial component is 90 ± 2 degrees relative to the longitudinal axis of the tibia.[1]

The ideal alignment is achieved through soft tissue releases aimed at balancing the collateral ligaments, and by placing the components in the correct orientation. If the proper alignment is not achieved, or if the ligaments are inadequately balanced, the components will be overloaded medially and subjected to excessive stresses, which may result in the eventual failure of the arthroplasty via either component loosening or accelerated wear. Intraoperatively, it is imperative to reassess each step of the soft tissue release so as not to overcorrect the deformity and create valgus instability.

PREOPERATIVE PLANNING

A careful physical examination of the knee should assess the range of motion, flexion contracture, degree of deformity, ligamentous stability, and muscle strength. Anterior cruciate ligament deficiency is a common finding in a degenerative knee, but it is not a surgical dilemma in total knee arthroplasty. In contrast, deficiency of the posterior cruciate ligament (PCL) is much less common. A more likely scenario is the situation of a fixed-varus deformity with a flexion contracture, which requires resection of the PCL for complete correction of the limb alignment and flexion contracture. For these cases, a PCL-substituting design should be utilized. In those cases with severe contracture requiring extensive soft tissue release, a constrained condylar implant should be available. This is more often the case for severe genu valgum and not for fixed-varus deformities.

A detailed assessment of preoperative radiographs should be made for accurate preoperative assessment. This includes weight-bearing anteroposterior (AP), lateral, and tangential patella radiographs, as well as a full length standing AP radiograph. Patella tracking should be noted on the tangential patella view, because this may suggest preoperatively the need for lateral retinacular release. Bony defects should also be noted, because prosthetic augmentation or bone grafting may be required. The mechanical axis, degree of deformity, and femoral valgus should also be noted. If an intramedullary instrumentation system is utilized in which the valgus orientation of the distal femoral cut can be adjusted, then knowledge of the deformity and anatomic femoral valgus can allow one to slightly increase the valgus orientation of the distal femoral cut. This would then facilitate ligamentous balancing in severe fixed deformities.

TECHNIQUE
Approach

The anterior midline approach, with a medial parapatellar arthrotomy, is preferred because this allows for adequate exposure in most knees. It is also extensile in nature and can easily be converted into a quadriceps snip[2,3] or V-Y turndown[4] when warranted by knees that are difficult to expose, such as post-osteotomy or in patella infera. An anterior incision also allows for exposure of both medial and lateral supporting structures, and obviates the need for additional incisions.

The anterior longitudinal skin incision is carefully placed medial to the tibial tubercle to avoid a tender scar postoperatively. Following this, a medial parapatellar arthrotomy is carried out through a straight incision extending over the medial one-third of the patella and is continued onto the tibia 1 cm medial to the tibial tubercle. The quadriceps expansion is peeled off of the anterior patella via sharp dissection. The synovium is divided in line with the arthrotomy, and the anterior horn of the medial meniscus is divided. Patellofemoral ligaments are released, and the patella is everted and dislocated laterally, while the knee is flexed up.

The anterior cruciate ligament, if present, should then be divided, as should the anterior horn of the lateral meniscus, which will facilitate eversion of the extensor mechanism. To avoid avulsion of the tibial tubercle, the patellar tendon should be dissected subperiosteally with a cuff of periosteum to the crest of the tibial tubercle. As much as one-third of the tubercle may be exposed, but this is rarely necessary. Lastly, the fat pad and synovium can be resected to help expose the lateral tibial plateau. This exposure is the most versatile and utilitarian of all the exposures for total knee arthroplasty.

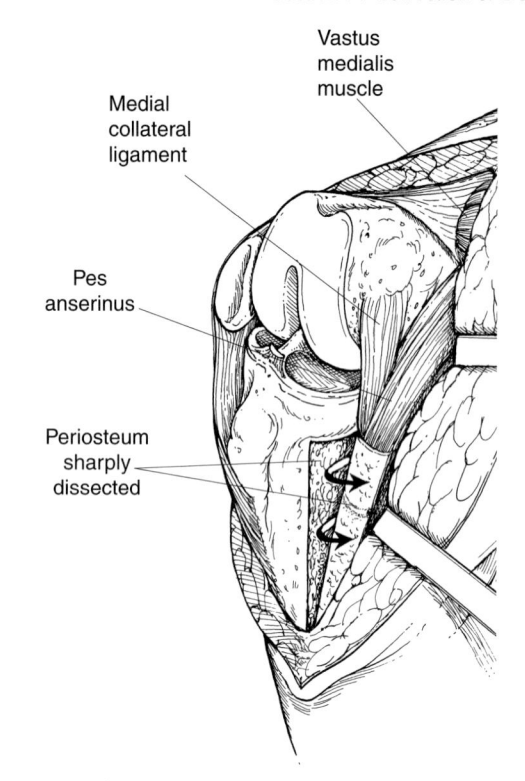

Figure 25.2. Subperiosteal sleeve sharply dissected from proximal anteromedial tibia, including superficial and deep MCL, along with the pes anserinus tendons, if needed.

Medial Release

To correct a fixed-varus deformity, progressive release of the tight medial structures is performed until they reach the length of the lateral supporting structures.[3] The release is begun with the knee in extension using sharp dissection of a subperiosteal sleeve from the proximal anteromedial tibia (Fig. 25.2). A periosteal elevator is useful in continuing this dissection to the midline. Care should be taken to pass the elevator deep to the superficial MCL. The elevator should be used at a level approximately 3 to 4 cm from the medial tibial plateau, where the medial metaphysis is curving to join the tibial diaphysis. It is at this location where the inferomedial geniculate artery may be seen (Fig. 25.3). A bent Hohmann retractor may then be placed, being sure that the tip is deep to the MCL (Fig. 25.4). Placement of this retractor allows for traction to be placed on the medial structures, thereby facilitating subperiosteal dissection.

With the knee in extension, a flat three-fourths inch osteotome is passed distally and deep to the superficial MCL (Fig. 25.5). A complete release requires that the osteotome be passed as much as 6 inches distal to the medial tibial plateau. Depending on the degree of release required, the pes anserinus can also be completely detached, or left partially attached as the osteotome el-

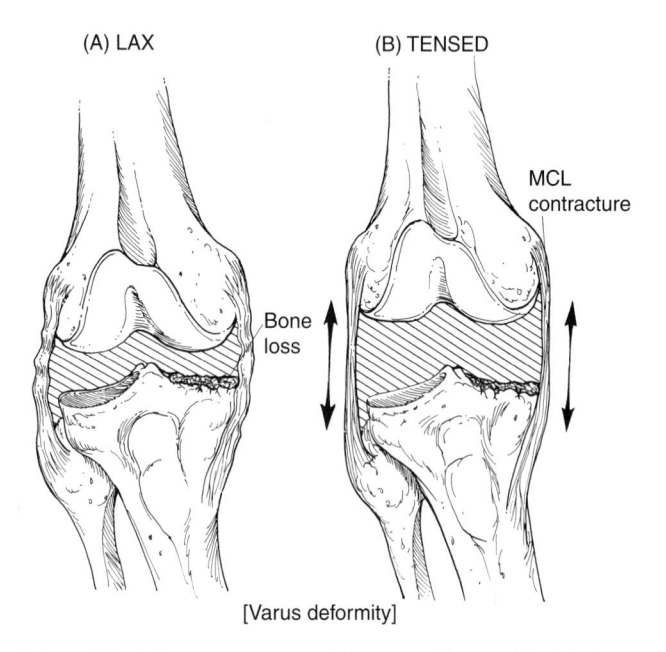

Figure 25.1. Genu varum usually caused by medial tibial bone loss and contractures of the medial soft tissue structures.

25. Medial Release for Fixed-Varus Deformity

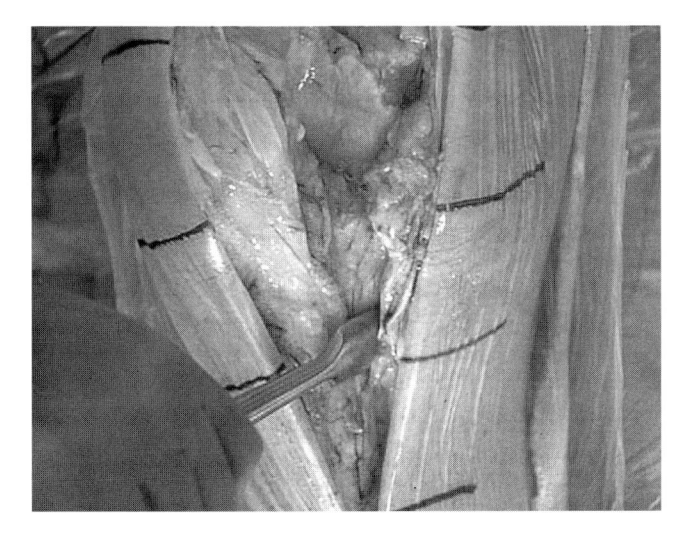

Figure 25.3. Subperiosteal sleeve continued posteriorly, using a periosteal elevator.

evates the MCL immediately posterior to the most anterior attachment of the pes tendons. Similarly, the osteotome can be used to release the deep attachment of the soleus muscle from the posteromedial tibial metadiaphysis.

Sharp dissection can then proceed superiorly to the level of the joint, which will elevate the deep MCL off of the tibia. Proceeding posteromedially with the lower leg externally rotated and the knee flexed, one can sharply elevate the semimembranosus off of the tibia, which often liberates fluid from the semimembranosus bursa (Fig. 25.6). In this way, the posteromedial tibia can be safely exposed to the midline. At this point, the tibia appears skeletonized (Fig. 25.7). Medial tibial osteo-

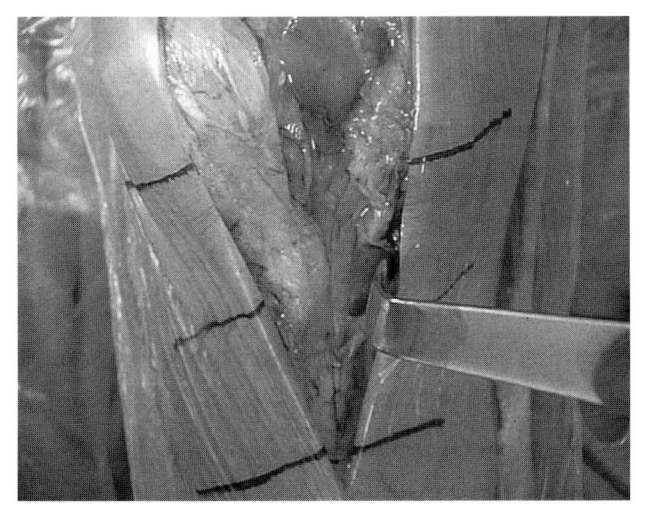

Figure 25.4. Hohmann retractor placed deep to subperiosteal sleeve places tension on structures, permitting further dissection.

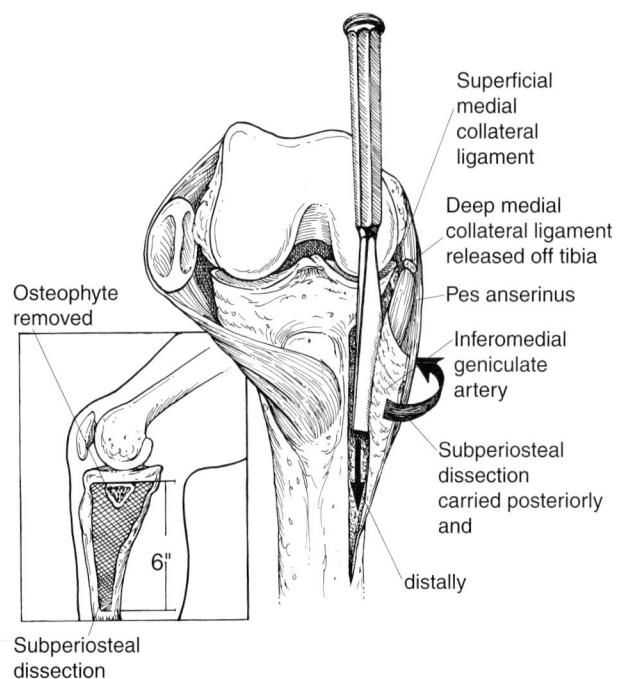

Figure 25.5. Osteotome inserted deep to periosteal flap or MCL, used to subperiosteally strip medial supporting structures from proximal tibia, while maintaining a continuous soft tissue sleeve.

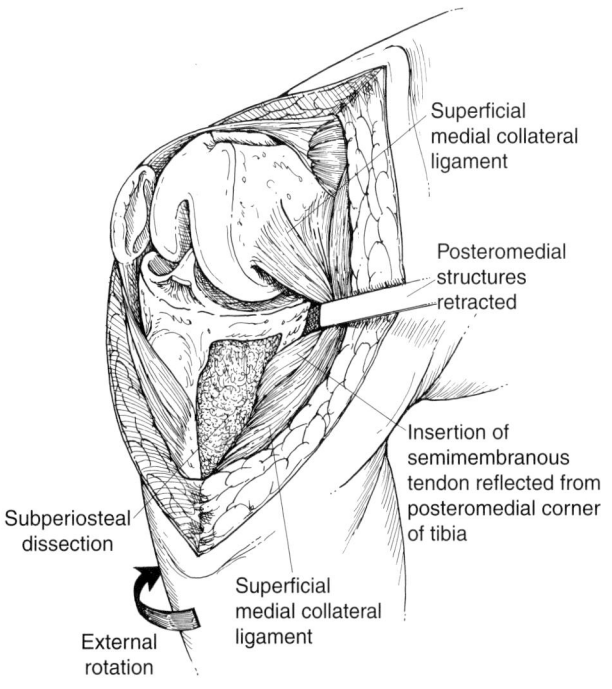

Figure 25.6. Semimembranosus insertion sharply dissected with tibia externally rotated.

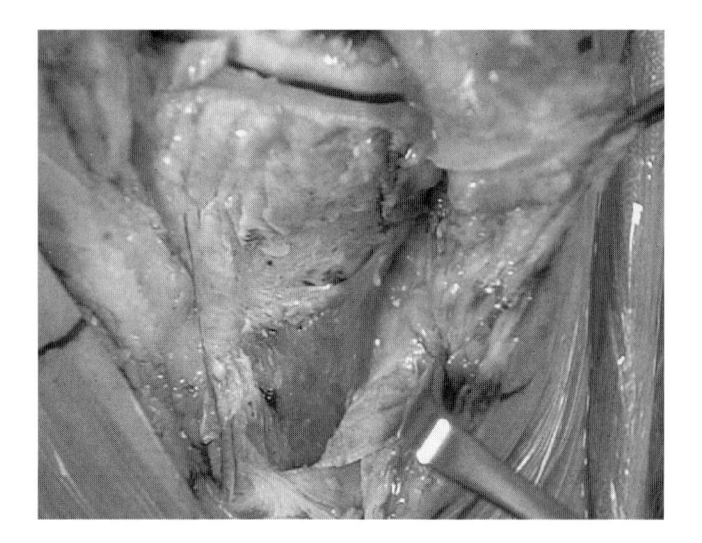

Figure 25.7. Skeletonized appearance of tibia after semimembranosus released.

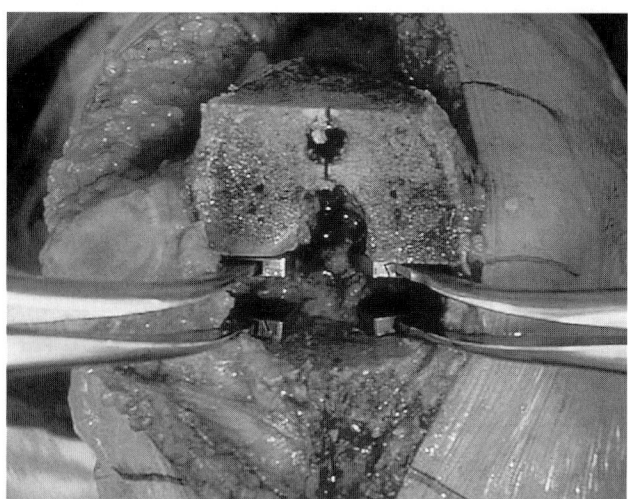

Figure 25.8. Laminar spreaders are useful in monitoring soft tissue balance and ligament releases.

phytes may serve to tighten the medial side, because the MCL is draped over the osteophytes. Thus, resection of the medial tibial osteophytes is the final step in releasing a fixed-varus knee. It is often useful to wait until a trial tibial component has been inserted before resecting the medial tibial osteophyte. In that way, one can use the trial component as a template and ensure that excessive bone is not excised.

Over release of the medial structures in a knee with even a mild deformity is usually not encountered, because this technique ensures that the MCL is not transected, but rather is maintained as a continuous sheet of tissue confluent with the periosteum. The extent of release can be monitored by placing the knee into full extension and exerting a valgus force. Alternatively, lamina spreaders can be gently inserted into the femorotibial articulation (Fig. 25.8) and the alignment judged with a plumb line.

The cruciate ligaments may inhibit correction and should then be resected. Attempts to retain the PCL in cases of severe varus deformity usually result in failure to adequately correct the deformity. Although it is attractive to some to progressively release the PCL and use a cruciate-retaining (CR) type of prosthesis, we prefer to sacrifice the PCL and use a posterior cruciate-substituting prosthesis. Furthermore, literature suggests that the PCL is often nonfunctional in CR knees, as evidenced by anterior translation of the femur on the tibia, or "rollforward."[3,5] Besides limiting correction, retention of a tight PCL can limit motion. In this case, the knee may fail to have the gliding and rolling that occurs with flexion and may open anteriorly like a book during flexion. Such phenomenon may account for component loosening in CR knees.[3]

When the medial release has been completed and proper alignment has been achieved, the standard bone cuts are then made. The distal femur is cut first with an intramedullary instrument that allows variation of the valgus orientation of the femoral component. For severe varus deformities, one may want to slightly increase the valgus orientation of the distal femoral cut to help facilitate soft tissue balancing. The femur is then sized and the appropriate cutting block is selected. The anterior and posterior surfaces of the femur are then cut with instrumentation that is rotationally aligned with the epicondylar axis[6,7] and that incorporates principles of anterior and posterior referencing into the same guide (Fig. 25.9). Care is taken to position this cutting guide so that the posterior condyles are not over- nor underresected, and that the femur is not notched anteriorly.

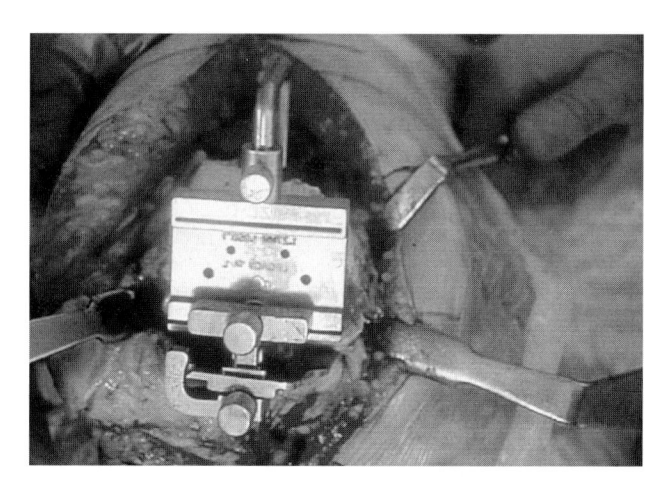

Figure 25.9. Anteroposterior femoral cutting guide is aligned along the epicondylar axis and incorporates principles of anterior and posterior referencing.

The remnants of the cruciate ligaments and menisci are then resected, as are the intercondylar osteophytes. Meticulous attention is then turned toward resection of posterior osteophytes because they may limit flexion. A curved three-fourths inch osteotome is used to resect this bone, as well as to perform a release of the posterior capsule off of the distal femur, when indicated (Fig. 25.10). This maneuver is particularly useful in correcting flexion contractures, but is also useful for releasing the medial gastrocnemius in knees with flexion contractures and fixed-varus deformities.

The tibial cut is then made utilizing an extramedullary guide adjusted to be perpendicular to the longitudinal axis of the tibial diaphysis, to match the posterior slope of the tibial plateau, and to resect approximately 1 cm of bone from the normal lateral tibial plateau. One should not resect the proximal tibia so as to eliminate any medial tibial bone defect that may exist, because this may be excessive.

The ligament balancing, as well as the overall limb alignment, is then assessed with the use of spacer blocks in flexion and extension. When performed in this manner, with soft tissue release preceding bony resection, the flexion and extension gaps are rectangular and are usually equal in magnitude (Fig. 25.11). Occasionally, the extension gap may be tighter than the flexion gap, necessitating re-cutting of the distal femur to equalize the flexion-extension gaps.

Alignment of the femoral cutting block with the epicondylar axis[6,7] is a more precise way of ensuring that the femoral component is externally rotated. This also helps to balance the collateral ligaments in flexion. Excessive external rotation of the femoral component should be avoided, because this will result in an asymmetric flexion space. Additionally, internal rotation of either the tibial component or the femoral component is to be avoided, because patellar instability may result.

The management of tibial bone defects is beyond the scope of this chapter. One suggestion that has been worthwhile is lateralization of the tibial component, because this may reduce the need for augmentation of a medial tibial defect.

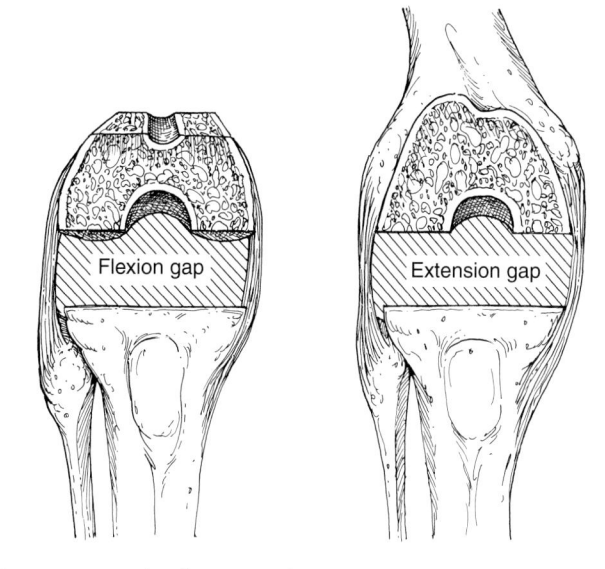

Figure 25.11. The flexion and extension gaps should be equal and rectangular in shape.

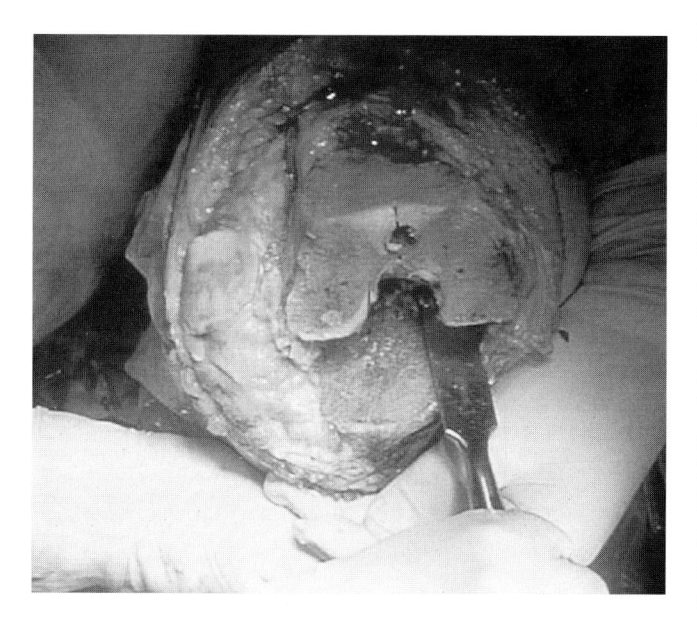

Figure 25.10. Curved osteotomes are used to remove posterior condylar osteophytes and recreate the posterior recess.

RESULTS

The technique described in this chapter for releasing the medial structures of the knee, balancing the ligaments, and restoring the normal alignment of the knee has proven to be successful. The survivorship data[8,9,10,11] and results of clinical and radiographic follow-up studies[1,12,13] have shown that this technique for medial release of fixed-varus deformities is both predictable and durable.

In a long-term follow-up of total condylar knees, the most senior author (JNI) and colleagues reported on 130 TKAs.[13] Of these, 63 (48%) had a varus deformity, including 23 (18%) who had a fixed-varus deformity of at least 10 degrees. At 10- to 12-years of follow-up, 88% had good to excellent results. Varus-valgus stability was maintained in all cases, except in one in which proper soft tissue balancing was not achieved, and varus instability recurred. In all, 81% had less than 5 degrees of instability to varus-valgus stress when tested in full extension.

Testing collateral stability in positions other than full extension is unreliable, because the lack of conformity in the prosthesis will allow some laxity with flexion. When the soft tissues are balanced meticulously, the released medial structures are usually not over-released, but rather remain contiguous with the medial tibial periosteum.

As stated earlier, it is our preference to sacrifice the cruciate ligaments and use a posterior cruciate-substituting prosthesis in correcting a fixed-varus deformity. Though it is our belief that PCL preservation may limit full correction of a fixed deformity, others have found that routine excision of the PCL is unnecessary, and that a CR knee can be used in cases of fixed-varus deformity.[14] Here, recession of the PCL must allow for correction of deformity, without creating posterior cruciate incompetence. This may be a formidable, if not impossible task, because fluoroscopic kinematic analysis of CR knees has demonstrated anterior sliding with flexion, secondary to PCL imbalance.[5]

COMPLICATIONS

Several complications can occur from the correction of fixed-varus deformities. These include instability of the tibiofemoral or patellofemoral articulations, or avulsion of the tibial tubercle.

Instability

Instability can occur in either extension or flexion, and can be either symmetric or asymmetric. Symmetric extension instability usually occurs from excessive resection of the distal femur, resulting in an extension gap that is inadequately filled by the components. Insertion of a thicker spacer may solve this problem, whereas creating a new one in that the flexion gap may now be too tight. A better solution is to build up the distal femur with the use of modular femoral augments.

Asymmetric extension instability is likely due to improper balancing of the collateral ligaments. This occurs when the contracted tight medial structures are inadequately released, or due to inadvertent division of the MCL. If the collateral ligaments cannot be balanced with soft tissue releases, or if the MCL is incompetent or transected, a constrained condylar implant may be needed.

Flexion instability may be asymmetric if the femoral component is malrotated into either internal rotation or excessive external rotation. Varus release balances the knee in extension, whereas external rotation of the femoral component creates a balanced, rectangular flexion gap. We prefer to set the rotational alignment of the femoral component along the epicondylar axis[6,7] to avoid excessive external rotation and internal rotation.

Symmetric flexion instability may paradoxically arise from insufficient resection of the distal femur. The tight extension gap then dictates a thin spacer, which inadequately fills the flexion gap, thereby creating flexion instability. The solution here would be to resect additional distal femur by an amount dictated by the difference in the thickness of the spacers used in flexion and extension (Fig. 25.12).

Downsizing may also create flexion instability because the posterior condyles are over-resected and re-

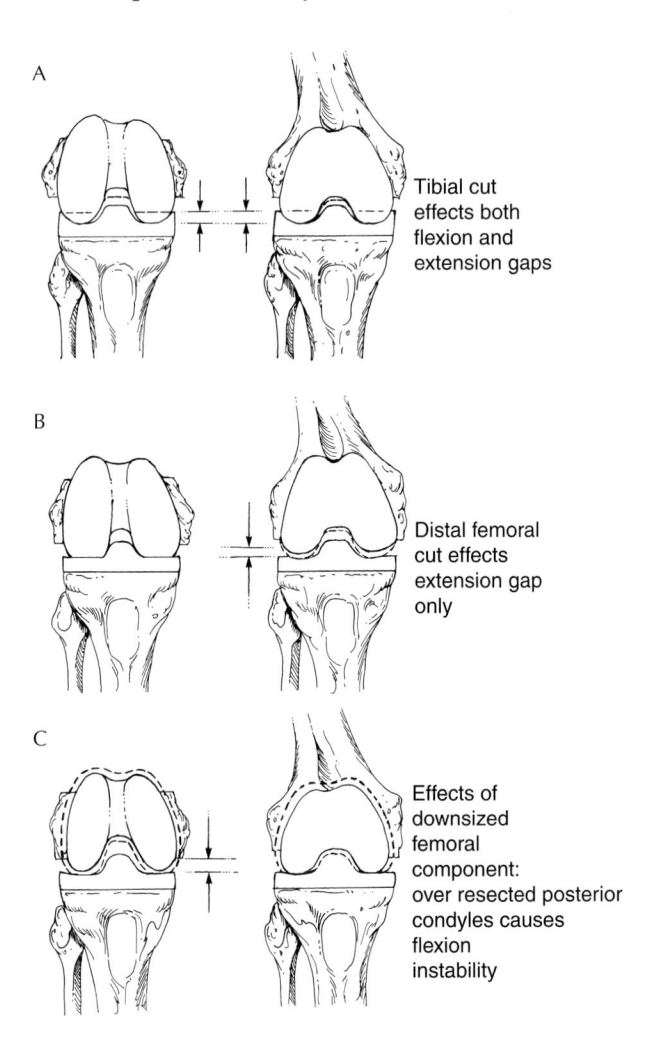

Figure 25.12. The effect of the bone cuts on prosthetic fit. (A) Tibial resection affects both flexion and extension gaps equally. (B) Distal femoral resection affects only the extension gap. In the case of extension instability, if the knee is too tight in flexion to admit a thicker tibial component, distal femoral augmentation is needed. (C) A downsized femoral component may inadequately fill the flexion gap, creating flexion instability. Use of a thicker tibial component may not help, because the knee may be too tight in extension. The solutions are to either use a larger-sized femoral component with posterior augments, or to resect additional distal femur and insert a thicker tibial component.

placed by a lesser amount of component (Fig. 25.12). In theory, a similar phenomenon may be encountered by instrumentation systems that rely on anterior referencing alone. The latest system of instruments that we use combines anterior and posterior referencing into the same guide as to minimize this dilemma.

Patellar Instability

Patellar instability more typically presents a challenge following correction of a fixed-valgus knee. However, even in a varus knee, attention to proper alignment and positioning principles is of paramount importance to ensure proper patellofemoral kinematics.

The femoral and tibial components must not be internally rotated, but rather externally rotated, as mentioned earlier. Internal rotation of the femoral component will create an asymmetric flexion space as mentioned earlier, but will also shift the lateral trochlea anteriomedially. This will increase the patellofemoral joint reaction force in a lateral vector, increasing the tendency for wear and/or subluxation. Internal rotation of the tibial component will shift the tubial tubercle laterally, in effect worsening the Q-angle and may result in patellar instability. The tibial and femoral component should also be lateralized, and the patellar component medialized, because this will improve tracking.

The "no thumbs" test of patellofemoral tracking has evolved to the use of a tenaculum clamp onto the quadriceps tendon through which a force is exerted in line with the rectus muscle. If tracking is still a problem intraoperatively, a lateral release should be performed, sparing the superior geniculate artery. On occasion, the artery may create a tether and should then be sacrificed. If tracking is still improper, a proximal realignment should be performed at the time of closure.[15]

Avulsion of the Tibial Tubercle

Avulsion of the tibial tubercle can easily occur during exposure of a stiff knee with a fixed-varus deformity. When the patella is everted and the extensor mechanism is dislocated laterally, considerable traction is exerted on the patella tendon, which risks being avulsed off of the tibial tubercle. Repairing a transverse rupture of the patellar tendon is a difficult and usually unsuccessful process, which is best avoided by meticulous technique during exposure of the knee.

The medial parapatellar arthrotomy should be continued onto the tibia to a point 1 cm medial to the tibial tubercle. This allows the patellar tendon to be dissected subperiosteally off of the medial third of the tibial tubercle with a long cuff of periosteum. Excessive tension on the extensor mechanism may pull the patellar tendon along with this periosteal sleeve farther away from the tibial tubercle, but maintains distal continuity of the soft tissues and prevents a horizontal tear.

The best method of preventing avulsion of the tibial tubercle is to avoid excessive tension on the tibial tubercle. In addition to subperiosteal dissection of a cuff of periosteum with the patellar tendon, one should use long skin incisions (8 to 10 cm proximal and distal to patella), extend the medial parapatellar arthrotomy far proximally into the quadriceps tendon, release completely the patellofemoral ligaments and excise the synovium from the lateral gutter, adjacent to the lateral tibial plateau. If after all of these measures there still exists excessive tension on the tibial tubercle, a quadriceps snip[2,3,16] or V-Y quadricepsplasty[4] should be performed.

References

1. Scuderi GR, Insall JN. The posterior stabilized knee prosthesis. *Orthop Clin North Am.* 1989; 20:71–78.
2. Garvin KL, Scuderi GR, Insall JN. Evolution of the quadriceps snip. *Clin Orthop.* 1995; 321:131–137.
3. Insall JN. Surgical techniques and instrumentation in total knee arthroplasty. In: Insall JN, ed. *Surgery of the Knee.* 2nd ed. New York: Churchill Livingstone; 1994: 739–804.
4. Trousdale RT, Hanssen AD, Rand JA, Cahalan TD. V-Y quadricepsplasty in total knee arthroplasty. *Clin Orthop.* 1993; 286:48–53.
5. Stiehl JB, Komistek RD, Dennis DA, Paxson RD, Hoff WA. Fluoroscopic analysis of kinematics after posterior-cruciate-retaining knee arthroplasty. *J Bone Joint Surg.* 1995; 77B:884–889.
6. Berger RA, Rubash HE, Seel MJ, Thompson WH, Crossett LS. Determining the rotational alignment of the femoral component in total knee arthroplasty using the epicondylar axis. *Clin Orthop.* 1993; 286:40–47.
7. Poilvache PL, Insall JN, Scuderi GR, Font-Rodriguez DE. Rotational landmarks and sizing of the distal femur in total knee arthroplasty. *Clin Orthop.* 1996; 331:35–46.
8. Colizza WA, Insall JN, Scuderi GR. The posterior stabilized total knee prosthesis. Assessment of polyethylene damage and osteolysis after a ten-year-minimum follow-up. *J Bone Joint Surg.* 1995; 77A:1713–1720.
9. Diduch DR, Insall JN, Scott WN, Scuderi GR, Font-Rodriguez D. Total knee replacement in young, active patients. Long-term follow-up and functional outcome. *J Bone Joint Surg.* 1997; 79A:575–582.
10. Scuderi GR, Insall JN, Windsor RE, Moran MC. Survivorship of cemented knee replacements. *J Bone Joint Surg.* 1989; 71B:798–803.
11. Stern SH, Insall JN. Posterior stabilized prosthesis. Results after follow-up of nine to twelve years. *J Bone Joint Surg.* 1992; 74A:980–986.
12. Insall JN, Hood JW, Flawn LB, Sullivan DJ. The total condylar knee prosthesis in gonarthrosis. A five- to nine-year follow-up of the first one hundred consecutive replacements. *J Bone Joint Surg.* 1983; 65A:619–628.
13. Vince KG, Insall JN, Kelly MA. The total condylar pros-

thesis. Ten- to twelve-year results of a cemented knee replacement. *J Bone Joint Surg.* 1989; 71B:793–797.
14. Tenney SM, Krackow KA, Hungerford DS, Jones M. Primary total knee arthroplasty in patients with severe varus deformity. *Clin Orthop.* 1991; 273:19–31.
15. Scuderi G, Cuomo F, Scott WN. Lateral release and proximal realignment for patellar subluxation and dislocation. A long-term follow-up. *J Bone Joint Surg.* 1988; 70A:856–861.
16. Scuderi GR, Insall JN. Fixed varus and valgus deformities. In: Lotke PA, ed. *Knee Arthroplasty.* New York: Raven Press; 1995: 111–127.
17. Scuderi GR, Insall JN. Total knee arthroplasty. Current clinical perspectives. *Clin Orthop.* 1992; 276:26–32.

CHAPTER 26
Lateral Release for Fixed-Valgus Deformity

Frankie M. Griffin, Giles R. Scuderi, and John N. Insall

VALGUS DEFORMITY IN TOTAL KNEE ARTHROPLASTY

Fixed-valgus deformity of the arthritic knee can be a difficult and challenging problem in total knee arthroplasty. Varus deformity is more commonly encountered, and therefore most surgeons are more comfortable with the surgical principles and releases used on the medial side of the knee. At our institution, at the time of knee replacement we encounter fixed-varus deformity (50 to 55%) three times more frequently than fixed-valgus deformity (10 to 15%). Ligament balancing and changes in boney anatomy of the valgus knee may be more difficult to correct than with varus deformity. In addition, the correct sequence and technique of release of the lateral structures remain controversial. Many different techniques to correct valgus deformity have been described, and they demonstrate the lack of a consensus among surgeons. Potential complications—including peroneal nerve palsy, flexion or extension instability, and patellar maltracking—also make correction of valgus deformity challenging.

PATHOPHYSIOLOGY

The normal knee is aligned with a femorotibial angle of 6 to 7 degrees valgus, has a full range of motion, and may be slightly more lax laterally in flexion. In arthritis of the knee, loss of bone and cartilage leads to instability, which can be classified as either symmetric or asymmetric. In response to the instability, adaptive changes occur. In fixed-valgus deformity the instability is asymmetric, and the surgeon is faced with deficiency of the lateral bone and cartilage, contracture of the lateral ligaments and capsule, stretching of the medial ligaments, and contracture of the iliotibial tract. The structures that may be "tight" include the lateral capsule, lateral collateral ligament, arcuate ligament, popliteus tendon, lateral femoral periosteum, distal iliotibial band, and lateral intermuscular septum[1]. In addition, there may be asymmetric wear of the posterior condyles with excessive wear of the posterolateral condyle. This wear has implications in surgical technique if the posterior condyles are utilized to reference femoral component rotational alignment[2]. Some authors have also reported external rotation deformity of the proximal tibia due to the tight iliotibial tract[3].

SURGICAL TECHNIQUES
Implant Selection

The successful results of total knee arthroplasty with the posterior-stabilized design are well documented in the literature[4]. In severe deformity, the PCL is often contracted and may limit correction of the deformity as described by Krackow's "cruciate limitation effect."[5] Even when an attempt at PCL-retention was made, Laurencian found that in 16% of knees he had to release the PCL[6]. Appropriate soft tissue balancing is much easier if the PCL is sacrificed. We believe it is much simpler to substitute a mechanical PCL for the diseased and contracted PCL in the severely deformed knee and that the results for the average surgeon will be better when the PCL is sacrificed routinely than when an attempt is made at soft tissue balancing with partial releases of the PCL and use of a posterior cruciate-retaining prosthesis. We therefore recommend use of the posterior-stabilized design.

In elderly low-demand patients, we prefer to use a constrained condylar knee to avoid the morbidity of extensive releases on the lateral side of the knee and to avoid the potential complications of peroneal nerve palsy and instability in flexion or extension. Bullek and associates (1996) evaluated the results of index-constrained condylar total knee arthroplasty in 28 patients with 34 TKAs.[7] The average age was 74.5 years, and the average preoperative deformity was 22 degrees valgus. No attempt at soft tissue balancing with lateral releases was made. Sixty-two percent required lateral retinacular releases for patellar tracking. All 34 TKAs (100%) had excellent (25 knees) or good (9 knees) results at an average follow-up of 3 years, and there was no evidence of early loosening or osteolysis. In younger patients, every attempt should be made to balance the knee and to avoid use of the constrained implant to eliminate the concern of early loosening in the more active, younger population.[8]

In some cases with bone deficiency, a modular implant with metal augments, offset stems, and variable tibial polyethelene thicknesses may be useful. In valgus deformity, patellar tracking is almost always an issue with lateral release rates reported from 62 to 100%.[7,8] Though one may speculate that the use of an implant that provides both left- and right-sided femoral components may improve patellar tracking, proper patellar preparation, and correct femoral component rotation are critically important.

Bone Cuts

Our preference is the medial parapatellar approach for all cases. Lateral osteophytes are often present and should be removed. The significance of the lateral osteophytes is debatable because the LCL's insertion on the fibular head takes the ligament away from the tibial rim, and therefore, lateral osteophytes do not typically bowstring the LCL the way that the medial osteophytes often impinge on the MCL.[9] However, Keblish and colleagues (1991) reported fewer LCL, popliteus, and capsule releases when the overhanging osteophytes were removed and a laminar spreader used to "tease" the joint apart in flexion and extension.[10]

Femoral component rotational alignment is important in the valgus knee to avoid flexion instability after lateral ligamentous release.[1] The surgical epicondylar axis may be helpful for rotational alignment of the femoral component in the valgus knee (Fig. 26.1).[11] Most current total knee instrumentation systems reference the rotation of the femoral cuts from the posterior condyles with some built-in "external rotation"—often around 3 degrees. However, in severe valgus deformity, the posterolateral condyle may be more worn, and therefore the amount of "external rotation" may need to be increased in reference to the posterior condyles. Because of the variability and posterolateral wear, the surgical epicondylar axis is a better reference for femoral component rotation than the posterior condyles—especially in valgus knees. In a recent study, we measured the posterior condylar angle (defined as the angle formed by the tangent to the posterior condyles and a line through the epicondyles as depicted in Figure 26.1) in 107 consecutive TKAs in 88 osteoarthritic patients and found the posterior condylar angle to be 3.29 ± 1.93 degrees for varus knees, 3.25 ± 2.25 for knees with no deformity, and 5.37 ± 2.29 for valgus knees. This led us to note that the posterior condylar angle was significantly greater in valgus knees compared to the other deformities ($p < 0.05$). The large standard deviations denote the variability of the posterior condylar angle in these osteoarthritic patients, and demonstrate that for valgus knees the surgical epicondylar axis is a more anatomic and consistent landmark.

The medial and lateral epicondyles are readily identified during routine exposure of the knee joint. The medial epicondyle is a horseshoe-shaped ridge on the medial femoral condyle that serves as the femoral attachment of the superficial fibers of the medial collateral ligament.[11] The center of the medial epicondyle is an indentation or sulcus where the deep fibers of the MCL insert (Figure 26.2).[11] In those knees where a sulcus is easily palpable, the center of the sulcus is marked. In those knees where the sulcus is not easily palpable, the fan-shaped origin of the MCL is identified on the medial femoral condyle and outlined with a marker. This forms a semicircle, which is then completed into a

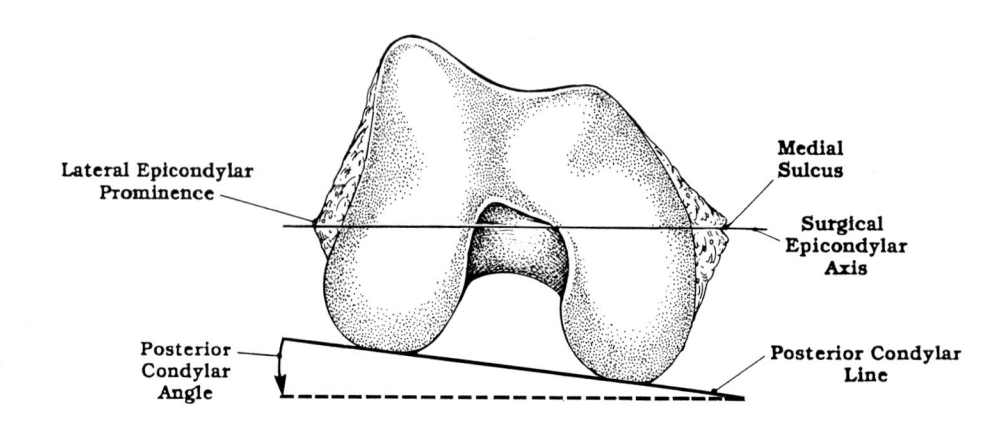

Figure 26.1. Surgical epicondylar axis posterior condylar angle.

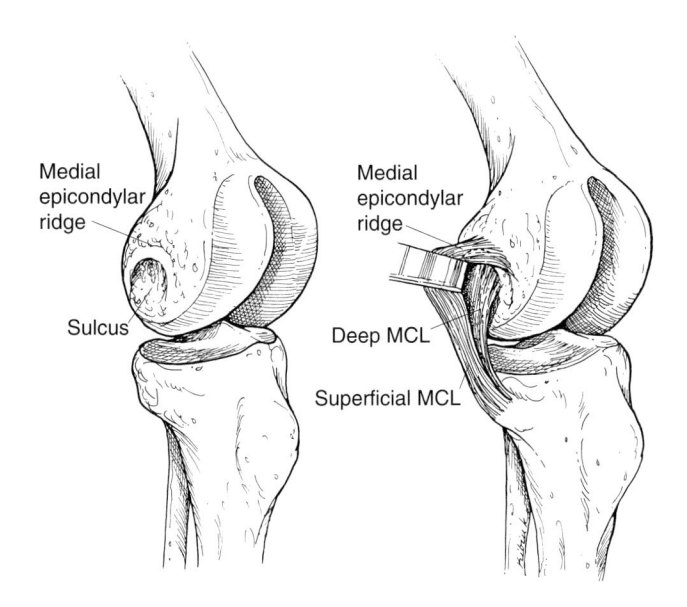

Figure 26.2. Medial epicondylar sulcus.

full circle. The center of the circle represents the sulcus and is the location of the medial epicondyle. The peak of the lateral epicondyle is more easily seen because it is the most prominent point on the lateral side. A line is drawn across the distal femur connecting those two points establishing the epicondylar axis.

The femoral component should be aligned with 5 to 7 degrees valgus angulation in the coronal plane and 0 to 10 degrees of flexion in the sagital plane.[12] Whitesides (1993) noted that appropriate placement of the femoral component is important to obtain appropriate joint line position in relation to the patella and to avoid damage to ligament attachments. Often the distal lateral femoral condyle is deficient and sclerotic.[3] Therefore, the distal femoral resection entails resection preferably from the medial femoral condyle and little or no bone resection from the lateral femoral condyle. In cases of severe genu valgum, the lateral femoral condyle may need to be bone grafted[3] or—as we prefer—built up with metal augmentation. By using this method of setting the distal femoral joint line, the joint line is not raised and ligament balancing in flexion and extension is achieved. This technique also helps to maintain the patellar height.

The tibial cut should be made at 90 ± 2 degrees to the long axis of the tibial shaft in both the coronal and sagital planes.[12] Whitesides has noted that over-resection of the proximal tibia to address a bony defect and create a flat surface for the tibial component may damage ligament attachments and may sacrifice excessive amounts of bone.[3] We have seen routine resection transect the popliteus tendon or detach the iliotibial band from the proximal tibia at Gerdy's tubercle. So caution must be taken when resecting the proximal tibia. The medial tibia is referenced and 10 mm of bone is resected. Bony defects can be addressed with cement, bone, or metal augments. The MCL must be protected during resection.

Soft Tissue Releases

The purpose of our release is to provide ligamentous balance with rectangular flexion and extension gaps (Fig. 26.3) while maintaining lateral side stability of the knee in flexion. The structures to be released may include the iliotibial tract, arcuate ligament, LCL, popliteus, biceps femoris, lateral gastrocnemius, lateral patellar retinaculum, PCL, and others. The release can be a full release, partial release, or Z-lengthening. Multiple soft tissue procedures have been described for use with valgus deformity with each of these structures.[3,6,8–10,13–21] The order of release varies among surgeons, and Table 26.1 shows the preferences of several surgeons as described in the literature.

Because access to the lateral supporting structures is easier, we prefer to perform the release after the tibial cut and distal femoral cut have been completed. Release is performed in a step-by-step controlled fashion and reassessed with laminar spreaders after each step. The endpoint of release is when the mechanical axis passes through the center of the knee and the flexion and extension gaps are equal and symmetrical.

Our preferred method of release is to begin by transversely cutting the posterolateral structures (arcuate ligament, posterolateral capsule, and reinforcing ligaments) just below the popliteus tendon from the corner of the cut surface of the tibia. Because the lateral meniscus has been removed, the popliteus tendon can be read-

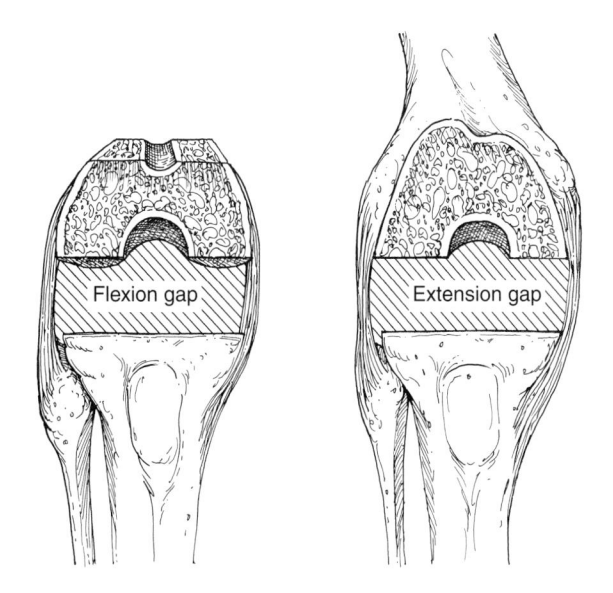

Figure 26.3. Flexion and extension gaps.

Table 26.1. Sequences of release

Author	First step	Second step	Third step	Final steps
Insall[17,18]	Posterolateral corner	Iliotibial tract	LCL, LIS	CCK
Ranawat[21]	Iliotibial tract transverse (2.5 cm)	Popliteus, LCL	Posterior capsule	LIS, lateral head of gastrocnemius
Keblish[10]	Lateral approach	Iliotibial tract multiple puncture	Posterolateral corner	Gerdy's tubercle, tibial tubercle elevation
Buechel[13]	Lateral approach	Iliotibial tract	LCL, popliteus	Fibular head excision
Clayton[14]	LCL, popliteus, lateral capsule	Posterolateral capsule, lateral head gastrocnemius, LIS	Iliotibial tract	Biceps femoris tendon Z-lengthening
Whitesides[3]	Iliotibial tract	Popliteus	LCL	Lateral head of gastrocnemius
Krackow[20]	Iliotibial tract	Popliteus	Posterolateral capsule, popliteus	Biceps femoris tendon, lateral head of gastrocnemius, MCL advancement in Type II

LIS = Lateral intermuscular septum
LCL = Lateral collateral ligament
CCK = Constrained condylar knee

ily identified and kept out of harm's way. When complete, the muscle belly of the popliteus and the lateral head of the gastrocnemius may be seen posteriorly. Soft tissue balance is rechecked with laminar spreaders, and occasionally release of the posterolateral structures alone is adequate. Usually with a fixed-valgus deformity, further release is necessary, and a "piecrust" release of the iliotibial tract and LCL is performed with a 15 blade by making multiple horizontal incisions in the iliotibial tract under direct visualization from inside to out (Fig. 26.4). It is helpful to keep the laminar spreaders in place during this release and to periodically squeeze them to stretch the lateral side. This works like a tensor and allows the lateral tissues to lengthen and slide with some degree of continuity. The incisions begin at the level of the joint line and are usually taken to a level approximately 10 cm proximal to the joint line. The release is carried further proximally if necessary. By this stage, a "pop" is usually felt and the valgus deformity is adequately corrected. The popliteus tendon should be preserved if possible to provide lateral stability in flexion. In our hands, release of the ITB and posterolateral corner corrects the majority of fixed-valgus deformities. If further release is still necessary, we proceed with a subperiosteal release of the remaining lateral structures including the lateral intermuscular septum to a point 7 to 8 cm from the joint line so that the whole "flap" is free to slide (Fig. 26.5). By this stage, almost all cases will have balanced, but if in the rare case further release is needed, we would release the lat-

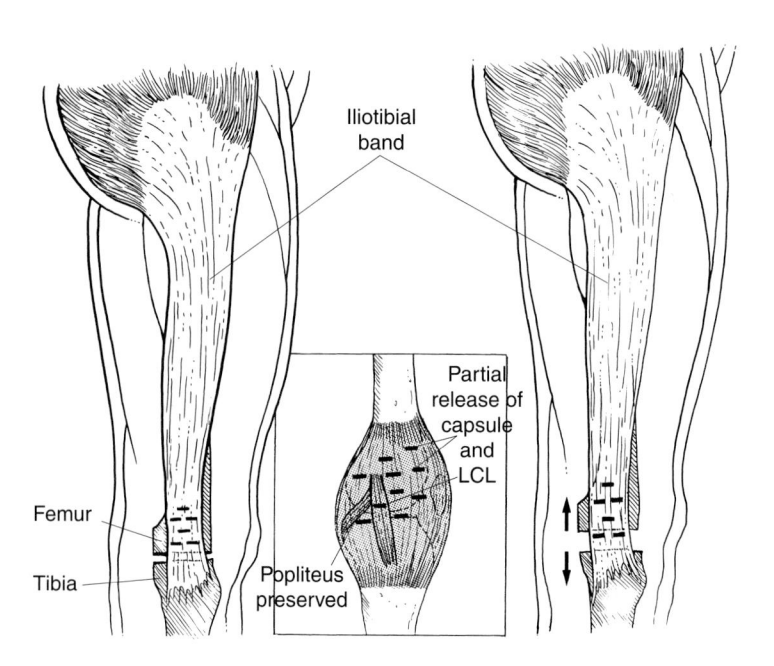

Figure 26.4. Piecrusting technique for valgus deformity.

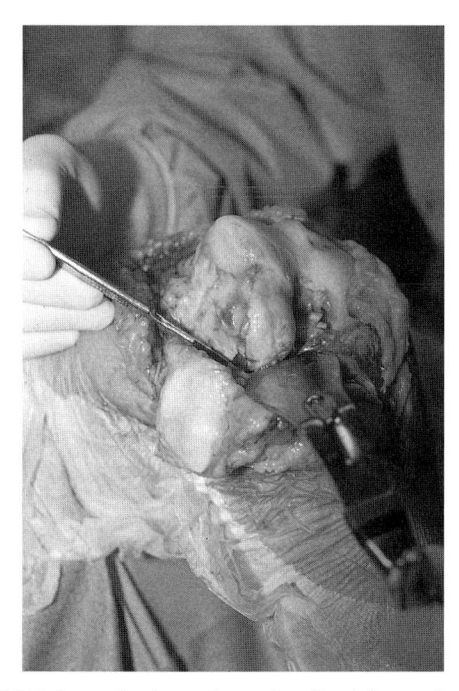

Figure 26.5. Lateral release from the distal femur for extreme valgus deformity.

eral head of the gastrocnemius from its femoral attachment. Release of the biceps femoris should be avoided if at all possible. If after complete release the medial ligament is too lax, then the ligament reconstruction procedures described by Krackow[5,20] should be considered, although we have limited experience with this option. Finally, if ligament stability cannot be achieved, a constrained condylar implant will be used.

Patellar maltracking is often associated with a valgus deformity. If present, a lateral retinacular release should be performed.

Postoperative Management

Patients who have undergone ligament releases for fixed-valgus deformity are managed in a manner similar to those who have had routine total knee arthroplasties. The knee is placed in a continuous passive motion (CPM) machine in the recovery room, because we have found CPM to decrease the rehabilitation period required to achieve 90 degrees of flexion.[22] To avoid a postoperative flexion contracture, we recommend use of a knee immobilizer during sleep for patients who have a tendency to flex their knee while sleeping. On the second postoperative day, patients are instructed to stand with assistance, and by the third postoperative day, they resume walking with full weight-bearing with crutches or a walker. Goals for hospital discharge include independent ambulation with crutches or a cane, ability to climb stairs, and attainment of 90 degrees of flexion.

COMPLICATIONS
Peroneal Nerve Palsy

With release of the lateral structures and correction of valgus deformity, some stretching of the peroneal nerve is unavoidable and some degree of postoperative ischemia can be predicted with this stretching. Peroneal nerve palsy has been reported in 3% of patients who underwent TKA with preoperative valgus deformity.[8] In addition to valgus deformity, risk factors that have been shown to increase the risk of peroneal nerve palsy include previous laminectomy and postoperative epidural anesthesia.[22] Some authors have described dissection of the peroneal nerve from its fascial sheath behind the fibular head and even fibular head resection in an attempt to avoid this complication.[10,13] However, a definitive benefit has not been shown and the possibility of direct injury is probably increased by the dissection. Therefore, we do not recommend direct exploration of the peroneal nerve. Idusuyi and associates (1996) reported that peroneal nerve palsy may present in a delayed fashion.[22] Placing the knee in a CPM machine in the recovery room reduces the tension on the peroneal nerve by allowing early flexion and by avoiding prolonged extension of the knee. If a peroneal nerve palsy is noted in the early postoperative period, the treatment is one of observation because the natural history of a postoperative peroneal nerve palsy is gradual partial or complete recovery. Stern and colleagues (1991) followed five patients with postoperative peroneal nerve palsies and noted that all tended to resolve over time, although all were left with some residual neurologic deficit.[8] Asp and Rand (1990) reported the natural history of 26 postoperative peroneal nerve palsies that occurred after 8998 TKAs.[23] In this group, they found that 18 had complete palsies and 8 had incomplete palsies with 23 combined motor and sensory deficits and 3 with only motor deficits. At an average of 5.1 years after TKA, 13 had complete recovery, 12 had partial recovery, and 1 had no improvement. Partial palsies had a better prognosis for complete recovery and had higher knee scores than those with complete palsies. Those with complete recovery also had higher knee scores than those whose recovery was incomplete. Krackow and associates (1993) reported the results of operative exploration and decompression of the peroneal nerve in 5 patients who developed peroneal nerve palsy-complicating TKA.[24] The procedure was performed 5 to 45 months after the index TKA, and the patients were graded pre- and postoperatively using a standard nerve palsy scale. They found that all 5 patients had improved nerve function and that 4 of the 5 patients had complete peroneal nerve recovery after the decompression. Thus, consideration should be given to surgical decompression of the peroneal nerve in cases that fail to respond to nonoperative measures.

Instability

Instability in extension can be described as either symmetric or asymmetric. Symmetric instability occurs when the extension gap is larger than the flexion gap resulting in residual laxity of the collateral ligaments in extension due to incomplete filling of the extension space by the prosthesis. Often this situation is caused by over-resection of the distal femur. Sometimes this problem can be solved by inserting a thicker tibial component. However, if the flexion gap is too tight to accommodate the thicker tibial component, the distal femur may need to be built up to make the extension gap smaller.[9] Asymmetric instability often is associated with inadequate release of a tight ligament. Therefore, ligament release in the stepwise fashion described earlier can be used to correct tight lateral ligaments. If asymmetric instability persists or if further release may result in overlengthening of the limb, a constrained condylar prosthesis should be utilized.

Resection of an insufficient amount of bone from the distal femur may also lead to flexion instability by forcing the surgeon to use a thinner tibial component to accommodate the smaller extension space.[9] Valgus release may also result in lateral instability in flexion. Preservation of the popliteus and a lengthened lateral soft tissue sleeve, when possible, may help to prevent this. In addition, use of the surgical epicondylar axis to rotationally orient the femoral component will ensure a more appropriate flexion gap based upon the patient's anatomy.

Patellar Instability

Lateral retinacular release is necessary in most severe valgus knees during total knee arthroplasty with surgeons reporting release rates of 62 to 100%.[7,8] Appropriate rotational alignment of the femoral component based upon the epicondyles with the surgical epicondylar axis or "external rotation" of the component—up to 5 or 6 degrees in relation to the posterior condyles—will improve patellar tracking. In addition the tibial component should be oriented by aligning the intercondylar eminence with the tibial crest. Proper rotational alignment of the components along with lateral retinacular release when necessary should diminish patellar complications. If the patella appears to be tracking laterally after lateral retinacular release, the rotational position of the components should be reevaluated, and if deemed correct, then a proximal patellar realignment should be performed during closure of the arthrotomy.

RESULTS

Total knee arthroplasty in the valgus knee provides reliable pain relief, correction of deformity, and good function. In general, the results have been only slightly inferior to the results obtained in standard total knee arthroplasty with a higher percentage of "good or excellent" results being "good" in the valgus knee and with more complications related to correction of deformity (peroneal nerve palsy, instability, patellar maltracking).

Stern and associates (1991) reviewed 134 TKAs in 98 patients with preoperative valgus deformities greater than 10 degrees with an average follow-up of 4.5 years.[8] Posterior-stabilized implants were used in the vast majority of cases (118 of 134), and valgus release consisted of release of the lateral structures from the lateral aspect of the femur. Postoperatively, the knees in their series had valgus alignment of 5 to 9 degrees, and a lateral retinacular release for patellar maltracking was required in 76% of cases. The authors reported 91% good or excellent results. However, only 71% were classified as excellent compared to 88% excellent in the standard TKA population.[25] Complications included peroneal nerve palsies in 5 knees (3%), aseptic loosening requiring revision in 3 knees, and one patient with chronic pain requiring revision.

Krackow and colleagues (1991) reviewed 99 TKAs in 81 patients with an average preoperative valgus deformity of 18 degrees.[20] They utilized a minimally constrained, PCL-sparing prosthesis, and divided the deformity into three types with all of their patients being either type I or II. The author defined type I (67 knees) knees as valgus deformity secondary to bone loss in the lateral compartment and soft tissue contracture without attenuation of the MCL, and type II (32 knees) knees as defined by obvious attenuation of the MCL. The mean preoperative tibiofemoral angle was 18.1 degrees in type I and 21.2 degrees in type II. The mean postoperative tibiofemoral angle was 4.8 degrees in type I and 5.9 degrees for type II. Releases used in type I deformities included the ITB, LCL, posterolateral capsule, popliteus tendon, biceps femoris tendon, and lateral head of gastrocnemius muscle. Type II was treated with medial ligament reconstruction. Results were 72% excellent, 18% good, 7% fair, and 2% poor.

Laurencin and associates (1992) reviewed 25 TKAs in 25 patients with average preoperative valgus deformities of 32 degrees.[6] To correct valgus deformity, they found it necessary to release the ITB at the level of the joint line in 76%, the popliteus and LCL in 56%, and biceps tendon just proximal to its fibular attachment in one case (3%). They made an attempt at cruciate retention in all patients, but 16% required sacrifice of the PCL for ligamentous balancing. All 25 patients required a lateral retinacular release for patellar tracking. The average postoperative alignment of the knees was 6 degrees valgus (range 0 to 10 degrees), and with an average follow-up of 5 years, there was no evidence of loosening and no revisions. Complications included three patellar stress fractures (two with osteonecrosis), one patellar dislocation, and one transient peroneal nerve palsy.

Whiteside reviewed 135 TKAs with mean preoperative valgus of 16 degrees.[3] His valgus release consisted of the ITB (at the joint line) initially, then the popliteus and lateral collateral ligament, and finally the lateral head of the gastrocnemius and the posterolateral capsule if necessary. Knees with greater than 25 degrees preoperative deformity all required release of the ITB, popliteus, and LCL, and 42% required release of the posterolateral capsule. He noted that this latter group had a tendency to have increased posterior laxity, which may have been related to the minimally constrained knee design that was implanted. When external rotational instability was present, he recommended a posterior-stabilized design. Because of femoral dysplasia or bone loss, 74% of knees with greater than 25 degrees valgus deformity had bone grafting of the lateral tibial plateau and 48% had grafting of the lateral femoral condyle. Six knees required medial ligament advancement. Because severe genu valgum is often associated with lateral patellar subluxation, it is not uncommon to have to realign the patella during TKA. In fact, in this series three knees with preoperative deformity greater than 25 degrees required tibial tubercle transfer in order to centralize the patella. The complexity of this deformity is substantiated by the related complications including eight knees with patellar component failure attributable to polyethylene wear, three knees with progressive posterior laxity (one symptomatically unstable), three knees with patellar dislocations (all during the first postoperative year), and five knees with postoperative wound hematomas.

There are some surgeons who prefer to approach the valgus knee from the lateral side in order to maintain the integrity of the extensor mechanism and theoretically improve patellar tracking. Keblish, in a review of 53 knees in 46 patients with preoperative valgus deformity averaging 22 degrees, utilized the lateral approach.[10] There was some variability in his implant selection. The low-contact stress (LCS) mobile-bearing knee system was used in 50 knees, and the kinematic rotating hinge was used in three. Of the LCS cases, 39 were meniscal-bearing cruciate-sparing (ACL and/or PCL) knees and 11 were rotating platform. Cementless "porocoat" LCS components were used in 41 knees. Because of the associated bony deficiencies, 48 of the 53 knees required bone grafting to the "lateral side." He reported 94% good or excellent results based on the New Jersey Orthopaedic Hospital scoring system at an average follow-up of 2.9 years. There was one transient sensory and one transient motor peroneal nerve palsy, and both recovered within 6 months without residual weakness or causalgia. As touted, there were no patellofemoral maltracking problems. Despite this experience, the lateral approach is not overwhelmingly popular because most surgeons are not familiar with the exposure and are concerned with closure.

SUMMARY

Fixed-valgus deformity can be a challenging problem for the reconstructive surgeon. The normal knee is aligned with a femorotibial angle of 6 to 7 degrees of valgus, and the goals of knee replacement surgery include a painfree knee with normal alignment and functional range of motion. We believe a posterior-stabilized prosthesis with sacrifice of the PCL will provide more reliable results for most surgeons in the valgus knee. The surgical epicondylar axis provides a reliable and reproducible landmark for appropriate rotational alignment of the femoral component, whereas the less involved medial femoral condyle and tibial plateau should be used to reference the distal femoral and proximal tibial cuts. Soft tissue balance should be achieved without modification of bone cuts. Sequential releases should be reassessed intermittently with laminar spreaders or a tensor. A variety of releases and sequences of release have been described, and our preferred method is described earlier in this chapter. Correctly balanced, 90 to 95% of patients with valgus deformity reportedly will have good or excellent results. Complications include peroneal nerve palsy, instability, and patellar maltracking.

References

1. Insall JN. *Surgery of the Knee*. 2nd ed.
2. Watanabe Y, Moriya H, Takahashi K, Yamagata M, Sonoda M, Shimada Y, Tamake T. Functional anatomy of the posterolateral structures of the knee. *Arthroscopy*. 1993; 9:57–62.
3. Whiteside, LA. Correction of ligament and bone defects in total arthroplasty of the severely valgus knee. *Clin Orthop*. 1993; 288:234–245.
4. Colizza WA, Insall JN. The posterior stabilized total knee prosthesis. *J Bone Joint Surg*. 1995; 77A(11):1713–1720.
5. Krackow KA. *The Technique of Total Knee Arthroplasty*. St. Louis: The C.V. Mosby Company; 1990.
6. Laurencin CT, Scott RD, Volatile TB, Gebhardt EM. Total knee replacement in severe valgus deformity. *The American Journal of Knee Surgery*. Summer 1992; 5(3):135–139.
7. Bullek DD, Scuderi GR, Insall JN. The constrained condylar knee prosthesis: an alternative for the valgus knee in the elderly. In: Insall JN, Scott WN, Scuderi GR, eds. *Current Concepts in Primary and Revision Total Knee Arthroplasty*. Philadelphia: Lippincott-Raven Publishers; 1996.
8. Stern SH, Moekel BH, Insall JN. Total knee arthroplasty in valgus knees. *Clin Orthop*. 1991; 273:5–8.
9. Scuderi GR, Insall JN. Fixed varus and valgus deformities. *Master Techniques in Orthopaedic Surgery*, Knee Arthroplasty. Lotke PA, ed. New York: Raven Press, Ltd; 1995.
10. Keblish PA. The lateral approach to the valgus knee: surgical technique and analysis of 53 cases with two-year follow-up evaluation. *Clin Orthop*. 1991; 271:52–62.

11. Berger RA, Rubash HE, Seel MJ, Thompson WH, Crossett LS. Determining the rotational alignment of the femoral component in total knee arthroplasty using the epicondylar axis. *Clin Orthop*. 1993; 286:40–47.
12. Scuderi GR, Insall JN. The posterior stabilized prosthesis. *Orthop Clinics North America*. 1989; 20(1):71–78.
13. Buechel FF. A sequential three-step lateral release for correcting fixed valgus knee deformities during total knee arthroplasty. *Clin Orthop*. 1990; 280:170–175.
14. Clayton ML, Thompson TR, Mack RP. Correction of alignment deformities during total knee arthroplasties: staged soft-tissue releases. *Clin Orthop*. 1986; 202:117–124.
15. Dorr LD, Boiardo RA. Technical considerations in total knee arthroplasty. *Clin Orthop*. 1986; 205:5–11.
16. Freeman MAR, Sculco T, Todd RC. Replacement of the severely damaged arthritic knee by the ICLH (Freeman-Swanson) arthroplasty. *J Bone Joint Surg*. 1977; 59B(1):64–71.
17. Insall JN. Modified technique of lateral release for valgus deformity. Personal communication.
18. Insall JN. TKA valgus deformity. Personal communication.
19. Insall JN, Scott WN, Ranawat CS. The total condylar knee prosthesis. *J Bone Joint Surg*. 1979; 61A(2):173–180.
20. Krackow KA, Jones MM, Teeny SM, Hungerford DS. Primary total knee arthroplasty in patients with fixed valgus deformity. *Clin Orthop*. 1991; 273:9–18.
21. Ranawat CS. Total-condylar knee arthroplasty for valgus and combined valgus-flexion deformity of the knee. *Techniques Orthop*. 1988; 3(2):67–75.
22. Idusuyi OB, Morrey BF. Personeal nerve palsy after total knee arthroplasty. Assessment of predisposing and prognostic factors. *J Bone Joint Surg*. 1996; 78A(2):177–184.
23. Asp JP, Rand JA. Peroneal nerve palsy after total knee arthroplasty. *Clin Orthop*. 1990; 261:233–237.
24. Krackow KA, Maar DC, Mont MA, Carroll C. Surgical decompression for peroneal nerve palsy after total knee arthroplasty. *Clin Orthop*. 1993; 292:223–228.
25. Insall JN, Lachiewicz PF, Burnstein AH. The posterior stabilized condylar prosthesis: a modification of the total condylar design. *J Bone Joint Surg*. 1982; 64A:1317.

CHAPTER 27
Medial and Lateral Ligament Advancement

Kenneth Krackow

INTRODUCTION

Considerable debate exists with respect to the need, hence propriety, of performing ligament advancement procedures in the midst of total knee arthroplasty surgery. Many extremely competent and experienced total knee replacement surgeons state that they have never found such techniques necessary. Others find that they have been necessary, or at least helpful.

The premises underlying the applicability of these techniques include the following points:

1. Not all severe varus or valgus deformities can be released to a satisfactorily corrected condition of normal tibiofemoral angulation with adequately balanced residual primary or secondary collateral soft tissue stabilizers. This statement may be most easily accepted in those cases of deformity in which the convex side of the knee (lateral in varus, medial in valgus deformities) has undergone significant stretching.
2. Even if adequate release could be performed, it would lead to undesirable lengthening and, in the case of valgus deformity especially, it could risk jeopardy to the peroneal nerve because it needs to span an elongated space.
3. The most common "stabilized" knee designs are posterior-substituting components that do not provide varus-valgus collateral stability to address the residual instability in severe cases.
4. One may simply have permanently positioned (i.e., cemented components) in place, and then may determine that collateral instability is not satisfactory. He or she may be in a situation in which an alternative level of prosthetic constraint is either not available, generally impractical, or otherwise contraindicated.
5. References to prior experience and lack of success with ligament reconstruction in total knee replacement and other comments about unsuccessful applications must be looked at more critically. Some of the experience cited does not involve simultaneous ligament advancement at primary total knee arthroplasty, but rather use of ligament advancement to treat existing, that is, later postoperative instability in total knee arthroplasty situations.

In my experience as well, such cases cannot reliably be managed by ligament reconstruction.

Other comments with respect to problematic experience from ligament advancement techniques need to be examined critically with respect to specifics of these techniques both intraoperative and postoperative. The techniques in after care are very particular. Unsatisfactory experience may be due largely to failure to address important technical and rehabilitative points. The main aspect to appreciate here is the general difficulty of achieving fixation of the advanced soft tissue element. This difficulty derives from the fact that the side (medial for valgus, lateral for varus) of advancement is the a priori convex side of the deformity. As such, this is bone that has generally been minimally stressed. A much higher proportion of weight is borne in the concave compartment. Reattaching the advanced soft tissue structures using ordinary soft tissue to bone-stapling techniques may not be expected to work reliably in this osteoporotic bone.

6. Even constrained intercondylar prostheses, which the author refers to as CIPs to avoid the brand connotations and very specific design particulars implied by the terms CCK and TC-3, have their limits. Most experienced referral total knee surgeons have seen cases of failures with these systems due to residual or developed soft tissue asymmetry, which allows the tibial component to drop away from the femur and for the intercondylar peg to become nonfunctional.

For all these reasons the author believes the techniques of soft tissue advancement and imbrication should be familiar to the total knee surgeon who takes on the difficult deformity cases. In rare situations these techniques may be helpful.

This last statement allows us to reemphasize that the overwhelming majority of total knee deformity situations will be adequately managed by "concave-side-release." The techniques described in this chapter are for the truly extraordinary, exceptional examples.

MEDIAL ADVANCEMENT

The technique of medial ligamentous advancement shown here is a proximal advancement on the femur. Published elsewhere are descriptions of distal advancement on the tibia. The author discarded this latter technique a number of years ago. In order for tissues to be advanced to provide capsular ligamentous tightness, this tissue needs to be freed from adjacent bone all the way to the joint line. The medial collateral ligament mechanism is more than just the superficial medial collateral ligament. It includes the posterior extension known as the posterior oblique ligament. Effective distal advancement requires elevation of the superficial medial collateral ligament and the entire soft tissue sleeve attached to the proximal posterior medial tibia with refixation of all of this distally.

The author felt that the dissection required and the difficulties attendant upon reattachment could be minimized by proximal advancement on the femur.

The medial collateral ligament mechanism on the femur has a type of "focal point" of origin at the medial epicondyle. The soft tissue dissection and elevation necessary to effect tightening are considerably less. And, re-fixation is addressed to a smaller region.

When medial collateral ligament tightening is elected, the actual fixation of soft tissue is undertaken only after final implantation of all total knee components, just before wound closure. The dissection to access the tissues can be performed at essentially any earlier point in the procedure. However, this dissection is easiest to do if either the tibial and femoral bone has not been resected or if trial or final components are in place. The resected bone ends without spacer effects if the components present a laxity situation with greater difficulty in performing the dissection described next.

The pre-capsular plane is developed as shown in Figure 27.1. The extent of this development is to a point approximately 1 cm posterior to the medial epicondyle, then extending slightly posterior as the development also leads distally to just below the joint line. One can palpate the medial epicondyle and the superficial medial collateral ligament, again, if the capsular plane is tight. An incision is made, as shown, that permits elevation of the medial collateral ligament attachment and development of a trapezoidal flap of tissue from the anterior border of the medial collateral ligament to the posterior border of the posterior oblique ligament. The flap is entirely elevated from the femur; it includes capsule, ligament, and synovium.

Adjacent, more proximal soft tissue, which is capsule and synovium, is elevated from the femur proximal to the medial epicondyle to the extent necessary to allow

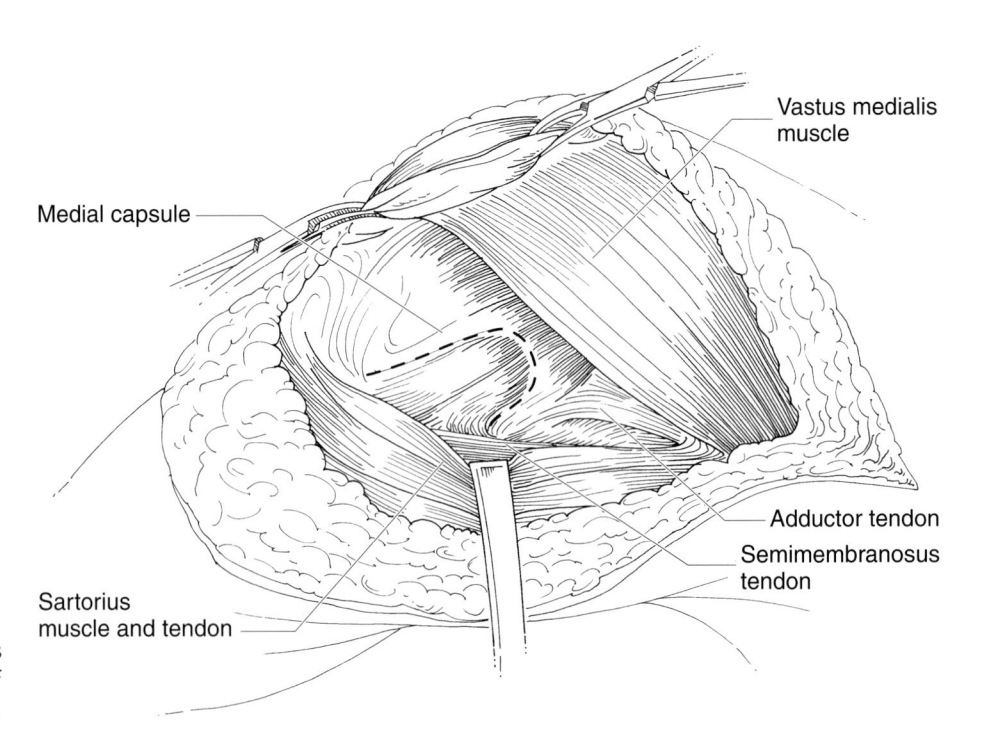

Figure 27.1. The broken line marks the incision for the development of the medial collateral ligament flap.

the advanced tissue to rest on bare bone. The proximal ligament advancement generally proceeds in a proximal and anterior direction. Although the proximal end of this flap obviously comes to lie above its original position at the epicondyle, the focal point of reapplication of the "advanced" ligament is still the epicondylar aspect of the femur. A soft tissue staple or ligament screw-washer device is used to provide application or contact of the medial collateral ligament back to this epicenter or apex point.

Prior to fixation of the soft tissue at the epicondyle, synovium is removed from the deep aspect of the flap and then specific ligament sutures are placed in the elevated tissue (Fig. 27.1B). Generally, heavy (#5) permanent suture material has been used, either as two separate sutures or a single doubled suture made from two strands (Fig. 27.2).

The real strength of fixation for the reconstructive complex is provided by these sutures and not by the staple or screw-washer element that applies tissue to the epicondyle (Fig. 27.3). These sutures are tied over a screw-washer arrangement positioned adequately proximal and anterior.

The author has not utilized suture anchors and would discourage their consideration. Again, a major feature of accomplishing secure fixation is recognition that the bone in this area is generally quite osteoporotic. The author fears that suture anchors would not hold well enough. The screw-washer complex may be preferred as well because a long screw can be directed to engage hard bone at the lateral aspect of the femur. Also, it can be directed in a proximal as well as a lateral direction so that this construct effects a partially longitudinal constraint position. If a somewhat similar screw were positioned from straight medial to lateral, it would not be as effective. It could lean or wobble in the soft tissue more readily and fail to provide better stabilization.

The advancement just described is performed without significant violation of the medial femoral cortex. To try to elevate a corticocancellous piece of bone and move this proximally, which leaves a void that may thwart fixation of the advanced element, William Healy (Boston, Mass) has developed an alternative technique in which the medial epicondyle is pulled into a counter sunken position, that is, essentially "deepening" the epicondyle. This is different from elevating and moving a bone "plug" proximally.

To the degree that the capsular ligamentous tissue is properly reattached to the region of the center of curvature and center of rotation at the medial aspect of the femur, the flexion extension ligament balance behavior of this reconstruction is quite good. Again, the reconstruction is not performed as a straight proximal advancement. In general, straight proximal would be expected to lead to relative laxity in flexion.

With the technique described, the amount of soft tissue dissection is really not excessive. The capsular ligamentous flap developed is quite thick and holds the suture material well.

Management at the lateral aspect of valgus knees will take two forms. If the medial advancement is planned at the outset, one might refrain from performing any lateral stabilizer release. In other cases, the lateral tissues may be seen as sufficiently contracted so that lateral re-

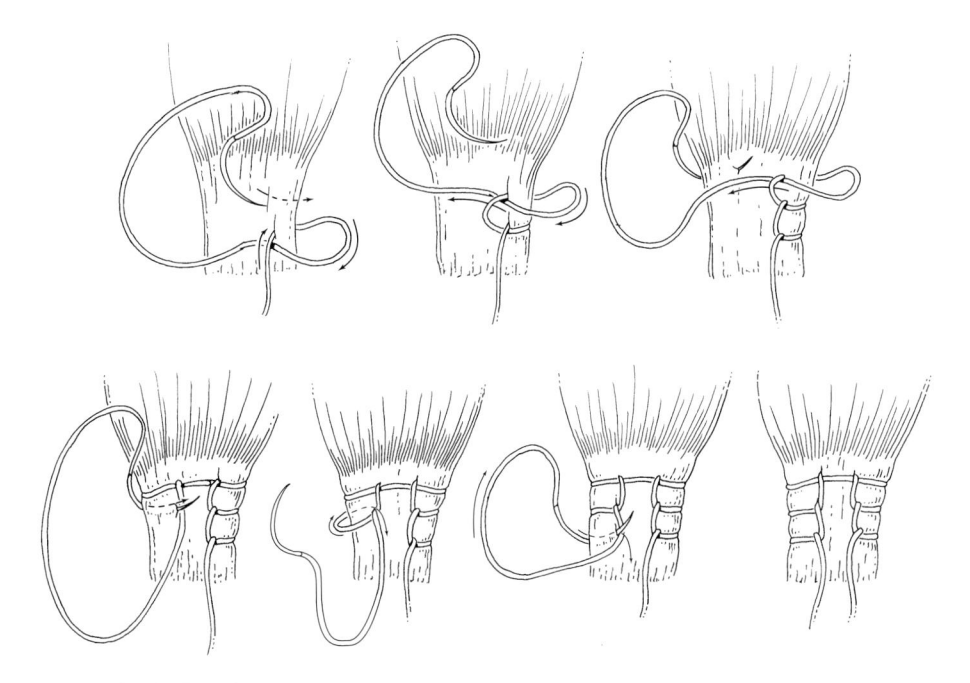

Figure 27.2. The locking loop ligament fixation suture prevents pull out and avoids tissue shortening.

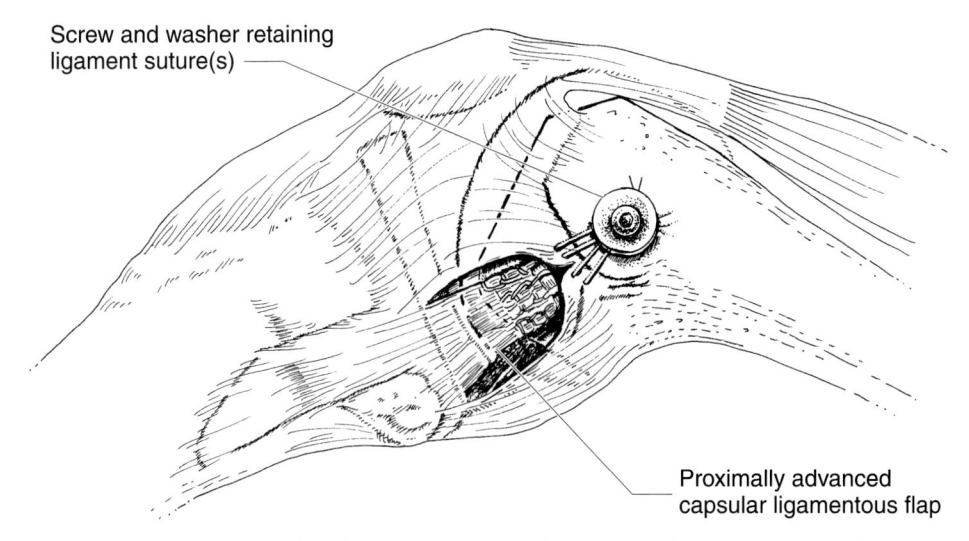

Figure 27.3. The staple is inserted at the desired center of rotation and the sutures over the screw and washer provide additional reinforcement.

lease is appropriate. As well, the medial plication may be undertaken because the lateral release, initially hoped to be adequate, was found to leave sufficient medial instability so that the medial advancement is performed.

LATERAL ADVANCEMENT

The lateral advancement technique described here is essentially identical to the proximal one described for the medial side. The initial experience also involved a distal advancement at the fibular head. Such an approach not only requires extensive additional exposure involving also attention to the peroneal nerve, but it left the situation of the distally advanced element, or the fibular head, connected to a proximally pulling "motor," the biceps femoris muscle. Active flexion therefore was pulling against the reconstruction. For both of these reasons, distal femoral advancement has been abandoned. Aside from total knee arthroplasty cases, however, distal advancement of the lateral collateral with the fibular head has still been used successfully in some complex tibial osteotomy cases with preoperative lateral instability.

The essence of proximal lateral advancement is shown in Figure 27.3. Again, a trapezoidal flap of capsule, ligament, and here, tendinous tissue is elevated and pulled proximally, also generally, proximally anteriorly. The procedure is analogous to that described by Hughston for posterolateral instability.

One or two locking loop ligament sutures are placed. The tissue is pulled taut; it is reapplied to the epicondylar center of rotation with a staple or ligament screw arrangement and the tails are secured more proximally, generally over a screw-washer combination.

Lateral ligamentous advancement is extremely rare in the author's experience. Most patients function quite well with some residual lateral laxity in varus cases; substantial lateral stretch is seen less often in varus cases; and, the most troublesome aspect of residual imbalance in varus cases may be addressed frequently by posterior-substituting components. This is a particular type of translational instability in the posterolateral direction (Fig. 27.4). This phenomenon is rare but can be seen with major medial stripping, residual lateral laxity, and a tibial component with a medium to low height intercondylar eminence. In this setting, what would seem to be a satisfactory degree of residual lateral laxity apparent on routine ligament testing with varus stress, in fact, permits posterolateral subluxation. Although posterior substituting or sacrificing knees do not provide direct lateral stabilization to varus stress, they do provide, to some degree, protection against this lateral translational instability.

AFTER CARE

The soft tissue to bone fixation described in this chapter for both lateral and medial reconstruction is secure but not optimal or perfect. It has been the author's practice to alter patients' postoperative courses to provide additional protection. Patients are immobilized in a straight knee immobilizer (velcro straps, canvas type of brace) for 3 weeks. They remove this brace or splint multiple times each day to perform active and gentle passive range of motion exercises, after which the brace is replaced. Weight-bearing is kept to a light partial weight-bearing mode (25% partial weight-bearing or less). At 3 weeks postop this splint or bracing is changed

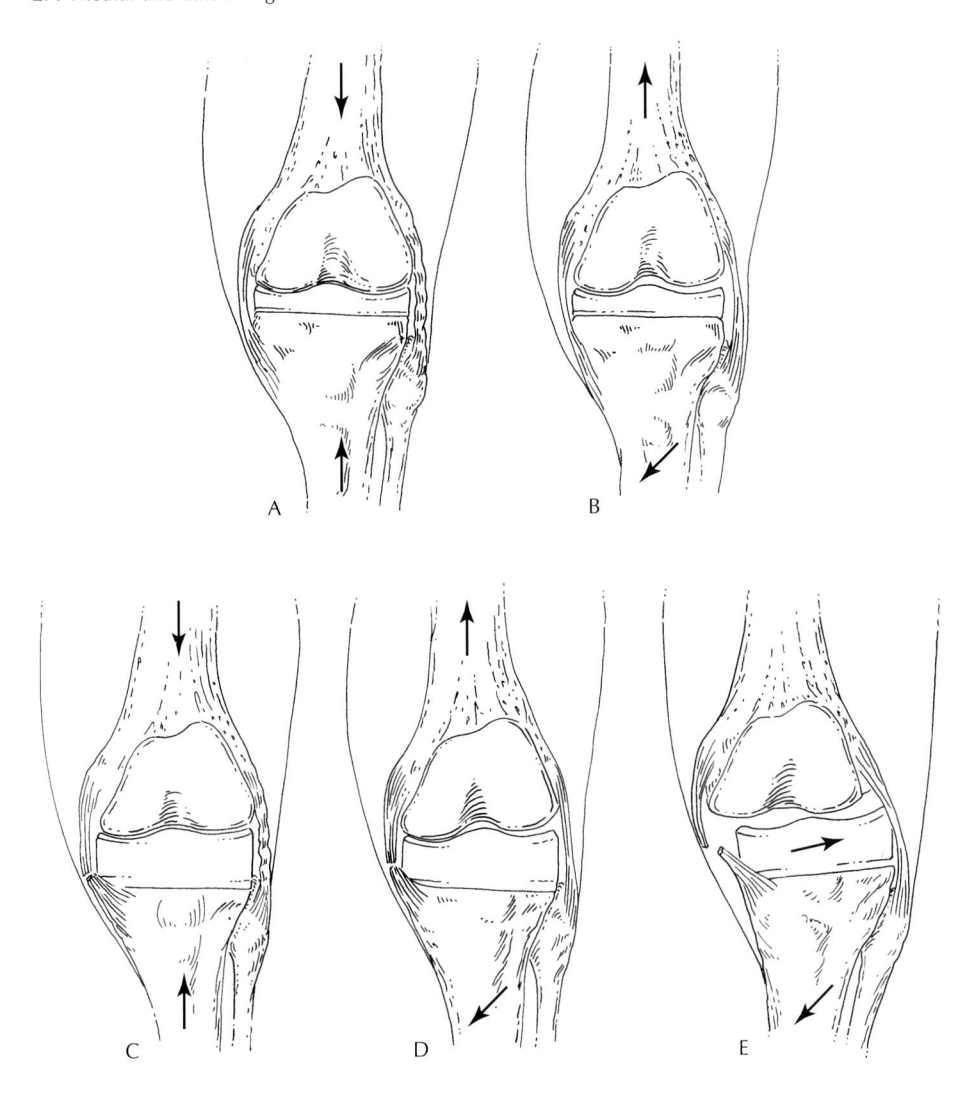

Figure 27.4. In A and B the residual lateral laxity in the varus knee is well tolerated. As the medial release is increased, there is more room for the lateral side to sublux despite the use of a thicker tibial component in C, D, and then E. There is not enough of a soft tissue component left in E to stop lateral displacement.

to use of a hinged long-legged splint so that range of motion can be accomplished throughout the day.

At 6 weeks and for the ensuing 6 weeks, that is, from 6 to 12 weeks postoperative, the patient wears a simple front laced, side hinged knee "cage." At all stages over the entire time, specific range of motion exercises are done with the patient out of all bracing or splinting. Splinting is undertaken to prevent unconscious, untoward movements at other times. It is presumed that these will not occur when the patient is concentrating on the knee during a specific range of motion exercise session.

At 3 months postoperative, no special precautions are instituted. CPM is generally not used in these patients. The author is concerned that especially in the first 2 to 5 days postoperatively, nursing or physical therapy staff may inadvertently disrupt the reconstruction in the process of "helping" the patient into or out of the CPM apparatus. In the absence of this concern, the author sees no disadvantage to CPM in these patients.

SUMMARY

The ligament advancement techniques described are rather infrequently indicated. Clearly, if patients' circumstances are such that one is confident introducing the level of constraint inherent in a CIP, these techniques are not necessary. For the quite elderly patient, such levels of constraint are most likely the treatment of choice. However, one may consider that such intrinsic prosthesis constraint is not appropriate in younger patients for whom concerns of loosening may prevail.

Finally, one may like to prepare to undertake ligament tightening if final components are in place, component alternatives are not readily available, and the ligamentous stability is judged unsatisfactory.

CHAPTER 28
Flexion Contracture in Total Knee Arthroplasty

Paul A. Lotke and R.G. Simon

Many patients requiring total knee arthroplasty will have a moderate flexion contracture that is fully corrected at surgery. However, when preoperative contractures are greater than 20 degrees, the deformity may become fixed and require special surgical consideration. This chapter will discuss these patients.

The deformity is a result of either a bone block and/or soft tissue contractures (Fig. 28.1). The proliferation of osteophytes in degenerative joint disease or prior trauma creates bone blocks that can occur in the anterotibial or posterofemoral condyles. They mechanically abut the intercondylar notch, or tether the posterior capsule, thus preventing full extension. The bone deformity may be slowly progressive and subsequently cause secondary soft tissue contracture of the posterior capsule and collateral ligaments.

Soft tissue contracture occurs in patients with long-standing deformities from a variety of disease states such as inflammatory arthritis, immobility, hemophilia, and neuromuscular disorders. These contractures can be static or progressive and can lead to increasing tightness in the posterior capsule, collateral ligaments, and hamstring muscles. Once the deformity exceeds 50 degrees, the collateral ligaments are inevitably involved.

Flexion of the knee is a response to inflammation, infection, or any condition that leads to joint swelling and increased intra-articular pressures. It has been demonstrated that increasing intra-articular pressure results in the knee assuming a 30- to 45-degree flexion position.[1]

Fixed flexion contractures decrease the patient's ability to walk. Velocity is slowed and energy costs are increased. Perry and associates[2] measured a 50% increase in work by the quadriceps at a given rate of ambulation in the presence of bilateral contractures of 30 degrees. The adjacent joints also assume abnormal posturing and increase the energy requirements with a corresponding reduction in endurance. Persons who have added disability of muscle weakness from disease atrophy or paralysis may lose their ability to walk.

Persistent flexion posture eventually leads to tightening of the posterior capsule and portions of the collateral ligaments. Normally these structures help prevent hyperextension and are at full length in extension. With a flexion contracture the collateral ligament and posterior capsule shorten, thereby preventing full extension. It is undetermined if the posterior cruciate ligament contributes to the persistence of flexion contracture, because this ligament lengthens with flexion.

The secondary soft tissue shortening of the capsule and portions of the collateral ligament makes it difficult to achieve ligament balancing during total knee replacement. At surgery we attempt to achieve an equal space between the femur and tibia in both flexion and extension (Fig. 28.2). This is referred to as a balanced flexion-extension gap. In a normal knee we use "measured resections" (i.e., removing equal amounts of bone from the femur and tibia that are to be replaced with prosthetic material). The flexion and extension gaps should be equal after the bony cuts are performed. Patients with long-standing flexion contractures will have a normal flexion gap, but a narrow gap in extension. This leads to persistence of the contracture. This imbalance can be corrected by releasing the soft tissue contracture and/or resecting more distal femur, thereby increasing the extension gap. As more bone is resected from the femur, the joint line is subsequently moved proximally. This creates alterations in the kinematics of the knee and in the contact points of the patella femoral joint. Occasionally it is necessary to take a few more millimeters of distal femur. However, the preferable method to achieve flexion-extension gap balance is to release the soft tissue structures.

In addition to the flexion contractures there is an attenuation in the extensor mechanism and anterior capsule.[3] Although this does not create intraoperative prob-

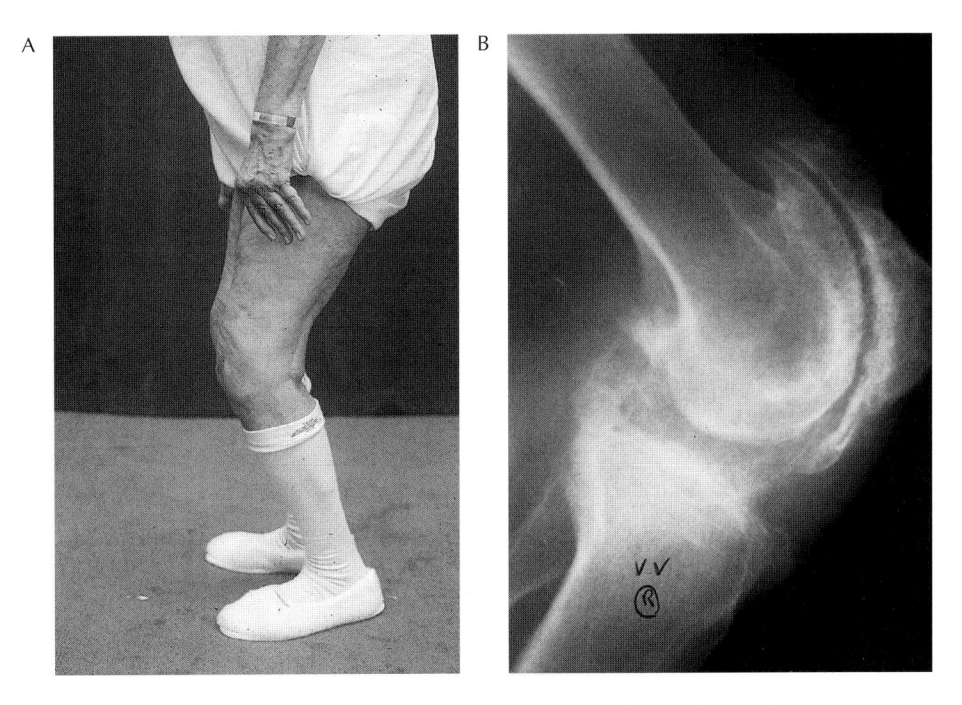

Figure 28.1. (A) Patient with rheumatoid arthritis and fixed flexion from soft tissue contracture. (B) X ray of patient with osteoarthritis and severe flexion contracture secondary to bone impingement preventing full extension.

lems, it may contribute to persistent extensor lag and some degree of persistent quadriceps weakness, and may inhibit the patient's ability to maintain full extension during the postoperative period. It is important to recognize this potential for prolonged extensor lag so that the knee can be protected from current deformity.

PREOPERATIVE EVALUATION

All patients should have the usual preoperative evaluations including medical history, functional history, and physical examinations. The standard standing anteroposterior X rays may be misleading because of the pos-

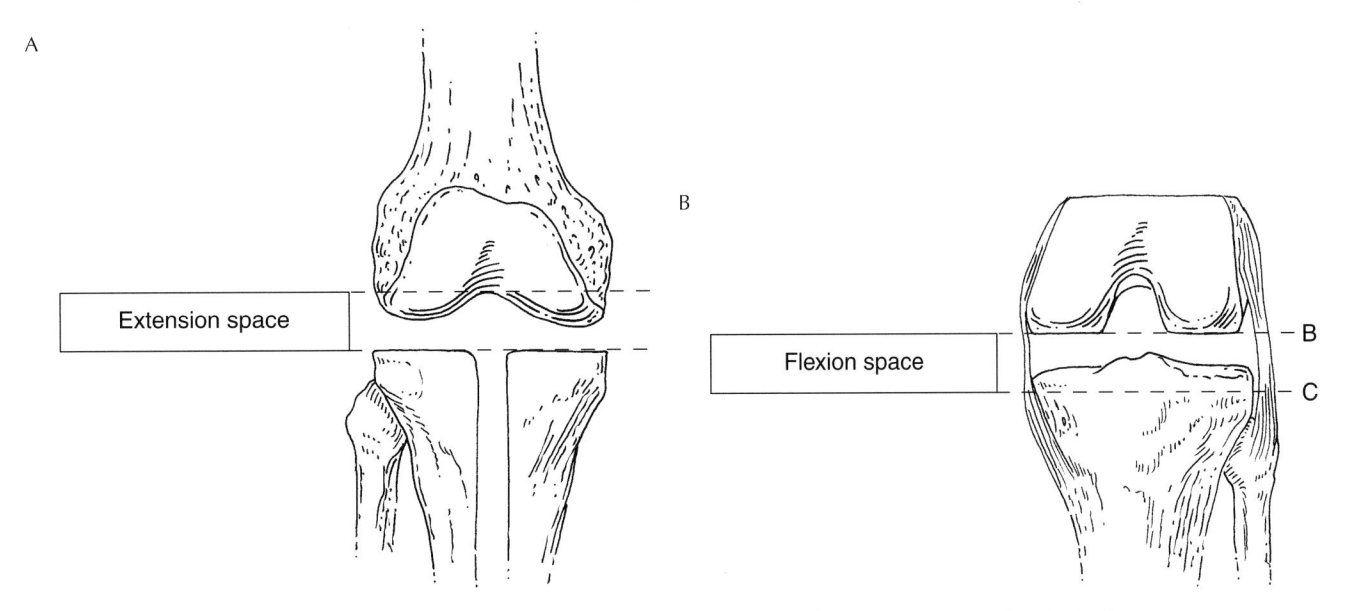

Figure 28.2. The space between the femur and tibia should be rectangular and equal in both flexion and extension with fixed flexion deformity. The extension space becomes too tight.

turing of the knee with a flexion contracture. This contracture will alter the apparent remaining joint space, because the X-ray beams may not be parallel to the joint line, and the joint space will appear to be obliterated. (Fig. 28.3). In addition, if there is external rotation of the knees when the X ray is taken, the apparent alignment will be misleading. Therefore, care should be taken to have the X rays taken parallel to the tibial plateau surface and with a true anteroposterior position. In addition to alignment and joint-space aberration there will also be increased magnification from X-ray beam parallax making the templating inaccurate. These variations should be recognized during preoperative planning.

Accurate preoperative anteroposterior X rays are important because a tangential X ray, which shows absence of joint space, is misleading and may suggest that an arthroplasty is required. If joint space remains and the principal abnormality is soft tissue contracture, then this knee could potentially be handled by soft tissue release alone. This would be particularly important in patients who have quiescent juvenile rheumatoid arthritis or immobility contractures with preservation of articular cartilage surface.

Some surgeons have recommended preoperative casting to reduce the contracture. This can potentially make the surgical procedures easier and avoid postoperative skin and nerve complications. If the contracture is of relative recent onset and there is a soft spring to the extension endpoint, indicating potential improvement in extension, then there may be some benefit from repeated preoperative casting to reduce the contracture.

Preoperative casting can be initiated with a knee manipulation under anesthesia and casting in the extended position. The cast must be very carefully applied with padding over the patella, achilles tendon, and posterior thigh. Pressure sores must be assiduously avoided.

In one study by Convrey and associates[4] 46 knees in 23 patients were treated with casts with an average correction of 60%. At follow-up averaging 41 months the patients showed a general tendency for the deformity to recur. However, the original deformity was maintained with a mean loss of only 5 to 11 degrees. The amount of correction that was obtained did not appear to be directly effected by the severity of joint destruction, precast deformity, or ambulatory status. The total degree of flexion was unchanged with the casting technique. The overall functional status was dependent on the deformity. The study acknowledged the difficulty in a retrospective review for multiple uncontrolled variables.

A variety of casting techniques have been described. These have included (1) serial casts with anesthesia; (2) removing a long anterior window from the foot, anterior tibia, and knee, with subsequently placing thicker soft padding behind the heel and calf; (3) hinges with turnbuckle extenders; and (4) traction. Most of these techniques have been described but not scientifically validated. They may or may not be appropriate for arthroplasty surgery.

There is very little written on casting for flexion contractures prior to joint arthroplasty. The number of patients that may require casting is relatively small, and there are a variety of disease processes with variable amounts of joint destruction. Therefore, it is difficult to make firm recommendations in this regard. However, our own preference is to consider casting for younger patients with recent contractures but not to utilize casting in patients who are older with fixed deformities and significant joint destruction.

SURGICAL TECHNIQUE

Standard total knee arthroplasty is initiated with "measured resection" in which the bone that is resected is the

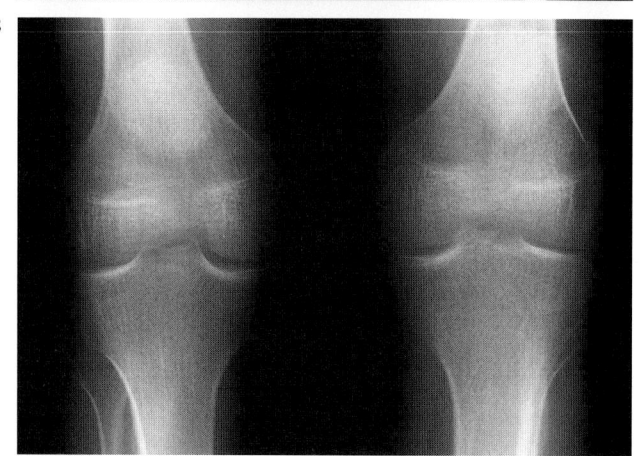

Figure 28.3. Patient with fixed flexion deformity. (A) Films taken in anteroposterior view with apparent obliteration of joint space. (B) X ray taken parallel to joint surface showing that good space remains.

same dimension as the prosthesis. In general, exposure is not a problem as these usually have good flexion. Once the measured resections are completed, osteophytes are carefully removed from all segments of the knee. We carefully remove osteophytes from the posterior femoral condyles and circumferentially around the tibial plateau with a curved osteotome and curette (Fig. 28.4). The knee is then evaluated for the space in flexion compared to the space in extension. There will be a wide variation in the discrepancy depending on the amount of deformity, rigidity of fixation, and age of the patient.

To equilibrate the flexion-extension space, a soft tissue release is carried out in stages, checking the extension gap after each step.[5-7] First, a periosteal elevator is used to elevate the capsule from the posterior femur (Fig. 28.5). Both the anterior and posterior cruciate attachments from the intercondylar notch of the femur are removed (Fig. 28.6) and the soft tissue capsular attachments in the posterior femur are dissected from the posterior femur (Fig. 28.7). The extension gap is again measured, and if more release is required, the dissection is carried more proximal releasing the gastrocnemius muscle origins from the femur. Again the extension gap is evaluated. If more release is required, we carefully dissect the medial and lateral corners approaching the posterior aspects of the medial and lateral collateral ligaments. We avoid resecting the collateral ligament attachments, although some authors completely skeletalize the distal femur. After all of the posterior capsule, gastrocnemius muscular origins, and posterior corners have been resected along with the posterior aspects of the collateral ligaments, if the extension gap remains too

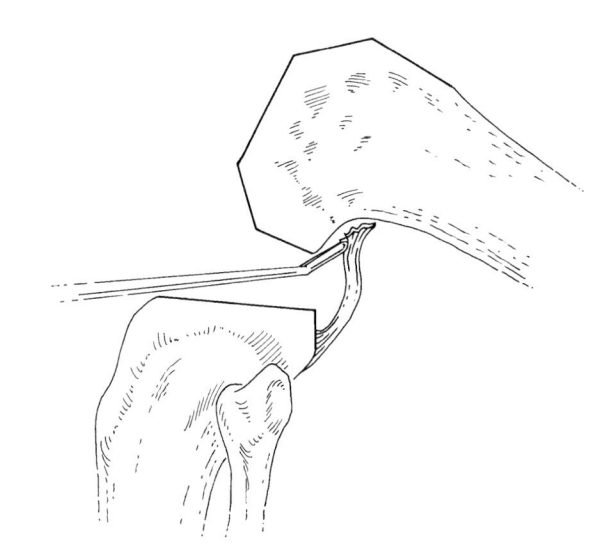

Figure 28.5. The posterior capsules become contracted and may require release from the femur.

tight, we will then resect more bone from the distal femur. The additional bone resection of the distal femur is done last because it significantly affects the joint mechanics by migrating the joint line proximally.

The soft tissue dissection of the posterior aspect of the joint and modest proximal migration of the joint line will correct most of the deformity and resolve the flexion-extension gap inequality. If the joint is still too tight in extension and/or too loose in flexion, the choice of a prosthesis with a high central trial spike, such as a total condylar III prosthesis, can be utilized in order to protect the knee from instability and subluxation. The inability to achieve full correction usually occurs in extremely disabled patients who have significant preoperative polyarticular deformity and who will not be achieving normal activity in the postoperative period.

Posterior femoral osteophyte
Posterior capsule

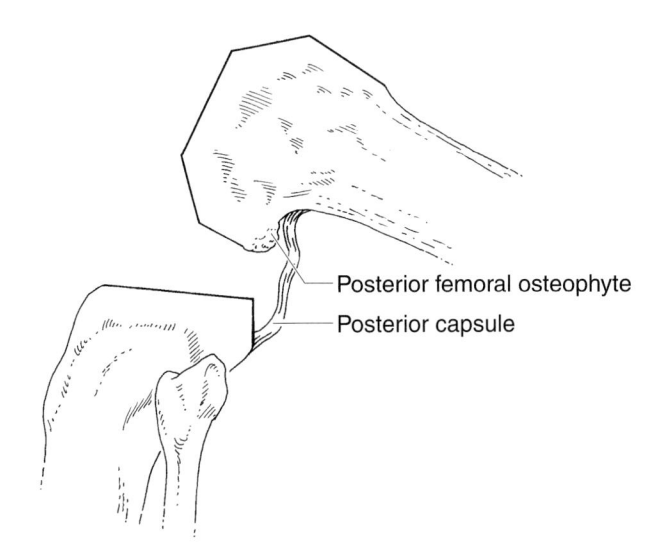

Figure 28.4. The osteophytes behind the posterior femoral condyles must be removed in order to prevent persistent flexion contracture from tethering of the posterior capsule.

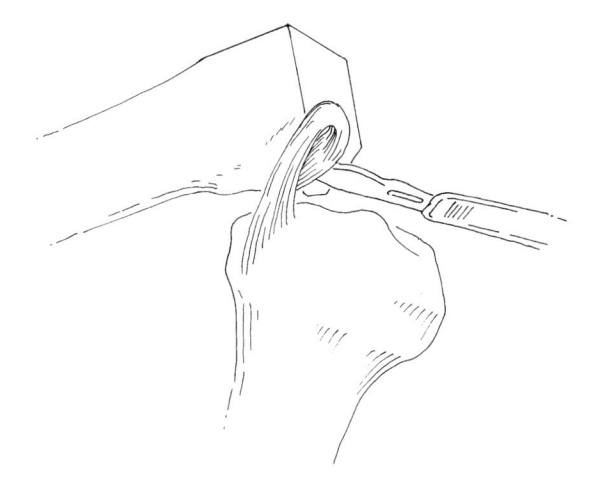

Figure 28.6. The cruciate ligaments will usually require releasing with large fixed flexion deformity.

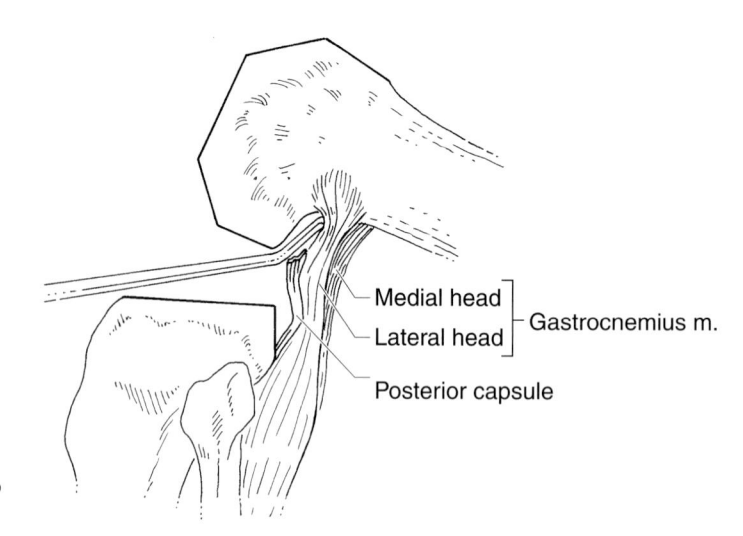

Figure 28.7. The gastrocnemius muscle insertion will also require release in severe fixed deformity.

Therefore this will not be a major functional compromise.

At the end of surgery we like to have almost all of the deformity corrected. With the lesser flexion contractures we expect the knee to come to full extension. With flexion contractures greater than 70 degrees a few degrees of flexion may remain at surgery.[8] In general, we work to avoid residual flexion contracture at the end of surgery.

POSTOPERATIVE MANAGEMENT

The degree of initial deformity affects the postoperative management. For the lesser deformities in which there is less anterior capsular stretching and quadriceps elongation with reasonable muscle tone, then routine care and management is all that is required. On the other hand, with a large preoperative deformity, the anterior capsular will be stretched, the quadriceps elongated, and there will be a prolonged extensor lag and subsequent tendency to develop recurrent deformity. These patients should be casted in full extension during the postoperative period. The duration of the casting will be determined by the deformity. The greater the deformity, the longer the postoperative cast. The duration of our postoperative casting will range from 3 to 28 days.

There is a tendency for the patients to assume the flexion position because of the extensor lag and muscle weakness. Physical therapy must insist that they obtain full extension passively every day in order to prevent fixation and recurrent deformity. It may be several months before patients can achieve full active extension. After discharge the patient should be carefully instructed on how to achieve full passive extension. If patients begin to develop recurrence of their flexion contracture, then a manipulation should be performed within the first few weeks. Occasionally a second manipulation will be required. However, it is very important not to allow a recurrent deformity to become fixed. The patient should always be able to maintain the degree of correction that was achieved at surgery.

In general, achieving motion in flexion in this group of patients is relatively easy and therefore attention should be carefully focused on the maintenance of full extension.

COMPLICATIONS

Releasing fixed flexion contractures during total knee arthroplasty has significant risks that increase with increasing deformity. The most serious ones include nerve and vascular injury. When recognized the knee should be immediately flexed and allowed to resume part of the preoperative deformity. Clayton reported that 2 of 20 patients with rheumatoid arthritis who had significant preoperative flexion contractures developed a peroneal nerve palsy.[5] Other soft tissue problems include poor wound healing, recurrent deformity, ligament instability, and residual laxity in flexion.

The possibility of posterior subluxation from instability in flexion is a mechanical problem that should be recognized intraoperatively and corrected with appropriate bone resections or prosthetic choice. If the imbalance persists, then a total condylar III style prosthesis should be selected to prevent subluxation.

RESULTS

Firestone and colleagues[9] evaluated their results of total knee arthroplasty in 51 knees that had flexion contractures greater than 20 degrees. A posterior cruciate-retaining device was used. The residual flexion contracture measured 3.1 degrees at the completion of the arthroplasty, 10.1 degrees at 3 months, and 7 degrees at 2 years. At 55 months postoperatively the average flexion contracture for the osteoarthritic group had improved from 25.5 degrees to 3.6 degrees, whereas the rheumatoid arthritis group improved from 28.7 degrees to 8.6 degrees. The average Knee Society Score for the osteoarthritic group was 89 as compared to 81 for the rheumatoid group. Knees that were left with greater residual flexion contracture at the completion of the arthroplasty were found to have greater residual flexion contractures at the latest review.

Some authors feel that it is not necessary to fully correct the flexion contracture at the time of surgery. McPhearson and associates[8] studied 29 patients who had relatively mild preoperative contractures, less than 30 degrees, but were not fully corrected to neutral following their total knee arthroplasty. They noted that the mean value of flexion contracture in the immediate postoperative period went from 10 degrees immediately postoperatively to 1 degree at 24 months. It may appear that complete intraoperative correction may not be necessary for small contractures up to 30 degrees.

Similar findings were noted by Tanzer and Miller.[10] Their study included 35 knees with less than 30 degrees of preoperative flexion contracture. All the patients had residual immediate postoperative contractures of 15 degrees. Eventually they went to an average of 2.9 degrees at their last follow-up. They felt that mild fixed flexion contractures do not have to be fully corrected at the time of arthroplasty and that intraoperative removal of excessive bone from the distal femur is not indicated. It should be emphasized that the reports are for mild contractures and probably not applicable to large contractures.

SUMMARY

The problems related to preoperative flexion contractures of the knee for total joint arthroplasty increase with increasing degree of deformity. In general, the lesser deformities will correct with less surgical dissection through removal of osteophytes and the release of the posterior capsule. The deformities that are extensive and fixed will require wide soft tissue releases posteriorly and collaterally, as well as some proximalization of the joint line with increased resection of the distal femur. Postoperatively the patient should be protected so they do not develop recurrent deformities. This can be accomplished with casting and manipulations if necessary. The most serious complications involve stretching the neurovascular structures and must be very carefully evaluated in the postoperative period.

Preoperatively, the patients with flexion contractures are so disabled with immobility states and significant restrictions in walking ability that, after surgery and full extension is achieved with a successful arthroplasty, they are amongst our most grateful patients.

References

1. Eyring EG, Murray WR. The effects of joint position on the pressure of intra-articular effusion. *J Bone Joint Surg*. 1964; 46A:1235–1241.
2. Perry J, Antonelli D, Ford W. Analysis of knee joint forces during flexed knee stance. *J Bone Joint Surg*. 1975; 57A:961–967.
3. Krackow KA. Flexion contracture. In: *The Techniques of Total Knee Arthroplasty*. St. Louis: Mosby; 1990; 282–294.
4. Convery FR, Conaty JP, Nickel VL. Flexion deformities of the knee in rheumatoid arthritis. *Clin Orthop*. 1971; 74:90–93.
5. Clayton ML, Thompson TR, Mack RP. Correction of alignment deformities during total knee arthroplasty. Staged soft tissue release. *Clin Orthop*. 1986; 202:117.
6. Colwell CW. Fixed flexion contracture. In: Fu F, Harner HD, Vince KG. *Knee Surgery*. Baltimore: Williams & Wilkins; 1994; 74:1391–1397.
7. Lombardi AL, Mallory TH. Dealing with flexion contractures in total knee arthroplasty. In: Insall J, Scott N, Scuderi GR, eds. *Current Concepts in Primary and Revision Total Knee Arthroplasty*. Philadelphia: Lippincott, Raven; 1996.
8. McPherson EJ, Kushner FD, Schiff CF, Friedman RJ. Natural history of uncorrected flexion contractures following total knee arthroplasty. *J of Arthroplasty*. 1994; 9:499–502.
9. Firestone TP, Krackow KA, Davis JD, Toeny SM, Hungerford DS. The management of fixed flexion contractures during total knee arthroplasty. *Clin Orthop*. 1992; 284:221–227.
10. Tanzer M, Miller J. Natural history of flexion contracture. *Clin Orthop*. 1989; 248:129–134.

CHAPTER 29
Correction of Combined Deformity

Paolo Aglietti and Roberto Buzzi

INTRODUCTION

Combined deformities can be defined as those that show deformity in both the frontal and the sagittal planes. In these knees a varus or valgus deformity is coupled with a significant flexion contracture. A flexion contracture up to 10 degrees is often present in varus or valgus arthritic knees. This degree of flexion contracture does not usually cause additional surgical difficulties and is corrected with standard bone cuts and medial or lateral release techniques. However, when the flexion contracture exceeds 10 degrees and does not decrease under anesthesia, additional maneuvers are often required to correct it.

Knees with combined deformities represent an advanced stage of the arthritic disease. Additional factors that increase the difficulties of surgery are often present. They include previous surgery, more often arthrotomy and joint debridement, osteotomy or open reduction, and internal fixation of a fracture. Joint stiffness with difficult joint exposure and bone loss are also encountered. Combined deformities are more difficult to correct and require extensive soft tissue releases. Postoperative complications including incomplete correction of the deformity, residual instability, restricted range of motion, and peroneal nerve palsy may occur.

INCIDENCE

In an effort to evaluate the incidence of combined deformities we reviewed a consecutive series of 516 total knee replacements. The preoperative diagnosis was osteoarthritis in 417 knees and rheumatoid arthritis in 99.

In the group of 417 arthritic knees, 337 (82%) had a varus alignment, 55 (13%) had a valgus alignment, and 25 (6%) had no deformity in the frontal plane. A flexion contracture over 10 degrees (average 22 degrees) was associated in 50 (15%) of the varus knees, in 6 (11%) of the valgus knees (average flexion contracture 19 degrees), and in 7 (28%) of the knees with no angular deformity (average flexion contracture 18 degrees).

In the group of 99 knees affected by rheumatoid arthritis 31 (31%) had a varus alignment, 38 (38%) had a valgus alignment, and 30 (30%) had no angular deformity in the frontal plane. A flexion contracture over 10 degrees (average 22 degrees) was present in 14 (45%) of the varus knees, in 17 (45%) of the valgus knees (average flexion contracture 30°), and in 13 (43%) of the knees without angular deformity (average 30 degrees).

From these data it can be observed that in arthritic knees the most frequent deformity was varus (82%), whereas in rheumatoid arthritis valgus was more common (38%), followed by varus (31%), and by knees with no angular deformity (30%). Combined deformities defined by the association of a flexion contracture over 10 degrees were present in 15% and 11% of the varus and valgus osteoarthritic knees, respectively. Combined deformities were more frequent in rheumatoid knees, where they reached 45% of both varus and valgus cases. We recognize that these data do not have an absolute value because they reflect the population of patients seen by a single center. We feel that the incidence of severe combined deformities may decrease because total knee replacement is becoming an accepted and reliable procedure and is offered earlier in the course of the disease. Nevertheless if the above data are accepted, combined deformities may be expected in 10 to 15% of the osteoarthritic knees and in almost half of the rheumatoid knees (Fig. 29.1) without major differences between knees with varus or valgus alignment.

SURGICAL PATHOLOGY

The surgical pathology of combined deformities contains elements of the varus or valgus knee and of the knee with flexion contracture. In the varus osteoarthritic knee the process begins with wear of cartilage and bone in the medial compartment and growth of osteophytes. A varus alignment of the lower limb, as measured according to the mechanical axes, may be present before the development of osteoarthritis and due to varus bow-

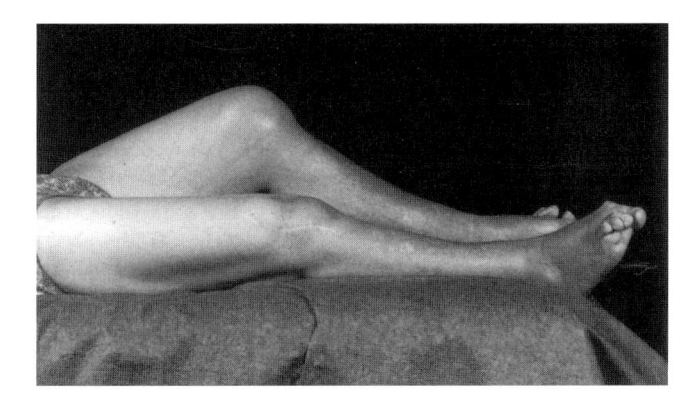

Figure 29.1. Rheumatoid patient with severe valgus and flexion contracture deformity of the left knee. The right knee has already received a total knee replacement with correction of the deformity.

ing of the tibia or femur. As the deformity increases, the medial ligamentous structures shorten due to the decreased distance between their insertion points and because of the tenting effect of the osteophytes. Lateral structures experience increasing tension and are progressively elongated.

In the valgus arthritic knee the same sequence of events occurs in the lateral compartment. The alignment of the lower limb may be valgus before the development of arthritis, due to valgus bowing of the tibia or, more frequently, of the femur. The process initiates with cartilage and bone wear and growth of osteophytes in the lateral compartment. The lateral ligamentous structures become shortened because of the decreased distance between their insertion points and because of the tenting effect of the lateral osteophytes. The medial structures are progressively stretched and may become elongated to a significant degree. In severe valgus knees an external rotation deformity of the tibia may be associated due to contracture of the iliotibial band (ITB). A lateral patellar subluxation with patellofemoral arthritis is present in most of the cases.

In mild varus or valgus osteoarthritic knees, the anterior cruciate ligament (ACL) is usually preserved and functional. In mild varus osteoarthritic knees with a preserved ACL, the deformity is usually correctable and tibial plateau erosion is localized anteriorly.[1] However, in severe angular or combined deformities, the ACL is often severely attenuated or absent. This fact leads to anterior subluxation of the tibia. Consequently, bone erosion in the tibial plateau is located more posteriorly. The posterior cruciate ligament (PCL) is present in most arthritic knees, although it may be attenuated in the worst deformities and in cases with previous surgery. The neural component area of the PCL of osteoarthritic knees has been found to be decreased compared to the PCL of normal knees,[2] which may have relevance for its proprioceptive function.

Surgical pathology of arthritic knees with a flexion contracture involves both the anterior and the posterior compartments. In the anterior compartment, growth of osteophytes in front of the tibial spine and around the anterior outlet of the intercondylar notch of the femur may limit extension. In the posterior compartment, the capsule shortens progressively and is tented by the osteophytes, which form around the posterior condyles. Cartilage and bone loss may involve the posterior aspect of the tibial plateau and femoral condyles. In rheumatoid knees with long-standing flexion contracture the posterior aspect of the femoral condyles may be severely eroded and acquire the peculiar "drumstick" appearance. Weakness of the quadriceps is often present in knees with a flexion contracture and contributes to the development of the deformity.

In combined deformities the above described factors are present in combination (varus plus flexion contracture or valgus flexion contracture) and in variable degrees. A clear understanding of the surgical pathology of these deformities is a key factor to their successful correction.

PREOPERATIVE PLANNING

The patient should be thoroughly evaluated preoperatively. The degree of angular deformity and the possibility to correct it with a manual stress are recorded. Loss of extension and maximum flexion are evaluated preoperatively as well under anesthesia. If the arc of motion is less than 90 degrees, especially in knees with previous surgery and patellar baja, difficulties of exposure are likely to be increased. The neurovascular status of the extremity is carefully evaluated including peripheral pulses and sensory and motor function. The strength of the anterolateral muscles of the leg (dorsiflexion and eversion of the foot) is tested and recorded. This aspect is particularly relevant in knees with valgus and/or flexion contracture deformity in which the peroneal nerve is at risk of postoperative palsy.

Preoperative radiographs should be obtained and carefully evaluated. However, their usefulness is limited in knees with significant flexion contracture. In these knees the angular deformity as visualized in the anteroposterior radiograph is strongly influenced by the rotational position of the limb. The image of the knee is also distorted by the flexed position and by the increased knee-cassette distance in the anteroposterior view. Therefore assessment of bone defects may be inaccurate.

The use of a posterior cruciate-substituting prosthesis is strongly recommended in knees with combined deformities. In a series of knees with fixed deformities greater than 15 degrees, the best results for alignment, residual flexion contracture, and maximum flexion were obtained with a PCL-substituting prosthesis compared with a PCL-saving implant.[3] A modular system with intramedullary stems, tibial wedges, and femoral augments should be available to treat bone defects. A prosthesis with intrinsic mediolateral stability should be also available if adequate stability cannot be restored by ligament releases. Our experience has been with the Insall-Burstein II total knee replacement system (Zimmer, Warsaw, Ind).

SURGICAL APPROACH

We approach these knees through a standard longitudinal midline skin incision with medial parapatellar arthrotomy and eversion of the patella. A medial tibial periosteal flap is raised and developed posteriorly to allow anterior subluxation of the tibia. If joint stiffness is present and patella eversion is difficult, the first step is the "quadriceps snip" (Insall, personal communication, 1993). It involves the proximal and lateral extension of the capsular incision through the rectus tendon. This maneuver usually allows sufficient mobility of the extensor mechanism to evert the patella. Further elevation of the medial periosteal flap around the posteromedial corner of the tibia, including detachment of the semimembranosus tendon, allows increased external tibial rotation and relaxation of the extensor mechanism. Intra-articular adhesions should be completely freed to recreate the suprapatellar pouch and the lateral gutters. Using these steps we are able to expose over 90% of the joints. After a "quadriceps snip," the postoperative course is not altered and there are no problems of postoperative quadriceps weakness.

In the knee with severe stiffness and patellar baja, a complete "quadriceps turndown" may be necessary to expose the joint. After the anteromedial arthrotomy, a second incision is performed from the apex of the quadriceps tendon distally through the rectus and vastus lateralis tendons. A complete flap including the patella can be everted. Lengthening of the quadriceps can be achieved by suturing the incision in a V-Y fashion with the knee in 20 to 30 degrees of flexion. The strength of the suture should be tested intraoperatively by flexing the knee until moderate resistance is felt and confirming that the suture does not disrupt. Postoperatively the knee is placed on a continuous passive motion device. Flexion is set at the level that was confirmed to be safe at surgery. Some quadriceps weakness is likely to persist for a few months postoperatively with 10 to 20 degrees of extension loss but eventually resolves in most of the joints.[4]

MEDIAL RELEASE

Some degree of medial release is routinely performed to expose the joint, as described above. If a varus deformity is to be corrected, the elevation of the medial periosteal flap should be continued in a distal and posterior direction until the length of the medial structures equals the lateral structures.

The first step in the medial release[5-7] is the elevation of the meniscotibial ligament all around the tibial plateau to the posteromedial corner of the tibia. A medial meniscectomy is performed. The femoral and tibial osteophytes are trimmed because they tent the medial capsular sleeve and cause a relative shortening of the medial structures. If this extent of release is not enough to correct the deformity, the second step is extension of the capsular release posteriorly to the midline of the knee including elevation of the semimembranous tendon. The third step includes elevation of the distal insertion of the medial collateral ligament from the anteromedial surface of the tibia. In the most deformed knees a periosteal flap is elevated from the anteromedial surface of the tibia down to its middle third. This is accomplished by sliding a three-fourths-inch wide periosteal elevator or osteotome below the pes tendons (Fig. 29.2). Proximal sliding of the entire flap allows correction of the deformity. Elevation of the pes tendons in itself is rarely useful and necessary.

It should be appreciated that balancing a severe varus deformity with an extensive medial release involves lengthening of the medial structures beyond their original length to match the length of the stretched lateral structures. In these conditions the PCL may become a significant deforming force and should be resected and substituted by a prosthesis with intrinsic posterior sta-

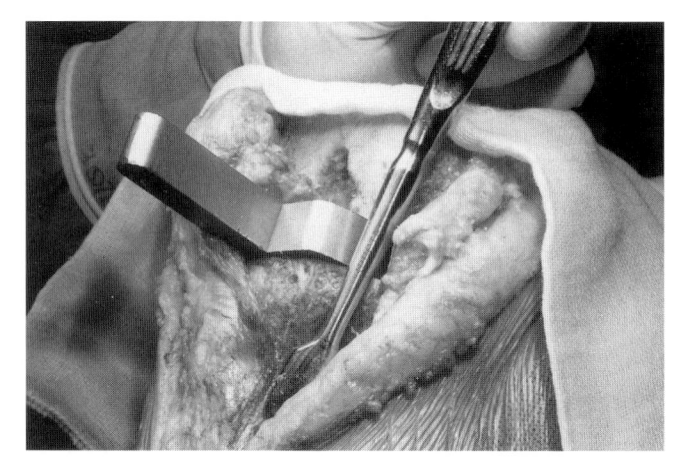

Figure 29.2. Medial release in a varus right knee. A periosteal elevator is directed along the anteromedial surface of the tibia, behind the pes tendons. It lifts a medial periosteal flap, which is allowed to slide proximally.

bility. The PCL is located in the center of the knee. Due to its position varus or valgus malalignments impose significant less stress on the PCL than on the peripheral structures. Therefore in varus deformities the PCL is usually less elongated than the lateral structures.

LATERAL RELEASE

Correction of a valgus deformity involves lengthening of the lateral structures until they reach the length of the medial structures. Stretching of the medial structures over their original length frequently occurs in severe deformities. Significant stretching of the medial structures in valgus knees is usually more frequent and severe than stretching of the lateral counterpart in varus knees. This can be probably attributed to the weaker dynamic support afforded by the pes tendons in comparison with the stronger ITB on the lateral side.

The first step that we use releasing the lateral structures[5-7] is detachment of the ITB from the lateral tibial plateau and Gerdy's tubercle. This maneuver is best accomplished with a sharp osteotome. At the same time the lateral meniscus is removed and femoral and tibial osteophytes are trimmed. The inferolateral genicular artery, which courses at the level of the joint line, should be coagulated. This release is usually sufficient to correct minor deformities. In moderate deformities we proceed to the second step, which involves releasing the lateral collateral ligament (LCL) and popliteus tendon (POP). These structures are detached from the lateral femoral condyle either using an osteotome to elevate a bone sliver or simply cutting them transversely. We prefer the second option. The third step of the lateral release is usually necessary to correct the worst deformities. It involves detachment of the posterior capsule and lateral head of the gastrocnemius from the back of the condyle. This can be achieved by sharp dissection with the knee at 90 degrees of flexion. A lateral parapatellar release is often required in valgus knees to correct lateral tracking of the patella. An attempt is made to save the superolateral genicular vessels to preserve a vascular supply to the patella.[8]

We have recently published the results of a series of 67 total knee replacements implanted in valgus knees.[9] The lateral ligamentous release was performed with the technique reported above. The Insall-Burstein posterior-stabilized total knee was used routinely. A lateral patellar release was necessary in half of the cases. We were able to review 51 knees (76%) with an average follow-up of 6 years. A satisfactory result according to the Knee Society rating system[10] was achieved in 92% of the knees. The average flexion was 105 degrees. Postoperative lateral instability was observed in only one knee. This may have been secondary to overrelease of the lateral structures.

More recently we have performed[11] the lateral release with the knee in extension (Insall JN, personal communication, 1993). After the distal femoral and the proximal tibial cut have been performed, the knee is extended and the extension gap is opened with laminar spreaders. The aim of the release is to lengthen the LCL, lateral capsule, ITB, and lateral parapatellar retinaculum using a single incision. The incision starts in the triangle defined by the resected surface of the tibia, LCL, and POP. It proceeds along the distal aspect of the POP tendon, which is saved, and releases the LCL, lateral capsule, the ITB, and the lateral patellar retinaculum if required (Fig. 29.3). The release can be accomplished simply by cutting through these structures obliquely or with a multiple puncture technique (Fig. 29.4). The latter technique seems advantageous because it affords a more gradual release. Furthermore it does not create a definite gap in the lateral structures, decreasing the potential of postoperative posterolateral instability. Preservation of the popliteus is also desirable in this sense. Performing the lateral release with the knee in extension is advantageous because it allows a more direct monitoring of the correction by opening the joint spreader. Saving the POP tendon is recommended because posterolateral instability is less likely to occur and the flexion gap tends to be more symmetric.

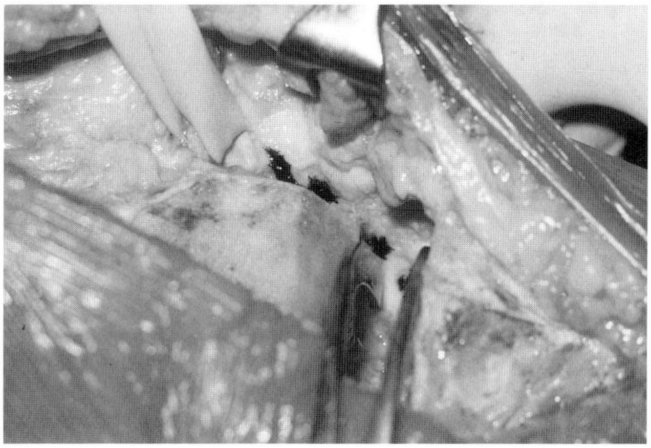

Figure 29.3. Lateral ligamentous release in a left knee with valgus deformity (feet on the right and head on the left of the figure). The knee is in extension and the joint line is opened with a laminar spreader. The superolateral genicular vessels have been isolated and a Penrose drain elevates them. The line of proposed release has been marked with methylene blue. The release begins on the tibial plateau, distal to the popliteus tendon. It parallels the popliteus tendon, which is saved. In a disto-proximal sequence the lateral collateral ligament, the lateral capsule, the iliotibial band and the lateral patellar retinaculum, if necessary, are released. The release may be performed cutting across these structures or with a multiple puncture technique.

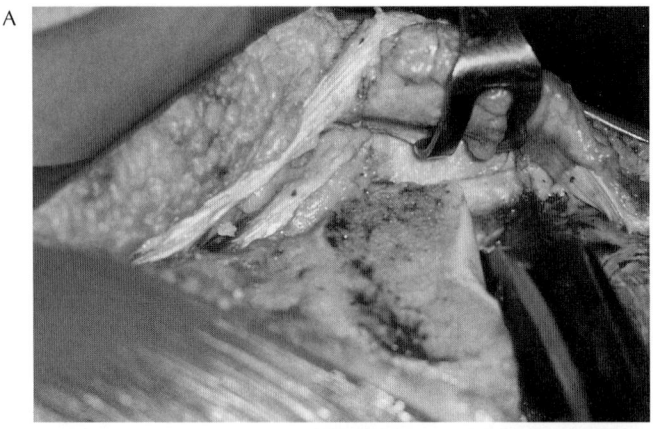

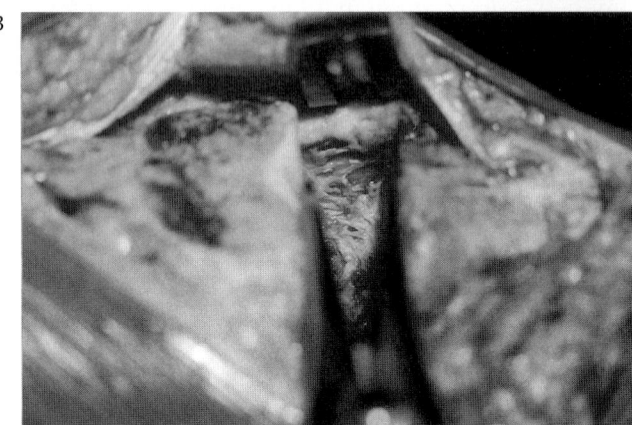

Figure 29.4. (A) Lateral ligamentous release in a left knee with valgus deformity. The joint line is opened with a spreader. The profile of the tight ITB is evident. The release was performed with a #11 blade and a multiple puncture technique. (B) After the release the joint line opens further. The multiple punctures are evident and the tight ITB profile has disappeared.

The PCL is frequently a deforming force in the correction of moderate to severe valgus knees and should be resected or released. Overdistraction of the joint is frequently necessary to correct severe deformities with stretching of the medial structures. This fact poses an additional threat on the peroneal nerve. Postoperative peroneal nerve palsy has been reported with a frequency of 3 to 4% in the literature.[12,13] If we feel that overdistraction is not desirable, we use an implant with intrinsic mediolateral stability (Constrained Condylar Knee, Zimmer, Warsaw, Ind) usually associated with retensioning of the medial structures.

Retensioning of the medial structures in valgus knees has been described[14] with implantation of a PCL-retaining prosthesis with a flat tibial component (PCA, Howmedica, Rutherford, New Jersey). The medial structures were detached on the femoral side, advanced proximally and fixed with nonabsorbable sutures around a screw and washer. A special stitch was developed to anchor the soft tissue flap.[15] We prefer to retension the medial structures on the tibial side. This seems advantageous for several reasons. First, moving the femoral insertion of the medial collateral ligament (MCL) may alter its center of rotation. It is more difficult to balance the tension of the ligament in flexion and extension. Moving the tibial insertion of the MCL does not cause problems in this respect. Second, it is easier to advance and fix a large medial tibial periosteal flap than to move the narrower femoral insertion of the MCL. We develop a wide medial periosteal flap in a manner similar to a medial release. Two Krachow stitches[15] are placed through the flap using a #2 nonabsorbable Ethibond suture (Ethicon, Pomezia, Italy). After fixation of the prosthesis, the sutures are tied around a cortical screw inserted in the anteromedial tibial cortex 6 to 8 cm distal to the joint line. The fixation is reinforced with a barbed staple (Fig. 29.5). Care should be taken to insert the screw and staple away from the peg of the tibial component.

BONE CUTS

We begin the operations with exposure of the joint and preliminary gradual ligament releases, as required from the deformity. Then we perform the bone cuts. The first cut to be performed is the distal femoral cut. We use an intramedullary guide that also has an extramedullary check. We aim at a cut perpendicular to the mechanical axis of the femur. The intramedullary guide is set at 6 to 7 degrees of valgus in varus deformities and at 3 to 4 degrees in valgus knees. The second cut is the anteroposterior femoral cut. The amount of bone removed

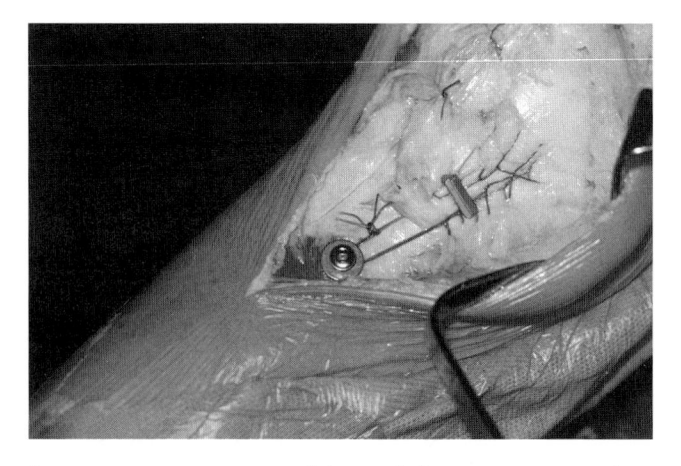

Figure 29.5. Retensioning of the medial structures in a right knee with valgus deformity. A medial osteoperiosteal flap is developed from the tibia. Two Krackow stitches are placed through the flap using #2 nonabsorbable sutures. The sutures are tied around a screw and washer, and fixation is reinforced with a barbed staple.

from the distal and posterior femoral condyles equals the thickness of the prosthesis to be inserted. A few (or 3) degrees of external rotation of the prosthesis in relationship to the posterior condylar line are desirable. This is useful to obtain a rectangular flexion gap. If the cut is performed parallel to the posterior condyles, the flexion gap is usually wider laterally. Some external rotation of the femoral component is also useful to improve patellar tracking. Extensive ligament releases as used in combined deformities may have an influence on the rotatory alignment of the femoral component. Medial releases tend to cause opening of the medial joint space in flexion and therefore reduce the need for external rotation of the femoral component. Lateral releases increase the opening of the lateral joint space in flexion and therefore require more external rotation to balance the flexion gap.

More recently the transepicondylar femoral axis has been proposed as a guide for the rotatory alignment of the femoral component.[16] The epicondyles are the insertion points of the collateral ligaments. Anatomical studies have shown that alignment of the femoral component along the transepicondylar axis imparts 3 to 5 degrees of external rotation in relationship to the posterior femoral condyles. Instruments have been developed to align the femoral component along the transepicondylar axis at surgery.

The third cut to be performed is the proximal tibial cut. If we implant a PCL-substituting device, 8–10 mm of bone are removed from the intact plateau.

At this point flexion-extension gaps have been created and they are sized with the spacers. Stability and alignment of the knee are evaluated in flexion and extension. Fine-tuning of the medial and lateral ligament releases is performed as necessary. The possibility to reach full extension is carefully checked with the spacers and with the trial prosthesis in place. If full extension cannot be achieved, a posterior release should be considered.

CORRECTION OF FLEXION CONTRACTURE

Minor degrees of flexion contracture, up to 10 degrees, are usually corrected with standard bone cuts, soft tissue releases, recreation of the posterior recesses, and removal of posterior osteophytes.[5–7,17,18] After the flexion gap has been created the posterior capsule is visualized using laminar spreaders. The posterior capsule is often adherent to the femoral condyles and it should be freed with a periosteal elevator. Posterior osteophytes are identified by finger palpation and should be removed using a curved osteotome and curette. Posterior osteophytes tent the posterior capsule and may be responsible for a flexion contracture.

If the flexion contracture is greater than 10 degrees and certainly if it is greater than 20 degrees, recreation of the posterior recesses and removal of posterior osteophytes are unlikely to fully correct the deformity. In these cases we release the capsule and the gastrocnemius heads from the back of the condyles using a periosteal elevator (Fig. 29.6). Care must be taken while working with sharp instruments in the back of the knee. Alternatively in knees with severe long-standing flexion contracture a formal posterior capsulotomy as described by Insall[5] can be successfully employed. The knee is flexed at 90 degrees and the posterior capsule is exposed and tensed with laminar spreaders. The PCL is removed. Two vertical incisions are performed at the posteromedial and posterolateral corners to divide the posterior capsule from the medial and lateral capsule. The posterior capsule is then cut transversely (Fig. 29.7) until the popliteal fat pad is exposed. Great care is exercised when cutting the capsule in the midline of the knee. The capsule may be grasped with a forceps and pulled distally and forward to make capsular incision safer. It has been our experience that with a posterior capsulotomy even severe deformities can be successfully corrected.

An alternative method to correct a flexion contracture is by increasing the thickness of the extension gap with further bone resection from the distal femur. Bone resection from the proximal tibia cannot be used because it widens both the flexion and extension gaps. We feel that further bone resection should not be routinely employed to correct a flexion contracture. First, it causes an unnecessary bone loss. Second, after further distal femoral resection full extension is achieved but stability is controlled by the posterior capsule in extension while

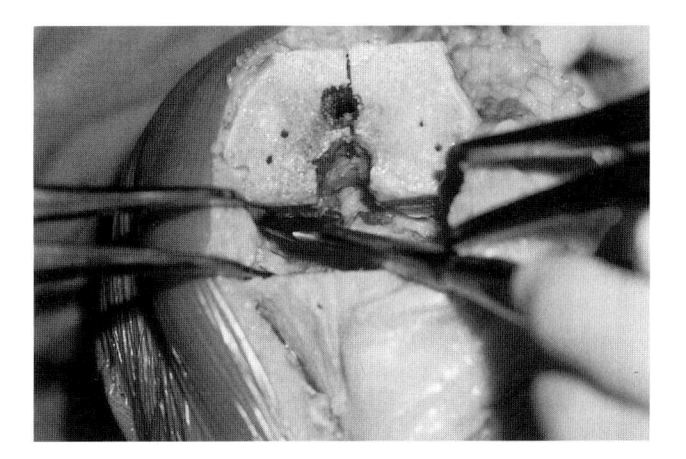

Figure 29.6. Posterior soft tissue release for correction of flexion contracture of the knee. After removal of the posterior osteophytes, the posterior capsule and gastrocnemius heads are detached from the back of the condyles using a periosteal elevator.

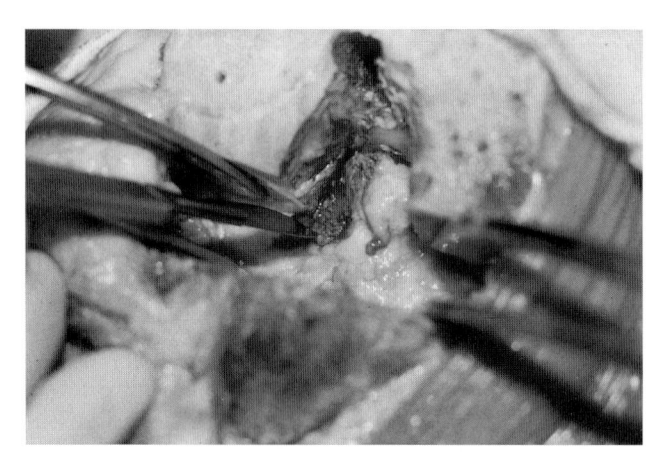

Figure 29.7. Transverse posterior capsulotomy to correct a flexion contracture of the knee. The posterior capsule is separated with two vertical incisions from the medial and lateral capsule. A transverse capsulotomy is performed with great care while cutting near the midline.

the collateral ligaments are lax. Therefore a kinematic abnormality is introduced and the quadriceps mechanism is relatively elongated. For these reasons we feel that distal femoral resection should not be the first line of defense in the treatment of a flexion contracture. However, it can be successfully employed in severe deformities in which posterior capsulotomy did not allow full extension. It can also be used in the occasional elderly patient in whom the additional trauma of a posterior release is undesirable.

POSTOPERATIVE TREATMENT

The patient is carefully evaluated for stability and motion at the end of the procedure. The limb is lifted from the heel. If the knee achieves full extension, a compressive bandage is applied and the limb is placed on a continuous passive motion device. However, if the knee requires some pressure to achieve full extension it is better to apply a cast with the knee in full extension. It has been our experience that if this is not done the patient will assume a flexed knee position as soon as he or she recovers from the anesthesia. The cast is worn for 24 hours and it is removed thereafter to allow flexion exercises. It is applied again during the nighttime, until the patient reaches full extension easily. It has been our experience that "off the shelf" braces are ineffective to correct a flexion contracture after a total knee replacement.

The neurovascular status of the limb is carefully monitored postoperatively. The peroneal nerve function is evaluated repeatedly. If decreased motor or sensory function is identified, the bandage or cast should be removed and the knee allowed to flex on a pillow. This complication may be more frequent in valgus knees.

Postoperatively attention is directed to complete correction of the flexion contracture utilizing stretching exercises and quadriceps strengthening. If the contralateral limb is shorter, a heel lift should be prescribed to avoid recurrence of flexion contracture in the operated knee. Rehabilitation is somewhat more difficult and prolonged in combined deformities because of the associated flexion contracture and frequent stiffness and because of the extensive surgery required.

COMMENTS

Combined deformities represent an advanced stage of the arthritic disease of the knee. A flexion contracture over 10 degrees is associated to varus or valgus deformity in 10 to 15% of the knees with degenerative disease, but is more frequent (45%) in the knees with rheumatoid disease. Correction of combined deformities by ligamentous releases requires a thorough understanding of the pathology. Extensive ligamentous releases are often required. Resection of the PCL and implantation of a PCL-substituting prosthesis may be advisable. Postoperative complications including peroneal nerve palsy, incomplete correction of the deformity, restricted range of motion, or postoperative instability may occur and should be prevented by careful surgical technique. Using adequate soft tissue releases to correct both the angular and flexion contracture deformities, a stable and well-aligned knee can be achieved in most of these demanding cases. A superstabilizing tibial insert to provide stability in both the frontal and the sagittal plane is rarely needed in primary cases.

References

1. White SH, Ludkowski PF, Goodfellow JW. Anteromedial osteoarthritis of the knee. *J Bone Joint Surg.* 1991; 73-B:582–586.
2. Franchi A, Zaccherotti G, Aglietti P. Neural system of the human posterior cruciate ligament in osteoarthritis. *J Arthroplasty.* 1995; 10(5):679–682.
3. Laskin RS, Rieger M, Schob C, Turen C. The posterior stabilized total knee prosthesis in the knee with a severe fixed deformity. *Am J Knee Surg.* 1988; 1(4):199–205.
4. Aglietti P, Windsor RE, Buzzi R, Insall JN. Arthroplasty for the stiff or ankylosed knee. *J Arthroplasty.* 1989; 4:1–5.
5. Insall JN. Surgical techniques and instrumentation in total knee arthroplasty. In: Insall JN, ed. *Surgery of the Knee.* New York: Churchill Livingstone; 1993:739–804.
6. D'Ambrosio F, Scott NW. Ligament releases in the arthritic knee. In: Scott NW, ed. *The Knee.* St. Louis: Mosby; 1993: 1199–1210.
7. Faris PM. In: Fu FH, Harner CD, Vince KG, eds. *Knee Surgery.* Baltimore: Williams and Wilkins; 1994:1385–1389.
8. Wetzner SM, Bezreh JS, Scott RD, et al. Bone scanning in

the assessment of patellar viability following knee replacement. *Clin Orthop*. 1985; 199:215–219.
9. Aglietti P, Buzzi R, Giron F, Zaccherotti G. The Insall-Burstein posterior stabilized total knee replacement in the valgus knee. *Am J Knee Surg*. 1996; 9:8–12.
10. Insall JN, Dorr LD, Scott RS, Scott WN. Rationale of the Knee Society rating system. *Clin Orthop*. 1989; 248:13–14.
11. Aglietti P, Giron F, Buzzi R. Ligament balancing in the valgus knee. In: Insall JN, Scott NW, Scuderi GR. *Current Concepts in Primary and Revision Total Knee Arthroplasty*. Philadelphia: Lippincott-Raven; 1996:183–190.
12. Stern SH, Moeckel BH, Insall JN. Total knee arthroplasty in valgus knees. *Clin Orthop*. 1991; 273:5–8.
13. Laurencin CT, Scott RD, Volatile TB, et al. Total knee replacement in severe valgus deformities. *Am J Knee Surg*. 1992; 5:135–139.
14. Krackow KA, Jones MM, Teeny SM, Hungerford DS. Primary total knee arthroplasty in patients with fixed valgus deformity. *Clin Orthop*. 1991; 273:9–18.
15. Krackow KA, Thomas SC, Jones LC. Ligament-tendon fixation: analysis of a new stitch and comparison with standard techniques. *Orthopedics*. 1988; 11:909.
16. Poilvache P, Insall JN, Scuderi GR, Font-Rodriguez DE. Rotational landmarks and sizing of the distal femur in total knee arthroplasty. Presented at the Interim Meeting of the Knee Society, February 1996, Atlanta.
17. Colwell CW. Fixed flexion contracture. In: Fu FH, Harner CD, Vince KG, eds. *Knee Surgery*. Baltimore: Williams and Wilkins; 1994:1390–1394.
18. Lombardi AV, Mallory TH. Dealing with flexion contractures in total knee arthroplasty. Bone resection versus soft tissue releases. In: Insall JN, Scott NW, Scuderi GR, eds. *Current Concepts in Primary and Revision Total Knee Arthroplasty*. Philadelphia: Lippincott-Raven; 1996:191–202.

SECTION 8
Component Position

CHAPTER 30
The Epicondylar Axis for Femoral Component Rotation

Pascal L. Poilvache

IMPORTANCE OF FEMORAL ROTATION

The importance of axial alignment in determining the longevity of a total knee arthroplasty was established in the seventies,[1,2] but the effect of rotational alignment received relatively less attention until recently. In the last few years, many authors stressed the critical influence of rotational alignment of the femoral component on the patellofemoral joint.

Malrotation of the femoral component on the femur may lead to patellofemoral dislocation or subluxation, to wear or loosening of the patellar component, or to fractures of the patella.[3-17] Malrotation of the femoral component may also induce an asymmetrical loading[18] and a torsional stress on the tibial component, which could lead to wear or loosening.[19-22]

The adverse effects of internal rotation of the femoral component have been observed clinically, and have been demonstrated experimentally. Rhoads and associates,[13] in a laboratory study using seven fresh anatomic knee specimens evaluated before and after total knee arthroplasty, demonstrated that internal rotation of the femoral component displaced and tilted the patella medially, as opposed to external rotation, which came closer to reproduce the patterns of patellar tracking of the intact knee.

Anouchi and colleagues[3] tested four fresh-frozen anatomic knee specimens for knee stability, patellar tracking, and patellofemoral contact points with the femoral component positioned in 5 degrees internal, 5 degrees external, or neutral axial rotational alignment of the femoral component referenced on the posterior femoral condyles. The externally rotated specimens provided varus-valgus stability of the knee that was closest to the normal control. Patellar tracking was also closest to normal in the externally rotated specimens.

The influence of rotation of the femoral component on valgus-varus stability and patellar tracking can be explained by the "gap" theory developed by John Insall.[9,23-25] The primary goal of a total knee replacement is to obtain a well-aligned and well-balanced knee both in flexion and in extension. In most normal knees, perpendicular resection of the upper tibial surface removes more bone from the lateral surface of the tibial plateau than from the medial surface, because the normal upper tibia has a 3 degree varus slope.[9,10,26-30]

Therefore, when resecting the upper tibia perpendicular to its long axis in a normal knee, with a 3-degree varus transverse axis, one would resect more off the lateral tibial plateau than off the medial tibial plateau, and more off the distal medial femoral condyle than off the distal lateral femoral condyle. In order to obtain a rectangular flexion gap, a larger amount of bone should be resected off the posterior medial femoral condyle than off the posterior lateral condyle.[9,10,31] If equal amounts are resected from the posterior femoral condyles, more bone would be resected from the lateral compartment of the knee in flexion than from the medial compartment, making the lateral compartment looser than the medial one. The situation is even worse if the posterolateral resection is larger than the posteromedial resection, thus when the femoral component is internally rotated on the femur.

In addition to creating valgus alignment and lateral laxity in flexion, internal rotation of the femoral component moves the groove portion of the femoral component medially, increasing the lateral force vector on the patella.[3,7,9,10,12,13,17,31,32] This effect on the position of the patellar groove is preponderant at its proximal end (Fig. 30.1).

In theory, this difficulty can be avoided, using the method recommended by Hungerford and Krackow.[33]

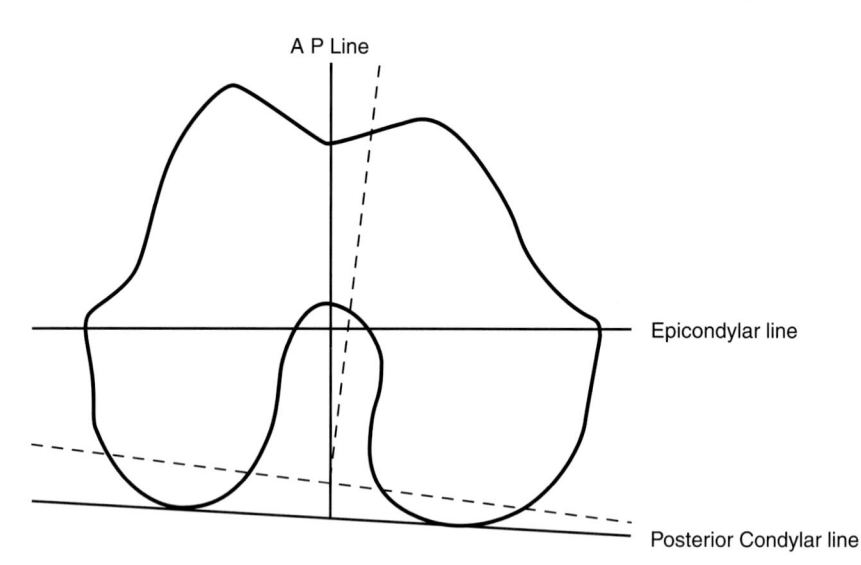

Figure 30.1. Diagram of the axial view of the distal femur. The dotted lines represent an internally rotated posterior cut, and its effect on the position of the prosthetic trochlear groove.

The tibial cut is made at a 3-degree medial slope, resecting equal amounts of the medial and lateral plateaus, and thus allowing a symmetrical distal femoral resection and a symmetrical posterior femoral resection. But this method does not provide the beneficial effect of moving the prosthetic sulcus laterally. Moreover, it will only be accurate in an ideal knee with a 3-degree varus transverse axis (Fig. 30.2).

The arthritic knee is usually not a standard knee with a 3-degree medial slope of the tibial plateau and a neutral mechanical axis. In arthritic knees, the normal anatomy can be distorted by the degenerative process,

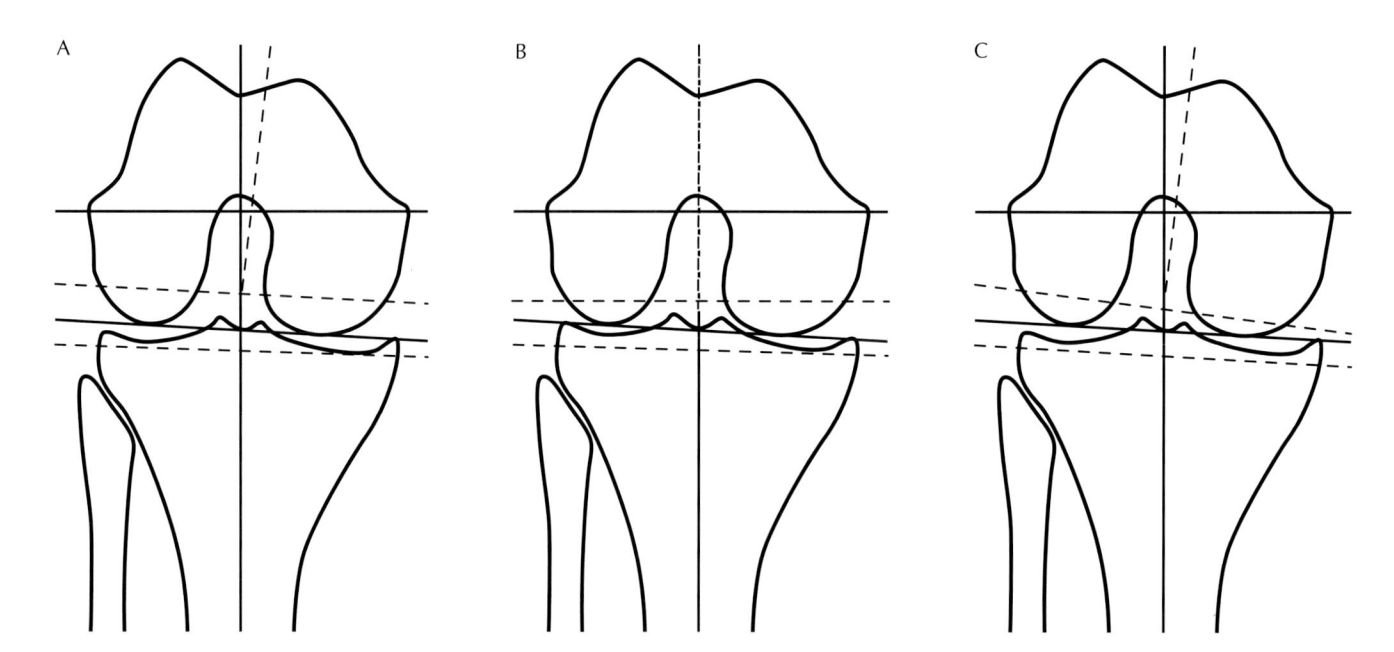

Figure 30.2. Three methods of resection in a knee with a 3-degree varus transverse axis. (A) The upper tibia is resected perpendicular to its long axis; the posterior condyles are cut parallel to the posterior condylar line. The flexion gap is trapezoïdal and the prosthetic sulcus is moved medially. (B) The upper tibia is resected perpendicular to its long axis; the posterior condyles are cut parallel to the transepicondylar line (± 3 degrees external rotation). The flexion gap is rectangular and the prosthetic sulcus is superimposed on the natural sulcus. (C) The upper tibia is resected with a 3-degree varus slope; the posterior condyles are cut parallel to the posterior condylar line. The flexion gap is rectangular but the prosthetic sulcus is moved medially.

and conversely the degenerative process can be caused by a distorted anatomy.

Eckhoff[34–37] showed that rotational malalignment, along with axial malalignment, should be considered as a mechanical cause of arthrosis. Cooke[38] described a group of varus knees with an excessive medial slope of the articular surfaces. In this group, geometric rotational disproportion of the distal part of the femur could have initiated the osteoarthritic changes.[39,40] If the intrinsic rotational deformity of the limb is not addressed, the durability of the arthroplasty may be compromised.[19,20,35,41–43]

To sum up, it clearly appears from the literature and from clinical experience that a certain amount of external rotation of the femoral component has to be set when performing a total knee arthroplasty with a perpendicular tibial cut, in order to balance the knee in flexion and to enhance patellar tracking. It also appears that the necessary external rotation is variable and has to be adjusted for every knee.

METHODS OF FEMORAL ROTATIONAL ALIGNMENT

Several methods have been proposed to establish rotational alignment of the femoral component. In the seventies, Insall[23,24] developed the flexion gap technique. In his original technique, the ligament releases are performed to correct fixed deformity, bringing the limb into appropriate alignment before the cuts are made. The proximal tibia is cut at right angles to the long axis of the tibial shaft in both anteroposterior and mediolateral planes. The posterior femoral condyles are resected, placing a tensor in the knee in flexion and rotating the femoral cutting block so that the posterior edge of the cutting block is parallel to the top of the tibia, in order to create a rectangular flexion gap. The knee is then extended and the ligaments are tensed. A distal femoral osteotomy is performed perpendicular to the mechanical axis, at the adequate level to obtain an extension gap exactly equal to the flexion gap.

The technique described by Stiehl,[44] using the tibial shaft axis, is very similar. The posterior femoral condyles are resected perpendicular to the extremedullary tibial shaft axis, combined with a perpendicular tibial cut. As a preliminary, soft tissues are tensioned using a laminar spreader.

The main objection to these techniques is the fact that they rely on the ligament release to rotate the femur, with a risk of malrotation in case of over- or underrelease. It may, therefore, be more reproducible to rely on anatomic landmarks in order to obtain proper rotational alignment of the femoral component. At least four bony landmarks are available for this purpose[9]—the posterior femoral condyles, the trochlear groove, the medial and lateral epicondyles, and the lateral ridge on the distal femoral metaphysis. The use of the posterior femoral condyles has already been discussed. In short, if the tibia is cut perpendicular to its long axis, a cut parallel to the posterior condyles will be incorrect most of the time, and a cut rotated externally by 3 degrees relative to the posterior condyles will be accurate only in the case of an ideal standard knee with a 3-degree varus transverse axis.

Whiteside[4,15] proposed a technique for using the trochlear groove to establish rotational alignment of the femoral component in the valgus knee. A line drawn from the deepest part of the patellar sulcus to the center of the intercondylar notch defined an anteroposterior axis. Examining 30 normal cadaveric femora, he stated that a line perpendicular to this anteroposterior axis was consistently approximated at 4 degrees of external rotation relative to the posterior condylar surfaces, and found that the transepicondylar line, connecting the two epicondyles, was more difficult to define, and was not as accurate. He significantly reduced the rates of tibial tubercle osteotomy and late patellar instability by using the anteroposterior axis for rotational alignment in a group of 107 valgus knees, compared to a reference group of 46 valgus knees done earlier, using the posterior femoral condyles as landmarks.[15]

In agreement with John Insall, we felt that the epicondyles were sound landmarks to ensure correct femoral rotational alignment, and we carried out a study in 100 knees undergoing a total knee replacement, in order to compare the different landmarks available.[45] The angles between the tangent line of the posterior condylar surfaces, the anteroposterior axis as described by Whiteside, the transepicondylar line and the trochlear line were measured. Also measured were the sulcus angle, the transepicondylar width, the height of the condyles, and the thickness of the various cuts (Fig. 30.3). Radiological measurements were made: the mechanical angle defined as the angle between the mechanical axis of the femur and the mechanical axis of the tibia,[27,30,43,46,47] the hip center-femoral shaft angle, the transcondylar angle, and the tibial plateau-tibial shaft angle (Fig. 30.4).

The mean values of these measurements were calculated, comparisons were made according to the sex and the mechanical angle, and correlations between the various measurements were calculated. The line perpendicular to the anteroposterior axis was at 3.08 degrees of external rotation relative to the posterior condylar surfaces; the epicondylar line was at 3.60 degrees of external rotation, close to the results of previous anatomical studies;[5,39,48,49] and the anteroposterior axis and the epicondylar line were roughly perpendicular to each

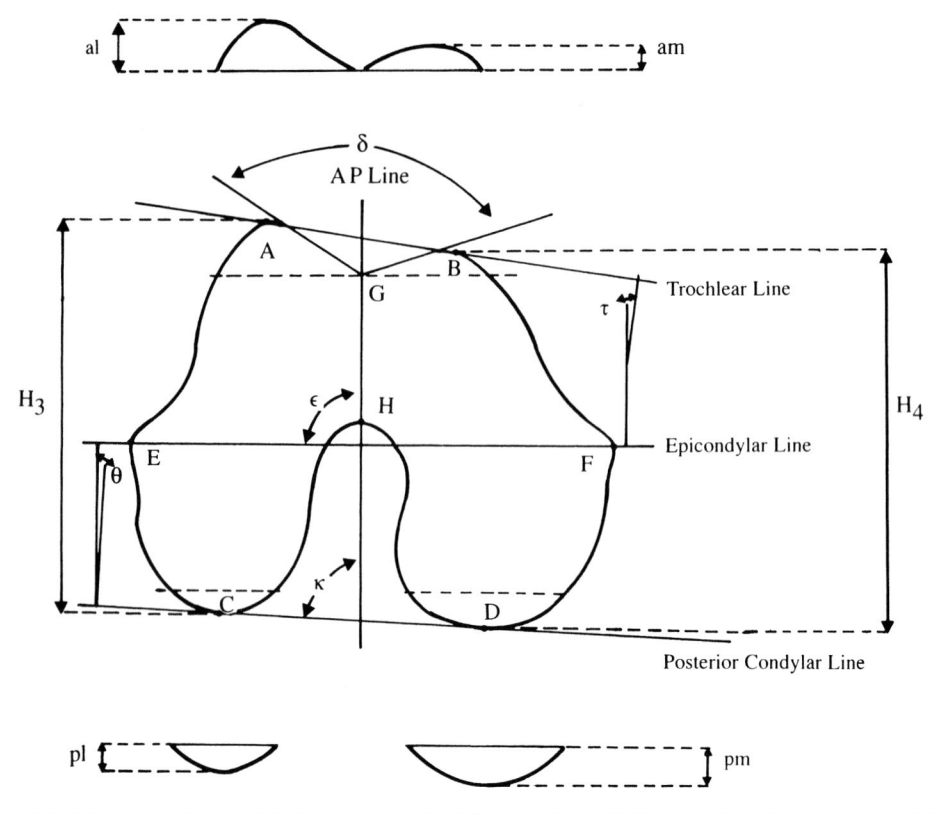

Figure 30.3. Diagram of the axial view or the distal femur. (From Poilvache, Insall, Scuderi et al.[45] by permission of *Clin Orthop*.)

A and B = the most anterior projections of the lateral and medial femoral condyles
C and D = the most posterior projections of the lateral and medial femoral condyles
E and F = the most prominent points of the lateral and medial epicondyles
G = the deepest part of the trochlar groove
H = the center of the intercondylar notch
AB = trochlear line
EF = epicondylar line
CD = posterior condylar line
GH = anteroposterior line
AGB = σ = sulcus angle
ϵ = anteroposterior (AP) line-epicondylar line angle
κ = anteroposterior (AP) line-posterior condylar line angle
θ = epicondylar line-posterior condylar line angle
τ = trochlear line-epicondylar line angle
H_3 = height of the lateral condyle
H_4 = height of the medial condyle
al = anterolateral cut   am = anteromedial cut
pl = posterolateral cut   pm = posteromedial cut

other (Table 30.1). The trochlear groove was angled somewhat externally relative to the epicondylar line in females, and somewhat medially in males (Table 30.1). The epicondylar line was externally rotated relative to the posterior condylar line by 3.51 degrees in varus or neutral knees, and by 4.41 degrees in valgus knees. If the rotation of the femoral component was set according to the anteroposterior axis, the amount of external rotation would be 2.73 degrees in varus or neutral knees, and 5.91 degrees in valgus knees (Table 30.2).

We felt that the anteroposterior axis was sometimes quite difficult to define, due to trochlear wear or to intercondylar osteophytes. In case of severe trochlear dysplasia, relying exclusively on the anteroposterior axis could induce excessive external rotation of the femoral component, as illustrated by the wide range (19 degrees) of the angles between the anteroposterior axis and the posterior condylar line. In some varus knees, relying on the anteroposterior axis could induce an internal rotation of up to 7 degrees. On the contrary, the range of the angles between the epicondylar line and the posterior condylar line was quite narrow (8 degrees, from 1 degree internal rotation to 7 degrees external rotation). The range of the angles between the anteroposterior axis and the epicondylar line was 14 degrees.

Several theoretical arguments support the use of the epicondyles as primary rotational landmarks. Kurosawa and associates[50] and Elias and colleagues[51] have shown that the posterior femoral condyles closely fit spherical surfaces, of 20 mm average radius, with a medial-lateral spacing of 46 mm. In a given knee, the radii can be slightly different for the medial and for the lateral condyle. Elias and colleagues[51] found that the femoral attachments of the medial collateral and posterior cruciate ligaments and of the lateral collateral and anterior cruciate ligaments were in the area of the center of the medial and lateral posterior femoral circles, respectively. This means that the axis of flexion of the knee is through the origin of the medial and lateral collateral ligaments. Yoshioka, Siu, and Cooke,[39,49] in a cadaver study of 32 normal femora, found that the mean transepicondylar line was at a right angle to the mechanical axis of the femur in the frontal plane, and that, with the knee flexed to 90 degrees, the transepicondylar line made a right angle with the long axis of the tibia as well. In this study[39,40] of the posterior extent of the condyles referred to the transepicondylar line showed wide variations, the posterior extent of the lateral condyle being smaller than that of the medial condyle. The transcondylar valgus angle, or the distal extent of the condyles to the transepicondylar line was also variable, the distal extent of the lateral condyle being again usually smaller than that of the medial condyle. More recently, Stiehl[44] confirmed Yoshioka's results and showed that the transepicondylar line was about 1 degree in a varus direction with regard to the mechanical axis of the femur, and that it was perpendicular to the tibial shaft both in flexion and in extension, and parallel to the knee flexion axis. This makes the transepicondylar line a sound landmark for rotational alignment of the femoral component

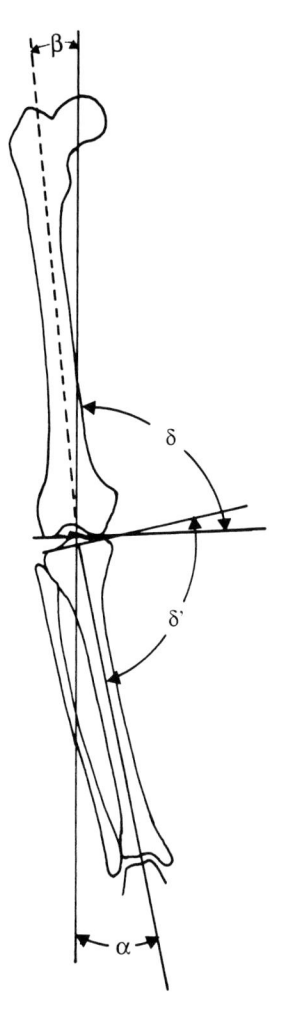

Figure 30.4. (From Poilvache, Insall, Scuderi, et al.[45] by permission of *Clin Orthop.*)
α = Mechanical axis of the femur - Mechanical axis of the tibia angle
β = Mechanical axis of the femur - Anatomical axis of the femur angle
δ = Mechanical axis of the femur - Distal condylar line angle
δ' = Tibial plateau - Tibial shaft angle.

Table 30.1. Angular measurements according to sex

Parameter	Group (N:100)	Male (N:46)	Female (N:54)	P
AP line— epicondylar line angle	90.33 [2.44]	91.2 [2.15]	89.59 [2.45]	0.001
AP line— posterior condylar line angle	86.92 [2.71]	88.07 [2.34]	85.94 [2.64]	<0.001
Epicondylar line— posterior condylar line angle	3.60 [2.02]	3.58 [2.16]	3.62 [1.93]	0.936

Average values expressed in degrees, with standard deviation in brackets.
(Source: Data from Poilvache, Insall, Scuderi, et al.[45])

Table 30.2. Angular measurements according to alignment

Parameter	Varus-neutral (N:89)	Valgus (N:11)	P
AP line—epicondylar line angle	90.53 [2.36]	88.73 [2.57]	0.047
AP line—posterior condylar line angle	87.27 [2.57]	84.09 [2.21]	0.001
Epicondylar line—posterior condylar line angle	3.51 [2.03]	4.41 [1.83]	0.15

Average values expressed in degrees, with standard deviation in brackets.
(Source: Data from Poilvache, Insall, Scuderi, et al.[45])

when resecting the proximal tibia at right angles to its mechanical axis.

However, it is not yet established whether the transepicondylar line should be perpendicular to the mechanical axis of the femur in every case. An exception that comes to mind is a femur with an acquired extra-articular deformity, like a malunion. In this situation, if the deformity is corrected intra-articularly at the time of the arthroplasty, the transepicondylar line will not be perpendicular to the mechanical axis of the femur nor to the long axis of the tibia in extension. If the posterior condyles are cut parallel to the transepicondylar line, making it perpendicular to the long axis of the tibia in flexion, it will be impossible to obtain proper ligament balance both in flexion and in extension. For this reason, a compromise is necessary in this specific case, or, if the deformity is severe, it should be corrected extra-articularly.

EPICONDYLAR AXIS: SURGICAL TECHNIQUE

In order to rotate the femoral component aligned with the epicondyles, the first step is to locate them precisely. This is an issue that is partly exposure and partly familiarity. On the lateral side, the patellofemoral ligament has to be divided in order to expose the lateral epicondyle. It appears as a discrete prominence that can be seen, felt, and marked (Fig. 30.5). On the medial side, the overlying synovium should be removed. The fan-shaped attachment of the medial collateral ligament is then visualized and outlined. The medial epicondyle is schematized as a circle and its center is located (Fig. 30.6). Berger[5] suggested using the sulcus of the medial epicondyle as a landmark, but we were unable to locate it reliably at surgery.

Next, using calipers, a line connecting the previously identified epicondyles is drawn on the distal femoral surface. A second line, parallel to the posterior condylar line is traced using a guide applied on the posterior condyles. The anteroposterior axis is also drawn through the deepest part of the patellar groove anteriorly and the center of the intercondylar notch posteriorly (Fig. 30.7). These two complementary lines serve as secondary landmarks, and allow to check the amount of external rotation produced by the epicondylar line. The anterior cut is then made parallel to the epicondy-

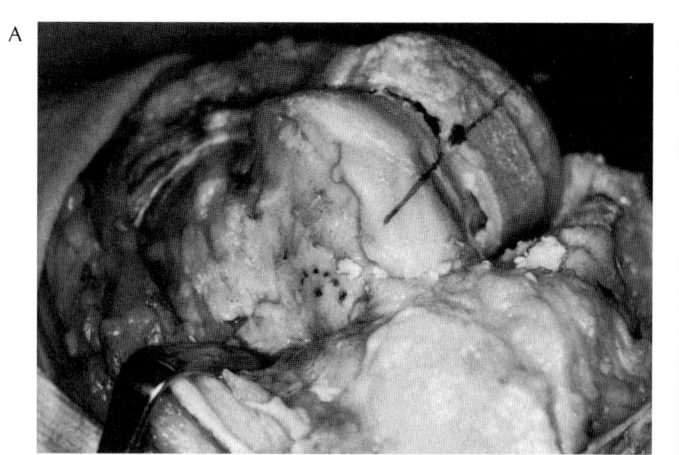

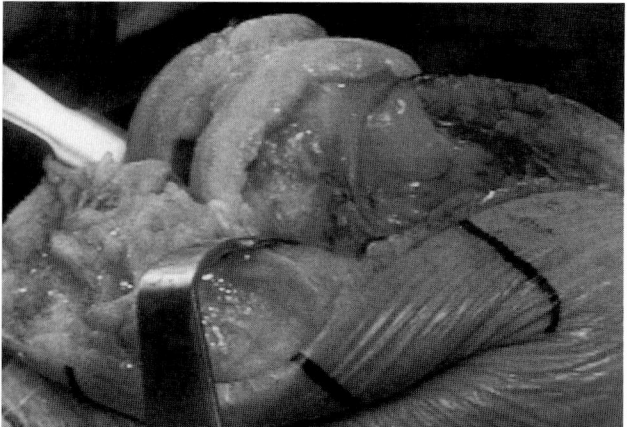

Figure 30.5. Intraoperative view of the lateral epicondyle.

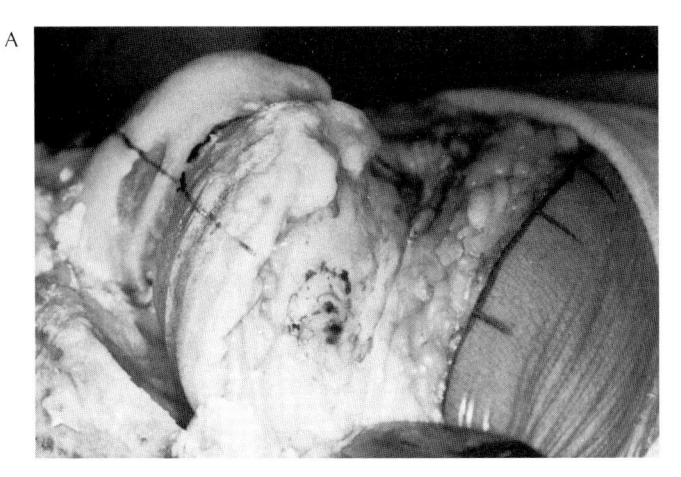

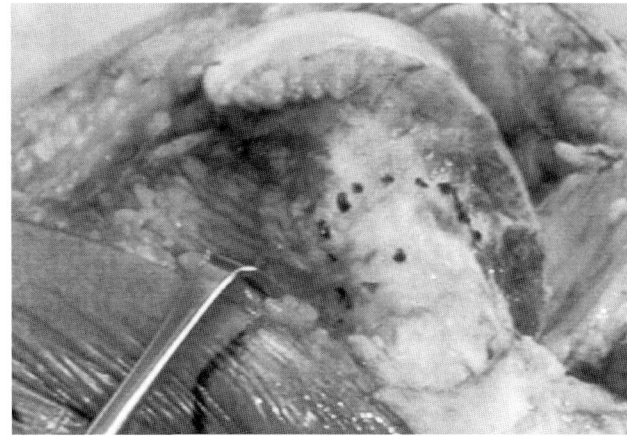

Figure 30.6. Intraoperative view of the medial epicondyle.

lar line, using the Dunn-Bertin intramedullary instrumentation, thus setting the rotation of the femoral component. The procedure then continues as usual.

Alternatively, Insall designed new instrumentation that allows to make the distal femoral cut first. A line is then drawn between the previously identified epicondyles, and a slot perpendicular to this line is cut into the femur, using a guide (Fig. 30.8). The anteroposterior cutting guide has a fin, which engages the slot in the femur. The guide can be moved in the slot in an anteroposterior direction. This possibility, combined with a 3-degree flexion of the distal femoral cut, allows a considerable anteroposterior adjustment without notching the anterior femur.

Finally, whatever the instrumentation system used, it is possible to make anteroposterior cuts parallel to a line connecting the epicondyles. The study we made in a consecutive series of 100 arthritic knees made us aware that the angle between the epicondylar line and the posterior condylar line is not constant. The low incidence of lateral retinacular releases (15 in 89 total knee replacements) in the group of neutral or varus knees suggests that "customizing" the amount of external rotation by using the epicondylar line can be useful even in primary total knee replacement.

From this study, it also appears that the trochlear groove is roughly perpendicular to the epicondylar line but that there can be considerable variation (range 14 degrees). Feinstein,[52] in a study of 15 cadaveric femora, obtained the same results (range 16 degrees). This implies that, even if rotation according to the epicondylar line will routinely produce symmetrical rectangular gaps, it will not solve all patellar problems. The design of the femoral component needs to accommodate vari-

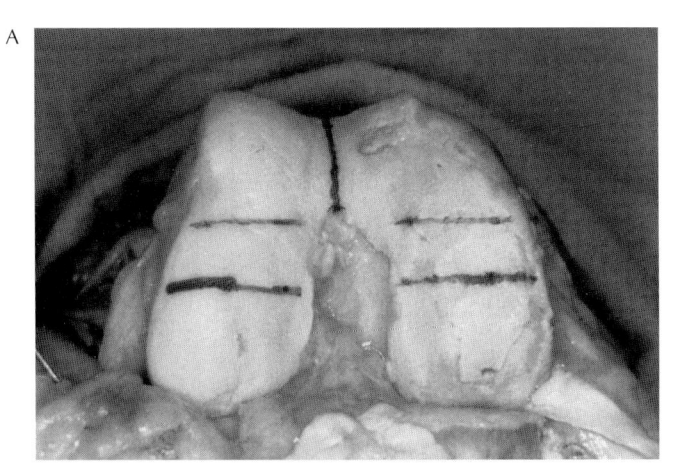

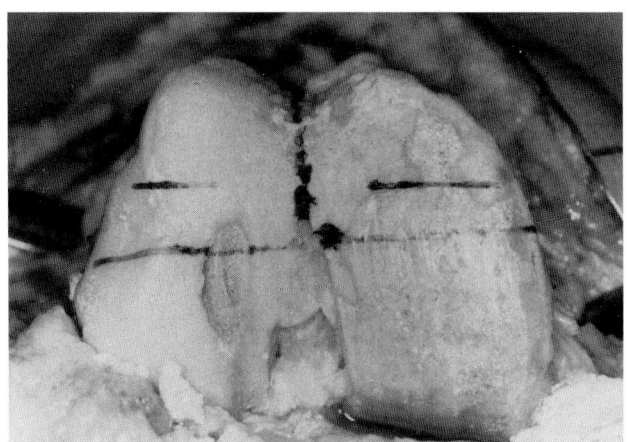

Figure 30.7. Intraoperative view of the distal femur. The anteroposterior line is drawn through the deepest part of the patellar groove, the transepicondylar line connects the epicondyles (lower line) and a line parallel to the posterior condylar line allows to check the amount of external rotation produced by the anteroposterior line and the transepicondylar line.

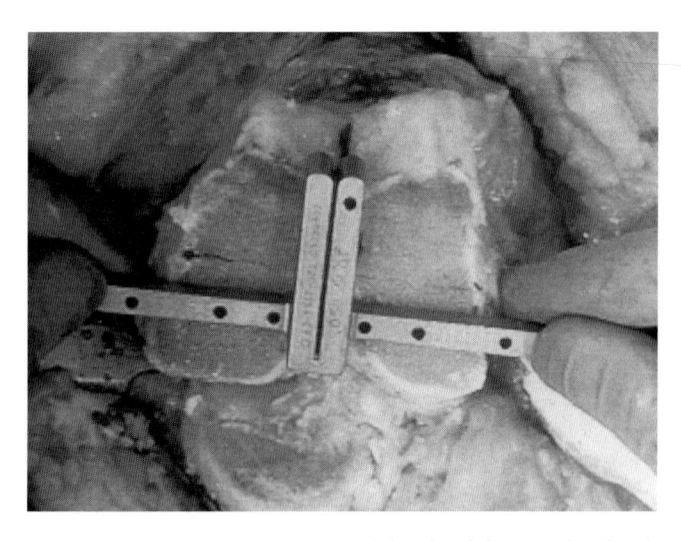

Figure 30.8. Intraoperative view of the distal femur. The distal femur is cut first. A line is drawn between the epicondyles. A special guide allows to cut a slot perpendicular to the transepicondylar line.

ations in orientation of the patellar groove. One should also be aware that contemporary design of femoral components with a laterally inclined trochlear groove create the risk, when externally rotating the femoral component, of patellar tilt and subluxation in the medial direction when the knee is extended.[53,54] Last, careful intraoperative adjustments of soft tissue tension still remain necessary to obtain proper patellar tracking.

References

1. Coventry MB. Two-part total knee arthroplasty. Evolution and present status. *Clin Orthop.* 1973; 145:29–36.
2. Lotke PA, Ecker ML. Influence of positioning of prosthesis in total knee replacement. *J Bone Joint Surg.* 1977; 59A:77–79.
3. Anouchi YS, Whiteside LA, Kaiser AD, et al. The effects of axial rotational alignment of the femoral component on knee stability and patellar tracking in total knee arthroplasty demonstrated on autopsy specimens. *Clin Orthop.* 1993; 287:170–177.
4. Arima J, Whiteside LA, McCarthy DS, et al. Femoral rotational alignment, based on the anteroposterior axis, in total knee arthroplasty in a valgus knee. *J Bone Joint Surg.* 1995; 77-A:1331–1334.
5. Berger RA, Rubash HE, Seel MJ, et al. Determining the rotational alignment of the femoral component in total knee arthroplasty using the epicondylar axis. *Clin Orthop.* 1993; 286:40–47.
6. Buechel FF. A sequential three-step lateral release for correcting fixed valgus knee deformities during total knee arthroplasty. *Clin Orthop.* 1990; 260:170–175.
7. Figgie HE, Golberg VM, Figgie MP, et al. The effect of alignment of the implant on fractures of the patella after total knee arthroplasty. *J Bone Joint Surg.* 1989; 71-A:1031–1039.
8. Goldberg VM, Figgie HE, Inglis AE, et al. Patellar fracture type and prognosis in condylar knee arthroplasty. *Clin Orthop.* 1988; 236:115–122.
9. Insall JN. *Surgery of the Knee.* 2nd ed. Vol. 2. New York: Churchill Livingstone; 1993: Chap. 26.
10. Moreland JR. Mechanisms of failure in total knee arthroplasty. *Clin Orthop.* 1988; 226:49–64.
11. Ranawat CS. The patellofemoral joint in total condylar knee arthroplasty. *Clin Orthop.* 1986; 205:93–99.
12. Rand JA. Patellar resurfacing in total knee arthroplasty. *Clin Orthop.* 1990; 260:110–117.
13. Rhoads DR, Noble PC, Reuben JD, et al. The effect of femoral component position on patellar tracking after total knee arthroplasty. *Clin Orthop.* 1990; 260:43–51.
14. Rosenberg AG, Andriacchi TP, Barden R, et al. Patellar component failure in cementless total knee arthroplasty. *Clin Orthop.* 1988; 236:106–114.
15. Whiteside LA, Arima J, McCarthy DS. Femoral rotational alignment in the valgus total knee arthroplasty based on the anterior-posterior axis. Presented at the 61st Annual Meeting of the American Academy of Orthopaedic Surgeons, New Orleans, Louisiana, February 24–March 1, 1994.
16. Tria AJ, Harwood DA, Alicea JO, et al. Patellar fractures in posterior stabilized knee arthroplasties. *Clin Orthop.* 1994; 299:131–138.
17. Scuderi GR, Insall JN, Scott WN. Patellofemoral pain after total knee arthroplasty. *J Am Acad Orthop Surg.* 1994; 2:239–246.
18. Stiehl JB, Komistek RD, Dennis DA, et al. Fluoroscopic analysis of kinematics after posterior-cruciate-retaining knee arthroplasty. *J Bone Joint Surg.* 1995; 77-B:884–889.
19. Eckhoff DG, Piatt BE, Gnadinger CA, Blaschke RC. Assessing rotational alignment in total knee arthroplasty. *Clin Orthop.* 1995; 318:176–181.
20. Eckhoff DG, Metzger RG, Vandewalle MV. Malrotation associated with implant alignment technique in total knee arthroplasty. *Clin Orthop.* 1995; 321:28–31.
21. Lewis P, Rorabeck CH, Bourne RB, et al. Postero-medial tibial polyethylene failure in total knee replacements. *Clin Orthop.* 1994; 299:11–17.
22. Wasielewski RC, Galante JO, Leighty RM, et al. Wear patterns on retrieved polyethylene tibial inserts and their relationship to technical considerations during total knee arthroscopy. *Clin Orthop.* 1994; 299:31–43.
23. Insall JN, Tria AJ, Scott WN. The total condylar knee prosthesis: the first 5 years. *Clin Orthop.* 1979; 145:68–77.
24. Insall JN, ed. *Surgery of the Knee.* New York: Churchill Livingstone; 1984: Chap. 20.
25. Insall JN, Binazzi R, Soudry M, et al. Total knee arthroplasty. *Clin Orthop.* 1985; 192:13–22.
26. Cooke TDV, Li J, Scudamore A. Radiographic assessment of bony contributions to knee deformity. *Orthop Clin North Am.* 1994; 25:87–93.
27. Cooke TDV, Bryant JT, Scudamore RA. Biomechanical factors in alignment and arthritic disorders of the knee. In: FU FH, Harner CD, Vince KG. *Knee Surgery.* Baltimore: Williams & Wilkins, 1994: 1061–1078.
28. Healy WL, Wilk RM. Osteotomy in treatment of the arthritic knee. In: Scott WN. *The Knee.* Vol. 2. St. Louis: Mosby; 1994: Chap. 57.

29. Kapandji IA. *The Physiology of the Joints.* 2nd ed. Vol. 2. New York: Churchill Livingstone; 1970: 74–75.
30. Moreland, JR, Bassett LW, Hanker GJ. Radiographic analysis of the axial alignment of the lower extremity. *J Bone Joint Surg.* 1987; 69-A:745–749.
31. Scuderi GR, Insall JN. The posterior stabilized knee prosthesis. *Orthop Clin North Am.* 1989; 20:71–78.
32. Laskin RS, Rieger MA. The surgical technique for performing a total knee replacement arthroplasty. *Orthop Clin North Am.* 1989; 20:31–48.
33. Hungerford DS, Krackow KA. Total joint arthroplasty of the knee. *Clin Orthop.* 1985; 192:23–33.
34. Eckhoff DG, Montgomery WK, Kilcoyne RF, et al. Femoral morphometry and anterior knee pain. *Clin Orthop.* 1994; 302:64–68.
35. Eckhoff DG. Effect of limb malrotation on malalignment and osteoarthritis. *Orthop Clin North Am.* 1994; 25:405–414.
36. Eckhoff DG, Johnson RJ, Stamm ER, et al. Version of the osteoarthritic knee. *J Arthroplasty.* 1994; 9:73–79.
37. Eckhoff DG, Kramer RC, Alongi CA, et al. Femoral anteversion and arthritis of the knee. *J Pediatr Orthop.* 1994; 14:608–610.
38. Cooke TDV, Pichora D, Siu D, et al. Surgical implications of varus deformity of the knee with obliquity of joint surfaces. *J Bone Joint Surg.* 1989; 71-B:560–565.
39. Yoshioka Y, Siu D, Cooke TDV. The anatomy and functional axis of the femur. *J Bone Joint Surg.* July 1987; 69-A:873–880.
40. Yoshioka Y, Cooke TDV. Femoral anteversion: assessment based on function axes. *J Orthop Res.* 1987; 5:86–91.
41. Yagi T. Tibial torsion in patients with medial-type osteoarthrotic knees. *Clin Orthop.* 1994; 302:52–56.
42. Moussa M. Rotational malalignment and femoral torsion in osteoarthritic knees with patellofemoral joint involvement. *Clin Orthop.* 1994; 304:176–183.
43. Harrison MM, Cooke TDV, Fisher SB, et al. Patterns of knee arthrosis and patella subluxation. *Clin Orthop.* 1994; 309:56–63.
44. Stiehl JB, Cherverny PM. Femoral rotational alignment using the tibial shaft axis in total knee arthroplasty. Presented at the Knee Society and AAHKS Specialty Day Program, Atlanta, Georgia, February 25, 1996.
45. Poilvache PL, Insall JN, Scuderi GR, et al. Rotational landmarks and sizing of the distal femur in total knee arthroplasty. *Clin Orthop.* 1996; 331:35–46.
46. Jiang C, Insall JN. Effect of rotation on the axial alignment of the femur: pitfalls in the use of femoral intramedullary guides in total knee arthroplasty. *Clin Orthop.* 1989; 248:50–56.
47. Chao EYS, Neluheni EVD, Hsu RWW, et al. Biomechanics of malalignment. *Orthop Clin North Am.* 1994; 25:379–386.
48. Mantas JP, Bloebaum RD, Skedros JG, et al. Implications of reference axes used for rotational alignment of the femoral component in primary and revision knee arthroplasty. *J Arthroplasty.* 1992; 7:531–535.
49. Cooke TDV. Letter to the Editor. *J Arthroplasty.* 1994; 9:225.
50. Kurosawa H, Walker PS, Abe S, et al. Geometry and motion of the knee for implant and orthotic design. *J Biomechanics.* 1985; 18:487–499.
51. Elias SG, Freeman AR, Gokcay EI. A correlative study of the geometry and anatomy of the distal femur. *Clin Orthop.* 1990; 260:98–103.
52. Feinstein WK, Noble PC, Kamaric E, et al. The anatomic alignment of the patellar groove. Presented at the Knee Society and AAHKS Specialty Day Program, Atlanta, Georgia, February 25, 1996.
53. Eckhoff DG, Montgomery WK, Stamm ER, et al. Location of the femoral sulcus in the osteoarthritic knee. *J Arthroplasty.* 1996; 11:163–165.
54. Eckhoff DG, et al. Location of the femoral sulcus. Presented at the Knee Society and AAHKS Specialty Day Program, Atlanta, Georgia, February 25, 1996.

CHAPTER 31
Tibial Shaft Axis for Femoral Component Rotation

James B. Stiehl

INTRODUCTION

Numerous authors have cited the importance of proper rotational alignment of the femoral component in total knee arthroplasty (TKA).[1-4] Position of the patellar groove and flexion gap stability are determined by the femoral component rotation. Improper alignment can lead to abnormal articulation with the tibial component as well as altered patellofemoral tracking.[5,6] Rotational malalignment may lead to an increase in the risk of a total knee clinical failure from the complications associated with the patellofemoral joint. Patellar subluxation, dislocation, patellar clunk, eccentric wear, and anterior knee pain have been described as complications of abnormal patellofemoral tracking.[2,7]

The axis of the posterior femoral condyles has normally been used as the reference for neutral rotation of the femur.[2,6,8,9] This was thought to be a reasonable landmark because the goal of TKA is to reestablish alignment of the anatomic femoral condyles.[10] However, recent biomechanical analyses have suggested that the transepicondylar axis (TEA) and not the posterior condylar axis parallels the primary center of rotation of the knee joint. Berger and associates[2] found that the angle between the posterior condylar surface and the surgical epicondylar axis, defined as the line connecting the lateral epicondylar prominence and medial sulcus of the medial epicondyle, was variable dependent upon sex. Mantas and colleagues[4] found a nearly constant relationship of 5 degrees external rotation of the TEA from the posterior condylar axis. The lateral epicondyle was closer to the joint line than the medial epicondyle in both extension and flexion.

In a previous study from the author's, laboratory measurements were made on 13 embalmed cadaver specimens to determine the relationship of the TEA to the longitudinal axis of the lower extremity in both extension and flexion.[11] The purpose of that study was to confirm whether or not the TEA could be used to reliably determine posterior condyle resection in TKA. The anatomical study clearly defined a constant relationship of the TEA to the transverse flexion axis of knee rotation and as a line perpendicular to the mechanical axis of the lower extremity. Most importantly, when the knee moves from extension to flexion, a perpendicular relationship is maintained from the TEA to the lower extremity centered on the midline of the talus. The mean tibial angle comparing the TEA to the mechanical axis was 0.4 degrees varus in extension and 0.43 degrees varus in flexion with no significant difference. It was also noted that the center of the knee, defined in the study as the lowest point of the intercondylar notch at the TEA, was located virtually on the mechanical axis of the leg as was the center of the tibial eminence. Based on these anatomical relationships, a technique was developed that allowed the femoral component rotation to be determined by lining up the posterior condylar cuts perpendicular with the longitudinal axis of the tibial shaft. By using the intramedullary femoral rod now available in most instrumentation sets, the posterior condylar cutting guide is attached to this rod, and a long axis rod simply aligns with the center of the ankle joint with the knee flexed.

SURGICAL TECHNIQUE

Standard knee exposure is done and it is important to identify the bone defects or ligamentous abnormalities present initially. As with "tibia cut first" methods, recommended for the total condylar or posterior-stabilized systems, ligamentous balancing must be done initially to the point of anatomical correction of an alignment problem. For example, for a typical varus deformity, this must be done by releasing the deep medial collateral ligament, posterior medial capsule, and the superficial medial collateral ligament as needed to create the anatomical femorotibial alignment of 5 to 7 degrees. For most standard posterior cruciate-retaining knee techniques, the next step is the appropriate intramedullary (IM) rod introduction. This rod must be inserted into the medullary canal to the level of the isthmus to confirm unobstructed passage. After this placement, a jig is placed on the distal femur for the distal femoral resection.

The next step is to cut the anterior and posterior femoral condyles. For the tibial shaft axis alignment, depending on the system, a long extramedullary (EM) rod was designed so it could be placed on the femoral IM alignment rod or the anteroposterior cutting block with the knee in flexion. (For the two systems studied, both had ancillary extramedullary rods available that could easily be adapted to make the anteroposterior femoral cutting jig align distally with the ankle joint.) This EM rod was used to determine the amount of external rotation required to balance the flexion gap based on the relationship of a perpendicular tibia cut to the lower limb axis. The EM alignment rod was attached to the femoral IM rod and rotation of the rod in the transverse plane was determined. The EM rod aligns distally to the center of the talar dome (Fig. 31.1). At this point, it is important to assess the amount of defect present and if significant flexion gap tensing will be needed to create a balanced flexion gap. This is usually done by inserting a lamina spreader(s) between the condyles for adequate spacing. If the gap is minimal, this tensing may be unnecessary. The appropriate anteroposterior cutting block is applied and the posterior condyles are resected with an oscillating saw based on a plane perpendicular to the mechanical axis of the lower limb, after which are made the anterior, posterior, and chamfer cuts.

Lateral Retinacular Release

After the femoral cuts are made, tibial cuts are made according to the standard protocol for the particular total knee system. Once all cuts are made, the knee is placed through a range of motion test in order to examine patellar tracking of the knee system. For knees in which tracking is not optimal (i.e., tendency of the patellar implant to lose medial prosthetic contact with the "no thumbs" assessment), a lateral release is performed for the purpose of improving patellar tracking. The extent of the lateral release will be dependent on the individual case.

CLINICAL RESULTS

One hundred consecutive primary total knee arthroplasties were performed by a single surgeon (JBS). The patient population data is given in Table 31.1. To determine the distal femoral component rotational alignment, the posterior condylar axis (which references femoral rotation parallel with the femoral condyles) was used as the reference for posterior femoral cuts in the first 54 consecutive knees and an extramedullary alignment rod was used in the next 46 knees. Four standard knee prostheses (Whiteside Ortholock, Wright Medical-Dow Corning, Arlington, Tenn; Axiom, Orthomet, Inc., Minneapolis, Minn; Genesis, Smith-Nephew-Richard's, Memphis, Tenn; Lacey, Wright Medical-Dow Corning, Arlington, Tenn) were used in this study (Table 31.1). Thirty-nine of the 54 (72.2%) patients who underwent TKA using the posterior condylar axis method for determining femoral component rotation had a lateral release performed, whereas only 13 of the 46 (28.3%) patients who underwent TKA using the extramedullary alignment rod had a lateral release performed. Results

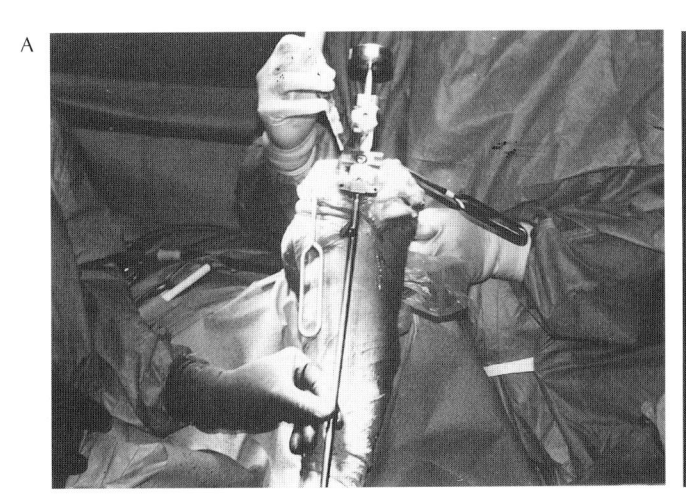

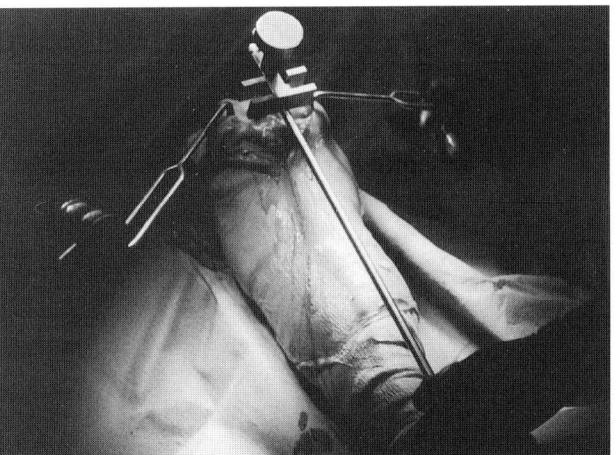

Figure 31.1. Femoral rotation alignment rod attached to an intramedullary rod and positioned to determine femoral component rotation and to align the anteroposterior cutting guide with the transepicondylar axis.

Table 31.1. Patient characteristics for two different techniques for femoral component rotational orientation

Variable	Posterior condylar axis method	Tibial shaft axis method
Patients		
Right TKA	25	26
Left TKA	29	20
Gender (%)		
Male	25.9	39.1
Female	74.1	60.9
Age (Years)		
Mean	66.6	65.1
Range	42–85	19–87
Preop Diagnosis		
Osteoarthritis	46	42
Rheumatoid Arthritis	7	3
Avascular Necrosis	1	1
Prosthetic Types		
Wright Medical Ortholock	21	10
Cemented	9	6
Cementless	16	11
Hybrid		
Orthomet Axiom	3	10
Cemented	—	—
Cementless	1	9
Hybrid		
Smith-Nephew Richard's Genesis	—	—
Cemented	—	—
Cementless	1	—
Hybrid		
Wright Medical Lacey	—	—
Cemented	—	—
Cementless	1	—
Hybrid		

Two of the patients underwent bilateral TKA on separate occasions so that equal posterior resection was used on one knee and extramedullary rotational alignment was undertaken on the contralateral knee.[11] Transverse computed tomographs of each knee were made at the level of the epicondyles and the angle of the prosthetic posterior condyles was measured in relation to the TEA. For the knees performed with equal posterior resection, the posterior condyle-TEA angle measured 5.0 and 4.0 degrees, respectively. For the knees performed with the extramedullary alignment rod, the posterior condyle-TEA angle measured 1.0 and 0.0 degrees, respectively (Fig. 31.2).

DISCUSSION

It is well known that optimum femoral component rotational orientation is essential for flexion gap balance, patellofemoral tracking, and normal kinematic function of the knee in TKA. From a previous anatomical study investigating the relationships of the TEA, we found that the perpendicular relationship of the TEA to the longitudinal axis of the lower extremity in 90-degree flexion allows the TEA to be used for posterior condylar resection.[11] By performing a perpendicular proximal tibial resection, the posterior condylar resection is parallel to the TEA. Thus, the ligaments can be appropriately balanced.

Both anatomical and biomechanical data point to the TEA as an important mechanical landmark as opposed to the posterior condylar axis.[1,2] Yoshioka and colleagues[12] have identified significant interspecimen variability of the

of a Chi-Square test with continuity correction (Yates correction) showed that the tibial shaft axis alignment method is associated with lower rates of lateral release ($p < 0.001$). Patellar fractures were found in 4 of the 54 (7.41%) knees using the posterior condylar axis method, whereas there were no patellar complications in the extramedullary alignment rod group. Due to the small number of patellar fractures, there was no statistical difference between the two groups.

All of the patellar fractures occurred in total knee replacements performed referencing the posterior condylar axis for posterofemoral resection. It is interesting to note that all of these patellar fractures occurred in female patients who underwent bilateral cemented (Wright Medical Ortholock) TKA. All of these cases had a lateral release performed and the contralateral knee replacements had satisfactory clinical results.

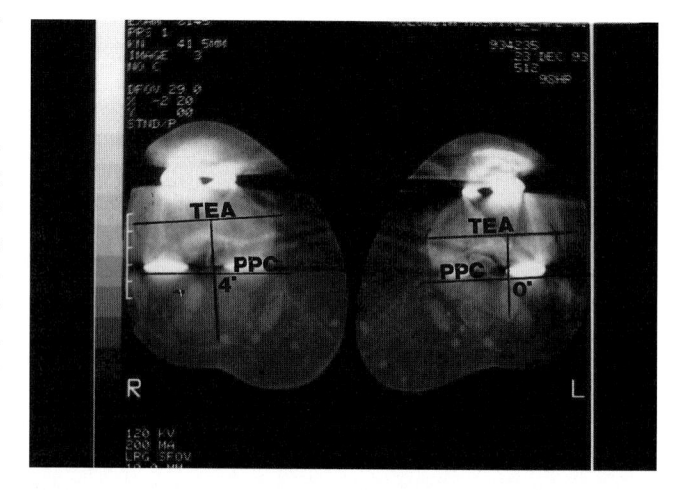

Figure 31.2. Transverse distal femoral computed tomograms at the level of the transepicondylar axis of a patient in which posterior condylar resection was undertaken on the right knee, parallel to the posterior condylar axis; and on the left knee, parallel to the transepicondylar axis using the femoral rotation alignment rod.

posterior condylar axis in comparison to the nearly constant relationship defined by the femoral shaft or hip center axis and the TEA. They suggest that the femoral component should be placed along a longitudinal axis that is centered at the knee, at the attachment of the PCL. To eliminate the need for finding the epicondyle peaks intraoperatively, we have used a long, extramedullary rod that can be attached to the IM femoral alignment guide to define the amount of external rotation required to balance the flexion gap. This concept is easily adapted to any standard total knee instrumentation.

Major patellar complications, such as patellar dislocation or fracture, have been reported in 1 to 12% of recent TKA cases and continue to be one of the leading causes of revision TKA.[7,13-15] Other minor problems, including anterior knee pain and patellar clicking, will occur even more frequently. The exact mechanism of patellar problems can be variable, but most may be attributable to malalignment of the prosthetic components, soft tissue imbalances, excessive valgus alignment, altered joint line, and tilted patellar cut.[7,14] If the lower extremity is aligned properly at the time of surgery, mild degrees of instability may be tolerated; however, if malalignment is created at the time of surgery, minor degrees of instability can lead to patellar subluxation. The author's experience would similarly indicate lateral release and femoral internal rotation as risk factors for patellar fracture.

In conclusion, a method is described that allows the anatomical amount of femoral component rotation based on the lower limb anatomical axis. Thus, appropriate posterior condyle resection can be performed in a manner that will allow a balanced flexion gap if the subsequent proximal tibial cut is made perpendicular to the same axis. Patellar fracture and the need for lateral retinacular release were diminished when this technique was compared with the posterior condylar axis method in similar implants.

References

1. Arima J, Whiteside LA, McCarthy DS, White SE. Femoral rotational alignment, based on the anteroposterior axis, in total knee arthroplasty in a valgus knee. *J Bone Joint Surg.* September 1995; 77-A:1331–1334.
2. Berger RA, Rubash HE, Seel MJ, Thompson WH, Crossett LS. Determining the rotational alignment of the femoral component in total knee arthroplasty using the epicondylar axis. *Clin Orthop.* January 1993; 286:40–47.
3. Insall JN. Total knee replacement. In: Insall JN, ed. *Surgery of the Knee.* New York: Churchill Livingston; 1984: 587–695.
4. Mantas JP, Bloebaum RD, Skedros JG, Hofmann AA. Implications of reference axes used for rotational alignment of the femoral component in primary and revision arthroplasty. *J Arthroplasty.* December 1992; 7:531–535.
5. Hsu HP, Garg A, Walker PS, Spector M, Ewald FC. Effect of knee component alignment on tibial load distribution with clinical correlation. *Clin Orthop.* November 1989; 248:135–144.
6. Moreland JR. Mechanisms of failure in total knee arthroplasty. *Clin Orthop.* January 1988; 226:49–64.
7. Figgie HE, Goldberg VM, Figgie MP, Inglis AE, Kelly M, Sobel M. The effect of alignment of the implant on fractures of the patella after condylar total knee arthroplasty. *J Bone Joint Surg.* August 1989; 71-A:1031–1039.
8. Jiang CC, Insall JN. Effect of rotation on the axial alignment of the femur. *Clin Orthop.* November 1989; 248:50–56.
9. Stiehl JB, Abbott B. A morphological analysis of the transepicondylar axis and the relationship to the mechanical axis of the leg. *J Arthroplasty.* 1995; 10:785–789.
10. Krakow KA. Rotational alignment. In: Krakow KA, ed. *The Technique of Total Knee Arthroplasty.* St. Louis: C. V. Mosby; 1990: 125–136.
11. Stiehl JB, Abbott B. Femoral component rotational alignment using the extramedullary tibial shaft axis: a technical note. *J Orthop Rheumatology.* 1995; 8:93–96.
12. Yoshioka Y, Siu D, Cooke DV. The anatomy and functional axes of the femur. *J Bone Joint Surg.* July 1987; 69-A:873–880.
13. Malkani AL, Rand JA, Bryan RS, Wallrichs SL. Total knee arthroplasty with the kinematic condylar prosthesis. *J Bone Joint Surg.* 1995; 77-A:423–431.
14. Rhoads DD, Noble PC, Reuben JD, Mahoney OM, Tullos HS. The effect of femoral component position on patellar tracking after total knee arthroplasty. *Clin Orthop.* November 1990; 260:43–51.
15. Scott W, Rubinstein M, Scuderi G. Results after total knee replacement with a posterior cruciate substituting prosthesis. *J Bone Joint Surg.* September 1988; 70-A:1163–1173.

CHAPTER 32
Alternatives for Rotational Alignment of the Femoral Component

Chitranjan S. Ranawat and José A. Rodriguez

INTRODUCTION

The goal of component position in total knee arthroplasty is proper alignment in all three planes, frontal, lateral, and axial. In this way the kinematics of the knee can be reproduced to achieve good range of motion without pain and so that the knee can remain stable throughout the range of motion. Most total knee implants are designed to fit a symmetrical flexion and extension space. As such the symmetry and balance of these spaces are crucial to the proper stability and function of the reconstructed knee, and could influence its long-term durability. The level of the joint line with respect to the attachments of the collateral ligaments should be maintained to optimize the range of motion, as well as the stability and tracking of the patella.

The anatomic variations in the normal human femur have been studied in detail by Yoshioka and associates in a cadaver study of 32 femora.[1] These authors found that the distal valgus angle of the articular surface of the femur to the epicondylar axis is an average of 4 degrees ±2 degrees. In assessing rotation of the distal femur, they noted that the posterior medial condyle projects an average 5 mm farther posteriorly than the lateral condyle.

Malalignment in femoral rotation has been studied in cadaver specimens by Anouchi and colleagues by altering the femoral component rotation and assessing the effect on stability and patellofemoral tracking.[2] They found that internal rotation of the femoral component produced a construct that was tight medially, and gapped open laterally in flexion. In addition, the patellofemoral tracking was closest to normal, and the contact pressures most evenly distributed on the patella with a component externally rotated 5 degrees. In a similar cadaveric study, Rhoades and associates noted that a femoral component placed 5 mm lateral to the center on the distal femur produced patellofemoral tracking closest to normal.[3]

Knees that have arthritis often have loss of anterior cruciate ligament and, in many cases, the posterior cruciate ligament is also not normal. Most of the remarks here, therefore, assume that the knee's stability following total knee replacement is provided by the soft tissue sleeve formed by the collateral ligament capsule in conjunction with scar tissue that is formed after surgery. This soft tissue sleeve in conjunction with the condylar geometry provides the stability to the knee throughout range of motion in most knees. The use of a posterior cruciate ligament-substituting knee device allows a reproducible point of rotation for proper kinematics and healing of the surrounding ligaments, capsule, and new scar tissue.

The patellofemoral joint should be aligned properly so it can track in the femoral groove. The following method of positioning of the femoral component in correct rotational alignment was designed using the instrumentation of the Modular PFC posterior cruciate-substituting knee replacement.

TECHNIQUE

After exposing the knee fully and sacrificing the remnants of the anterior and posterior ligaments, the proximal and medial side of the tibia is mobilized, and the tibia is delivered in front of the femur. The patellofemoral ligament is released so that the patella can be everted. This exposes the proximal tibia fully and allows it to be visualized completely. With the appropriate extramedullary tibia cutting device, the proximal tibia is cut between 8 to 10 mm from the least-affected condyle. For example, in a varus deformity, 8 to 10 mm of the lateral tibial plateau will be removed. The tibial cut is created at 90 degrees to the long axis of the tibia and is not sloped posteriorly, whereas with the PFC modular knee there are 4 degrees of posterior tilt built into the tibial plateau insert. The amount of tibial resection is a few millimeters greater when the knee has a flexion contracture and is a few millimeters less when there is a hyperextension deformity.

Attention then is directed to the distal cut of the femur. The distal femoral condyles are cut equal to the thickness of the femoral component, which is an average of 8 to 10 mm. The distal femoral cut of 8 to 10 mm is made using an extra- or intramedullary cutting device so that 8 to 10 mm of least involved condyle is cut. A provisional cut of the anterior surface of the femur is sometimes made to allow the distal femoral cutting guide closer to the femur and minimizing error in the distal femoral cut. After making the proximal tibial and distal femoral cuts, the gap between the two cut surfaces is assessed using the appropriate spacer.

The balance of the ligaments is then tested. If the medial soft tissue sleeve is tighter, such as in the varus knee, the medial side will be narrower than the lateral side. In this situation, soft tissue release of the posteromedial capsule from the tibia is carried out. This release, along with removal of the osteophytes, is sufficient to correct most varus deformities. Occasionally, the superficial medial collateral ligament insertion must be released subperiosteally in a gradual manner to create a balanced knee with an extension gap of 20 mm. Very rarely, selective lengthening of the pes anserinus tendon insertion is performed.

Let us now assume that the release of the medial structures is appropriate and the knee is balanced in extension. The criterion for good soft tissue sleeve on either side is judged by having 2 to 4 mm of gapping both medially and laterally with the appropriate spacer in place, while applying a varus or valgus stress. When such soft tissue balance is achieved, the release on the medial side is complete. No additional releases are necessary. The next cut is for anterior femoral and posterior femoral condyle.

At this time, the anteroposterior femoral cutting block is applied to the cut surface of the distal femur. This block requires adjustment in three different directions: (1) anterior and posterior, (2) lateromedial, and (3) axial rotation. The cutting block is first lateralized so that the lateral margin of the block matches the cut surface of the lateral femoral condyle. The anterior and posterior placement is gauged based on the stylus which will tell the location of the block in the front or back direction.

At this stage, the block is secured with the provisional pin in the lateral femoral condyle. A provisional femoral pin is then inserted on the medial part of the block to create a parallel surface with the proximal tibial cut. A laminar spreader is then applied to the posterior margin of the block with the knee at 90 degrees of flexion. This brings the soft tissue sleeve medially and laterally under tension (Fig. 32.1A). The space created between the posterior cutting slot and the cut surface of the tibia should be 20 mm and parallel to the tibia. If this has not been achieved, the provisional pin from the femoral side is removed and the block is externally rotated further, or internally rotated, depending on the condition present (Fig. 32.1B). The object is to create a 20 mm gap with the laminar spreader in place. The tension applied to the laminar spreader will approximate the tension in the soft tissues following reconstruction in this position. Once this is achieved, the block is secured to the distal femur with the two interlocking pins (Fig. 32.2). The anteroposterior femoral cuts are then carried out. In ap-

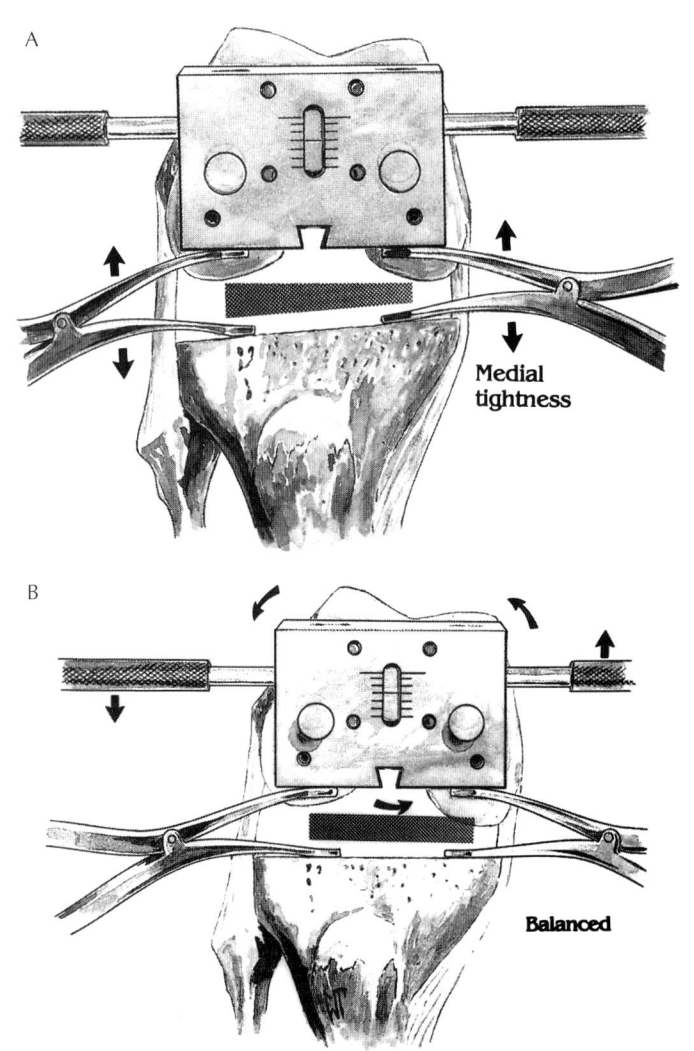

Figure 32.1. With the knee at 90 degrees of flexion a laminar spreader places the medial and lateral soft tissues under tension (A). If the cutting block is not parallel to the resected tibial surface, the femoral cutting guide is externally rotated (B).

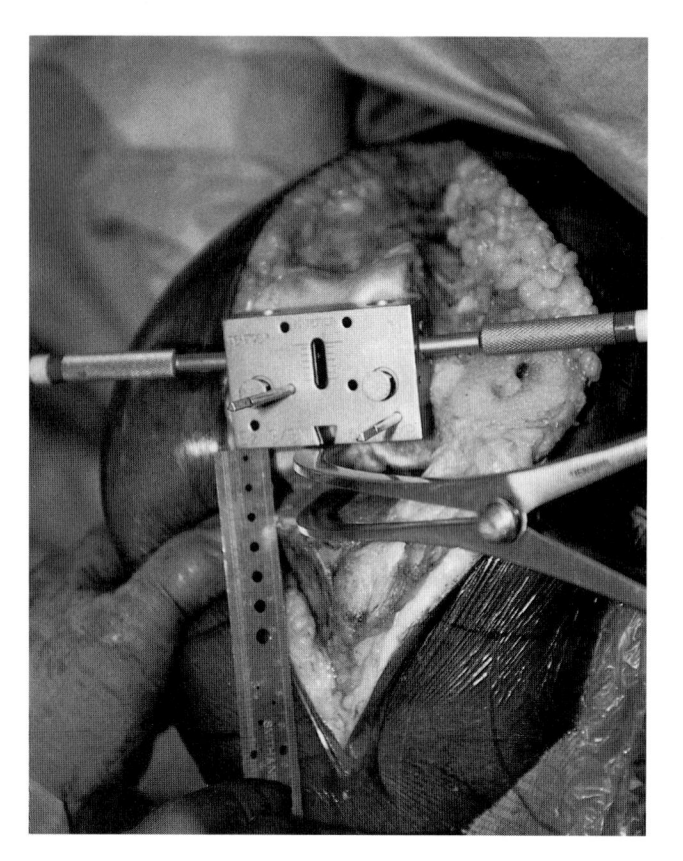

Figure 32.2. Once the flexion gap is determined to be symmetrical, the femoral cutting block is secured to the femur. The object is to create a 20 mm gap with the laminar spreader in place.

plying this cut, it is common to have an asymmetrical section of the distal femoral condyle, with more bone removed on the medial side than the lateral.

DISCUSSION

Most other techniques of positioning the femoral component in total knee replacement attempt to restore the posterior femoral joint line to its normal level using bony cuts, and subsequently balance the soft tissues. The posterior femoral condyles are a frequently used landmark for femoral rotation.[4,5] Laskin noted that an average of 3 degrees of external rotation of the femoral cutting guide with respect to the posterior condyles was necessary to create a rectangular flexion space.[5] However, this technique presumes no bony deformity in the posterior part of the femoral condyles, and may be insufficient to create a rectangular gap. Additional release at that point would also affect the previously balanced extension gap.

The transepicondylar axis, defined as a line joining the attachment of the lateral and medial collateral ligaments to the femur, has also been used as a landmark for rotating the femoral component.[6] However, this landmark is not always easily identified intraoperatively. Even in the controlled environment of the laboratory with cadaver specimens, the interobserver variation in defining this axis was 4 degrees.[6] Another landmark suggested for femoral component rotation is the femoral trochlear sulcus. The deepest part of the trochlear groove is marked on the bone as it intersects with the medullary canal of the femur, and a perpendicular line drawn on the cut distal surface of the femur sets the rotation.[7] Once again, this technique presumes no bony deformity, and is likely to result in errors in cases of deformity. One additional technique involves creating the tibial cut at 90 degrees to the shaft axis, and generically creating the posterior femoral cut parallel to the tibial cut.[8] This does not take into account any soft tissue laxity or tightness that may have been present preoperatively. With experience each of these techniques will probably yield identical positioning of the femoral component in straightforward cases without bony or soft tissue deformity.

Our technique creates the soft tissue balance in extension, and uses this balanced soft tissue sleeve to guide the rotational positioning of the femoral component. It is reproducible and applicable to cases of bony and soft tissue deformity. In this way, the soft tissue tension and balance will be identical in flexion and extension, creating optimal collateral ligament function and kinematics. At the same time, the femoral component will be externally rotated appropriately to reduce the risk of maltracking of the patella.

References

1. Yoshioka Y, Sui D, Cooke DV. The anatomy and functional axes of the femur. *J Bone Joint Surg.* 1987; 69A:873–880.
2. Anouchi YS, Whiteside LA, Kaiser AD, Milliano MT. The effects of axial rotational alignment of the femoral component on knee stability and patellar tracking in total knee arthroplasty demonstrated on autopsy specimens. *Clin Orthop.* 1993; 287:170–177.
3. Rhoads DD, Noble PC, Reuben JD, Mahoney OM, Tullos HS. The effect of femoral component position on patellar tracking after total knee arthroplasty. *Clin Orthop.* 1990; 260:43–51.
4. Insall JN. Surgical techniques and instrumentation in total knee arthroplasty. In: Insall JN, Windsor RE, Scott WN, Kelly MA, Aglietti P, eds. *Surgery of the Knee.* 2nd Ed., Vol. 1. New York: Churchill Livingstone; 1993.
5. Laskin RS. Flexion space configuration in total knee arthroplasty. *J Arthroplasty.* 1995; 10:657–660.
6. Berger RA, Rubash HE, Seel MJ, Thompson WH, Crossett LS. Determining the rotational alignment of the femoral component in total knee arthroplasty using the epicondylar axis. *Clin Orthop.* 1993; 286:40–47.
7. Whiteside LA. Rotation of the femoral component in total knee replacement. Video demonstration of technique. Annual Meeting of the Knee Society, Atlanta, Georgia, February 25, 1996.
8. Stiehl JB, Cherveny PM. Femoral rotational alignment using the tibial shaft axis in total knee replacement. Annual Meeting of the Knee Society, Atlanta, Georgia, February 25, 1996.

# CHAPTER 33
Tibial Component Position

Lawrence S. Crossett and Harry E. Rubash

INTRODUCTION

The placement of the component in total knee arthroplasty (TKA) can profoundly influence the functional result of the surgical procedure. The position of the tibial component may directly affect pain relief, patellofemoral function, and the longevity of fixation. Depending on the surgical technique used, the tibial position may indirectly influence the femoral component positioning, especially rotation. These direct and indirect influences of tibial position will be reviewed in this chapter and their impact on knee arthroplasty function explained in detail.

TECHNIQUE OF TOTAL KNEE ARTHROPLASTY

Two surgical techniques of TKA have evolved over time. As the influence of the tibial component position can vary depending on the technique employed, an understanding of the differences is helpful. The *flexion-extension gap* technique arose from the use of posterior cruciate ligament-sacrificing or substituting implants, but is applicable to cruciate-retaining designs. With this method the proximal tibia is resected perpendicular to the tibial shaft, which is coincident with the mechanical axis of the tibia (Fig. 33.1). Soft tissue releases are performed so that the knee is axially aligned in extension. The knee is flexed to 90 degrees and distracted, recreating the ligament tension determined in extension (Fig. 33.2). The proper sized femoral anteroposterior cutting guide is placed on the end of the femur, rotated to create a rectangle, and the cuts are completed. The flexion gap is measured and a matching sized gap is created in extension with the distal femoral cut (Fig. 33.3). The theoretical advantage of this method is the formation of equally balanced gaps in flexion and extension and a well-aligned extremity. Two potential disadvantages of this method exist. First, if the tibia is inadvertently cut in varus, the resulting femoral cut is in relative internal rotation, a position not well tolerated by the patella (Fig. 33.4). Also, if an inappropriate large flexion gap is created, over-resection of the distal femur must be performed to match the extension gap. This will lead to elevation of the joint line and a relative patellar baja, negatively impacting patellofemoral function. Despite these concerns, long-term results of this surgical technique have documented reproducible excellent results.[3–5]

The second method is the *anatomic measured resection* technique. This method has evolved in an attempt to re-create normal knee anatomy and function and has been popularized by the posterior cruciate-retaining prosthesis, in which joint line position is of critical importance. Initially the technique required a tibial cut in 3 degrees of varus in reference to the tibial shaft (but perpendicular to the vertical axis) (Fig. 33.5). The femur and tibia were resected independent of one another and the amount of resected bone reflected the thickness of the respective components. Rotation of the femur was based on the posterior femoral condyles in an anatomic manner. Many systems at present recommend a tibial resection at 90 degrees to the tibial shaft, and 3 degrees of external rotation of the femur is required to maintain an appropriately rectangular flexion space. The advantages of this technique are its ease, and the fact that any error in ligament balance or tibial resection will not influence the femoral cuts. Ligament balance is performed near the end of the procedure with the tibial components in place. Although equally balanced flexion and extension gaps are not assured, long-term results for this technique are also excellent.[6,7]

Most knee systems available today have combined aspects of both the flexion extension gap technique and the measured resection technique. Measured resection of most bony cuts helps to maintain the joint line position regardless of the style of knee. Femoral rotation can be determined by many methods including femoral anatomy, spacer blocks, or soft tissue tensioning devices. The role of the tibial cut, in determining femoral rotation or soft tissue balance must be understood by the sur-

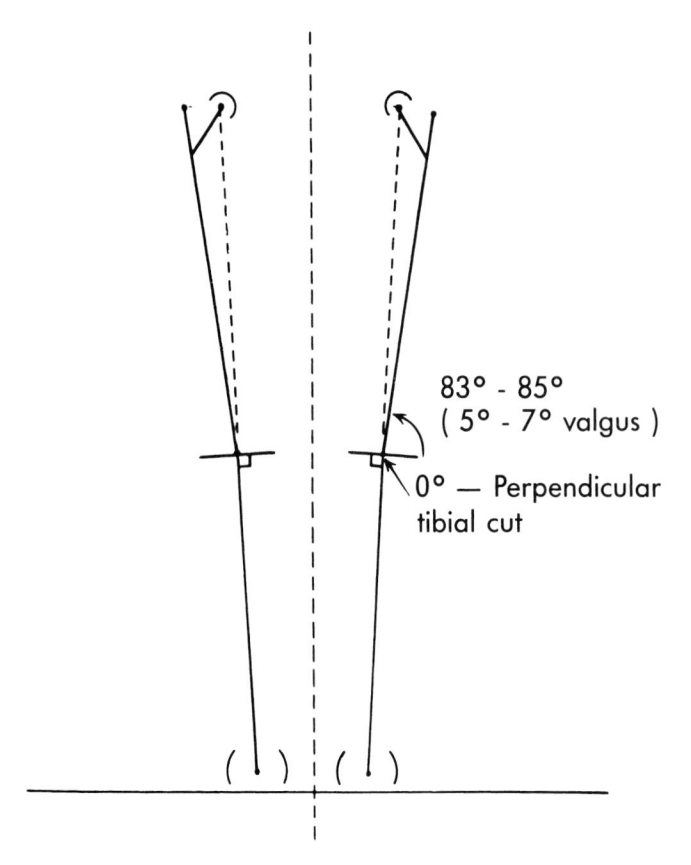

Figure 33.1. The classic alignment. Note that the tibial joint line is perpendicular to the mechanical axis extending from the center of hip to the center of the ankle. (From Krackow,[1] by permission of The C.V. Mosby Company.)

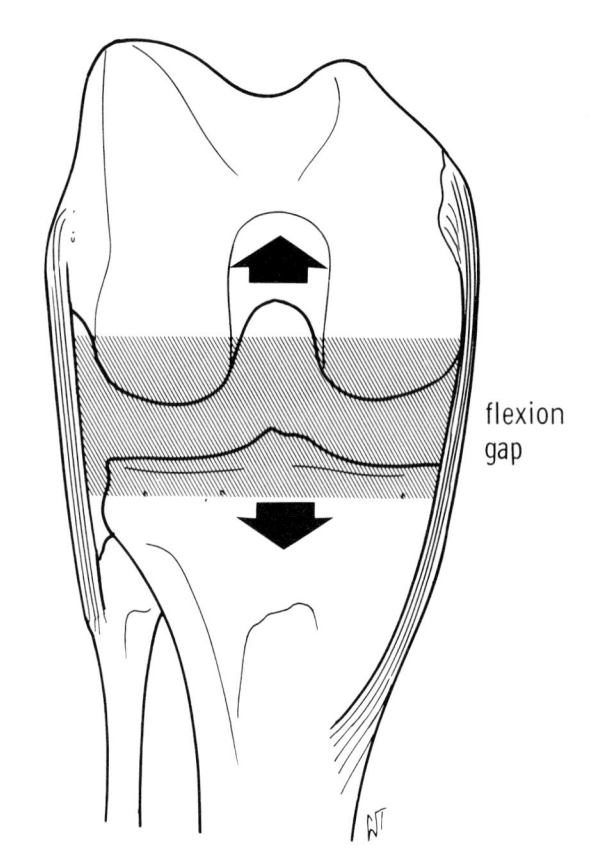

Figure 33.2. Following appropriate ligament releases, the knee is flexed and distracted creating equal ligament tension. The anteroposterior femoral cutting guide should be rotated parallel with the cut surface of the tibia creating a rectangular flexion gap. (From Insall,[2] by permission of Churchill Livingstone.)

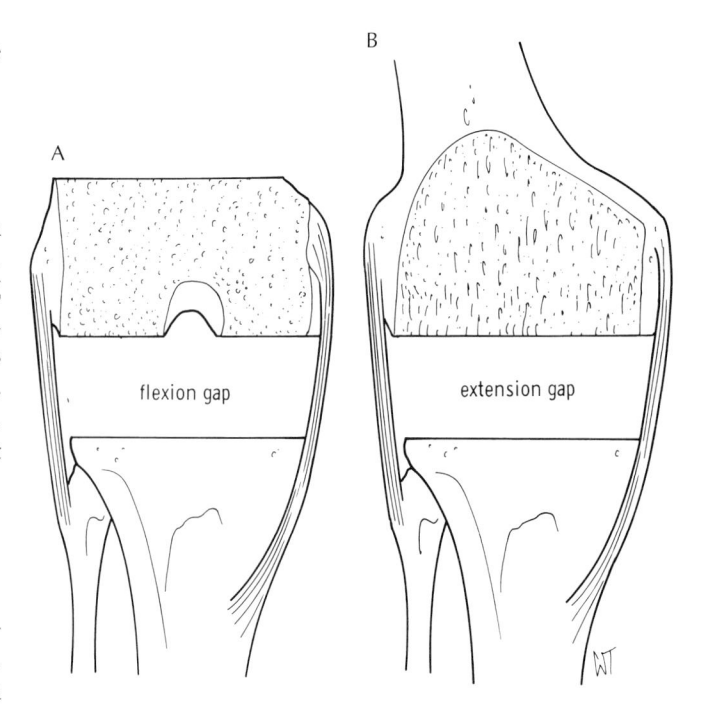

Figure 33.3. The extension gap is created to equal the flexion gap. (From Insall,[2] by permission of Churchill Livingstone.)

geon so that intraoperative decisions can be made accurately.

POSITION

To accurately describe tibial component position in TKA, 6 degrees of positional freedom must be defined. Three translational planes exist along the X, Y, and Z axes: anteroposterior position, mediolateral position, and proximal-distal position. Three rotation planes exist around these translational axes: varus-valgus, internal-external rotation, and flexion-extension (Fig. 33.6). Each one separately influences tibial component position and may, at times, influence another.

VARUS-VALGUS

The proximal tibial resection determines the varus-valgus and flexion-extension plane of the tibial component. For that reason, careful consideration should be given to the establishment of this cut. Intramedullary and extramedullary tibial cutting guides are available. Al-

33. Tibial Component Position

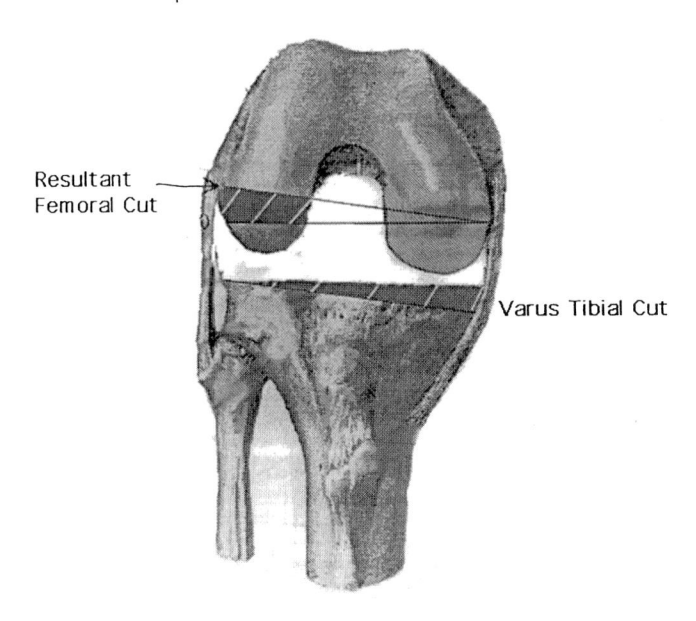

Figure 33.4. If the tibia is cut in varus and the posterior femoral cut is positioned to parallel the tibial cut, the result will be an internally rotated femoral component. Note the change in femoral position with an appropriate tibial cut (see shaded areas).

femoral component is not beneficial to patellar tracking (Fig. 33.8).

FLEXION-EXTENSION

As mentioned earlier, the proximal tibial resection will establish the varus-valgus *and* flexion-extension orientation of the tibial component. A tibial cut in extension must be avoided because any rollback during flexion will tighten the flexion gap and restrict flexion of the knee regardless of the knee arthroplasty design.

Many knee designs, especially cruciate-retaining designs, attempt to recreate the 10-degree posterior slope of the normal tibia. As the minimal amount of polyethylene required in TKA has increased, additional bony resection of the proximal tibia is required. This additional bony resection, coupled with a 10-degree posterior slope, may compromise the attachment of the posterior cruciate ligament (PCL). Increasing congruency between the femur and polyethylene articulation has al-

though the use of intramedullary guides have been supported through several studies, others have shown some limitation of this technique, especially in the valgus knee.[9–11] The intramedullary rod must be of sufficient length to reach the distal tibial epiphyseal scar and the proximal entry point must be accurate. Extramedullary tibial cutting guides are more commonly used and the limitations are well documented. The tendency for a varus cut is common, whereas a valgus cut is rare. Proximally the cutting guide must be placed snugly against the tibial tubercle. Excessive adipose tissue and reflected patellar tendon at this area may displace the guide medially. Distally, most guides tend to align with the crest of the tibia. The center of the talus (ankle mortice) lies several millimeters medial to the central point between the malleoli. For this reason, medial displacement of the distal tibial alignment guide may be considered (Fig. 33.7).

The accuracy of the varus-valgus alignment of the tibial cut is important to assure adequate axial alignment of the knee and to balance forces across the joint. If using the flexion-extension gap technique, this cut becomes more critical because the varus tibial cut will reflect itself in internal rotation of the femur (Fig. 33.4). Although the thickness and balance of the gaps will be equal, the position of the flexion gap will be in slight varus with resultant internal rotation of the femur. As stated earlier, this position of the

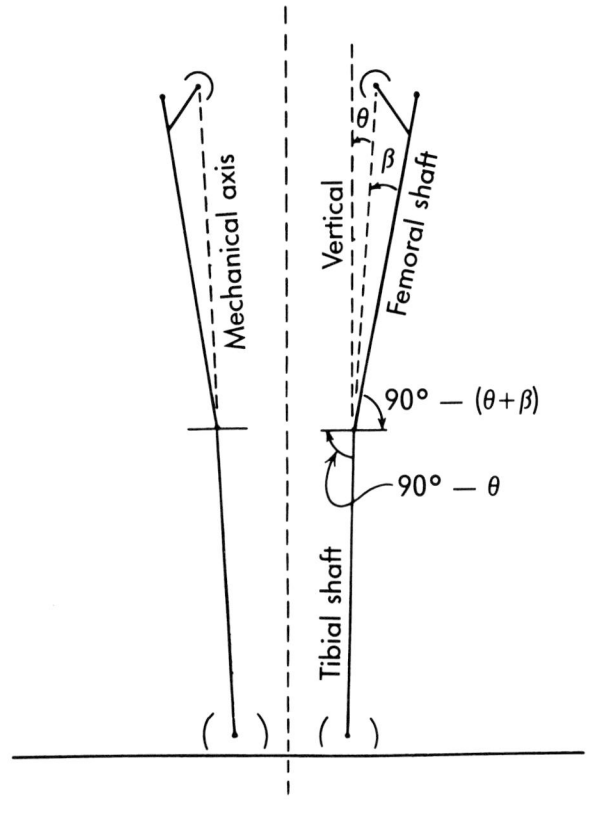

Figure 33.5. The anatomic alignment. As compared to the classic alignment, the tibial joint line is now positioned parallel to the ground while in the stand phase. This position required a tibial cut in 3 degrees of varus. (From Krakow,[1] by permission of The C.V. Mosby Company.)

Translocations

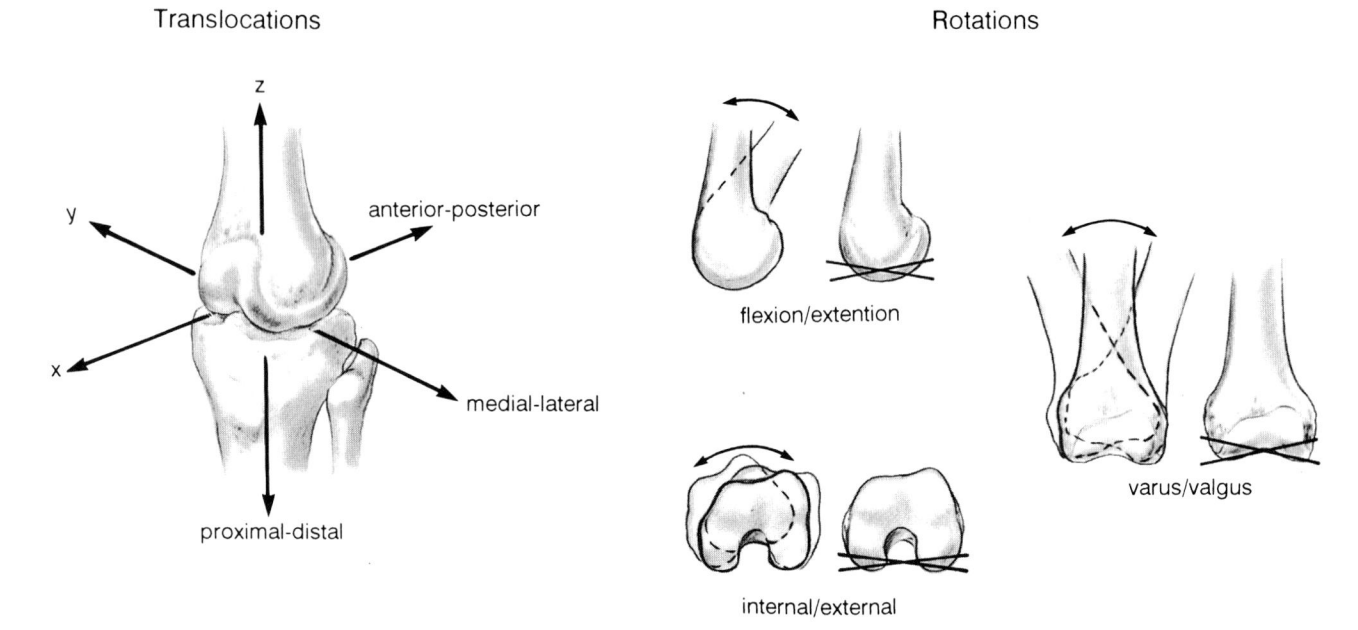

Rotations

Figure 33.6. The three transitional axes are noted by X, Y, and Z. For the tibia, the flexion-extension plane rotates about the Y axis, the varus-valgus plane rotates about the X axis, and the internal-external plane rotates about the Z axis. (From Rand,[8] by permission of Raven Press.)

lowed some designs to incorporate several degrees of posterior slope within the polyethylene insert, limiting the amount of posterior slope of the bony resection. Also, some systems incorporate the posterior slope into its cutting block, whereas others require a distal adjustment of the tibial cutting guide (Fig. 33.9). The surgeon must be familiar with the system and must create the correct posterior slope. Although rotation of the tibial component will be discussed later, the rotational orientation of the proximal tibial cut must be considered in the discussion of the flexion-extension plane. With any degree of posterior slope to the tibial cut, rotational malalignment of the tibial guide will tend to lead to varus or valgus obliquity of the cut. Consider a tibial resection performed at 90 degrees to the axis of the tibia with a 10-degree posterior slope built into the cut. If the cutting guide is inadvertently externally rotated (as could happen with the cutting guide oriented anteriorly over the tubercle as opposed to its medial surface), the resulting cut will be directed in flexion from anterior lateral to posterior medial as opposed to directly anterior to posterior (Fig. 33.10). Even if the correct rotational position of the component is chosen, a mild varus orientation of the tibial component will be noted (higher anterolateral: lower posteromedial). With lesser degrees of posterior slope, this error will be less apparent; however, this mild varus deformity, coupled with a mild varus cut and/or a slightly internally rotated tibial component will all contribute to increasing conflict in the kinematic and mechanical function of the knee arthroplasty.

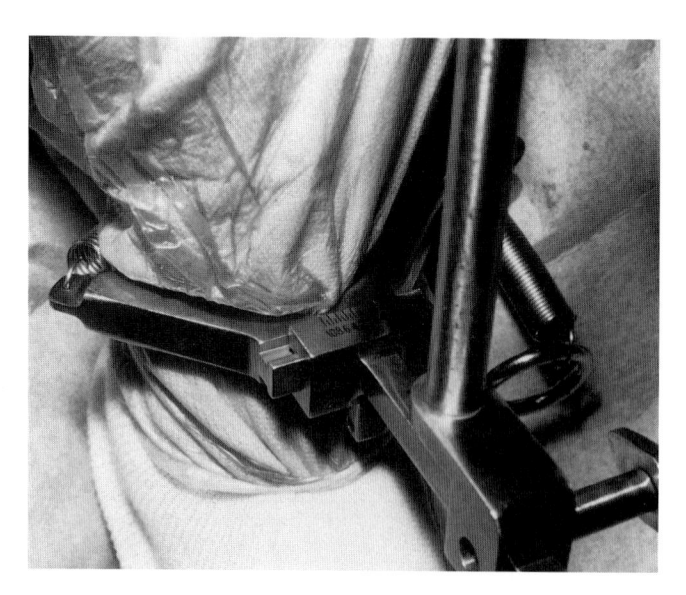

Figure 33.7. Medial displacement of the distal aspect of the tibial alignment guide is useful to avoid the common error of a varus tibial cut.

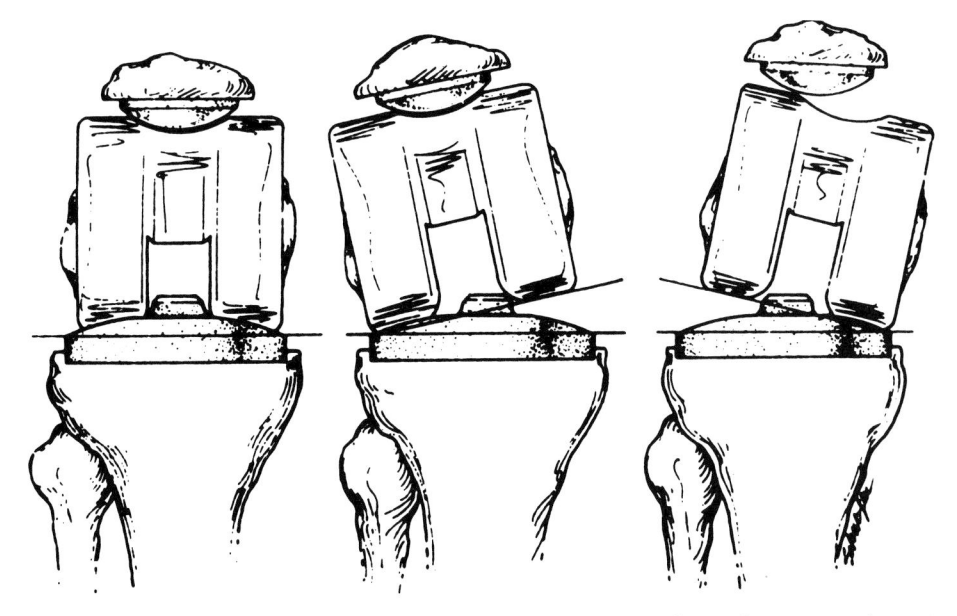

Figure 33.8. Illustrated is the relative effect of femoral rotation on patella tracking. Neutral position and an externally rotated position are well tolerated by the patella. Internal rotation of the femur moves the trochlear groove medially and contributes to patellofemoral maltracking. (From Figgie,[12] by permission of *Journal of Bone and Joint Surgery*.)

MEDIAL-LATERAL/ANTERIOR-POSTERIOR

These two degrees of positional freedom will be discussed together because the final rotational position of the tibial component simultaneously determines the mediolateral and anteroposterior position. With the many sizes of tibial components available today, the goal of mediolateral and anteroposterior positioning is to maximize proximal tibial coverage while avoiding any significant overhang. Medial overhang will cause painful irritation of the medial collateral ligament (Fig. 33.11). Lateral overhang is better tolerated due to positioning of the lateral collateral insertion on the fibular head, but still should be avoided. A limited amount of posterolateral tibial overhang seems to be tolerated well (Fig. 33.12). By accepting this overhang, internal rotation of the tibial component can be avoided. An asymmetric tibial component may avoid this posterolateral overhang but may not add to maximal proximal tibial coverage.[12]

Historically, posterior positioning of the tibial component of the resected tibial surface was recommended.[13] With the increasing number of tibial sizes available, maximal coverage of the tibia is the primary goal of the surgeon. The optimal size of the tibial component will minimize the forces of the bone-cement-metal interfaces. The use of larger tibial components may preclude posterior displacement of the component on the tibial bone.

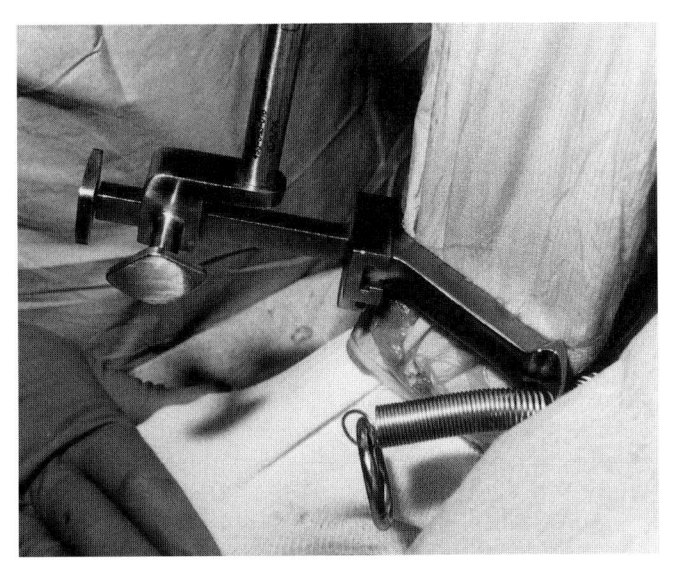

Figure 33.9. Several tibial alignment guides require distal adjustments to assure posterior slope of the tibial cut and to avoid extension in this cut.

PROXIMAL-DISTAL

A goal of the proximal tibial resection is to maintain the anatomic position of the joint line. Over-resection of the

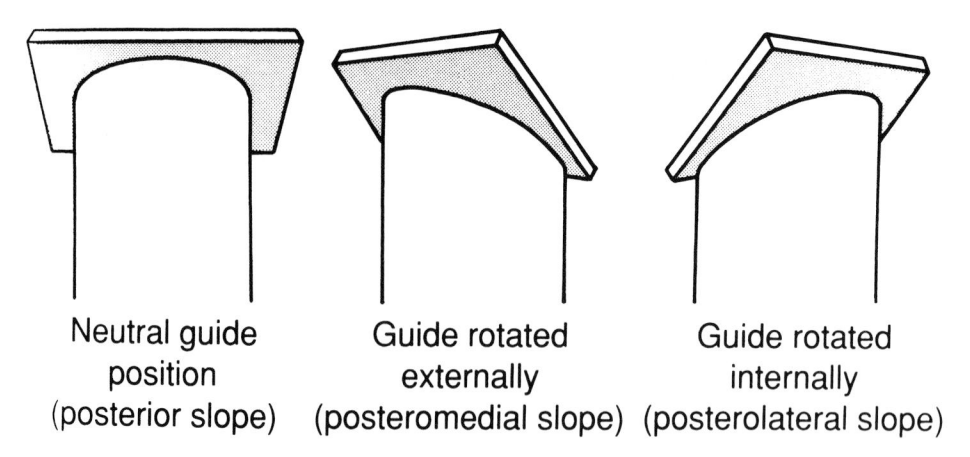

Neutral guide position (posterior slope)   **Guide rotated externally (posteromedial slope)**   **Guide rotated internally (posterolateral slope)**

Figure 33.10. Inadvertent rotation of the tibial cutting guide may lead to a varus (externally rotated guide) or valgus (internally rotated guide) orientation of the tibia cut. (From Insall,[2] by permission of Churchill Livingstone.)

joint line can be compensated for by insertion of a thicker tibial polyethylene. However, an increasing distal tibial resection may lead to two problems. First, the strength of the tibial bone diminishes rapidly as you go distal from the strong subchondral bone. Placement of the tibial component in this weaker supporting bone may compromise tibial fixation. Second, due to the funnel shape of the proximal tibia, distal resection will provide a smaller surface area of tibia and a smaller tibial component. Although many systems allow the use of different sizes of tibial and femoral components, the situation could lead to either a smaller articular contact surface area (with noncongruent articular designs) or the use of a polyethylene insert that overhangs the metal base plate (with congruent articular designs) (Fig. 33.13).

Proximal positioning of the tibial component (inadequate tibial resection) can lead to several problems. To maintain correct joint line position, an inadequate thickness of polyethylene has been used in the past. The accelerated wear and catastrophic polyethylene failure associated with minimal polyethylene thickness precludes their use (Fig. 33.14).

If a minimum standard of 8 to 10 mm of metal and polyethylene is used in the tibial component, the problem caused by an inadequate resection of the proximal tibial bone will depend on the surgical technique used. If a measured resection technique is used, the femur is resected independently of the tibia. After insertion of the tibial components, the knee will be tight in flexion *and* extension. The knee will not reach full extension and will be noted to roll back excessively in flexion (or the tibial polyethylene trial may be seen to lift off anteriorly) (Fig. 33.15). Additional tibial resection will correct the problem. If erroneously thought to be a problem of a tight PCL, resection of the PCL alone will be unlikely to resolve the problem. If a flexion-extension gap technique is used by the surgeon, the likely sequelae of inadequate tibial resection is compensatory over-resection of the distal femur and an elevation of the joint line. Although a slight rise in

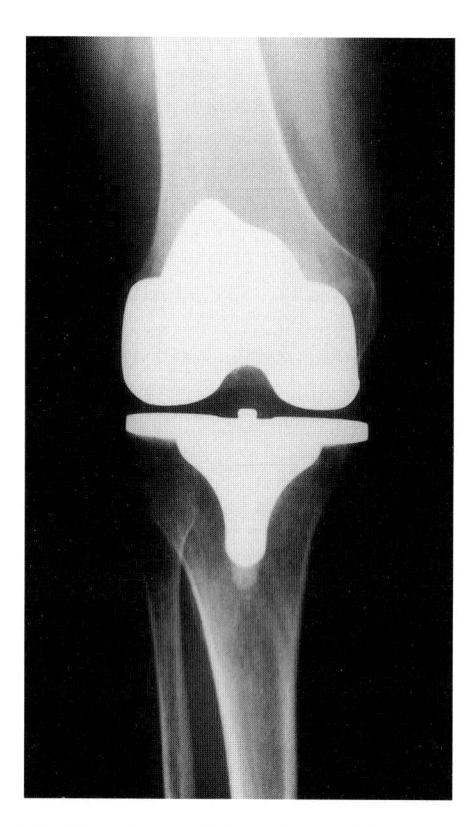

Figure 33.11. Note the medial overhang of the prosthesis on the proximal tibia. The patient's complaints of pain were significant and were localized anatomically to that area. The patient was revised to a smaller tibial component with prompt resolution of symptoms.

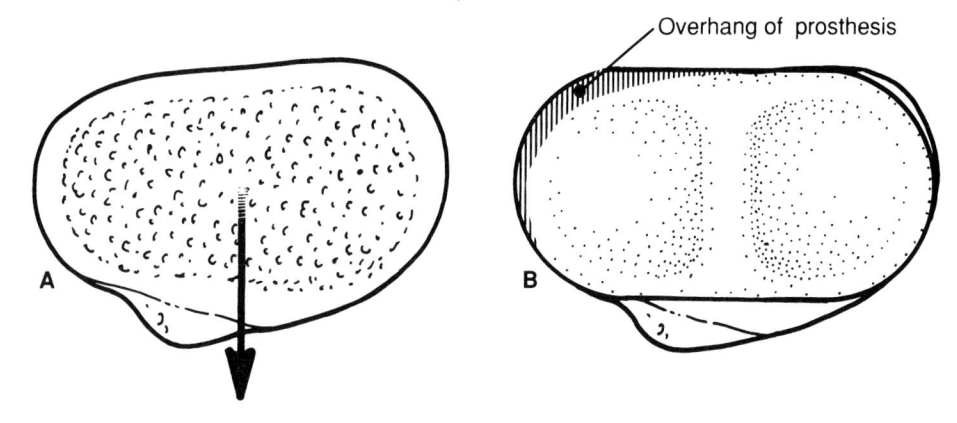

Figure 33.12. Limited amounts of posterolateral overhang of tibial prosthesis appears to be tolerated well and will help to avoid internal rotation of the tibial component. (From Insall,[2] by permission of Churchill Livingstone.)

the joint line position is tolerated well with cruciate-sacrificing or substituting knee designs, proximal positioning of the joint line and lowering of the patellar height has been shown to limit the functional result of the knee arthroplasty.[13–15]

Finally, with either surgical technique, the problem may be misinterpreted as an error in extension only. Additional distal femoral resection will result in a full extension, but the joint line will be moved proximally and flexion will likely be limited (Fig. 33.16).

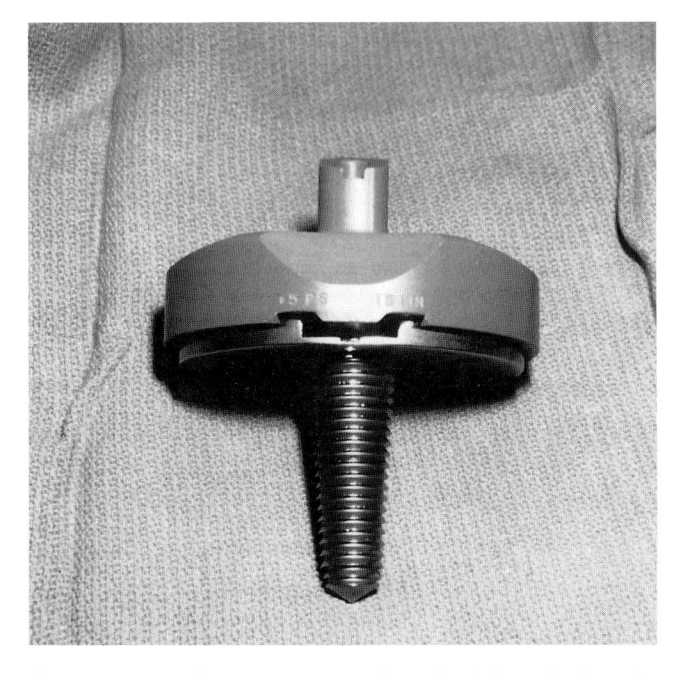

Figure 33.13. With congruent articular polyethylene designs, the polyethylene insert must match the size of the femoral component. The use of a smaller tibial component may require the use of a larger polyethyelene insert leading to overhang.

ROTATION

Internal rotation of the tibial component in TKA has long been appreciated as a cause of patellar instability. Internal rotation of the tibial articular surfaces places the tibial tubercle in a relatively externally rotated position. This effectively increases the Q-angle of the extensor mechanism increasing the likelihood of patellar maltracking or instability (Fig. 33.17). Although recognized as a potential problem, tibial rotation has not been reliably documented by radiographic or clinical means.

Recent work at our institution with computerized tomographic scanning (CT scan) has resulted in the radiographic measurement of tibial component positioning (Fig. 33.18). A preliminary study of patients with normal knees has demonstrated an angle of approximately 18 degrees of internal rotation between the orientation of the tibial articular surface and the *center* of the tibial tubercle. This angle, measured in patients undergoing successful TKA, reliably orients the tibial articular surface along the medial one-third of the tibial tubercle, supporting the clinical use of this long-standing anatomic landmark.

We have recently studied a group of patients with isolated patellofemoral failure following patellofemoral complications following TKA. These patients have documented adequate axial alignment, were not loose or infected, and had no apparent reason for their failure. CT evaluation of these patients demonstrated internal rotation of the tibia and/or femur in every case. More importantly, the severity of the clinical problem increased with the amount of additive internal rotation of the tibial and femur.[16] Although the study does not resolve all issues regarding component in TKA, it does document the influence of component malrotation on patellofemoral instability and provides a method of quantitat-

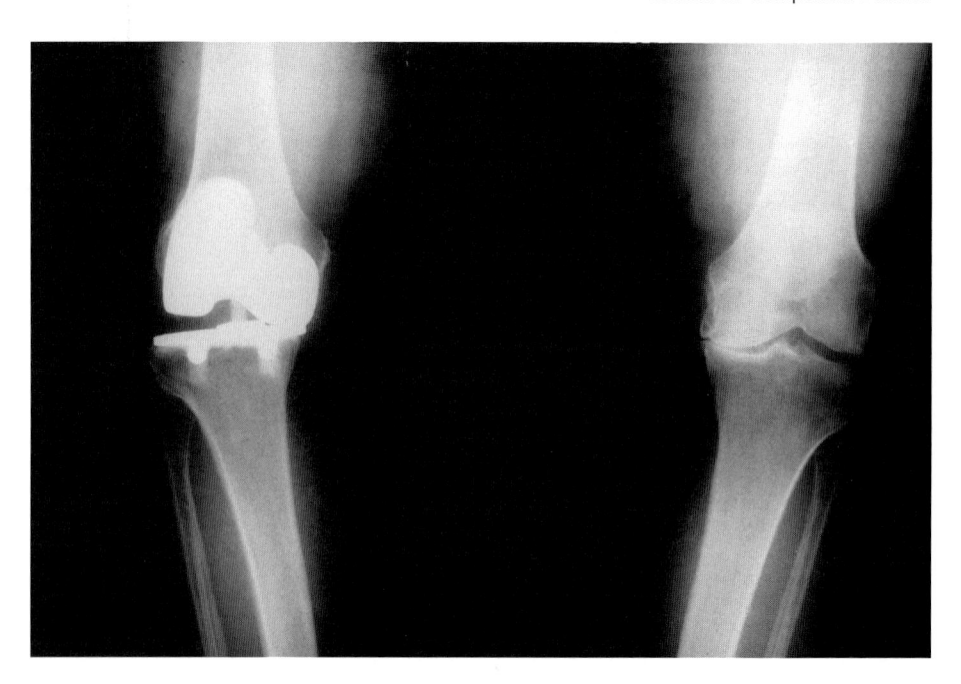

Figure 33.14. Catastrophic polyethylene wear associated with thin polyethylene bearing surfaces.

ing the relative rotational position of the tibial and femoral component following TKA.

The clinical method of determining the rotational position of the tibial component rotation during TKA has been debated. Two options include the selection of a fixed position based on anatomic landmarks or allowing the tibial trial to "float" and seek its own rotation position through a range of motion. Flat, unconstrained polyethylene would be most influenced by residual imbalance of the ligamentous structures and not likely to select an appropriate position. With increasing polyethylene congruency, the "floating" trial would be most influenced by the rotational position of the femoral component, especially in extension where conformity is usually highest. If the femoral position is correct, this method of tibial positioning would optimally align the

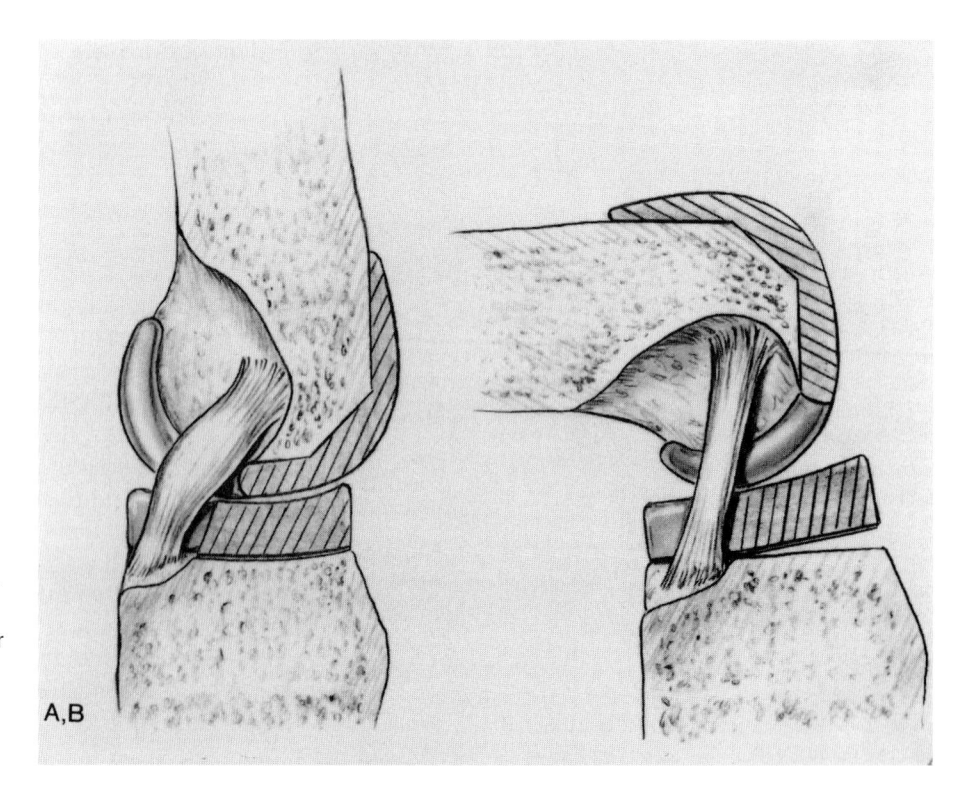

Figure 33.15. While commonly associated with a tight posterior cruciate ligament (PCL), the situation of excessive tibial rollback and anterior liftoff of the tibial trial may also be seen with an "overstuffed" flexion space. (From Rand,[1] by permission of Raven Press.)

33. Tibial Component Position

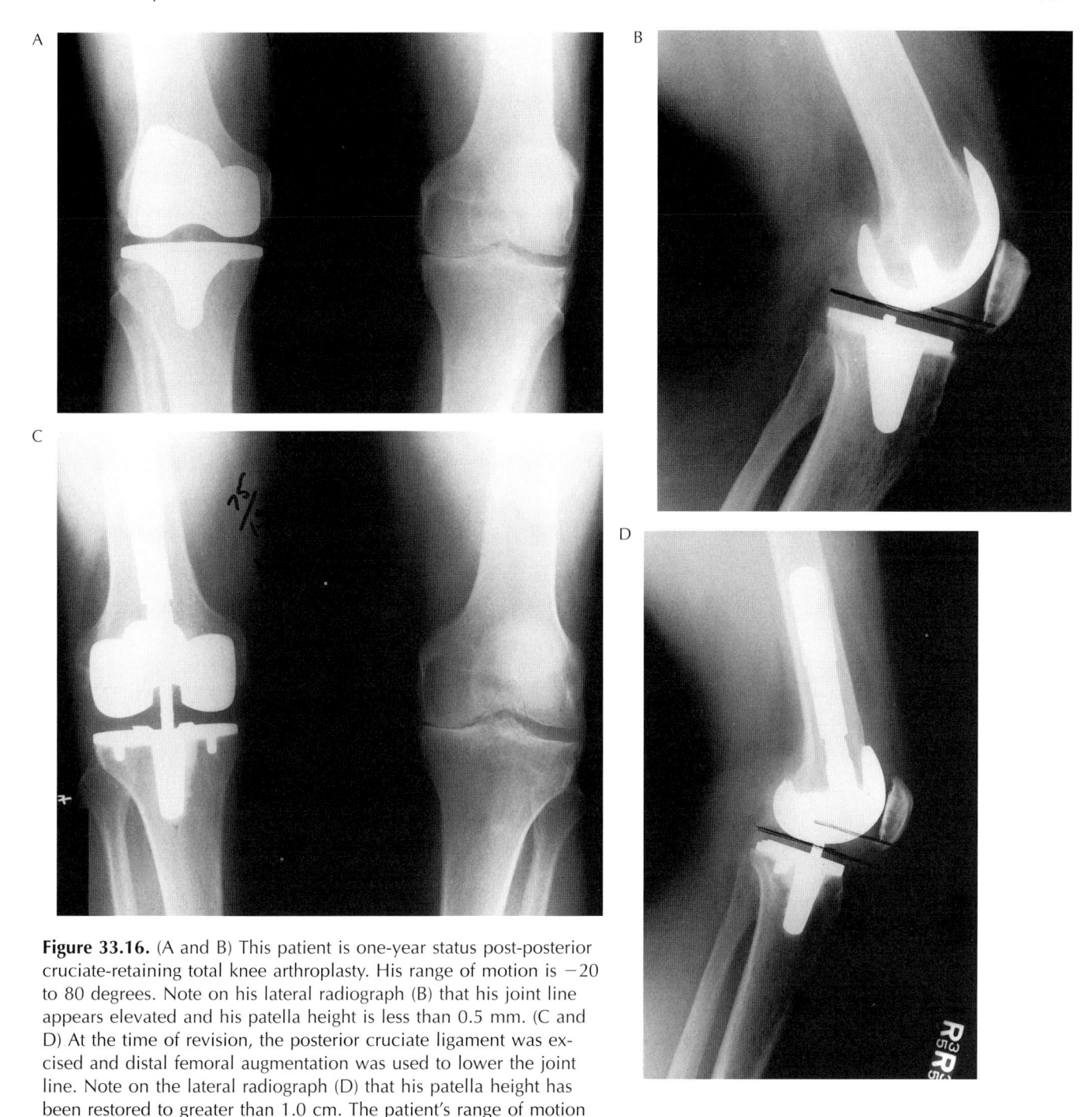

Figure 33.16. (A and B) This patient is one-year status post-posterior cruciate-retaining total knee arthroplasty. His range of motion is −20 to 80 degrees. Note on his lateral radiograph (B) that his joint line appears elevated and his patella height is less than 0.5 mm. (C and D) At the time of revision, the posterior cruciate ligament was excised and distal femoral augmentation was used to lower the joint line. Note on the lateral radiograph (D) that his patella height has been restored to greater than 1.0 cm. The patient's range of motion at four-months post-revision is −5 to 105 degrees.

components within a well-balanced soft tissue sleeve. If the femoral component position is incorrect (and internal rotation is the more common error), the tibial component position would mirror this error and select the position of matching internal rotation. As mentioned earlier, the additive error in component malrotation can adversely affect patellofemoral function.

The tibial rotational position can be determined and fixed by a trial. The final determination of the rotational position can be influenced by the trial reduction. If patellofemoral maltracking is noted during the range of motion with the trials, component malposition should be suspected. Any apparent conflict between the femoral and tibial position can be more easily noted in extension. Review of the rotational position of both components may reveal an error, and soft tissue tension should be inspected to assure equal and balance gaps. If using an instrument system em-

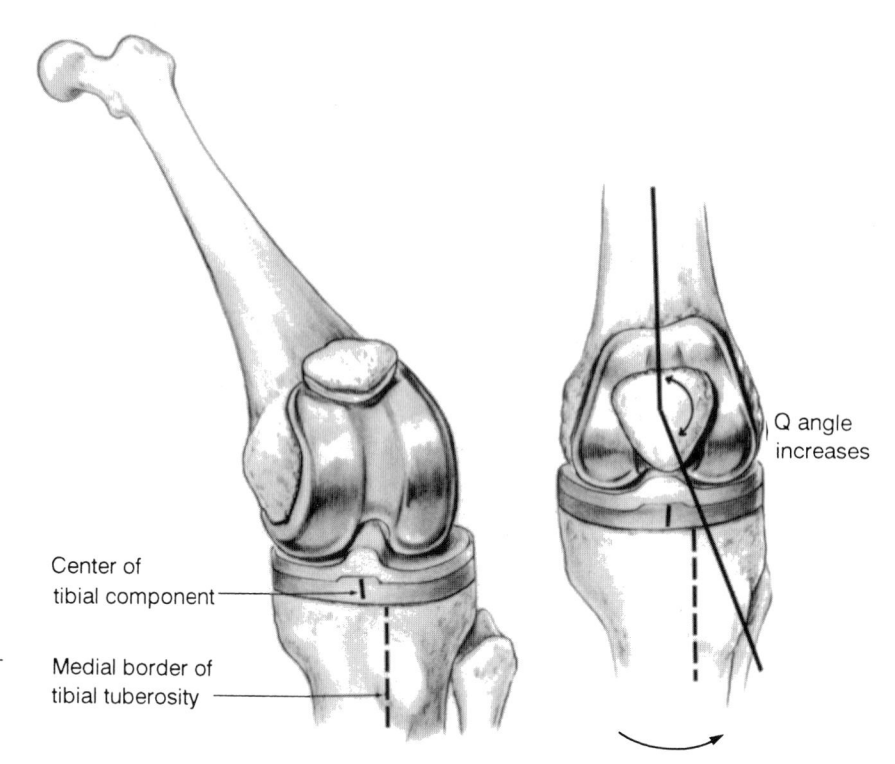

Figure 33.17. Internal rotation of the tibial component effectively increase the Q-angle leading to potential patellar instability. (From Rand,[1] by permission of Raven Press.)

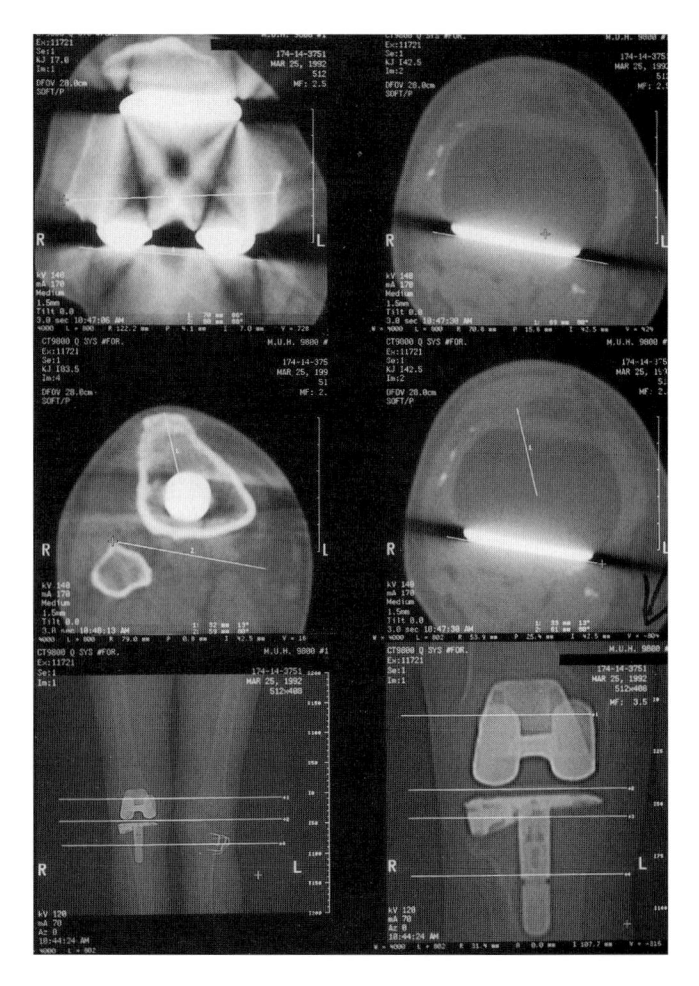

Figure 33.18. This patient complained of patellar instability following total knee arthroplasty. He had previously undergone a high tibial osteotomy. Rotational analysis of his femoral component shows internal rotation of the femoral component by 6 degrees (as referenced from the posterior condyles of the femoral component and the epicondylar axis, using the prominence of the lateral epicondyle and the sulcus of the medial epicondyle). Rotational analysis of the tibial component showed it to be 23 degrees internally rotated from the center of the tibial tubercle. The reference points for the tibial component are a line perpendicular to the transverse axis of the tibial component (direction of the tibia articular surface) and a line through the center of the tibial tubercle.

ploying a flexion-extension gap technique, a varus tibial cut should be suspected. Following the systematic review of the knee and observing the patellofemoral tracking, the final position of the tibial component can be determined.

Several anatomic landmarks have been used to aid in the selection of the tibial rotational position. The transverse axes of the tibial plateau, the tibial tubercle, the transmalleolar axis of the ankle, and the positioning of the second ray of the foot have all been described. The transmalleolar axis varies significantly between zero and 45 degrees and may not be reliable. The position of the second ray may be altered by pronation of the foot commonly noted when the knee is flexed during surgery. The transverse axis of the proximal tibial *and* the tibial tubercle should be used together to determine the tibial component rotation. A trial tibial component placed in the proper medial lateral and anteroposterior position and rotated appropriately should be directed over the medial one-third of the tubercle. No *single* anatomic landmark can be used exclusively. Extensive posterior tibial osteophytes or previous trauma can alter the appearance of the tibial plateau. Congenital patellofemoral dysplasia or previous surgery such as a Maquet or Hauser procedure can alter the position of the tibial tubercle. As is commonly the case, the appropriate decision is best made only after review of the appropriate surgical history, inspection of all anatomic landmarks, assessment of ligamentous balance, and observation of the trial components during range of motion.

References

1. Krackow KA. *The Technique of Total Knee Arthroplasty*. Philadelphia: CV Mosby Company; 1990.
2. Insall JN, et al. *Surgery of the Knee*. 2nd ed. New York: Churchill Livingstone; 1993.
3. Stern SH, Insall JN. Posterior stabilized prosthesis: results after follow-up of nine to 10 years. *J Bone Joint Surg*. 1992; 74A:980.
4. Lombardi AV, Sydney SV, Mallory TH, et al. Six-year survivorship analysis of the Insall-Burstein posterior stabilized knee: a clinical and radiographic evaluation. *Orthop Trans*. 1988; 12:711.
5. Ranawat CS, Boachio-Adjel O. Survivorship analysis and results of total condylar knee arthroplasty: eight–eleven year follow-up period. *Clinic Orthop*. 1988; 226:6–12.
6. Cobb AC, Ewald FC, Gordon NH, et al. The kinematic knee survivorship analysis of 1,943 knees. Proceedings of the Annual Meeting of the British Orthopeadic Assoc. *J Bone Joint Surg*. 1990; 72-B:542.
7. Ritter MA, Campbell E, et al. Long-term survival analysis of the posterior cruciate condylar total knee arthroplasty: A ten year evaluation. *J Arthroplasty*. 1989; 4:293–296.
8. Rand JA. *Total Knee Arthroplasty*. New York: Raven Press; 1993.
9. Bono JV, Roger DJ, Laskin RS, et al. Tibial intramedullary alignment in total knee arthroplasty. *Amer J Knee Surg*. 1985; 8(1):7–11.
10. Simmons ED, Sullivan JA, et al. The accuracy of tibial intramedulary alignment devices in total knee arthroplasty. *J Arthroplasty*. 1991; 6(1):45–50.
11. Evans TD, Marshall PD, et al. Radiographic study of the accuracy of a tibial intramedullary cutting guide for knee arthroplasty. *J Arthroplasty*. 1995; 10(1):43–46.
12. Incado SJ, Ronchetti PJ, et al. Tibial plateau coverage in total knee arthroplasty. *Clin Orthop*. 1994; 299:81–85.
13. Figgie HE, Goldberg VM, Heiple KG, Moller HD, Gordon NH. The influence of tibial-patellofemoral location of function of the knee in patients with the posterior stabilized condylar knee prosthesis. *J Bone Joint Surg*. 1986; 68-A:1035–1040.
14. Martin JW, Whiteside LA. The influence of jointline position on knee stability at the condylar knee arthroplasty. *Clin Orthop*. 1990; 259:146–156.
15. Sidles JA, Matsen SA, Garbini JL, et al. Total knee arthroplasty: functional effects of tibial resection level. *Trans Orthop Res Soc*. 1986; 11:263.
16. Berger RA, Crossett LS, et al. Component malrotation causing patella-femoral complication in total knee arthroplasty. AAOS, New Orleans, Louisiana 1994.

SECTION 9
Fixation

CHAPTER 34
Cement in Primary Total Knee Arthroplasty

Alfred J. Tria, Jr.

INTRODUCTION

The concept of resurfacing or replacing the knee joint was first entertained in the late 1860s.[1-4] By 1940 to 1950 the designs were improving significantly but the problem of fixation became a serious barrier to further progress. Before Charnley and his associates developed polymethylmethacrylate (PMMA), knee arthroplasty was limited to partial replacements of the joint surfaces and hinge designs that relied upon ligament stability and simple bone-metal contact to keep the prosthetic device in the planned position.[5,6] The early replacements did not include the patella. The membrane arthroplasties,[1,2,4] GUEPAR hinge,[6] and the MacIntosh interpositional arthroplasty[5] represented attempts to replace the surface and to relieve discomfort. The early results were encouraging; however, subsequent loosening and progression of the arthritis in other areas of the knee led to prosthetic failure.

In 1969, Charnley's laboratory developed PMMA for use in total hip arthroplasty.[7] Gunston applied the same technology to the polycentric knee and was able to resurface the tibiofemoral articulation and space the cruciate ligaments.[8] The prosthetic device was implanted with some simple guides and permitted better range of motion while preserving stability of the joint. Knee designs improved rapidly during the 1970s and 1980s in good part due to the more reliable fixation that the cement provided.

MONOMER, POLYMER, AND POLYMERIZATION

PMMA is a derivative of acrylic acid that is formed by the combination of a monomer liquid mixed with polymer powder that leads to an exothermic reaction with change into a solid state. The solid powder consists of polymethylmethacrylate polymer and methylmethacrylate-styrene copolymer. The liquid monomer (methylmethacrylate) leads to polymerization and bonds the spherical copolymer molecules in a polymethylmethacrylate matrix. Barium sulfate is often added to produce radiopacity for roentgenographic evaluation of the bone cement and metal cement interfaces. Although this addition does change the properties slightly, the ability to visualize the interfaces is of great importance.

All cements are not identical. The polymerization process takes several minutes with the change from the liquid state through a doughy period to a solid material. The sequence can be divided into three phases: the initial liquid period, the period of time as a doughy material, and the period of time from the doughy state to the solid phase. The time required for the monomer and the polymer to mix and become one liquid material ("wetting" stage) is usually quite short for all cement types; however, there can be some slight variation in the ease of the early mixing. It is difficult for the surgeon to change the first phase to any significant extent. The second phase from the liquid to the doughy state is much more susceptible to outside factors. The polymerization time can be altered by changing the temperature of either the liquid monomer or the powder polymer. Because the liquid monomer holds the temperature for a longer period of time than the powder, cooling the monomer has a much greater effect on the setup process. The total time required for the cement mixture to solidify is temperature dependent and is, therefore, affected by the ambient temperature of the operating room area. Humidity in the room also has a similar affect but to a lesser extent. The lower temperature inhibits the monomer-polymer reaction and less monomer is allowed to evaporate, leading to a higher concentration of free monomer and to a prolongation of the handling time.[9] Lower temperature and humidity combine to lengthen the setup time from the liquid to the doughy state. The particle size of the powder varies slightly from one manufacturer to another. The larger particle size prolongs the liquid phase and slows the changeover from the doughy to the solid state.[10]

Mixing the cement in a vacuum environment removes incorporated air more thoroughly and shortens the time from the liquid to the doughy state.[11] In a similar fashion the cement can be centrifuged to remove all of the air impurities and improve the overall consistency; however, this will also lead to a more rapid change from the liquid to the doughy state by increasing the viscosity.[12] The vacuum and centrifugation can increase the fatigue life of the cement by up to 136%.[13-15] Hansen examined nine different cements with both chilling and vacuum.[9] The data showed that vacuum alone shortened the setting time and preserved a higher viscosity during the handling time. Prechilling lowered the viscosity and prolonged the setting time. Combining the prechilling and the vacuum allowed a longer period to manage the cementing process in the operating room with a lower viscosity that permitted greater penetration into the bone. It is still important to note that both Burke and Hansen found significant variations between different manufacturers' cements.

The thickness (viscosity) of the cement after the monomer and polymer become liquid can also be controlled by the manufacturer. "Low-viscosity" cements remain liquid for a longer period of time with a thinner consistency that permits increased penetration into the bone surface. The prolongation of the liquid phase usually decreases the doughy phase time and requires slightly different handling in the operating room. In the liquid phase the mixture is more adherent to surfaces and tends to be "sticky" to palpation. Syringes and injection guns are often necessary to handle the cement in the liquid state.[16]

The final stage is from the doughy state to the solid cement. Similar to the first stage of the liquid mixing (wetting), this final stage is not significantly affected by outside factors such as temperature, humidity, vacuum, and centrifuging. This period of time does, however, vary slightly from one brand of cement to another.

Each manufacturer's cement tends to have its own unique properties that the surgeon must understand before changing from one to another. The viscosity of the initial liquid phase, the length of time for the liquid phase, the length of time for the doughy phase, and the time from doughy state to the solid state can all vary. The surgeon may prefer one over the other according to the requirements of his own primary arthroplasty technique; or, the surgeon may use the same cement for all arthroplasty cases with individual adjustments in temperature, vacuum, centrifuging, and his associated surgical technique. Most surgeons prefer one type of cement for all of the cases and make adjustments accordingly.

Palacos, CMW, Simplex, and Zimmer Regular represent just a few of the common cements that are available on the market. Palacos is commonly used in Europe with the addition of antibiotics.

Bone penetration can be a two-edged sword depending upon the needs of the surgeon. The first question that should be addressed is the ideal thickness of the cement mantle around the prosthesis. How much cement is necessary for ideal fixation? It is possible to have too little or too great a thickness? The total hip literature has a good deal of discussion concerning the mantle and in general implies that the ideal thickness is 2 to 5 mm.[17] The knee literature is not as clearly defined and the femoral and tibial sides are significantly different. The femoral components cover the distal femur and transfer compressive forces well. There are valid arguments that the cement is unnecessary on the femoral side.[18,19] On the tibial side, there can be significant rotational and bending forces that require a firm application to the underlying bone. On this side of the knee joint, a cement mantle is certainly desirable; however, the ideal thickness is probably suspect to a multitude of variables. Greater penetration can theoretically lead to firmer fixation and less chance of loosening of the prosthesis over time; however, the exothermic reaction that occurs as the cement sets within the bone may lead to bone necrosis and possible loss of the interstitial complex in the bone.[20] The death of the bone at the bone-cement interface is thought to occur from either the mechanical cutting devices (saws, rotary blades) that elevate the temperature as they shape the bone cut, or from the cement polymerization, or from leakage of the monomer into the surrounding bone.

Protein denatures at 56°C. The coagulation temperature of bone collagen is at least 70°C Jefferis recorded temperatures as high as 72°C in the greater trochanter in the cadaveric specimen.[21] However, in vivo the temperatures were between 53°C and 65°C at the bone-cement interface of the distal femur and the proximal tibia of the knee joint. Thus, it appears unlikely that there is significant matrix degeneration during the cemented implant process. However, this does not rule out the possibility of cellular death. Monomeric polymethylmethacrylate is toxic and does leach out from the cement mass during the polymerization process. It is still not clear if the monomer has a significant affect upon the surrounding bone.[22]

Ryd has published data that shows there is a temperature elevation with the use of power instruments. He reports a temperature of 47°C as the critical temperature for the induction of bone necrosis. Eight oscillating sawblades were tested on ox bone in the laboratory and led to temperatures of 34°C to 450°C. In vivo he recorded temperatures from 45°C to 100°C. Thus, it is possible that the exothermic reaction or the mechanical instruments can lead to necrosis at the bone-cement interface.[23] Yet, the data from Schultz shows negligible effect upon small tubular bones[24] and the data from Boss indicates no necrosis of the bed of the implant and shows a thin fibrous membrane alternating with bone and osteoid.[20] At this time it is safe to conclude that the thermal effects of the cemented total knee arthroplasty are not clinically significant.

PMMA PROPERTIES

After the cement has set up in the bone environment, it must interact with the prosthesis and with the bone as a form of intermediary. The cement is not an adhesive agent and performs best under conditions of compression. Young's modulus in compression for the PMMA is lower than that of cortical bone and of the metallic prostheses. The PMMA modulus is higher than the modulus of cancellous bone and slightly higher than the modulus of the polyethylene. Because the bone-cement interface is more critical than the prosthetic cement interface, it is best if the modulus of the cement is closer to that of the underlying bone. The present cements do have a close differential modulus but also have an order of 100 to 200 times less than the overlying prosthesis. Thus, the cement is acceptable but not ideal.[25]

The vacuum effect during cement preparation leads to fewer voids and an increase in the viscosity. The cement can also be subjected to centrifugation. This process leads to less aeration of the final solid material and to a more solid substrate. Davies showed that the centrifuged cement had greater fatigue properties when subjected to repeated tension compression testing. At physiologic strain levels, he found that 8 of the 11 uncentrifuged specimens fractured before undergoing 10 million cycles. The average number of cycles to failure was 1.8 million. All 11 centrifuged specimens remained intact at 10 million cycles.[12]

ADDITIVES

The most common additive to the cement mixture is an antibiotic. In the setting of the primary total knee, antibiotics are not usually added to the cement. The addition is more common in the revision total knee replacement or after a previous infection. Although the properties of the cement do change with this addition, the fatigue properties are not changed at all. Askew showed that the porosity of the tobramycin-cement complex was doubled; however, there were no significant differences in bending strength of any of the specimens.[26] If the antibiotic is added in the powder form, the cement properties are only slightly changed. Addition in the liquid form has greater effect and is not recommended. When antibiotics are added, each individual cement leaches the drug out to the surrounding soft tissues at a different rate partially related to the particle size of the powder that is used. Thus, it is again critical that the surgeon understands the properties of the specific cement that he is using.

CEMENT TECHNIQUE

The author presently cements all components in the total knee arthroplasty with a posterior-stabilized knee design. The cement is mixed in two separate stages some 2 to 3 minutes apart. Many surgeons cement all of the components with a single mix of cement. This technique can represent both a cost- and time-saving approach; however, it is much more demanding to set all of the components at once and does leave more possibility for malpositioning.

We presently use Simplex cement because the liquid, doughy, and final setup times are about the same. The patellar component is cemented at the same time as the femoral. The femoral cement is used in the doughy stage once the mixture is no longer "sticky." The patella is held in place in the bone bed with a clamp and the femoral component is impacted onto the distal femur with the cement placed on the exposed bone surface and with some cement placed on the posterior runners of the actual component. The posterior aspect of the femur is often obscured by the component itself and contact there is important. Therefore, we place cement on the runner itself to ensure full coverage. When the component is impacted onto the bone surface, there is a common tendency to place the component in the flexed position, especially because the cement covers the bone surface. The tendency is less common when the component design includes short condylar pegs; however, not all systems have the pegs. Thus, it is probably best to hand place the component onto the distal femur and adjust the early position before using mechanical impaction.

The two cement mixings are timed to allow for removal of the exposed cement from the femoral side without waiting for the complete setting of the cement. This usually requires a separation time of 2 to 3 minutes. It is important to observe the femoral side while turning direction to the tibial side to ensure that the femoral component does not lift off during the final setup stage and that it is not pulled off the bone surface in an overzealous attempt to expose the tibia for the cementing.

The tibial side is cemented last when a posterior-stabilized component is used. We prefer that this cement is slightly more liquid to allow for better penetration into the proximal tibia. The cement is hand applied and the intramedullary peg hole is manually "pressurized" with thumb pressure to block off the upper hole and force the cement into the metaphyseal bone. This technique develops a cement "bulge" about the distal intramedullary stem. The chief criticism of the "pressurization" technique for the tibial stem is the greater difficulty of removal of the complex with an increase in loss of bone substance. The author has performed approximately 1000 arthroplasties with this technique and has had 3 tibial loosenings (in the same series we have about 6 femoral loosenings). Less than 5 tibial components have required removal because of infection, and no significant bone compromise has occurred with the extraction of the tibial tray and the cement. The author does, however, agree that the technique for tibial component cementing remains controversial.

After the excess peripheral cement is removed from the tibial tray, the knee is located and extended with slight manual pressure to compress the components onto the bony surfaces. When the bone is osteoporotic (such as in the rheumatoid knee), the extension maneuver should be performed with care to avoid collapse of the underlying bone and loss of fixation of the components. We again remove excess cement before it is completely set up and hold tourniquet release until the cement is solid in order to preserve the bone-cement interface.

Our technique is individualized to our own prosthetic line and prosthetic design. At the present time in the United States there are more cruciate-retaining total knees performed than posterior-stabilized. The cruciate-retaining knees are often performed as "hybrid" replacements. The tibial and patellar components are cemented first, and the femoral component is impacted onto the distal femur with a cementless design. This technique requires only one portion of cement but also requires a slightly more expensive femoral component for cementless application. Thus, the cementless component does save some time but the cost benefit is questionable.

There are several variations for the cementing of the tibial component depending upon the design of the tibial tray. Some trays include a central intramedullary stem of 3 to 4 cm in length. Most surgeons cement the undersurface, including the stem. However, European surgeons often cement the undersurface and leave the stem uncemented and without a special surface for ingrowth. The latter technique is not recommended by most designers but is at the decision of the operating surgeon. The short intramedullary stem is designed to share load with the surrounding metaphyseal bone and performs this function best, if there is some bone ingrowth or if there is a cement mantle around the stem to transfer load over to the bone. If the stem is cemented or fully coated for bone ingrowth, revision surgery will certainly be more difficult and will probably lead to greater bone loss. Yet, poor fixation leads to loosening and a certain revision.

Other trays are designed with four short pegs of approximately 10 mm in width and length that can all be cemented with the undersurface of the tray. Some new designs are returning to the all-polyethylene tibial component because of cost concerns. In this setting the entire component should be cemented, including the short intramedullary stem.

SUMMARY

At the present time, total knee surgeons are still faced with the decision concerning the type of fixation that they will rely upon for knee arthroplasty. The two camps have well-established theories. Cementless fixation has long-term results that are equal to those of the cemented prostheses. Studies out to 15 years and now approaching 20 years clearly document reliable results.[27-30] The well-ingrown total knee should remain fixed for a lifetime with just the possibility of polyethylene wear as the only consequence. The major problem with the cementless technology is the early loosening. Almost all studies report a 1% incidence most commonly on the tibial side. The loosening may be the result of surgical failure to establish full, acceptable surface contact. If this is the case, improvement in surgical technique should help to decrease loosening rates. There are new cutting instruments (such as milling devices) and guides that may improve surgical accuracy and increase contact. However, the loosening can be a result of micromotion at the interface that may be unavoidable if one expects to move the joint early after surgery to maintain range of motion. In this scenario, loosening may represent a persistent problem.

The cemented prostheses also have an excellent long-term history with similar 15- to 20-year results. The early loosening rate is well below 1% and is a rare occurrence. However, there is the lingering question concerning ultimate failure of the cement mantles. Thus far, this ultimate failure rate has not presented itself at the 15- to 20-year mark. Some investigators believe that the failure is inevitable. However, the surgeon must presently choose between a well-known early loosening rate with the cementless design or a theoretical concern for the future that has not as yet presented itself as a significant problem.

In light of this discussion, the author remains dedicated to cement fixation with an open eye toward the improvement of the cementless technology.

References

1. Verneuil AS. Affection articular du genou. *Arch med.* 1863.
2. Baer WS. Arthroplasty with the aid of animal membrane. *Am J Orthop Surg.* 1918; 16:1–29, 171–199.
3. Campbell WC. Arthroplasty of the knee: Report of cases. *Am J Orthop Surg.* 1921; 19:430–434.

4. Brown JE, McGaw WH, Shaw DT. Use of cutis as an interposing membrane in arthroplasty of the knee. *JBJS*. 1958; 40:1003–1018.
5. MacIntosh DL. Arthroplasty of the knee in rheumatoid arthritis (abstract). *JBJS*. 1966; 48:179.
6. Mazas FB, GUEPAR. GUEPAR total knee prosthesis. *Clin Orthop*. 1973; 94:211–221.
7. Charnley J. The reaction of bone to self-curing acrylic cement: a long-term histological study in man. *J Bone Joint Surg*. 1970; 52B:340–353.
8. Gunston FH. Polycentric knee arthroplasty: prosthetic simulation of normal knee movement. *JBJS* Br. 1971; 52: 272–277.
9. Hansen D, Jensen JS. Prechilling and vacuum mixing not suitable for all bone cements. *J Arthroplasty*. 1990; 5:287–290.
10. Bloch B, Haken JK, Hastings GW. Evaluation of cold curing acrylic cement for prosthesis stabilization. *Clin Orthop*. 1970; 72:239.
11. Wixson RL, Lautenschlager EP, Novak MA. Vacuum mixing of acrylic bone cement. *J Arthroplasty*. 1987; 2:141–149.
12. Davies JP, O'Connor DO, Burke DW, Harrigan TP, Harris WH. The effect of centrifuging bone cement. *J Bone Joint Surg*. 1989; 71B:39–42.
13. Burke DW, Gates EI, Harris WH. Centrifugation as a method of improving tensile and fatigue properties of acrylic bone cement. *J Bone Joint Surg*. 1984; 66:1265–1273.
14. Lidgren L, Drar H, Moller J. Strength of polymethylmethacrylate increased by vacuum mixing. *Acta Orthop Scand*. 1984; 55:536.
15. Robinson RP, Wright TM, Burstein AH. Mechanical properties of polymethylmethacrylate bone cements. *J Biomed Mater Res*. 1981; 15:203.
16. Miller J, Krause WR, Krug WH, Eng B, Kelebay L. Low voscosity cement. *Clin Orthop*. 1992; 276:4–6.
17. Ebramzadeh E, Sarmiento A, McKellop HA, Llinas A, Gogan W. The cement mantle in total hip arthroplasty. Analysis of long term radiographic results. *J Bone Joint Surg*. 1994; 76:77–87.
18. Homsy CA, Cain TE, Hessler FB, Anderson MS, King JW. Porous implant systems for prosthesis stabilization. *Clin Orthop*. 1972; 89:220–235.
19. Cook SD, Thomas KA, Haddad RJ. Histologic analysis of retrieved human porous-coated total joint components. *Clin Orthop*. 1988; 234:90–101.
20. Boss JH, Shajrawi I, Dekel S, Mendes DG. The bone cement interface: histological observations on the interface of cemented arthroplasties within the immediate and late phases. *J Biomater Sci Polym Ed*. 1993; 5:221–230.
21. Jefferis CD, Lee AJC, Ling RS. Thermal aspects of self-curing polymethylmethacrylate. *J Bone Joint Surg*. 1975; 57:511–518.
22. Dahl OE, Garvik LJ, Lyberg T. Toxic effects of methylmethacrylate monomer on leukocytes and endothelial cells in vitro. *Acta Orthop Scand*. 1994; 65:147–153.
23. Toksvig-Larsen S, Ryd L, Lindstrand A. Temperature influence in different orthopaedic sawblades. *J Arthroplasty*. 1992; 7:21–24.
24. Schultz RJ, Johnston AD, Krishnamurthy S. Thermal effects of polymerization of methylmethacrylate on small tubular bones. *Int Orthop* 1987; 11:277–282.
25. Swanson SAV, Freeman MAR. Methylmethacrylate as a bonding agent. In: *The Scientific Basis of Joint Replacement*. New York: Wiley and Sons; 1977: 151–152.
26. Askew MJ, Kufel MF, Fleissner PR, Gradisar IA, Salstrom SJ, Tan JS. Effect of vacuum mixing on the mechanical properties of antibiotic impregnated polymethylmethacrylate bone cement. *J Biomed Mater Res*. 1990; 24:573–580.
27. Scuderi GR, Insall JN, Windsor RE, Moran MC. Survivorship of cemented knee replacements. *J Bone Joint Surg*. 1989; 71:798–803.
28. Stern SH, Insall JN. Posterior stabilized prosthesis. Results after follow-up of nine to twelve years. *J Bone Joint Surg*. 1992; 74:980–986.
29. Moran CG, Pinder IM, Lees TA, Midwinter MJ. Survivorship analysis of the uncemented porous-coated anatomic knee replacement. *J Bone Joint Surg*. 1991; 73:848–857.
30. Whiteside LA. Cementless total knee replacement. Nine to 11 year results and 10 year survivorship analysis. *Clin Orthop*. 1994; 309:185–192.

CHAPTER 35
Cementless Total Knee Arthroplasty

Aaron A. Hofmann and David F. Scott

INTRODUCTION

Cementless total knee arthroplasty presently enjoys a success rate equal to cemented designs. Clinical results of early cementless total knee replacements had both design and development problems,[1-3] similar to early cemented systems.[2,4] Some early cementless knee series had suboptimal results, especially with metal-backed patellas.[5-10] Likewise, just as cemented total knee designs and clinical results improved,[11,12] so too have the evolution and clinical results of cementless total knee replacements. Cemented and cementless total knee arthroplasty are similar in respect to requirements for alignment, ligament balancing, and precise bone cuts. In order to achieve durable fixation, cementless fixation may require greater surgical precision than cemented TKA, and is optimized by certain prosthetic design modifications. Cementless fixation may provide several advantages, especially for the younger and more active patient. With increasing life expectancy, a more durable interface would be desirable, especially if bone rather than fibrous tissue attachment could be reproducibly assured. If porous-coated stems and pegs are avoided in the majority of primary total knee replacements, potential future revisions are more bone-sparing.

A number of recent reports indicate that excellent results can be obtained with cementless total knee arthroplasty,[13-17] especially if design considerations are coordinated with surgical technique. The authors' 7- to 11-year experience demonstrates that primary cementless fixation in an appropriately selected patient group provides results comparable to cemented TKA with the advantage of conserving bone stock and eliminating the potential problems of methylmethacrylate fixation.[18]

CEMENTLESS IMPLANT DESIGN

There are several important design and surgical considerations for cementless total knee arthroplasty components. These include biological issues such as the type of coating utilized to promote bone ingrowth, the routine use of morselized autogenous bone chips, and careful patient selection. Other considerations include the geometry of the components, and their alignment and kinematics after implantation.

CEMENTLESS IMPLANT DESIGN: BIOLOGIC CONSIDERATIONS

Patient Selection

We treat a relatively young (average age of TKA patient: 64 years) and very active patient population with osteoarthritis or well-controlled rheumatoid arthritis, and consequently select almost 90% for cementless fixation. Older, sedentary patients with poor bone quality or major medical problems are selected for cemented fixation.

Porous Coating

Although some early designs included femoral components fabricated from treated titanium alloy with a titanium alloy-polyethylene articulation, most femoral components are now fabricated from cobalt chrome for improved polyethylene wear and resistance to third body wear. Our choice for the porous coating is commercially pure titanium sintered to a cobalt chrome alloy substrate. This has been shown to provide excellent bone ingrowth.[19] Our preference for the femoral component is a bimetal design, combining the superior wear properties of cobalt chrome with polyethylene, and the biocompatibility of titanium.[20] This coating has an average pore size of 400 μm and a porosity of 55%, compared to a beaded surface porosity of about 35% regardless of bead size.

Porous-coated pegs and stems are avoided to minimize stress-shielding of the interface and improve bone preservation during revision. Porous-coated pegs may cause a starburst pattern of bone ingrowth, which stress shields the remaining interface and causes significant bone loss if revision is required.

Autogenous Bone Chips as a Biologic Cement

Analysis of the resected proximal tibia reveals that the cortical bone surface area is an average of 6% of the total tibial surface, and that cancellous bone accounts for 18% of the total area, with bone marrow space comprising 76% of the remaining surface area.[21] The implication is that some form of "cement" is required to increase the surface attachment between the tibial component and the resected cancellous bone, and thus eliminate loosening and subsidence and provide durable fixation. The authors advocate the routine use of autograft cancellous bone chips[22–25] as a biologic "cement" to improve bone ingrowth by reconstructing the subchondral bone region creating a dense neocortex at the implant interface, and to increase the cancellous bone surface attachment of porous-coated tibial components to host bone.[24,25] The autologous bone chips are prepared using the patellar reaming instruments on the cut surface of the tibial wafer.

The use of morselized autogenous bone chips appears to enhance the fixation of cementless components. An experimental study was performed in which paired porous-coated devices were implanted with and without the addition of morselized autogenous bone chips into the contralateral medial femoral condyle of patients undergoing the first stage of bilateral total knee arthroplasty.[25] The devices were removed *en bloc* at the second total knee arthroplasty. Backscattered electron imaging revealed significantly more bone in the implant with autogenous bone chips. Tetracycline labeling demonstrated that this was living bone. In a postmortem retrieval study[23] of tibial components implanted with and without supplementary morselized autograft bone chips, the tibial components implanted with bone chips had a clear advantage in bone ingrowth and bone apposition to the porous-coated surface. Postmortem retrieval analysis of 10 porous-coated tibial components implanted with autograft cancellous bone chips revealed bone in contact with 64% of the porous-coated interface, and backscattered electron imaging revealed bone ingrowth within 8 to 22% of the porous coating by volume[24] (Fig. 35.1).

CEMENTLESS IMPLANT DESIGN: GEOMETRY

Femoral and Tibial Component Design

An anatomic design with near-normal kinematics is required for successful cementless total knee arthroplasty. Smooth pegs are preferred for all three components. If a tibial stem is required, it should also possess a non-porous surface. The femoral component is a bimetal design as discussed previously. A deep trochlear groove is desirable because it improves range of motion, and minimizes patellar subluxation or dislocation,[2] and prevents excess wear and load on the patellar component. It should be angled 6 degrees as in the normal distal femur for proper tracking. A deep trochlear groove avoids functional shortening of the extensor mechanism seen in knee systems that have shallow grooves.[2]

The proximal tibia is 5 to 6 mm smaller on the lateral side than on the medial side.[26] An asymmetric replacement will provide the best coverage of the proximal tibia and avoid soft tissue impingement. With symmetric replacements, the only options are undersizing the medial side or overhanging the lateral side.[27–29] It has been suggested that tibial coverage is inadequate with a symmetric tibial baseplate without overhang.[27,28] Tibial fixation and initial stability is also enhanced with two 6.5 mm titanium alloy cancellous bone screws that augment the components' four peripherally placed smooth pegs. A smooth central stem is recommended when fixation is required in softer bone (i.e., rheumatoid arthritic patients, osteoporotic females).[30]

Patellar Component Design

Failure of metal-backed patellar components has been attributed to insufficient polyethylene thickness around the periphery of the metal backing and the absence of an anatomically deep trochlear inset in the femoral component. Our preferred patellar component[31] has a modified dome-shaped polyethylene button that has a minimum 3 mm thickness around the periphery, and no overhanging polyethylene (Fig. 35.2). Patellar component fixation is augmented by three integral peripherally placed smooth pegs inserted into a planed flat bed. The thickness of the metal-backed patellar component can be accommodated without over-thickening the patella-implant complex by countersinking the implant 2 to 3 mm into the reamed bone bed. This is an essential surgical step in order to prevent the recent problems with metal-backed patellar components.

CEMENTLESS IMPLANT ALIGNMENT AND KINEMATICS

Restoration of Normal Alignment

Anatomic and radiographic studies reveal that the normal joint line is oriented horizontally. An average of 6 degrees of overall tibiofemoral valgus is produced by an average of 8 to 9 degrees of distal femoral valgus combined with an average of 2 to 3 degrees of proximal tibial varus (range: 0 to 6 degrees),[32] and the joint line is parallel to the floor. Following this orientation during total knee arthroplasty provides an anatomic alignment.

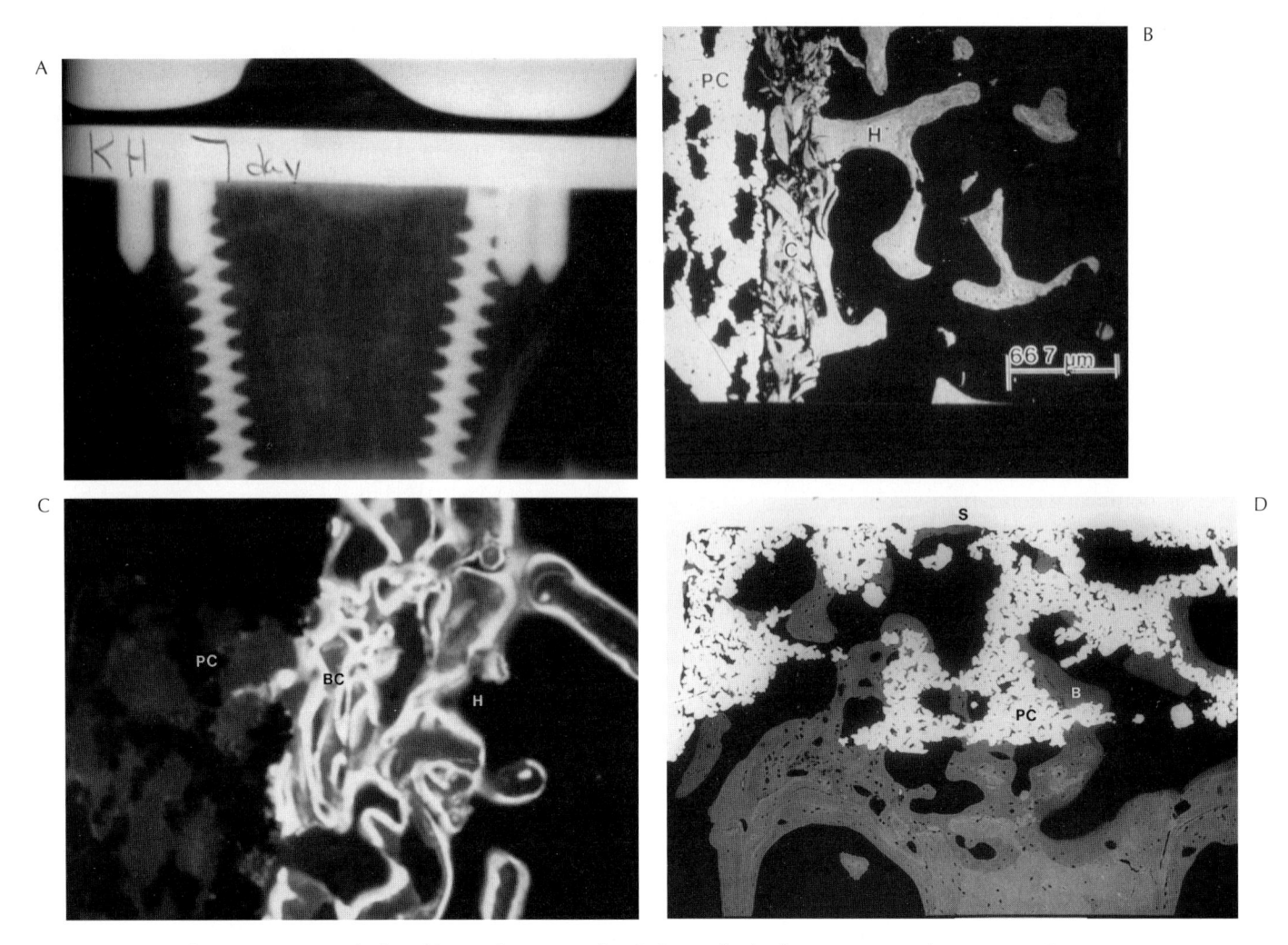

Figure 35.1. [A] "Blush" of bone chips immediately beneath tibial component 7-days postop. [B] Backscattered electron imaging showing the bone chips interposed between the porous coating (PC) and the host tissue (H). Three-week postmortem retrieval. [C] Tetracycline-labelled bone chips (BC) interposed between the porous coating (PC) and host bone (H) demonstrating viability and incorporation of bone chips at 12 weeks. Human in vivo plug model. [D] Bone ingrowth into retrieved tibial component 6-years postimplantation showing excellent bone ingrowth (B) into porous coating (PC). Osteointegration of bone and porpus coating demonstrated. Substrate (S).

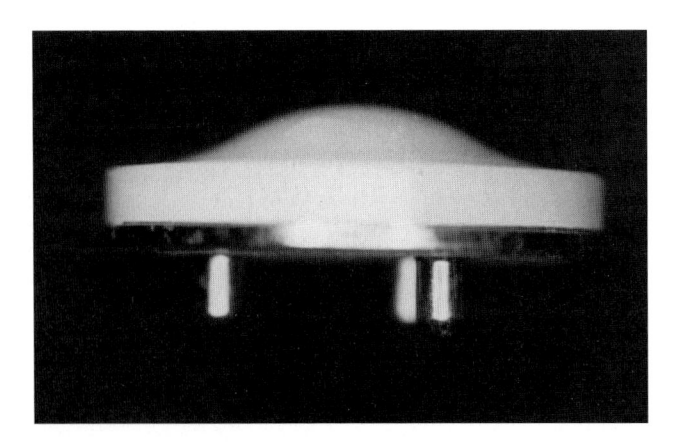

Figure 35.2. Photograph of metal-backed Natural-Knee™ patellar component demonstrating minimum 3 mm peripheral polyethylene thickness.

This places the mechanical axis slightly into the medial compartment providing an even distribution of forces across an asymmetric tibial tray. No external rotation of the femoral component is required for this method.

Most total knee instrumentation produces a slightly different joint line, which is oriented perpendicular to the mechanical axis (from the center of the femoral head to the center of the ankle), due to a tibial resection that is perpendicular to the long axis of the tibia. The joint line produced is generally 2 to 3 degrees from parallel to the floor. Krakow has referred to this alignment approach as *classical* alignment.[33] Externally rotating the femoral component 3 degrees is recommended to compensate for the iatrogenic soft tissue imbalance that this creates (Fig. 35.3).

Our preference is to reestablish the normal anatomy

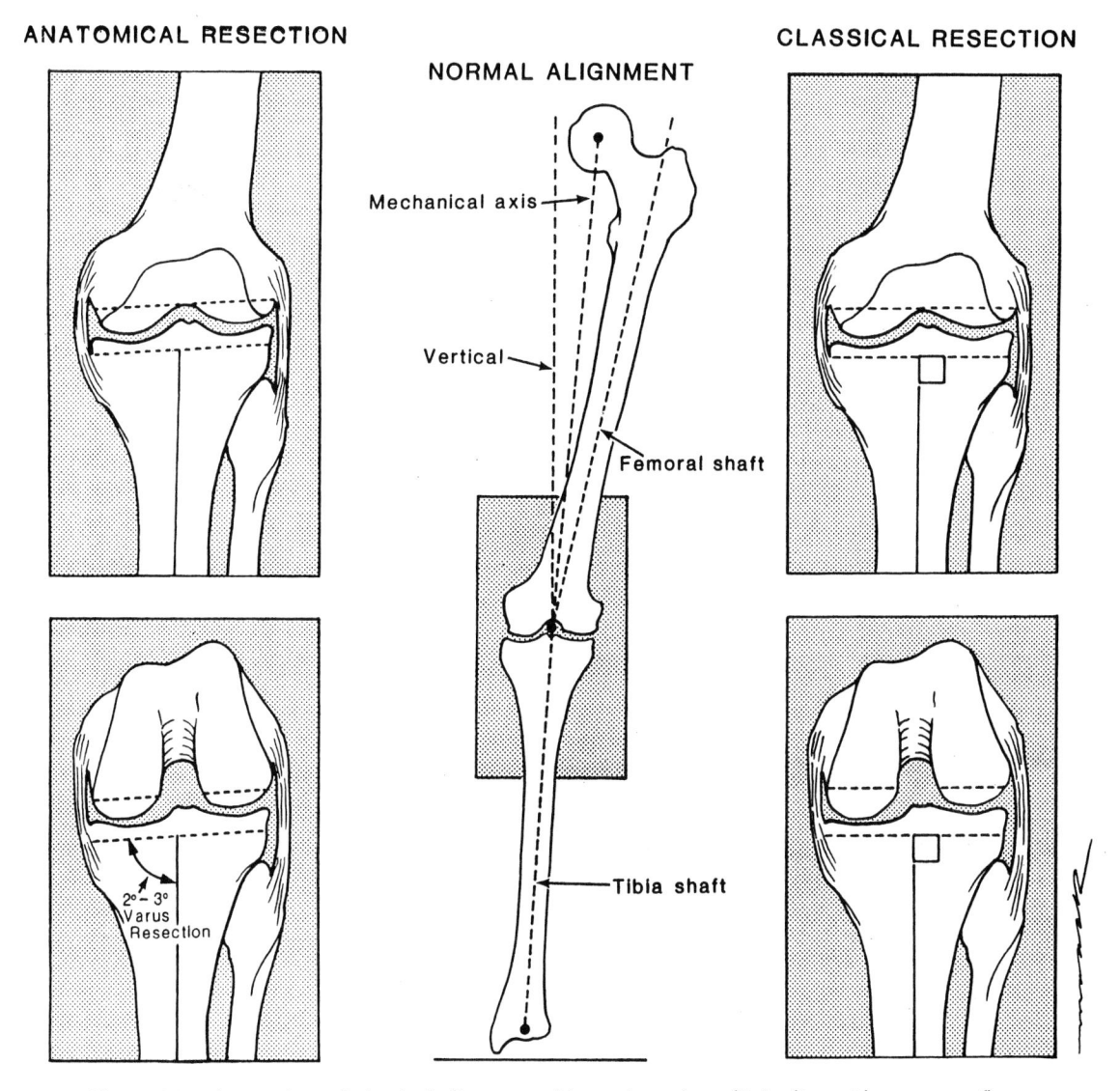

Figure 35.3. Anatomic and classical alignments. Note orientation of joint line with respect to floor.

as closely as possible, in order to achieve the goal of normal kinematics. Correct positioning of the implants is usually accomplished by cutting the tibia perpendicular for the valgus knee, or in slight varus in the frontal plane for the varus knee, and by cutting the distal femur in 6 degrees of valgus from the anatomic axis. This accomplishes an overall alignment of 4 to 6 degrees of valgus with better patellar tracking. A standard 6-degree valgus cut of the femur is recommended, although the instruments allow 4, 6, or 8 degrees. The anatomic-mechanical axis angle can be measured from a radiograph, but it may be inaccurate by 1 to 2 degrees because of rotational inconsistency. The true anatomic axis may be off with all intramedullary instruments if the starting point on the distal femur is too medial or lateral, or if the medullary rod is not perfectly centered in the medullary canal.

Restoration of Anatomy

A measured resection technique[33] is used for resurfacing the knee by referencing the least-diseased portion of the femoral condyle, the least-involved portion of the tibial plateau, and the thickest portion of the medial facet of the patella. The resected bone is replaced millimeter for millimeter with implant. This restores bony anatomy and the anatomic joint line. Knee rotation testing and computer modeling have shown that the level of resection relative to the amount replaced by the prosthesis on the distal femur plays an important role in knee kinematics and ligament balance. Resection of bone followed by an equal amount of prosthetic replacement will provide the knee with near normal varus-valgus and rotational stability throughout the full range of motion and excellent clinical results.

The level of the trochlear groove on the femur is anatomically restored by a stepped anterior chamfer cut that allows the bone to be resected and replaced with a deeply grooved femoral component. As a result, patellofemoral joint stability is achieved, making lateral release infrequent and, when required, less extensive. Increased patellofemoral compressive forces are avoided by maintaining the patellofemoral joint line, which reduces wear and patellar breakage and failure.

The tibial cut is made parallel to the joint line in the sagittal plane. Because the normal posterior tilt of the tibia is not at a fixed angle (range 4 to 12 degrees), this cut must be adjustable to reproduce each individual's normal posterior slope.[34] If the posterior slope is fixed at a single angle, the normal kinematics of the knee will not be simulated, because the PCL will be either too loose or too tight. Furthermore, cutting the tibia parallel to the patient's natural posterior slope greatly improves the load-carrying capacity of the supporting bone. A 40% improvement in ultimate compressive strength was noted when bone cuts were made parallel to the joint versus those made perpendicular to the tibial shaft axis.[34] Clinically, anterior subsidence is avoided if the tibial cut closely matches the anatomic posterior slope. Recent basic science investigations conducted in our research labs utilizing stereoscopic analysis have shown that when the bone is resected parallel to the natural anatomical slope, the trabeculae are oriented parallel to the resultant load.[35] This study provides a morphological explanation for the increased biomechanical strength measured in our previous study.[34]

For marked anatomic variation (i.e., malunion), an external alignment tower pointing toward the preoperatively marked femoral head can be utilized.

PCL Retention or Substitution

The authors argue that PCL retention better preserves the normal kinematics of the knee with maintenance of femoral rollback, clearance of the femur for increased range of motion and quadriceps strength, increased stair-climbing ability, fewer patellar complications, and reducing anteroposterior shear forces thus reducing bone-prosthesis interface shear stress.[36–41]

Balancing of the flexion and extension gaps is critically dependent upon the preoperative state of the posterior cruciate ligament. If the PCL is contracted in valgus knees or knees with fixed flexion deformities, flexion-extension balancing is difficult, and the PCL should be sacrificed. The PCL is often inadequate or absent in cases of inflammatory arthritis, as well as in some cases of advanced degenerative arthritis. When the PCL is sacrificed or incompetent, stability of the knee depends upon PCL substitution.[42–44] In traditional PCL-substituting TKA systems, a central polyethylene post of the posterior middle portion of the tibial insert articulates with a transverse cam on the femoral component. As the knee flexes to 75 degrees, the post and cam come into contact, preventing the tibia from subluxating posteriorly and maintaining femoral rollback. Although this design has proven useful, it is not without problems and complications including post failure and dislocation. In order to improve results with posterior stabilization, a more congruent (ultracongruent) tibial polyethylene insert was designed[45] (Fig. 35.4). The insert is designed with an anterior buildup of 12.5 mm, and a more congruent articular surface to stabilize the femur in the anteroposterior plane, and has proven clinically successful for over 5 years.[45]

Patella Medialization

Patellar maltracking problems in total knee arthroplasty have ranged from 1 to 20% in the literature, and up to 50% of knee revisions are due to patella-related complications.[4,46,47] Multiple causes of patellar maltracking have been cited, including excessive postoperative valgus, internally rotated tibial or femoral components, malposition of the tibial or femoral component in the coronal plane, and malposition of the patellar component.[48–54] Correction of patellar maltracking has traditionally involved the use of a lateral retinacular release. Problems related to lateral retinacular release include increased postoperative pain and wound-healing complications, delayed rehabilitation, and compromised patellar blood supply.[15–17,19,27] Work at our institution has

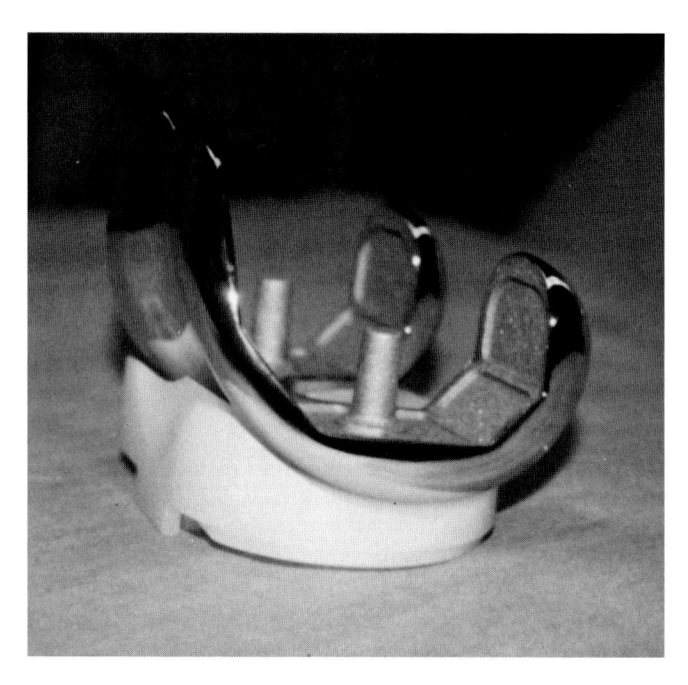

Figure 35.4. Photograph of the ultracongruent polyethylene insert with standard primary femoral component.

found that lateral retinacular release is required in 46% of patients whose patellar component is centralized on the patella, and in only 17% of patients whose patellar component is relatively medialized by centering over the anatomical high point or sagittal ridge.[55] This technique is described next in the techniques section. It must be emphasized that the previous design and combined surgical procedure, as mentioned before, must be followed to limit patellar complications.

SURGICAL TECHNIQUES

Surgical Approach

The subvastus approach is preferable for many total knee arthroplasties,[56] and is used by the senior author in 80% of cases. The subvastus approach should be avoided in situations that may make patellar eversion difficult, such as with previous lateral compartment scarring (tibial osteotomy), obesity, and patients with a prior medial arthrotomy. With a subvastus approach, the deep fascia of the thigh overlying the vastus medialis is incised in line with the skin incision. Using blunt dissection, this fascia is elevated off the vastus medialis obliquus (VMO). The inferior edge of the vastus is identified and lifted off the intermuscular septum using blunt dissection. The vastus medialis muscle belly is then lifted anteriorly. While under tension, the transverse tendinous insertion to the medial capsule is cut at the level of the midpatella, leaving the underlying synovium intact.

The arthrotomy is then performed vertically adjacent to the patella and the patellar tendon. The fat pad is incised at the medial edge to minimize bleeding and is not excised unless redundant. The patella is then carefully everted and dislocated as the knee is maximally flexed to provide generous exposure of the distal femur. If the patella is difficult to evert, a partial lateral release can be performed here for the heavy patient or the valgus leg with subluxating patella. The patella insertion device can be placed on the patella to facilitate eversion.

Preliminary proximal release of the tibial soft tissue is performed and should extend to the posteromedial corner of the tibia. All osteophytes are removed to identify true bony landmarks and dimension. If a marked deformity is present, further soft tissue release may need to be performed prior to making the bone cuts. However, this can usually be best titrated once the trials are in place.

Bone Cuts

Bone resorption and connective tissue formation occur when bone is surgically traumatized and heated to above 47°C for longer than one minute.[57] To control thermal injury, the sawblade is cooled by constant irrigation when making bone cuts. Without irrigation, any sawing or drilling can quickly raise the temperature of the bone to 170°C. All bone cuts should be made with a new sawblade coupled with a precisely toleranced saw capture. Sharp sawblades will decrease both operating time as well as trauma to the bone.

To ensure that a near perfect flat surface has been created, the saw capture is removed and all bone cuts sighted (in two planes) against the cutting blocks. A central high spot near the intercondylar notch of the femur may persist and will require additional planing. The high spot must be eliminated to keep the femoral component from becoming "high centered" when it is implanted. The high spot is eliminated by making a few extra passes with the sawblade using a slight upward spring of the blade against the bone. The flatness can also be checked using an auxiliary cutting block.

PCL Preservation

To preserve the PCL, it can be recessed 8 to 9 mm using a small knife blade, and protected by placing a small one-fourth-inch osteotome just anterior and deep to the ligament, preventing the sawblade from going too posterior.

Measured Resection Technique

Proper positioning of the joint line is essential for normal kinematics. The distal femoral alignment guide is applied and further stabilized by dialing the medial or lateral adjustable screw down to the defective distal femoral condyle. If both condyles are defective (i.e., with rheumatoid arthritis), both adjustable screws are dialed down slightly to compensate for the lost cartilage (2 to 3 mm). This maneuver avoids elevation of the joint line.

If the patient has normal proximal tibial varus, which ranges from 0 to 6 degrees,[32] it is preferable to make a 2-degree varus cut to allow resection of a more symmetrical wedge of proximal tibia. This will significantly improve soft tissue balancing and allow for proper orientation of the joint line. A caliper is used to measure the resected tibia in areas of relatively normal cartilage. Adding 1 mm to this measurement for bone loss from the saw blade will predict the thickness of the tibial replacement.

Before making any bone cuts, the maximum thickness of the patella is determined using a caliper. The total patellar resection should equal the thickness of the patellar insert, except in cases of severe patellar wear. Increasing the overal thickness of the patella-prosthesis construct will increase the patellofemoral joint forces and cause tracking problems and excessive wear, necessitating a lateral release. For improved fixation of the patella, countersinking the 10 mm components 2 to 3 mm is a routine procedure in our clinical practice.

Tibial Sizing

The surgeon should select the largest size tibial baseplate that does not overhang. Medial overhang is a recognized source of pes bursitis[58] and should be avoided. Sizing of the tibia is optimized by the use of an asymmetric tibial tray to obtain maximum coverage of the resected bone surface.

Patella Medialization

Using a one-eighth-inch drill, the middle of the highest portion of the sagittal ridge of the patella is drilled perpendicular to the articular surface to a depth of approximately 12 mm. A patellar osteotomy is then made at the osteochondral junction, removing 7 mm of bone. The previously drilled hole is then identified, and used as the landmark for centering the patellar implant. This acts as a guide for proper medialization of the patella. The patellar sizer is then used to identify the correct size of patellar component that can be centered over the drill hole to reproduce the position of the patient's original high point, and allow a continuous rim of bone around the implant (Fig. 35.5). Eccentric placement of the patella 3 to 4 mm toward the medial facet utilizing this technique allows for better tracking and improved clinical results as discussed previously.

Trial Reduction

Prior to trial reduction, posterior osteophytes on the femur are removed using a three-fourth-inch curved osteotome while lifting the femur with a bone hook. Osteophyte removal is essential for maximum knee flexion.

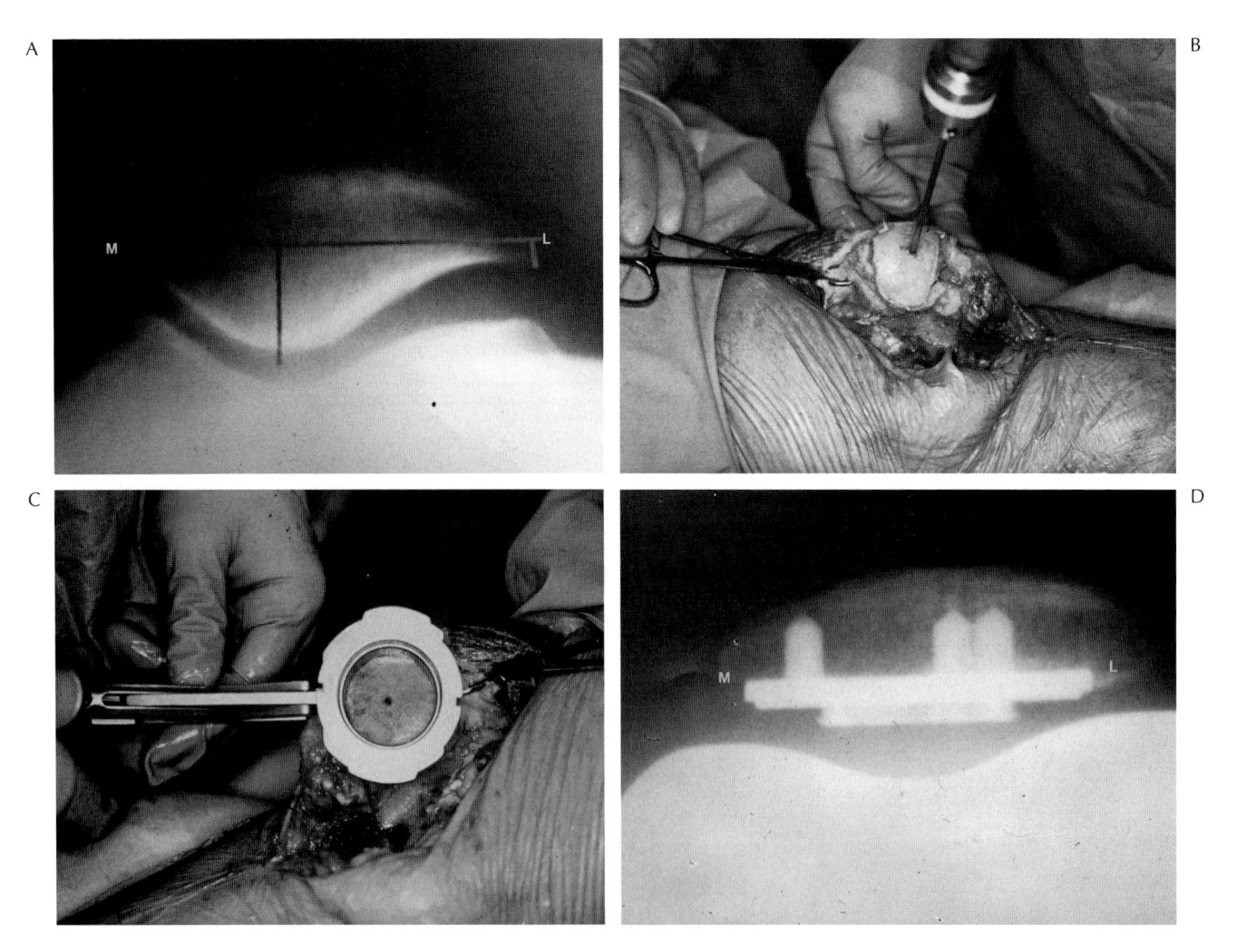

Figure 35.5. (A) Preoperative radiograph illustrating medial position of sagittal ridge of patella. (B) Drilling at the midpoint of sagittal ridge to mark the patella for medialization of the component. (C) Centering patellar reamer over the drill mark. (D) Postoperative radiograph of a medialized patellar component.

Stability is checked in full extension, 20 degrees of flexion, and full flexion. If the PCL is intact, slight medial and lateral laxity should be allowed. Full extension must be obtained on the operating table. The femur should track in the center of the tibial tray. If the PCL is absent, the next thicker size tibial insert must be selected. The slight flexion deformity this creates will stretch out over the first 6 months. It is suggested that the PCL be resected intentionally if the patient has more than 10 degrees varus or valgus deformity or more than a 10- to 15-degree flexion contracture preoperatively.

Implantation of Components-Morselized Autogenous Bone Grafting

A slurry of cancellous bone is obtained from the cut undersurface of the tibial wafer (Fig. 35.6). The patellar reamers are utilized for this purpose. This biologic bone "cement" is applied to every surface on the tibia, femur, and patella. In a routine varus knee, the bone is more porotic on the lateral side, and care is taken to spread additional bone slurry on the lateral tibial plateau to improve the contact between the implant porous coating and bone. This also serves to reinforce the bone in this region and rebuild the subchondral plate.

CLINICAL RESULTS

The early clinical results of cementless total knee arthroplasty were variable, with some reports not comparing favorably to the results of later cemented TKA designs.[1-3,59] However, with the development of instrumentation that allows precise bone preparation, and prostheses based upon sound biomechanical designs, the results of several different series of cementless TKA are now comparable to the best results of cemented TKA in the first 10 years of follow-up.

Whiteside[13] reported the 10-year survivorship analysis of a series of 265 cementless total knee components. One knee loosened during the 9- to 11-year follow-up period and was revised, and five knees were revised for infection. Five knees had revision of the patellar and tibial components for wear that began with the patella and later involved the tibia. Including infection as a mode of failure, the 10-year survivorship in this group was 94%. Ten years after surgery, 83.7% of the patients had no pain, 6.1% had mild pain, 8.2% had moderate pain, and 2% had severe pain. Knee flexion was 110 degrees preoperatively, and increased to 115 degrees at 2 years postoperatively and remained unchanged during the entire follow-up period.

Laskin[14] reported the 2-year results of 96 cementless total knee arthroplasties done using the Tricon-M prosthesis. Each patient was matched for age, body habitus, and diagnosis to a patient with a cemented total knee arthroplasty. There was no statistical difference between the two groups with respect to pain, range of motion, stability, or patient satisfaction.

Rosenburg and colleagues[15] reported the 3- to 6-year results of 132 cementless and 139 cemented Miller-Galante prostheses. The fixation technique was based on patient age, bone quality, and ability to delay full weight-bearing. Eight cemented knees and six cementless knees required component revision. No cemented knee failures were due to loosening, and two cementless knees were revised for tibial loosening.

Buechel and associates[60] reported the results of 147 cementless total knee arthroplasties with condylar femoral components, rotating metal-backed patellar components, and either meniscal-bearing or rotating-platform tibial components. The 6-year survival rate of the bicruciate-retaining meniscal-bearing implant was 100%. The 6-year survival rate of the posterior cruciate-retaining meniscal implant was 97.9%, and the 6-year survival rate of the rotating platform was 98.1%. In a second report of 80 cementless total knees of the above designs, 96.3% had a good to excellent clinical outcome at 12 years.[61]

The senior author (AAH)[31,62] has reported the 6- to 10-year results of cementless TKA. Between 1985 and 1989, 302 consecutive cementless posterior cruciate-sparing TKAs were performed at the authors' institution. The implant used was the titanium alloy porous-coated Natural Knee™ (Intermedics Orthopedics, Inc. Austin, Texas). This implant system has a deep trochlear grooved femoral component with two smooth pegs and a metal-backed patella with three smooth pegs. The tibial tray is fixed with four smooth pegs and two fully threaded 6.5 mm cancellous screws. The tibial tray is asymmetrically designed to conform to the anatomy of

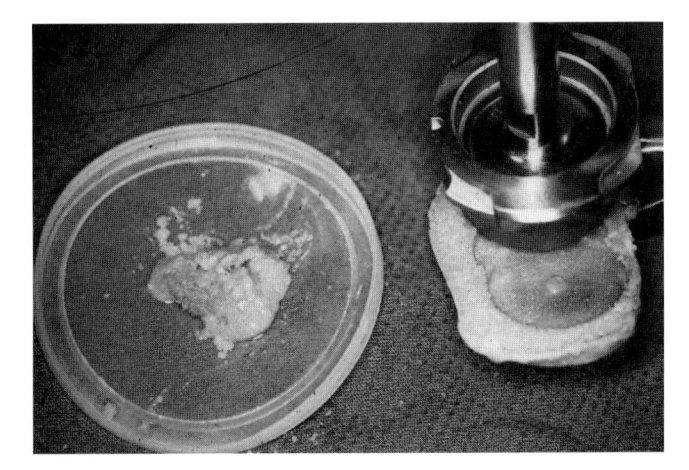

Figure 35.6. Preparation of bone slurry from the undersurface of a tibial wafer. Patellar reamer is shown reaming the undersurface of the resected tibial wafer. The autograft bone paste is seen in the plastic tray.

the normal tibia, with the lateral side 4 mm smaller than the medial. At a 6- to 10-year follow-up, 59 patients had died and 31 were lost to follow-up, resulting in 212 knees available for long-term review. Radiographic evaluation obtained at each clinic visit include fluoroscopically assisted views to allow for precise evaluation of the implant interface[63,64] (Fig. 35.7). The mean preoperative modified HSS knee score was 58, with a mean flexion of 105 degrees. Postoperatively, the mean HSS knee score plateaued at 99, and mean flexion was 122 degrees, excluding the scores of the patients requiring reoperation. There was no evidence of component subsidence or loosening requiring revision. There have been a total of 15 reoperations to date. Nine knees were revised for development of PCL insufficiency, necessitating polyethylene exchange to an ultracongruent insert. Two knees were revised for infection, and two were revised for tibial component oversizing. Nine patellar components were revised incidentally at the same time to a newer design metal-backed component with thicker polyethylene. Two revisions were specifically for patellar complications, one for maltracking and one for component wear. Overall component survivorship at 6- to 10-year follow-up is as follows: femoral component 98%, tibial component 98%, polyethylene tibial insert 95%, and metal-backed patellar component 96%.

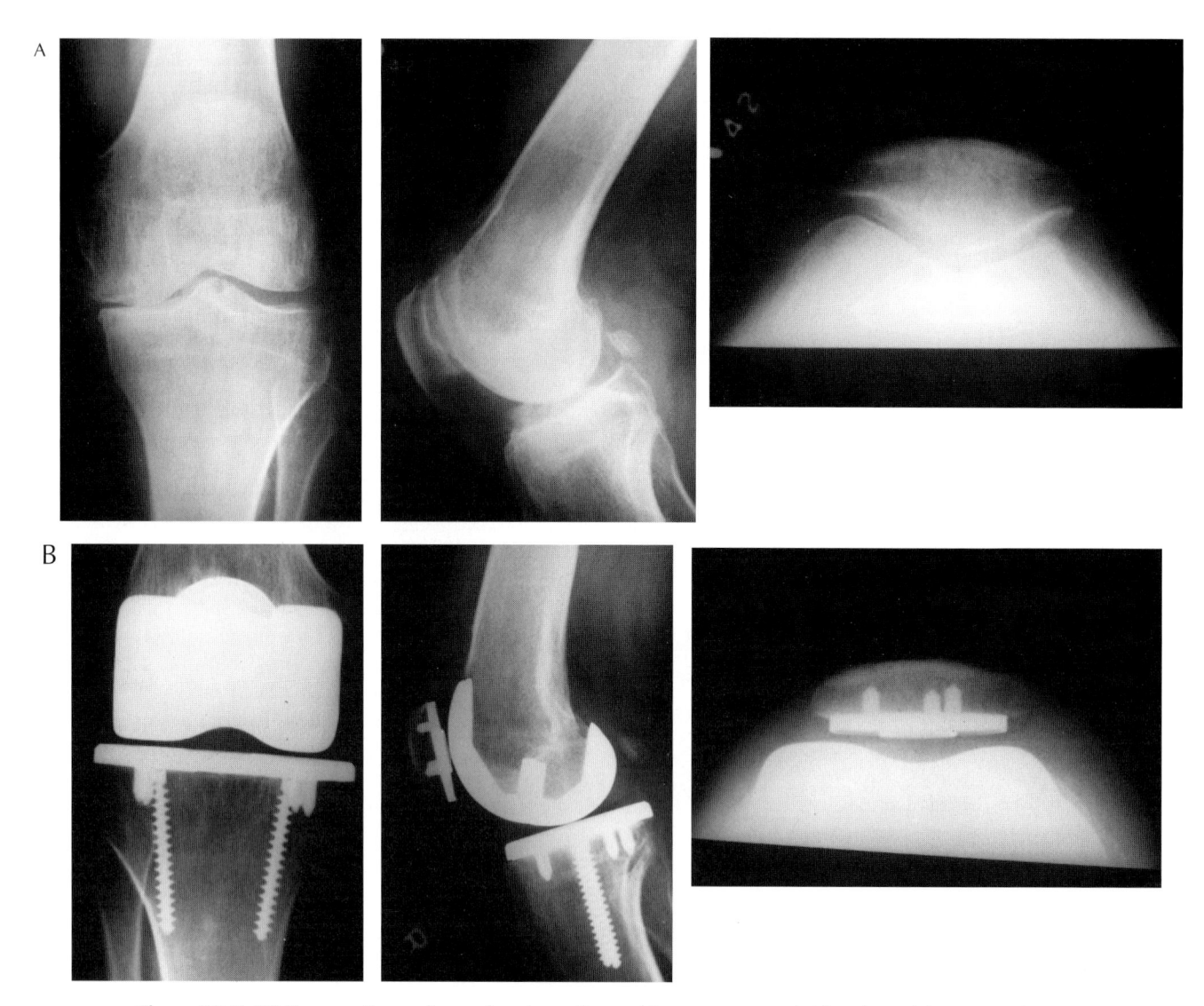

Figure 35.7. (A) Preoperative radiographs of a patient with varus osteoarthritis selected for cementless TKA. (B) Nine-year follow-up radiographs of cementless TKA revealing good position of components and no radiolucencies. Note preservation of polyethylene thickness of a patella component on skyline view, and tibial interface with an excellent bone apposition.

CONCLUSIONS

Recent reports with up to 10-year clinical follow-up have demonstrated that cementless total knee arthroplasty can yield excellent results in young, active patients when sound implant design principles and surgical techniques are followed. Intimate apposition of the prosthesis to host bone is achieved with instrumentation that allows precise bone resection, and by the routine application of morselized autogenous bone chips to the cut surfaces. Revision of cementless total knee components without porous-coated pegs, keels, or stems has proven to be bone-sparing, which is an important consideration in the younger patient who may outlive their prosthesis. The authors believe that cementless fixation is a superior alternative to cemented fixation for primary total knee arthroplasty in younger patients with higher functional demands and good bone stock.

References

1. Hungerford DS, Krakow KA. Total joint arthroplasty of the knee. *Clin Orthop*. 1985; 192:23–33.
2. Moreland JR. Mechanisms of failure in total knee arthroplasty. *Clin Orthop*. 1988; 226:49–64.
3. Ranawat CS, Johanson NA, Rimnac CM, Wright TM, Schwartz RE. Retreival analysis of porous-coated components for total knee arthroplasty. A report of two cases. *Clin Orthop*. 1986; 209:244–248.
4. Insall JN, Hood RW, Flawn LB, Sullivan DJ. The total knee prosthesis in gonarthrosis. A five- to nine-year follow-up of the first one hundred consecutive replacements. *J Bone Joint Surg*. 1983; 65A:619–628.
5. Anderson H, Carsten E, Frandsen P. Polyethylene failure of metal-backed patellar components. *Acta Orthop Scand*. 1991; 62:1–3.
6. Baech J, Kofoed H. Failure of metal-backed patellar arthroplasty. *Acta Orthop Scand*. 1991; 62:166–168.
7. Bayley JC, Scott R, Ewald F, Holmes G. Failure of the metal-backed patellar component after total knee replacement. *J Bone Joint Surg*. 1988; 70-A:668–673.
8. Lombardi A, Engh G, Volz R, Albrigo J. Fracture/dissociation of the polyethylene in metal-backed patellar components in total knee arthroplasty. *J Bone Joint Surg*. 1988; 70-A:675–679.
9. Rosenberg A, Andriacci T, Barden R, Galante JO. Patellar component failure in total knee arthroplasty. *Clin Orthop*. 1988; 236:106–114.
10. Stulberg D, Stulberg B, Hamati Y, Tsao A. Failure mechanisms of metal-backed patellar components. *Clin Orthop*. 1988; 236:88–105.
11. Davies JP, Jasty M, O'Conner DO, Burke DW, Harrigan TP, Harris WH. The effect of centrifuging bone cement. *J Bone Joint Surg*. 1989; 71B:39–42.
12. Miller J. Fixation in total knee arthroplasty. In: Insall J, ed. *Surgery of the Knee*. New York: Churchill Livingstone; 1984: 717–728.
13. Whiteside LA. Cementless total knee replacement. Nine- to eleven-year results and 10-year survivorship analysis. *Clin Orthop*. 1994; 309:185–192.
14. Laskin RS. Tricon-M uncemented total knee arthroplasty. A review of 96 cases followed for longer than two years. *J Arthroplasty*. 1988; 3:27–38.
15. Rosenberg AG, Barden RM, Galante JO. Cemented and ingrowth fixation of the Miller-Galante prosthesis. Clinical and roentgenographic comparison after three- to six-year follow-up studies. *Clin Orthop*. 1990; 260:71–79.
16. Mont MA, Mathur SK, Krakow KA, Loewy JW, Hungerford DS. Cementless total knee arthroplasty in obese patients. A comparison with a matched control group. *J Arthroplasty*. 1996; 11:153–156.
17. Whiteside LA. Fixation for primary total knee arthroplasty: cementless. *J Arthroplasty*. 1996; 11:125–127.
18. Jones LC, Hungerford DS. Cement disease. [Review]. *Clinical Orthopaedics & Related Research*. 1987; 225:192–206.
19. Leland RH, Hofmann AA, Bachus KN, Bloebaum RD. Biocompatibility and bone response of human osteoarthritic cancellous bone to a titanium porous-coated cobalt chromium cylinder. *Transactions of the Society for Biomaterials*. 1991; 14:153 (abstract).
20. Hofmann AA. Response of human cancellous bone to identically structured commercially pure titanium and cobalt chromium alloy porous coated cylinders. *Clin Mater*. 1993; 14:101–115.
21. Bloebaum RD, Bachus KN, Mitchell W, Hoffman G, Hofmann AA. Analysis of the bone surface area in resected tibia. Implications in tibial component subsidence and fixation. *Clin Orthop*. 1994; 309:2–10.
22. Bloebaum RD, Bachus KN, Momberger NG, Hofmann AA. Mineral apposition rates of human cancellous bone at the interface of porous coated implants. *J Biomed Mater Res*. 1994; 28:537–544.
23. Bloebaum RD, Rhodes DM, Rubman MH, Hofmann AA. Bilateral tibial components of different cementless designs and materials: microradiographic, backscattered imaging, and histologic analysis. *Clin Orthop*. 1991; 268:179–187.
24. Bloebaum RD, Rubman MH, Hofmann AA. Bone ingrowth into porous-coated tibial components implanted with autograft bone chips: analysis of ten consecutively retrieved implants. *J Arthroplasty*. 1992; 7:483–493.
25. Hofmann AA, Bloebaum RD, Rubman MH, Bachus KN, Plaster R. Microscopic analysis of autograft bone applied at the interface of porous-coated devices in human cancellous bone. *Int Orthop*. 1992; 16:349–358.
26. Krug WH, Johnson JA, Souaid DJ, Miller JE, Ahmed AM. Anthropomorphic studies of the proximal tibia and their relationship to the design of knee implants. *Trans Orthop Res Soc*. 1983; 8:402 (abstract).
27. Branson PJ, Steege J, Wixson RL, Stulberg SD. Rigidity of initial fixation in noncemented total knee tibial components. *Trans Orthop Res Soc*. 1987; 12:293 (abstract).
28. Dupont JA, Weinstein AM, Townsend PR. Tibial plateau coverage in total knee replacement. Tenth Annual Meeting Society for Biomaterials 1984; Washington, DC (abstract).
29. Westrich GH, Haas SB, Insall JN, Frachie A. Resection specimen analysis of proximal tibial anatomy based on 100

total knee arthroplasty specimens. *J Arthroplasty*. 1995; 10: 47–51.
30. Lee RW, Volz RG, Sheridan DC. The role of fixation and bone quality on the mechanical stability of tibial knee components. *Clin Orthop*. 1991; 273:177–183.
31. Evanich CJ, Tkach TK, von Glinski S, Camargo MP, Hofmann AA. Six to ten year experience using countersunk metal-backed patellae. *J Arthroplasty*. 1996; In Press.
32. Moreland JR, Bassett LW, Hanker GJ. Radiographic analysis of the axial alignment of the lower extremity. *J Bone Joint Surg*. 1987; 69-A:745–749.
33. Krakow KA. *The Technique of Total Knee Arthroplasty*. St. Louis: C.V. Mosby; 1990:118–137.
34. Hofmann AA, Bachus KN, Wyatt RWB. Effect of the tibial cut on subsidence following total knee arthroplasty. *Clin Orthop*. 1991; 269:63–69.
35. Bachus KN, Harman MK, Bloebaum RD. Stereoscopic analysis of trabecular bone orientation in proximal human tibias. *Cells Mater*. 1992; 2:13–20.
36. Andriacchi TP, Galante JO, Rermier RW. The influence of total knee replacement design on walking and stair climbing. *J Bone Joint Surg*. 1982; 64-A:1328–1335.
37. Ewald FC, Jacobs MA, Miegel RE. Kinematic total knee replacement. *J Bone Joint Surg*. 1984; 66-A:1032–1040.
38. Kelman GJ, Biden EN, Wyatt MP, Ritter MA, Colwell CW. Gait laboratory analysis of a posterior cruciate-sparing total knee arthroplasty in stair ascent and descent. *Clin Orthop*. 1989; 248:21–25.
39. Ranawat CS, Hansraj KK. Effect of posterior cruciate sacrifice on durability of cement-bone interface. *Orthop Clin N Amer*. 1989; 20:63–69.
40. Dorr LD, Ochsner JL, Gronley J. Functional comparison of posterior cruciate-retained versus cruciate-sacrificed total knee arthroplasty. *Clin Orthop*. 1988; 236:36–43.
41. Shoji H, Wolf A, Packard S, Yoshino S. Cruciate-retained and excised total knee arthroplasty. *Clin Orthop*. 1994; 305: 218–222.
42. Insall JN, Lachiewcz PF, Burstein AH. The posterior stabilized condylar prosthesis: a modification of the total condylar design. *J Bone Joint Surg*. 1982; 64-A:1317–1323.
43. Scott WN, Rubenstein M, Scuderi G. Results after knee replacement with a posterior cruciate-sparing prosthesis. *J Bone Joint Surg*. 1988; 70-A:1163–1173.
44. Scuderi GR, Insall JN. The posterior stabilized knee prosthesis. *Orthop Clin N Amer*. 1989; 20:71.
45. Hofmann AA, Tkach TK, Evanich CJ, Camargo MP. Posterior stabilization in total knee arthroplasty with use of an ultracongruent polyethylene insert. *Orthopedic Transactions*. 1996; (abstract).
46. Cameron HU, Federhow DM. The patella in total knee arthroplasty. *Clin Orthop*. 1982; 165:196–199.
47. Clayton ML, Thirpathy R. Patellar complications after total condylar arthroplasty. *Clin Orthop*. 1982; 170:152–155.
48. Brick GW, Scott RD. The patellofemoral component of total knee arthroplasty. *Clin Orthop*. 1988; 231:163–178.
49. Anouchi YS, Whiteside LA, Kaiser AD, Milliano MR. The effects of axial rotational alignment of the femoral component on knee stability and patellar tracking in total knee arthroplasty demonstrated on autopsy specimens. *Clin Orthop*. 1993; 287:170–177.
50. Briard JL, Hungerford DS. Patellofemoral instability in total knee arthroplasty. *J Arthroplasty*. 1989; S87–S97.
51. Grace JN, Rand JA. Patellar instability after total knee arthroplasty. *Clin Orthop*. 1988; 237:184–189.
52. Merkow RL, Soudry M, Insall JN. Patellar dislocation following total knee replacement. *J Bone Joint Surg*. 1985; 67-A:1321–1327.
53. Nagamine R, Whiteside LA, White JE, McCarthy DS. Patellar tracking after total knee arthroplasty: the effect of tibial tray malrotation and articular surface configuration. *Clin Orthop*. 1994; 304:263–271.
54. Rhoads DD, Noble PC, Reuben JD, Mahoney OM, Tullos HS. The effect of femoral component position on patellar tracking after total knee arthroplasty. *Clin Orthop*. 1990; 260:43.
55. Hofmann AA, Tkach TK, Evanich CJ, Camargo MP, Zhang Y. Patellar component medialization in total knee arthroplasty. *J Arthroplasty*. 1997; 12(5):155–160.
56. Hofmann AA, Plaster RL, Murdock LE. Subvastus (southern) approach for primary total knee arthroplasty. *Clin Orthop*. 1991; 269:70–77.
57. Krause WL. Temperature elevations in orthopaedic cutting operations. *J Biomech*. 1982; 15:267–275.
58. Scott RD, Santore RF. Unicompartmental replacement for osteoarthritis of the knee. *J Bone Joint Surg*. 1981; 63A:536–544.
59. Collins DN, Heim SA, Nelson CL, Smith P. Porous-coated anatomic total knee arthroplasty. A prospective analysis comparing cemented and cementless fixation. *Clin Orthop*. 1991; 267:128–136.
60. Buechel FF, Pappas MJ. Long-term survivorship analysis of cruciate-sparing versus cruciate-sacrificing knee prostheses using meniscal bearings. *Clin Orthop*. 1990; 260:162–169.
61. Beuchel FF. Cementless meniscal bearing knee arthroplasty: 7- to 12-year outcome analysis. *Orthopedics*. 1994; 17:833–836.
62. Tkach TK, Evanich CJ, Hofmann AA, Camargo MP, Zhang Y. Six to ten year follow-up with cementless fixation. *Orthopedic Transactions*. 1996; (abstract).
63. Magee FP, Weinstein AM. The effect of position on the detection of radiolucent lines beneath the tibial tray. *Trans Orthop Res Soc*. 1986; 11:357 (abstract).
64. Mintz AD, Pilkington CA, Dip T, Howie DW. A comparison of plain and fluoroscopically guided radiographs in the assessment of total knee arthroplasty. *J Bone Joint Surg*. 1989; 71A:1343–1347.

CHAPTER 36
Hybrid Total Knee Arthroplasty

Michael W. Becker

INTRODUCTION

Total knee arthroplasty has proven to be highly successful in relieving pain and improving function in properly selected patients. All modern implant designs have evolved from the total condylar prosthesis introduced in 1970. Long-term results of this design, despite the disadvantages of limited implant-sizing options and relatively primitive instrumentation, have been excellent and provide the standard for subsequent comparisons.[1–14] Fixation of total knee arthroplasties with polymethylmethacrylate (PMMA) has proved lasting in multiple implant designs including the total condylar knee.[2,6–8,12] It has been argued, however, that cementless fixation has theoretical advantages in the long term over the use of bone cement, and this has led to the development of porous-coated implants. Early experience with this technology has produced mixed results.[1,3,13,15–24] The major problem areas with porous knee implants have been with the tibial and patellar components. Femoral components inserted without cement have proven as reliable as their cemented counterparts in numerous clinical studies. Techniques including roentgen stereophotogrammetric analysis (RSA) used to study possible mechanisms of implant failure have therefore focused on the tibial side.[22,25–29] Hybrid total knee arthroplasty offers the theoretical advantages of cementless fixation on the femoral side with the reliability and clinical safety of cement fixation of tibial and all polyethylene patellar components. This technique is presented here as a reasonable alternative to an entirely cemented total knee arthroplasty.

PUBLISHED RESULTS

Published series of hybrid total knee arthroplasties began to appear in 1990. Wright and colleagues[30] reviewed 114 press-fit condylar knee arthroplasties at an average of 2.8 years after surgery. Good to excellent results were seen in 93% of patients. Thirty percent of the femoral components had a radiolucent line in at least one zone two-thirds of which were present immediately after surgery. These radiolucent lines undoubtedly relate to the accuracy of the femoral cuts during surgery. Some initial radiolucencies were found to disappear in subsequent radiographs. The Miller-Galante prosthesis utilizing hybrid fixation has also been reviewed in several centers. Kraay and associates[31] followed 29 hybrid Miller-Galante total knee arthroplasties. The average Knee Society Knee Score at 2 years was 93. Fluoroscopically guided radiographs were obtained to examine the interfaces and no significant or progressive radiolucencies were seen. Adverse bone remodeling, such as the lytic appearance in the distal femur attributed to stress shielding, was not seen under any of the porous femoral components. Kobs and Lachiewicz[32] reviewed 41 hybrid Miller-Galante knees followed between 2 and 5 years. An average postoperative knee score of 90 was observed. Metal-backed patellar components were used in this series. Six of 41 failed during the study period and this represented the major problem for these patients. Nonprogressive radiolucencies were seen about 15% of the femoral components.

Because the initial results of hybrid total knee arthroplasties only began to appear in the literature around 1990, long-term follow-up is still lacking. Long-term review is available for completely cemented knee implants and to a lesser extent for cementless knee replacements. Cementless femoral components have performed well in the cementless studies, the major problems occurring with the cementless tibial and patellar components.[1,5,16,20,21,23,24,32–35] Cement fixation of the tibia in total knee arthroplasty, however, has proven reliable and durable in multiple long-term reviews with both cruciate-sacrificing and cruciate-retaining designs.[4,8,9,12,14] The reasonable argument then is that hybrid total knee arthroplasties with a cementless femur, cemented tibia, and cemented all-polyethylene patella should last in a similar fashion to a completely cemented implant.

OSTEOLYSIS

The major problems with joint replacements in early designs were implant fracture and loss of fixation. Although these problems have not been solved, implant technology has advanced to the point where failure along these lines will usually occur less quickly if at all. This has allowed more time after arthroplasty to observe new problems, often more complex and difficult to repair than the earlier failures. Osteolysis has become a disconcerting observation and major clinical problem in joint replacement surgery. In early knee replacement studies, bone loss was attributed to mechanical wear from a loose implant and stress shielding adjacent to rigidly fixed implant component.[6,14,24,36] The biological response to implant materials is now emphasized as the adverse effects of polyethylene debris have become apparent. The important concept of "access disease" has been reviewed by Smalzreid and colleagues.[30,37,38] Particulate matter must have access to bone within the "effective joint space" in order to incite the biological responses visible later as loss of bone or "osteolysis." This physiological concept must be kept in mind in future implant designs, instrumentation, and modes of fixation. Whatever its drawbacks, cement provides a "seal" at the interface thus limiting the "effective joint space" protecting against the phenomenon of osteolysis. With fixation of tibial implant to bone less reliable with cementless technique, an incomplete "seal" should be expected. An impressive and disturbing demonstration of this issue was published by Peters and associates in 1992,[39] in which 174 consecutive total knee arthroplasties performed without cement were reviewed. Osteolysis was diagnosed in 27 knees (16%) within 3 years of surgery. More than half of these were revised within the next year. The medial tibial plateau was the most frequent area where osteolysis occurred. The distal femur had obvious osteolysis in only two of their patients. This and multiple other studies emphasize that it is much more difficult to create an effective "seal" of the metaphyseal bone with a cementless tibia than it is with a cementless femur in total knee arthroplasty surgery.

INDICATIONS FOR HYBRID FIXATION/CEMENTLESS FIXATION OF THE FEMORAL COMPONENT

There are no true indications for fixation type in knee arthroplasty surgery. Completely cemented, completely cementless, and hybrid fixation have been used successfully and each have their advantages and disadvantages, both practical and theoretical. With cementless technique, however, only femoral fixation has been reliable across multiple implant designs in achieving durable success without increased loosening and wear.

There are several reasons why this would be expected to occur. A more extensive surface area for bony ingrowth is available on the femoral side and the quality of bone in the distal femur may in fact be better. Strength in compression of femoral metaphyseal bone increases with the depth of resection. The opposite is true for the tibia.[32] Firm press fit alone, even with less than ideal bony ingrowth, probably suffices for clinical success on the femoral side. A relative indication for hybrid technique is the younger patient requiring knee replacement. The potential benefits of cementless fixation are more important under these circumstances. That being said, advanced patient age does not preclude using cementless technique. What is important in choosing a cementless femoral component and thereby a hybrid knee arthroplasty is firm press fit of the femoral component onto a distal femur with good bone quality accepting no gaps at the interfaces between metal and bone (see Fig. 36.1). This will more likely seal the interface, avoid possible pain from micromotion, and provide for a satisfactory and durable clinical outcome. This can occur in patients of all ages and with a variety of preoperative diagnoses. Agreed, there is a certain "forgiveness"

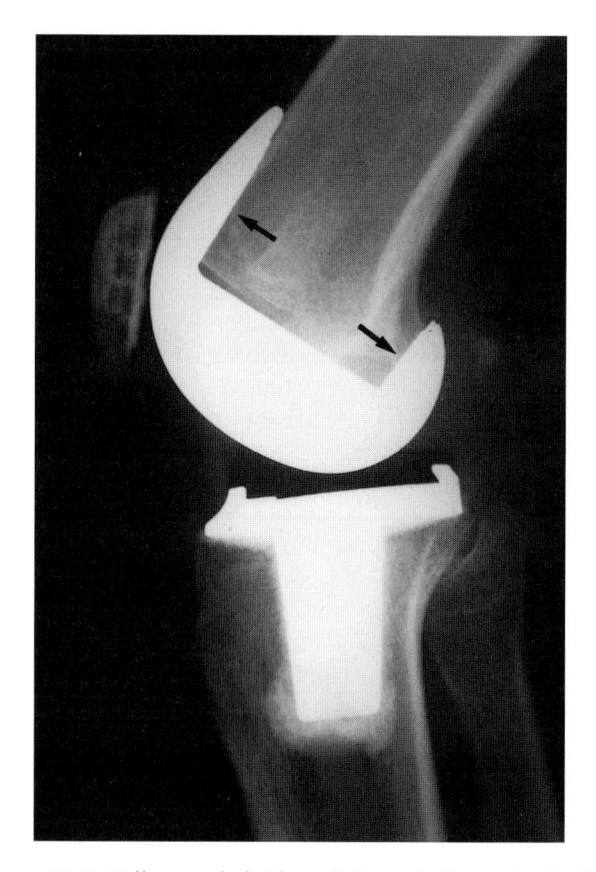

Figure 36.1. Follow-up hybrid Insall-Burstein II prosthesis. Satisfactory interfaces are seen anteriorly and posteriorly (arrows). The notch of the femoral component precludes review of the distal interfaces.

from a technical perspective with early cementless femurs inserted with gaps at the interfaces achieving good clinical results (see Fig. 36.2). These knees undoubtably did well due to adequate press fit. Less stringent criteria, however, for implanting a cementless femur makes no intuitive sense considering the excellent longevity of the cemented femoral component and the potential problems with cementless fixation with imprecise distal femoral cuts. Imprecise fit should be considered the true contraindication to cementless femoral component fixation in total knee arthroplasty. Precise distal femoral cuts should occur more commonly with recent advances in instrumentation. The fewer the cutting guides required to cut the distal femur, the fewer the chances for imprecise fit, and the newer systems available are clearly following this principle.

Cost has become a major topic of discussion in joint replacement surgery. Porous-coated implants are typically more expensive than their nonporous counterparts to be used with cement. Other factors need to be considered, however, such as operative time used and other materials required during surgery. All of these costs vary from institution to institution and even at the same location from surgeon to surgeon and ultimately needs to be reviewed by each surgeon individually.

CONCLUSION

If attention is given to precise surgical technique, excellent results in the long term may be expected with a hybrid total knee arthroplasty. Although hybrid fixation has been described with various combinations including cemented tibia cementless femur, cemented femur cementless tibia, and cemented or cementless patella, the hybrid knee arthroplasty recommended in this review includes cemented tibial, cementless femoral, and cemented all-polyethylene patellar components. This is suggested because it incorporates the clear advantages of cement for the tibia and patella with the possible advantages or at least clear clinical predictability of the cementless femur. With this configuration, clinical and/or radiographic loosening of the arthroplasty should mirror the excellent long-term published results of entirely cemented total knee arthroplasties. A proper "seal" should occur between all three components and their respective bones limiting the "effective joint space" and thus protecting against osteolysis if and when polyethylene wear occurs.

References

1. Collins DN, Heim SA, Nelson CL, Smith P 3d. Porous-coated anatomic total knee arthroplasty. A prospective analysis comparing cemented and cementless fixation. *Clin Orthop.* June 1991; (267):128–136.
2. Insall JN, Kelly M. The total condylar prosthesis. *Clin Orthop.* 1986: 205–243.
3. Kavolus CH, Ritter MA, Keating EM, Faris PM. Survivorship of cementless total knee arthroplasty without tibial plateau screw fixation. *Clin Orthop.* December 1991; (273): 52–62.
4. Malkani AL, Rand JA, Bryan RS, et al. Total knee arthroplasty with the kinematic condylar prosthesis. *J Bone Joint Surg Am.* 1995; 77:423–431.
5. Moran CG, Pinder IM, Lees TA, et al. Survivorship analysis of the uncemented porous-coated anatomic knee replacement. *J Bone Joint Surg Am.* 1991; 73:848–857.
6. Ranawat CS, Boachie-Adjei O. Survivorship analysis and results of total condylar knee arthroplasty. Eight to 11 year follow-up period. *Clin Orthop.* 1988; 226:6–13.
7. Ranawat CS, Flynn WF Jr, Deshmukh RG. Impact of modern technique on long-term results of total condylar knee arthroplasty. *Clin Orthop.* 1994; (309):131–135.
8. Ranawat CS, Flynn WF Jr, Saddler S, et al. Long-term results of the total condylar knee arthroplasty: a 15-year survivorship study. *Clin Orthop.* 1993; (286):94–102.
9. Ritter MA, Herbst SA, Keating EM, et al. Long-term survival analysis of a posterior cruciate-retaining total condylar total knee arthroplasty. *Clin Orthop.* 1994; (309):136–145.
10. Scuderi GR, Insall JN, Windsor RE, et al. Survivorship of cemented knee replacements. *J Bone Joint Surg Br.* 1989; 71:798–803.
11. Stern SH, Insall JN. Posterior stabilized prosthesis: results after follow-up of nine to twelve years. *J Bone Joint Surg Am.* 74:980–986.
12. Vince KG, Insall JN, Kelly MA. The total condylar prosthesis 10 to 12 year results of a cemented knee replacement. *J Bone Joint Surg Br.* 1989; 71:793.
13. Whiteside LA. Cementless total knee replacement: nine- to 11-year results and 10-year survivorship analysis. *Clin Orthop.* 1994; (309):185–192.

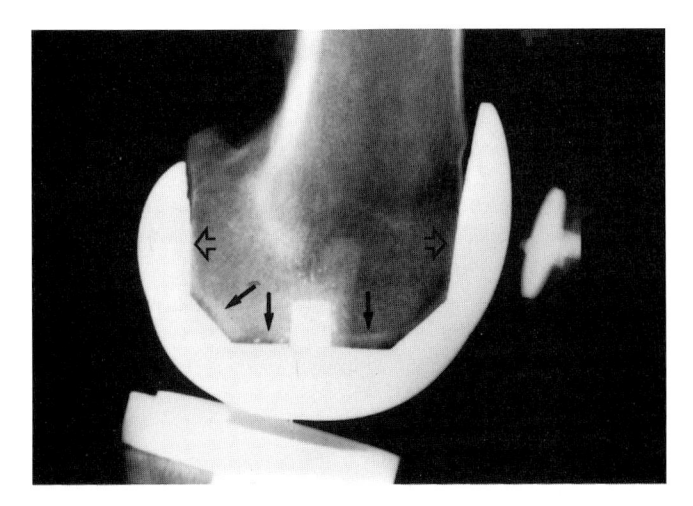

Figure 36.2. The 4-year follow-up radiograph demonstrating areas of fibrous interface (closed arrows) and areas of satisfactory bone implant contact (open arrows). Bead dissociation suggests micromotion at least in the early postoperative period. Gaps like these, if seen at surgery with the trial components, should support cementing the femur.

14. Wright J, Ewald FC, Walter PS, Thomas WH, Poss R, Sledge CB. Total knee arthroplasty with the kinematic prosthesis. *J Bone Joint Surg Am*. 1990; 72:1003–1009.
15. Cadambi A, Engh GA, Dwyer KA, et al. Osteolysis of the distal femur after total knee arthroplasty. *J Arthroplasty*. 1994; 9:579–594.
16. Engh GA, Parks NL, Ammeen DJ. Tibial osteolysis in cementless total knee arthroplasty. A review of 25 cases treated with and without tibial component revision. *Clin Orthop*. December 1991; (273):170–176.
17. Lewis PL, Rorabeck CH, Bourne RB. Screw osteolysis after cementless total knee replacement. *Clin Orthop*. December 1995; (321):173–177.
18. Lewonowski K, Dorr LD. Revision of cementless total knee arthroplasty with massive osteolytic lesions. *J Arthroplasty*. December 1994; 9(6):661–663.
19. Moran CG, Pinder IM. Osteolysis around cementless porous-coated knee prostheses [letter; comment]. *J Bone Joint Surg Br*. July 1995; 77(4):667–668.
20. Rand JA. Cement or cementless fixation in total knee arthroplasty? *Clin Orthop*. December 1991; (273):52–62.
21. Rosenberg AG, Barden RM, Galante JO. Cemented and ingrowth fixation of the Miller-Galante prosthesis. Clinical and roentgenographic comparison after three- to six-year follow-up studies. *Clin Orthop*. November 1990; (260):71–79.
22. Shimagaki H, Bechtold JE, Sherman RE, Gustilo RB. Stability of initial fixation of the tibial component in cementless total knee arthroplasty. *J Orthop Res*. January 1990; 8(1):64–71.
23. Sumner DR, Kienapfel H, Jacobs JJ, Urban RM, Turner TM, Galante JO. Bone ingrowth and wear debris in well-fixed cementless porous-coated tibial components removed from patients. *J Arthroplasty*. April 1995; 10(2):157–167.
24. Young-Hoo K, Jeong-Hwan O, Seung-Hwan O. Osteolysis around cementless porous-coated anatomic knee prostheses. *J Bone Joint Surg Br*. March 1995; 77(2):236–241.
25. Hilding MB, Xunhua Y, Ryd L. The stability of three different cementless tibial components. A randomized radiostereometric study in 45 knee arthroplasty patients. *Acta Orthop Scand*. 1995; 66(1):21–27.
26. Kraemer WJ, Harrington IJ, Hearn TC. Micromotion secondary to axial, torsional, and shear loads in two models of cementless tibial components. *J Arthroplasty*. April 1995; 10(2):227–235.
27. Rorabeck CH, Bourne RB, Lewis PL, et al. The Miller-Galante knee prosthesis for the treatment of osteoarthrosis: A comparison of the results of partial fixation with cement and fixation without any cement. *J Bone Joint Surg Am*. 1993; 75:402–408.
28. Nilsson KG, Karrholm J, Linder L. Femoral component migration in total knee arthroplasty: randomized study comparing cemented and uncemented fixation of the Miller-Galante I design. *J Orthop Res*. 1995; 13:347–356.
29. Rand JA. Comparison of metal-backed and all-polyethylene tibial components in cruciate condylar total knee arthroplasty. *J Arthroplasty*. 1993; (8):307–313.
30. Ryd L, Albrektsson B, Carlsson L, Herberts P, Lindstrand A, Regner L, Dansgaard F, Toksvig-Larsen S. Roentgen stereophotogrammetric analysis (RSA) as a predictor of mechanical loosening. *J Bone Joint Surg Br*. 1995. In press.
31. Schmalzried TP, Jasty M, Harris WH. Periprosthetic bone loss in total hip arthroplasty. Polyethylene wear debris and the concept of the effective joint space. *J Bone Joint Surg Am*. July 1992; 74:849–863.
32. Kraay JM, Meyers SA, Goldberg VM, Figgie HE 3d, Conroy PA. "Hybrid" total knee arthroplasty with the Miller-Galante prosthesis. A prospective clinical and roentgenographic evaluation. *Clin Orthop*. December 1991; (273):32–41.
33. Kobs JK, Lachiewicz PF. Hybrid total knee arthroplasty. Two- to five-year results using the Miller-Galante prosthesis. *Clin Orthop*. January 1993; (286):78–87.
34. Dannenmaier WC, Haynes DW, Nelson CL. Granulomatous reaction and cystic bony destruction associated with high wear rate in a total knee prosthesis. *Clin Orthop*. 1985; (198):224–230.
35. Mitsui H. Hybrid total knee arthroplasties in rheumatoid arthritis. *Bull Hosp Jt Dis*. Summer 1993; 53(3):19–20.
36. Wright RJ, Lima J, Scott RD, Thornhill TS. Two- to four-year results of posterior cruciate-sparing condylar total knee arthroplasty with an uncemented femoral component. *Clin Orthop*. November 1990; (260):80–86.
37. Schmalzried TP, Jasty M, Harris WH. Polyethylene wear debris and tissue reactions in knee as compared to hip replacement prostheses. *J Applied Biomat*. 1994; (5):185–190.
38. Schmalzried TP. Osteolysis in cemented total knee arthroplasties. *J Arthroplasty*. 1995; (10):118–119.
39. Peters PC Jr, Engh GA, Dwyer KA, Vinh TN. Osteolysis after total knee arthroplasty without cement. *J Bone Joint Surg Am*. July 1992; 74(6):864–876.
40. Callahan CM, Drake BG, Heck DA, et al. Patient outcomes following tricompartmental total knee replacement: a meta-analysis. *JAMA*. 1994; (271):1349–1357.

CHAPTER 37
Hydroxyapatite

Matthew J. Kraay, Victor M. Goldberg

Aseptic loosening of early cemented total joint prostheses and the perception of polymethylmethacrylate as the weak link in this method of fixation has stimulated investigation into alternative methods of implant fixation to the underlying bone. The potential for biologic fixation by bone ingrowth into porous-surfaced implants has subsequently been studied extensively. Animal and human investigations have demonstrated that under the appropriate circumstances, stable fixation by tissue ingrowth into porous implants is possible.

Improvements in cemented and uncemented, porous-surfaced total knee arthroplasty designs and surgical techniques have significantly reduced the incidence of fixation-related failure with both of these methods. Concern still exists, however, regarding the longevity of cemented total knee arthroplasty in the young, active patient with advanced arthrosis of the knee.[1,2] As a result, the clinical use of uncemented total knee prostheses and the search for a method of permanent biologic fixation has continued. A successful cementless total knee prosthesis must provide satisfactory long-term pain relief, preservation of bony structure without bone loss due to stress shielding, bony integration of the implant with a stable interface that can resist significant in vivo loads, and an interface that will provide a satisfactory barrier to particulate wear debris from the articular surface.

The basic science and historical development of biologic fixation with porous-coated implants has been well summarized.[3–5] Bone ingrowth fixation is a complex process requiring an appropriate porous surface structure, adequate osteogenic potential, close proximity of the implant to the underlying bone, and limitation of motion across the developing bone-implant interface. Although the orthopedic alloys most commonly used for total joint implants possess the necessary mechanical properties and biocompatibility for implant integration, direct bonding of bone-to-metal (which is thought to be desirable) does not occur.[6] Bone has been demonstrated, however, to form strong, intimate bonds with various calcium phosphate ceramics, resulting in the laboratory investigation and clinical use of these biomaterials to enhance cementless implant fixation.

BASIC SCIENCE OF HYDROXYAPATITE AND RELATED CALCIUM PHOSPHATE CERAMICS

The two most extensively studied, and hence clinically used, calcium phosphate ceramics are hydroxyapatite ($Ca_{10}(PO_4)_6(OH)_2$) and tricalcium phosphate ($Ca_3(PO_4)_2$). Tricalcium phosphate can exist in several different states (isomorphs) that are identical chemically but have different crystallographic structures (e.g., alpha-tricalcium phosphate and beta-tricalcium phosphate) and slightly varied properties. The environmental conditions and methods used during the manufacture of these calcium phosphate ceramics affects the chemical composition, crystalline structure, porosity, solubility, and other critical properties of these materials. Implant coatings of hydroxyapatite and tricalcium phosphate have been shown to be osteoconductive,[7–11] biocompatible,[12–16] and bioactive.[17] Hydroxyapatite appears to provide effective osteoconductive and osteophilic properties to encourage bone to attach directly to orthopedic implants without an intervening fibrous layer, and provide a method of enhancing bony ingrowth across gaps. Osteoblasts anchor, attach, spread, and proliferate on the surface of a wide variety of calcium phosphate ceramics in vitro.[18] Calcium phosphate ceramics do not appear however to be osteoinductive or to stimulate osteogenesis.

The most widely accepted mechanism of bonding between bone and implants coated with calcium phosphate ceramics has been proposed by Legeros[19] and appears to first involve partial dissolution of the ceramic macrocrystals at the surface of the coating. This results in the liberation of calcium and phosphate into the surrounding microenvironment, followed by formation of carbonate apatite microcrystals. These microcrystals then associate with an organic matrix of bone, resulting in the formation of bone. Accepting the above, the dissolution characteristics of a calcium phosphate ceramic coating are likely to affect the precipitation of the carbonate-apatite at the interface. Clearly, some critical amount of coating dissolution is essential to obtain rapid bone bonding. A potential conflict might exist, however, between obtaining rapid bonding to bone and the manufacture of a slowly resorbing, stable calcium phosphate ceramic coating.

The solubility of these calcium phosphate ceramics are the principal determinants of their bioresorption. Tricalcium phosphate is considerably more soluble than hydroxyapatite, and thus is resorbed relatively quickly and extensively after implantation. Although this promotes early union with the surrounding bone, the effects of complete early dissolution of the coating on long-term implant fixation are uncertain. If the ceramic is completely or significantly resorbed, a new interface must be formed between bone and the surface underlying the ceramic. The characteristics and stability of this resultant interface are unknown. Tricalcium phosphate coatings would intuitively be most useful in directing early ingrowth into porous-coated implants, which already have considerable inherent potential for biologic fixation.

As a result of their reduced solubility, hydroxyapatite (HA) coatings would be expected to have enhanced long-term stability compared to tricalcium phosphate coatings. The degradation of hydroxyapatite coatings can be reduced further by increasing the degree of crystallinity of the coating material during the manufacturing process. Theoretically, both of these factors may be associated with a reduced potential for early osteointegration, if calcium and phosphate are insufficiently liberated into the surrounding area of the developing interface. Despite these concerns, the use of HA coatings with high degrees of crystallinity has not been associated with early ingrowth failures clinically.

Despite their relative stability, slow, but progressive, resorption of hydroxyapatite coatings applied to smooth microstructured implants may ultimately occur and the properties of the resultant interface formed between the bone and the underlying metal substrate after long-term implantation are unknown. Sandwich coatings consisting of a deep layer of stable high crystallinity HA and a surface layer of rapidly dissolving tricalcium phosphate, or coatings with a mixed composition of HA and tricalcium phosphate, may allow the advantages of both HA and tricalcium phosphate to be realized clinically. In the case of HA/tricalcium phosphate coating of porous-surfaced implants, the resulting macro-interlock of implant to bone via ingrowth into the porous surface would likely persist, but patterns of loading and bone remodeling might change.

APPLICATION OF COATINGS

Hydroxyapatite and tricalcium phosphate are typically applied to orthopedic implants using plasma flame-spraying techniques.[20] This results in a dense, strongly adherent coating with a maximum thickness of 100 μm. Coatings can be quickly and easily applied to implants with complex shapes using this technique. Because the plasma-spraying process is associated with heating of the implant substrate to less than 300°C, there is no associated deterioration of the mechanical properties of the metal substrate. Other potentially useful application techniques under investigation include high-velocity oxygen fuel spraying and magnetron sputter-coating.[21]

The optimal thickness of hydroxyapatite coatings appears to be in the range of 30 to 100 μm. Bioresorption appears to be excessively rapid with coatings less than 30 μm and coatings greater than 100 μm appear to be prone to fatigue fractures.[21,22] Bonding strength between hydroxyapatite coatings and their underlying metal substrate appears to be significantly increased with titanium, as compared to cobalt chromium, and may be due to chemical as well as mechanical bonding of the hydroxyapatite to titanium.[9,23] Porosity of the applied hydroxyapatite also affects the mechanical properties of the coating and excessively porous coatings should be avoided.[24]

The composition of the coating material may be altered during the plasma-spraying process, resulting in a final product that is chemically or structurally different than the starting material. Composition, purity, crystallinity, thickness, and porosity of the applied coating can, and need to be, controlled during the application process.

ANIMAL INVESTIGATIONS OF HYDROXYAPATITE IMPLANT COATINGS

The potential advantages of hydroxyapatite in enhancing implant fixation have been documented in numerous experimental studies. The strength of attachment of bone to hydroxyapatite-coated porous-surfaced implants has been shown to be increased for up to 1 year after implantation, compared to uncoated porous-surfaced implants.[25–27] Use of hydroxyapatite-coated implants also appears to promote osteointegration between implant and host bone across gaps of 1 mm, which should result in more reliable biologic implant fixation, especially in compromised situations (e.g., revisions, osteopenia).[25–28]

Soballe and associates compared the interface properties of titanium and porous hydroxyapatite-coated implants subjected to stable (unloaded) and unstable mechanical conditions.[29] The situation of implant instability was simulated by an implanted dynamic loading device, which produced controlled motions of 500 μm. Under stable conditions, the shear strength of HA-coated implants was 250% stronger than titanium porous-coated implants and had five times as much bone ingrowth as the titanium implants. Although there was no difference in the amount of bone ingrowth between the two types of implants under unstable conditions, the shear strength of the hydroxyapatite-coated implants was five times greater than that of unstable titanium implants. Gap healing was significantly improved with stable hydroxyapatite implants, but neither implant showed any appreciable gap healing in an unstable situation.

Our previous investigations of calcium phosphate ceramic coating of orthopedic implants have focused on the enhancement of osteointegration of commercially pure titanium fiber-metal porous surfaced implants, coated with hydroxyapatite and tricalcium phosphate.[30,31] We believe this to be an attractive material couple for the surface of total joint prostheses because a thin plasma-sprayed coating of hydroxyapatite-tricalcium phosphate does not obstruct the pores of the surface, and because the porous fiber metal surface has been demonstrated to have considerable inherent potential for biologic fixation and resultant mechanical interlock with bone.

The majority of studies investigating cementless fixation with calcium phosphate ceramics have not utilized implants placed in a cancellous bone environment. Although previous models employing intramedullary or intracortical implants may simulate those conditions occurring following total hip arthroplasty, implantation into a cancellous bone environment is probably more representative of the conditions present following total knee replacement. Although it might be anticipated that cancellous bone would provide a more biologically responsive site for this process than cortical bone, conflicting results have been reported.[32-34] In some cases, higher interface shear strength and increased bone ingrowth has been described in intramedullary or intracortical placement, as compared with intracancellous placement. In other studies, extensive ingrowth has been observed in in-

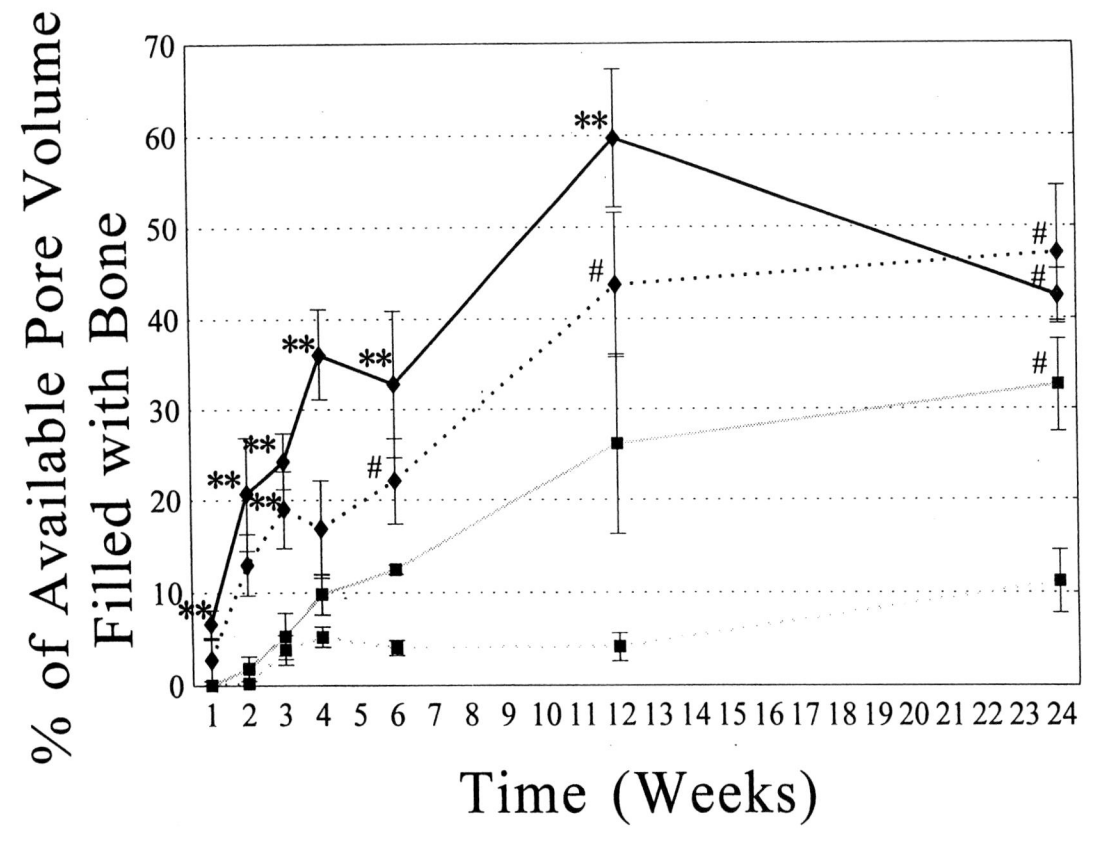

Figure 37.1. Percentage of available pore volume filled with bone. Comparison of intramedullary and intracancellous placement of HA-TCP-coated and noncoated fiber-metal implants. Dependent variable: % of available pore volume filled with bone. Solid lines indicate HA-TCP coating; dotted lines indicate smooth surfaces. Intramedullary implants are represented by ■; intracancellous implants are identified by ◆. Data expressed as means of groups ± SEM. # Greater than noncoated intramedullary implants, $p < 0.05$; ** Greater than all intramedullary implants, $p < 0.05$.

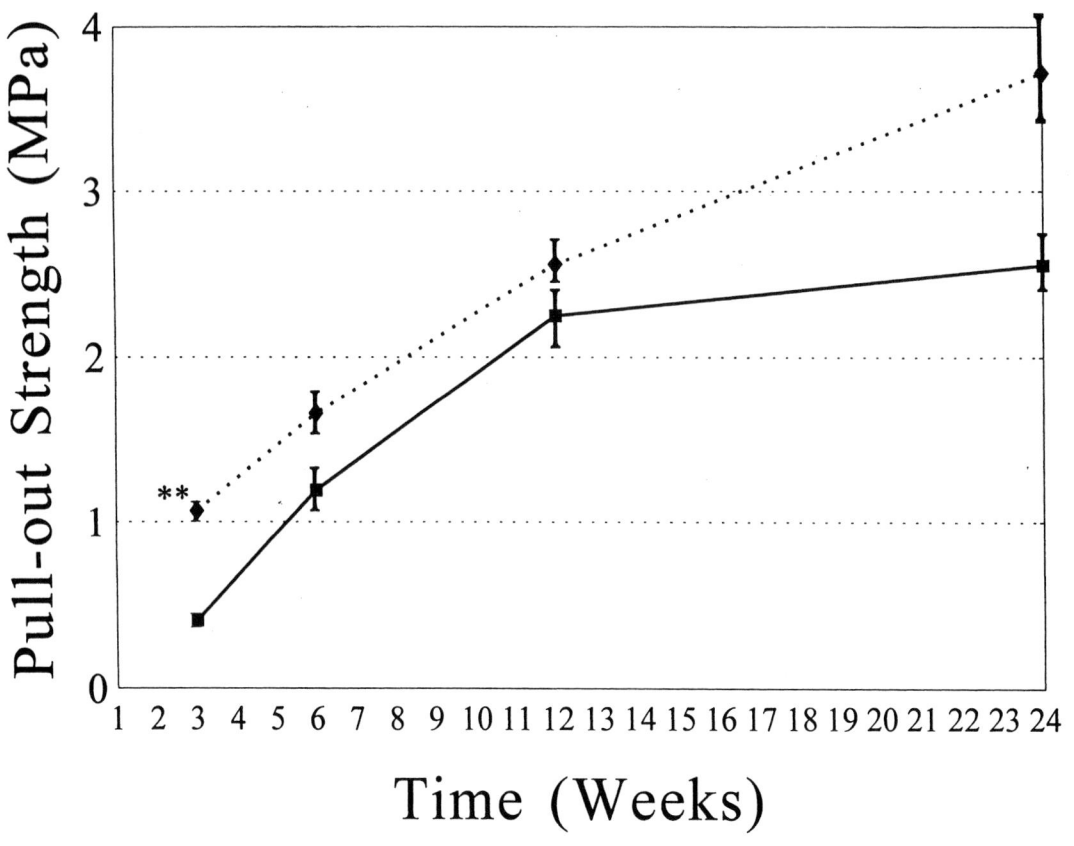

Figure 37.2. Pull-out strength in megapascals. Comparison of intramedullary and intracancellous placement of HA-TCP-coated and noncoated fiber-metal implants. Dependent variable: pull-out strength. Solid lines indicate HA-TCP coating. Intramedullary implants are represented by ■; intracancellous implants are identified by ◆. Data expressed as means of groups ± SEM. ** Greater than all intramedullary implants, $p < 0.01$.

tracancellous implantation sites. Some of the inconsistencies in these animal studies may result from difficulties of modeling implant-implantation site interaction, as well as the inherent variables of surgical technique, fit, initial stability, and loading. We have attempted to isolate the biological interactions between the implant surface treatment and the implantation site using otherwise identical hydroxyapatite and tricalcium phosphate-coated and noncoated titanium implants in non-weight-bearing intramedullary and intracancellous sites in the rabbit distal femur.[30,31]

Ceramic-coated implants in these studies had a 75 to 100 μm thick layer of plasma flame-sprayed hydroxyapatite-tricalcium phosphate $[Ca_{10}(PO_4)_6(OH)_2]$ applied to the surface of the titanium fibers.[22] The composition of the ceramic layer based on X-ray diffraction was 65% hydroxyapatite and 35% beta- and alpha-tricalcium phosphate. These implants were not subjected to early axial loading, which would produce micromotion typically observed in clinically or experimentally implanted total joint prostheses.[4,35]

Hydroxyapatite-tricalcium phosphate significantly enhanced bone apposition to both the perimeter and the internal surfaces of coated implants in comparison to the noncoated implants. Implantation site was the major determinant of bone formation within the available pore volume and of pull-out strength (Figs. 37.1 and 37.2). At almost all time periods both hydroxyapatite-tricalcium phosphate-coated and noncoated intracancellous implants had greater percentages of their available pore volume filled with bone than intramedullary implants, whether hydroxyapatite-tricalcium phosphate-coated or not. Among hydroxyapatite-tricalcium phosphate-coated implants, intracancellous placement appeared to further enhance the amount of bone in contact with the perimeter of the implant. The kinetics of bone formation on the perimeter and internal surface lengths are presented in Figures 37.3 and 37.4. The amount of bone apposed to both perimeter and internal surfaces of hydroxyapatite-tricalcium phosphate-coated implants increased rapidly from 1 to 6 weeks and stabilized thereafter. Intracancellous placement accelerated bone formation and significantly increased the amount of bone apposed to the surface of hydroxyapatite-

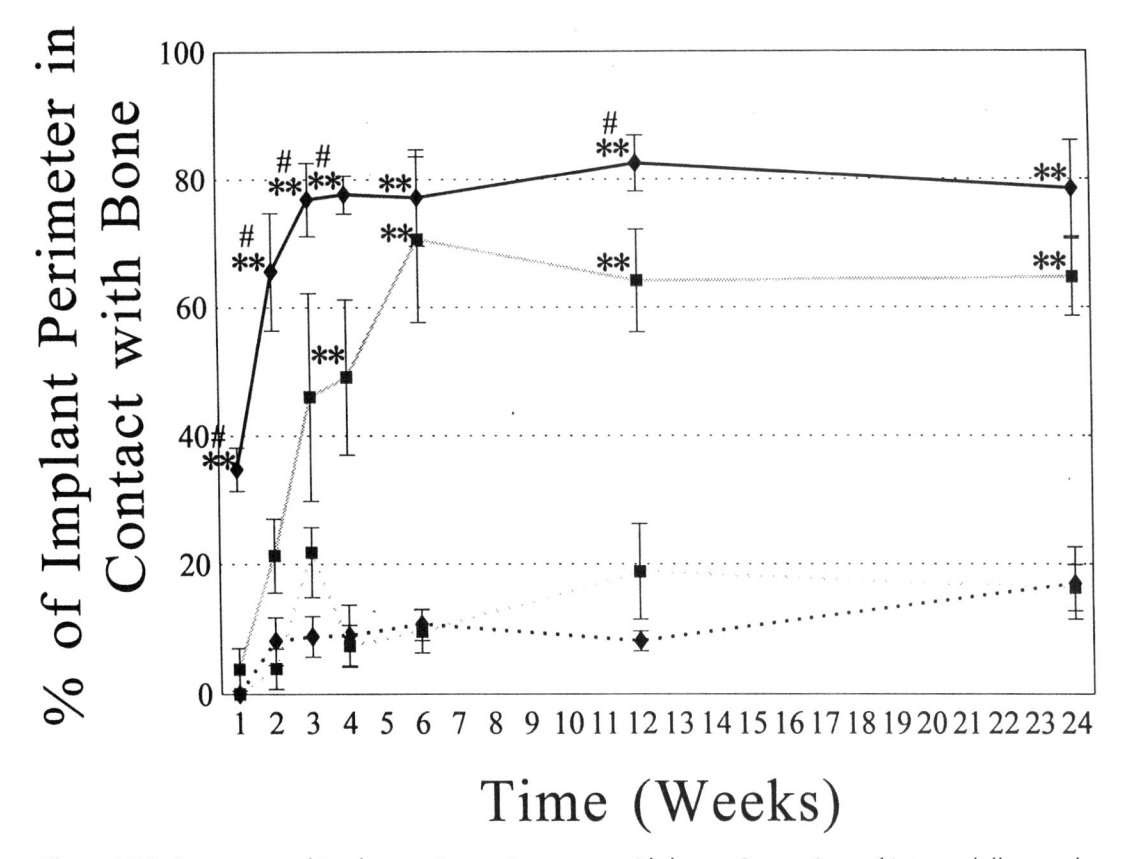

Figure 37.3. Percentage of implant perimeter in contact with bone. Comparison of intramedullary and intracancellous placement of HA-TCP-coated and noncoated fiber-metal implants. Dependent variable: % of implant perimeter in contact with bone. Solid lines indicate HA-TCP coating. Intramedullary implants are represented by ■; intracancellous implants are identified by ◆. Data expressed as means of groups ± SEM. # Greater than HA-TCP-coated intramedullary implants, $p < 0.05$; ** Greater than all noncoated implants, $p < 0.01$.

tricalcium phosphate-coated implants from 1 to 4 weeks after implantation.

Scanning electron microscopic backscatter analysis showed that new bone formed directly on hydroxyapatite-tricalcium phosphate-coated fibers without tissue interposition (Fig. 37.5). Bone ingrowth in noncoated implants was rarely in direct contact with the smooth titanium fibers. No significant obstruction of the fiber-metal pores by the thin hydroxyapatite-tricalcium phosphate coating was noted.

Abundant, progressive, lamellar bone formation had occurred in hydroxyapatite-tricalcium phosphate-coated implants by 4 to 6 weeks when placed in the intracancellous site and by 12 weeks in the intramedullary site (Fig. 37.6). This lamellar bone formation was in intimate contact not only with the surfaces of peripheral fibers coated with hydroxyapatite-tricalcium phosphate, but also with those deeper internal fibers not coated with hydroxyapatite-tricalcium phosphate during the plasma-spraying process. Bone formation, although lamellar, was minimal in noncoated implants from 4 to 6 weeks onward.

CLINICAL EXPERIENCE WITH HYDROXYAPATITE AND RELATED COATINGS

The vast majority of clinical experience with hydroxyapatite-tricalcium phosphate-coated implants in total joint replacement has occurred as a result of its use in total hip arthroplasty.[6,17,36] Recent reports suggest that the application of hydroxyapatite and tricalcium phosphate to the surface of metal implants creates an intimate bond between the bone, coating, and metal, and results in successful integration of implants.[6,17,30,37] Early reports at an average follow-up of 5 years suggest that hydroxyapatite-coated total hip replacements have provided successful implant fixation and interfaces.[38] Autopsy retrievals of hydroxyapatite-coated hip pros-

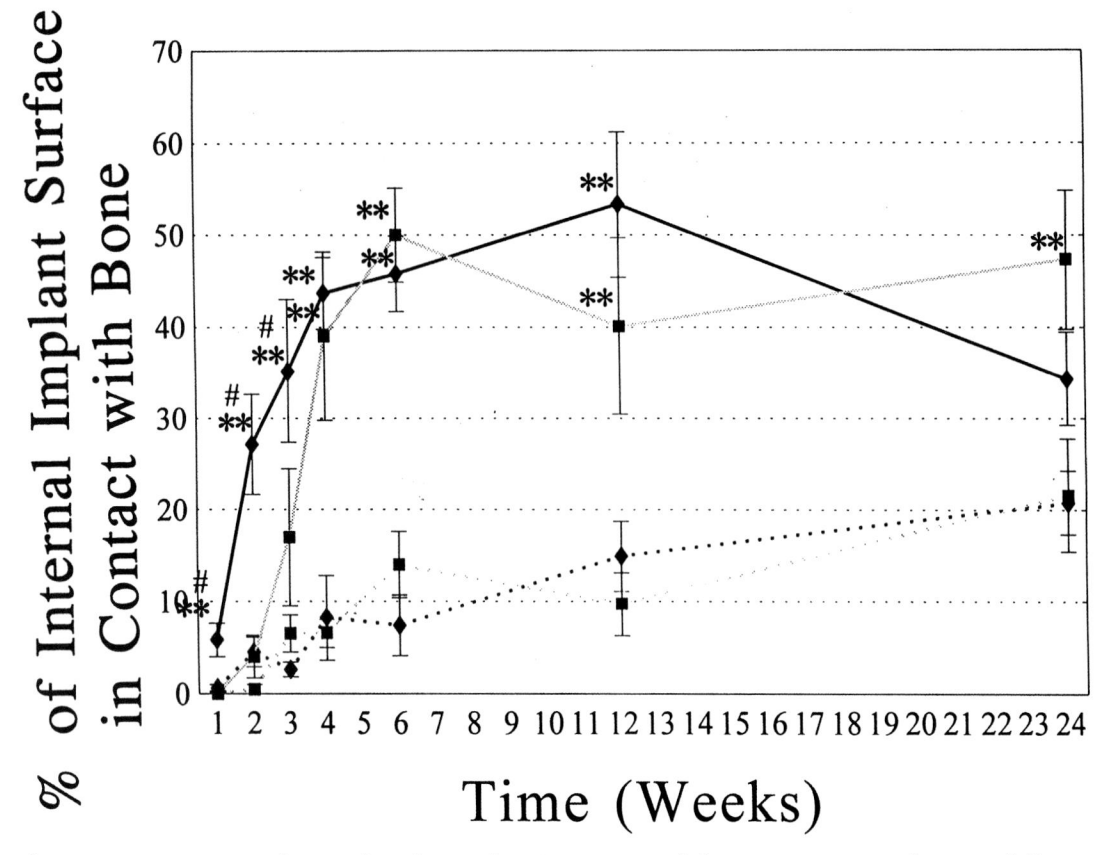

Figure 37.4. Percentage of internal implant surface in contact with bone. Comparison of intramedullary and intracancellous placement of HA-TCP-coated and noncoated fiber-metal implants. Dependent variable: % of internal implant surface in contact with bone. Solid lines indicate HA-TCP coating; dotted lines indicate smooth surfaces. Intramedullary implants are represented by ■; intracancellous implants are identified by ◆. Data expressed as means of groups ± SEM. # Greater than HA-TCP-coated intramedullary implants, $p < 0.05$; ** Greater than all noncoated implants, $p < 0.01$.

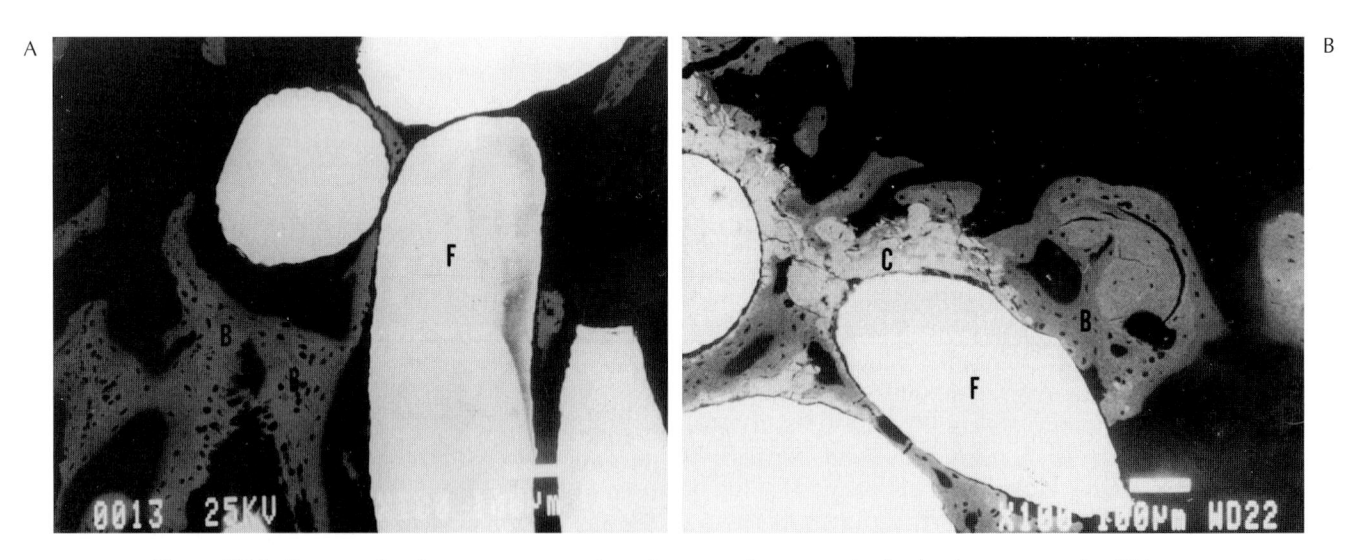

Figure 37.5. Four weeks after surgery, scanning electron microscopy in the backscatter mode, OM 100×. [A] Intramedullary, noncoated. The spaces between bone and the surface of the fibers (F) are readily apparent in this electron micrograph. Sometimes these spaces were difficult to see by light microscopy because of the shadows and profiles resulting from the thickness of the section and the depth of focus of the microscope. [B] Intracancellous, HA-TCP coated. Bone (B) was intimately entwined with HA-TCP coating (C) on the surface and also seemed directly to abut even fiber-metal (F) surfaces without discernible HA-TCP coating.

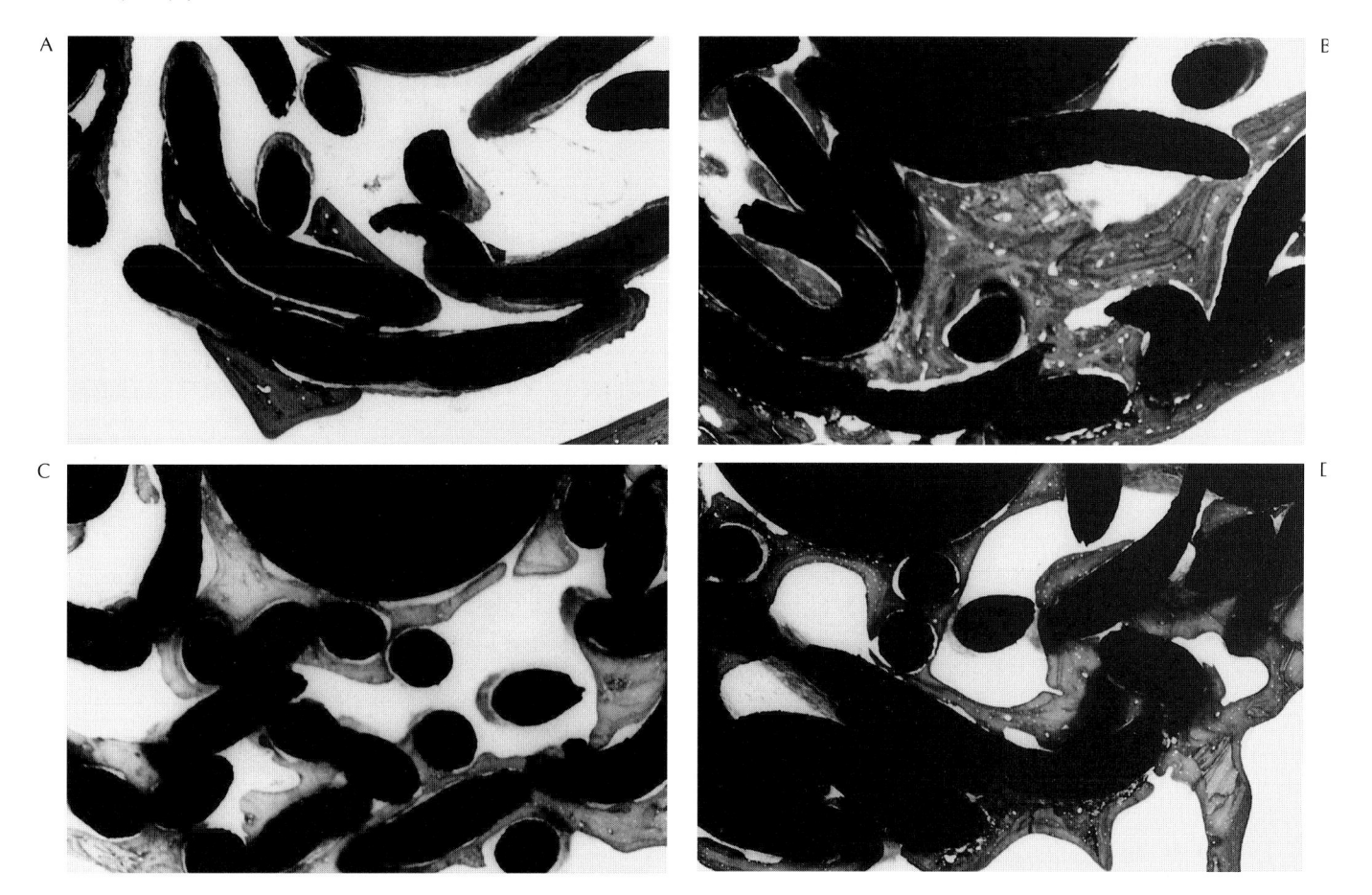

Figure 37.6. Twelve weeks after surgery. Toluidine blue stain, OM 10×. (A) Intramedullary noncoated. Lamellar bone has formed in the pores of the implant. (B) Intramedullary, HA-TCP coated. Abundant lamellar bone has formed in the pores of and along the surface of this HA-TCP-coated implant. Note the apposition of bone to ceramic. (C) Intracancellous, noncoated. Pore filling of noncoated implants was almost as complete as that of HA-TCP-coated implants although a space can be seen between bone and fiber surfaces. (D) The peripheral and internal surfaces are covered with bone and the pores of this HA-TCP-coated implant are filled with woven and lamellar bone.

theses have shown that these implants provide excellent degrees of osteointegration, even in older-aged patients. Further, radiographic analysis of hydroxyapatite-coated implants showed excellent quality of bone around implants without any radiolucencies around the coated segments of the component. However, long-term performance of these implants must be determined in order to establish the role of hydroxyapatite for fixation of total hip replacements.

In order to evaluate the in vivo bone response to hydroxyapatite-coated implants, Carlsson and associates[39] inserted small conical titanium implants into the proximal tibiae of 8 patients (11 knees) 3 to 6 months prior to scheduled total knee arthroplasty. Each knee received an implant with a smooth finish, a grit-blasted finish and a plasma-sprayed coating of hydroxyapatite. Fit and insertion of the implants were carefully controlled to obtain a similar degree of "press-fit." At the time of total knee arthroplasty, these implants were removed en bloc and evaluated histologically. Stable fixation was reliably obtained with approximately 40 to 50% bone apposition in both the grit-blasted and the hydroxyapatite-coated implant groups, but not in the smooth titanium implant group. At 6 months, there was a tendency for more bone apposition in the hydroxyapatite-coated group, however, small sample sizes precluded meaningful statistical evaluation of this trend.

Reports documenting the clinical results of hydroxyapatite in total knee arthroplasty are extremely limited. Verhaar reported the short-term results of a series of 26 cementless knee arthroplasties using the Osteonics Omnifit prosthesis plasma-sprayed with hydroxylapatite.[40] The average age of the patients was 61 years and average follow-up was 12 months. Complications were minimal and significant improvements in Hospital for Special Surgery (HSS) and Knee Society Knee score were seen postop, similar to those seen with cemented total knee replacement. Only one reoperation was performed because of patella complications. No knees were revised for loosening and no knees were radiographically loose. Radiographic evaluation indicated similar findings to total hip replacements with radiolucent and sclerotic lines demonstrated adjacent to uncoated areas. Verhaar concluded that "HA-coated total knee prostheses do better than pressfit uncoated prostheses."

Nilsson and colleagues reported a case of early failure of the hydroxyapatite coating of a tibial component in a total knee arthroplasty.[41] The hydroxyapatite coating had a purity of 98%, porosity of 20%, and thickness of 200 μm. At the time of revision, the coating appeared to have separated from the underlying titanium substrate and large amounts of hydroxyapatite crystals were found in histiocytes and giant cells within the thickened interface membrane. Serial roentgen stereophotogrammeric analysis (RSA) performed postoperatively demonstrated satisfactory initial implant stability, with progressive component migration noted after the 6-week period. The authors suggested that this was indicative of at least limited early bonding of implant to bone, with later failure at the hydroxyapatite-implant interface due to a combination of insufficient amount of bonding of the implant to bone, implant overloading, and suboptimal properties of the relatively thick, porous hydroxyapatite coating. The authors concluded that although HA coating has the potential for substantially improving the initial fixation of cementless prostheses, the optimum characteristics of such a coating need to be more completely established.

CONCLUSIONS

Our growing understanding and favorable clinical experience with hydroxyapatite and related calcium phosphate ceramic implant coatings in orthopedics suggest that these materials may be a significant development in the search for a permanent method of biologic implant fixation. Research at the authors' institution and the work of numerous others suggest that hydroxyapatite, tricalcium phosphate and several other bioactive ceramics facilitate adhesion, attachment, and spreading of osteoblasts, resulting in an enhancement of the quality and quantity of implant osteointegration.

Although several different strategies for the use of hydroxyapatite and tricalcium phosphate coatings have been utilized previously, we have considered these coatings to be adjuncts for enhancing the fixation of porous-surfaced joint replacement implants, which have already been demonstrated to have considerable inherent potential for biologic fixation. In this situation, dissolution of calcium phosphate serves to direct early bone apposition and ingrowth. Assuming that with the passage of time, complete dissolution of any bioactive ceramic coating may likely occur regardless of its biologic stability, the underlying porous coating may constitute a second line of defense against loosening.

Successful long-term biologic implant fixation is a complex process with numerous prerequisites including an appropriate implant surface, adequate host osteogenic potential, close fit and proximity of the implant to the underlying bone, and sufficient initial implant stability to limit motion across the developing bone-implant interface. Despite their potential advantages, the influences of operative technique, implant design, and other related parameters probably overwhelm the potential contribution of calcium phosphate ceramic coatings in obtaining successful implant fixation. Even the optimum calcium phosphate ceramic surface coating will fail to result in successful implant osteointegration and a stable implant-bone interface if the underlying prosthesis is poorly implanted or poorly designed.

Enhanced bone apposition and implant osteointegration appears to be the result of early, more effective attachment of bone-forming cells to the surface of these bioactive ceramic coatings. Enthusiasm for this exciting and promising technique of implant fixation must, however, be tempered by concerns regarding the material and mechanical properties of these coatings, their change with the passage of time, and the ultimate remodeling and integration of the entire implant surface. Further laboratory and clinical investigation is necessary to establish the role of these calcium phosphate ceramic coatings as a primary method of implant fixation, and whether these coatings do indeed represent a substantial development in the search for a method of permanent biologic fixation of joint replacement prostheses.

References

1. Ranawat CS, Boachie-Adjei O. Survivorship analysis and results of total condylar knee arthroplasty. *Clin Orthop.* 1988; 226:6–13.
2. Stern SH, Bowen MK, Insall JN, Scuderi GR. Cemented total knee arthroplasty for gonarthrosis in patients 55 years old or younger. *Clin Orthop.* 1990; 260:124–129.
3. Haddad RJ, Cook SD, Thomas KA. Current concepts review: biological fixation of porous-coated implants. *J Bone Joint Surg.* 1987; 69A:1459–1466.
4. Spector M, Shortkroff S, Sledge CB, Thornhill T. Advances in our understanding of the implant-bone interface: factors affecting formation and degeneration. *Instructional Course Lectures.* 1991; 40:101–113.
5. Spector M. Historical review of porous coated implants. *J Arthroplasty.* 1987; 2: 163–177.

6. Geesink RGT. Hydroxylapatite-coated hip implants. *Thesis*. Rijksuniversiteit Limburg te Maastricht, Maastricht, the Netherlands, 1988.
7. Daculsi G, Passuti N, Martin S, Deudon C, Legeros RZ, Raher S. Macroporous calcium phosphate ceramic for long bone surgery in humans and dogs. Clinical and histological study. *J Biomed Mater Res.* 1990; 24:379–396.
8. Geesink RGT, deGroot K, Klein C. Chemical implant fixation using hydroxyl-apatite coatings: the development of a human total hip prosthesis for chemical fixation to bone using hydroxyl-apatite coatings on titanium substrates. *Clin Orthop.* 1987; 225:147–170.
9. Geesink RGT, deGroot K, Klein C. Bonding of bone to apatite-coated implants. *J Bone Joint Surg.* 1988; 70B:17–22.
10. Heughebaert M, Legeros RZ, Gineste M, Guilhem A, Bonel G. Physicochemical characterization of deposits associated with HA ceramics implanted in nonosseous sites. *J Biomed Mater Res.* 1988; 22 (3 suppl):257–268.
11. Jarcho M, Kay JF, Gumaer KI, Doremus RH, Drobeck HP. Tissue, cellular, and subcellular events at a bone-ceramic hydroxylapatite interface. *J Bioeng.* 1977; 1:79–92.
12. Dutton R, Dawson E, Ackerman D, Dickstein H. Preliminary observations in segmental femoral substitution with porous hydroxyapatite implants in the dog. *Orthop Trans.* 1981; 5:267 (abstract).
13. Grundel R, Chapman M, Yee T. The evaluation of a biphasic calcium phosphate ceramic in diaphyseal defects in the canine ulna and metaphyseal defects in the canine humerus. *Trans Orthop Res Soc.* 1987; 12:218.
14. Grundel RE, Chapman MW, Yee T, Moore DC. Autogeneic bone marrow and porous biphasic calcium phosphate ceramic for segmental bone defects in the canine ulna. *Clin Orthop.* 1991; 266:244–258.
15. Kato K, Aoki H, Eng D, Tabata T, Ogiso M. Biocompatibility of apatite ceramics in mandibles. *Biomater Med Devices Artif Organs.* 1979; 7:291–297.
16. Nade S, Armstrong L, McCartney E, Baggaley B. Osteogenesis after bone and bone marrow transplantation. The ability of ceramic materials to sustain osteogenesis from transplanted bone marrow cells: preliminary studies. *Clin Orthop.* 1983; 181:255–263.
17. Geesink RGT. Hydroxyapatite-coated total hip prostheses. Two-year clinical and roentgenographic results of 100 cases. *Clin Orthop.* 1990; 261:39–58.
18. Bagambisa FB, Joos U. Preliminary studies on the phenomenological behavior of osteoblasts cultured on hydroxyapatite ceramics. *Biomaterials.* 1990; 11:50–56.
19. Legeros RZ, Orly I, Gregoire M, Daculsi G. Substrate surface dissolution and interfacial biological mineralization. In: Davies JE, ed. *The Bone-Biomaterial Interface.* University of Toronto Press; 1991: 76–88.
20. Serekian P. Process application of hydroxylapatite coatings. In: Geesink RGT, Manley MT, eds. *Hydroxylapatite Coatings in Orthopaedic Surgery.* New York: Raven Press; 1993: 81–87.
21. deGroot K, Jansen JA, Wolke JGC, Klein CPAT, vanBlitterswijk CA. Developments in bioactive coatings. In: Geesink RGT, Manley MT, eds. *Hydroxylapatite Coatings in Orthopaedic Surgery.* New York: Raven Press; 1993: 49–62.
22. deGroot K, Geesink R, Klein CP, Serekian P. Plasma sprayed coatings of hydroxylapatite. *J Biomed Mater Res.* 1987; 21:1375–1381.
23. Filiaggi MJ, Coombs NA, Pilliar RM. Characterization of the interface in the plasma-sprayed HA coating/Ti-6Al-4V implant system. *J Biomed Mater Res.* 1991; 25:1211–1229.
24. Manley MT, Cook ST, Dalton JE. A compositional, mechanical, and histological comparison of hydroxyapatite. *Trans Orthop Res Soc.* 1993; 18:467.
25. Cook SD, Thomas KA, Dalton JE, Volkman T, Kay JF. Enhancement of bone ingrowth and fixation strength by hydroxylapatite coating porous implants. *Trans Orthop Res Soc.* 1991; 16:550.
26. Cook SD, Thomas KA, Dalton JE, Volkman T, Whitecloud TS, Kay JF. Hydroxylapatite coating of porous implants improves bone ingrowth and interface attachment strength. *J Biomed Mater Res.* 1992; 26:989–1001.
27. Dalton JE, Cook SD, Thomas KA, Kay JF. The effect of operative fit and hydroxyapatite coating on the mechanical and biological response to porous implants. *J Bone Joint Surg.* 1995; 77A:97–110.
28. Soballe K, Hansen ES, Brockstedt-Rasmussen H, Hjortdal VE, Juhl GI, Pedersen CM, Hvid I, Bunger C. Gap healing enhanced by hydroxyapatite coating in dogs. *Clin Orthop.* 1991; 272:300–307.
29. Søballe K, Hansen ES, Rasmussen HB, Jorgensen PH, Bünger C. Tissue ingrowth into titanium and hydroxyapatite-coated implants during stable and unstable mechanical conditions. *J Orthop Res.* 1992; 10:285–299.
30. Tisdel CL, Goldberg VM, Parr JA, Bensusan JS, Staikoff LS, Stevenson S. The influence of a hydroxyapatite and tricalcium-phosphate coating on bone growth into titanium fiber-metal implants. *J Bone Joint Surg.* 1994; 76A:159–171.
31. Dean JC, Tisdel CL, Goldberg VM, Parr J, Davy D, Stevenson S. Effects of hydroxyapatite tricalcium phosphate coating and intracancellous placement on bone ingrowth in titanium fibermetal implants. *J Arthroplasty.* 1995; 6:830–838.
32. Clemow AJ, Weinstein AM, Klawitter JJ, Koeneman J, Anderson J. Interface mechanics of porous titanium implants. *J Biomed Mater Res.* 1981; 15:73–82.
33. Ducheyne P, Hench LL, Kagan A 2nd, Martens M, Bursens A, Mulier JC. Effect of hydroxyapatite impregnation on skeletal bonding of porous coated implants. *J Biomed Mater Res.* 1980; 14:225–237.
34. Sandborn PM, Cook SD, Spires WP, Kester MA. Tissue response to porous-coated implants lacking initial bone apposition. *J Arthroplasty.* 1988; 3:337–346.
35. Callaghan JJ, Dysart SH, Savory CF, Hopkinson WJ. Assessing the results of hip replacement. A comparison of five different rating systems. *J Bone Joint Surg.* 1990; 72B:1008–1013.
36. Jaffe WL, Scott DF. Total hip arthroplasty with hydroxyapatite-coated prostheses. *J Bone Joint Surg.* 1996; 78A:1918–1934.
37. Søballe K, Brockstedt-Rasmussen H, Hansen ES, Bünger C. Hydroxylapatite coating modifies implant membrane formation. *Acta Orthop Scand.* 1992; 63:128–140.

38. D'Antonio JA, Capello WN, Crothers OD, Jaffe WL, Manley MT. Early clinical experience with hydroxyapatite-coated femoral implants. *J Bone Joint Surg.* 1992; 74A:995–1008.
39. Carlsson L, Regner L, Johansson C, Gottlander M, Herberts P. Bone response to hydroxyapatite-coated and commercially pure titanium implants in the human arthritic knee. *J Orthop Res.* 1994; 12:274–285.
40. Verhaar J. Early clinical results of hydroxylapatite-coated total knee replacements. In: Geesink RGT, Manley MT, eds. *Hydroxylapatite Coatings in Orthopaedic Surgery.* New York: Raven Press; 1993: 297–304.
41. Nilsson KG, Cajander S, Karrholm J. Early failure of hydroxyapatite-coating in total knee arthroplasty. *Acta Orthop Scand.* 1994; 65(2):212–214.

SECTION 10
Bone Defects

CHAPTER 38
Autogenous Bone Grafting for Tibial Deficiency

Thomas P. Sculco and William O'Connor

BONE GRAFTING FOR TIBIAL DEFICIENCY

When severe malalignment occurs in destructive knee joint disease, the articular surface is devastated and associated changes result in underlying bone and soft tissues. Bone loss takes place on both the tibial and femoral surfaces of the knee joint in association with severe angular deformity. In the varus knee bone loss tends to be greater on the tibial surface and in valgus deformities the bone loss tends to be more symmetrical on the tibial and femoral surfaces. The extent of bone deficiency is usually more marked on the posterior aspect of the tibial plateau because often flexion contractures are concomitant with these marked deformities. There is associated asymmetry of soft tissues about the joint that complicate the management of these deformities and most commonly soft tissue releases will be necessary on the concave side of the deformity to balance lax soft tissues on the convex side of the deformity.

The management of bone deficits on the tibial surface are varied depending upon the extent and location of the loss of bone. Methylmethacrylate can be used as a filler in smaller defects with or without screw reinforcement. It is not recommended for larger defects because fracture and fragmentation of large unsupported methylmethacrylate columns may lead to implant failure. In the most severe bone deficits, augmentation can be effected by using additions to the implant itself or autogeneous bone grafting.

The area of bone loss on the tibial surface has a significantly sclerotic bed. The tibial rim is usually destroyed as the deficiency occurs and the femur subluxes (Fig. 38.1). This produces a deficiency that is concave at its floor and often has a wedge configuration. Defects may be seen with an intact tibial rim but these are much less common. In deficiencies that are 6 to 12 mm in depth, resection of 10 mm of upper tibia will generally remove most of the sclerotic bed. If deficits remain after resection of the tibia that are less than 5 mm, these can be fenestrated with a drill and filled with methylmethacrylate to support the tibial component.

Bone grafting is the preferred technique in defects that are greater than 12 to 15 mm in depth. Wedge augments (Fig. 38.2) may be added to the undersurface of the tibial component to fill these areas, but there are a number of disadvantages to this technique. Wedge augments tend to add expense to the cost of the implant and the locking mechanism of the wedge augment to the undersurface of the tibial plate usually requires screws that may produce fretting and abrasive metallic debris. These metallic particles may produce an inflammatory reaction similar to polyethylene debris and potentially lead to osteolysis. Additionally limited sizes and configurations of wedges are available and these may not fit the deficit. Most importantly, however, wedges do not restore bone that has been lost by the arthritic destructive process. Attempts should be made to restore bone that has been lost and reconstruction with a biologic augmentation, autogenous bone, is readily available from the distal femur and can be shaped to fit the area of bone deficiency. Additionally incorporation occurs and this restores bone stock to the upper femur if revision surgery should be necessary.

TECHNIQUE OF AUTOGENOUS BONE GRAFTING FOR TIBIAL DEFICIENCY

The initial tibial proximal bone cut is made utilizing a standard tibial cutting guide in the usual fashion. This tibial cut is conservative and about 8 mm of bone is resected from the more preserved tibial plateau. An oscillating saw is then used to create an oblique osteotomy on the side of the tibial defect (Fig. 38.3). Angled tibial wedge instruments may be used to make this osteotomy. The bony bed of the concave side of the defect is usu-

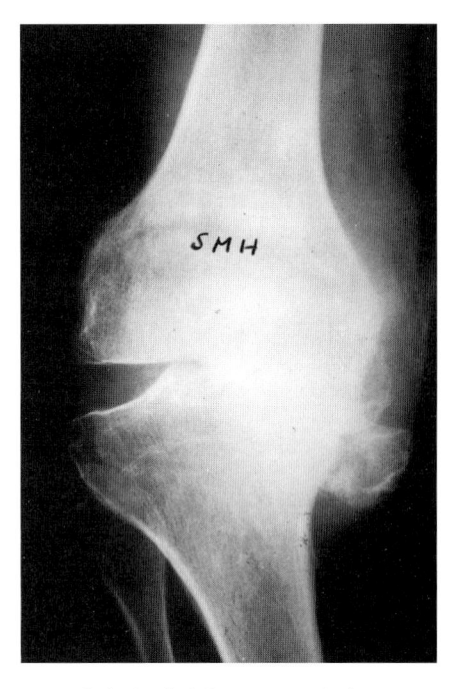

Figure 38.1. Medial tibial deficiency with destruction of peripheral rim and joint subluxation.

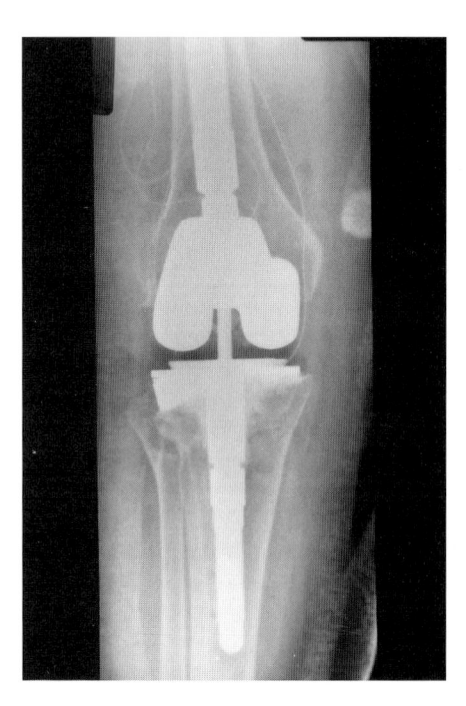

Figure 38.2. Tibial wedge augment fixed to tibial baseplate with screws.

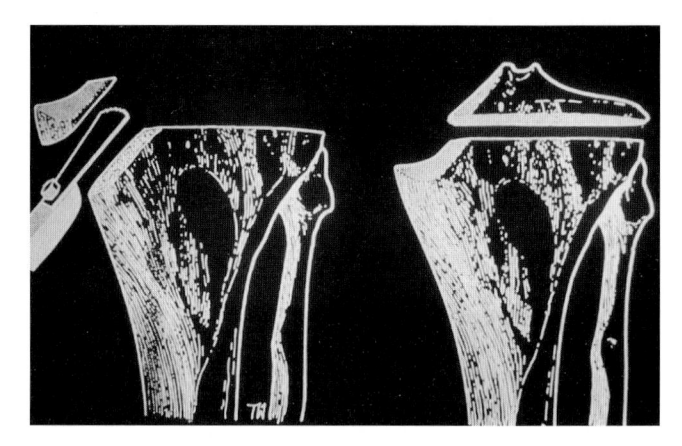

Figure 38.3. Oblique osteotomy of upper tibial surface to remove sclerotic tibial bed.

ally very sclerotic and this surface should be resected. The deep surface of the tibial bed should be 80 to 90% cancellous bone after this oblique osteotomy has been performed. There may be cystic areas in this bed once the sclerotic surface has been removed, and these may be curetted and filled with cancellous bone that is available from bone resection. It is important to remove this sclerotic bone and to expose cancellous bone otherwise consolidation of the graft will be impeded and failure of the graft may occur.[1] The osteotomy should be planar and flat so that a femoral condylar graft will fit intimately with the cancellous bed.

If the implant to be used has a stem for fixation, then the peg hole should be made after preparation of the defect bed. This will ensure that when the fixation screws are inserted into the graft the stem hole will not be entered. For implants with peripheral fixation peg holes, this step is of less importance.

The next step is to remove the distal femoral bone. Generally, the resected distal medial femoral condyle is larger than the lateral condyle and therefore tends to be the better graft material. Having resected the distal femoral condyle, this segment of bone is rotated so that its cancellous surface is coapted against the cancellous surface of the recipient bed (Fig. 38.4). The defect should

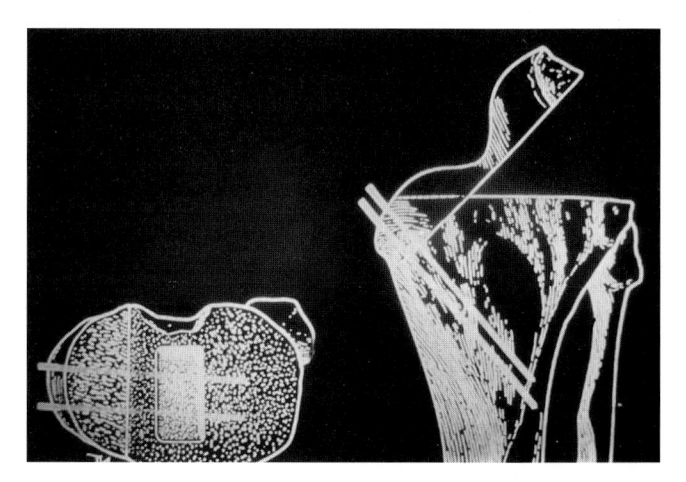

Figure 38.4. Resected femoral condyle being apposed to the tibial bed.

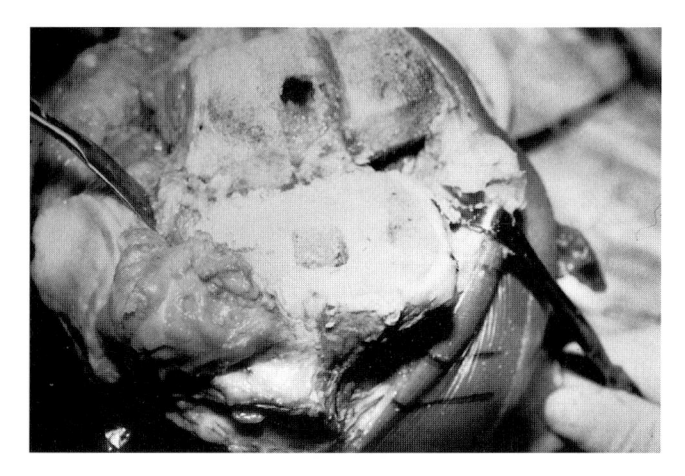

Figure 38.5. Reconstitution of the upper tibial surface after resection of redundant graft.

be completely filled with bone graft. There will be an overhanging segment of bone that protrudes above the cut surface of the tibia when the femoral condyle is placed on the upper tibial surface to fill the defect and this will be resected. If there is any gapping between the bone graft and the recipient bed, the bed must be further resected to create a flat cancellous surface. Once coaptation is precise, two screws are inserted to stabilize the graft to the proximal tibia. They should be inserted from the periphery and not make contact with the metal tibial baseplate. Care must be taken to not crack the graft as the screws are inserted. After the graft has been fixed in position, the overhanging bone should be removed using the resected tibial plateau surface as a guide. At this point the proximal tibia has been reconstituted. On observing the tibia from its upper surface, the subchondral bone of the femoral conydlar bone graft will act as the peripheral tibial bone of the upper tibia (Fig. 38.5).

Cortical screws are generally used to fix the graft and these can be overdrilled proximally to allow a lag effect when inserted. It is of utmost importance that cement not be allowed to enter the interval between the graft and recipient bed. An excellent method of preventing this from occurring is to cement the femoral component first and use a small portion of doughy cement to caulk the upper surface of the tibia along the line of the graft and host bone. This will harden so that when the tibial cement is inserted it will not penetrate into the graft-tibial bed interface. In the first patient in whom this technique was used, this caulking technique was not used and cement spread into a segment of the interface between graft and tibia. The graft became sclerotic but there was some consolidation in the depth of the graft so that neither collapse nor prosthetic settling occurred (Fig. 38.6).

Postoperative rehabilitation for these patients is the same as for those patients without bone grafting. The tibial implant support is maintained on the more normal side of the tibia and because the graft is securely fixed to the tibia, weight-bearing has not been limited in these patients. Continuous passive motion is employed on the first postoperative day in a manner analogous to that in patients without bone grafting.

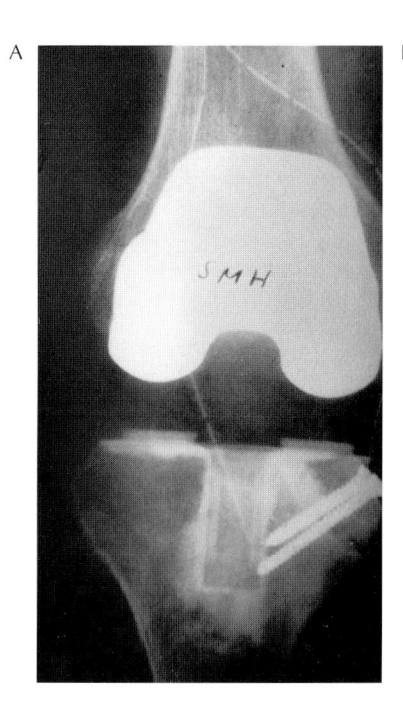

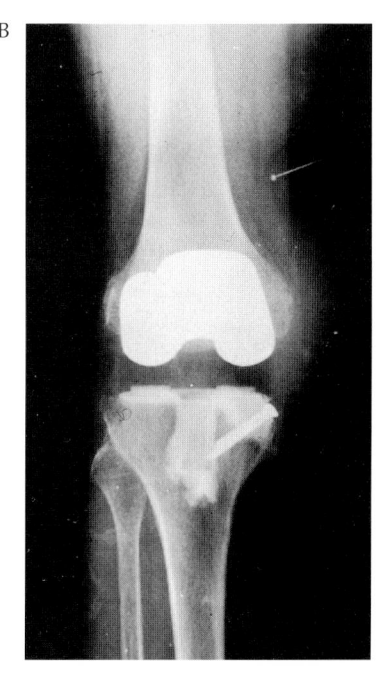

Figure 38.6. Radiographs immediate postoperative and at 12-years postoperative demonstrating methylmethacrylate in interface between graft and bed.

RESULTS

Forty autogeneous bone grafts to the upper tibia have been performed over the past 15 years using the technique outlined in this chapter. The results to date have been excellent with no patient experiencing collapse of the graft and/or loss of implant position (Fig. 38.7). Peripheral resorption of the graft has occurred in 15% of patients but structural support to the tibial component has not been lost in any patient to date. Because of the complex nature of these knee deformities, a more constrained prosthesis was used in 15 of these knees. The greatest deformities treated included patients with 25 degrees of varus and 30 degrees of valgus. Revision surgery was necessary in one patient because of an incompetent medial collateral ligament after trauma to the knee 5 years after the primary arthroplasty. This patient was reoperated for the severe recurrent valgus deformity and the graft was examined at the time of the procedure and was noted to be completely consolidated at the interface. Early results with this series were reported by Altchek and colleagues.[2]

Dorr and associates[3] described 24 total knee arthroplasties with proximal tibial defects treated with autogeneous bone grafting. In a follow-up period of 3 to 6 years, union and revascularization was demonstrated in 22 of 24 cases by tomogram, bone scan, and bone biopsy. In the two instances in which nonunion occurred, the first was attributed to insufficient preparation of the bony bed, and the second failure and eventual collapse of the graft was caused by postoperative varus alignment. Clinically, 20 of the 24 postoperative knees had good or excellent results on the Hospital for Special Surgery knee score.

Windsor and colleagues[4] used the femoral condylar grafting method described here and in addition described a technique developed by Insall that utilizes a self-locking principle in which the bone graft is shaped into a trapezoid. The graft is then keyed into a created trapezoid defect on the upper tibial surface. K-wires are used to hold the bone block in place during cementing, but are subsequently removed. Over a 5- to 7-year follow-up period, clinical and radiographic results have proved excellent with no radiolucency or collapse in any case.

Scuderi and associates[5] examined autogenous inlay bone grafting of tibial defects using the Insall technique in 26 total knee arthroplasties. The average Hospital for Special Surgery knee score postoperatively was 89 points with 25 of 26 knees demonstrating a good or excellent result and only one patient had a fair result. All grafts were incorporated within the first year with cross trabeculation between the proximal tibial bone and graft, based on serial roentgenograms. Two knees showed radiolucent lines underneath the tibial component, one of which was due to collapse of the graft, but both were less than 2 mm and nonprogressive.

Similar results were obtained by Aglietti and colleagues,[6] who described 17 patients with large medial tibial bony defects who underwent autologous bone

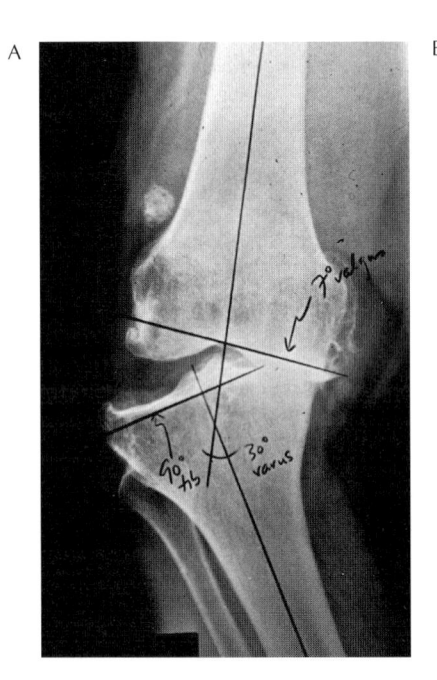

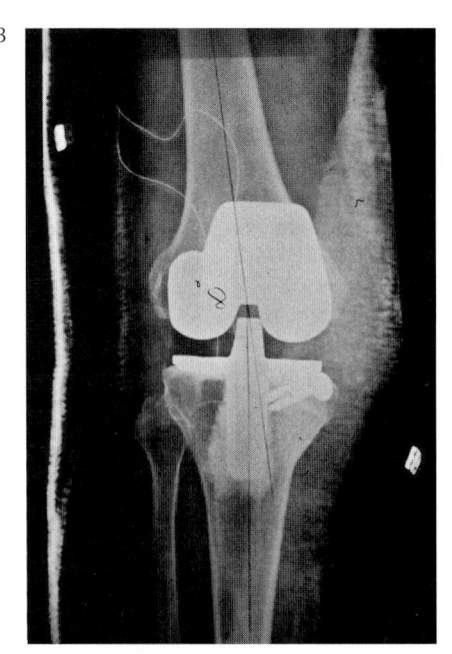

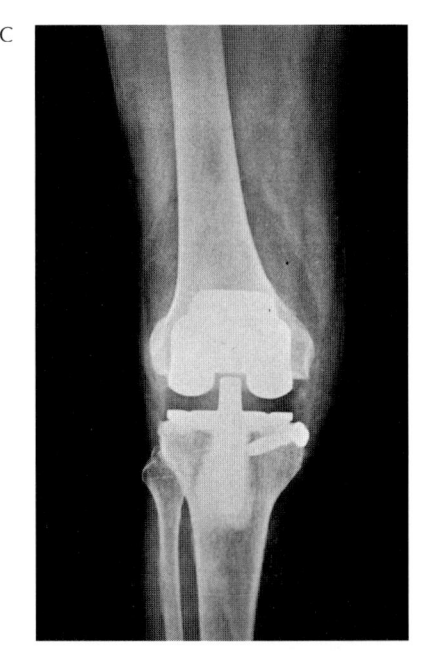

Figure 38.7. Preoperative, immediate postoperative, and 10-years postoperative demonstrating incorporation of bone graft.

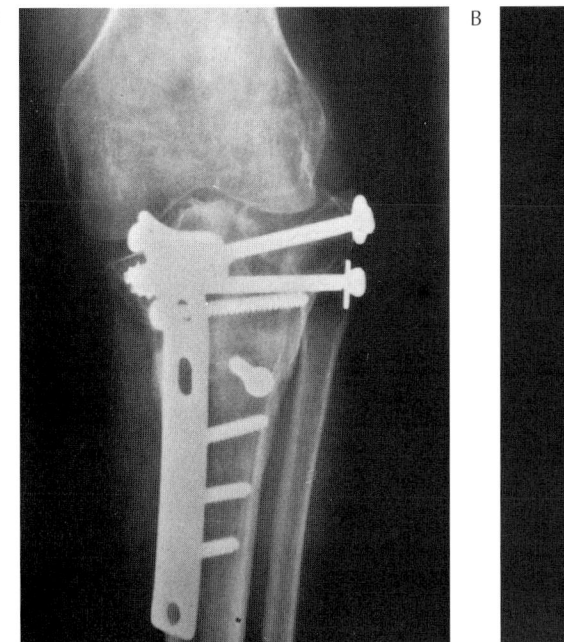

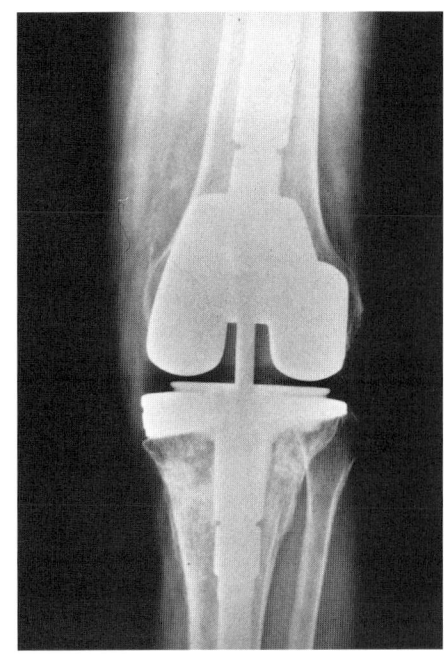

Figure 38.8. Tibial plateau fracture treated with plate fixation and postoperative radiograph demonstrating bone grafting and stem fixation to bypass the screw holes of the plate.

grafting during total knee arthoplasty. Bone resected from the distal condyles was used to fill the defect and later permanently fixed using one or two cancellous screws. The knees were reviewed over an average of 4 years. The radiographs showed complete union in 14 knees and a partially fibrous union in 3 cases with no evidence of necrosis or collapse, confirmed by bone scans and tomograms. The knee scores demonstrated good or excellent results on 16 of 17 knees, with 1 poor result due to aseptic loosening of the femoral component attributed to excessive postoperative valgus alignment.

Laskin[1] had inferior results in comparison to those reported previously in a technique that employed the posterior femoral condyles rather than the distal femoral bone as the graft material. Twenty-six patients with tibial defects were reported with a 67% success after 5-years follow-up utilizing tomograms and bone biopsy, with 4 knees demonstrating complete collapse and 4 showing radiolucency between the proximal tibia and the graft. However, the sclerotic bed was not removed when the bone graft was inserted, which may explain the inferior results. Also the author stated that the high failure rate may have been due to excessive use of subchondral and cortical bone rather than cancellous bone. The posterior condyles of the femur consist of a predominant amount of this type of bone rather than cancellous bone seen in distal femoral condylar bone.

Tibial deficiency is almost always seen with severe deformity and particularly if it is biplane or triplane.

The area of bone deficiency may be managed in a number of ways depending upon the extent and depth of the defect. Bone grafting is the preferred choice for deficiency that is greater than 12 mm. The distal femoral condyle offers signficant cancellous bone for grafting and because of its subchondral surface the upper tibial

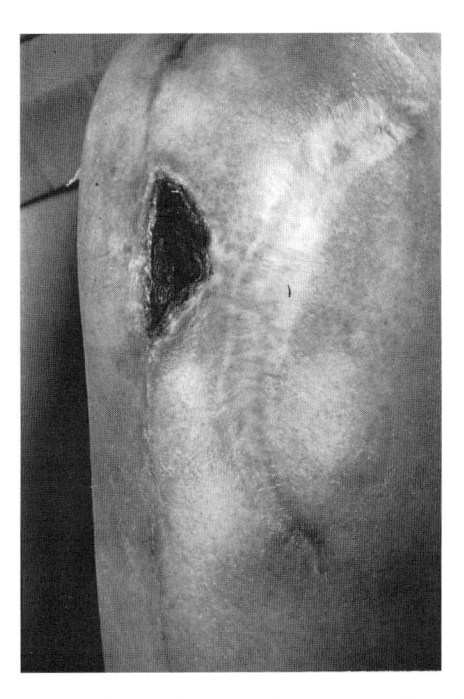

Figure 38.9. Wound slough in area between previous incision for plateau fixation and arthroplasty incision.

rim may be reconstituted as part of the grafting process. Bone augmentation by grafting allows an improved bony substrate if revision surgery should be necessary. The autogenous bone can be shaped to fill the defect but it is important to the success of the technique that cancellous bone be exposed by excision of sclerotic bone at the tibial bed. Coaptation must be precise between graft and underlying bed. If the surgical technique is accurately performed, bone-grafting techiques for tibial deficiency have demonstrated excellent long-term results in a large number of patients.

TIBIAL BONE LOSS IN PLATEAU FRACTURE

Tibial bone loss may be significant when plateau fracture occurs and despite internal fixation techniques subsequent tibial surface collapse occurs. Arthritic changes complicate the deformity present on the upper tibial surface. The areas of tibial loss in these patients may be complex and involve both the plateau itself and the tibial rim. Significant areas of depression may persist in these fractures and the tibial surface may be split. Internal fixation plates further complicate the management of these patients.

MANAGEMENT OF TIBIAL DEFICIENCY AFTER PLATEAU FRACTURE

If the previous incision is not excessively posterior, it is incorporated in the knee arthroplasty incision. Depending upon whether a medial or lateral plateau fracture is present, a medial or lateral parapatellar incision is used proximally. The plate is removed after exposure of the proximal tibia. There is usually significant scar in the involved compartment, which must be resected as part of the exposure of the knee joint.

The proximal tibial osteotomy is made in the usual fashion and areas of irregular bone loss will be corrected as part of this procedure. If the remaining deficiency is primarily in the plateau surface and the rim is intact, cancellous bone can be taken from the intercondylar area or the femoral condyles and morsellized and impacted into the depressed plateau deficit areas. If the peripheral cortical rim of the tibia has also been damaged, then distal femoral bone grafting may be used as outlined in the previous section. If autogenous bone is not available to fill both the central plateau and rim defect, a wedge may be used in addition to the impaction grafting of the central plateau deficiency (Fig. 38.8).

An intramedullary press fit stem is recommended to bypass the screw holes of the internal fixation plate if one is removed. The upper surface of the tibia should be caulked with methylmethacrylate and allowed to harden before inserting the tibial component to prevent cement interdigitating with the bone graft.

The major difficulty with these reconstructions has been wound healing especially if narrow skin flaps are created as part of the exposure. If at all possible a single incision should be used in these patients (Fig. 38.9). Reconstitution of the upper tibial surface with bone grafting in post-traumatic knees has been successful in most patients. Incorporation of the graft has occurred without exception in my experience.

References

1. Laskin RS. Total knee arthroplasty in the presence of large bony defects of the tibia and marked knee instability. *Clin Orthop.* 1989; 248:66–70.
2. Altchek D, Sculco TP, Rawlins B. Autogeneous bone grafting for severe angular deformity in total knee arthroplasty. *J Arthroplasty.* 1989; 4 (2):151–155.
3. Dorr LD, Ranawat CS, Sculco TP, McKaskill B, Oriesek BS. Bone grafting for tibial defects in total knee arthroplasty. *Clin Orthop.* 1986; 205:153–165.
4. Windsor RE, Insall JN, Sculco TP. Bone grafting of tibial defects in primary and revision total knee arthroplasty. *Clin Orthop.* 1986; 205:132–137.
5. Scuderi GR, Insall JN, Haas, SB, Becker-Fluegel MW, Windsor RE. Inlay autogenic bone grafting of tibial defects in primary total knee arthroplasty. *Clin Orthop.* 1989; 248:93–97.
6. Aglietti P, Buzzi R, Scrobe F. Autologous bone grafting for medial tibial defects in total knee arthroplasty. *J Arthroplasty.* 1991; 6(4):287–294.

CHAPTER 39
Bone Grafting in Primary Femoral Deficiency

Thomas P. Sculco

FEMORAL BONE DEFICIENCY AND BONE GRAFTING

Angular deformity results in loss of bone both on the femoral and tibial surfaces, and this must be addressed during total knee arthroplasty. The most common type of bone loss encountered is tibial plateau deficiency on the medial and posterior tibia as the result of severe varus and flexion deformity. There is associated femoral bone loss in the varus knee but it tends to be less in the distal medial femur and greater in the posterior condylar aspect of the femur. Therefore, in the author's experience, bone grafting is rarely necessary on the femoral side of the knee joint even in the most severe varus deformities. However, tibial grafting, which has been presented previously, is commonly necessary in these patients.

In the severe valgus deformity the pathologic findings are somewhat different than in the varus knee. The distal lateral femoral condyle tends to be deficient to a greater extent as well as the posterior lateral condylar bone. Bone loss on the femoral side tends to be proportionally similar to what is found on the tibial side in the valgus knee. These distal and posterior surfaces of the femur tend to be extremely sclerotic and frank depression centrally may be present. Soft tissue contracture tends to be more complex on the lateral side of the joint and both tibial and femoral releases may be necessary.

Management of distal femoral bone loss in angular deformity varies depending on the extent of bone deficiency. If the deficiency is less than 10 mm additional bone may be removed on the opposite femoral condyle and this will often allow insertion of the femoral component without augmentation of the deficient condyle. As in tibial defects, methylmethacrylate can be used to fill small areas of bone deficiency. However, whenever possible, it is preferable to achieve coaptation of the implant to the bony surface of the femur. When resecting additional bone from the femur it is important to remember the location of the joint line. In a review that the author performed of 50 osteoarthritic knees the distal articular face of the femur was 18 to 20 mm distal to the lower border of the collateral ligament origin. If this distance is maintained when the implant is inserted, then the joint line will be at approximately its correct level and the surgeon can feel confident that he or she has restored the joint line.

Increased amounts of distal femoral deficiency (greater than 12 to 15 mm) should be reconstructed by augmentation techniques. Autogenous bone grafting may be performed by utilizing bone from the opposite femoral condyle. The femoral condylar bone is resected from the less-affected femoral condyle as it would be normally and this bone is transferred to the deficient side. This grafted bone can be held in place by two screws directly into the condylar graft. Because contact may occur between the femoral component and screws, compatible metals must be used. Care must be taken to ensure that the recipient bed is primarily cancellous and that close apposition is present at the graft site. For small grafts in this area K-wire fixation alone may be sufficient. By employing this technique cancellous bone is apposed to a cancellous surface and this ensures high probability of consolidation to the underlying femur. The implant can then be placed directly on the condylar surface of the resected femoral condylar graft (Fig. 39.1).

Modular implants can be used as an alternative method to deal with distal and posterior femoral bone loss. Augments are currently available that can be added to the femoral component in thicknesses to 10 mm. When deficiency is greater the author has cemented augments together to increase their thickness to 20 mm. When deficiency is of a greater magnitude, combina-

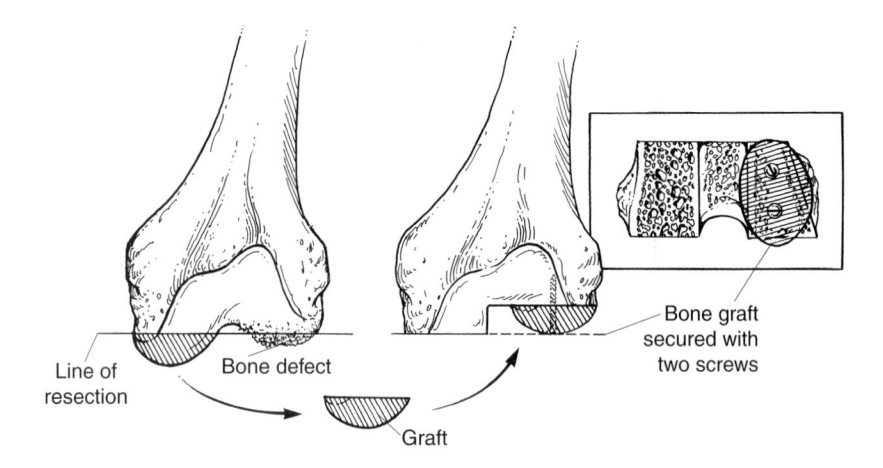

Figure 39.1. Femoral bone graft transferred from a lesser involved condyle.

tions of distal femoral grafting and augments may be used. Augments also allow for posterior augmentation when deficiency exists. Rehabilitation has not been altered when either bone grafting or modular augmentation has been used.

Aside from arthritic angular deformity, bone loss occurs on the femoral side in other clinical circumstances that are amenable to bone-grafting techniques. Osteonecrosis of the femoral condyle may produce significant areas of bone destruction. Usually most of the necrotic area is resected with the distal femoral osteotomy but significant bone defects may persist. These are usually managed with morsellized cancellous bone that can be impacted into these defective areas. When the defect is significant, larger segments of cancellous bone can be harvested from the intercondylar area of the femur, particularly if a cruciate-substituting prosthesis is being used (Fig. 39.2). This cancellous graft can be fashioned to fill these large cavities and impacted into place. The distal femoral surface can then be recreated by using a saw to smooth out the irregular surface. In employing this technique, the distal femur can be restored and its face can be prepared for the femoral component.

In patients undergoing total knee replacement after prior supracondylar osteotomy or fracture, bone grafting is usually necessary to the femur if a blade or screw plate composite has been used for fixation. When these are removed from the supracondylar area, large defects may be present extending to just above the area where the implant is fixed to bone. If the internal fixation is quite cephalad in the bone, it may be left in place and the implant resurfacing may occur below it. However, if the placement of the screw or blade has been lower, then a stress riser is created when the device is removed and dealing with bone deficiency must be performed. The area where the device is removed can be filled with cancellous bone taken from the intercondylar area or from bone resected from the tibia. The cancellous graft is impacted into these defective supracondylar areas. An intramedullary stem should be used to bypass the weakened area of bone in the supracondylar zone and also

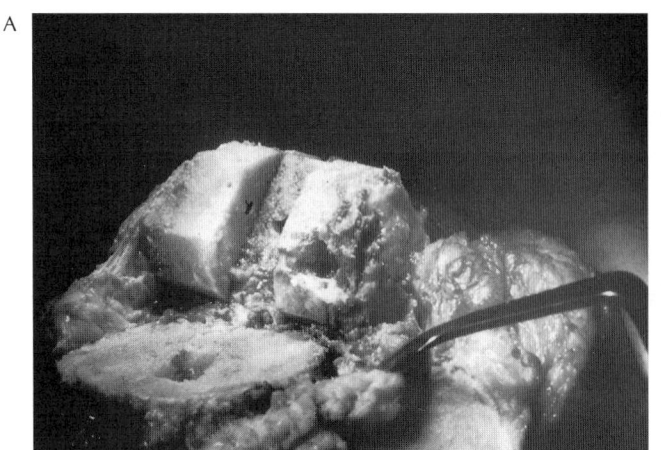

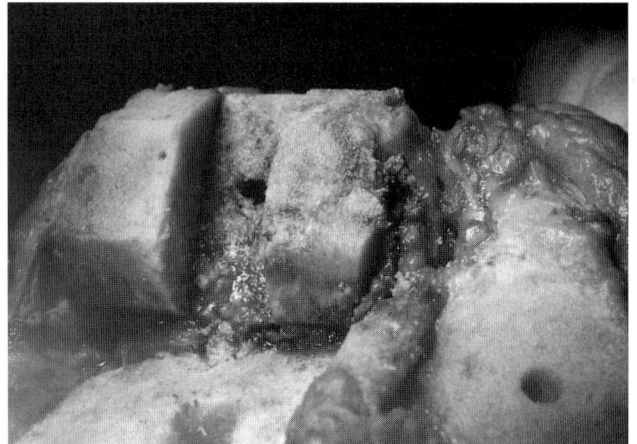

Figure 39.2. Large area of osteonecrosis treated with autogenous cancellous grafting.

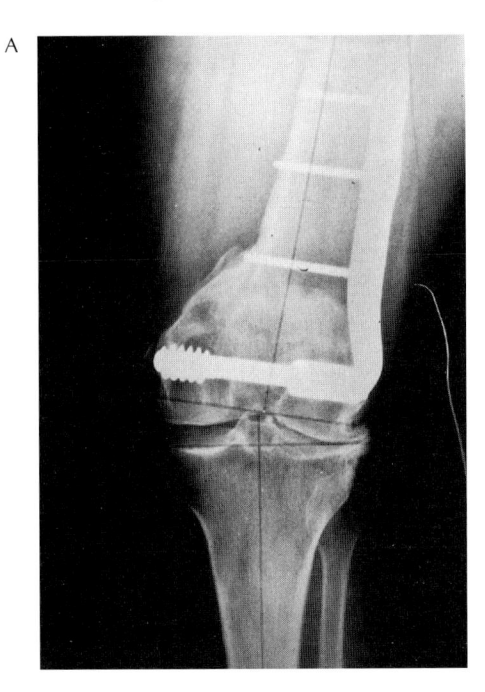

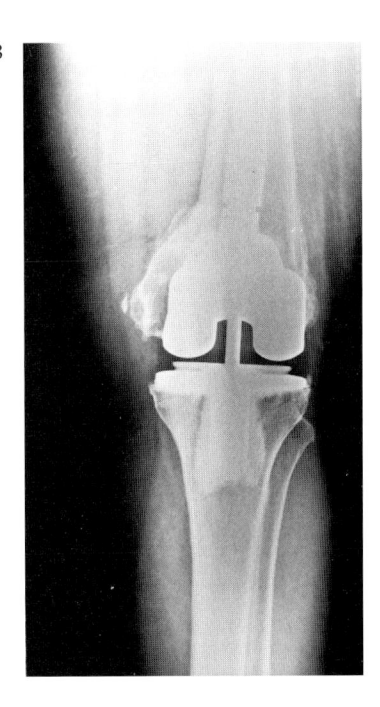

Figure 39.3. Supracondylar screw plate device removed and treated with femoral grafting and stemmed implant.

to traverse the bone that has been fixed with screws. Bone graft tends to incorporate readily in these patients in the author's experience (Fig. 39.3).

Bone loss on the femoral side in the primary knee tends to be less common than tibial deficiency. The principles are similar for both tibial and femoral bone loss. If defects are small and cystic, cancellous impaction techniques can be performed. If defects are larger and more extensive, structural autogenous grafting is necessary to provide support to the implant and effect restoration of bone stock. These structural grafts may be used alone or in combination with modular augmentation to the femoral component. Success in consolidation of these grafts requires careful technique to ensure excellent fixation of the graft and a viable bed onto which the graft is apposed. Autogenous bone is available in the primary knee, which is not the case in the revision setting in which allografting is an inferior technique to prosthetic augmentation.

SECTION 11
Patellar Preparation

CHAPTER 40
Onset Patella

Lisa Nason and Michael A. Kelly

INTRODUCTION

Resurfacing of the patella in total knee arthroplasty is commonly if not routinely performed with present total knee arthroplasty designs. Despite improved surgical techniques and implant designs, patellofemoral problems remain a frequent source of complaint following total knee arthroplasty.[1–4] These complaints may be attributed in large part to poor extensor mechanism kinematics secondary to faulty surgical technique. Two primary patellar resurfacing implant types and techniques have evolved over the past decade consisting of onset and inset patellar designs. We have favored the onset patellar implant techniques, whereas others have reported successful results with the inset designs. This chapter will focus on the surgical principles and priorities involved in performing a successful onset patella in total knee arthroplasty. These technical points are not design specific but generic to the principles of an onset patellar component.

Patellar Preparation

It is commonly assumed that restoration of the native patellar thickness is most desirable. Increasing patellar thickness during resurfacing may have detrimental effects on total knee function and contribute to anterior knee pain and decreased knee flexion (Fig. 40.1). Conversely, diminished patellar thickness following resurfacing has been postulated to lead to an increased incidence of patellar fractures.[2,5] Similarly, a recent biomechanical study by Reuben and coworkers demonstrated increased patellar strains when patellar osteotomy resulted in a bony patella thickness of less than 15 millimeters, suggesting a possible clinical concern for fractures in this group.[6] Greenfield and associates demonstrated improved patellar tracking with a marked reduction in the rate of lateral retinacular release following onset patellar resurfacing when slightly diminishing overall patellar thickness (average 1.58 millimeters).[7] The variation in patellar thickness in this series routinely leads to a residual bone thickness less than 15 millimeters (Fig. 40.2). A recent review of this original cohort of patients was evaluated at an average follow-up of three years by Geary.[8] This review demonstrated only a single patellar fracture in 121 patients. Our recommendation is to restore or slightly diminish the composite patellar thickness with onset resurfacing techniques when possible.

Patellar Osteotomy

The patellar osteotomy should create a symmetric patellar resection.[9] The line of bony resection should extend from the margin of the medial facet to the margin of the lateral facet. All too frequently an asymmetric resection is performed placing the component obliquely on the lateral facet. This should be avoided and may contribute to maltracking of the patellar component. The resection may be accurately performed using a reciprocal saw and "eyeball technique," or one may utilize a variety of calibrated cutting guides allowing a measured resection. These guides have been designed utilizing either a saw cut or reaming systems for bone resection (Fig. 40.3).

Onset Component Placement

Yoshi and coworkers have studied the effect of patellar button placement and femoral component design on patellar tracking in total knee arthroplasty.[10] A medialized position on the patellar undersurface is recommended for optimal patellar tracking[10–12] (Fig. 40.4). Additionally, we favor, when possible, a superior position for the onset component. The majority of present onset patellar designs favor three small peripheral pegs for fixation. Guide systems allow for proper positioning of these peg holes in a superomedial position. Complete coverage of the patella with an onset component is not necessary to achieve optimal results. We prefer no bony overhang of the patellar component.

Component Fixation

Our present recommendations are to utilize an all-polyethylene component. The problems are well chron-

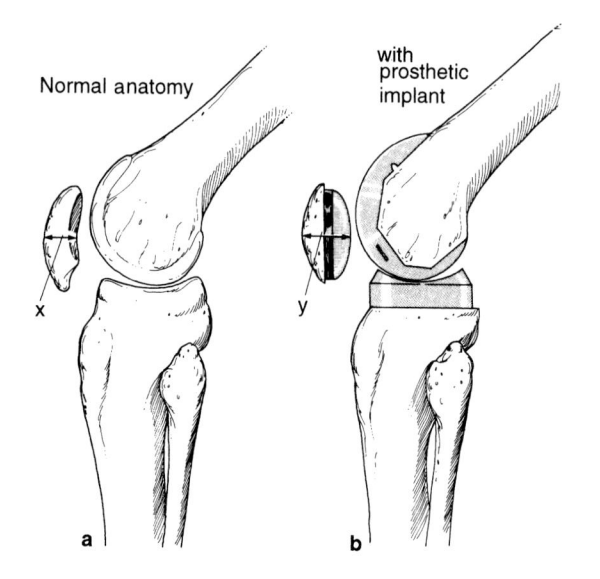

Figure 40.1. Patellar thickness.

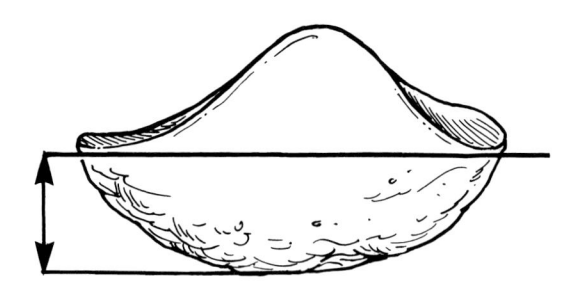

Figure 40.2. Level of patella resection.

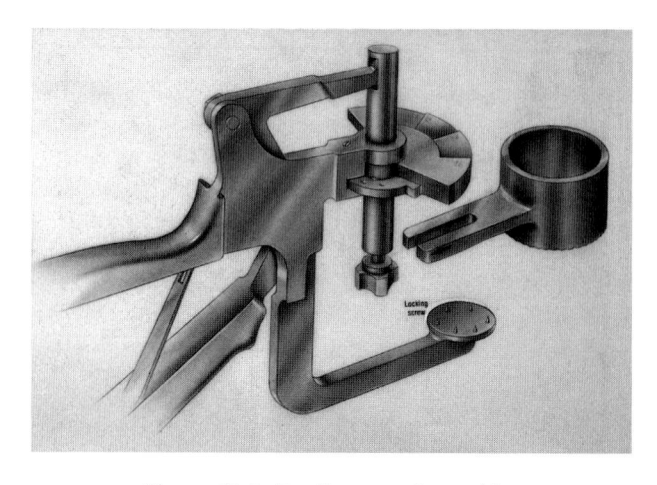

Figure 40.3. Patellar resection guide.

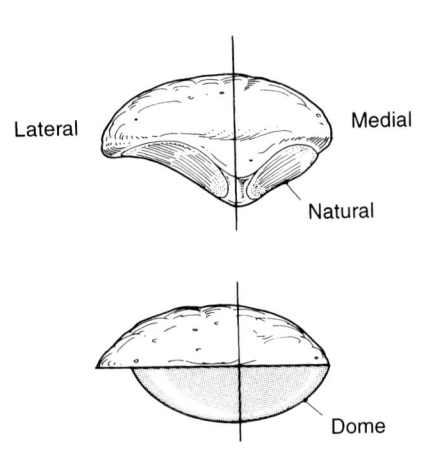

Figure 40.4. Medialized position.

icled and not recommended for routine use.[13,14] Most present designs utilize two or three peripheral pegs for implant fixation. Previously, designs had utilized a large central fixation lug. However, this has been felt to contribute to an increased incidence of patellar fracture and has been largely abandoned.[1,2,5,8] Cement is routinely utilized for fixation. The bone surface is prepared with thorough lavage and cement is applied in a doughy state. No attempt is made to pressurize the cement during application. A patellar clamp is utilized to secure the patellar component while the cement is hardening and excess cement is removed. After all the components are well fixed, the knee is reduced. We utilize a modified no thumbs technique to evaluate patellar tracking.[15,16] Additional detail of these considerations are provided in Chapter 43 as well as the indications for lateral retinacular release. Finally, the peripatellar soft tissues including the synovium and fat pad are evaluated. Typically, the synovial tissue in the area along the undersurface of the distal quadriceps is excised. This tissue has been implicated in the occasionally encountered patellar clunk syndrome, and it is important to remove it at the time of patellar resurfacing.[3,4,12]

DISCUSSION

Proper surgical technique is critical to successful patellar resurfacing in total knee arthroplasty. We have outlined the important issues in the surgical technique utilizing an onset patellar design for resurfacing. These techniques are not design specific and when utilized with the general principles regarding total knee arthroplasty will minimize patellar complications following resurfacing.

References

1. Brick GW, Scott RD. The patellofemoral component of total knee arthroplasty. *Clin Orthop*. 1988; 231:163–178.

2. Clayton ML, Thirupathi R. Patellar complications after total condylar arthroplasty. *Clin Orthop*. 1982; 170:152–155.
3. Insall JN, Haas SB. Complications of total knee arthroplasty. In: Insall JN, Windsor RE, Scott WN, Kelly MA, Aglietti P (eds). *Surgery of the Knee*. New York: Churchill Livingstone; 1993:902–922.
4. Vince KG, McPherson EJ. The patella in total knee arthroplasty. *Orthop Clin North Am*. 1992; 23(4):675–686.
5. Barnes CL, Scott RD. Patellofemoral complications of total knee replacement. Instructional Course Lectures. American Academy of Orthopaedic Surgeons. 1993; 42:303–308.
6. Reuben JD, McDonald CL, Woodard PI, Hennington LJ. Effect of patella thickness on patella strain following total knee arthroplasty. *J Arthroplasty*. 1991; 6(3):251–258.
7. Greenfield MA, Insall JN, Case GC, Kelly MA. Instrumentation of the patellar osteotomy in total knee arthroplasty. *Am J Knee Surg*. 1996; 9(3):129–132.
8. Geary SP. Personal communications.
9. Ranawat CS. The patellofemoral joint in total condylar knee arthroplasty. Pros and cons based on five- to ten-year follow-up observations. *Clin Orthop*. 1986; 205:93–99.
10. Yoshii I, Whiteside LA, Anouchi YS. The effect of patellar button placement and femoral component design on patellar tracking in total knee arthroplasty. *Clin Orthop*. 1992; 275:211–219.
11. Hofman AA, Tkach TK, Evanich CJ et al. Patellar component medialization in total knee arthroplasty. *J Arthroplasty*. 1997; 12(2):155–160.
12. Insall JN. Surgical techniques and instrumentation in total knee arthroplasty. In: Insall JN, Windsor RE, Scott WN, Kelly MA, Aglietti P (eds). New York: Churchill Livingstone; 1993:767–772.
13. Bayley JC, Scott RD, Ewald FC et al. Failure of the metal-backed patellar component after total knee arthroplasty. *J Bone Joint Surg*. 1988; 70-A:668–674.
14. Stulberg SD, Stulberg BN, Hamati Y et al. Failure mechanisms of metal-backed patellar components. *Clin Orthop*. 1988; 236:88–105.
15. Ewald FC. Leg-lift technique for simultaneous femoral, tibial, and patellar prosthetic cementing: "Rule of no thumb" for patellar tracking, and steel rod rule for ligament tension. *Techniques Orthop*. 1991; 6:4446.
16. Scott RD. Prosthetic replacement of the patellofemoral joint. *Orthop Clin North Am*. 1979; 10:129–137.

CHAPTER 41
Inlay Technique

Richard S. Laskin

When the surgeon elects to resurface the patella during a total knee arthroplasty, there are two techniques that are available. One method, called the onset technique, entails resecting the articular surface and subarticular patellar bone to form a level surface on which the implant is seated. The implant that is used usually has supplemental central peg(s) to enhance fixation on this flat surface. The second method is the inlay technique. Here, a central recess is reamed into the patellar bone and the implant is seated into the bone rather than on the cut surface. Most inlay implants likewise have a supplemental central peg to enhance cement fixation.

This chapter will deal with the inlay technique of inserting a patellar implant, its history, its rationale, and its evaluation both clinically and biomechanically. It is the method of patellar implantation that the author has been using for total knee replacement for the past 15 years.

HISTORICAL DEVELOPMENT OF THE INLAY TECHNIQUE

The original total knee implants used during the late 1960s and early 1970s were truly not "total knee replacements." In almost all cases, the patellofemoral articulation was not replaced and attention was focused only on the tibial and femoral articular surfaces. The earliest attempts at performing an arthroplasty of the patellofemoral surfaces occurred when a trochlear flange was added to the femoral prosthesis. The unresurfaced patella articulated against this metal flange. In the early 1970s, Gschwend[1] described a patellar implant that was inset into the patella. The total knee prosthesis that he used (the G.S.B.) for the femoral tibial arthroplasty was an articulated implant. As with many articulated fixed axis implants of the 1970s there were many associated problems related to wear and loosening. Interestingly enough, however, there were few problems that were attributable to the inset patellar implant.

As part of the evolution of his many prostheses, Freeman began using an inset patellar implant in the 1980s. The implant covered only the most central portion of the patella and had a concave surface that articulated with a trochlear femoral surface. This Freeman-Samuelson implant[2] was fixed without acrylic cement, relying instead on a press fit of the implant in the bone and a supplemental flanged polyethylene fixation peg on the back of the implant.

In 1981, Dr. Hugh Cameron in Toronto, Canada, and the author began biomechanical and clinical studies of an inset polyethylene patellar implant. Its articular surface was symmetrical and dome shaped. Its fixation in the patellar bone was augmented by a flanged polyethylene peg, identical to that used by Freeman. We began using this implant, the Tricon-P, in 1982 and continued with it for 18 months. At the same time we began studies using an implant with a similar articular surface and flanged polyethylene fixation peg but with a porous-coated cobalt-chrome metal baseplate. We used this implant, the Tricon-M, for the subsequent 6 years.

Early in 1988, the author began implantation of an inset patellar implant as part of the Genesis total knee prosthesis. This implant was biconvex in shape with a short central peg to augment cement fixation. Within the last year, the articular surface of this inset patellar implant has been redesigned to match the new articular geometry of the Genesis II total knee prosthesis. This is the inlay or inset patellar implant that the author is now using.

BIOMECHANICAL STUDIES ON INLAY PATELLAR IMPLANTS

A major consideration when designing any prosthetic joint implant is how the prosthesis will affect the strength of the bone. Indeed, there had been some early concerns that insetting an implant into the patella would cause it to weaken and increase the potential for fracture.

Gomes, Bechtold, Sherman, and Gustilo[3] studied patellar strength using both the inset and inset techniques of implant insertion. For their studies they used 10 cadaver legs, studying both patellae from each cadaver.

In one patella from each cadaver they used a flat reamer to obtain a flat surface. In the other patella they used a convex reamer reaming into the center of the bone. In both cases, the thickness of the patella remaining was such that the combined thickness of the resultant bone and implant would equal that of the patella before preparation. The cemented implants that were used were the Genesis© Biconvex, and the Genesis© Three Pegged Flat protheses. Ten clinical situations were studied (Table 41.1). Each patellar sample was tested in a three-point bending mode, the end point being fracture of the bone.

Their testing demonstrated that the three-point bending strength (as measured in Newton-centimeters) of those patellae that were reamed flat (as for preparation of an onset patellar implant) were statistically equal to the contralateral intact control patella (Pair 4). Subsequent cementing of a flat button on the flat surface did not further increase, nor decrease the bending strength (Pair 9) over the intact patella.

The three-point bending strength of those patella that were reamed (as for preparation of an inlay patellar implant) was statistically diminished as compared to the contralateral intact control patella (Pair 4). However, when they then cemented an inlay biconvex patellar implant in the bone (Pair 10), there was a statistically significant increase in the bending strength by more than 50% over that of the intact patella.

It was likewise noted that the fracture patterns that were eventually seen in both types of patellar preparation differed. The fracture pattern in the patellae with an inlay biconvex implant was longitudinal, whereas that in the flat cut patella with an onlay implant was transverse. Theoretically, one might argue that a longitudinal fracture would cause less disruption of the extensor mechanism than would a transverse fracture and might have less deleterious sequellae. Because of the small numbers of patellar fractures that do occur, an appropriate power value for this type of study would require several thousand knee replacements, and at this point, that study has not been performed.

SURGICAL TECHNIQUE FOR USING AN INSET PATELLA

Normally the patellar is prepared for its implant only after the femur and tibia have been resected and their trial components inserted. All the peripheral osteophytes are removed as a first stage. Often these osteophytes mask the true shape and size of the patella and can lead to erroneous placement of the implant.

The patella is grasped with a reaming clamp, the midpoint of which is oriented with the center ridge of the patella. The center ridge is located medially on the articular surface, which is essentially the patellar implant on the bone. Such medialization enhances patellar tracking. The reaming clamp that we are presently using has parallel jaws so that it will not shift as the locking mechanism is secured.

The thickness of the patella is now measured. In actuality one is measuring the combined thickness of the patellar bone, its articular cartilage, and a very thin layer of pre-patellar retinaculum and associated bursa.

Normally, the amount of cartilage and bone removed should equal the thickness of the implant to be used. A measuring template is used and a stop is set on the reamer to assure this depth of reaming. The patella is reamed to the limit of the depth stop. This technique is applicable to almost all osteoarthritic knees.

The situation is somewhat modified in patients with inflammatory arthritis, especially those in whom there has been marked patellar erosion so that the measuring template does not have a "normal" surface off which to

© Smith and Nephew Orthopaedics, Memphis, Tenn.

Table 41.1. Bending strength of the patella with two methods of reaming and two designs of patellar prosthesis

Pair 1:	Flat reamed no implant	Biconvex reamed no implant
Pair 2:	Flat reamed no implant	Flat reamed flat button implant
Pair 3:	Flat reamed no implant	Biconvex reamed biconvex implant
Pair 4:	Flat reamed no implant	Intact patella
Pair 5:	Biconvex reamed no implant	Flat reamed flat button implant
Pair 6:	Biconvex reamed no implant	Biconvex reamed biconvex implant
Pair 7:	Biconvex reamed no implant	Intact patella
Pair 8:	Flat reamed flat button implant	Biconvex reamed biconvex implant
Pair 9:	Flat reamed flat button implant	Intact patella
Pair 10:	Biconvex reamed biconvex implant	Intact patella

key. Scott has shown that this thickness is fairly consistent, measuring approximately 26 mm in males and 23 mm in females. Consequently in eroded patellae we arbitrarily aim for a combined bone-implant thickness of this size.

After the prosthetic implant is fixed into its bony bed, we remove any large protruding ridges and any remaining osteophytes. Overzealous removal of peripheral bone should not be performed lest the bony rim about the implant be inadvertently fractured.

CLINICAL STUDIES

The Knee Society and H.S.S. rating systems[4] do not specifically address problems that may be related to the patella and its implant. For this reason a supplemental evaluation was used in the studies to be described. Patients were specifically queried about the presence of anterior knee pain as distinct from pain on other areas of the knee. Pain was determined related especially to ascending and descending stairs. Likewise a determination was made about whether or not there was pain on compression of the patella against the femoral condyle. The standard roentgenographic evaluation included an anteroposterior, lateral and patellar tangential view, the latter taken with the knee in 30 to 45 degrees of flexion.

As a baseline for comparison for patients having an inlay patellar implant, we evaluated 50 patients who had undergone a total knee replacement using an onset patellar implant. Using the clinical criteria described above, 11% of the patients with an onset patella implant had some degree of anterior knee pain 2 years after surgery.

Study 1: All Polyethylene Inset Patellar Implant: Uncemented

During 1982 and 1983, 63 domed all-polyethylene patellar implants were used in 63 osteoarthritic patients as part of a tricompartmental total knee arthroplasty. The patellar components had a short flanged polyethylene peg and were inserted cement-free into the reamed recess in the patella. The femoral and tibial were cemented Richards Maximum Contact (RMC)© prostheses. All the surgeries were performed in a horizontal laminar flow environment with body exhaust suits. All patients were maintained on prophylactic antibiotics for 48 hours and Coumadin for 10 days.

Postoperatively, the patients were begun on continuous passive motion on the second postoperative day and allowed to bear weight with support in two hands on the second day as well. They continued with bimanual support for 6 weeks after which they used a cane in the contralateral hand for an additional 6 weeks.

Fifty-seven of the 63 patients have been followed for at least 10 years after surgery. The mean Knee Society Score in these patients at 10 years was 86 with a range of from 76 to 98. Anterior knee pain was found in 11% of the knees. There were 6 knees with patellar tilt, 2 cases of patellar subluxation, and no case of frank dislocation.

Four of the knees had been revised prior to the 10-year evaluation; in all four the indication for revision was tibial component loosening. None of the revised patients had anterior knee pain. At the time of revision (4, 7, 8, and 8.2 years after the index arthroplasty) the patellar component was routinely evaluated and removed. In all four cases there was a large patellar meniscus present with less than 10 mm diameter of polyethylene uncovered by the membrane. When the meniscus was removed, each of the implants was noted to demonstrate some motion within the patella. The implant was removed and a new patellar implant cemented in placed.

Examination of the undersurface of the removed implants revealed mild abrasive wear. The fibrous tissue between the implant and the bone histologically contained fibrocytes. Only rarely did we find macrophages or giant cells. The patellar meniscal tissue was found to be fibrous in nature with no neural elements.

Study 2: Metal-Backed Polyethylene Inset Patellar Implant: Uncemented

Beginning in 1983, we began inserting metal-backed domed inset patellar implants. The implants were 30 mm in diameter and were symmetrical in configuration. The polyethylene surface was prolonged through the metal baseplate as a flanged peg. The polyethylene was 8.5 mm thick, with no metallic endoskeleton, while the metal baseplate was 1.6 mm thick. The undersurface of the base plate was covered with a multi-level surface of sintered cobalt-chrome-molybdenum beads enclosing pores of approximately 250 microns in diameter.

In 1990[5] Bucknell and the author reported a joint series of 425 knee replacements in which this metal-backed patellar implant was inserted cement-free. The mean follow-up at that point was four years with all patients reported having been followed for at least 3 years. At that time we had 7 patients with subluxation of the patella and 2 with gross dislocation, both of whom required a recentralizing procedure. There had been no case of implant dissociation nor of wear through of the polyethylene to the metal baseplate. None of the patients had a boggy synovitis nor any retro-patellar squeaking. This series was being reported at the time

© Smith and Nephew Orthopaedics, Memphis, Tenn.

that other series using metal-backed patellar implants were demonstrating a high incidence of polyethylene wear through and metal-on-metal synovitis.[6–8]

We felt at that time that the absence of a metal endoskeleton enabled us to maximize the polyethylene thickness used, and that the insetting of the implant, distanced the metal from any potential contact with the metal trochlear surface of the femoral component.

The author has now personally followed 245 patients with this inset metal-backed patellar component for up to 10 years after their surgery. Over 70% of the patients had osteoarthritis. The femoral and tibial components were Tricon-M© implants and were inserted cement-free.[9] The postoperative physical therapy regimen, as well as the operative suite and perioperative regimen remained because it had been in the all-polyethylene series preceding it.

At 10 years after surgery, 10% of the patients had anterior pain. There were 19 cases with patellar tilt and 6 cases with subluxation laterally. The mean Knee Society Knee Score was 84. There were two knees with patellar fractures; one was a nondisplaced inferior pole fracture and the other a nondisplaced longitudinal fracture. In both cases the fractures were treated nonoperatively and eventually clinically healed.

Although at the 4-year follow-up we had not seen any "wear-throughs," by the seventh year after implantation these began to be evident. At this point we have had to revise four patients in whom the patellar polyethylene wore down to the metal (1.8%). These problems occurred at 6.5, 7.2, 7.5, and 8 years, respectively, after the original operation. Each patient had rheumatoid arthritis and had developed moderate instability of the knee many years after the original arthroplasty with a significant enlargement of the flexion space associated with dislocation of the patella laterally. In each case the arthroplasty had been performed with retention of the posterior cruciate ligament. At the time of revision, it was found that in each case the posterior cruciate ligament had ruptured and autolyzed allowing anteroposterior and rotatory instability and patellar dislocation. The dislocating patella then developed a rapid wear-through of the polyethylene down to the metal baseplate.

It appeared that even with an inset implant with thick polyethylene, the metal baseplate was at risk for contact with the femoral trochlear flange if the patella did not remain centralized in the femoral groove. Although we have not yet seen this problem in any of our osteoarthritic patients, there is the potential for wear-through in these cases as well should lateral instability occur.

© Smith and Nephew Orthopaedics, Memphis, Tenn.

Study 3: All Polyethylene Biconvex Inset Patellar Implant: Cemented

Beginning in 1988 we began evaluating a type of inset patellar component that had initially been designed by Gustilo as part of the Genesis total knee prosthesis. The implant was all polyethylene and was biconvex with a small 3 mm central fixation peg. It was inserted in the patella using instruments similar to those used for the previous two Tricon patellar implants, but with the reamer modified so as to create an appropriate central concave recess in the patella for the implant. We have at this point inserted 814 biconvex patellae. In 205 knees, the femoral and tibial prostheses were uncemented Genesis components, while in the remaining cases they were cemented Genesis components.[10]

In this series of patients the physical therapy was modified as compared to the previous two series. We now allowed the patients to begin motion of the knee with a continuous passive motion machine on the day of surgery. Patients were allowed to ambulate on the second postoperative date with support in two hands, and advanced to a single cane on the sixth or seventh postoperative day. The majority of the patients had their surgery performed under epidural anesthesia, with a continuous epidural PCA infusions used for two days after surgery.

Two hundred and twenty-one implants have been followed for at least 4 years after implantation. The incidence of anterior knee pain has been 2.3%. There have been 2 cases of lateral subluxation of the patella, and 13 cases with patellar tilt on Merchant X-ray views. There has been only one patellar fracture, which occurred in a patient who fell down a basement staircase 9 months after surgery. The fracture was longitudinal, the quadriceps mechanism was intact, and the patient did not require surgery.

Because of the convex configuration of the underside of the implant, it is not possible to align the X-ray beam parallel to the complete undersurface. Radiolucent line evaluation, therefore, is much less accurate than in a flat patellar implant. We have noted, however, no patient who has had a global radiolucency in the patellar implant and no case of gross loosening of the implant.

Study 4: Inset vs. Onset Cemented Implants

Rand and Gustilo have reported on a study of 250 total knee replacement arthroplasties using the Genesis total knee prosthesis in which the cemented femoral and tibial components were identical; however, two types of cemented patellar implants were used, inset and onset. The mean follow-up was 2.3 years.

Patellar tilt was measured on Merchant view of the knee. For the onset resurfacing patellar implants the mean patellar tilt was 3.5 degrees whereas for the biconvex inset implants it was 0.6 degree. The difference was statistically significant ($p < .001$). Seventy-nine percent of the knees with the resurfacing implant required lateral release, whereas only 28% of the knees with the inset biconvex implant did ($p < .01$). Furthermore, the incidence of residual lateral subluxation at two years was 6% in the resurfacing group, whereas it was 3% in the inset group ($p < .02$). It would appear that using a technique to inset the patellar implant resulted in a better ability to centralize the extensor mechanism.

Study 5: Inset Patellar Component in Cases of Severe Patellar Bone Loss

There are two clinical situations in which an inset patellar implant may be the only method available for resurfacing of the patella. In both of these situations there has been severe patellar bone loss, in one from advanced rheumatoid arthritis and the other in a patient requiring a revision arthroplasty.

In reviewing the last 100 cases in which a total knee arthroplasty was performed in patients with inflammatory arthritis, there were 16 cases in which there was severe central erosion of the patella centrally. This erosion was most marked in valgus rheumatoid knees with lateral subluxation of the patella. For these knees, it was not possible to resect the patella to obtain a flat base for an onset implant, lest the bone be severely thinned. An inset implant, however, was applicable without further diminishing patellar bone stock and obviates the problems attendant with the alternative or a patellectomy or patelloplasty.

A similar situation was noted in revision surgery, especially in those cases in which an uncemented porous ingrowth patellar implant was being revised. The availability of an inset implant allowed patellar resurfacing in all but one such case over the past two years.

THE PATELLAR MENISCUS

The patellar meniscus is a fibrous ring of tissue that is often seen about the periphery of the patellar implant at the time of arthroscopy or revision of the total knee patient. It has been alleged that it is the cause of anterior knee pain in some patients after a knee arthroplasty; however, these reports are usually apocryphal and undocumented.

We have noted the presence of a patellar meniscus in over 90% of all total knees that we have revised; knees in which both an onlay and an inlay implant was used. In the overwhelming majority of these knees, the patients had no patellofemoral symptoms or anterior knee pain prior to the surgery, the operation being performed mainly for tibial loosening and/or component malposition. Microscopic examination of a removed fibrous meniscus revealed well-differentiated fibrous tissue. There were no neural elements demonstrable in the meniscal tissue. It does not seem plausible, therefore, that the meniscus is the cause of anterior knee pain after a total knee replacement. Likewise arthroscopic surgery to remove this meniscus in an attempt to alleviate postsurgical anterior knee pain appears to be worthless.

The meniscus can form only in areas in which the patellar implant does not contact the femoral trochlear surface. The meniscus increases the contact area between the patella and the trochlear flange. Its presence probably diminishes patellofemoral contact stresses, stresses which in vitro are normally higher than the deformation point of polyethylene. The formation of the meniscus over the peripheral rim of bone around an inlay patellar implant eliminates contact between the rim and the trochlear flange as well.

SUMMARY

Our experience over the past fifteen years indicates that an inset patellar implant has yielded excellent results when used in both cemented and uncemented modes. There are theoretical and clinical benefits to insetting the implant that include obtaining a stronger composite of bone and prosthesis, a decreased incidence of patellar tilt, and the ability to perform a patellar arthroplasty is cases of severe patellar erosion and bone loss, as in the rheumatoid or revision patient.

The only potential drawback of this type of patellar preparation is that the reamed-out bone is weaker than the intact patella. Care must be taken therefore not to unduly traumatize the reamed bone until the permanent implant is cemented in place, at which point its strength markedly increases. It is for that reason that we prepare the patella only after the femur and tibia have been prepared.

It has been alleged that disruption of the intraosseous vascular supply of the patella by reaming into it, when combined with disruption of some or all of the extrinsic genicular blood supply, would lead to an increased incidence of osteonecrotic fracture of the bone. This has not been seen despite using this technique for over 15 years.

References

1. Gschwend N. The GSB knee: a further possibility, principles, results. *Clin Orthop.* 1976; 132:170–176.

2. Freeman MAR, Samuelson KM, Elias Marrorenzi LJ, Gokcay EI, Tuke M. The patello-femoral joint in total knee arthroplasty-design considerations. *Journal of Arthroplasty.* 1989; (Supple):69–74.
3. Gomes LSM, Bechtold JE, Gustilo RB. Patellar prosthesis positioning in total knee arthroplasty. *Clin Orthop* 1988; 236:72–81.
4. Ewald FC. The Knee Society total knee arthroplasty roentgenographic evaluation and scoring system. *Clin Orthop.* 1989; 248:9–15.
5. Laskin RS, Bucknell A. The use of a metal-backed patellar prosthesis in total knee arthroplasty. *Clin Orthop.* 1990; 260:52–55.
6. Bayley JC, Scott RD. Further observations on metal-backed patellar component failure. *Clin Orthop.* 1988; 236:82–87.
7. Bayley JC, Scott RD, Ewald FC, Holmes GB. Failure of the metal-backed patellar component after total knee replacement. *J Bone Joint Surg.* 1988; 70:66–674.
8. Lombardi AV Jr, Engh GA, Volz RG, Albrigo JL, Brainard BJ. Fracture/dislocation of the polyethylene in metal-backed patellar components in total knee arthroplasty. *J Bone Joint Surg.* 1988; 70:675–679.
9. Laskin RS. Tricon-M uncemented total knee prosthesis. *Techniques in Orthopedics.* 1987; 18–30.
10. Laskin RS. Modular total knee replacement with posterior cruciate retention. A three year follow up study. *The Knee.* 1994; 1:46–53.

CHAPTER 42
Rotating Patella

Frederick F. Buechel

INTRODUCTION

A congruent-contact, metal-backed, rotating-bearing patellar prosthesis was developed and first used clinically in 1977.[1] This bispherical bearing has an anatomically designed larger lateral facet than medial facet and tracks congruently into the deep sulcus femoral groove of the femoral component. The bearing surface is formed by a single surface of revolution that creates a common generating curve for all articulating surfaces of the knee replacement (LCS ® Knee Replacement System-Depuy, Warsaw, Indiana) (Fig. 42.1).

The rotation of the bearing is limited by a pin-in-slot arrangement that allows 90 degrees of total motion to provide normal axial rotation and to allow for significant surgical malalignment (Fig. 42.2). The fixation of the thin, metal-anchoring plate is provided by cruciform fins that are porous coated (Porocoat ®- Depuy, Warsaw, Indiana) for cementless fixation or bead-blasted for cemented fixation. The cruciform fins structurally reinforce the thin metal-anchoring plate against torsional stresses while also reinforcing the patella remnant against fractures.[2]

SURGICAL TECHNIQUE: (MEDIAL APPROACH) PATELLAR RESECTION

After a medial parapatellar approach and routine placement of the femoral and tibial components with a tibial bearing that provides equal flexion and extension tension, the patella is everted laterally and the articular surface is resected at the level of the quadriceps tendon insertion. A towel clip in the medial retinaculum may be used to facilitate and stabilize the everted patella. A thin, wide oscillating sawblade can be used to rest on the quadriceps tendon-superior pole patella junction after the synovial rim has been sharply exposed (Fig. 42.3). The saw should leave a patellar remnant that parallels the quadriceps-patellar tendons and has equal medial-lateral as well as superior-inferior thickness that generally ranges from 12 to 15 mm (see Fig. 42.4).

SURGICAL TECHNIQUE: (LATERAL APPROACH)

After a lateral parapatellar approach and routine placement of the femoral and tibial components, the patella is everted medially and the articular surface is resected at the level of the quadriceps tendon insertion similar to the medial approach. The handle portion of the patellar template is reversed, however, to allow the long limb of the cruciate-fixturing channel to be in the proper lateral position for the burr. Reversing the position of the patellar template is the only technical difference in patellar preparation, although the fat pad may be retained and mobilized for lateral retinacular defect coverage as previously described.[3]

PATELLAR TRIAL

Place the appropriate size patellar template over the femoral component and perpendicular to the long axis of the extremity with pegs pointing upward. Reduce and press the resected patella onto the template engaging the pegs in the resected patellar surface. Flex the knee and assure that the patellar template remains perpendicular to the long axis of the extremity and parallel to the prosthetic joint line.

With the knee extended, evert the patella while pressing the template into the patellar remnant. The handle of the template will usually lie approximately 30 to 45 degrees downward from the perpendicular. Mark the cross for the trial patellar component with the cautery or a marking pen.

Remove the template and press the trial patellar component onto the resected patellar surface with the pins located at the ends of the cruciate mark.

Reduce the patella. While flexing and extending the knee, evaluate patellar tracking. The metal portion of the patella should remain parallel with the knee joint. Thumb pressure should be used to hold the patellar component congruently in the femoral groove. If lateral displacement occurs despite thumb pressure, then per-

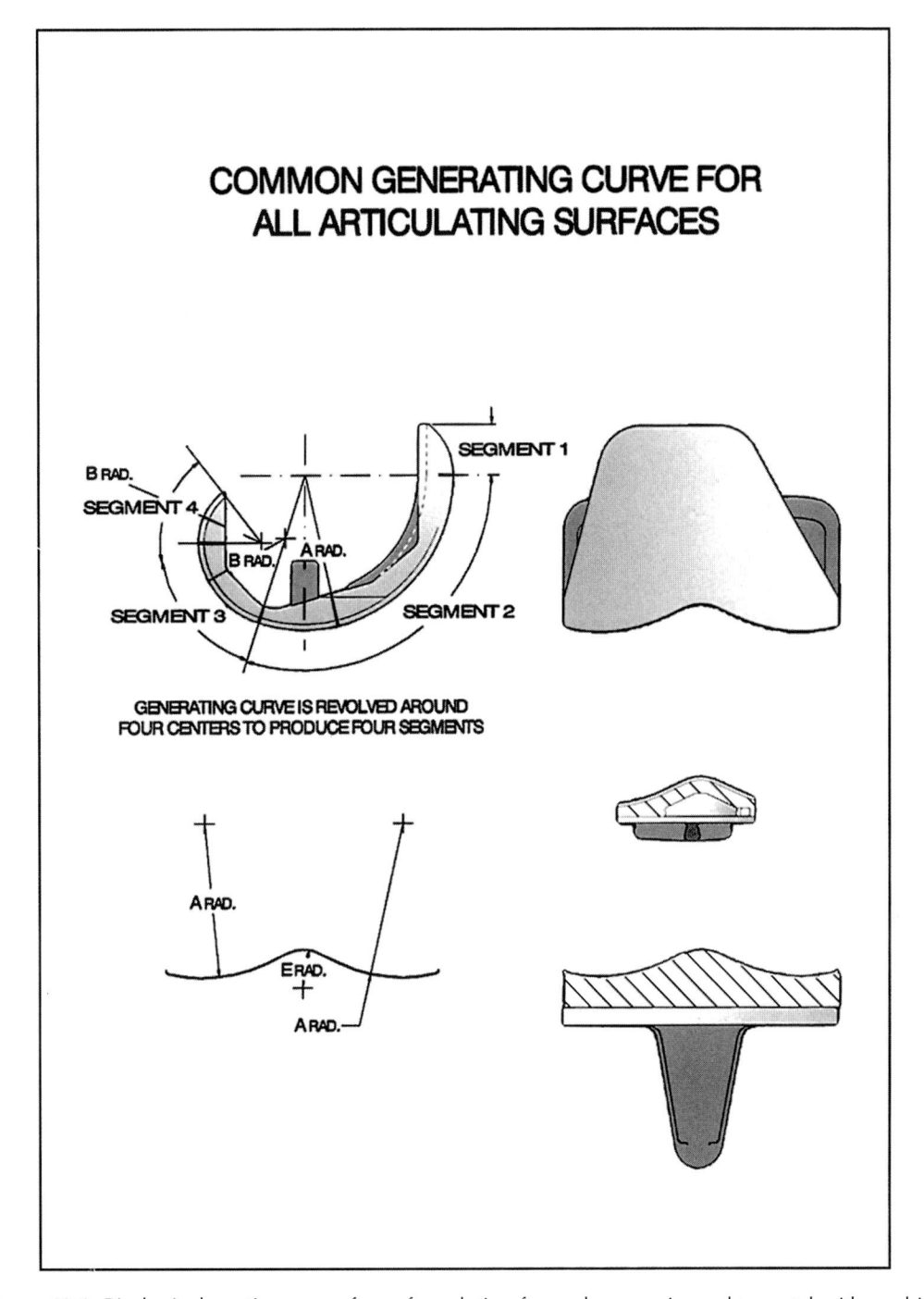

Figure 42.1. Bispherical continuous surface-of-revolution femoral groove is used to match either a bispherical congruently tracking patellar component or the natural patella.

form a sequential lateral release beginning at the lateral rim of the patella, followed by the distal, then the proximal retinacula.

PATELLAR PREPARATION

Once more align the appropriate size and type of patellar template over the mark on the patellar remnant representing proper alignment. A hard bone template for sclerotic bone, and a standard template for osteoporotic bone are available. Use the hard bone template when cementing. Prepare the cruciate channels using the patellar burr through the slot in the template. Ensure that the channels are sufficiently deep to avoid any resistance to the fixturing fins of the final patellar component.

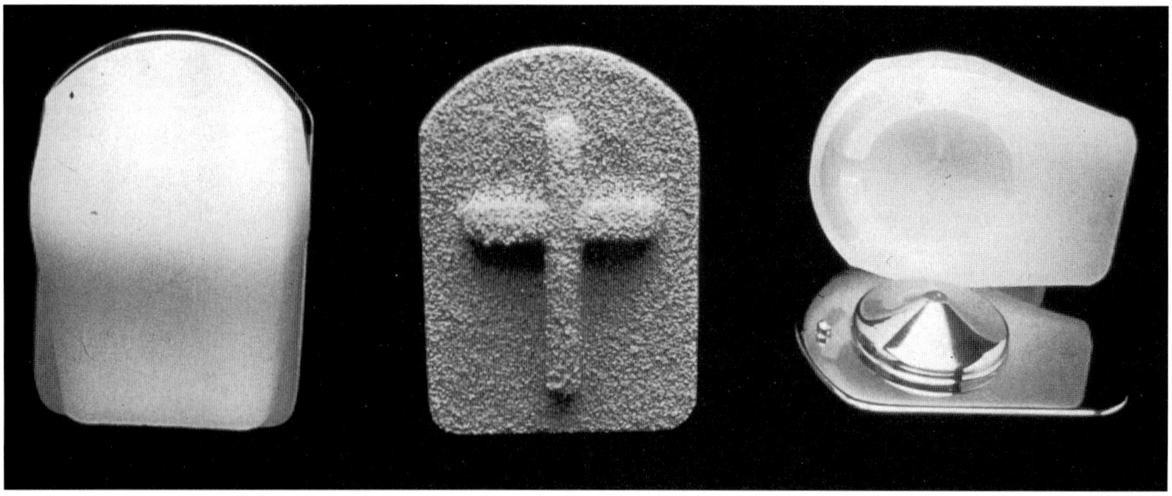

Figure 42.2. Uncoupled rotating patella prosthesis demonstrating the conical trunion connection and the 90-degree rotational stop.

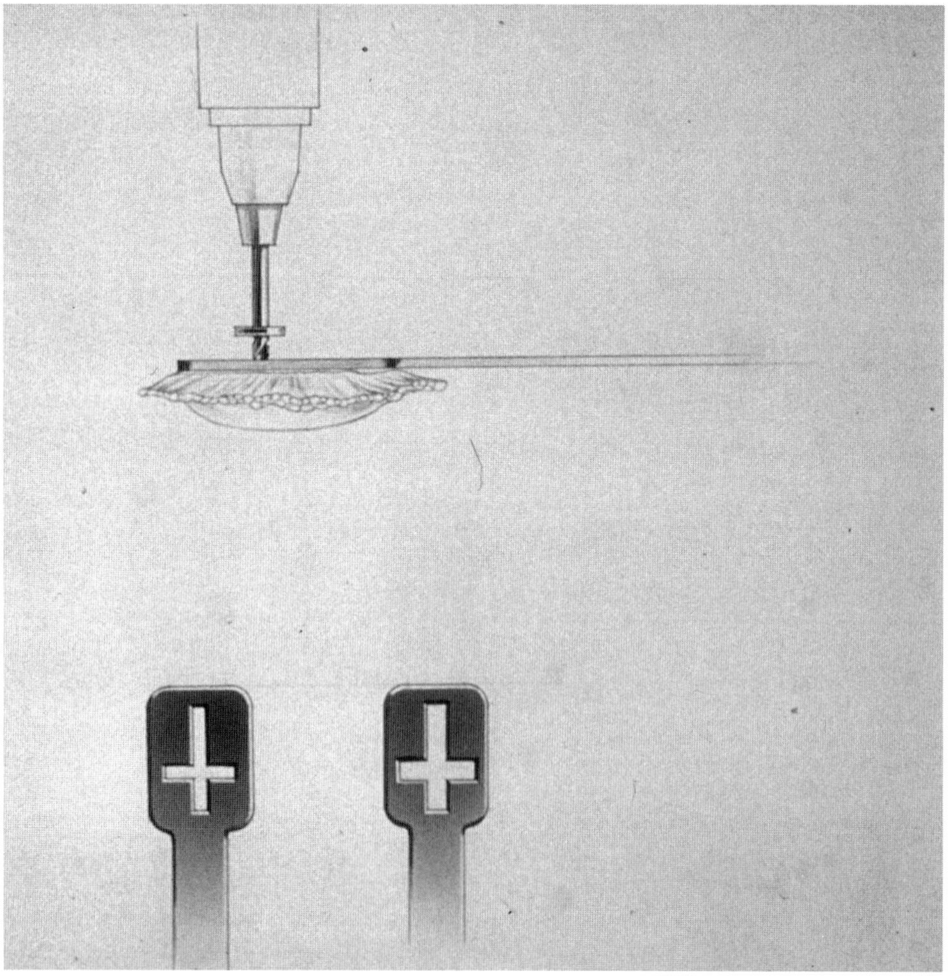

Figure 42.3. Everted patella with thin, wide sawblade resting on the quadriceps tendon prior to resection.

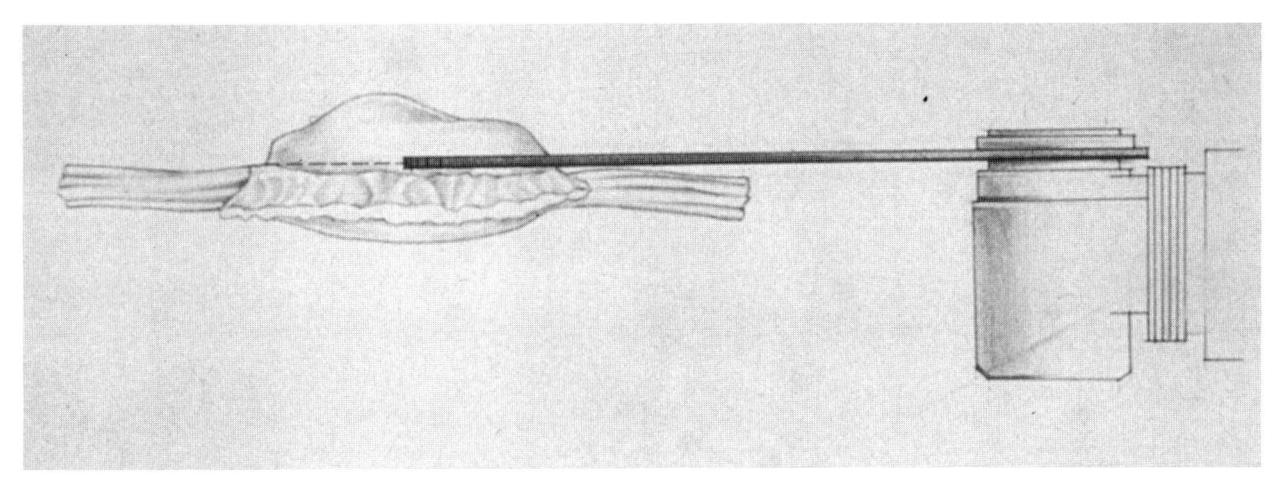

Figure 42.4. Power saw cutting the patella parallel to the quadriceps-patellar tendons.

FINAL PATELLAR IMPLANTATIONS

Align the cruciate-fixturing fins and press the patellar-anchoring plate flat against the resected bone surface using the patellar clamp. Reduce the patella and evaluate motion and tracking. Final soft tissue and bony resection should be performed to ensure free bearing movement and central patellar tracking.

If cement is used, copiously irrigate and dry the bony surfaces prior to cementation. Be sure all extra cement is removed from the nonfixation surfaces of the bone and that no cement particles remain on the bearing surfaces.

POSTOPERATIVE REHABILITATION

Cemented and cementless rotating patellar replacements are treated the same postoperatively and are integrated into the LCS total knee rehabilitation protocol.[2]

SURVIVORSHIP OF ROTATING PATELLAR PROSTHESES

Previous long-term studies of this metal-backed, rotating-bearing patellar prosthesis have documented overall failure rates of less than 1% and mechanical failures of less than 0.5% after 11 years.[2,4–6]

More recent evaluation of 515 rotating patellar replacements initially followed for 11 years[2] and now followed for 19 years demonstrates an overall survivorship of 98.1% using revision of any component for any reason as the end point. Specific causes of failure requiring revision occurred in 4 knees. Two displaced patella fractures in revision cases required implant removal. One dislocated patella in a multiply-operated knee became infected and the knee was fused. One patella bearing fractured after 10 years in active, multiply-operated cross-country cyclist and required replacement with a new bearing without disturbing the cementless fixation plate.

Survivorship of at least 90% at the 10-year interval, using an end point of revision of any component for any reason, has been recommended as an FDA standard for new prosthetic joint replacement designs.[7] The rotating patellar replacement described in this chapter meets and exceeds this requirement out to the 19-year interval, thus demonstrating superior wear, fixation, and functional capabilities.

Counterface improvements and enhanced polyethylene quality may allow similar patellar devices to enjoy demanding long-term use in the future if the insertion techniques presented are embraced.

References

1. Buechel FF, Pappas MJ. New Jersey Low Contact stress knee replacement system. Ten-year evaluation of meniscal bearings. *Orthop Clin NA*. 1989; 20:147–177.
2. Buechel FF, Rosa RA, Pappas MJ. A metal-backed, rotating-bearing patellar prosthesis to lower contact stress. An 11-year clinical study. *Clin Orthop*. 1989; 248:34–49.
3. Buechel FF. A sequential three-step lateral release for correcting fixed valgus knee deformities during total knee arthroplasty. *Clin Orthop*. 1990; 260:170–175.
4. Buechel FF, Sorrels B, Pappas MJ. New Jersey Rotating Platform total knee replacement: clinical, radiographic, statistical, and survivorship analyses of 346 cases performed by 16 surgeons. Food and Drug Administration Panel Presentation, Gaithersburg, Md, November 22, 1991.
5. Buechel FF, et al. New Jersey LCS Posterior Cruciate Retaining total knee replacement: clinical, radiographic, sta-

tistical, and survivorship analyses of 395 cementless cases performed by 13 surgeons. Food and Drug Administration Panel Presentation. Rockville, Md, June 1, 1990.
6. Buechel FF, et al. New Jersey LCS Unicompartmental knee replacement: clinical, radiographic, statistical and survivorship analyses of 106 cementless cases performed by 7 surgeons. Food and Drug Administration Panel Presentation. Rockville, Md, August 16, 1991.
7. Buechel FF, Pappas MJ, Greenwald AS. Use of survivorship and contact stress analyses to predict the long term efficacy of new generation joint replacement designs: a model for FDA device evaluation. *Orthop Rev*. 1991; 20:50–55.

SECTION 12
Extensor Mechanism Alignment

CHAPTER 43
The Intraoperative Assessment of Patellar Tracking

Mark W. Pagnano and Michael A. Kelly

INTRODUCTION

The decision to resurface the patellofemoral joint during total knee arthroplasty has historically been controversial. The impetus to incorporate patellar resurfacing in condylar knee designs was provided by clinical data suggesting that as many as 24 to 50% of patients with an unresurfaced patella after TKA experienced anterior knee pain.[1-17] The introduction of condylar knee prostheses with an anterior femoral flange for articulation with a patellar button changed the nature of problems at the patellofemoral joint following TKA. Resurfacing the patella has proved reliable in reducing the incidence of post-arthroplasty anterior knee pain, but resurfacing has introduced its own set of complications. Patellofemoral instability, fracture, loosening, component wear or failure, patellar clunk syndrome, and patellar ligament and quadriceps tendon disruption have all been associated with technical errors in the performance of patellar resurfacing. Complications arising from the resurfaced patellofemoral articulation have varied in incidence from 5 to 50% of TKAs and have been implicated as the cause of up to 50% of the revision TKA procedures currently performed.[1,5,8,9,12,15,21-28]

Several reports in the literature have focused on the intraoperative technical aspects of patellar resurfacing.[29-33] Unsatisfactory tracking of the patellofemoral articulation can lead to patellofemoral pain, instability, loosening, wear or failure.[1,5,8,9,12,14,20,24,32,34-36] Satisfactory tracking of the patellofemoral joint is essential to the success of total knee arthroplasty with or without patellar resurfacing.[14] Few reports, however, specifically address the intraoperative assessment of patellar tracking. This chapter presents a comprehensive approach to the assessment of patellar tracking in total knee arthroplasty including a focused review of the preoperative X rays, specific techniques to intraoperatively assess tracking, and a checklist approach should a tracking problem be encountered intraoperatively.

PREOPERATIVE ASSESSMENT

A brief, focused review of the patient's preoperative radiographs is an invaluable adjunct to the intraoperative assessment. The merchant view reveals both the thickness and symmetry of the native patella and thus aids in orienting the patellar osteotomy to produce a symmetric patellar bone remnant (Fig. 43.1). Particular note is made of the patellar high point as intraoperative efforts are directed at slightly medializing or at least reproducing that high-point location[37] (Fig. 43.2). The merchant view also provides an opportunity to note the presence of patellar tilt or subluxation. The lateral view may reveal the presence of patellar baja (Fig. 43.3). Exposure problems may be anticipated in cases with marked baja and the surgeon should be prepared to make a more extensile exposure by utilizing a quadriceps snip or tibial tubercle osteotomy.[38,39] The full-length standing and anteroposterior views of the knee are used to evaluate limb alignment. Valgus angulation increases the Q-angle and predisposes to patellar instability. Distal femoral bone loss from the lateral condyle in the valgus knee can lead the surgeon to inadvertently cut the distal femur in excessive valgus (Fig. 43.4). If the surgeon then adds a mild varus cut to the tibia, the overall alignment of the limb may in fact be satisfactory. The problem, of course, is that inappropriately positioned components, even in a well-aligned limb, will predispose to patellar problems. One must also plan for bone loss from the posterior aspect of the lateral femoral condyle in the valgus knee. Total knee systems that reference femoral component rotation based on the posterior condyles will lead to excessive internal rotation of the femoral component in the valgus knee.

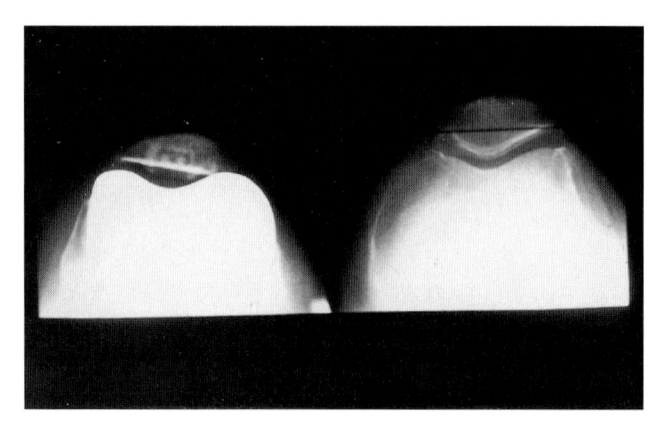

Figure 43.1. The merchant view of the patella can serve as a guide to orient both the direction and thickness of the patellar osteotomy.

INTRAOPERATIVE ASSESSMENT

The intraoperative assessment of patellar tracking begins after the bone cuts and soft tissue releases have been performed to balance the knee in flexion and extension. Trial components are then assembled and stability and overall limb alignment are verified. Attention is then turned to patellar tracking.

Preferred Technique

Our preferred technique in the assessment of patellar tracking involves placement of a towel clip through the medial edge of the quadriceps tendon 8 cm proximal to the superior pole of the patella[38] (Fig. 43.5). Gentle traction is then directed proximally, in line with the pull of the quadriceps musculature, to eliminate any slack in the extensor mechanism. We specifically avoid placing any medial or lateral traction on the quadriceps tendon. The knee is then slowly flexed and the behavior of the patellofemoral articulation is observed. Acceptable tracking includes contact of the patellar component with both the medial and lateral femoral condyles with no tendency for patellar tilt or subluxation (Fig. 43.6). Particular attention is given to the behavior of the patella as the knee progresses from 60 to 90 degrees of flexion because this is the range at which subluxation and tilt are most evident.

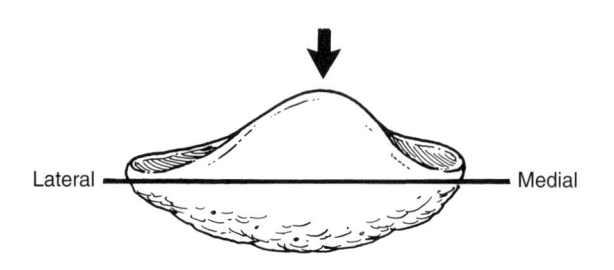

Figure 43.2. Note the medial position of the high point in the typical patella.

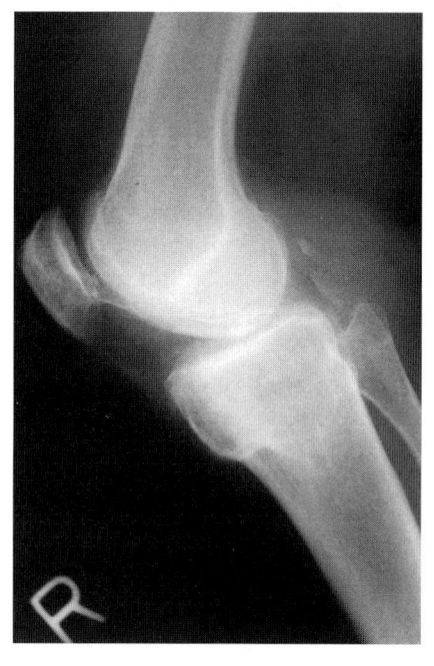

Figure 43.3. Patellar baja, in this case mild and a result of previous surgery, should be noted preoperatively. Exposure difficulties may be encountered in such cases and a quadriceps snip or tubercle osteotomy may be required.

Alternative Techniques

Several other intraoperative techniques have been suggested to help assess patellar tracking and guide the need for lateral release. The most widely utilized technique is the so-called "rule of no thumb" proposed by Scott.[14] In this technique, if the patella tracks well without closing the capsule and without the surgeon holding the patella located with his thumb, then no lateral release is needed. Should the patella demonstrate a tendency to subluxate without counteracting pressure from the thumb, then a lateral retinacular release is recommended. Our thought has been that the "rule of no thumb" tends to overestimate the need for lateral release.

A variation of the "one-stitch test" involves the use of a single towel clip to reapproximate the capsule (Fig. 43.7). Similarly, one towel clip placed above the patella and one below the patella has been proposed as a method to simulate the soft tissue tension attained with formal capsular closure. Both of these "towel clip closures" facilitate visualization of the patellofemoral articulation to allow assessment of patellar tracking.

Rae and associates have proposed a "one-stitch test."[40] A single suture is placed adjacent to the patella to close the capsule and the knee is brought into deep

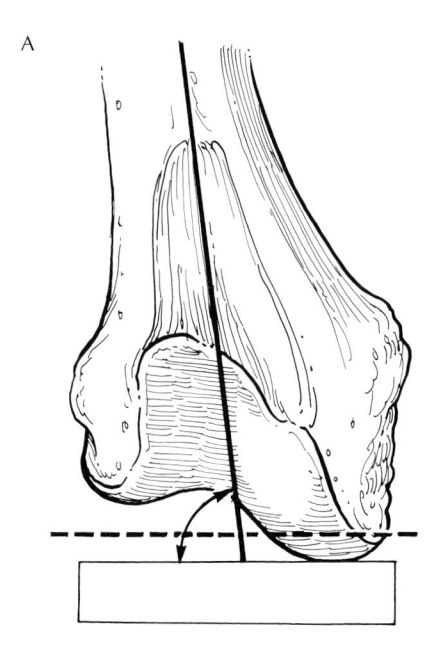

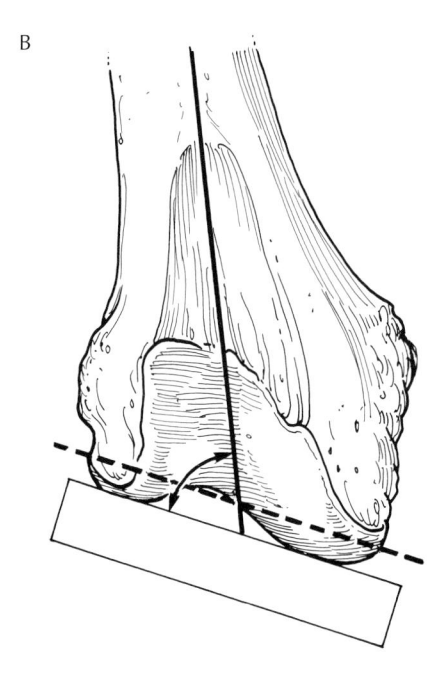

Figure 43.4. In the valgus knee, distal bone loss from the lateral femoral condyle dictates that the distal femoral cutting block should rest in air distal to the lateral condyle (A). Attempts to make the distal cutting block rest on both femoral condyles results in a distal femoral cut in excessive valgus (B).

flexion (Fig. 43.8). If that suture cuts out of the capsule, then a lateral release is indicated. The test is then performed again after the lateral release to verify appropriate tracking of the patella.

Significance of a Patellar-Tracking Problem

An intraoperative patellar-tracking problem at the time of trial reduction should serve as a red flag to the surgeon. Patellar-tracking abnormalities are often the manifestation of a technical error in the performance of the arthroplasty. The surgeon who chooses to ignore this red flag and proceeds directly with a lateral retinacular release may well improve patellar tracking but may miss the opportunity to correct rotational, translational, and orientation errors in the arthroplasty that may affect the longevity of the implant. In addition, the surgeon may needlessly subject the patient to potential problems such as hematoma and wound compromise associated with lateral retinacular release.[41] Therefore, a tracking problem should prompt the sur-

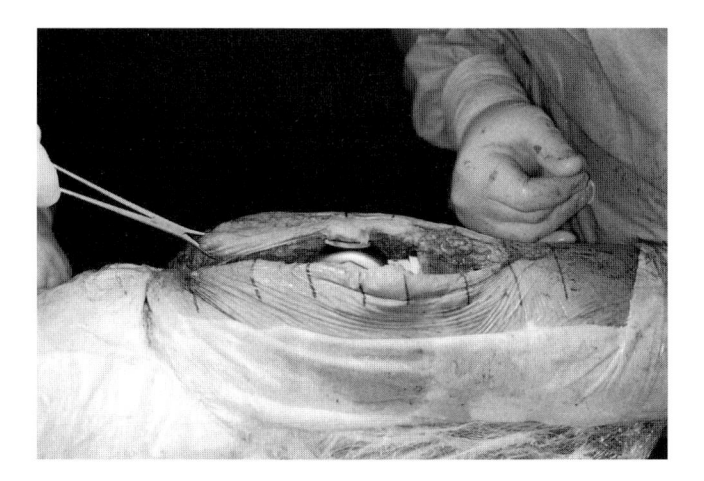

Figure 43.5. We prefer to assess patellar tracking by placing a towel clip through the medial edge of the quadriceps tendon 8 cm proximal to the patella. Gentle longitudinal traction is applied to take the slack out of the tendon and then the knee is placed through a range of motion.

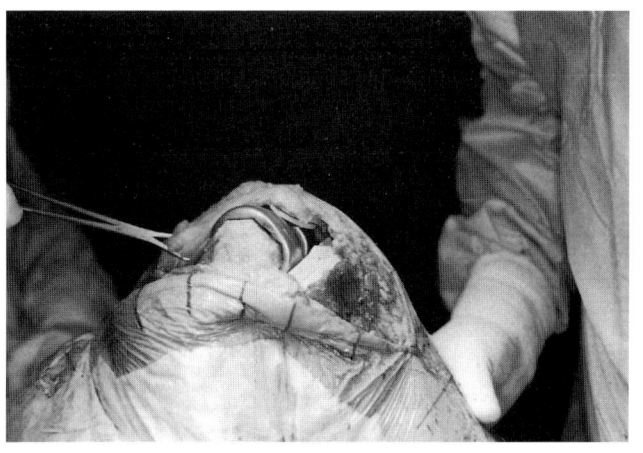

Figure 43.6. Requirements for acceptable tracking include contact of the patellar component with both the medial and lateral condyles and no tendency for tilt or subluxation.

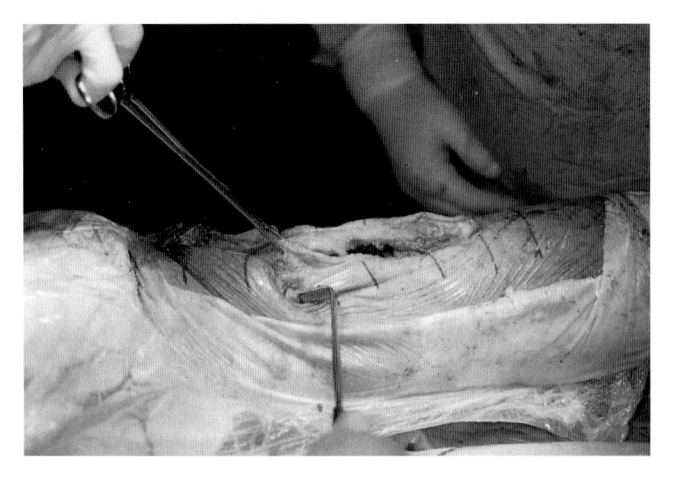

Figure 43.7. The so-called "towel clip test" has been proposed as a method to assess patellar tracking. A towel clip is placed at the superomedial aspect of the patella to reapproximate the extensor mechanism and the knee is then placed through a range of motion.

geon to conduct a brief, focused review of several key steps in the arthroplasty.

To limit patellar-tracking problems, preoperative and intraoperative attention should be focused on obtaining a femoral component that is sized appropriately in the anteroposterior plane, rotated neutrally with respect to the transepicondylar axis, and translated slightly laterally; a tibial component that is aligned close to the tibial crest and avoids excessive internal or external rotation; and a patellar bone-prosthesis composite that is slightly thinner than the native patella and in which the patellar high point is slightly medialized. A minority of TKAs in which those criteria are met will require lateral retinacular release. Our recent experience suggests a need for lateral retinacular release in less than 10% of the cases.

INTRAOPERATIVE CHECKLIST

When a patellar-tracking problem is encountered intraoperatively, we suggest that the surgeon undertake a focused review of the position and orientation of all three components of the TKA. Only when that review has been completed and appropriate component position is verified should lateral retinacular release be carried out. The following checklist can serve as an aid to the intraoperative assessment of component position.

Patellar Thickness

The goal is a patellar composite thickness equal to or 1 to 2 mm less than the native patella. The native patella should be measured with a caliper and its thickness noted prior to osteotomy (Fig. 43.9). The aim should be to slightly reduce the overall thickness of the patella-prosthesis composite compared to the native patella. In a recent study, Greenfield and colleagues were able to reduce the incidence of lateral release from 55 to 12% by ensuring that the patellar composite thickness was less than or equal to that of the native patella.[42] Although a previous biomechanical study[43] has suggested that a minimum bony thickness of 15 mm be maintained, Greenfield and colleagues found no clinical problems despite routine residual bony thicknesses un-

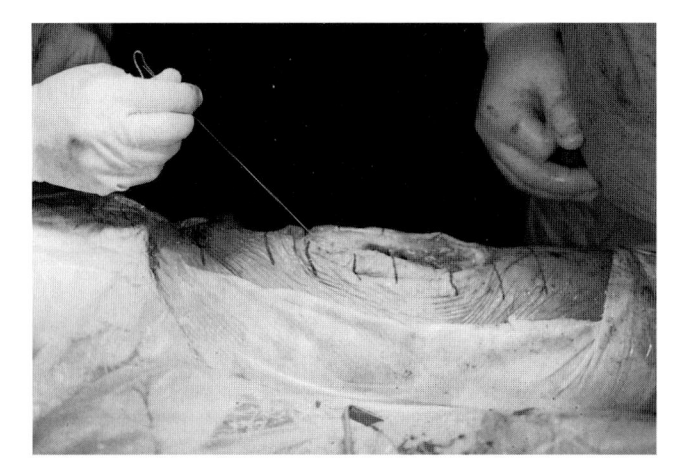

Figure 43.8. The "one-stitch test" utilizes one suture placed adjacent to the superomedial corner of the patella. If that suture cuts out of the capsule as the knee is brought into flexion, then a lateral release is indicated.

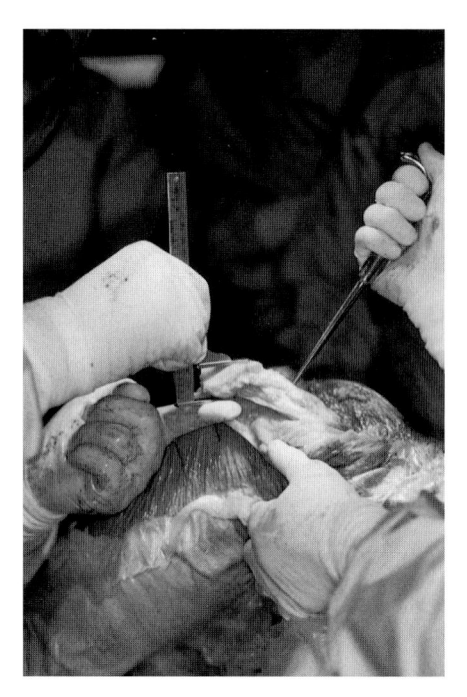

Figure 43.9. The native patella should be measured with a caliper prior to osteotomy.

der 15 mm. If an intraoperative tracking problem is encountered, the surgeon should remeasure the patellar composite thickness. We have encountered situations in which a 1 to 2 mm increase in patellar composite thickness has precipitated a tracking problem. That situation is easily remedied by recutting the patella to produce a thinner composite.

Patellar Symmetry

The goal is a symmetrical patellar bone remnant. The normal patella has an asymmetric contour with the medial facet notably thicker than the lateral facet. Inadvertent asymmetric resection of the patella arises from a failure to recognize that aspect of patellar anatomy (Fig. 43.10). Most often asymmetric resection occurs during an attempt to remove equal amounts of bone from both the medial and lateral facets. That type of resection in the normal patella results in a bone remnant that is often too thick medially and too thin laterally. Asymmetric resurfacing has been noted in numerous reports from experienced surgeons, and its deleterious effect on the midterm results of TKA has been highlighted recently.[12,29,31,44] Manual palpation of the patellar bone remnant is an excellent means of assessing the symmetry of the resection. The patella should be recut if asymmetry is noted intraoperatively.

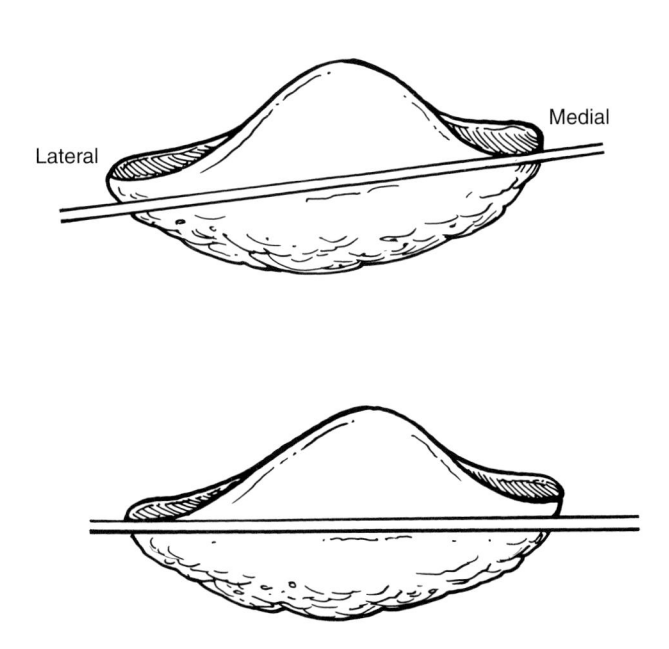

Figure 43.10. The normal patella has an asymmetric contour with the medial facet notably thicker than the lateral. Inadvertent asymmetric patellar resection may occur from an attempt to remove equal amounts of bone from both the medial and lateral facets.

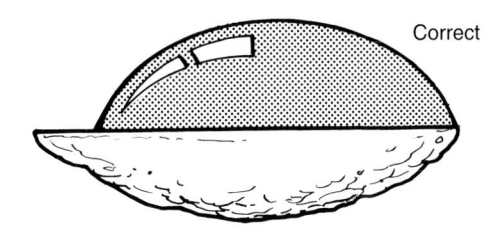

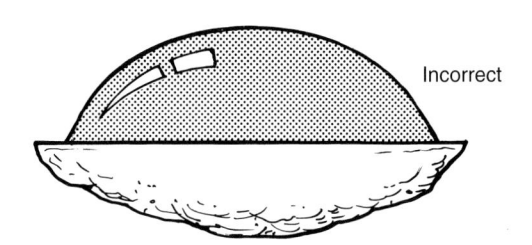

Figure 43.11. Medial position of a dome-shaped patella will provide more normal tracking. A slightly smaller dome-shaped patella is often required to create a medial high point and thus one must accept a slight amount of uncoverage of the lateral facet bone.

Patellar Button Position

The goal is a patellar high point that is slightly medial. There is moderate variability in the position of the patellar high point amongst patients. Compared to a central high-point position, medial placement of a dome-shaped patella will provide more normal tracking of the patella.[33] A slightly smaller patellar component is often required to create a medial high-point position (Fig. 43.11). One must accept slight uncoverage of the lateral facet bone when the smaller, dome-shaped component is utilized. Anatomically shaped patellar components can re-create the medial high point with more uniform bone coverage, but these components have a drawback in that they are sensitive to rotational malposition.[18] Malrotation of an anatomically shaped patellar button itself can contribute to tracking problems. Intraoperative discovery of a lateral high point can be corrected by redrilling the centering holes and repositioning the patellar button medially.

Femoral Rotation

The goal is neutral rotation with respect to the transepicondylar axis. The transepicondylar axis has recently been shown to represent the functional axis of the knee in the flexion-extension arc[19] (Fig. 43.12). Any TKA instrumentation system that sets femoral component rotation based on the posterior condyles will tend to place the femur in a mean of 3 degrees of internal rotation rel-

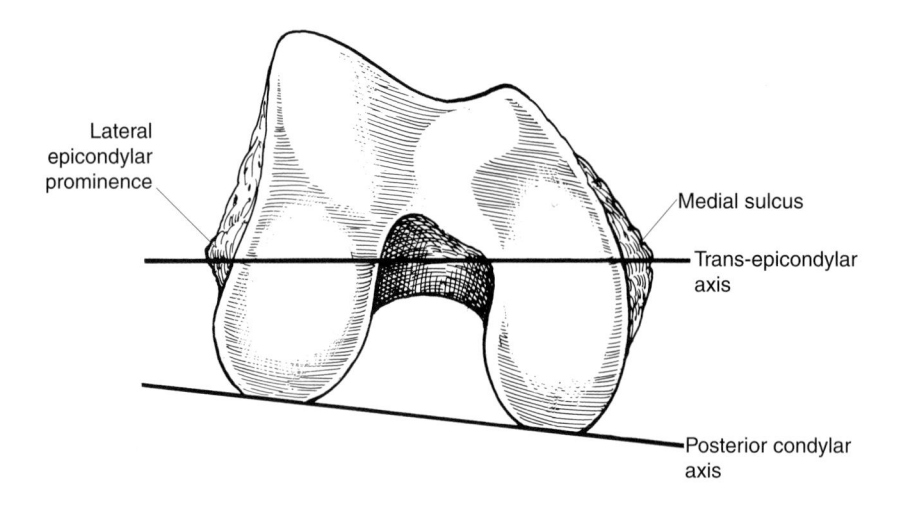

Figure 43.12. The transepicondylar axis is used to set femoral component rotation. The appropriate surgical landmarks are the lateral epicondyle and the sulcus within the medial epicondyle.

ative to the transepicondylar axis.[45] For that reason, posterior condylar referencing systems gave rise to the clinical axiom to "slightly externally rotate" the femoral component. The problem lies with the variability in the relationship between the posterior condylar axis and the transepicondylar axis. Although the mean difference is indeed 3 degrees of internal rotation, the range is from 0 to 10 degrees of internal rotation.[45] Given that variability, we feel that femoral component rotation is more reliably set by identifying the medial and lateral epicondyles and by aligning the component parallel to the line that joins those two points.

Femoral Translation

The goal is a lateralized femoral component. Lateral translation of the femoral component has been demonstrated to improve patellar tracking compared to central or medial positioning.[46] Clinically we make an effort to position the lateral shoulder of the femoral prosthesis flush with the lateral edge of the anterior femoral cut (Fig. 43.13). This achieves slight lateralization of the component while avoiding component overhang that could lead to soft tissue impingement.

Femoral Axial Alignment

The goal is 5 to 7 degrees of valgus. Excessive valgus limb alignment will increase the Q-angle and contribute to patellar-tracking problems. A limb in which the femoral component is in excess valgus and the tibial component is in varus may achieve acceptable overall alignment but it remains predisposed to patellar problems. Knees with preoperative valgus deformity are particularly prone to femoral component malalignment. Most TKA instrumentation systems use a cutting block attached to an intramedullary guide rod that rests on the distal femoral condyles to set the valgus orientation of the femoral component. Bone loss from the distal aspect of the lateral femoral condyle is typical in the valgus knee. To achieve the typical 5- to 7-degree valgus orientation, this bone loss dictates that while the distal femoral cutting block rests on the medial femoral condyle it remains suspended in air distal to the lateral femoral condyle (Fig. 43.4). Impaction of the distal femoral cutting guide so that it makes contact with both femoral condyles will result in an excessive valgus cut of the distal femur.

Tibial Position

The goal is to avoid excess internal or external rotation. Both excessive internal rotation and external rotation of the tibial component have been associated with clinical problems. With the current emphasis on increasing tibiofemoral conformity, close matching of the motion arcs of the femur and tibia is mandatory. Excessive tibial polyethylene wear has been suggested in cases in which the tibial component has been placed in exces-

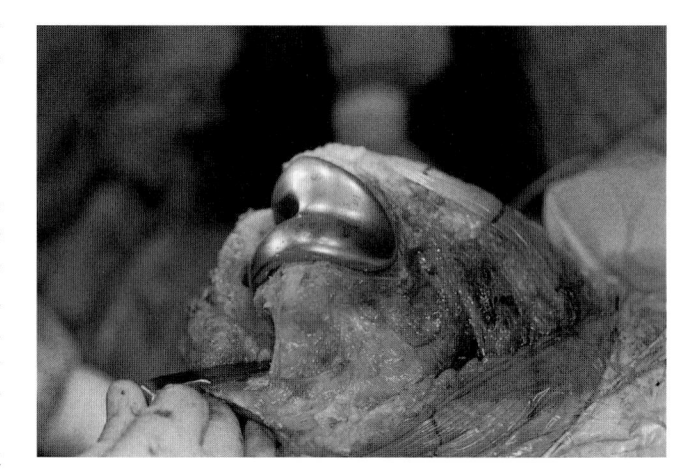

Figure 43.13. Lateralizing the femoral component can improve patellar tracking. Clinically we position the lateral shoulder of the prosthesis flush with the lateral edge of the anterior femoral cut.

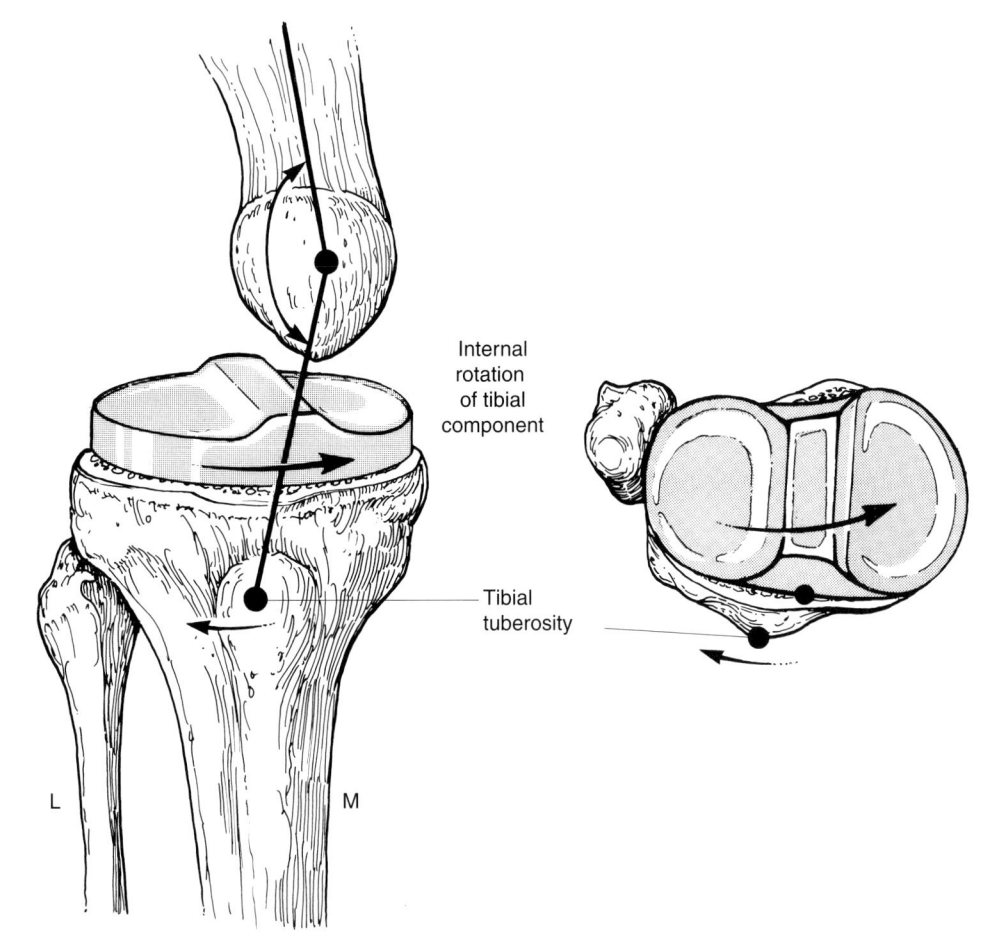

Figure 43.14. Because it increases the Q-angle, internal rotation of the tibial component can cause patellar instability.

sive external rotation. Internal rotation of the tibial component has been clinically implicated as a leading cause of patellar instability and has biomechanically been shown to increase patellofemoral forces (Fig. 43.14). Typically the tibial baseplate should be aligned with the anterior tibial crest, which is colinear with the medial third of the tibial tubercle. Use of a stemless tibial tray during trial reduction has been advocated as a means to determine appropriate rotation. By placing the knee through a full range of motion several times, the tibial component will "seek its own correct rotational alignment." This dynamic positioning of the tibial component may accommodate small errors in femoral component alignment and ligament balance. When dynamic positioning suggests that the tibial tray be oriented medial to the tubercle's medial third or lateral to its middle third, then a reassessment of femoral component orientation should be undertaken. Our approach has been to set femoral component rotation based on the transepicondylar axis and then align the tibial baseplate with the tibial crest as suggested by Merkow and associates.[24]

Soft-Tissue Releases

The goal is to release the patellofemoral ligaments. Occasionally a mild intraoperative patellar-tracking problem can be eliminated by sectioning of the patellofemoral ligaments alone. We routinely release the lateral patellofemoral ligaments as part of the initial exposure. Release of those ligaments facilitates eversion of the patella and at the same time eliminates their tendency to pull the patella laterally and contribute to tracking problems. Before a formal lateral retinacular release is considered the surgeon should ensure that the patellofemoral ligaments have been fully divided and then reassess patellar tracking. Similarly, we have occasionally encountered instances in which mild patellar-tracking problems can be eliminated by a limited subfascial dissection of the skin and subcutaneous tissue overlying the patella. This more commonly occurs in obese patients and this simple subfascial release of adherent skin and subcutaneous tissue may be enough to eliminate the need for formal lateral retinacular release.

CONCLUSION

Although total knee arthroplasty is a remarkably successful procedure, the patellofemoral articulation remains its weak link. Complications related to the patellofemoral joint are clearly multifactorial and involve an interplay between prosthetic design considerations, patient demands, and surgical technique. Careful preoperative planning and intraoperative attention to detail, however, can eliminate many patellofemoral problems. A patellar-tracking problem noted intraoperatively serves as a warning sign and should prompt the surgeon to reassess each component of the arthroplasty. Correction of technical errors in component position, orientation, and alignment can eliminate the need for lateral retinacular release and contribute to the long-term success of the arthroplasty. When the components of the arthroplasty are well placed and a tendency for tilt or subluxation of the patella persists, then lateral retinacular release is an effective procedure to improve patellofemoral tracking.

References

1. Clayton M, Thirupathi R. Patellar complications after total condylar arthroplasty. *Clin Orthop*. 1982; 170:152–155.
2. Eftekhar N. Total knee replacement arthroplasty. Results with the intramedullary adjustable total knee prosthesis. *J Bone Joint Surg*. 1983; 65A:293–309.
3. Enis J, Gardner R, Robledo M, Latta L, Smith R. Comparison of patellar resurfacing versus nonresurfacing in bilateral total knee arthroplasty. *Clin Orthop*. 1990; 260:38–42.
4. Evanski P, Waugh T, Orofino C, Anzel S. UCI knee replacement. *Clin Orthop*. 1976; 120:33–38.
5. Freeman M, Todd R, Bainert P, Day W. ICLH arthroplasty of the knee 1968–1977. *J Bone Joint Surg*. 1978; 60B:339–344.
6. Insall J, Scott W, Ranawat C. The total condylar knee prosthesis: a report of 220 cases. *J Bone Joint Surg*. 1979; 61A: 173–180.
7. Kaufer H, Matthews L. Spherocentric arthroplasty of the knee. *J Bone Joint Surg*. 1981; 63A:545–559.
8. Mochizuki R, Schurman D. Patellar complications following total joint arthroplasty. *J Bone Joint Surg*. 1979; 61A: 879–883.
9. Moreland J, Thomas R, Freeman M. ICLH replacement of the knee: 1977 and 1978. *Clin Orthop*. 1979; 145:47–59.
10. Murray D, Webster P. Variable axis knee prosthesis. Two year follow-up study. *J Bone Joint Surg*. 1981; 63A:687–694.
11. Picatti G, McGann W, Welch R. The patellofemoral joint after total knee arthroplasty without patellar resurfacing. *J Bone Joint Surg*. 1990; 72A:1379–1382.
12. Ranawat C. The patellofemoral joint in total condylar knee arthroplasty: pros and cons based on 5–10 year follow-up observations. *Clin Orthop*. 1986; 205:93–99.
13. Ranawat C, Insall J, Shine J. Duo-condylar knee arthroplasty. *Clin Orthop*. 1976; 120:76–82.
14. Scott R. Prosthetic replacement of the patellofemoral joint. *Ortho Clin North Am*. 1979; 10:129–137.
15. Sledge C, Ewald F. Total knee arthroplasty: experience at the Robert Breck Brigham Hospital. *Clin Orthop*. 1979; 145:78–84.
16. Sledge C, Stern P, Thomas W, Ewald F, Poss R, Scott R. Two year follow-up of the duo-condylar total knee replacement. *Orthopedic Trans*. 1978; 2:193 (abstract).
17. Vanhegan J, Dabrowski W, Arden G. A review of 100 Attenborough stabilized gliding knee prostheses. *J Bone Joint Surg*. 1979; 61B:445–450.
18. Bayley J, Scott R, Ewald F, Holmes GJ. Failure of the metal-backed patella component after total knee replacement. *J Bone Joint Surg*. 1988; 70A:668–674.
19. Berger R, Rubash H, Seel M, Thompson W, Crossett L. Determining the rotational alignment of the femoral component in total knee arthroplasty using the epicondylar axis. *Clin Orthop*. 1993; 286:40–47.
20. Doolittle KH, Turner RH. Patellofemoral problems following total knee arthroplasty. *Orthop Rev*. 1988; 17:696–702.
21. Haberman E, Hungerford D. *Total Knee Arthroplasty: A Comprehensive Approach*. Baltimore, MD: Williams and Wilkins, 1984.
22. Hungerford D, Krackow K. Total joint arthroplasty of the knee. *Clin Orthop*. 1985; 192:23–33.
23. Leblanc J. Patellar complications in total knee arthroplasty: a literature review. *Orthop Rev*. 1989; 18:296–304.
24. Merkow R, Soudry M, Insall J. Patellar dislocation following total knee replacement. *J Bone Joint Surg*. 1985; 61A: 1321–1327.
25. Scott R, Turoff N, Ewald F. Stress fracture of the patella following duopatellar total knee arthroplasty with patellar resurfacing. *Clin Orthop*. 1982; 170:147–151.
26. Simison A, Noble J, Hardinge K. Complications of the Attenborough knee replacement. *J Bone Joint Surg*. 1986; 68B:100–105.
27. Thomas W, Ewald F, Poss R, Sledge C. Duo-patella total knee arthroplasty. *Orthopedic Trans*. 1980; 4:329 (abstract).
28. Thompson M, Hood R, Insall J. Patellar fracture in total knee arthroplasty. *Orthop Trans*. 1981; 5:490 (abstract).
29. Gomes L, Bechtold J, Gustilo R. Patellar prosthesis positioning in total knee arthroplasty: a roentgenographic study. *Clin Orthop*. 1988; 236:72–81.
30. Marmor L. Technique for patellar resurfacing in total knee arthroplasty. *Clin Orthop*. 1988; 230:166–167.
31. Rand J. Patellar resurfacing in total knee arthroplasty. *Clin Orthop*. 1990; 260:110–117.
32. Rand J, Gustilo R. Technique of patellar resurfacing in total knee arthroplasty. *Techniques in Orthopedics*. 1988; 1:33–57.
33. Yoshii I, Whiteside L, Anouchi Y. The effect of patellar button placement and femoral component design on patellar tracking in total knee arthroplasty. *Clin Orthop*. 1992; 275: 211–219.
34. Brick GW, Scott RD. The patellofemoral component of total knee arthroplasty. *Clin Orthop*. 1988; 231:163–178.
35. Dennis D. Patellofemoral complications in total knee arthroplasty: a literature review. *Am J Knee Surg*. 1992; 3: 156–166.
36. Lynch A, Rorabeck C, Bourne R. Extensor mechanism complications following total knee arthroplasty. *J Arthroplasty*. 1987; 2:135–140.

37. Hoffman AA, Kane KR, Tkach TK, Camargo MC. Patellar component medialization in total knee arthroplasty. *Scientific Exhibit: American Academy of Orthopedic Surgeons.* February 1995, Orlando, FL.
38. Insall J. Surgical techniques and instrumentation in total knee arthroplasty. In: Insall JN, Windsor RE, Scott WN, eds. *Surgery of the Knee*. New York: Churchill Livingstone; 1993: 739–804.
39. Whiteside L, Ohl M. Tibial tubercle osteotomy for exposure of the difficult total knee arthroplasty. *Clin Orthop.* 1990; 260:6–9.
40. Rae P, Noble J, Hodgkinson J. Patellar resurfacing in total condylar knee arthroplasty. *J Arthroplasty.* 1990;5: 259–265.
41. Johnson D, Eastwood D. Lateral patellar release in knee arthroplasty: effect on wound healing. *J Arthroplasty.* 1992; 7:427–431.
42. Greenfield M, Insall J, Case G, Kelly M. Instrumentation of the patellar osteotomy in total knee arthroplasty: the relationship of patellar thickness and lateral reinacular release. *Am J of Knee Surgery.* 1996; 9: 129–131.
43. Reuben J, McDonald C, Woodard P, Hennington L. Effect of patella thickness on patella strain following total knee arthroplasty. *J Arthroplasty.* 1991; 6:251–258.
44. Pagnano M, Trousdale RT. Asymmetric patella resurfacing in total knee arthroplasty. *Am J of Knee Surgery.* 2000; 13: 228–233.
45. Poilvache P, Insall J, Scuderi G, Font-Rodriguez D. Rotational landmarks and sizing of the distal femur in total knee arthroplasty. *Clin Orthop.* 1996; 331:35–46.
46. Rhoads D, Noble P, Reuben J, Tullos H. The effect of femoral component position on the kinematics of total knee arthroplasty. *Clin Orthop.* 1993; 286:122–129.

CHAPTER 44
Benefits and Pitfalls of Lateral Patella Release

Fred D. Cushner and W. Norman Scott

INTRODUCTION

Despite numerous advances in the technique of total knee arthroplasty (TKA), problems of patella component tracking and instability remain a concern. Although improvements have occurred in component design, fixation, and surgical technique, the complication rate attributed to the patellofemoral joint articulation remains quite high. Brick and associates noted 50% of all complications noted in their series to the patellofemoral joint with 19 knees requiring reoperation.[1] Other authors have noted patellofemoral complications including instability, fracture, loosening, and component failure.[1-5] The etiology of these complications is multifactorial, with component design, component malalignment, patella avascularity, and increased patellofemoral stresses secondary to technique, all being implicated as causes of patellofemoral dysfunction.[6-8]

Many of the above factors have been addressed in previous chapters of this text. Although Chapter 42 focused on assessment of the patellofemoral tracking, this chapter will focus on the indications and surgical technique of patella lateral release. The relationship between lateral release and the above complications will also be discussed.

BLOOD SUPPLY OF THE PATELLA

Before any discussion on the technique of lateral patella release, a firm understanding of the patella's blood supply is needed. The vascular anatomy of the patella consists of both an extensive prepatellar arterial network as well as an intraosseous plexus and has been well described by numerous authors[9,10] (Fig. 44.1). This network consists of an extraosseous arterial ring and can be divided into superior and inferior portions. The plexus has intraosseous branches that enter the center and lower poles of the patella forming an intraosseous plexus as well.

The extraosseous blood supply can be divided into two portions, the superior and inferior portions. The superior portion consists of the superior lateral and superior medial genicular arteries as well as the supreme genicular artery, while the inferior medial and inferior lateral genicular arteries as well as the anterior tibial recurrent artery form the inferior portion. The superior medial genicular artery and superior lateral genicular artery both arise from the popliteal artery. Each runs forward around its respective femoral condyle supplying the condylar region prior to reaching the level of the patella. The inferior medial and lateral genicular arteries also arise from the popliteal artery just distal to the posterior joint line. These vessels run deep to the collateral ligaments, supply their respective tibial plateau as well as the capsule, collateral ligaments, and patella tendon. Other areas supplied include the anterior aspect of the anterior cruciate ligament as well as the tibial epiphysis and metaphysis. The anterior tibial recurrent artery arises from the anterior tibial artery at the level of the fibular neck.[9,10]

Superiorly, the medial and lateral superior genicular arteries run along the superior border of the patella and anastomose with the supreme genicular artery just anterior to the quadriceps insertion. Inferiorly, the medial and lateral inferior genicular arteries divide into three branches before reaching the patella tendon. These branches include the ascending parapatellar artery, oblique prepatellar artery, and the transverse infra-patellar artery. The ascending parapatellar branches run superiorly along the lateral patella margin and join the descending branches of the superior genicular arteries, while the oblique prepatellar branches converge on the anterior surface of the patella. The transverse infra-patellar branches

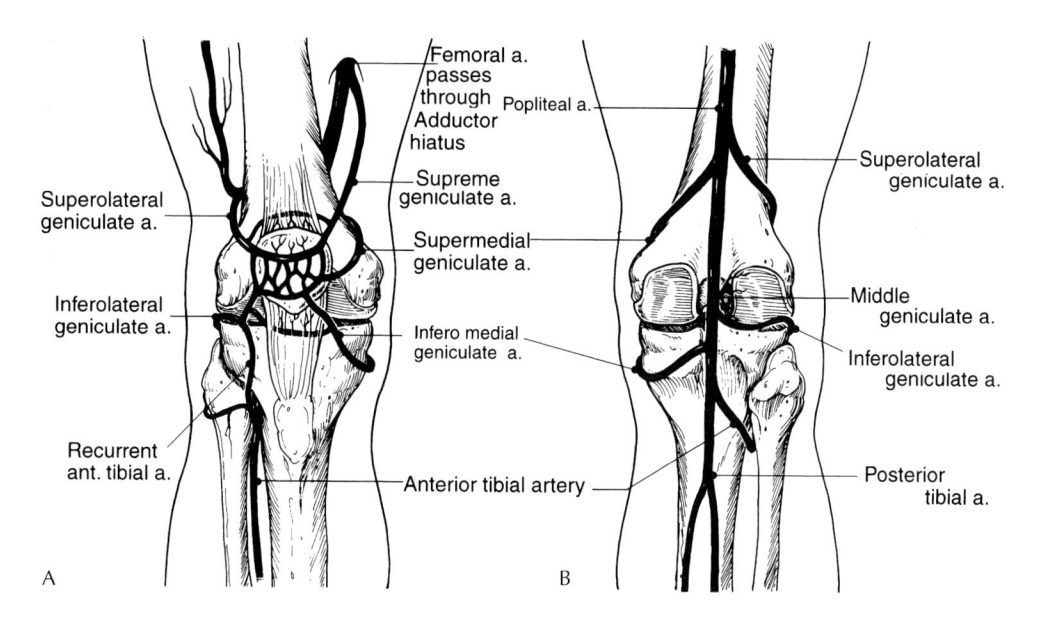

Figure 44.1. Vascular anatomy of the patella. (A) Anterior view. (B) Posterior view.

anastomose behind the patella and enter the inferior pole of the patella.

The intraosseous vessels consist of two separate systems. The first system consists of mid-patella vessels that enter through a vascular foramen at the middle one-third of the anterior patella, whereas the second vascular system consists of the infrapatellar osseous branches mentioned previously.

Bjorkstrom and Goldie[11] describe an intratendinous blood supply. These authors demonstrated arteries that penetrate the superior pole of the patella from within the quadriceps tendon. With advancing age these vessels were noted to become less developed.

Thus, it can be seen that a vascular plexus exists giving the patella an extensive extraosseous and intraosseous blood supply.

THE TECHNIQUE

The Approach

We favor a medial parapatellar incision in performing a total knee arthroplasty. Although other options exist (subvastus, midvastus, and lateral approach), they will be considered in other chapters of this text. This approach splits the quadriceps tendon proximally and goes through the medial retinaculum distally. Therefore, as a result of this approach the medial superior genicular artery flow as well as the medial inferior genicular artery flow is disrupted (Fig. 43.2). At this point in the procedure the patella vascular supply is primarily from the lateral genicular vessels.

Patella Evaluation

As noted in the previous chapter patella tracking is evaluated and based on the patella prosthesis articulation with the femoral component, and no thumbs test[12] (Fig. 43.2). At this time a decision is made on whether to proceed with a lateral patella release. It should be noted that a patella release will aid in patella tracking when a tight retinaculum exists and further soft tissue balance of the patellofemoral joint is needed.

Causes of Patella Maltracking

Many factors can play a role in the need for performing a lateral release. Valgus alignment of greater than 10 degrees or more than 7 degrees of valgus of the femoral component can lead to maltracking.[13] This, in essence, causes a surgical increase in the Q-angle of the limb resulting in a lateral quadriceps vector. Numerous other

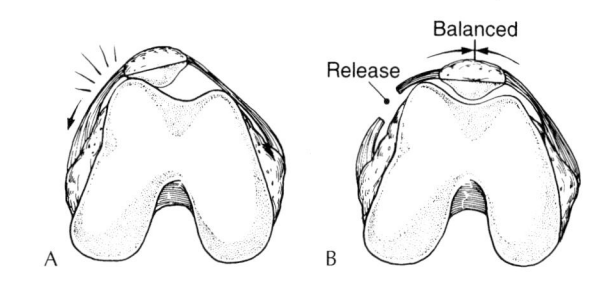

Figure 44.2. Patellofemoral joint balancing. (A) Tight lateral capsule indicating a need for a lateral release. (B) Balanced.

factors can cause relative lateral retinacular tightness. Medial displacement of the femoral component as little as 5 mm[14,15] as well as internal rotation of the femoral component[14] increases lateral tracking of the patella. Lateralization of the patella prosthesis on the osteotomized patella can also lead to lateral retinacular tightness if the prosthesis impinges on the lateral trochlea flange, thus, increasing contact stresses. Therefore, medialization of the patella component on a lateralized femoral component is recommended to relieve retinacular stresses and improved patella tracking.[14–17] Internal rotation of the tibial component can also lead to a tight lateral retinaculum causing maltracking of the patella component (Fig. 44.3).

Other important factors include the patella anatomy as well as the femoral component design. Although a deep trochlear groove and a high lateral ridge may serve to constrain the patella component; conversely, a flat trochlea surface may cause a tendency of lateral tracking even with physiologic valgus stresses. A surgeon must not only rely on design constraints to maintain essential patella tracking because if the soft tissues are not properly balanced, dynamic patella stresses may occur leading to early failure.

Patella prosthesis shape[18,19] as well as patella prosthesis composite thickness can also influence patella tracking. At our institution, Greenfeld and colleagues[20] evaluated the role of patella thickness on a lateral release rate. Using the same primary surgeon and identical indications for lateral release, the lateral release rate decreased from 55 to 12.4% when the patella prosthesis composite was equal or slightly less than the original patella width (Fig. 44.4). Although Ruben and associates[6] noted increased stress at the patella prosthesis with an osteotomized patella thickness of less than 15 mm, no fractures were noted in this series. By utilizing new instrumentation at our institution referencing the epicondylar axis,[21] the lateral release rate has been reduced to 2% (Fig. 44.3).

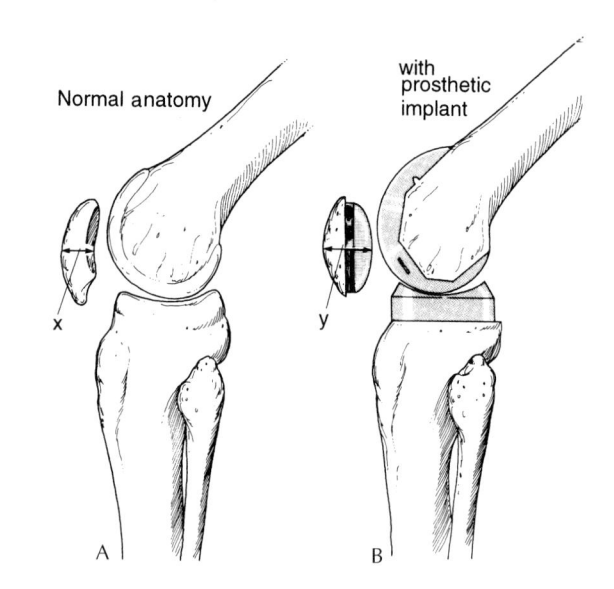

Figure 44.4. (A) Patella and (B) patella prosthesis thickness. Measurement "x" and measurement "y" should be equal.

Other factors leading to lateral patella tracking would include rupture of the medial retinacular repair[1] or secondary to a contracted lateral retinaculum in a valgus knee even after the leg is returned to physiologic valgus. Dynamic forces may also favor lateral patella tracking, but unfortunately, these may not be detectable in the operating room theater.[22]

The Release

When indicated, a lateral retinacular release is performed in a stepwise approach. The lateral retinacular release begins with release of the patellofemoral ligament. Although often release is part of the exposure for the patella osteotomy, this area is reinspected for any remaining tight bands.

Attention is then turned to the lateral retinaculum itself. We prefer an all-inside technique for several reasons. The first is the avoidance of a large lateral cutaneous flap.[12] By avoiding a large cutaneous flap, possible vascular injury to the skin from a thin flap is avoided especially in the multiply operated knee. A second advantage of the all-inside technique is the maintenance of an adequate postoperative joint seal. With an all-inside release we feel the postoperative hemarthrosis is better contained in the joint helping to avoid wound problems. Should a superficial wound infection occur, a direct connection to the joint is not present with the all-inside technique. Finally, utilizing the all-inside

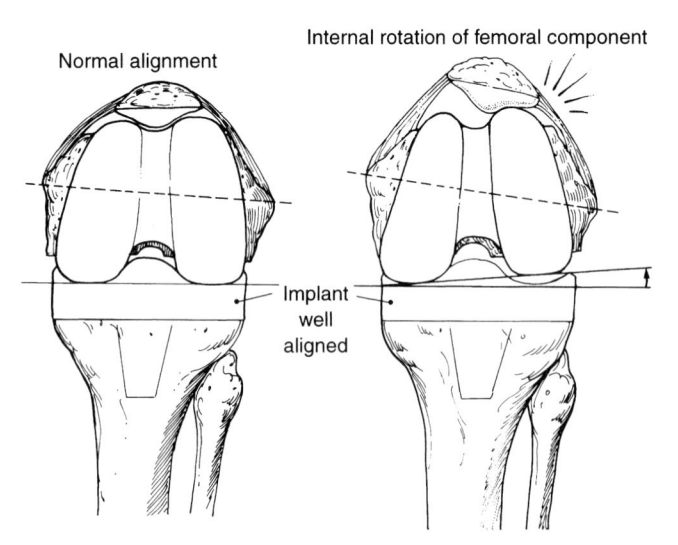

Figure 44.3. Internal tibial component rotation as a cause for lateral retinacular tightness.

technique allows preservation of the superior lateral genicular artery. Although preservation of the superficial lateral genicular artery will be discussed in the following discussion, we find it beneficial to preserve this vessel.

Therefore, once a decision is made to perform a lateral retinacular release, the all-inside technique is utilized. The first step is for localization of the superior lateral genicular artery. Soiffer and colleagues[20,23] at our institution evaluated 15 consecutive total knee arthroplasties in order to help provide adequate landmarks for evaluating and protecting this vessel. This study concluded that the most reliable identification for the location of the lateral superior genicular artery was the superior pole of the patella with the artery located a mean of 1.5 mm from this landmark.[24]

Once located, blunt dissection is utilized to further isolate the vessels. A one-fourth inch penrose drain is then placed around the vessel so gentle superior and inferior traction can be performed as needed (Fig. 44.5). The lateral release is then performed approximately 1 to 2 cm from the lateral patella margin. Using gentle inferior traction on the vessels, the release is extended superiorly and can involve the lower fibers of the vastus lateralis as needed. Gentle superior traction is then applied and the release is carried distally to the level of the joint. An oblique incision can be used in the lateral retinaculum to avoid the inferior lateral genicular artery. In rare cases, the vessels must be sacrificed if they act as a tether to the patella.

Closure of the standard parapatellar arthrotomy should be done carefully to ensure not only adequate closure, but to measure continued acceptable patella tracking. Motion should be checked throughout the closure, and the authors prefer a slight proximal advancement to help avoid postoperative patellar baja. At the end of closure, gentle range of motion is performed to ensure the integrity of the medial repair.

DISCUSSION

Although the technique itself to perform a lateral release is quite simple, much debate exists about the morbidity involved with the above technique. Some of this concern is over disrupting the patella blood supply. The medial parapatellar approach along with a lateral retinacular release compromises geniculate and anastomotic ring leaving only the intratendinous circulation intact to vascularize the patella until revascularization occurs. Scuderi and associates[7] reviewed 36 knees to evaluate patella viability following total knee arthroplasty. Of the 36 knees, 16 patellas required a lateral release secondary to patella maltracking. No attempt was made to preserve the genicular blood flow laterally. Bone scans were obtained within seven days and these authors noted that 56.3% of the lateral release group demonstrated a vascular insult to the patella compared to 15% in the nonlateral release group. One clinically insignificant fracture was noted in the lateral release group. It appears that the lateral release may negatively effect patella viability, but factors other than disruption of the lateral blood supply may also be involved. Thermal necrosis and anatomic variations may explain the incidence of three "cold" patellas in the nonlateral release group. This data differs from that presented by Scuderi and associates[24] when younger patients (mean age 23) were evaluated following iliotibial band anterior cruciate ligament reconstruction. This technique also involved medial and lateral genicular disruption, but only 14% developed "cold" patellas. Perhaps this is secondary to no patella bone resection being performed for this procedure. It appears that the intratendonous circulation was adequate enough in this younger population to preserve patella circulation. This data is supported by Bjorkstrom and colleagues[11] who noted thinner intratendonous arteries and terminal arterial endings that did not reach the articular surface when patients were over 60 years of age.

Although radionuclide avascularity of the patella is common, the correlation with eventual patella fracture from the avascularity is of major concern. McMann and associates[25] noted evidence of "cold" patella following lateral release, but no correlation with patella fractures could be found.

Tria and colleagues[26] reviewed 504 total knee arthroplasties done over an 11-year period noting a patella fracture rate of 3.6%. All fractures were associated with

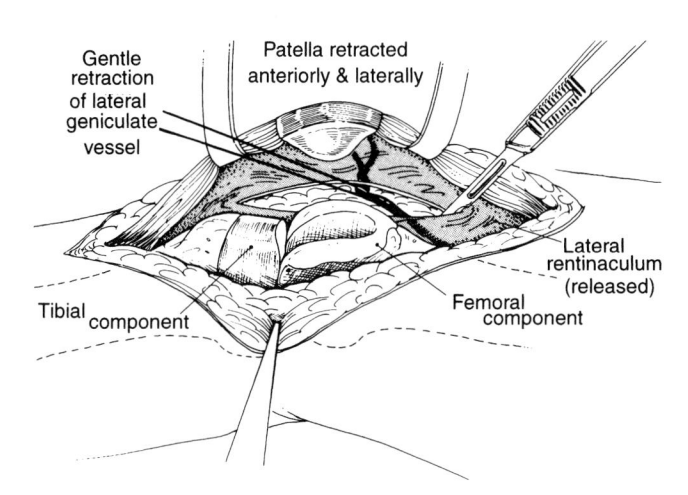

Figure 44.5. The lateral release is performed with preservation of the lateral superior genicular artery. The release is performed 2 to 3 cm from the lateral patella border.

knees in which a lateral release was performed. It should be noted that the lateral release rate for this series was 82%, and no attempt was made to preserve the genicular vessels. Significant malalignment was not present in this series to account for the occurrence of these patella fractures, and these authors concluded that attempts should be made to preserve the lateral superior genicular artery.

Ritter and associates[27] also looked at the relationship between lateral release and patella fractures. In this series 84 knees in which a lateral release was performed with no attempt at genicular preservation was compared to 471 knees in which no lateral release was performed. It was interesting to note that the fracture rate was actually higher in the nonlateral release group (3.6%) compared to the lateral release group (1.5%). These fractures in the nonrelease group were thought to be secondary to residual retinacular tightness and its effect on the bone remaining laterally to the patella prosthesis. A lateral release rate for this series was 15%, and these authors concluded that perhaps more generous indications for a lateral release should be considered.

As a matter of fact, these authors did increase their lateral release rate in a 1996 reported study on 1,205 arthroplasties performed at their institution using a cruciate-sparing prosthesis (AGC. Biomet, Warsaw, Indiana) rather than the posterior cruciate condylar prosthesis utilized in the original study.[28] The lateral release rate was 35% and in 75% of these lateral releases the genicular artery was saved. In this study, lateral release had no effect on patella subluxation, dislocation, or loosening, but was associated with more patella fractures. The nonrelease group conversely had less fractures but a higher radiolucency rate. No benefit was noted from the superior lateral genicular artery preservation with regards to radiolucency loosening or fracture rate but there was a significantly greater occurrence of a radiographically subluxed patella in the superior lateral genicular artery preserved group. These authors remained concerned about the patella avascularity, but based on these results, felt that preserving the superior lateral genicular artery was not necessary.

Although benefit of preserving the superior lateral genicular artery to decrease fracture incidence can be debated, other indications for preservation of this vessel should be considered. Johnson and associates[29] evaluated the effect of lateral release on wound healing. These authors found an increased incidence of wound discoloration and superficial wound infections with the genicular artery sacrificed. Perioperative transcutaneous measurement of skin oxygen tension was used and demonstrated an objective reduction in lateral wound edge skin viability following the lateral release.

In conclusion, the literature is mixed in regards to a lower incidence of patella fractures following lateral release without the preservation of the lateral superior genicular artery. This study gives some objective benefit in regards to wound healing to justify genicular preservation.

RESULTS OF LATERAL RELEASE

Several studies have evaluated postoperative tilt and subluxation following total knee arthroplasty. Bindelglass and colleagues[22] evaluated 234 postoperative total knee arthroplasties and noted central tracking in only 54.7% of these examined. Although 31.2% of the patellas were tilted and 14.5% displaced, no relationship was noted between patella position and pain scores or function. It is interesting to note that no improvement was noted when a lateral release was performed in regards to patella position on X ray. Laughlin and colleagues[30] also evaluated patella tilt following total knee arthroplasty and found a similar incidence of patella tilt. Unlike the previous study, patella tilt was found to be dynamic over time. A medially tilted patella tended to move to a more neutral position with the passage of time, whereas a laterally tilted patella, greater than 5 degrees, actually worsened with time. This may be secondary to the fact that the knee kinematics perform a lateral vector with quadriceps strength laterally greater than the medial quadriceps strength. Once again, no difference was noted in the lateral release group suggesting the success of performing a lateral release when indicated.

CONCLUSION

Lateral release is a successful tool to provide soft tissue balance to the patellofemoral joint. Lateral release does have its limitations and will not substitute for poor surgical technique. We recommend preservation of this lateral superior genicular artery when possible, not only for patella avascularity, but also for the potential benefits with wound healing. Utilization of the all-inside technique not only allows for vessel identification, but also avoids a large lateral skin flap that could also interfere with wound healing.

References

1. Brick GW, Scott RD. The patellofemoral component of total knee arthroplasty. *Clin Orthop*. 1988; 231:163.
2. Clayton ML, Thirupathi R. Patella complications after total condylar arthroplasty. *Clin Orthop*. 1982; 170:152.
3. Grace JM, Sim FH. Fracture of the patella after total knee arthroplasty. *Clin Orthop*. 1988; 230:168.
4. Ranawat CS. The patellofemoral joint in total condylar knee arthroplasty: pros and cons based on 5–10 year follow-up observations. *Clin Orthop*. 1986; 205:93.

5. Rand JA. Patella resurfacing in total knee arthroplasty. *Clin Orthop*. 1990; 200:110.
6. Reuben JD, McDonald L, Woodard PL, Hennington LJ. The effect of patella thickness on patella strain following total knee arthroplasty. *J Arthroplasty*. 1991; 6:251.
7. Scuderi G, Scharf SC, Meltzer LP, Scott WN. The relationship of lateral releases to patella viability in total knee arthroplasty. *J Arthroplasty*. 1987; 2:209.
8. Windsor RE, Scuderi GR, Insall JN. Patella fractures in total knee arthroplasty. *J Arthroplasty*. 1989; 4(Suppl):63.
9. Scapinelli R. Blood supply of the human patella. *J Bone Joint Surg*. 1967; 9B:563.
10. Shim SS, Leury G. Blood supply of the knee joint. A microangiographic study in children and adults. *Clin Orthop*. 1986; 208:119–125.
11. Bjorkstrom S, Goldie IF. A study of the arterial blood supply of the patella in the normal state, in chondromalacia patellae and in osteoarthritis. *ACTA Orthop Scand*. 1980; 51:63.
12. Scott RD. Prosthetic replacement of the patellofemoral joint. *Clin Orthop North Am*. 1979; 10:129–137.
13. Spitzer AI, Vince KG. Patellar considerations in total knee replacement. In: *The Patella*. New York: Springer-Verlag, 1995:309–331.
14. Rhoades DP, Noble PC, Reuben JD, et al. The effect of femoral component position on the kinematics of total knee arthroplasty. *Clin Orthop*. 1993; 286:122–129.
15. Rhoades DP, Noble PC, Reuben JD, et al. The effect of femoral component position on patella tracking after total knee arthroplasty. *Clin Orthop*. 1990; 260:43–51.
16. Yoshi I, Whiteside LA, Anouchi YS. The effect of patella button placement and femoral component design on patellar tracking in total knee arthroplasty. *Clin Orthop*. 1992; 275:211–219.
17. Briard JL, Hungerford PS. Patellofemoral instability in total knee arthroplasty. *J Arthroplasty*. 1989; 4 (Suppl):87–97.
18. Flandry F, Hardy AF, Kester MA. A chronically dislocating prosthetic patella; a case report. *Orthopedics*. 1988; 11:457–460.
19. MacCrollum MS, Karpman RR. Complications of the PCA Anatomic Patella. *Orthopedics*. 1989; 12:1423–1428.
20. Greenfeld MA, Insall JN, Case GA, Kelf MA. Instrumentation of the patellar osteotomy in total knee arthroplasty. The relationship of patellar thickness and lateral retinacular release. *Am J Knee Surg*. 1996; 9(3):129–132.
21. DeMuth BL, Scuderi GR, Insall JN. The effect of the epicondylar axis on patella tracking in total knee arthroplasty. Knee Society and American Association of Hip and Knee Surgeons Combined Meeting. San Francisco, California, February, 1997.
22. Bindelglass DF, Cohen JL, Dorr LA. Patellar tilt and subluxation in total knee arthroplasty, relationship to pain, fixation and design. *Clin Orthop*. 1993; 286:103–109.
23. Soifer TB, Gavin MD, Insall JN. Localization of the superior lateral genicular artery. *Am J Knee Surg*. 1993; 6(4):163–166.
24. Scuderi GR, Scharf SC, Meltzer L, Nisonson B, Scott WN. Evaluation of patella viability after disruption of the arterial circulation. *Am J Sports Med*. 1987; 15(5):490–493.
25. McMahon MS, Scuderi GR, Glashow JL, Scharf SC, Meltzer LP, and Scott WN. Scintigraphic determination of patella viability after excision of the infrapatellar fat pad and/or lateral release in total knee arthroplasty. *Clin Orthop*. 1990; 260:10.
26. Tria AJ, Harwood DA, Alicea JA, Cody RP. Patella fractures in posterior stabilizer knee arthroplasties. *Clin Orthop*. 1994; 299:131–138.
27. Ritter MA, Campbell ED. Postoperative patella complications with or without lateral release during total knee arthroplasty. *Clin Orthop*. 1987; 219:163–168.
28. Ritter MA, Herbst SA, Kelly M, Faris PM, Meding JB. Patellofemoral complications following total knee arthroplasty—effect of lateral release and sacrifice of the superior lateral genicular artery. *J Arthroplasty*. 1996; 11(4):368–371.
29. Johnson DP, Eastwood DM. Lateral patella release in knee arthroplasty. Effect on wound healing. *J Arthroplasty*. 1992; 7:427–431.
30. Laughlin RT, Werries RA, Verhulst SJ, Hayes JM. Patella tilt in TKA. *Am J Orthopaedics*. 1996; XXV(4):300–304.

CHAPTER 45
Proximal Patellar Realignment for Recurrent Patellar Instability

Jonathan Archer and Giles R. Scuderi

Dysfunction of the patellofemoral joint still exists as a source of failure in total knee arthroplasty. Historically, prior to the advent of patella resurfacing, anterior knee pain existed in approximately 40 to 58% of patients.[1] Insall and associates found that in several early total knee designs the source of residual pain was in the patellar compartment.[2] At times, when pain interfered with function, patellectomy was recommended. This was considered as a salvage option due to the sequelae, including quadriceps weakness[3] and patient dissatisfaction with cosmesis. Subsequent total knee designs introduced patella resurfacing. Patellar resurfacing has generated a new source of problems. In a recent review, Dennis has delineated a variety of complications specific to the patellofemoral articulation, including patellar fractures, component loosening, component failure, tendon rupture, patella clunk syndrome, and patellofemoral instability.[4]

In a prior review, Grace and Rand[5] noted that the incidence of patellar instability ranged from less than 1% to nearly 50%. A host of factors have been implicated in the problem of patellofemoral instability such as trauma, quadriceps muscle imbalance, component placement, component constraint, genu valgum, and errors in surgical technique.[5–12] The most common causes of patellar instability are errors in surgical technique and muscle imbalance.[5] Merkow and colleagues also found that the most prevalent etiology for patellar dislocation after total knee arthroplasty was technical error.[13]

The key to avoiding patellar instability is to recognize the potential pitfalls either preoperatively or intraoperatively. Preoperative evaluation should identify those patients with severe valgus deformity, congenital patellar dislocation, and/or patellofemoral subluxation.[14] A tangential radiograph of the patellofemoral joint, such as the Merchant view, will permit preoperative evaluation of patellar position. The information gathered preoperatively should be utilized at the time of arthroplasty.[24] Because the position of all these components impact patellofemoral stability, special attention must be taken at the time of the index procedures.[14] Internal rotation of the femoral and tibial components must be avoided. Though it is beyond the scope of this chapter, and component position has been addressed elsewhere, we have found the epicondylar axis to be the most reliable reference for rotational positioning of the femoral component. Our preference also includes lateralization of the femoral and tibial components with medialization of the patellar component. Patellar preparation has been discussed elsewhere, but restoration of the patellar thickness with the bone component composite has improved patellar tracking.

EVALUATION

Determining the cause of late patellar instability can be difficult. The onset of patellar instability after total knee arthroplasty in different series has ranged from an average of 5 to 11 months, but has occurred as early as 3 days and as late as 54 months.[5,13,15] The time of onset may give a clue to the etiology, such as a fall with hyperflexion of the knee early in the postoperative period, which may disrupt the medial capsular closure causing instability. In the study by Merkow and colleagues, all patients with patellar dislocation had anterior knee pain.[13] Other symptoms include difficulty with stair climbing and weakness. Physical exam findings may include subluxating or dislocating patellae, decreased flexion, or an extensor lag.

The use of plain radiographs in the evaluation of patellar instability should include anteroposterior, lateral, and Merchant or tangential views. These radiographic views are useful for determining axial limb alignment, patellar height, patellar thickness, and patellar position.[16] In order to evaluate rotational malalignment, computerized tomography (CT) can be much more helpful. Crossett and associates advocate the use of CT to evaluate failed total knee arthroplasty because rotatory malalignment of the femoral and/or tibial components can be determined.[17] With this in mind all knees being revised for patellar instability are evaluated with a preoperative CT scan to determine the rotational position of the femoral component (Fig. 45.1). If the femoral component is internally rotated greater than 5 degrees, relative to the epicondylar axis, femoral component revision to correct this malrotation should be contemplated.

SURGICAL TECHNIQUE

Once the etiology of patellar instability or dysfunction has been determined, surgical correction needs to be performed. Any significant rotational malalignment should be addressed with component revision. If the components are correctly positioned, extensor mechanism instability can be addressed with soft tissue techniques. As previously discussed, a lateral retinacular release may be sufficient to correct a lateral patellar tilt. However, should this not correct the problem or if the instability persists, proximal patellar realignment has been advocated by Insall as an effective procedure for correcting patellar instability and dislocation.[13] This procedure acts to redirect the "resultant force vector of the quadriceps."

The knee is approached through the prior skin incision, which is usually a straight midline skin incision, followed by a medial parapatellar arthrotomy. This arthrotomy extends in a straight line through the quadriceps tendon from the upper edge of the vastus medialis, over the medial patella, and down the medial margin of the patellar tendon to the tibial tubercle. A lateral retinacular release extending through the synovial membrane and into the inferior fibers of the vastus lateralis is performed prior to medial advancement. The lateral superior geniculate artery is usually cut during the lateral retinacular release, so it is important to identify this vessel and to cauterize it. The proximal realignment involves medial capsular tightening and advancement of the vastus medialis. This is accomplished by overlapping the medial capsule and vastus medialis on the quadriceps tendon and patella approximately 1 cm. The advancement of the medial structures is directed laterally and distally in the direction of the fibers of the vastus medialis obliques (Fig. 45.2).

The advancement is held with several provisional sutures so that the position and tracking of the patella can be assessed. The amount of overlap is variable and depends on the preoperative patella position. The patella is determined to be centralized if it tracks entirely with the anterior phlange of the femoral component with no medial or lateral tilt through a full range of motion. Care should be taken not to overtighten the medial capsule or rotate the patella at the time of closure. Once the correct position and tension has been determined, the arthrotomy is closed with multiple horizontal mattress stitches utilizing no. 0 absorbable sutures. Distally along the patella tendon, there is little advancement and the closure tends to be side to side. The subcutaneous tissue and skin incision are closed in a routine fashion and a soft milky dressing is applied.

Postoperatively, the patient is placed in a compressive dressing and continuous passive range of motion is initiated in the recovery room. Physical therapy is started on the first postoperative day consisting of passive and active-assist range of motion exercises. Full weight-bearing as tolerated is permitted and ambulation improves as muscle control of the lower extremity improves.

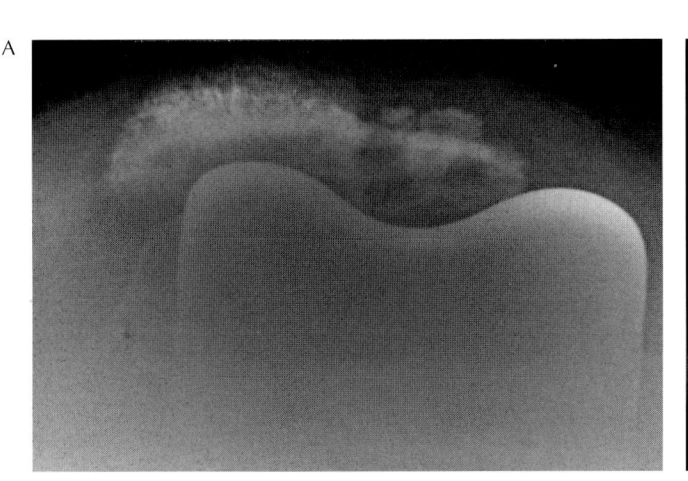

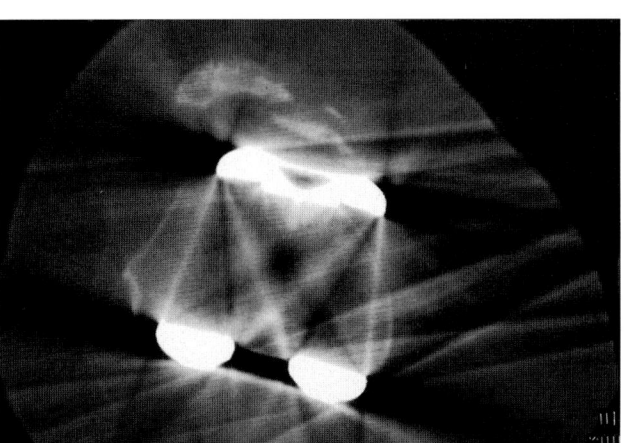

Figure 45.1. Merchant view showing a transverse patella fracture with lateral displacement of the major fragment. (A) The patella component is still in the trochlear groove. (B) The CT scan reveals similar findings and is useful for determining the rotational position of the femoral component.

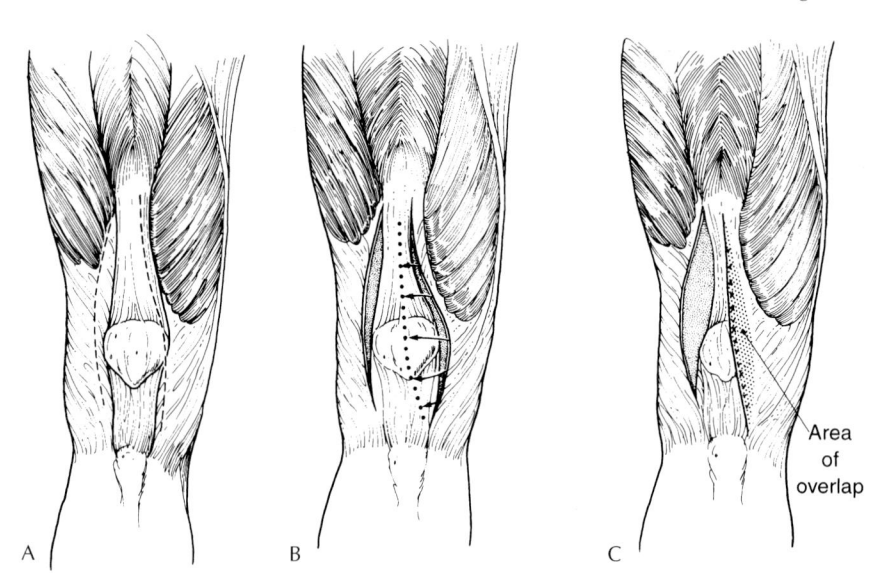

Figure 45.2. (A) The proximal patella realignment utilizes a medial parapatellar arthrotomy and lateral retinacular release. (B) The medial flap, which includes the vastus medialis and medial capsule, is advanced laterally over the patella. (C) Once these structures are secured in place, the patella should track centrally.

RESULTS

In 1985, Merkow and associates[13] published their results for treating patellar dislocation after total knee arthroplasty. Their study included 12 knees in 11 patients with an average age of 62 years. The average interval from total knee arthroplasty to patellar instability was 5 months (range, 1 to 18 months). The instability occurred in 9 primary arthroplasties and in 3 revision cases. Of the 12 knees, 10 were managed with proximal realignment as previously described, 1 with lateral release only, and 1 with proximal realignment combined with revision of components. No patient had recurrent patellar instability and the average Hospital for Special Surgery knee score improved by 27 points from 62 to 89.

Grace and Rand[5] reviewed the results of 25 knees that had operative realignment for patellar instability. The average age was 72 years at time of realignment. Fifty-two percent of knees had previous surgery prior to the index total knee arthroplasty. Fourteen knees underwent proximal patellar realignment, 9 had combined procedures consisting of a proximal patellar realignment and a distal realignment and 2 with complete component revision. The average Hospital for Special Surgery knee score improved by an average of 19 points from 56 to 75. There was no significant difference in knee scores between those who had proximal patellar realignment alone, a combined procedure, or those who had component revision. Their study advocated against the routine use of the combined procedure because 22% (2 of 9) of these knees had patellar tendon ruptures. Although recurrent instability occurred in 20% (5 of 25) of the knees, the authors noted that 28.5% (4 of 14) of knees that underwent proximal patellar realignment alone continued to have instability. This suggests that component malposition may have continued to be a contributing factor.

In a review delineating patellofemoral problems after total knee arthroplasty, Doolittle and Turner[20] found a 28.5% (10 of 350) incidence of patellar instability. Eight of the 10 knees underwent surgical patellar realignment including 2 Roux-Goldthwaite type, 2 Hauser type, and 7 proximal patellar realignments. They found an overall 80% satisfactory result. However, 3 patients required multiple revisions for patellar instability. Because one patient with a Roux-Goldthwaite procedure developed a patellar tendon rupture, the authors recommended and preferred a proximal patellar realignment for patellar instability, if component orientation is correct.

Jiang and associates[15] found a 4.4% (13 of 294) incidence of patellar instability after total knee arthroplasty in another series. The average time from index procedure to the development of instability was 8 months. Six knees, 2 dislocators and 4 subluxators, underwent proximal patellar realignment, whereas the remaining 7 had conservative treatment. The authors reported that at last follow-up, no knee had evidence of further instability, and recommend that proximal patellar realignment should be entertained if the patient fails a 6-month course of nonoperative treatment.

The results of TKA in chronic patellar dislocation were reviewed by Bullek and coworkers.[24] They recommend realignment of the chronically dislocated patella at the time of arthroplasty with a proximal patellar realignment and lateral retinacular release. This is similar to the experience of Hanssen and Rand.[25] Though this may not be universally accepted,[26] we have found realignment of the extensor mechanism possible, allowing restoration of both quadriceps strength and normal knee kinematics.

COMPLICATIONS

Complications involving a proximal patellar realignment procedure can be related to the lateral release component of the reconstruction. With a lateral release, it has been advocated by Scott[21] that one should attempt to preserve the superior lateral geniculate artery if possible. In a study by Scuderi and associates evaluating the vascularity of the patella after a lateral release, they found a 56.4% incidence of vascular compromise of the patella utilizing radionuclide scanning.[22] Nevertheless, there was only one clinical complication that was a patellar fracture successively treated nonoperatively. Ritter and Campbell[23] found no increased complication rate in knees in which a lateral release sacrificing the superior lateral geniculate vessels. There was no increased incidence of osteonecrosis, patellar fracture, or radiolucency around the patella. They did note an increased frequency of patellar fracture in those patients who had not had a lateral release. They found no difference in clinical outcome in regards to pain, ambulation, or range of motion. Merkow and colleagues[13] had one complication related specifically to the proximal patellar realignment, which was a superficial skin necrosis that healed with local wound care. None of the patellae in their study redislocated. Grace and Rand[5] had a 28.5% (4 of 14) rate of recurrent instability after proximal realignment alone. This was attributed to quadriceps imbalance because these four patients had no evidence for trauma, component malposition, or abnormal axial alignment. Jiang[15] reported no recurrent instability in those patients treated with proximal realignment alone. They also had no infections, fractures, or evidence for loosening of the patellar component. Though there is potential for complication resulting from devascularization of the patella from a lateral release, it has been well accepted that "patellar equilibrium must take precedence over concern about vascularity."[14]

Though there is a theoretical concern that overtightening of the medial capsule and medial musculature may pull the patella too far medially, there have been no reported cases of medial dislocation following a proximal patella realignment.

SUMMARY

Patellar instability following total knee arthroplasty still exists as a complication. The most common cause appears to be related to technical errors during the index arthroplasty. Malrotation or malalignment of either femoral, tibial, or patellar component may result in patellar instability. If component orientation is found to be correct, then muscle imbalance should be suspected as the cause for instability. Proximal realignment has been advocated as the treatment of choice for instability should conservative measures fail.[5,13,15,20] The use of distal realignment procedures is advocated with caution because there have been reports of patellar tendon rupture postoperatively.[5,20]

References

1. Picetti GD, McGann WA, Welch RB. The patellofemoral joint after total knee arthroplasty without patellar resurfacing. *J Bone Joint Surg*. 1990; 72(A):1379–1382.
2. Insall JN, Dethmers DA. Revision of total knee arthroplasty. *Clin Orthop*. 1982; 170:123–130.
3. Kaufer H. Mechanical function of the patella. *J Bone Joint Surg*. 1971; 53(A):1551–1560.
4. Dennis DA. Patellofemoral complications in total knee arthroplasty. In: Callaghan JJ, Dennis DA, Paprosky WG, et al., eds. *Orthopaedic Knowledge Update: Hip and Knee Reconstruction*. Rosemont, IL: AAOS; 1995: 238–289.
5. Grace JN, Rand JA. Patellar instability after total knee arthroplasty. *Clin Orthop*. 1988; 237:184–189.
6. Buchanan JR, Greer RB, Bowman LS, et al. Clinical experience with the variable axis total knee replacement (Abstract). *J Bone Joint Surg* 1982; 64(3):337–346.
7. Cameron HU, Fedorkow DM. The patella in total knee arthroplasty. *Clin Orthop*. 1982; 165:197–199.
8. Clayton ML, Thirupathi R. Patellar complications after total condylar arthroplasty. *Clin Orthop*. 1982; 170:152–155.
9. Goldberg VM, Henderson BT. The Freeman-Swanson ICLH total knee arthroplasty: complications and problems. *J Bone Joint Surg*. 1980; 62(A):1338–1344.
10. Insall JN, Hood RW, Flawn LB, et al. The total condylar knee prosthesis in gonarthrosis: a five- to nine-year follow-up of the first one hundred consecutive replacements. *J Bone Joint Surg*. 1983; 65A:619–628.
11. Jones EC, Insall JN, Inglis AE, et al. GUEPAR knee arthroplasty results and late complications. *Clin Orthop*. 1979; 140:145–152.
12. Moreland JR, Thomas RJ, Freeman MAR. ICLH replacement of the knee. *Clin Orthop*. 1979; 145:47–59.
13. Merkow RL, Soudry M, Insall JN. Patellar dislocation following total knee replacement. *J Bone Joint Surg*. 1985; 67(A):1321–1327.
14. Briard JL, Hungerford DS. Patellofemoral instability in total knee arthroplasty. 1989; (suppl):S87–S97.
15. Jiang C, Yip KM, Liu D. Patellar thickness in total knee replacement. *J Formos Med Assoc*. 1994; 93:17–20.
16. Ghelman B. Imaging of total knee replacements. In: Insall JN, Scott WN, Scuderi GR, eds. *Current Concepts in Primary and Revision Total Knee Arthroplasty*. Philadelphia: Lippincott-Raven, 1996: 227–234.
17. Crosset LS, Rubash HE, Berger R. Computerized tomography in total knee arthroplasty. In: Insall JN, Scott WN, Scuderi GR, eds. *Current Concepts in Primary and Revision*

Total Knee Arthroplasty. Philadelphia: Lippincott-Raven; 1996: 235–248.
18. Madigan R, Wissinger HA, Donaldson WF. Preliminary experience with a method of quadriceps plasty in recurrent subluxation of the patella. *J Bone Joint Surg*. 1975; 57(A):600–607.
19. Freeman BL, III. Recurrent dislocations. In: Crenshaw AH, ed. *Campbell's Operative Orthopaedics*. St. Louis: Mosby; 1992: 1391–1464.
20. Doolittle KH, Turner RH. Patellofemoral problems following total knee arthroplasty. *Orthopedic Review* 1988; 17: 696–702.

# CHAPTER 46
Distal Realignment for Recurrent Patellar Instability

Leo A. Whiteside

Between January 1980 and January 1994, 15 knees with a valgus angle of more than 12 degrees and 16 knees with revision total knee arthroplasty had lateral patellar subluxation that could not be corrected with lateral patellar release and vastus medialis advancement. All underwent distal quadriceps realignment. Eighteen knees had medial tibial tubercle transfer done by elevating the tibial tubercle and proximal 6 cm of the tibial crest through a lateral approach that left the medial periosteum intact. Three cases had medial transfer of the medial one-half of the patellar tendon. Ten cases had modified the Roux-Goldthwait procedure.

Neither late patellar subluxation nor dislocation has occurred in any case with distal realignment. Three cases of medial tibial tubercle transfer developed hematomas and two required surgical evacuation. Neither fracture nor displacement of the tubercle fragment has occurred. No significant patellar complication has occurred with the patients who have had the modified Roux-Goldthwait procedure or those with medial transfer of the medial one-half of the patellar tendon. One year after surgery, mean knee flexion was 113 degrees and four knees had a flexion contracture of 5 degrees. None of the knees had a quadriceps lag.

INTRODUCTION

Abnormal patellar tracking, patellar tilt, and quadriceps malalignment are some of the most persistent yet poorly defined complications of total knee arthroplasty. These abnormalities may be caused by imbalance between the medial and lateral muscle forces on the patella, medial displacement of the patellar groove, shallow or incompetent patellar groove, or lateral displacement of the tibial tubercle. Internal rotation of the femoral component can be responsible for the majority of these disorders, and is especially likely to occur in revision total knee arthroplasty. A simple lateral patellar release and vastus medialis advancement are often insufficient to correct mechanical abnormalities and to prevent progressive subluxation. Success with these procedures would require that the vastus medialis maintain its shortened length for the lifetime of the knee arthroplasty regardless of the forces that continually pull the patella and the quadriceps mechanism laterally. It may be possible to remedy the situation in some cases by revising the femoral component and rotating it externally to position the patellar groove under the quadriceps mechanism, but this may adversely affect the stability of the knee in flexion. Another alternative is to realign the quadriceps pull to form a nearly straight line through the patella between the tibial tubercle and the quadriceps muscle group. This would correct the mechanical abnormalities responsible for lateral patellar subluxation by diminishing the lateralizing forces. Thus it would likely not apply abnormally high forces to the vastus medialis. This study reviews 31 cases of distal realignment of the patellar tendon, and describes the three surgical techniques for managing patellar-tracking disorders occurring in total knee arthroplasty.

MATERIALS AND METHODS
Surgical Procedure
Modified Roux-Goldthwait Procedure
For knees with moderate-to-severe malalignment and a Q-angle measuring greater than 15 degrees, a modification of the Roux-Goldthwait procedure consistently cor-

Reprinted with permission from Lippincott-Raven. In: "Distal realignment of the patellar tendon to correct abnormal patellar tracking," Clin Orthop 344:284–289, 1997, by Leo A. Whiteside, MD.

rected the tracking abnormality intraoperatively, and held the patella in tight apposition to the femoral surface throughout the arc of flexion.

The lateral one-half of the patellar tendon was detached distally from the tibial bone surface, and the patellar tendon was split longitudinally to the patellar attachment proximally. The lateral segment of the patellar tendon then was folded over the top of the medial one-half of the patellar tendon, leaving intact the attachments to the synovial membrane and to the fat pad. The patella was released enough laterally under direct vision to allow the patellar tendon segment to be fully transferred anteriorly over the top of the medial one-half of the patellar tendon without excessive tension in the retinaculum or synovial membrane. The distal end of the lateral tendon segment was sutured directly beneath the medial capsular edge just medial to the distal attachment of the medial segment of the patellar tendon. The medial capsule then was closed with multiple interrupted sutures to both segments of the patellar tendon. The lateral defect also was closed to seal the joint cavity (Fig. 46.1).

These patients all were mobilized in a normal fashion postoperatively, beginning with a continuous passive motion machine in the recovery room and full weight-bearing the day after surgery. The physical therapist was advised not to manipulate the knee, nor ask the patient to do straight-leg lifts with weights or knee bend exercises while standing in order to avoid stretching the quadriceps mechanism.

Medial Transfer of the Medial One-Half of the Patellar Tendon

When the patellar tendon was partially avulsed distally from its bony attachment, and the patellar-tracking abnormality was moderate, the medial one-half of the patellar tendon was transferred medially. The lateral attachment was left intact, and the portion of the patellar tendon that was avulsed was separated with a straight incision from the lateral half of the tendon, while leav-

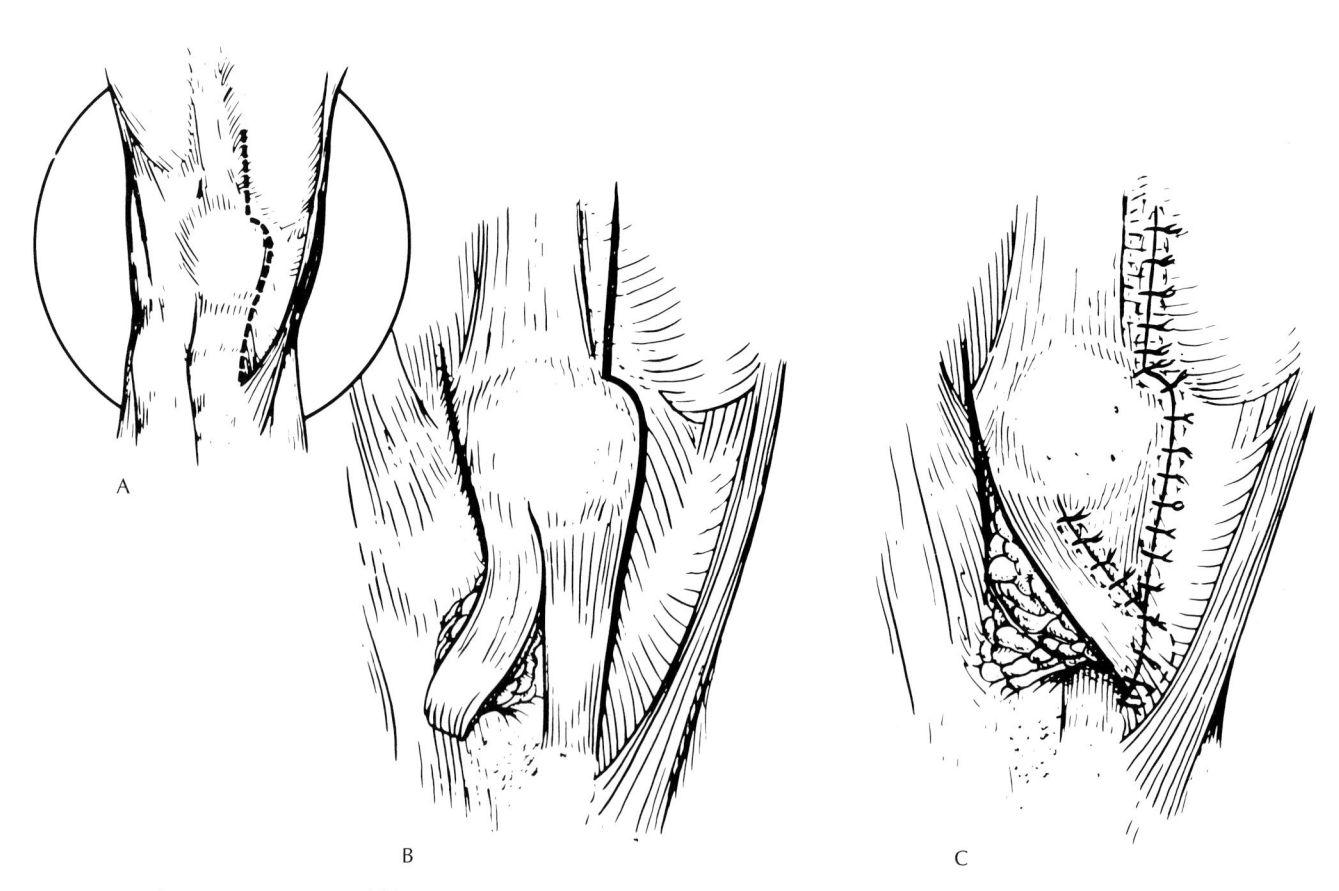

Figure 46.1. Roux-Goldthwait procedure. (A) Standard medial parapatellar incision is made. (B) During closure, the lateral half of the patellar tendon is detached from the tibial tubercle and separated up to the patella. Lateral patellar release is done extrasynovially, and the superior lateral genicular artery is preserved. (C) With the fat pad attachments left intact, the lateral half of the patellar tendon is crossed over the medial half, and its distal end is sutured under the medial capsular flap. Other sutures are added to secure its attachment.

ing it attached to the patella proximally. Tissue attachments to the fat pad were left intact, and the medial one-half of the patellar tendon was transferred medially under the medial capsular flap and sutured in place with multiple absorbable sutures (Fig. 46.2). Patellar tracking then was checked through the full range of motion.

Medial Tibial Tubercle Transfer

The tibial tubercle was transferred medially in cases with severe patellar subluxation and persistent dislocation. The subcutaneous tissue was dissected from the tubercle and from the anterior tibial crest. An oscillating saw was used to make a cut angled cephalad in the tibial crest approximately 6 cm across from the top of the tibial tubercle. A curved half-inch osteotome was used to penetrate the lateral cortex of the tibial tubercle and tibial crest, then the osteotome was passed beneath the tibial tubercle to osteotomize the medial tibial cortex. The medial periosteum and attachments of the pes anserina around them were left attached to the bone fragment. The fragment and the patellar tendon were elevated, the fat pad was detached from the anterior tibia but left intact to the patellar tendon, and the medial 1 to 1.5 cm of periosteum was elevated from the medial tibial cortex. Care was taken to avoid damage to the superficial medial collateral ligament at its attachment to the tibia. The undersurface of the tibial tubercle and crest fragment was debrided of loose cancellous bone with a ronguer. The tubercle then was shifted medially and placed directly atop the edge of the medial tibial cortical surface. Although the tibial tubercle was held in its new position, patellar tracking was checked through the full range of motion. The lateral patellar ligament and scarred synovium were released to allow the patella to follow the new Q-angle. The tubercle then was secured with a combination of wires and screws (Fig. 46.3). In 10 knees the tubercle was held with two or three screws passed through the lateral one-third of the tubercle fragment and through the medial tibial cortex. The tibial tubercle was secured with a combination of screws and wires in 8 knees because the large tibial stem did not allow screws to pass through the medial cortex. Rather, titanium wires were passed through drill holes in the medial tibial cortex that skirted the stem. These drill holes were made along the lateral edge of the tibial tubercle, then the distal ends of the wires were passed

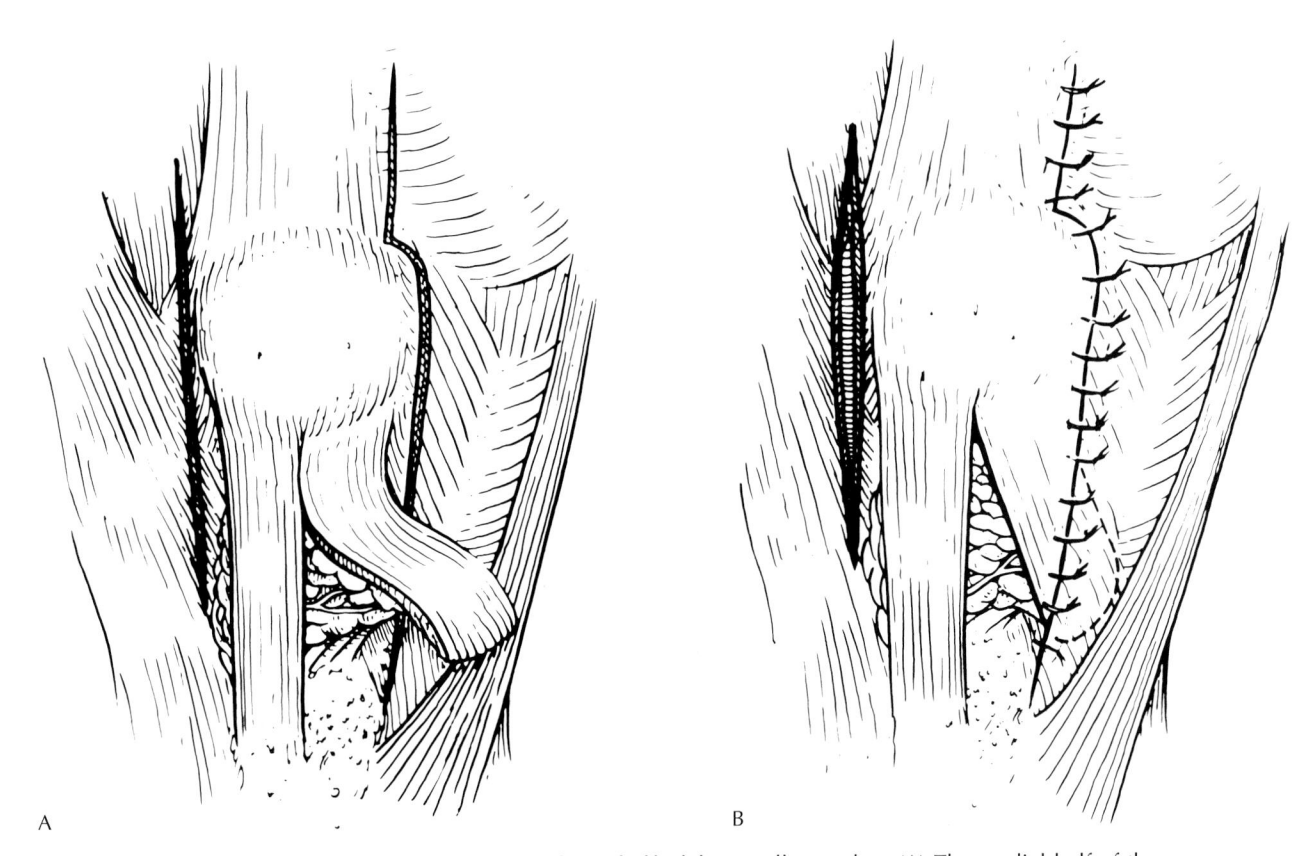

Figure 46.2. Medial transfer of the medial one-half of the patellar tendon. (A) The medial half of the patellar tendon has avulsed spontaneously from the tibial tubercle. It is separated up to the patella, but the fat pad attachments are left intact. The lateral retinaculum has been released extrasynovially. (B) The medial half of the patellar tendon has been transferred medially, and the distal end is sutured under the medial capsular flap. Other sutures are added as needed to secure the medial tendon.

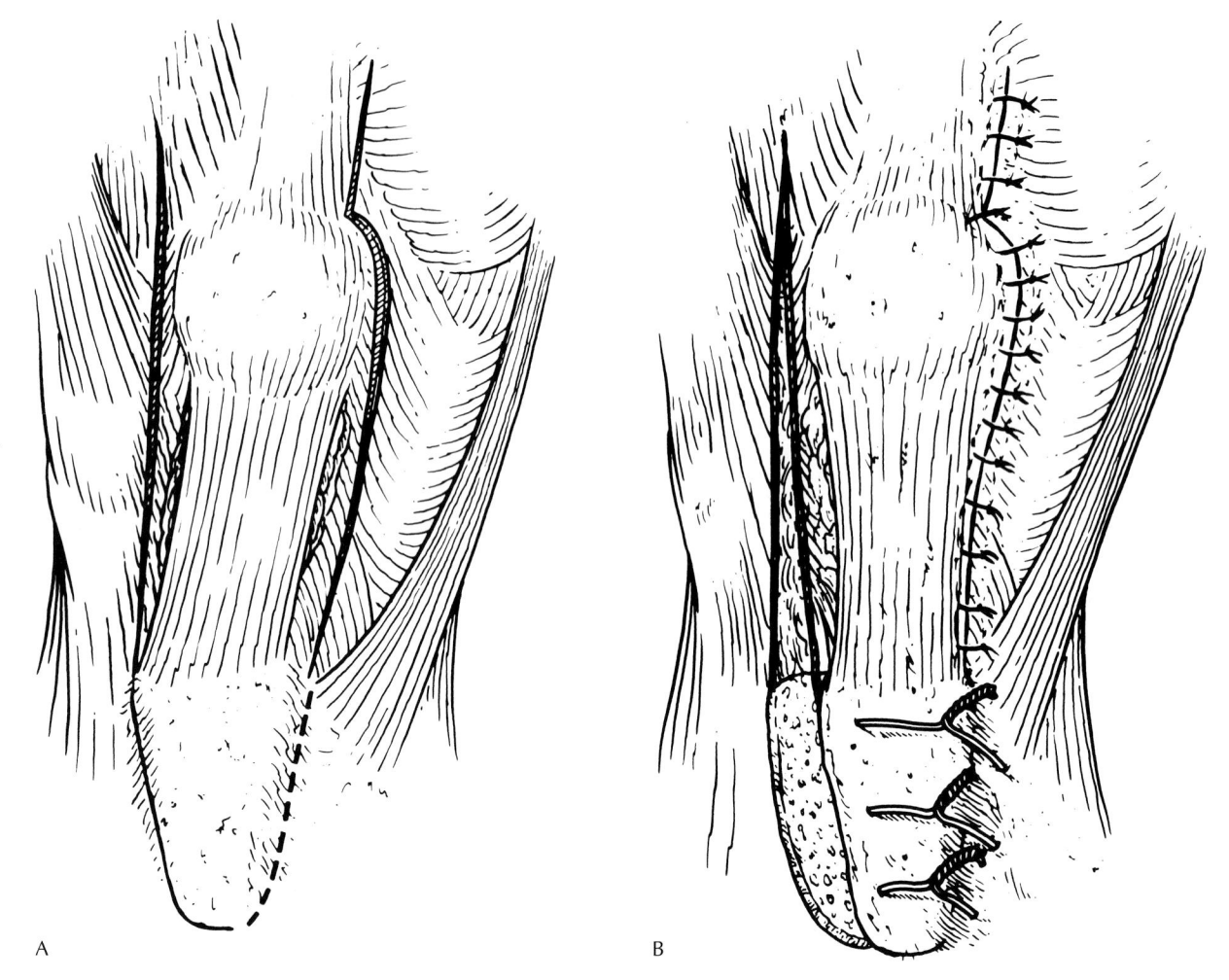

Figure 46.3. Medial tibial tubercle transfer. (A) The tibial tubercle is osteotomized from laterally, and the medial periosteal attachments are left intact. A lateral patellar release has been done to facilitate medial shift of the patella and patellar tendon. A thin strip of tissue has been resected from the tendon of the vastus medialis and medial retinaculum to maintain medial tension. (B) The tibial tubercle has been shifted medially, and the medial capsular structures have been sutured. The lateral release has opened slightly to accommodate the medial shift of the quadriceps mechanism.

through the periosteal pedicle and were twisted together and tightened to firmly secure the tubercle fragment to the tibial surface. A single screw was passed proximally through the lateral edge of the tubercle and then through the medial tibial cortex to control rotational position and micromotion of the fragment. The screw hole was drilled carefully so that it was not placed in the center of the fragment near the proximal end of the tibial tubercle in which fracture could occur.

These patients were treated with active mobilization postoperatively, but they were splinted in full extension during weight-bearing, and were not allowed straight-leg raising exercises in a seated position for the first 6 weeks. The splint was discontinued after 6 weeks and full active rehabilitation of the quadriceps mechanism was begun.

Clinical Cases between January 1980 and January 1994

Fifteen knees with a valgus angle greater than 12 degrees and 16 knees with revision total knee arthroplasty had lateral patellar subluxation that could not be corrected with extensive lateral patellar release. In all of these cases it was apparent from direct observation that the Q-angle was excessive and that the mechanical disturbance that caused the tracking abnormality was not excessively lax medial capsular structures. The distal quadriceps was realigned in all cases: 18 knees had medial tibial tubercle transfer, 10 had modified Roux-Goldthwait procedure, and 3 had medial transfer of the medial one-half of the patellar tendon.

RESULTS

The patellar-tracking abnormalities were corrected with these procedures. Neither late patellar subluxation nor dislocation has occurred in any case as a result of distal realignment. However, other complications have occurred. Three patients with medial tibial tubercle transfer developed hematomas. Two required surgical intervention, one of which developed late onset infection that required removal of the implants, debridement, and revision arthroplasty. Neither fracture nor displacement of the tibial tubercle has occurred. No significant patellar complication has occurred in those patients who have had the Roux-Goldthwait procedure, and none of them has had significant wound complications. The same is true of the patients with medial transfer of the medial one-half of the patellar tendon.

One year after surgery mean knee flexion was 113 degrees. No knees had flexion less than 90 degrees. Four knees had flexion contracture of 5 degrees. None of the knees had quadriceps lag.

DISCUSSION

Patellar abnormalities are among the most common complications after total knee arthroplasty, but relatively little information is available in the orthopedic literature to guide the practicing orthopedic surgeon. The most common recommendation for correction of tracking abnormalities is an extensive lateral patellar release and medial reefing.[1] However, when an abnormally large Q-angle is the underlying problem, the patella is still at risk of subluxation. A more appropriate procedure is to correct the abnormality of alignment and to leave intact the normal structures and circulation to the extensor mechanism. Distal realignment of the quadriceps mechanism has been used successfully to solve this problem, but it involves some risk to the patellar tendon.[1] A detailed description of the technique and presentation of the results with this procedure is lacking in the literature. Krackow mentioned this procedure in his book and included an illustration of the procedure.[2] The section on handling patellar-tracking abnormalities did not mention proximal procedures, but described only the medial transfer of the tibial tubercle for recalcitrant patellar-tracking abnormalities. Goldberg identified this procedure as a solution to patellar-tracking abnormalities caused by rotational malalignment of the tibial component, but suggested that tibial component revision likely would be necessary in most cases.[3] Goldberg also suggested that soft tissue procedures are usually inadequate for rotational malalignment in a femoral component, and that femoral component revision and realignment are necessary.[3] Habermann mentioned medial transposition of the tibial tubercle in a single case, but did not give surgical details.[4]

Most proximal realignment procedures have a relatively poor record for solving patellar-tracking problems associated with osteoarthritic knees. Chrisman reported a 17% redislocation rate with the Hauser procedure and a 5% rate with the Roux-Goldthwait procedure.[5] DeCesare reported a 7% dislocation rate with the Hauser procedure,[6] whereas Crosby and Insall reported a 19% redislocation rate with distal realignment of the quadriceps mechanism, and a 25% rate with proximal realignment.[7] Persistent problems with patellar tracking continue in many knees treated for osteoarthritis because the underlying cause is dysplasia or damage to the femoral surface. In total knee arthroplasty, however, the femoral aspect of the patellofemoral mechanism has been reconstructed, so that the only abnormality that remains to be corrected is quadriceps mechanism alignment.

Although proximal realignment procedures were once the mainstay for reconstruction of patellofemoral abnormalities, such has not always been the case. Roux's original description for treatment of this condition entailed a medial transfer of the medial attachment of the patellar tendon, and it had excellent early results.[8] However, the Hauser procedure, as it was commonly performed, often caused severe problems secondary to patellar baja.[5] Proximal realignment then was favored for some time, but Hughston and Walsh still recommended distal realignment if the Q-angle was greater than 10 degrees.[9]

Goldthwait's original operation for lateral patellar dislocation was presented at the annual meeting for the American Orthopaedic Association in 1895.[10,11] He described transferring the lateral half of the patellar tendon beneath the medial half and into the medial capsule and pes anserina. We have modified this procedure to simplify it, and to provide a passive restraint to lateral tilt of the patella. When the lateral half of the tendon is passed under the medial half, it tends to lift the medial half of the patella. However, when it is transferred over the anterior surface of the medial patellar tendon, it depresses the patella and gently presses the medial edge of the patella against the femur. This is easier to do, and the fat pad attachments to the medial half of the patella tendon can be left intact.

This series is too small to make reliable predictions regarding recurrence rate and complications with distal realignment of the patella mechanism. However, it was done only in severe cases—those with major abnormalities of the Q-angle—and this group of patients was selected from more than 2,000 arthroplasty procedures done during the same time period.

Although distal realignment of the quadriceps is not often necessary, these simple procedures appear to offer a reliable solution to an otherwise difficult problem. Even the most ardent supporters of proximal realignment do not advocate it for moderate or severe patellofemoral malalignment problems. Goldberg and co-authors advocated proximal soft tissue realignment procedures for mild tracking abnormalities, but when true anatomical abnormalities are present, they discourage simple soft tissue procedures and advocate distal realignment.[3] However, supporting data are absent from their review article, and a dearth of reliable clinical data remains in the orthopedic literature about this important issue. Because the modified Roux-Goldthwait and medial one-half patellar tendon transfer procedure seem to be reliable, and add little to the operative time, they are used more frequently in our practice for less-severe tracking abnormalities because they do not require extensive work on the quadriceps mechanism that would devascularize the patella and scar the muscles and tendons above the patella.

Although proximal lateral release and medial quadriceps and capsular advancement may solve the immediate intraoperative appearance of patellar instability, that approach is anathema to the prevailing philosophy of independent tracking of the patella. The "no thumbs test" is considered the standard by which most orthopedic surgeons judge intraoperative patellar tracking. If the patella cannot be made to track without closing the medial capsular incision, it will also be unstable once the patient is awake and using the extremity. Although this complication is difficult to document in the literature, it is equally difficult to ignore because most arthroplasty surgeons have learned this by experience.[12,13]

ACKNOWLEDGMENT

The author thanks Diane Morton, BA, for editorial assistance in the preparation of this manuscript.

References

1. Grace J, Rand J. Patellar instability after total knee arthroplasty. *Clin Orthop.* 1988; 237:184–189.
2. Krackow K. *The Technique of Total Knee Arthroplasty.* St. Louis: Mosby, 1990.
3. Goldberg V, Figgie H III, Veregge P, et al. Surgical considerations in patellar replacement. In: Goldberg V, ed. *Controversies of Total Knee Arthroplasty*. New York: Raven Press; 1991:155–165.
4. Habermann E. Revision arthroplasty for failed total knee replacement. In: Hungerfold D, Krackow K, Kenna R, eds. *Total Knee Arthroplasty: A Comprehensive Approach.* Baltimore: Williams & Wilkins; 1984:219–257.
5. Chrisman O, Snook G, Wilson T. A long-term prospective study of the Hauser and Roux-Goldthwait procedures for recurrent patellar dislocation. *Clin. Orthop.* 1979; 144:27–30.
6. DeCesare W. Late results of Hauser procedure for recurrent dislocation of the patella. *Clin Orthop.* 1979; 140: 137–144.
7. Crosby E, Insall J. Recurrent dislocation of the patella. Relation of treatment to osteoarthritis. *J Bone Joint Surg.* 1976; 58A:9–13.
8. Roux C. Recurrent dislocation of the patella: operative treatment. Revue de Chirurgie, 1888. *Clin Orthop.* 1979; 144:4–8.
9. Hughston J, Walsh W. Proximal and distal reconstruction of the extensor mechanism for patellar subluxation. *Clin Orthop.* 1979; 144:36–42.
10. Goldthwait J. Dislocation of the patella. *Trans Am Orthop Assoc.* 1895; 8:237.
11. Goldthwait J. Permanent dislocation of the patella. *Ann Surg.* 1899; 29:62.
12. Merkow R. Patellar dislocation following total knee replacement. *J Bone Joint Surg.* 1985; 61A:1321–1327.
13. Scott R. Treatment of patellar instability associated with total knee replacement. *Tech Orthop.* 1988; 3:9–14.

SECTION 13
Evaluation of the Painful Total Knee Arthroplasty

CHAPTER 47
Clinical Evaluation

Aaron G. Rosenberg and Richard A. Berger

Although total knee arthroplasty has taken its place in the orthopedic armamentarium as one of the most successful of surgical procedures, it remains a commonplace of orthopedic practice to encounter patients with complaints of pain related to their joint replacement. Appropriate evaluation of these patients remains an important function of any surgeon who performs knee replacement. The patient with complaints referable to their total knee arthroplasty represents a broad spectrum of possible clinical scenarios. Such an individual may present with a rather simple problem, easily evaluated and relatively easily treated, such as an implant placed many years ago that had given excellent results and is now painful and radiographically loose. On the other end of the "difficulty" spectrum is the patient with persistent complaints of pain and who has by all objective appearances a well-performed, well-fixed, and well-functioning arthroplasty. This chapter will review the principles involved in the clinical evaluation of these patients, and the following chapter will outline ancillary imaging studies that may be appropriate in the evaluation of these patients.

Exploration of the painful total knee arthroplasty without an adequate preoperative diagnosis has been documented to result in a high percentage of patients with persistent complaints. Thus one of the most important principles in evaluation and management of the patient with complaints referable to their total knee arthroplasty is to avoid surgical intervention until a diagnosis is made and rational therapy can be formulated.

Of equal importance to the clinician is to establish the degree of disability engendered by the patient's complaints and the degree to which additional findings may warrant intervention. Any decision about intervention, ranging from surgical exploration to simple diagnostic testing by X ray, requires the clinician to weigh the multiple variables of risk to benefit in the proposed intervention before proceeding. Thus establishing the degree of disability and the severity of complaint is an essential task in determining the advisability of further diagnostic or therapeutic intervention.

The mainstay of all medical diagnosis is the history. No less so in the evaluation of the patient with complaints referable to their total knee arthroplasty, the history provides the clinician with an opportunity to understand the patient's point of view, to establish a relationship of trust and mutual rapport and to obtain the information that will direct the physician's effort at further data collection. Although all of these are important, we will focus our attention on the aspect of the history that provides information for the development of alternative hypotheses that explain the patient's symptoms and may lead to a treatment plan.

The main purpose of initial information accumulation of the history is to aid in the development of the differential diagnosis. The differential diagnosis in actuality becomes the focus for a process in which hypothesis generation occurs. The generation of hypothesis is followed by a period of additional data gathering. The clinician must then decide which additional diagnostic examinations (further questions, physical examinations, and other tests) are appropriate to evaluate the hypothesis (diagnosis) chosen. This data will either serve to confirm or refute the diagnoses in the differential and, depending on the degree of confidence in the findings, may lead to alternative hypotheses generation, which then serves to stimulate another round of data accumulation in the forms of questions, physical examination, and additional laboratory study (Fig. 47.1).

Although the actual cognitive process that clinicians use to derive accurate diagnosis remains unknown, there are various models that have been used to describe the process. The linear model presupposes that as new information is acquired it assumes a positive or negative weight, with the eventual sum of the information accumulated leading to acceptance or discard of the hypothesis. The Bayesian model presupposes that each new piece of information must be weighed against the background of the previous information accumulated as

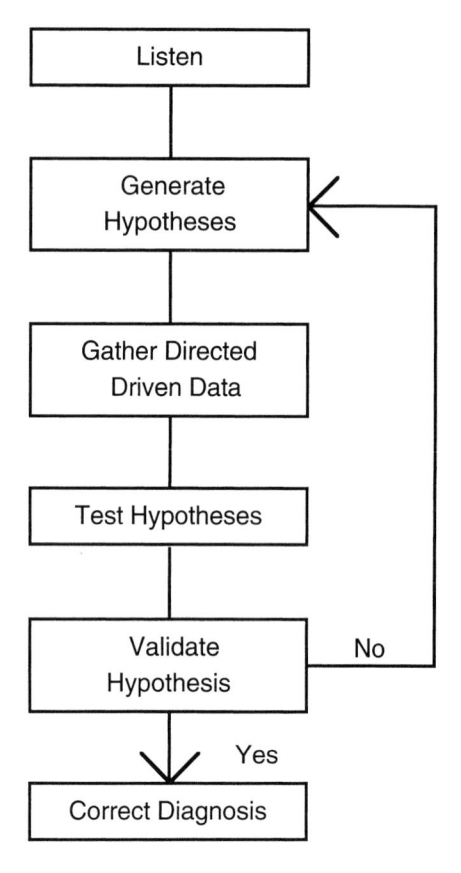

Figure 47.1. Algorithm for determining the diagnosis.

well as the relative incidence of the process in the population from which the patient originates. The algorithmic model presupposes that the physician uses a branching and screening process with a predetermined internal logic, either self-generated from experience or learned, in order to test a given hypothesis. Although these models differ in their ability to account for several features of the cognitive process clinicians use to arrive at diagnoses, it is useful to review several principles common to the process of differential diagnosis generation and diagnosis confirmation as they relate to the evaluation of the patient with complaints referable to their total knee arthroplasty.

PRINCIPLES OF DIAGNOSIS

First, the differential diagnosis should be based on the twin principles of probability and importance. The principle of probability takes into account the adage that "common diseases are common" and thus the differential diagnosis should take into account the disease processes that most commonly account for the symptoms expressed. As this relates to the painful total knee, the complaint of pain with weight-bearing but relief with rest would suggest mechanical loosening of the prosthesis as a more probable diagnosis. The finding of pain at rest or at night in addition to activity-related pain would suggest an inflammatory or infectious process. This latter diagnosis may also serve to illustrate the point of "importance" in the differential diagnosis. The clinician should consider those diagnoses for which failure to treat would lead to serious disability or a missed opportunity for cure by which disease progression may account for substantial morbidity. Such may be the case in the acute infection, for which failure to diagnose may result in the need for prosthetic removal, and for which early diagnosis may lead to component salvage.

A second principle is that when hypotheses are difficult to generate, it may be appropriate to revert to a different diagnostic approach. The diagnostic search may be helped by either a more detailed review of complaints, to think of categories of disease, or to think of anatomic structures rather than specific diagnoses as being responsible for the patient's complaints. Anatomic categories would include such items as bone, muscle, nerve, connective tissue, ligament, extensor mechanism, etc. Disease categories may be inferred from the differential diagnosis list noted in Table 47.1 but would in-

Table 47.1. Differential diagnosis of complaints referable to total knee arthroplasty

Surgical diagnosis	Nonsurgical diagnoses
Prosthetic loosening—component failure	Referred pain
	Hip
Component wear	Thigh
Component overhang	Calf
Deformity	Reflex sympathetic dystrophy—causalgia
Instability	
Sepsis	Stress fracture
Progressive bone loss	Bursitis—tendonitis
Arthrofibrosis-inadequate motion	Pes anserine bursitis
Patellofemoral malfunction	Patellar tendonitis
Clunk syndrome	Hamstring tendonitis
Subluxation/dislocation	Persistent crystalline deposition
Recurrent intra-articular soft tissue impingement	Gout
	CPPD
Recurrent effusion	Neurovascular problems
Persistent synovitis	Neuropathy
Rheumatoid arthritis	Radiculopathy
Other primary inflammatory synovial diseases	Sciatica
	Spinal stenosis
	Vascular claudication
	Thrombophlebitis—DVT
	Fibromyalgia—fibrositis
	Expectation/result mismatch
	Multiply-operated failed knee syndrome
	Depression
	Unrealistic expectations
	Minimal preoperative arthritic change

clude the classical listing of inflammatory, infectious, tumor, trauma, etc.

Although evaluation of the patient usually proceeds from the chief complaint, the development of a complete line of questioning in all possible areas involved in the total knee arthroplasty is rarely performed. In most cases of evaluation, the need for as detailed a process as outlined here will be superfluous. Rather the questioning process is selective and follows a branching and screening process as described above. However, the review to follow will demonstrate the type of information that would be acquired in the complete evaluation of the patient who presents with complaints referable to their total knee arthroplasty.

THE HISTORY

The chief complaint is occasionally described by the patient in "classical fashion," but more often needs reinterpretation by the clinician as new information is developed, and this best occurs by the development of a dialogue between patient and physician. Thus, complaints of fatigue may mask the real symptom of pain, or complaints of pain may be masking an actual complaint of instability. Additionally, pain localization by the patient may be based on personal beliefs rather than according to established anatomic referral patterns.

Most appropriate after establishing the chief complaint is to develop an accurate perception of the time course of the patient's complaints. Even though these may be succinct and easily communicated, frequently the time course of the disease process is more complex and will require repeated questioning until an accurate picture can be established. Thus, query into the patient's history prior to the onset of current symptoms is usually appropriate. The surgeon should inquire into developmental disorders associated with the knee or trauma prior to the current arthroplasty. An understanding of the patient's symptoms prior to the most recent surgical intervention is also appropriate. In particular, a prior surgical history is invaluable and the time course of symptoms prior to arthroplasty, the postoperative course, and the interval between that intervention and the current onset of symptoms may need careful evaluation. Particular attention should be focused in terms of wound problems, drainage, and return to function after the initial arthroplasty. The physician should assess how long, if at all, the arthroplasty was functioning well without pain. In the multiply-operated patient, this may be a time-consuming process but is almost always worthwhile. Should a history of complications in the postoperative course be obtained, these may require a more detailed evaluation that can usually be improved by a review of medical records. In the complex case, these may be essential in obtaining accurate information. Establishing a relationship between activity, trauma, or another intercurrent illness and the onset of knee symptoms may be helpful in establishing both diagnosis and etiology, though the clinician should also be aware of the propensity of patients to convert temporal relationships to causative ones in an attempt to explain their symptoms.

Close questioning on methods previously recommended or used to relieve discomfort as well as on prior testing is essential. Previous treatment attempts and diagnostic tests may have been performed and the clinician should avoid being embarrassed by recommending a test or treatment that has recently been performed elsewhere. Close questioning of the patient in terms of previous consultations, diagnostic tests, and attempts at treatment are also essential in order to assess the patient's current status and may provide valuable information in formulating the differential diagnosis list.

SYMPTOMS

Perhaps of greatest concern, and most troubling to the patient, is the symptom of pain. The patient should be carefully questioned about the nature of the pain; is it burning, stabbing, aching, or catching. Where is the pain located? Is it diffuse or in a specific area? Questions on pain should also include its radiation to or from additional anatomic sites juxtaposed or unrelated to the knee. Activities that exacerbate the pain and that relieve the discomfort should be elicited. The patient should be asked whether or not the pain disturbs sleep or is improved with rest. Any other relationships should be noted between the pain and activities.

A sharp catching pain usually indicates mechanical etiology. Pain at rest is not usually mechanical in origin. Pain after activity is characteristic of synovial irritation or tendonitis.

Because the orthopedic diagnosis is so often dependent on an accurate anatomic assessment of pain localization, it is usually helpful to have the patient actually point to and demonstrate those areas that are perceived as being the course or location of the painful sensation. This may give the clinician clues to the actual source of the patient's problem and can allow for more detailed focus during the physical examination.

Detailed information about pain radiation may lead the clinician to consider extra-articular sources of pain in certain cases. This should lead naturally to the development of the history of adjacent joints such as the hip or the lumbar spine.

Finally, the patient should be questioned about other regions of musculoskeletal pain. In some cases of referred pain this will lead to the ultimate diagnosis, and in other cases may simply provide the clinician with a better picture of the overall health and musculoskeletal status of the patient.

An important part of the assessment of pain and disability is the functional status of the patient as well as the need for medication. Whether or not the patient is currently taking NSAIDS or narcotic pain medication and whether or not these have been attempted in the past should be elicited. Careful questioning about all other medications taken may reveal the use of antidepressants or anxietiolytic medication. The use of these drugs may give some clues about the presence of any undisclosed underlying psychotropic disorder, which may in part be responsible for some of the patient's perceptions or complaints referable to their knee. An additional important line of questioning in these patients regards their sleep patterns, including the presence of pain at rest, at night, or awakening the patient. Disturbed sleep is not uncommonly seen in fibromyalgia and associated disorders that may require ancillary antidepressant medication for treatment regardless of any problems requiring surgical intervention.

The patient should be asked about the stability of the knee and of the patella. If instability is present, is it objective, associated with giving out, or subjective? Does the patient have a sensation of weakness? With all activities, or only in certain activities? Does the patient have a history of injury or trauma to the knee? In addition, questions should be asked of any audible sounds that may be associated with the knee.

The physician should determine what the patient is able or unable to do functionally. Is there disability in particular activities? Functional status is best determined from standard questioning regarding the average and maximum distance walked. The ambulatory tolerance should be obtained both without pain, until pain begins, and despite pain. The need for assistive devices and the ability to navigate uneven terrain should be assessed. The patient should be questioned about ascending and descending stairs and arising from a chair. Interference with any other activities of daily living should also be determined. For the patient with complaints of instability, further questioning may be required to determine the situations in which and the frequency with which this instability takes place.

Although in most cases the answer to these questions will provide a sufficient background to understand the actual disability of the patient, in many cases it may be worthwhile to actually develop a formal rating score such as the Hospital for Special Surgery or Knee Society scores in order to determine a more "accurate" appraisal of the patient's disability. This is particularly true when the patient's complaints seem out of proportion to findings and little "objective" evidence of disability is encountered. In discussing pain out of proportion to evidence, the physician should think of reflex sympathic dystrophy, which is discussed later.

Additional questioning regarding the general medical and surgical history is also important. In particular the presence of diabetes mellitus, vascular or neurologic problems should be evaluated. In the diabetic patient, a history of or symptoms consistent with peripheral neuropathy may be important. Other neurologic disorders may also present with limb pain and problems with low-back pain or previously experienced lower extremity radiation is not uncommon in patients in this age group. Vascular claudication may mimic periarticular knee pain and confirmation of the status of the lower extremity vascular supply should be part of every exam of the patient with complaints referable to a total knee arthroplasty.

PHYSICAL EXAMINATION

A "final" working diagnosis is arrived at by combining features of the history, physical examination, and ancillary imaging or other studies as needed. When the diagnosis is straightforward, the physical examination may be limited to those aspects that provide sufficient information for the diagnosis and any preoperative planning that may be needed should surgery be the treatment of choice. However, when the diagnosis is not forthcoming, a more detailed and thorough examination may be required. In either case, the clinician must integrate the findings from each arena of the investigation (history, physical, etc.) in order to link those significant findings that represent the "diagnostic findings."

Although every clinician eventually develops a personal routine in the physical exam, consistency in the performance of one's routine is essential in order to minimize the possibility of missing an important finding. A reasonable routine is to begin with the knee itself and then move to peripheral joints, neurovascular status, and finally functional evaluation.

The physical examination should take place with both lower extremities, from the pelvic girdle to the feet, easily exposed to the examiner. Access to the back should be available if there is any question of lumbosacral spine pathology presenting as leg pain.

Evaluation of the patient's knee generally begins with inspection. Erythema, swelling, and gross deformity may be noted. View the knee from the front, side, and back with the patient standing to achieve a better perspective. Have the patient sit, again view the knee from the front and side. Specific areas of periarticular swelling as well as evidence of effusion should be noted. It is important to differentiate effusion, intra-articular from periarticular swelling. Any discoloration, blemishes, or bruises should be noted as well.

Palpation should be systematic and include a careful evaluation of those areas claimed as painful by the patient. These should include medial and lateral joint lines, peripatellar tissues, patellar tendon, pes tendons, as well as the popliteal space and the hamstring tendons. If peritendinous tenderness is noted, it may be helpful to attempt to elicit pain via resisted motion to establish a periarticular tendonitis as the source of pain. Alternatively, local Xylocaine injection may also help clinch this diagnosis. Although peripatellar or joint line tenderness may be nonspecific, particular patterns of tenderness may correspond to particular facets of the patient's history or with subtle X-ray findings that might not otherwise be considered as problematic or as the potential source of symptoms, such as small degrees of component overhang or lateral patellar facet contact with the femoral condyle.

Patellofemoral compression and general patellar mobility can also be evaluated by palpation. In particular, the patient with long-standing complaints of pain referable to the knee, with no other objective findings of pathology should be evaluated by palpation for peripheral neuromata, which can be evaluated by careful palpation about the knee and by an attempt to elicit a Tinel's sign. The examiner should also note the presence and location of scars about the knee as well as palpating for tenderness about the scars themselves.

The extensor mechanism should be evaluated for competence along with general quadriceps strength and muscle bulk. Measuring the thigh circumferential is very helpful. Range of motion should be noted. This should be active and passive. The presence of any extensor lag or flexion contracture should be assessed. Patellar tracking may be evaluated by both visual inspection and palpation during range of motion. In particular, any complaints referable to the extensor mechanism such as crepitation and/or "clunk" should lead to careful evaluation of the extensor mechanism during active motion. The Q-angle should be measured with the leg in extension and then in flexion.

Evaluation of limb alignment is important. Varus or valgus alignment can be noted clinically but is more accurately measured with standing mechanical axis radiographs. Unfortunately rotational malalignment of the knee is a common problem following arthroplasty but this may be difficult to evaluate on physical examination. Excessive external rotation of the foot may be indicative of internal rotation of the tibial or femoral components. This may be the cause of patellofemoral problems such as subluxation, dislocation, or loosening. The angle between the tibial tuberosity and the foot is useful in assessing the rotational position of the tibial component. In general, rotational malposition of the components are best evaluated with CT scanning.

Joint stability must be evaluated by careful examination, and this should be done in the standard fashion. That is, medial and lateral joint opening under valgus or varus stress should be done with the knee fully extended as well as with the knee in varying degrees of flexion. The examiner should be careful to avoid the false perception of mediolateral stability with the knee in full extension when that stability is provided by tight posterior capsular structures. As the knee is brought into flexion, the posterior structures relax and more realistic evaluation of the medial and lateral ligamentous structures may be carried out. Anteroposterior stability can be evaluated through standard drawer tests but should be interpreted in light of the patient's artificial knee status. Most total knees are implanted with resection of the anterior cruciate, and a "positive" anterior drawer sign is a common finding in normal total knees. Significant posterior drawer or sag should generally not occur, and such findings need to be correlated with both clinical complaints as well as lateral radiographs of the knee, which can be obtained during weight-bearing if there is any question about instability during stance.

The remainder of the physical exam is confined to evaluation of the gait as well as evaluation of the adjacent joints and the lumbar spine. We have previously evaluated patients who were scheduled for total knee revision surgery, who had well-functioning knees, but who had severe undiagnosed hip arthritis. It is not uncommon for patients with hip pathology to have little in the way of classic hip pain and significant complaints referable to the knee. Careful evaluation of hip range of motion, and any associated discomfort, should always be performed in patients with complaints of pain in the knee.

Although the foot or ankle is rarely the source of patient complaints following total knee arthroplasty, it is not uncommon for significant foot or ankle deformity to affect the knee. In most cases, significant valgus or pes planus type deformity may shift the ground reaction force to the lateral aspect of the knee and result in a significant valgus or abduction moment at the knee. When severe enough and of sufficient duration, this may lead to substantial medial ligamentous laxity and valgus instability of the knee. If unaccounted for at the time of primary or revision surgery, such deformity may result in persistent complaints of instability or recurrent deformity.

The patient's neurologic and vascular status is an important part of the evaluation of the patient with complaints referable to their total knee arthroplasty. Absent or diminished pulses may identify intermittent vascular claudication as the source of the patient's symptoms and workup of the extent of vascular insufficiency will be required if any surgical revision is contemplated. Alterations in the neurologic status of the limb may lead the clinician to a more careful evaluation of the lumbosacral spine or may demonstrate evidence of peripheral neuropathy or local neuromata, which can be responsible for pain complaints.

Pain out of proportion to the physical findings should make the physician suspicious of reflex sympathetic dystrophy. The four cardinal signs of reflex sympathetic dystrophy are pain, swelling, stiffness, and discoloration. Pain is the most notable symptom of reflex sympathetic dystrophy. The pain is often characterized as burning or deep aching. The pain is exacerbated by motion or cold temperatures. This pain is diffuse, global to the knee. It is often difficult for the patient to indicate the source of pain. Stiffness is also a common complaint. Stiffness results from pain caused by motion. At times the motion loss is substantial. If long-standing, arthrofibrosis will result. Swelling is not usually intra-articular but periarticular instead. Discoloration of the skin around the knee, leg, and foot may present as dusky or cyanotic. This discoloration may increase during exposure to cold. Secondary findings include decreased skin temperature and skin atrophy.

Last, the diagnosis of infection requires a high index of suspicion. The time to diagnosis of infection following arthroplasty is very variable. The early, acute, fulminate infection is easily diagnosed but is infrequently encountered. An early infection often demonstrates only mild elevation in temperature and prolonged serous drainage from the wound. Cultures are often useless because they only show skin colonization of the wound rather than the true deep infection. Chronic low-virulence infections are more common. Chronic low-virulence infections, especially anaerobic infections, may present as persistent pain with or without small effusions. The physician must pursue an extensive evaluation to determine if sepsis is present. Persistent, unexplained pain, effusion, erythemia, prolonged wound drainage, or failure of primary wound healing should raise suspicion of deep wound infection. Finally, the diagnosis of infection is often only made when the physician thinks of infection. A painful total knee arthroplasty, unexplained by other mechanisms, must be evaluated with a high index of suspicion of infection. Failure to diagnose the acute infection may result in the need for prosthetic removal, whereas early diagnosis may lead to component salvage.

CHAPTER 48
Imaging of the Painful TKR

Kevin R. Math and Robert Scheider

INTRODUCTION

Diagnostic imaging plays a central role in the evaluation of the patient with a painful total knee replacement (TKR). Following a thorough clinical evaluation, a tailored approach to imaging these patients starting with conventional radiographs will usually enable the orthopedist to diagnose the cause of the patient's symptoms.

The standard radiographic examination should include AP, lateral, and tangential axial views of the knee. The imaging workup is dependent on the specific diagnosis in question (e.g., loosening, infection, and prosthetic malposition), and includes plain films, nuclear imaging, computed tomography (CT), and arthrography. The role of magnetic resonance imaging (MRI) is significantly limited by the substantial metallic artifact caused by the prosthetic components.

CONVENTIONAL RADIOGRAPHY—ROUTINE ASSESSMENT

The alignment of the femoral and tibial components is readily evaluated on a standard AP radiograph. More complete assessment of the mechanical axis can be achieved by obtaining a standing AP view of the entire lower extremity from hip to ankle on a long film cassette. Some surgeons advocate obtaining a short film of the knee and an additional view of the pelvis rather than a full-length film.[1,2] However, this appears to be a matter of personal preference. Alignment of the femoral and tibial components relative to the anatomic axis of the respective bones, as well as the alignment of the components relative to each other, should be assessed on AP and lateral views. On the AP view (normal position) (Fig. 48.1), the femoral component should be in slight (4–11 degrees, optimally 7 degrees) valgus relative to the anatomic axis of the femur,[3,4] and the tibial component should approximate the normal tibial articular surface, aligned perpendicular to the tibial shaft on the AP view.[5] Alignment at the femorotibial joint should be about 5–7 degrees of valgus (no greater than 10). The prosthetic joint space at the medial and lateral compartments should be roughly equivalent on an AP view. However, variability in the joint space is common, strongly dependent on technical factors and the degree of knee flexion; one should avoid presuming that asymmetry in the prosthetic joint space reliably indicates polyethylene wear. On the lateral view (Fig. 48.2), the femoral component should be nearly parallel to the long axis of the femur, and the posterior aspect of the anterior flange of the femoral component should be flush with the underlying anterior cortex of the distal femur.[4,5] Mild radiolucency may normally appear between the prosthesis and bone at the anterior flange due to stress shielding (Fig. 48.3). The tibial component on the lateral view should be perpendicular to the long axis of the tibia or can be posteriorly tilted by up to 10 degrees.[6]

Patellar height or the vertical distance from the lower patella to the joint line should measure 10–30 mm, and the joint line should not be altered by more than 8 mm. The Insall-Salvati ratio is the most widely used method of assessment of the vertical height of the patella.[8,9] The length of the patellar tendon (as measured from the lower patella to the tibial tubercle) divided by the greatest diagonal length of the patella should equal 1.02 ± 20%. Therefore, a ratio of >1.2 or <0.8 is considered to be abnormal, and is termed patella alta or patella baja (or infera), respectively. Patella baja following TKR is not uncommon, owing to elevation of the joint line. Patella alta suggests patellar tendon disruption, whereas significant patella baja can be seen in quadriceps tendon tears.

Abnormalities of the patellofemoral joint account for the majority of painful TKRs, comprising up to half of all TKR complications.[10,11] Therefore, it is important to

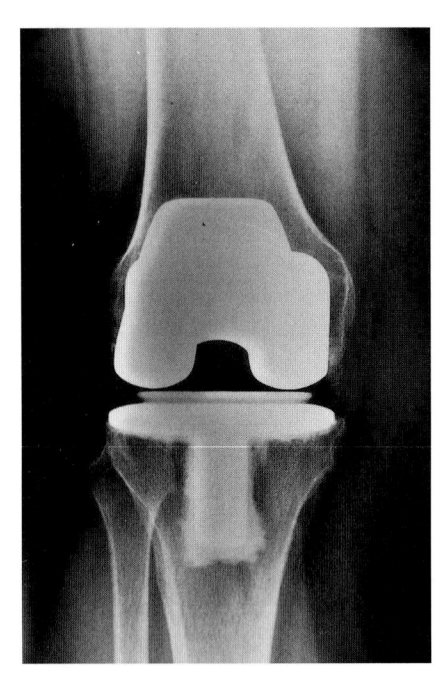

Figure 48.1. AP View—Normal TKR
The components well aligned, and there is not radiolucency at any of the interfaces.

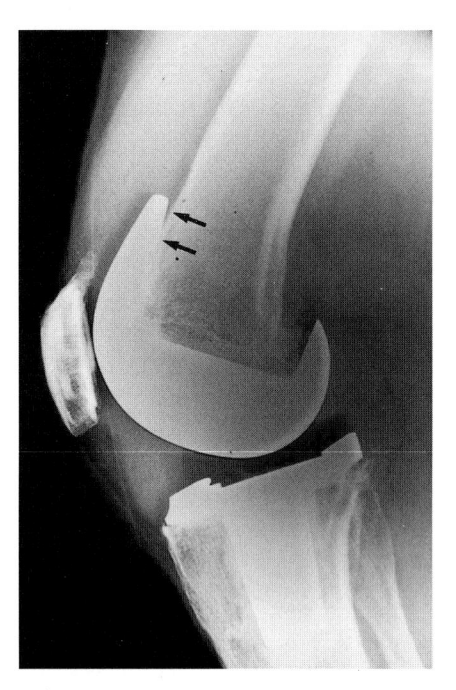

Figure 48.3. Stress Shielding
Lateral view of asymptomatic TKR. There is a small area of lucency beneath the anterior flange of the femoral component (arrows). This finding is not uncommon, and is consistent with stress shielding.

routinely obtain a tangential axial (Merchant) view on all follow-up studies[12] (Fig. 48.4). This view is ideal for assessment of patellofemoral tracking, patellar component loosening, and polyethylene wear over the patella. By convention, this view is taken with the knee flexed 45 degrees; excessive flexion should be avoided, because as patellofemoral malalignment is best seen at earlier degrees of flexion, and abnormal tracking may be undetected if this view is not properly obtained. Although other tangential axial views have been described, the Merchant view is in most common usage.[13,14]

On all views, the interface between the prosthesis and cement or prosthesis and bone (for uncemented components) should be routinely assessed for any radiolucency. Radiolucent lines at these interfaces can occur in asymptomatic TKRs and are not necessarily abnormal. Wider radiolucencies (>2 mm) or progressive widening from one exam to the next should be viewed with suspicion, because this may represent component loosening (Fig. 48.5). In an attempt to promote uniformity of radiographic assessment, the Knee Society has developed a standardized system of radiographic evaluation and scoring of total knee arthroplasty.[15] In addition to assessing the alignment of the components and the implant–bone surface area, this system provides a highly specific and reproducible analysis of radiolucencies around the components (Fig. 48.6).

COMPLICATIONS OF TOTAL JOINT ARTHROPLASTY

The most common complications of total knee arthroplasty necessitating revision surgery are component

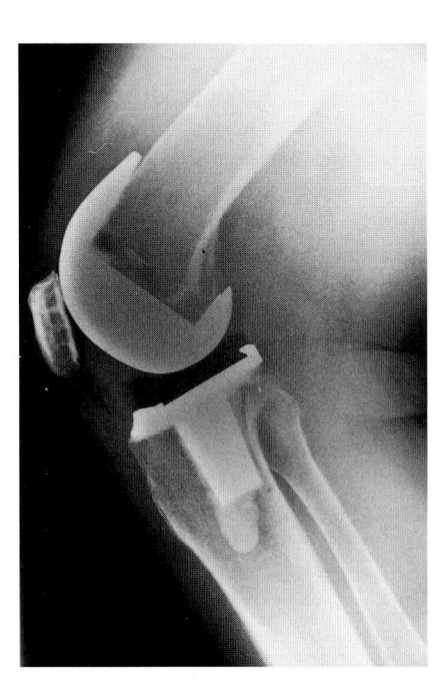

Figure 48.2. Lateral View—Normal TKR
Component alignment, patellar height and all interfaces are normal.

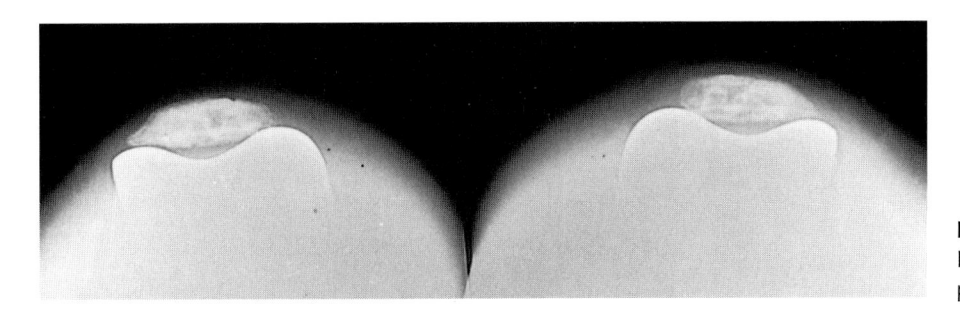

Figure 48.4. Merchant View Bilateral TKRs with normal patellofemoral alignment.

loosening, polyethylene wear, infection, and instability (Fig. 48.7); other causes of prosthesis failure include fracture, osteolysis, and component malposition.

Loosening

Prosthetic component loosening most commonly involves the tibial component. Radiographic signs of loosening are usually evident on radiographs;[4,16] however, they are often subtle and sometimes absent. These signs include:

1. A wide area of radiolucency between the prosthesis and bone (usually beneath the medial tibial tray) or progressive increase in this lucency from one exam to the next (Fig. 48.8). In femoral component loosening the abnormal lucency characteristically occurs at the posterior condyles, and is seen to best advantage on the lateral view.

2. A shift in position of the component. When the implant sinks into the bone, it is termed "subsidence"; this is clearly seen on an AP view of the knee (see Fig. 48.8). Femoral component loosening typically results in a shift of the femoral component into flexion on the lateral view (Fig. 48.9), whereas loose tibial components usually shift into varus alignment (Fig. 48.10). Loose patellar implants can partially dissociate from the patella, and can eventually migrate into the joint (Fig. 48.11).

3. Fracture of the cement mantle.

Occasionally, routine radiographic views fail to demonstrate the important but subtle radiolucency at the prosthesis–bone interface. Fluoroscopically obtained views, in which the interface is positioned directly tangent to the X-ray beam under fluoroscopic visualization and coned down views are obtained, can reveal a radiolucent zone beneath the prosthesis, not evident on routine views (Fig. 48.12). This study can be helpful for those patients with clinically suspected loosening and normal radiographs.[16,17]

The clinical significance of a thin radiolucent line at the prosthesis–bone interface is controversial. Although asymptomatic TKRs often display this finding, it may also be abnormal, sometimes the only sign of a symptomatic loose prosthesis. The Knee Society has developed a scoring system that describes the precise location of these radiolucent lines relative to the components (see Fig. 48.6). These lines should be routinely assessed on early radiographs and follow-up studies for progression. Some investigators have reported an association of increased radionuclide uptake on bone scans in

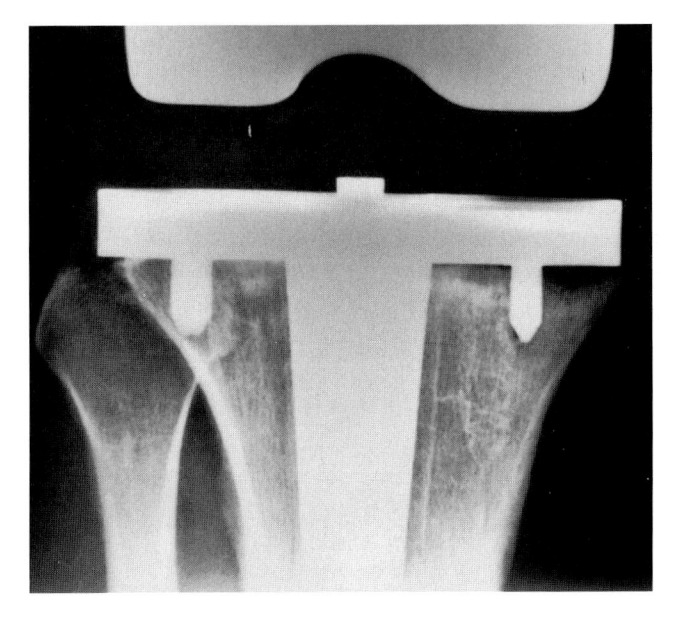

Figure 48.5. Loose Tibial Component
There is osteolysis beneath the medial tibial tray and a wide zone of radiolucency at the medial margin of the tibial stem.

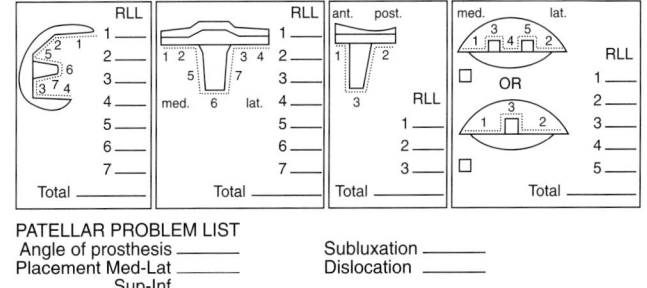

Figure 48.6. Knee Society Radiographic Scoring System

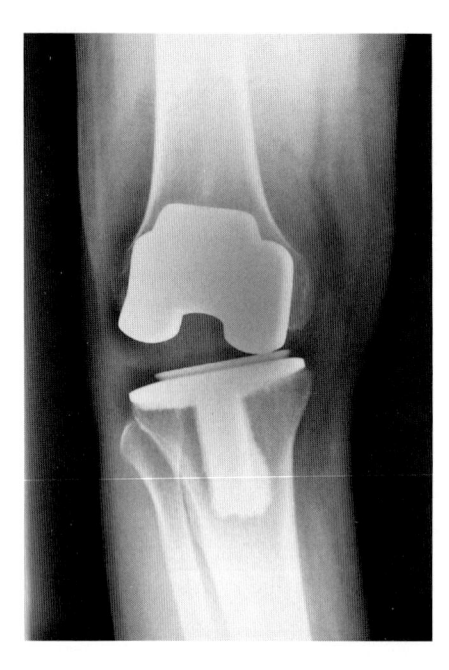

Figure 48.7. Lateral Instability
There is varus alignment at the knee with widening of the lateral joint compartment on this standing view indicating instability.

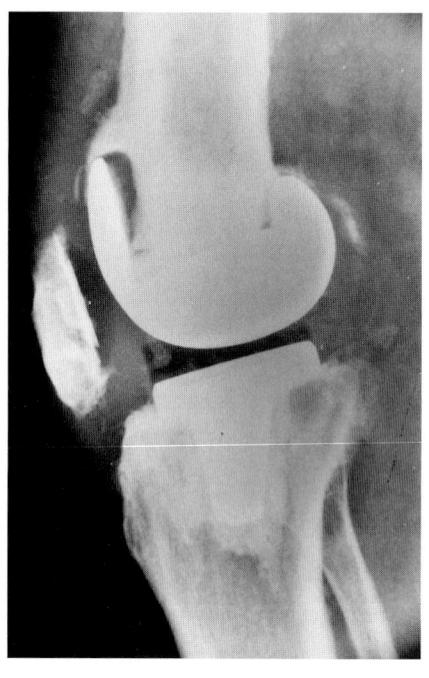

Figure 48.9. Loose Femoral Component
There is significant bony resorption beneath the anterior flange of the femoral component. This is much more than would be expected with stress shielding, and the loose femoral component has shifted into mild flexion.

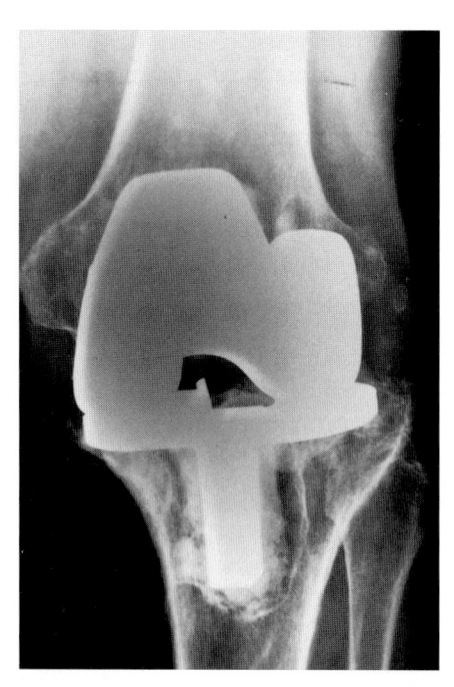

Figure 48.8. Loose Tibial Component
There is a wide zone of lucency at the cement–bone interface around the tibial stem, combined with subsidence of the tibial component.

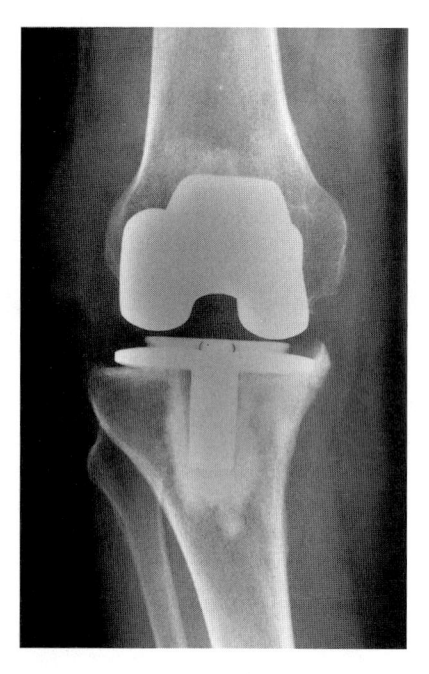

Figure 48.10. Loose Tibial Component
This aseptically loose tibial component has shifted into varus alignment, with lucency at the lateral aspect of the tibial stem and subsidence at the medial tibial plateau.

nificance, arthrography can provide objective evidence that this lucency truly represents loosening.[20,21] Iodinated contrast material is injected into the knee joint under fluoroscopic observation. Any flow of this contrast into the lucency at the interface signifies loosening. However, failure to demonstrate this finding does not exclude loosening; viscosity and particle size of the contrast material may be too great to allow flow into the interface. Some authors advocate supplementing routine arthrography with a radionuclide arthrogram in evaluating suspected loose joint prostheses.[22–25] This technique is most often utilized for total hip replacements but can also be utilized for TKRs. This requires no additional needle puncture, and simply entails the injection of a small amount of a radiopharmaceutical (e.g., technetium 99m-sulfur colloid) into the joint through the needle previously placed for routine arthrography. The

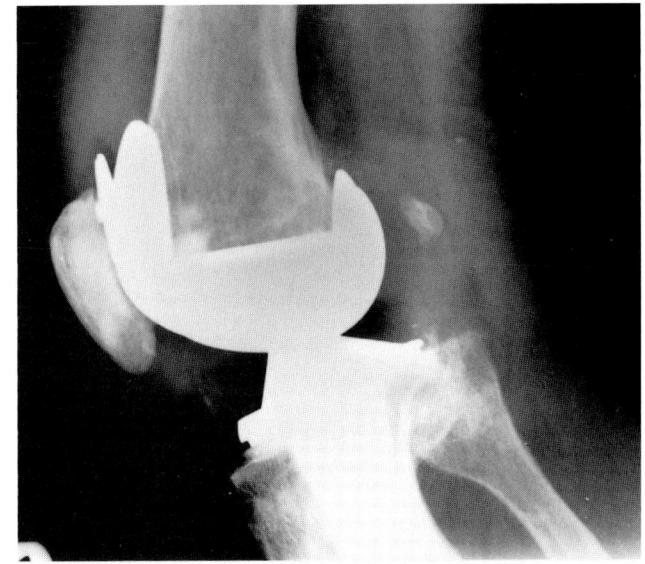

Figure 48.11. Loose Patellar Component
(A) There is loosening of the metal-backed patellar component, shifting superiorly relative to the patella. (B) Two years later there is complete dissociation of the patellar implant, with migration into the suprapatellar pouch.

patients exhibiting these radiolucencies, but others have refuted this.[18,19]

Even though comparing the width of the radiolucency on sequential exams can help to determine its sig-

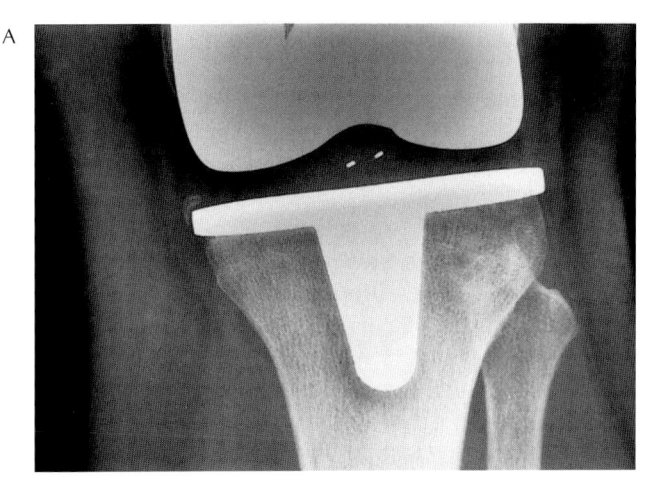

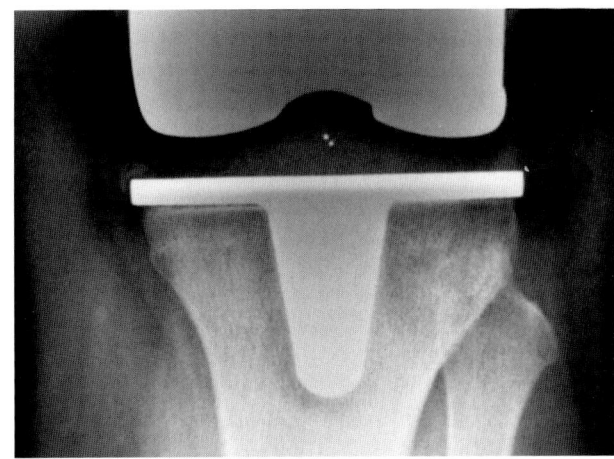

Figure 48.12. Value of Fluoroscopic Views of the TKR
(A) AP view of a painful aseptically loose tibial component. The prosthesis–bone interfaces appear normal. (B) Fluoroscopically obtained AP view: The knee was positioned under fluoroscopy to bring the X-ray beam tangent to the prosthesis. Note the mild (but significant) radiolucency beneath the medial tibial tray.

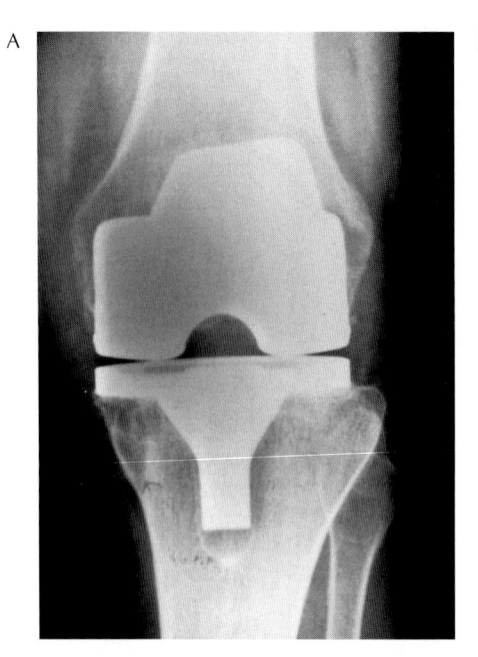

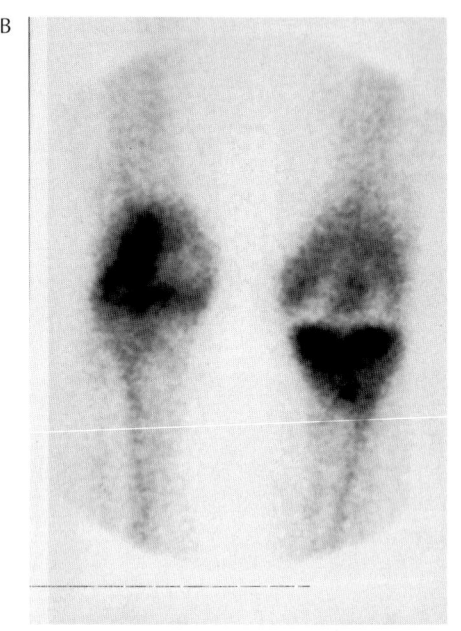

Figure 48.13. Loose Tibial Component—Osteolysis
(A) There is a focal area of osteolysis beneath the medial tibial tray. This area has well-defined margins, a feature distinguishing it from stress shielding. (B) The radionuclide bone scan reveals disproportionate increased activity around the entire tibial component, indicating loosening.

patient is subsequently imaged under a gamma camera to assess for activity surrounding a loose component; all radionuclide activity should be limited to the joint cavity. The small particle size and relatively low viscosity of this agent may allow demonstration of activity around a loose prosthesis not evident on routine arthrography. Again, a negative study does not exclude loosening, but renders it considerably less likely.

Loosening of the femoral component is much less common than tibial component loosening, and is much more difficult to appreciate radiographically. Visualization of the interfaces around the implant is obscured by these relatively large opaque metal prostheses; this especially limits assessment on the AP view.

The radionuclide bone scan (RNBS) can sometimes help in evaluating for suspected component loosening in TKR. Unfortunately, the specificity of this study for diagnosis of loosening is limited by the prolonged increased radionuclide activity around normal asymptomatic TKR components. Unlike total hip arthroplasty, in which activity typically returns to normal 6 to 12 months after surgery,[26] increased periprosthetic uptake following TKR can persist indefinitely, significantly limiting the utility of this modality.[27–29] Rosenthal and colleagues reported increased periprosthetic uptake around 89% of tibial components and 63% of femoral components more than one year after surgery.[29] This renders interpretation of a "hot" bone scan relatively nonspecific for diagnosing loosening or infection. Analogous to the radiolucency at the prosthesis–bone interface on plain films, a progressive increase in radionuclide uptake on sequential bone scans is much more informative than its mere presence on a single study. However, it is not practical nor cost effective to obtain a baseline bone scan on all patients.

Although component loosening most commonly occurs as a result of mechanical loosening or infection, this complication can also occur as a result of bone destruction by osteolysis or "particulate disease." This condition typically results from a foreign body reaction in-

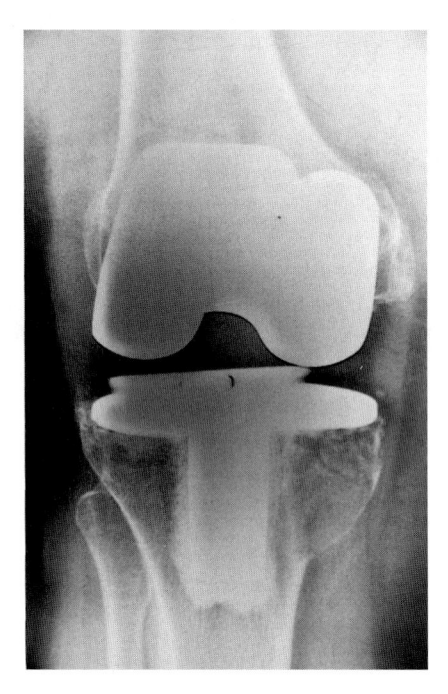

Figure 48.14. Osteolysis with Pathologic Fracture
There is a large area of osteolysis at the medial tibial plateau, with a subtle fracture line extending through it. The patient was asymptomatic until sustaining this fracture.

cited by particulate wear debris (usually polyethylene), giving rise to synovitis and potential bone resorption around the components.[30,32] These focal areas of lucency are readily seen on conventional radiographs, and can result in secondary loosening (Fig. 48.13) or fracture (Fig. 48.14). Computed tomography (CT) can precisely delineate the size and extent of these lesions and can effectively display cortical and soft tissue involvement and the proximity of the lytic area(s) to the prosthesis (Fig. 48.15). Using state-of-the-art CT scanners, metal artifact at the level of the tibial prosthesis does not significantly interfere with imaging, though visualization of the patellar and femoral component interfaces remains limited.

Polyethylene wear occurs most commonly at the tibial and patellar components and is manifested radiographically as asymmetrically narrowed prosthetic joint spaces, or an interval decrease in this space on sequential studies. This finding is best appreciated on weight-bearing views, and is usually radiographically occult. Advanced polyethylene wear can result in metal-on-metal contact and resultant metal debris ("metallosis") (Fig. 48.16).[33,34] Arthrography is much more sensitive than conventional radiography for detection of polyethylene wear; the polyethylene at the patellar component and tibiofemoral joint is outlined by contrast, and any thinning or cracks can be readily detected (Fig. 48.17).

Infection

Most cases of late infection following TKR occur after several months, and are due to septic hematogenous seeding from a distant source. The overall incidence of deep infection is about 1% to 2% with a range of 1.1% to 12.4%.[35–37] The incidence is greater for revision surgery than primary cases, and is increased in rheumatoid arthritis, psoriatic arthritis, and diabetes mellitus.[35,38]

Differentiation of mechanical loosening from infectious loosening cannot be made based solely on conventional radiographs. Furthermore, an infected TKR often presents with normal radiographs save for the presence of soft tissue swelling or a joint effusion. Ra-

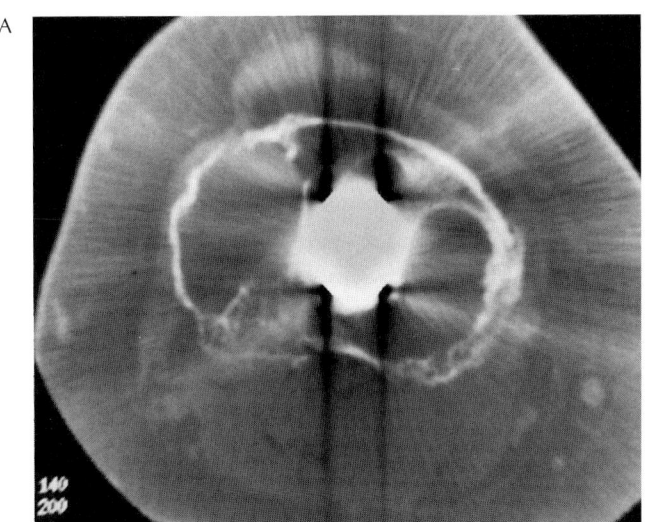

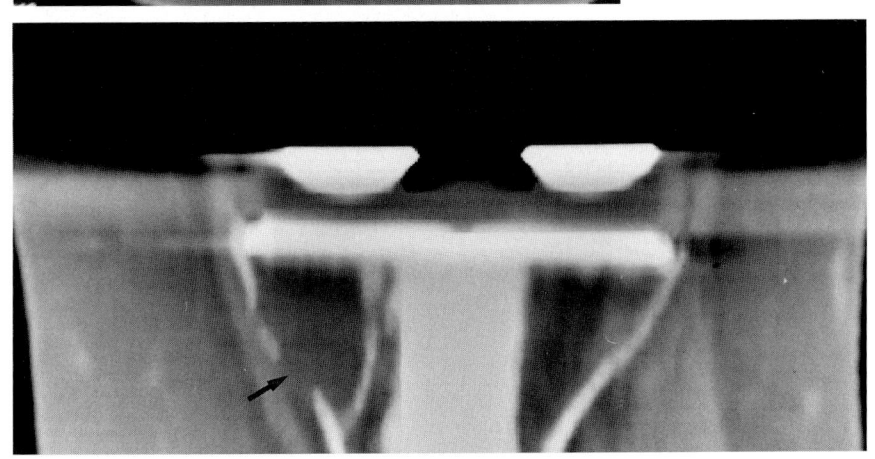

Figure 48.15. Osteolysis—CT (A) An axial image through the level of the metallic tibial stem reveals extensive osteolysis on either side of the stem. (B) Different patient: 2-dimensional coronal reformatted image reveals a focal osteolytic lesion beneath the medial tibial tray with an area of cortical penetration at the medial metaphysis (arrow).

ture, sensitivity, gram stain, cell count). However, the clinical, laboratory, and plain film diagnosis of infection is frequently equivocal or nonspecific.[27,28,39–41] Nuclear imaging can play a key role in increasing or decreasing the diagnostic likelihood of infection and can assist in the clinical management of these patients. Nuclear imaging is an ideal imaging modality for patients with total joint arthroplasty where utilizing MRI is virtually precluded by extensive artifacts.

The three phase bone scan is the most commonly used modality (following plain films) for the evaluation of suspected osteomyelitis; in patients without a history of prior surgery, trauma, or other preexisting pathology, its sensitivity and specificity are in the neighborhood of 95%.[42–44] Unfortunately, in the TKR patient population, the bone scan, while maintaining a high sensitivity, suffers from poor specificity for infection. Reing and colleagues reported the sensitivity and specificity of bone scintigraphy alone for diagnosing an infected joint replacement to be 100% and 15%, respectively.[45] Increased periprosthetic uptake can be seen in aseptic loosening or infection, and is also common in asymptomatic patients following TKR. Nuclear imaging with inflammation-specific agents (radiolabeled leukocytes, Gallium-67 citrate) has been shown to dramatically improve the specificity for assessment of suspected infected joint arthroplasty.[46–54]

Leukocytes (WBCs) can be labeled with either technetium 99m (Tc-99m) or Indium-111; the advantage of the former is that Tc-99m images have better spatial resolution than Indium images, and patients can be imaged a few hours after injection rather than the 24 hours re-

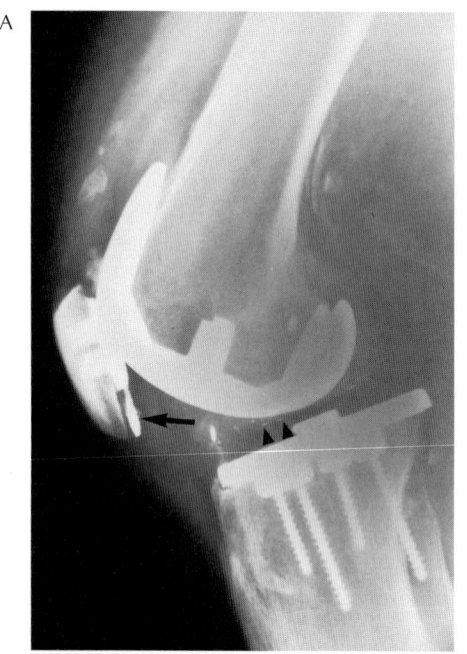

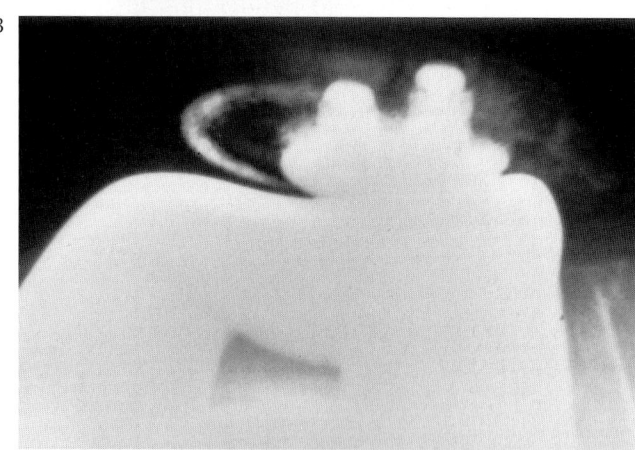

Figure 48.16. Severe Polyethylene Wear with Metallosis
(A) Lateral view of the knee reveals marked narrowing of the patellofemoral joint space with metal-on-metal contact between the metal-backed patellar component and the femoral component. This resulted in liberation of metal debris into the joint and coating of the posterior aspect of the patellar polyethylene (arrow). Small metal particles also outline the tibial polyethylene (arrowheads). (B) Merchant view: The metal debris gives an "arthrogram effect" with a crescentic arrangement of metal particles outlining the rim of remaining polyethylene at the medial facet of the patella.

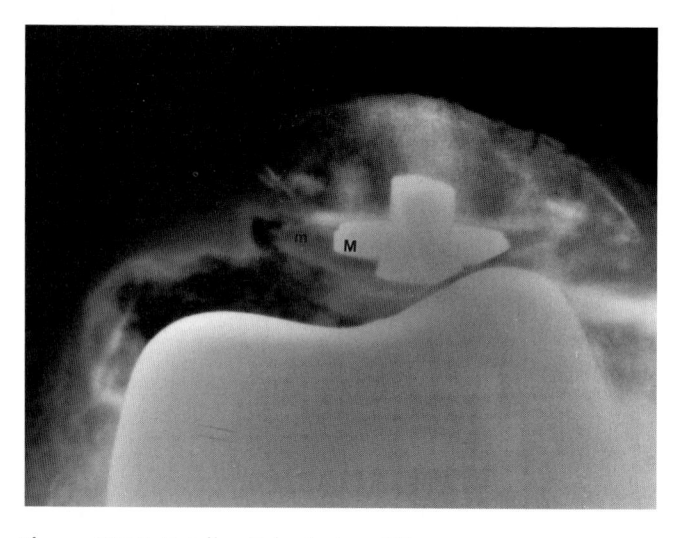

Figure 48.17. Patellar Polyethylene Wear
This double contrast arthrogram gives an air-contrast view of the patellar polyethylene. Polyethylene thickness over the medial facet (M) is maintained, while there is severe wear over the lateral facet, and associated lateral patellar subluxation.

diographic findings of an infected joint replacement include bone resorption at the interfaces, periosteal reaction, soft tissue swelling, and/or gas and component loosening (Figs. 48.18–48.21). The diagnosis of an infected TKR is often made clinically, through history and physical examination, and by laboratory evaluation of peripheral blood (leukocyte count, erythroid sedimentation rate, C-reactive protein) and synovial fluid (cul-

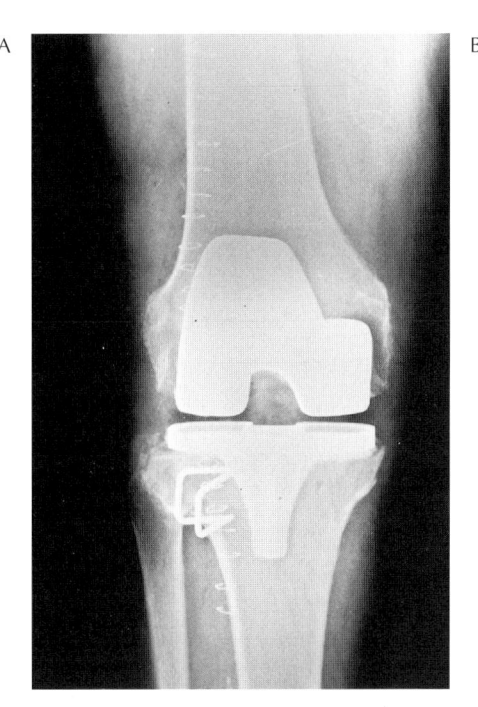

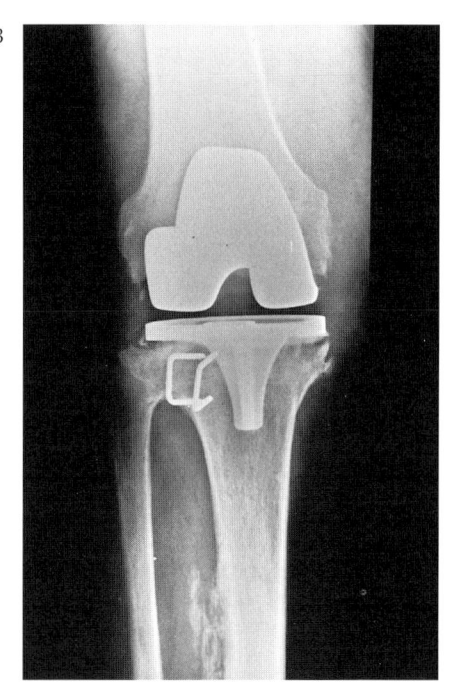

Figure 48.18. Infected TKR—Bone Resorption
(A) Immediate postoperative and (B) 4 years postoperative AP views reveal interval development of radiolucent zones beneath the medial and lateral tibial prosthesis. These bony resorptive changes were due to infection.

quired by Indium. Indium labeling of WBCs is in more common usage than technetium labeling for imaging suspected arthroplasty infection, probably due to personal preference and more experience with the former. Infection results in increased accumulation of radiolabeled WBCs in the marrow, visualized as areas of increased activity around the prosthesis. For arthroplasty infection, the sensitivity and specificity of the Indium–WBC scan alone is highly variable ranging from 50% to 100% and 23% to 100%, respectively.[46,47] Cur-

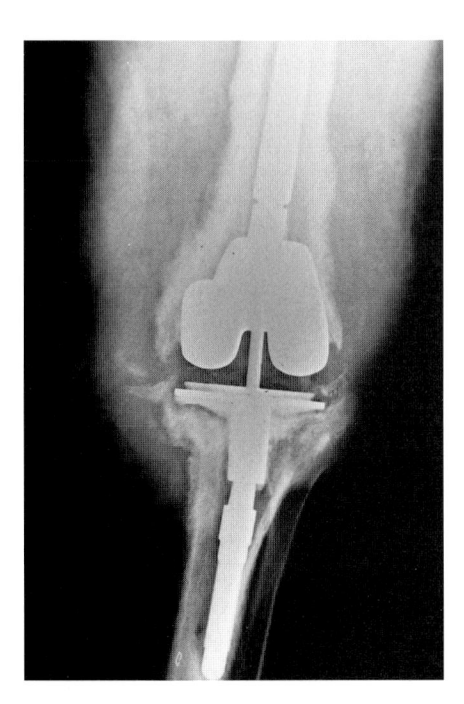

Figure 48.19. Infected TKR—Component Loosening and Periosteal Reaction
AP view of the knee shows radiographic evidence of a loose tibial component with wide areas of lucency at the prosthetic interfaces and subsidence. There is wavy periosteal reaction at the distal femur indicating osteomyelitis.

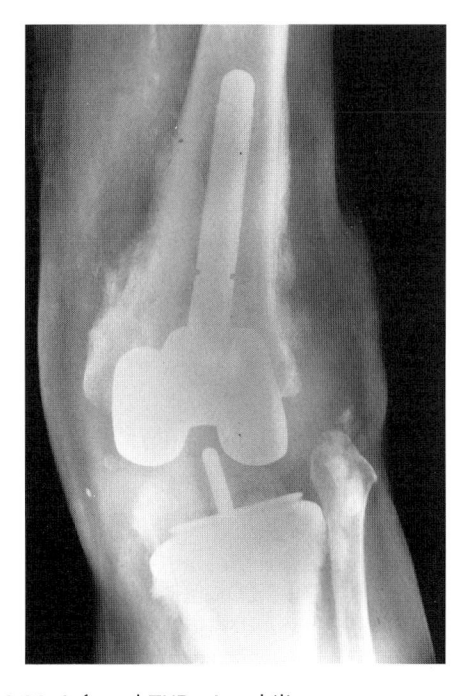

Figure 48.20. Infected TKR—Instability
AP view of the knee reveals accentuated valgus alignment with widening of the medial compartment indicating medial instability. The periosteal reaction at the distal femur is secondary to osteomyelitis.

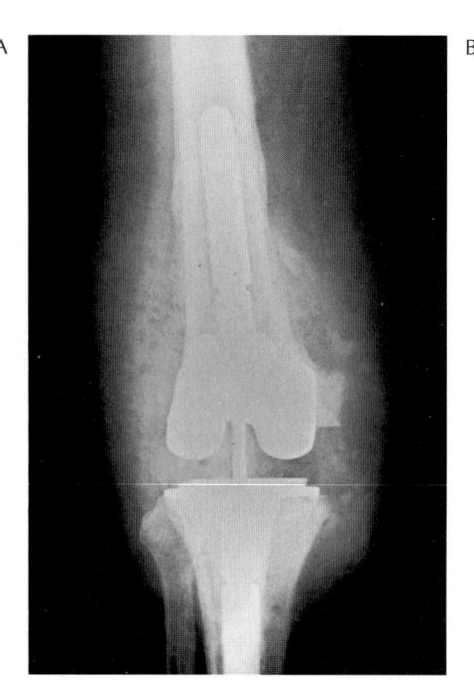

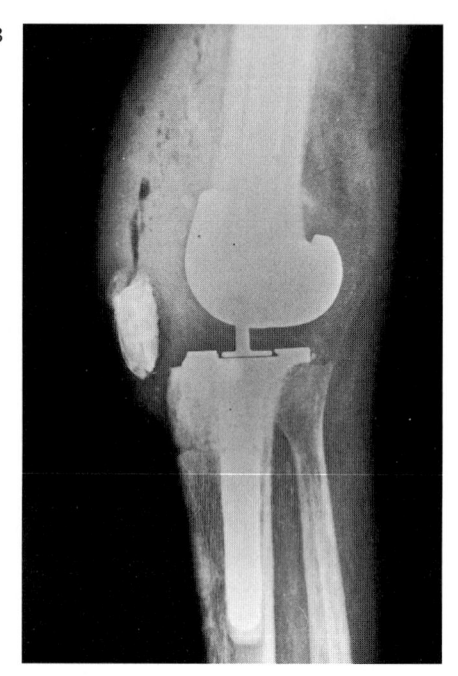

Figure 48.21. Infected TKR—Intra-articular Gas
(A) AP and (B) lateral views of the knee show gas bubbles and soft tissue swelling in the suprapatellar pouch, consistent with abscess formation. There is osteomyelitis of the distal femur, as well.

rently, radiolabeled WBC imaging is virtually universally preferred over gallium imaging due to the suboptimal accuracy and specificity and poorer image quality of the later agent.[43,48,50] A normal Indium–WBC scan excludes infection with a high degree of certainty; Johnson and colleagues reported negative predictive value of 100%.[41] The same study reported a positive predictive value (PPV) of only 47%. The variable specificity of Indium–WBC imaging (and resultant poor PPV) can be explained by the normal accumulation of radiolabeled WBCs in the aberrant marrow normally present around joint prostheses. Indeed, up to 50% of uninfected total knee replacements will exhibit periprosthetic WBC activity on these scans.[40,47,54] The diagnostic utility of Indium–WBC scans is dramatically improved when combined with a bone scan or a Tc-99m-sulfur colloid marrow scan. Interpretation of the Indium–WBC scan in conjunction with a bone scan has been shown to markedly improve the specificity for infection from 45% to 85% in one series, and from 50% to 95% in another.[41,52]

The third phase of the bone scan and the images from the WBC scan are compared with relation to sites and degree of increased activity. Areas of increased uptake on the WBC scan that are normal on the bone scan or "hotter" on the WBC scan than the bone scan are considered to be "incongruent" and are consistent with infection (Fig. 48.22). Matching areas of increased uptake (sites and degree) on both scans are "congruent" and are unlikely to be infected. Interpretation of dual scans of this nature has consistently proved to be highly accurate, with accuracy ranging from 85% to 93%.[41,46,50–52]

An important limitation of dual scanning with In-dium–WBCs and three-phase bone scans is the risk of falsely positive incongruent scans that may result from the normal postoperative marrow distribution following TKR. Labeled WBCs will accumulate wherever active cellular marrow exists, and there is a known alteration in this marrow distribution following TKR marked by a regional increase in cellular marrow elements around the prosthesis components. This aberrant, but normal, marrow will display white cell activity and can result in a mismatch when compared with the routine bone scan (which reflects bone rather than marrow conditions). Palestro and colleagues contend that diagnostic accuracy and specificity are improved if dual scanning is performed by pairing the Indium–WBC scan with a Tc-99m-sulfur colloid scan rather than a routine bone scan.[46,47] The rationale for sulfur colloid scanning is as follows: Sulfur colloid will accumulate at areas of active cellular marrow in the same manner as Indium–WBCs,[55] resulting in matching scans in the normal state. Infection will result in increased accumulation of WBCs in the marrow (and resultant increased Indium activity) and will inhibit sulfur colloid accumulation.[56,57] Discordant or incongruent scans ("hot" on Indium scan, normal on sulfur colloid scan) are 95% to 97% accurate for the diagnosis of infected total joint arthroplasty, with sensitivities and specificities consistently exceeding 90% (Fig. 48.23).[45,46,53,54,58] These studies suggest that when infection is suspected, dual scanning with Indium–WBC and technetium-sulfur colloid scans offer the highest diagnostic utility when compared to other combinations. Note that if the Indium–WBC scan is normal, infection is effectively excluded, and the

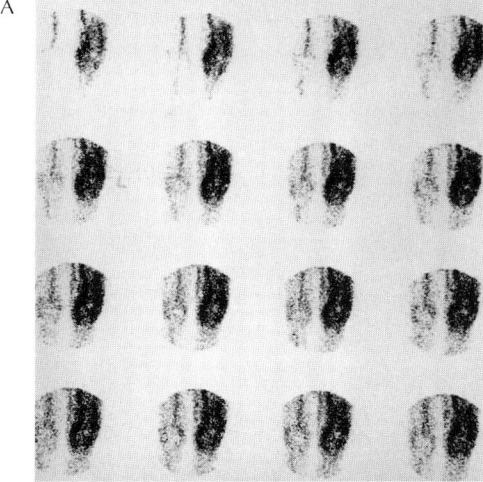

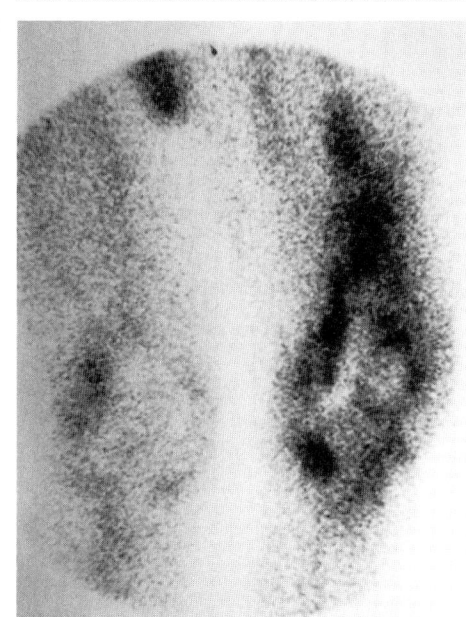

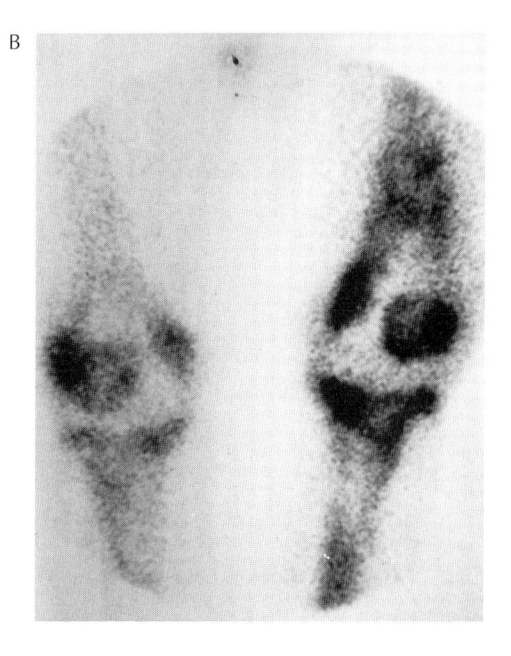

Figure 48.22. Infected TKR—Incongruent Scans
(A) First and (B) third phases from a radionuclide bone scan. There is marked hyperemia to the distal left femur on the first phase of the scan, with increased uptake around all three components on the delayed (third) phase. Note the extension of abnormal uptake proximally in the distal femur. (C) Indium-labeled leukocyte scan: The abnormal white cell uptake at the distal femur is more extensive and greater in degree than the uptake on the bone scan. This "incongruence" or mismatch is consistent with infection.

sulfur colloid scan is unnecessary. Those patients who present with a draining sinus can be imaged using sinography. The sinogram is done by injecting contrast material through the draining site using a small catheter. Under fluoroscopic evaluation the opacified tract can be assessed as to its depth, and for the presence of any associated abscess cavity or intra-articular involvement (Fig. 48.24).

MALPOSITION/MALROTATION OF COMPONENTS

Abnormal internal rotation of the femoral component is an important, often overlooked, cause of a painful TKR.[59–61] Rotational malalignment of the femoral component can give rise to patellar fracture, patellofemoral maltracking, and extensor mechanism dysfunction[62] (Figs. 48.25–48.26).

The epicondylar axis appears to be a reliable reference for determining the femoral component rotation and position. The epicondyles of the distal femur are clearly visualized on cross-sectional images.[63] The medial epicondyle has the appearance of two ridges with an intervening sulcus, while the lateral epicondyle is a single steeply peaked ridge. A line drawn from the medial sulcus to the peak of the lateral epicondyle represents the *epicondylar axis*. The angle between the epicondylar axis and a line drawn tangent to the posterior margins of the femoral condyles (the posterior condylar line) is termed the *posterior condylar angle*. Berger and colleagues[61] reported that the posterior condylar angle averages 3.5 degrees (external rotation) in males and 0.3 degrees (internal rotation) in females. The femoral prosthesis should be aligned to approximate the epicondylar axis of the distal femur. An internally rotated femoral

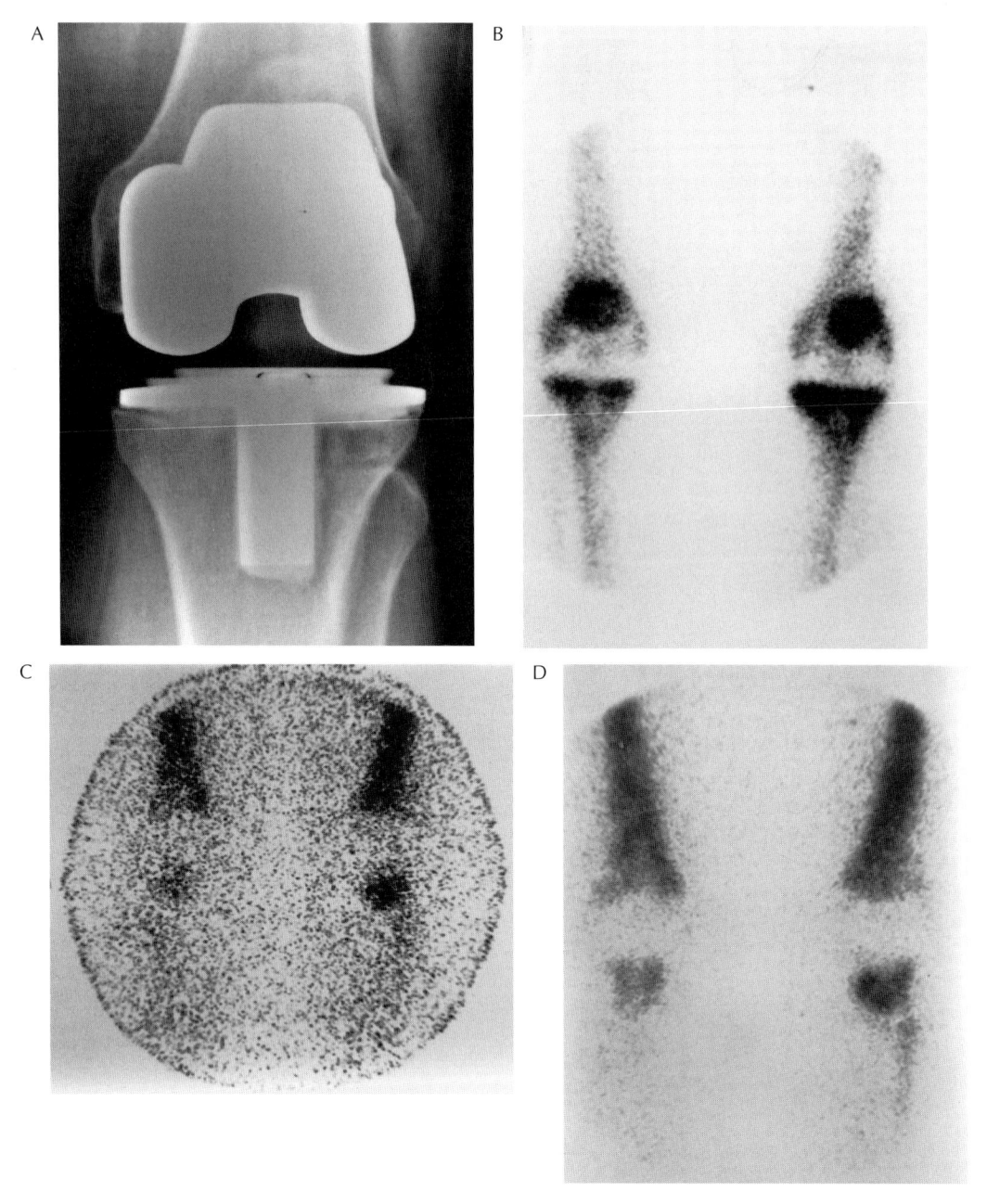

Figure 48.23. False-Positive Indium Scan: Value of Marrow Scan
(A) AP view of the knee: There are new mild bony resorptive changes beneath the medial and lateral tibial prosthesis suggesting loosening in this symptomatic patient. (B) Radionuclide bone scan of same patient with bilateral TKRs shows asymmetric increased uptake at the symptomatic left tibial component, representing loosening. (C) Indium leukocyte scan shows significant focal uptake at the proximal left tibia in a different distribution to the bone scan (mismatch). This was interpreted as infection, though the clinical index of suspicion was low. (D) Sulfur colloid marrow scan reveals increased uptake at the proximal tibia that matches the uptake on the indium scan in distribution and degree. This correlates with areas of aberrant marrow around the tibial prosthesis rather than infection. Aseptic loosening was present at surgery with negative cultures and an uneventful year following the revision.

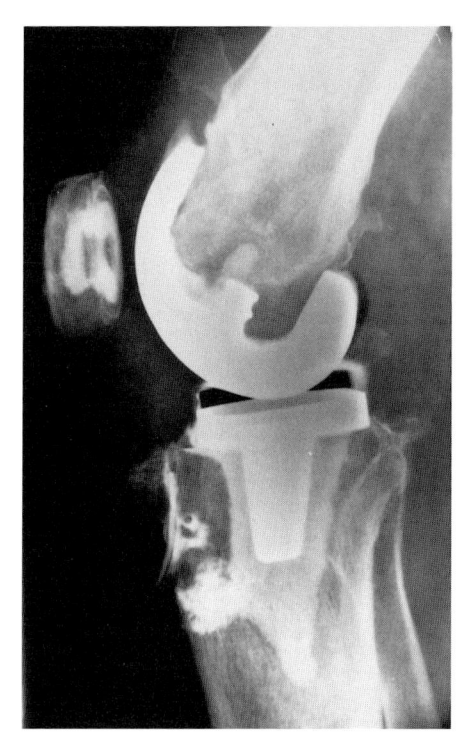

Figure 48.24. Infected TKR—Sinogram
A catheter was placed in a draining sinus at the anterior tibial tubercle and iodinated contrast was injected. The tract is opacified, and the contrast extends intra-articulary, coating the tibial polyethylene. This indicates communication of the sinus tract with the joint cavity.

component can result in patellar fracture, abnormal patellofemoral tracking, polyethylene wear, and pain. The degree of rotation of the femoral component is easily assessed on CT.[61-63] Axial 5-m-thick sections are obtained through the knee at the level of the distal femur and the angle between the posterior margins of the condylar component and the epicondylar axis can be measured.

Although CT evaluation of metallic implants is limited by "beam hardening" artifact from the prosthesis, this artifact does not significantly hinder visualization of the epicondyles and alignment of the prosthesis.

The degree of rotation of the tibial component relative to the tibial tubercle can also be readily assessed on CT. Excess internal rotation of the tibial component can also give rise to patellar instability.[64]

EXTENSOR MECHANISM DISRUPTION

Extensor mechanism disruption following TKR can usually be diagnosed by physical exam and assessment of patellar height on conventional radiographs. Patellar fracture is the most common cause of extensor mechanism disruption, occurring in 1.5% to 5.4% of cases[65-68] (Fig. 48.27).

Quadriceps and patellar tendon tears are much less common than patellar fracture, each occurring with an incidence of about 1%,[69-71] these injuries often result in patella baja and patella alta, respectively. However, partial tears may not significantly affect patellar height and may be difficult to diagnose clinically. MRI, while highly sensitive for assessing the integrity of these structures following athletic injury, cannot be effectively used due to significant artifact from the prosthesis. In experienced hands, ultrasound is an effective method of assessing for tendinous continuity. The quadriceps and patellar tendons, being relatively superficial structures, are well visualized using a

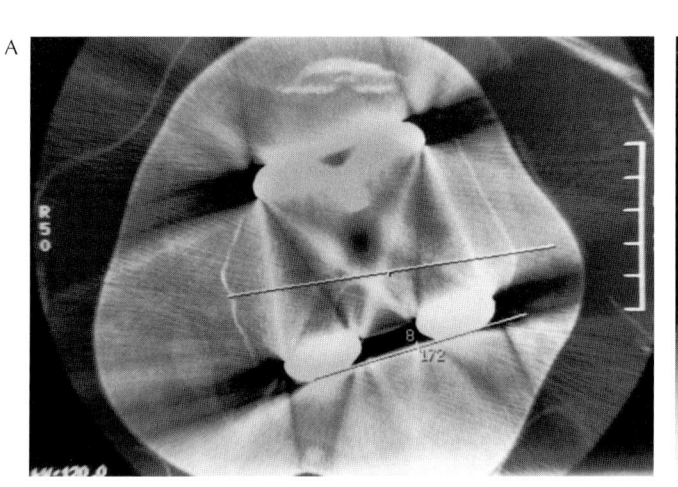

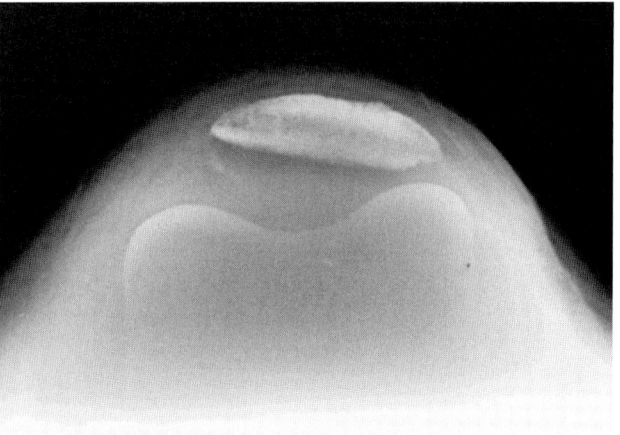

Figure 48.25. Femoral Component Rotational Malalignment
(A) CT scan through the femoral component of a patient with patellofemoral symptoms: The femoral component is internally rotated by 8 degrees relative to the epicondylar axis. (B) Mild, but symptomatic, patellar malalignment is seen on the Merchant view.

Figure 48.26. Femoral Component Malrotation—Patellar Dislocation There is bilateral lateral patellar dislocation in this patient with internally rotated femoral components.

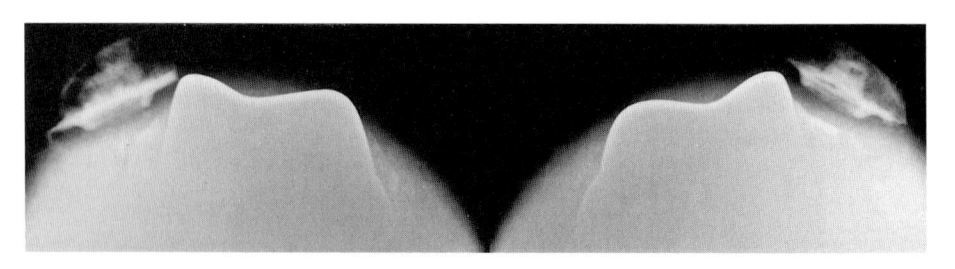

high-frequency transducer, and tendon tears can be reliably diagnosed. Ultrasound is strongly user-dependent, and the accuracy of these studies directly correlates with the experience and expertise of the examiner.

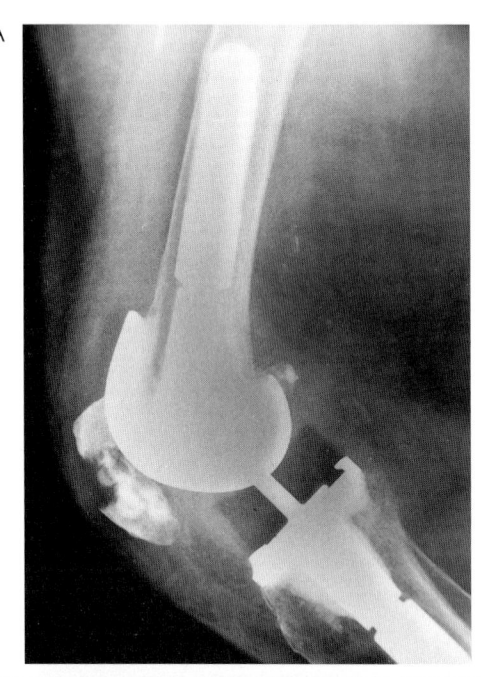

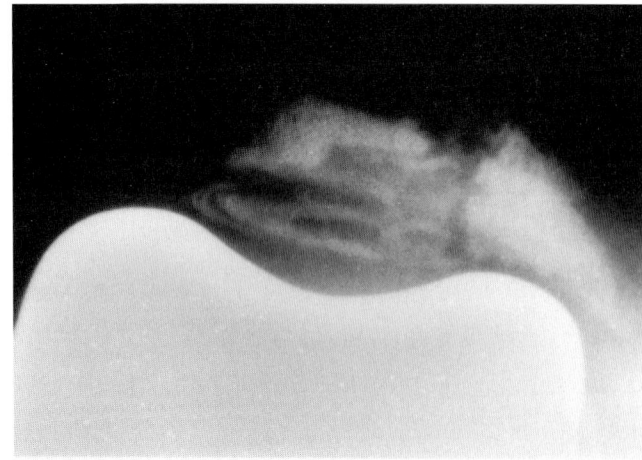

Figure 48.27. Patellar Fractures
(A) Transverse and (B) longitudinal patellar fractures. The lateral fragment in "B" is markedly sclerotic, indicating osteonecrosis.

FRACTURE

Periprosthetic fractures most commonly occur at the patellar component, seen in up to 1% of cases. These injuries are usually readily apparent on routine conventional radiographs. In difficult cases, CT may be useful in assessing for fractures, especially at the level of the patella and tibia where metal artifact is less pronounced. A radionuclide bone scan may also be useful; fractures are manifested by a focal area of intense uptake.

REFLEX SYMPATHETIC DYSTROPHY

Reflex sympathetic dystrophy (RSD) is an uncommon, yet potentially debilitating complication of TKR. The classical clinical presentation of limited flexion, constant pain unrelated to physical activity and cutaneous hypersensitivity in the absence of sepsis or radiographic loosening should lead the surgeon to consider this diagnosis. Katz and colleagues, in a series of 662 primary total knee arthroplasties, reported this complication in 0.8%.[72] Conventional radiographs often reveal osteopenia in advanced stages of RSD[73] and are useful as an initial imaging modality primarily for ruling out other pathologic processes such as loosening. The radionuclide bone scan is a useful imaging tool for confirming cases of clinically suspected RSD. The reported sensitivity for detection of RSD ranges from 83% to 100%,[73,74] and is higher for advanced cases than early cases. The specificity and positive and negative predictive values range from 80% to 98%, 54% to 88%, and 99% to 100%, respectively.[75] The classical picture of increased radionuclide activity on all three phases of a triple phase bone scan is seen in most patients. The third (delayed) phase is most specific, because the uptake is in a typical periarticular distribution. Scintigraphic abnormalities may involve an entire extremity, but are most commonly seen at the hand or foot. Lumbar sympathetic blockade is a highly effective procedure for both diagnosis and therapy of this disorder.[72,76,77]

CONCLUSION

The imaging workup of a painful total knee replacement should be based on a focused, problem-directed approach. Conventional radiographs, including AP, lateral, and tangential axial views are mandatory in all patients. Although interpretation of nuclear imaging studies may be challenging following total knee arthroplasty, these scans are often very valuable and diagnostic, especially when they are normal. For suspected infection, the authors suggest obtaining an Indium-labeled leukocyte scan and three-phase bone scan. A normal Indium scan essentially excludes infection, while matching uptake on the two scans renders infection highly unlikely. A mismatch on the two scans (hot on Indium scan, normal on bone scan) is consistent with infection. Those patients whose scans are equivocal or where the clinical index of suspicion does not correlate with the findings on the scans often benefit from a bone marrow scan.

When occult fracture or reflex sympathetic dystrophy is suspected, a radionuclide bone scan should be ordered following conventional radiographs.

The rotational alignment of the femoral and tibial components is effectively assessed on CT, which can be utilized despite the presence of metal artifact.

The metal composition of prosthetic components results in significant degradation of MR images, and limits the utility of this modality in this patient population; however, MR imaging software is currently being investigated that attempts to minimize metal artifact.

References

1. Patel DV, Ferris BD, Aichroft PM. Radiologic study of alignment after total knee replacement: Short radiographs or long radiographs? *Int Orthop* (Germany). 1991; 15: 209–210.
2. Ranawat CS, Rodriguez JA. Malalignment and malrotation in total knee arthroplasty. In: Insall JN, Scott WN, Scuderi GR (eds). *Current concepts in primary and revision total knee arthroplasty*. Philadelphia: Lippincott-Raven Publishers; 1996:115–122.
3. Peterson TL, Engh GA. Radiographic assessment of knee alignment after total knee arthroplasty. *J Arthroplasty*. 1988; 3:67–72.
4. Allen AM, Ward WG, Pope TL Jr. Imaging of total knee arthroplasty. *Radiol Clin North Am*. 1995; 33:289–303.
5. Benjamin JB, Lund PJ. Orthopedic devices. In: Hunter TB, Bragg DG (eds). *Radiological guided to medical devices and foreign bodies*. St. Louis: Mosby; 1994:348–385.
6. Weissman BN. Radiographic evaluation of total joint replacement. In: Sledge CB, Ruddy S, Harris ED Jr et al. (eds). *Arthritis surgery*. Philadelphia: WB Saunders; 1994: 846–907.
7. Figgie HE III, Goldberg VM, Heiple KG et al. The influence of tibial-patellofemoral location on function of the knee in patients with the posterior stabilized condylar knee prosthesis. *J Bone Joint Surg (Am)*. 681035–40, 1986.
8. Insall JN, Salvati E. Patella position in the normal knee joint. *Radiology*. 1971; 101:101–104.
9. Scuderi GR. Radiographic assessment of patellar length, thickness and height. Presented at the American Academy of Orthopaedic Surgeons Annual Meeting. Washington, DC, 1992.
10. Goldberg VM, Figgie HE III, Figgie MP. Technical considerations in total knee surgery: Management of patella problems. *Orthop Clin North Am* 1989; 20:189–199.
11. Briard JL, Hungerford DS. Patellofemoral instability in total knee arthroplasty. *J Arthroplasty*. 4 (suppl): 1989; S87–S97.
12. Merchant AC, Mercer RL, Jacobs RH et al. Roentgenographic analysis of patellofemoral congruence. *J Bone Joint Surg (Am)*. 1974; 56:1391–1396.
13. Math KR, Ghelman B, Potter HG. Imaging of the patellofemoral joint. In: Scuderi BR. *The patella*. New York: Springer-Verlag Inc; 1995:83–125.
14. Fulkerson JP. Imaging the patellofemoral joint. In: Fulkerson JP. *Disorders of the patellofemoral joint*. Baltimore: Williams & Wilkins; 1997:73–104.
15. Ewald FC. The Knee Society total knee arthroplasty roentgenographic evaluation and scoring system. *Clin Orthop Rel Res*. 1989; 248:9–12.
16. Weissman BN. Radiographic evaluation of total joint replacement. In: Sledge CB, Ruddy S, Harris ED Jr et al. (eds). *Arthritis surgery*. Philadelphia: WB Saunders; 1994: 846–907.
17. Mintz AD, Pilkington CAJ, Howie DW. A comparison of plain and fluoroscopically guided radiographs in the assessment of arthroplasty of the knee. *J Bone Joint Surg (Am)*. 1989; 9:1343–1347.
18. Rozing PM, Bohne WH, Insall JN. Bone scanning for the evaluation of knee prostheses. *Acta Orthop Scand*. 1982; 53:291–295.
19. Duus BR, Boeckstyns M, Kjaer L et al. Radionuclide scanning after total knee replacement: Correlation with pain and radiolucent lines. A prospective study. *Invest Radiol*. 1987; 22:891–895.
20. Gelman MI, Dunn HK. Radiology of knee joint replacement. *Am J Roentgenol*. 1976; 127:447–455.
21. Freiberger RH. Techniques of knee arthrography. In: Freiberger RH, Kaye JJ (eds.). *Arthrography*. New York: Appleton-Century-Crofts; 1979:5–30.
22. Uri G, Wellman H, Capello W et al. Scintigraphic and x-ray arthrographic diagnosis of femoral prosthesis loosening: Concise communication. *J Nucl Med*. 1984; 25:661–663.
23. Oyen WJG, Lemmens AM, Claessens RAM et al. Nuclear arthrography: Combined scintigraphic and radiographic procedure for diagnosis of total hip prosthesis loosening. *J Nucl Med*. 1996; 37:62–70.
24. Miniaci A, Bailey WH, Bourne RB et al. Analysis of radionuclide arthrograms, radiographic arthrograms and sequential plain radiographs in the assessment of painful hip arthroplasty. *J Athroplasty*. 1990; 5:143–146.
25. Swan JS, Braunstein EM, Wellman HN et al. Contrast and nuclear arthrography in loosening of the uncemented hip prosthesis. *Skeletal Radiol*. 1991; 20:15–20.
26. Utz JA, Lull RJ, Galvin EG. Asymptomatic total hip prosthesis: Natural history determined using Tc-99m MDP bone scans. *Radiology*. 1986; 61:509–514.
27. Schneider R, Hood RW, Ranawat CS. Radiographic eval-

uation of knee arthroplasty. *Orthop Clin North Am.* 1982; 13:225–244.
28. Schneider R, Soudry M. Radiographic and scintigraphic evaluation of total knee arthroplasty. *Clin Orthop.* 1986;205: 108–120.
29. Rosenthal L, Lisbona R, Hernandez M et al. Tc-99m-PP and Ga67 imaging following insertion of orthopedic devices. *Radiology.* 1979; 133:717–721.
30. Peters PC, Engh GA, Dwyer KA et al. Osteolysis after total knee arthroplasty without cement. *J Bone Joint Surg (Am).* 1992; 74:864–876.
31. Knezevich S, Vaughn BK, Lombardi AW et al. Failure of the polyethylene tibial component of a total knee replacement associated with asymptomatic loosening secondary to polyethylene and metallic wear debris. *Orthopedics.* 1993; 16:1136–1140.
32. Tucker WF Jr, Rosenberg AF. Osteolysis following total knee arthroplasty. In: Insall JN, Scott WN, Scuderi GR (eds). *Current concepts in primary and revision total knee arthroplasty.* Philadelphia: Lippincott-Raven; 1996:131–146.
33. Weissman BN, Scott RD, Brick GW et al. Radiographic detection of metal-induced synovitis as a complication of arthroplasty of the knee. *J Bone Joint Surg (Am)* 1991; 73: 1002–1007.
34. Quale JL, Murphey MD, Huntrakoon et al. Titanium-induced arthropathy associated with polyethylene-metal separation after total joint replacement. *Radiology.* 1992; 182:855–858.
35. Masini MA, Maguire JH, Thornhill TS. Infected total knee arthroplasty. In: Scott WN. *The knee.* St. Louis, Missouri: Mosby-Year Book, Inc.; 1994:1261–1278.
36. Rand JA, Bryan RS. Reimplantation for the salvage of an infected total knee arthroplasty. *J Bone Joint Surg (Am).* 1993; 65:1081–1086.
37. Rand JA, Bryan RS, Morrey BF et al. Management of infected total knee arthroplasty. *Clin Orthop.* 1986; 205:75.
38. Cameron HU, Hunter GA. Failure in total knee arthroplasty: Mechanisms, revisions and results. *Clin Orthop.* 1982; 170:141–146.
39. Magnuson JE, Brown ML, Hauser MF et al. In-111-labeled leukocyte scintigraphy in suspected orthopedic prosthesis infection: Comparison with other imaging modalities. *Radiology.* 1988; 168:235–239.
40. Palestro CJ, Swyer AJ, Kim CK et al. Infected knee prosthesis: Diagnosis with In-111 leukocyte, Tc-99m sulfur colloid, and Tc-99m MDP imaging. *Radiology.* 1991; 179:645–648.
41. Johnson JA, Christie MJ, Sandler et al. Detection of occult infection following total joint arthroplasty using sequential technetium 99m HDP bone scintigraphy and indium-111 WBC imaging. *J Nucl Med.* 1988; 29:1347–1353.
42. Howie DW, Savage JP, Wilson TG et al. The technetium phosphate bone scan in the diagnosis of osteomyelitis in childhood. *J Bone Joint Surg (Am).* 1983; 65:431–435.
43. Lisbona R, Roenthall L. Observations on the sequential use of 99m Tc-phosphate complex and 67-Ga imaging in osteomyelitis, cellulitis and septic arthritis. *Radiology.* 1977; 123:123–127.
44. Schauwecker DS. The role of nuclear medicine in osteomyelitis. In: Collier BD Jr, Fogelman I, Rosenthall L (eds.). *Skeletal nuclear medicine.* St. Louis, Missouri: Mosby-Year Book, Inc.; 1996: 182–203.
45. Reing CM, Richin PF, Kenmore PI. Differential bone scanning in the evaluation of a painful total joint replacement. *J Bone Joint Surg Am.* 1979; 61:933–936.
46. Palestro CJ, Kim CK, Swyer AJ et al. Total hip arthroplasty: periprosthetic indium-111-labeled leukocyte activity and complementary technetium-99m sulfur colloid imaging in suspected infection. *J Nucl Med.* 1990; 31:1950–1955.
47. Palestro CJ, Swyer AJ, Kim CK et al. Infected knee prosthesis: Diagnosis with In-11 leukocyte, Tc-99m sulfur colloid and Tc-99m MDP imaging. *Radiology.* 1991; 179:645–648.
48. LaManna MM, Garbarino JL, Berman AT et al. An assessment of technetium and gallium scanning in the patient with painful total joint arthroplasty. *Orthop.* 1983; 6:580–582.
49. Merkel KD, Brown ML, Fitzgerald RH Jr. Sequential technetium-99m HMDP-gallium-67 citrate imaging for the evaluation of infection in the painful prosthesis. *J Nucl Med.* 1986; 27:1413–1417.
50. Merkel KD, Brown ML, Dewanjee MK et al. Comparison of indium-labeled leukocyte imaging with sequential technetium-gallium scanning in the diagnosis of low-grade musculoskeletal sepsis. *J Bone Joint Surg (Am).* 1985; 67: 465–476.
51. McKillop JH, McKay I, Cuthbert GF et al. Scintigraphic evaluation of the painful prosthetic joint: A comparison of gallium-67 citrate and indium-111 labeled leukocyte imaging. *Clin Radiol.* 1984; 35:239–241.
52. Wukich DK, Abreu SH, Callaghan JJ et al. Diagnosis of infection by preoperative scintigraphy with indium-labeled white blood cells. *J Bone Joint Surg (Am).* 1987; 69:1354–1360.
53. King AD, Peters AM, Stuttle AWJ et al. Imaging of bone infection with labeled white blood cells: Role of contemporaneous bone marrow imaging. *Eur J Nucl Med.* 1990; 17:148–151.
54. Palestro CJ. Radionuclide imaging after skeletal interventional procedures. *Semin in Nucl Med.* 1995; 25:3–14.
55. Datz FL, Taylor A Jr. The clinical use of radionuclide bone marrow imaging. *Semin Nucl Med.* 1985; 15:239–259.
56. Feigin DS, Strauss HW, James AW. The bone marrow scan in experimental osteomyelitis. *Skeletal Radiol.* 1976; 1:103–106.
57. Rao S, Solomon N, Miller S et al. Scintigraphic differentiation bone infarction from osteomyelitis in children with sickle cell disease. *J Pediatr.* 1985; 107:685–688.
58. Seabold JE, Nepola JV, Marsh JL et al. Postoperative bone marrow alterations: Potential pitfalls in the diagnosis of osteomyelitis with In-11-labeled leukocyte scintigraphy. *Radiology.* 1991; 180:741–747.
59. Anouchi YS, Whiteside LA, Kaiser AD et al. The effects of axial rotational alignment of the femoral component on knee stability and patellar tracking in total knee arthroplasty demonstrated on autopsy specimens. *Clin Orthop.* 1993; 287:170–177.

60. Rhoades DD, Noble PC, Reuben JD et al. The effect of femoral component positioning on patellar tracking after total knee arthroplasty. *Clin Orthop*. 1990; 260:43–51.
61. Berger RA, Seel MJ, Rubash HE et al. Determining the rotational alignment of the femoral component in total knee arthroplasty using the epicondylar axis. *Clin Orthop*. 1992; 186:40–47.
62. Crossett LS, Rubash HE, Berger R. Computerized tomography in total knee arthroplasty. In: Insall JN, Scott WN, Scuderi GR (eds). *Current concepts in primary and revision total knee arthroplasty*. Philadelphia: Lippincott-Raven: 1996: 235–248.
63. Math KR, Griffin F, Scuderi GR, Insall JN. Imaging of the epicondylar axis of the distal femur: Utility in the evaluation of the painful total knee arthroplasty. Presented at The Radiological Society of North America Scientific Assembly, 12/97, Chicago, Illinois.
64. Merkow RL, Soudry M, Insall JN. Patellar dislocation following total knee replacement. *J Bone Joint Surg (Am)*. 1985; 67:1325–1328.
65. Cameron HU, Fedorkow DM. The patella in total knee arthroplasty. *Clin Orthop*. 1982; 165:197–199.
66. Gomes LSM, Bechtold JE, Gustilo RB. Patellar prosthesis positioning in total knee arthroplasty. A Roentgenographic study. *Clin Orthop*. 1988; 236:72–81.
67. Goldberg VM. Patella fracture type and prognosis in condylar total knee arthroplasty. *Clin Orthop*. 1988; 236: 115–122.
68. Clayton M, Thiripathi R. Patellar complications after total condylar arthroplasty. *Clin Orthop*. 1982; 170:131–140.
69. Booth RE Jr. Patellar complications in total knee arthroplasty. In: Scott WN (ed). *The knee*. Mosby-Year Book: 1325–1332.
70. Rand JA, Morrey BF, Bryan AS. Patellar tendon rupture after total knee arthroplasty. *Clin Orthop*. 1989; 244: 233–238.
71. Lynch AF, Rorabeck CH, Bourne RB. Extensor mechanism complications following total knee arthroplasty. *J Arthroplasty*. 1987; 2:135–140.
72. Katz MM, Hungerford DS, Krackow KA et al. Reflex sympathetic dystrophy as a cause of poor results after total knee replacement. *J Arthroplasty*. 1986; 1:117–124.
73. Kozin E, Soin JS, Ryan LM et al. Bone scintigraphy in the reflex sympathetic dystrophy syndrome. *Radiology*. 1981; 138:437–441.
74. Holder LE, Cole LA, Myerson MS. Reflex sympathetic dystrophy in the foot: Clinical and scintigraphic criteria. *Radiology*. 1992; 184:531–537.
75. Holder LE, Mackinnon SE. Reflex sympathetic dystrophy in the hands: Clinical and scintigraphic criteria. *Radiology*. 1984; 152:517–524.
76. Cameron HU, Park YS, Krestow M. Reflex sympathetic dystrophy following total knee replacement. *Contem Orthop*. 1994; 29:279–281.
77. O'Brien SJ, Ngeow J, Gibney MA et al. Reflex sympathetic dystrophy of the knee: Causes, diagnosis and treatment. *Am J Sports Med*. 1995; 23:655–659.

CHAPTER 49
Arthroscopic Management of Problematic Total Knee Arthroplasty

David R. Diduch and Giles R. Scuderi

INTRODUCTION

The role of arthroscopy in evaluating and treating problematic total knee replacement is evolving. Few references exist in the literature prior to 1989 with the exception of descriptions of the use of arthroscopy for lysis of adhesions in arthrofibrosis.[1–3] Since descriptions by Hozack and Insall of patella clunk syndrome,[4,5] numerous papers have helped to establish arthroscopy as a tool to manage soft tissue impingement.[6–8] In addition to arthrofibrosis and the patella clunk syndrome, arthroscopy has been described for debridement of impinging soft tissue problems elsewhere in the knee,[9–11] for diagnosis of component wear,[12,13] and polyethylene fracture[14–16] to perform lateral release for patella maltracking[9,10,17] and to remove loose patella buttons.[18] Arthroscopy has also been described to treat acute infections following knee replacement, although this is generally not recommended.[19]

We recently examined the efficacy of arthroscopy according to the particular diagnoses to better define its role.[20] Arthroscopy confirmed the diagnosis in 39 of 40 knees (97.5%), demonstrating the diagnostic effectiveness of arthroscopy in a problematic knee replacement. This included 14 knees with only a nonspecific diagnosis of pain preoperatively, which were identified in all but one case to have some type of soft tissue impingement at arthroscopy. Therapeutically, arthroscopy effectively relieved symptoms in 73% of knees. Arthroscopy was most effective at relieving soft tissue impingement symptoms such as a clunk or a retained posterior cruciate ligament stump.

No arthroscopy-related infections or complications were noted in our series or in other series in the literature with the exception of one report.[21] Thus, arthroscopy has been shown to be efficacious both diagnostically and therapeutically, and to be a safe procedure in the patient with a problematic knee replacement.

PATIENT EVALUATION

The preoperative workup of a patient with a problematic knee replacement should include an appropriate history and physical examination. The examiner must pay close attention to evidence of patella component problems such as loosening, maltracking, or instability. Radiographs, including standing anteroposterior views, lateral views, and Merchant or sunrise views should be obtained to look for component loosening or malposition. Range of motion should be documented both actively and passively for evidence of arthrofibrosis.

It is important to rule out an occult infection in the problematic knee replacement prior to the consideration of arthroscopy. The radiographic evaluation includes X rays as listed above as well as bone scans and gallium scans. Appropriate laboratory evaluation should include white blood cell count with differential, erythrocyte sedimentation rate, and C-reactive protein. Aspiration of the knee should be performed in a sterile manner with fluid sent for aerobic and anaerobic culture as well as gram stain. Analysis can also be made for polyethylene wear debris as well as fluid chemistry and cell counts. In general, the aspiration and blood work are performed on at least two separate occasions to confirm that they are negative prior to considering arthroscopy for a painful knee replacement without a specific diagnosis.

The patient presenting with soft tissue impingement problems may describe the patella clunk syndrome. A patella clunk refers to a buildup of fibrous tissue that becomes trapped between the patella and femoral components.[4,5,7] The patient experiences a painful "snap" or "clunk" sensation during active extension. Soft tissue impingement elsewhere in the knee may only produce symptoms of pain and intermittent effusions. In some instances, mechanical complaints of catching may be noted referable to the area of impingement. We feel that when one can establish an area of mechanical soft tissue impingement preoperatively, the anticipated results of arthroscopic debridement are best. The orthopedic surgeon should be careful about taking a patient with a painful knee replacement to arthroscopy without a specific diagnosis or surgical plan.

INDICATIONS

After infection, component wear, loosening, or malposition have been excluded as reasons for pain in a problematic knee replacement, the surgeon may elect arthroscopic intervention with the following indications:

1. Soft tissue impingement under the patella consistent with a clunk.[6–8,20]
2. Soft tissue impingement elsewhere in the knee, such as hypertrophic synovitis.[9–11]
3. Retained posterior cruciate ligament stump impinging in the notch.[20]
4. Removal of loose body, including a loose patella component in a low-demand individual not desiring revision.[10,18]
5. Confirmation of clinically suspected but radiographically undetermined component wear or fracture.[12–15]
6. Patella lateral subluxation to be addressed with arthroscopic lateral release.[9,10,17]
7. Lysis of adhesions for arthrofibrosis to be performed in conjunction with manipulation under anesthesia. In general, this is indicated more than 3 months after initial arthroplasty when adhesions may be more consolidated potentially risking fracture if forceful manipulation is performed without lysis of adhesions.[1–3]

ARTHROSCOPIC TECHNIQUE

Surgical arthroscopy is performed through two or three standard peripatellar portals with routine instrumentation. In-flow may be attached to the arthroscopic cannula or through a separate suprapatellar portal. Mirror reflection off the metal component should be anticipated. Extreme care should be exercised to avoid iatrogenic damage to prosthetic components, especially the polyethylene patella and tibial articulation that could potentially generate wear debris and eventual loosening. Each compartment is inspected statically and during knee range of motion for possible impinging soft tissue. We routinely use a tourniquet for hemostasis but this is optional. A leg holder or post is not utilized to minimize risk of periprosthetic fracture.

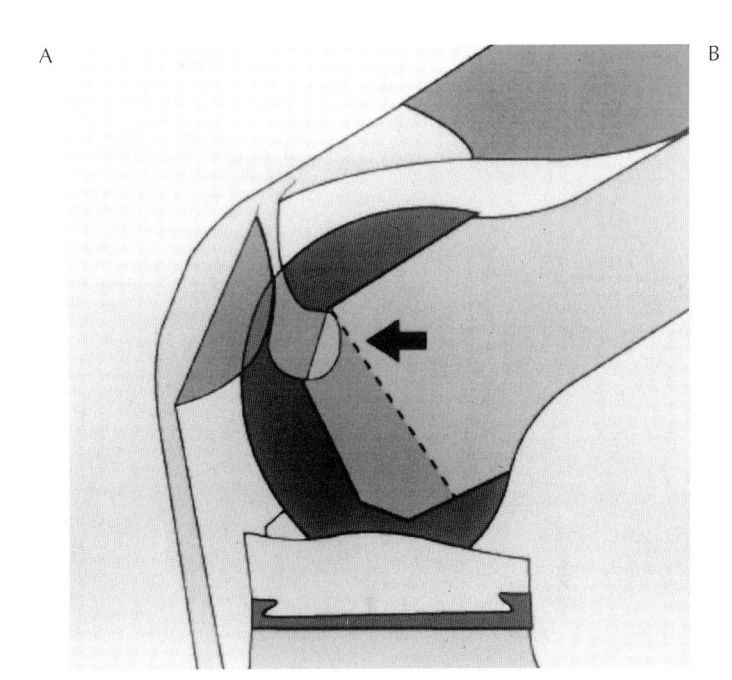

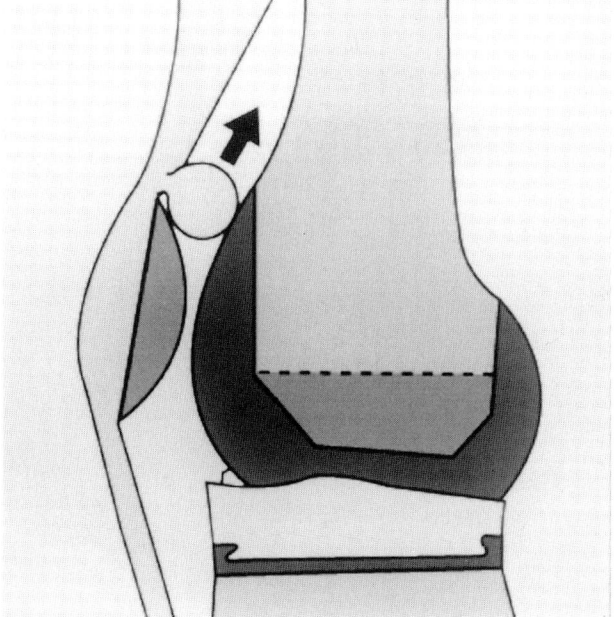

Figure 49.1. (A) Diagram of a clunk. The buildup of fibrous tissue becomes trapped between the patella component and the femoral notch (arrow). (B) During active knee extension, the fibrous tissue suddenly exits the notch into the suprapatellar pouch (arrow) producing a painful "clunk" sensation.

SOFT TISSUE IMPINGEMENT

Soft tissue impingement is the diagnosis most successfully treated arthroscopically in the problematic knee replacement.[20] Impingement may occur throughout the knee, including the patellofemoral articulation, the femoral-tibial articulation, and within the notch in the cam mechanism of a posterior-stabilized knee replacement.

A patella clunk refers to a buildup of fibrous tissue at the superior pole of the patella that hypertrophies with time and becomes trapped between the patella and femoral components. The patient experiences a painful "snap" or "clunk" sensation during active knee extension (Fig. 49.1). Clunks have been noted to be more common after knee replacement with a posterior-stabilized design, probably due to early designs with a shallow femoral surface and a sharp transition into a deeper femoral box.[4,6,7] Nonoperative management includes quadricep strengthening utilizing a stationary bike in the hope of mechanically softening and autodebriding the impinging soft tissue with repetitive motion. Should these exercises as well as therapy modalities prove unsuccessful, arthroscopy is indicated.

Upon insertion of the arthroscope, the surgeon may see a large soft tissue nodule under the patella that impinges in the notch (Fig. 49.2). As the knee is taken through a range of motion this may be seen snapping as it exits the notch during knee extension. Because the clunk is often quite firm and fibrotic, arthroscopic debridement usually must begin with forceps or scissors followed by the motorized shaver (Fig. 49.3). As debridement continues, the undersurface of the patella component becomes more visible. Extreme care must be taken to avoid iatrogenic damage to the polyethylene patella button. Commonly, a lip of fibrous tissue is noticed to be overlying the rim of the patella component. This can be removed with arthroscopic biting forceps followed by gentle use of the motorized shaver (Fig. 49.4). At the completion of the debridement, the contour of the undersurface of the extension mechanism should be smooth without impinging soft tissue as the patella is visualized during knee range of motion (Fig. 49.5).

Impinging hypertrophic synovitis may occur elsewhere in the knee. This may occur at the inferior pole of the patella in the region of the infrapatellar fat pad and may also become entrapped in the notch (Fig.

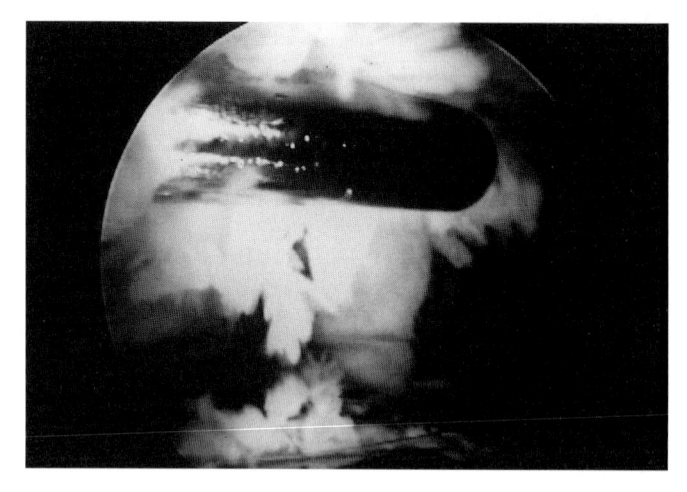

Figure 49.3. Debridement of a clunk. The motorized shaver is seen at the beginning of debridement of the clunk.

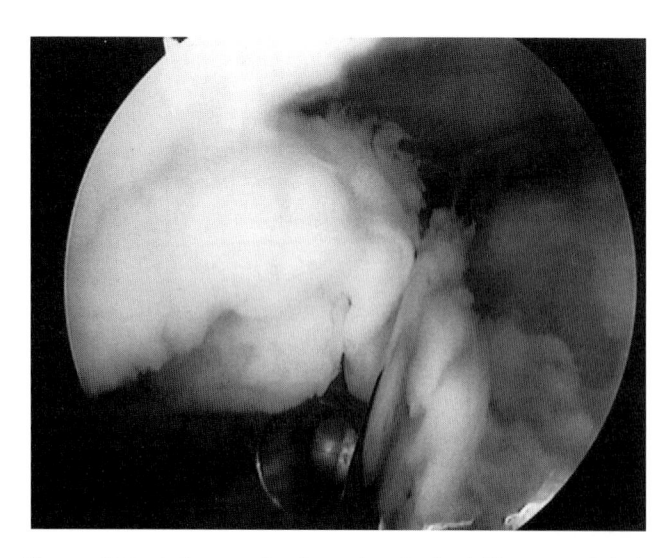

Figure 49.2. Arthroscopic view of a clunk. A fibrous nodule is trapped within the femoral notch and obscures the patella from view.

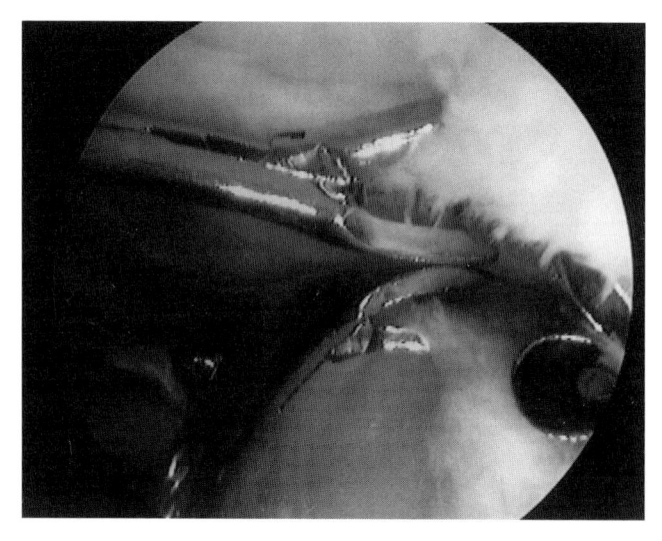

Figure 49.4. Fibrous tissue overlying the rim of the patella. An arthroscopic forceps is seen grasping and biting through the fibrous tissue that obscures the rim of the patella component circumferentially.

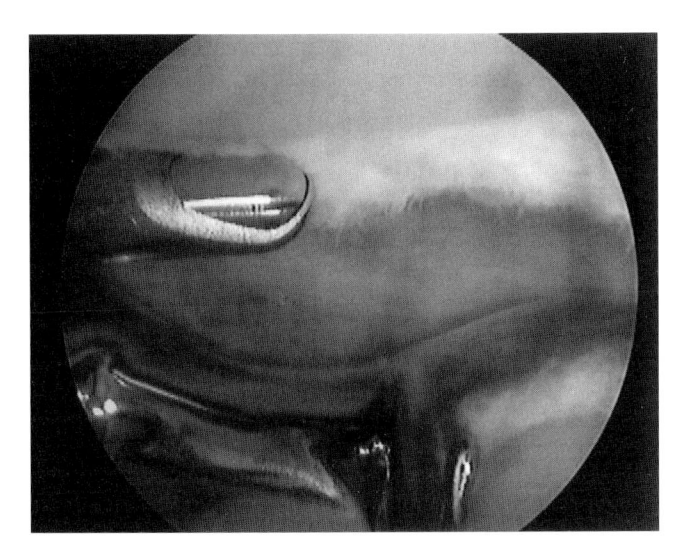

Figure 49.5. Arthroscopic view of the clunk at the conclusion of debridement. The motorized shaver is seen adjacent to the patella component in the suprapatellar pouch.

49.6A). This is addressed arthroscopically in a manner similar to a clunk with forceps and the motorized shaver (Fig. 49.6B). Other common locations of impingement include hypertrophic synovitis between the femoral and tibial components, which have been termed the pseudomeniscus.[10] Whether this represents inadequate debridement of the meniscus at the time of initial arthroplasty or later hypertrophy of the synovium is unclear.

Another location of soft tissue impingement is a retained posterior cruciate ligament stump within the femoral notch. This is a complication unique to posterior-stabilized designs. The retained PCL stump can impinge against the tibial polyethylene component of the cam mechanism. Symptoms include pain, especially in flexion, and recurrent effusions. Arthroscopic management involves debridement using the motorized shaver until impingement is relieved (Fig. 49.7).

Arthroscopic debridement of impinging soft tissue has been most successful for the diagnosis of a clunk. Symptoms were relieved by arthroscopy in our study for 14 of 17 patients.[20] Other authors have reported similar results.[6–9] Debridement of a retained posterior cruciate ligament stump relieved symptoms in 3 of 4 knees. Debridement of impinging soft tissue problems other than a clunk or retained PCL stump was only effective in 3 of 6 knees.[20]

PROSTHESIS WEAR

Prosthetic polyethylene wear may be responsible for painful effusions in the problematic knee replacement. Usually this can be documented radiographically by evidence of loosening or joint-space asymmetry on weight-bearing anteroposterior views of the knee. Another mechanism for diagnosis utilizes laboratory analysis of the joint aspirate for polyethylene particles. When these methods are unsuccessful but prosthetic wear is suspected, arthroscopy is a relatively noninvasive method to establish the diagnosis prior to committing to total knee revision.[12,14–16]

Arthroscopy offers visual inspection of articular surfaces for evidence of wear or fracture. Findings may include deformation of the surface in a smooth pattern

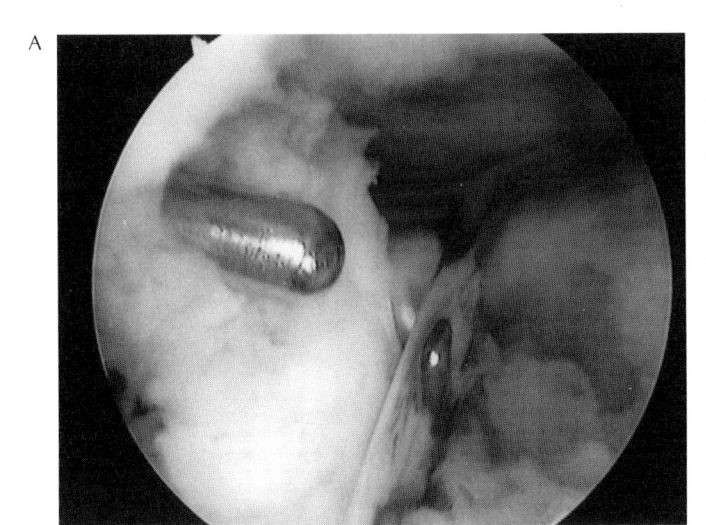

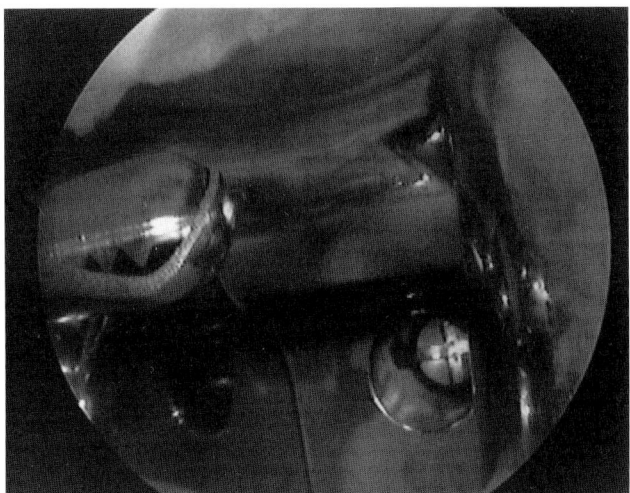

Figure 49.6. Soft tissue impingement elsewhere in the knee. (A) Hypertrophied soft tissue originating from the infrapatellar fat pad at the distal pole of the patella is seen completely occupying the notch of the femoral component. A motorized shaver is shown at the initiation of debridement. (B) The same arthroscopic view now shows the femoral notch after completely removing the impinging soft tissue.

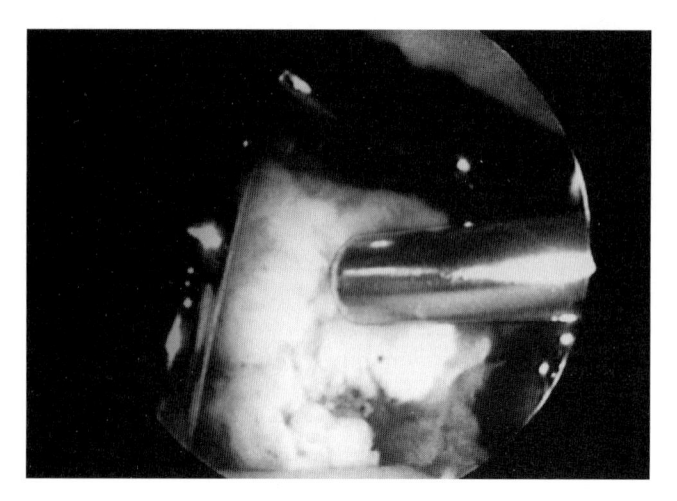

Figure 49.7. Arthroscopic view of debridement of a retained posterior cruciate ligament stump in the femoral notch using the motorized shaver.

without delamination consistent with cold flow changes that generally do not require revision. Alternatively, one may see gross fragmentation or delamination consistent with true polyethylene wear and generation of debris that may lead to loosening (Fig. 49.8). When one observes fissures or cracking of the polyethylene, revision orthoplasty should be considered.

PATELLA PROBLEMS

Patients with patella component maltracking, subluxation, or loosening frequently complain of pain anteriorly in the knee that is accentuated by deep flexion or stair climbing. Effusions may or may not be present. Instability or maltracking can often be determined by physical examination. Merchant radiographs may offer radiographic confirmation.

A maltracking, laterally subluxed patella may be addressed arthroscopically with a lateral release. This may be performed with a combination of the arthroscopic hook knife or scissors. These manual instruments may be safer than use of the arthroscopic bovie cautery because of the risk for electrical conduction through the metal knee component.[10] Arthroscopy also offers the opportunity to visualize patella tracking after the release to confirm correction. If maltracking persists, consideration is given to proximal realignment or patella revision to a smaller, thinner more medially located patella component.[13]

Loosening of the patella component is usually diagnosed radiographically (Fig. 49.9). However, at times the patella may be loose but still attached to its bed making radiographic diagnosis equivocal. In this case, arthroscopy may be used to visually inspect the patella and assess its stability using a probe. If the patella component is loose, then one may proceed to arthrotomy for revision. Alternatively, and especially in low-demand individuals who do not desire a major open surgical procedure, simple excision of the patella component may be performed. A miniarthrotomy is used to facilitate

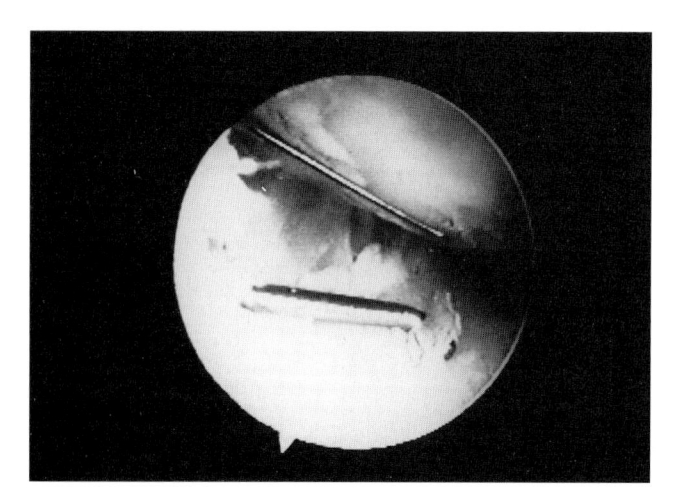

Figure 49.8. Arthroscopic view of polyethylene wear. The probe is seen lifting up areas of delamination of the tibial polyethylene surface.

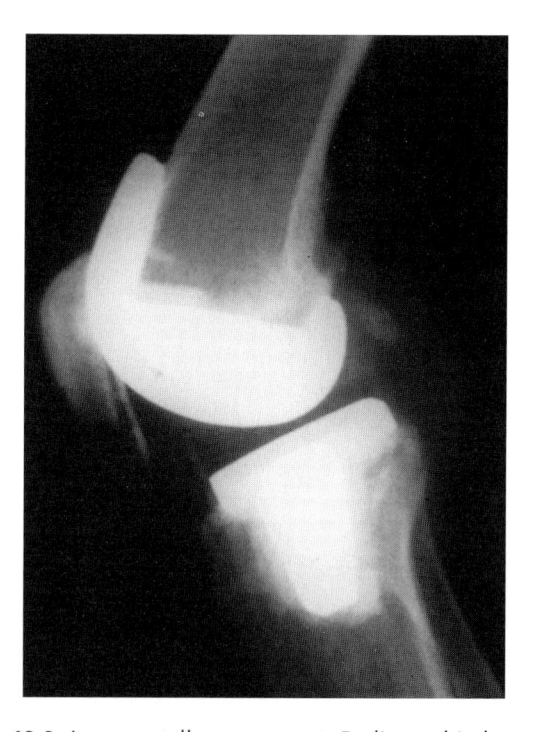

Figure 49.9. Loose patella component. Radiographic lateral view of a loose patella component is seen as demonstrated by the sclerotic line at the inferior pole of the patella. This patient elected not to have revision of the patella component. Instead, she had arthroscopic removal of the loose patella button through a miniarthrotomy.

arthroscopic removal of the patella button with a grasper. An arthroscopic high-speed burr or motorized shaver may then be utilized to smooth the undersurface of the remaining patellar bone to perform a patelloplasty. We successfully treated three patients in our series in this manner.[20]

ARTHROFIBROSIS

Arthrofibrosis can be a very disabling problem following total knee replacement. In the vast majority of cases, manipulation under anesthesia can be performed without need for arthroscopic intervention. Over an 8-year period at our institution, we found that arthroscopic lysis of adhesions was necessary in 8% of our manipulations under anesthesia. Generally, arthroscopy is reserved for manipulations performed greater than at least 3-months post-knee replacement. When contracture due to arthrofibrosis has been present for longer periods of time, excessive force may be needed even with anesthesia to accomplish the manipulation. Because of concerns about creating an iatrogenic periprosthetic fracture, arthroscopic lysis of adhesions can be performed prior to a manipulation. The manipulation should then require less force.

The surgical technique involves three and occasionally four peripatellar portals. Reestablishment of the suprapatellar pouch and medial and lateral gutters is initially performed with arthroscopic forceps and the motorized shaver. Upon initial introduction of the arthroscope in the knee, very limited space is available for visualization and great care must be taken to avoid damaging the prosthetic surfaces. Visualization becomes easier with time as the pouch and gutters are redeveloped. In addition to lysis of the adhesions in the gutters and the suprapatellar pouch, debridement of impinging soft tissue in the notch may be necessary due to hypertrophy of the intrapatellar fat pad remnant. At the conclusion of the arthroscopic lysis of adhesions, a gentle manipulation is performed.

Over an 8-year period in our study, we performed arthroscopic lysis of adhesions on 8 patients an average of 7.4 months after initial knee replacement. Maximum flexion was improved from a mean of 73 degrees preoperatively to a mean of 99 degrees postoperatively, for an average improvement in flexion at follow-up of 26 degrees.[20] Other authors report similar gains in flexion, although extension was minimally improved.[1,2]

POSTOPERATIVE MANAGEMENT

Patients are admitted overnight to allow 24 hours of perioperative intravenous antibiotics for infection prophylaxis. If the diagnosis was of arthrofibrosis preoperatively, a continuous passive motion machine is started in the recovery room and continued at home upon eventual discharge. The patients are referred to physical therapy for quadricep and hamstring strengthening to parity as well as range-of-motion exercises and modalities as needed. Those patients who have had problems with impinging soft tissue such as a clunk under the patella generally benefit from further work on a stationary bicycle. The repetitive motion may help to prevent recurrence of impinging soft tissue in addition to quadricep strengthening.

COMPLICATIONS

With the exception of one study, there have been no reported arthroscopy-related infections in the literature. Sisto and associates reported a 6% incidence of infected total knee replacements following arthroscopy.[21] His patients received only one preoperative dose of antibiotics as opposed to the 24 hours of intravenous antibiotics we routinely administer and are used in other studies in the literature. Therefore, we feel overnight admission for 24 hours of intravenous antibiotics is an important factor in preventing infections.

There have been no other reported arthroscopy-related complications to the best of our knowledge in the literature. Recurrence of symptoms, however, has been noted. In our study of 40 arthroscopies in 38 patients, symptoms were resolved in 29 of 40 knees (73%). Therefore, approximately one-fourth of patients either did not experience relief of symptoms or had recurrence of symptoms.

SUMMARY

Arthroscopy has been demonstrated to be helpful in the management of the problematic total knee replacement with soft tissue impingement, including the clunk syndrome, impinging soft tissue elsewhere in the knee, and a retained posterior cruciate ligament stump. Furthermore, arthroscopy is helpful in diagnosing polyethylene wear, in removing a loose patella button in a patient not desiring patellar revision, and for lysis of adhesions in arthrofibrosis to facilitate a more gentle manipulation. One must be cautioned, however, to complete a thorough preoperative evaluation for identifiable causes for the problematic knee replacement before performing arthroscopy. A specific therapeutic or diagnostic goal should be established first. Once such a plan is in place, we have shown that arthroscopy demonstrated a therapeutic efficacy of relieving symptoms in 73% of knees.[20] Arthroscopy is most effective at relieving soft tissue impingement symptoms such as a clunk.

Therefore, arthroscopy is effective in the management

of problematic total knee replacements, and can be performed safely without excessive complication risk. For properly selected problems, arthroscopy may avoid the need for arthrotomy or revision arthroplasty.

References

1. Del Pizzo W, Fox JM, Friedman MJ, Snyder SJ, Ferkel RD. Operative arthroscopy for the treatment of arthrofibrosis of the knee. *Contemporary Orthop.* January 1985; 10(1):67–72.
2. Campbell ED Jr. Arthroscopy in total knee replacements. *Arthroscopy.* 1987; 3(1):31–35.
3. Sprague NF, O'Connor RL, Fox JM. Arthroscopic treatment of postoperative knee fibroarthrosis. *Clin Orthop.* 1982; 166:165–172.
4. Insall JN, Lachiewicz PF, Burstein AH. The posterior stabilized condylar prosthesis: a modification of the total condylar design. *J Bone Joint Surg.* 1982; 64-A:1317–1323.
5. Hozack WJ, Rothman RH, Booth RE, Bladerston RA. The patella clunk syndrome. *Clin Orthop.* 1989; 241:203–208.
6. Vernace JV, Rothman RH, Booth RE, Balderston RA. Arthroscopic management of the patellar clunk syndrome following posterior stabilized total knee arthroplasty. *J Arthroplasty.* 1989; 4(2):179–182.
7. Beight JL, Yao B, Hozack WJ, Hearn SL, Booth RE. The patella "clunk" syndrome after posterior stabilized total knee arthroplasty. *Clin Orthop.* 1994; 299:139–142.
8. Lintner DM, Bocell JR, Tullos HS. Arthroscopic treatment of intra-articular fibrous brands after total knee arthroplasty. *Clin Orthop.* 1994; 309:230–233.
9. Bocell JR, Thorpe CC, Tullos JH. Arthroscopic treatment of symptomatic total knee arthroplasty. *Clin Orthop.* 1991; 271:125–134.
10. Johnson DR, Friedman RJ, McGinty JB, Mason JL, St. Mary EW. The role of arthroscopy in the problem total knee replacement. *Arthroscopy* 1990; 6(1):30–32.
11. Johnson DR, McGinty JB, Mason JL, St. Mary E. Arthroscopy of total knee replacements. A preliminary report. *Arthroscopy* 1988; 4(2):140.
12. Mintz MD, Tsao AK, McCrae CR, Stulberg SD, Wright T. The arthroscopic evaluation and characteristics of severe polyethylene wear in total knee arthroplasty. *Clin Orthop.* 1991; 273:215–222.
13. Scuderi GR, Insall JM, Scott WN. Patellofemoral pain after total knee arthroplasty. *J Am Acad of Orthop Surg.* 1994; 2(5):239–246.
14. Havel PE, Giddings JD. Fracture of polyethylene tibial component in total knee arthroplasty diagnosed by arthroscopy. *Orthopedics.* 1994; 17(4):357–359.
15. Wasilewski SA, Frankl U. Fracture of polyethylene of patella component in total knee arthroplasty diagnosed by arthroscopy. *J Arthroplasty.* 1989; (suppl)5:19–22.
16. Wasilewski SA, Frankl U. Arthroscopy of the painful dysfunctional total knee replacement. *Arthroscopy.* 1989; 5(4): 294–297.
17. Yoshii I, Whiteside LA, Anouchi YS. The effect of patella button placement and femoral component design on patellar tracking in total knee arthroplasty. *Clin Orthop.* 1992; 275:211–219.
18. Diduch DR, Insall JN, Scott WN, Scuderi GR, Font-Rodriquez D. Total knee replacement in young, active patients: long term follow up and functional outcome. *J Bone Joint Surg.* 1997; 79-A(4):575–582.
19. Flood JN, Kolarik DB. Arthroscopic irrigation and debridement of infected total knee arthroplasty. Report of two cases. *Arthroscopy.* 1988; 4(3):182–186.
20. Diduch DR, Scuderi GR, Scott WN, Insall JN, Kelly MA. The efficacy of arthroscopy following total knee replacement. *Arthroscopy.* 1997; 73(2):166–171.
21. Sisto DJ, Cook DL. Infection following knee arthroscopy in joint replacement patients. *Arthroscopy.* 1996; 12(3): 350–351.

SECTION 14
Revision Arthroplasty

CHAPTER 50
Component Removal

Paul N. Smith and Cecil H. Rorabeck

INTRODUCTION

The surgeon performing revision total knee joint arthroplasty will face a wide variety of revision scenarios ranging from the situation in which the prosthetic complex virtually falls out of the wound to that in which major difficulties in removal of both component and cement are encountered. As a general rule resurfacing design components proves less difficult to remove than more exotic designs that incorporate longer stems either or both on the tibial or femoral sides. The situation is often made more difficult when cement has been used with longer stemmed components, presenting removal challenges similar to those encountered in revision hip surgery on the femoral side. Many revisions are undertaken in the face of existing severe damage to bone stock. Great care must be taken to ensure removal of the prosthetic joint with as little damage to bone stock as possible in order to minimize the complexity of the subsequent reconstruction.

PREOPERATIVE ASSESSMENT AND PLANNING

The total knee replacement may fail in a number of ways. These include infection, loosening of femoral, tibial, or patellar components, wearing of the polyethylene insert, patellar maltracking, or dislocation and instability of the prosthetic complex (Fig. 50.1). In the great majority of cases, failure of the total knee arthroplasty will lead to progressive damage and loss of bone stock, and therefore with time one encounters a more difficult revision scenario. In this light, early diagnosis of failure is important and patients should be followed conscientiously at regular intervals to monitor the status of their arthroplasties and enable early detection of a problem.

The patient with a failed arthroplasty must be carefully evaluated with a view to identifying the reason or reasons behind the failure of the prosthesis. Diagnosis of infection is most important. A careful history and physical examination of the patient is undertaken. Particular note is taken of problems with wound healing, episodes of infection at other sites, and multiple operations on the knee in question. The temporal relation of onset of symptoms or of failure of the arthroplasty to the initial operation is important. Infection often is an early postoperative problem, whereas failure due to component loosening and/or polyethylene wear is mainly a later phenomenon. Careful note should be taken of the location of surgical scars about the knee and any incision planned must take these into consideration in order to avoid potential problems with skin necrosis. Should infection be suspected, routine blood screens for infection including ESR and CRP are performed. Aspiration of joint fluid is undertaken, with fluid analyzed for organisms and white blood cells, and sent for both aerobic and anaerobic culture.

Thorough preoperative planning must be undertaken, not only to anticipate problems in the removal of the prosthesis but to prepare for the endoprosthetic reconstruction. The type of existing prosthesis must be identified by reference to the patients previous records. If the patient had the prior surgery in another institution, it is important to access those records for reasons of prosthesis identification but also to find out if any problems in either surgery or postoperative recovery were encountered. Many component systems have customized instruments that enable easy disassembly of modular componentry. It is a simple matter to access these instruments from the respective manufacturer and they often save both time and effort in removal of parts. Similarly, some older hinged designs are formally linked and may need special instruments to uncouple the components to facilitate their removal.

Preoperative templating enables estimation of bone stock loss that may be found in the revision and hence allows planning of bone grafting and prosthetic augmentation in advance of surgery (Fig. 50.2). In revision surgery it is important to expect the worst and be prepared for it. There should be very few surprises in the operation and one should be well armed to meet any

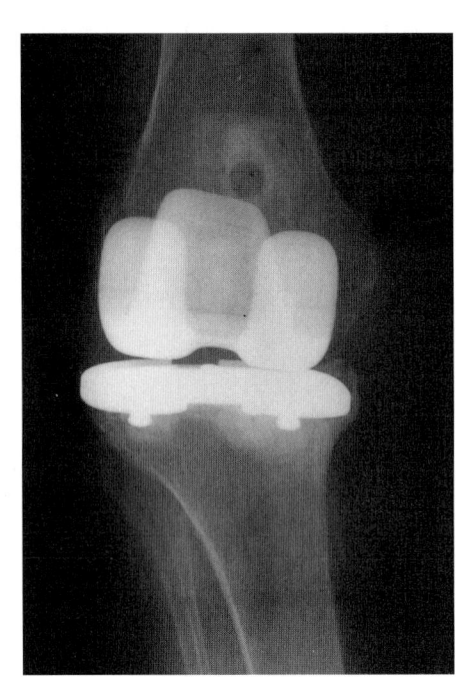

Figure 50.1. Failure of arthroplasty with collapse of the tibial component into varus.

unexpected eventuality. Modern revision systems have an enormous range of implant options, having various stem sizes and lengths, and augmentations or wedges to meet virtually any scenario. Rarely, customized components are required to deal with a specific deformity.

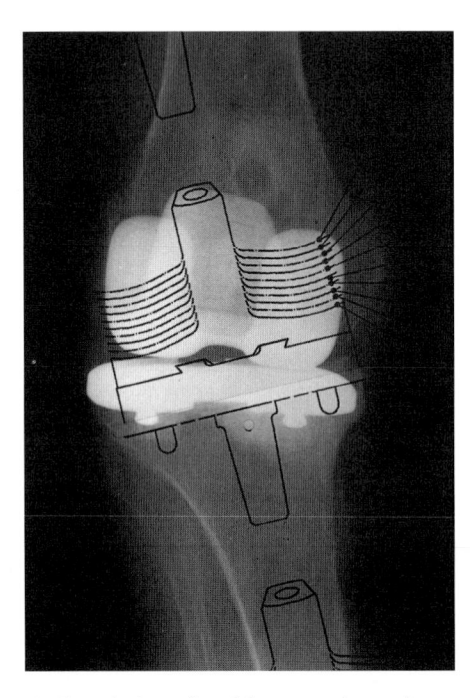

Figure 50.2. Templating of revision to estimate bone resection level and need for augmentation of implant or bone grafting.

EXPOSURE OF THE FAILED PROSTHESIS

As alluded to above, many cases with failed total knee prostheses have multiple incisions about the knee. We prefer a straight anterior skin incision wherever possible, and if an incision of this type has been previously used then it should be used again (Fig. 50.3). One should avoid creating tram-tracks on the front of the knee. Insall[1] has described the technique of using a so-called "sham" incision when skin viability is in doubt. In cases in which complex skin incision patterns create doubt about skin viability, then early consultation with the vascular and plastic surgical services is of assistance.

The tissues of the previously operated knee are often thickened and less compliant than normal. Hence a longer incision through skin, subcutaneous tissue, and extensor mechanism is needed to obtain adequate exposure than in the virgin knee. One often encounters a degree of tethering of the quadriceps mechanism, with or without patellar baja, rendering the patella difficult or impossible to reflect in the usual fashion. Routinely, the author utilizes the medial parapatellar approach to the knee. An important point in this exposure is to dissect tissues subperiosteally off the medial tibial plateau around to the posteromedial corner of the tibia. This allows external rotation of the tibia and aids in anterior subluxation of the proximal tibia in exposing the joint.

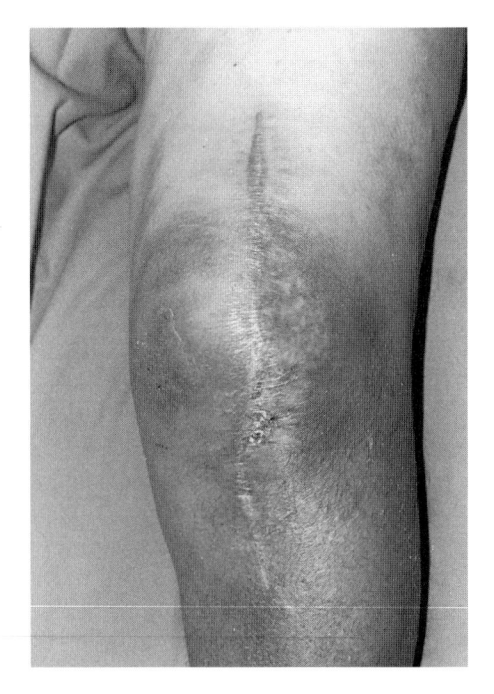

Figure 50.3. Anterior skin incision. This patient had an early infection of her arthroplasty and wound-healing problems with skin slough over the inferior pole of the patella. The wound healed without the need for grafting; however, further problems in subsequent surgery were inevitable.

In addition, this maneuver helps to reduce tension on the quadriceps mechanism, thus protecting the patellar tendon insertion. It is vital that adequate exposure is achieved to enable ready visualization of the interfaces to facilitate component removal. The patella must be reflected to this end, and, if there is tethering of the quads mechanism or patellar infera, the act of reflection of the patella will place the insertion of the patellar tendon at considerable risk. Avulsion of the patellar tendon must be avoided at all costs, and if there is any difficulty in achieving a safe reflection of the patella, one must proceed to either a tibial tubercle osteotomy[2–4] (Fig. 50.4) or quadriceps snip[5] or V-Y turndown.[6,7]

Once satisfactory exposure of the implant has been achieved, the next step is to fully display the bone-cement or bone-prosthesis interfaces. This enables thorough inspection of the interfaces for assessment of components for loosening in the cases in which implants are not obviously loose on radiological grounds alone. In addition, implant removal in a safe, controlled manner is only possible when all interfaces can be visualized and taken down under direct vision by whatever means appropriate to that situation. Display of the interfaces is facilitated by a thorough debridement of tissue and synovium contaminated by metal and polyethylene debris during exposure of the implants (Fig. 50.5).

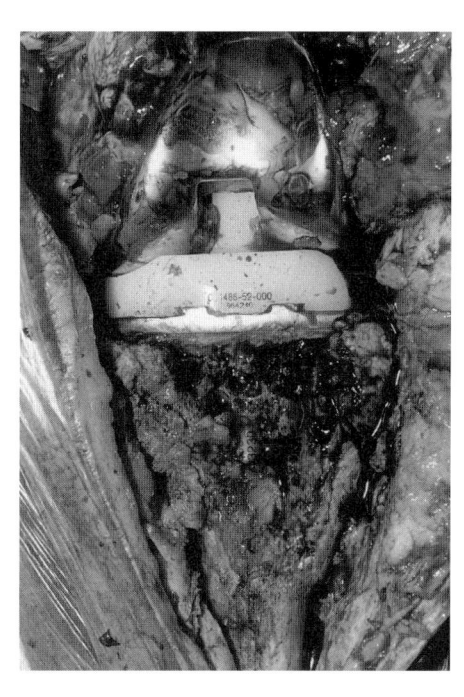

Figure 50.5. Contamination of tissues with debris and exuberant synovitis. Synovectomy and thorough debridement allows satisfactory display of interfaces.

REMOVAL OF THE FEMORAL COMPONENT

The femoral component is removed first because its removal will render exposure of the tibial component and therefore its removal simpler. Following identification of the cement-bone or prosthesis-bone interfaces, the aim is to take down the interface with as little damage to bone stock as possible (Fig. 50.6). The prosthesis must be freed from bone as completely as one is able before removal is attempted. Severe damage to bone in the form of either fracture of the femoral shaft or condyle or avulsion of a large segment of bone from the remaining metaphysis may occur if removal is attempted without first freeing the component from the bony bed.

In order to take down the interface, several strategies can be employed. Narrow, flexible osteotomes can be driven between the prosthesis and bone or between prosthesis and cement. These are effective and have the advantages of being available in a number of blade widths and being disposable, because damage to an osteotome used in component removal is almost inevitable. Their flexibility can also be a disadvantage in that the osteotome can skive off at an angle from that intended into bone, causing unplanned damage. Therefore, care must be taken in the use of these instruments, with caution taken not to use too much force because it is in this situation that the instrument can wander from its intended path.

Power instruments such as the Midas Rex or Anspach can be similarly used to dissect the interface. Although

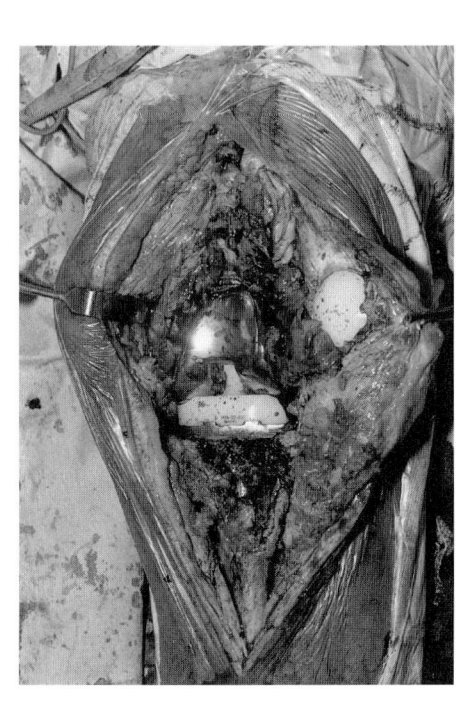

Figure 50.4. Wide exposure of failed infected TKR. Note the long skin incision. This patient had initial revision surgery using a tibial tubercle osteotomy that was too short—only 6 cm. This had failed to unite and assisted us in exposure in this instance.

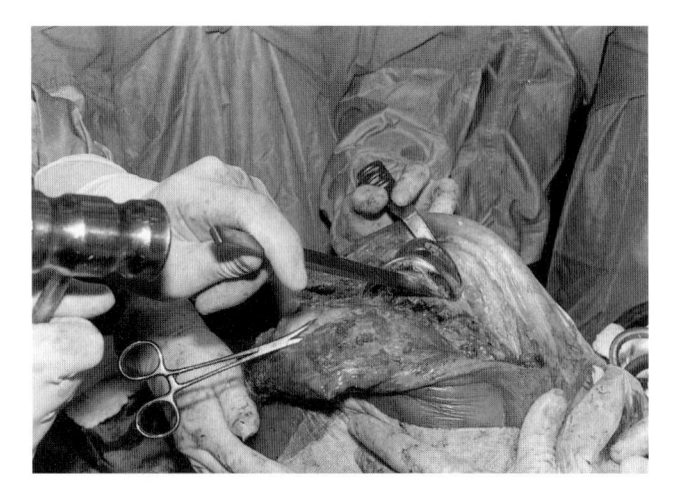

Figure 50.6. Use of osteotome to break down the bone-cement interface of the femoral component.

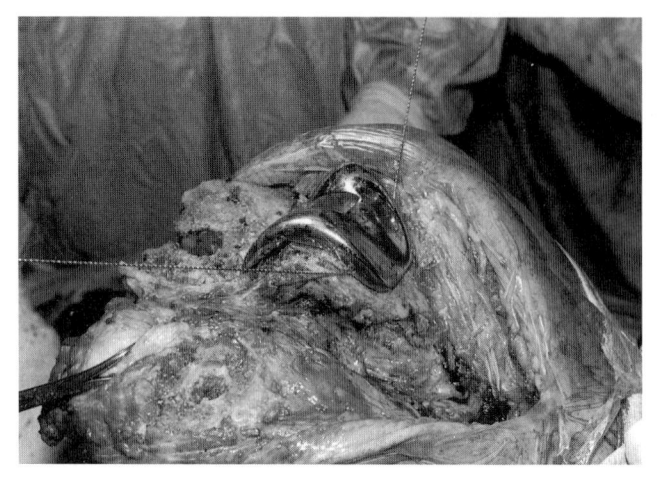

Figure 50.8. The Gigli saw is most effective in taking the interface bond down. It is drawn back and forth with steady force rather like two people sawing a log.

effective, these instruments are expensive and the cutting bits are single use and may be damaged in the course of the procedure, necessitating the use of several such bits—also a consideration in these days of cost containment (Fig. 50.7). Not every institution has access to such technology and many prefer to use the more standard oscillating saws with varying blade sizes to remove the implant.

The Gigli saw is another valuable adjunct in the removal of the femoral component (Fig. 50.8). The Gigli saw can be drawn from proximal to distal beneath the front of the femoral component down to the level of either the stem of the component if present, or the fixation lugs. This method allows good control of the removal process, minimizing damage to bone stock. Similarly, the Gigli saw can be passed behind the posterior flange of the component using a curved instrument and then drawn anteriorly, again as far as the stem

or lugs. This maneuver is made easier if the tibial component is modular and the polyethylene liner can be removed, thus providing more room for exposure at the back of the knee.

Great pains are taken to free the component as far as possible. When the femoral component is a standard resurfacing design, a combination of the above will give satisfactory mobilization of the component. Once the component has been mobilized, an extraction device can be attached to remove the component (Fig. 50.9). Many systems have their own such devices; however, a simple punch or similar tool for gently disimpacting the component is equally effective (Fig. 50.10).

Occasionally one is confronted with the scenario of a femoral component with a well-fixed cemented stem. In

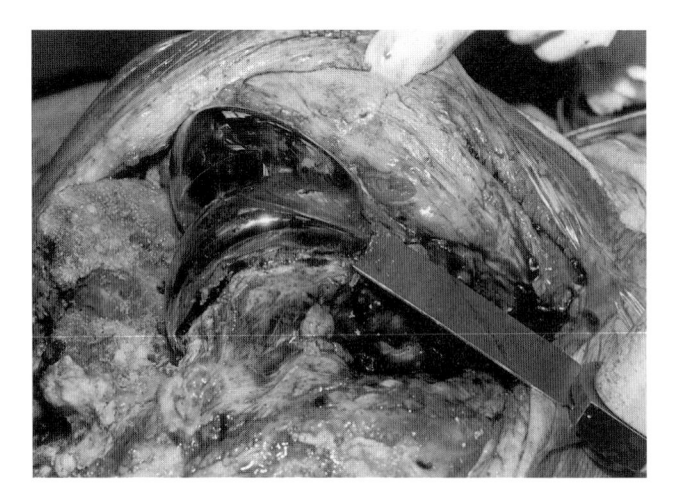

Figure 50.7. A power saw carefully directed can rapidly take down an interface.

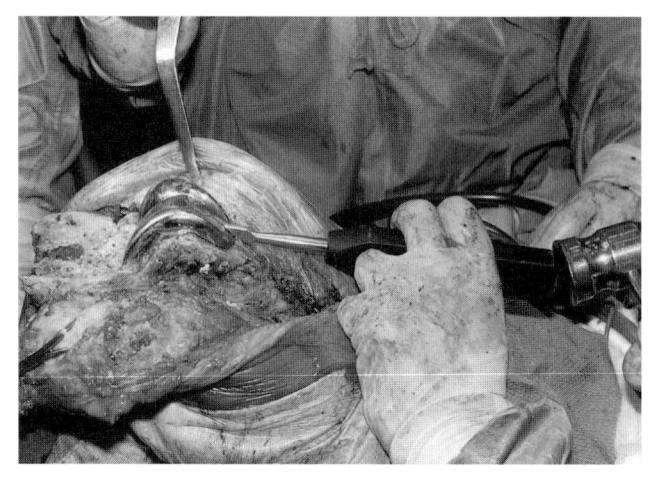

Figure 50.9. The extraction punch is used after the interfaces are broken down as far as possible. Care is taken not to use too great a force as fracture may occur with over vigorous hammering.

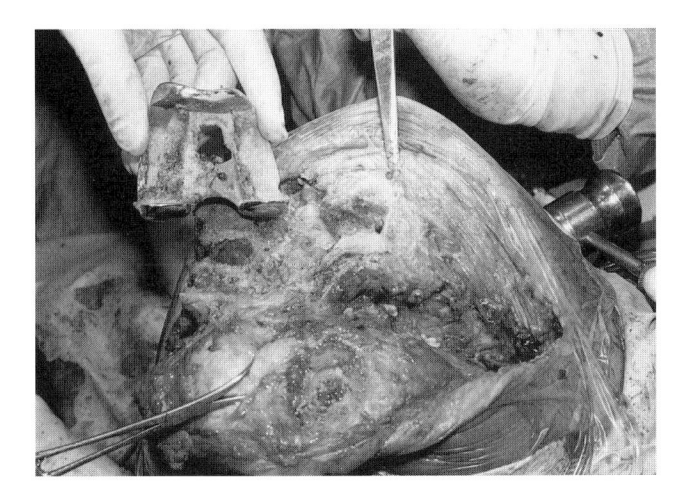

Figure 50.10. The objective is to remove the femoral component with minimal damage to bone stock.

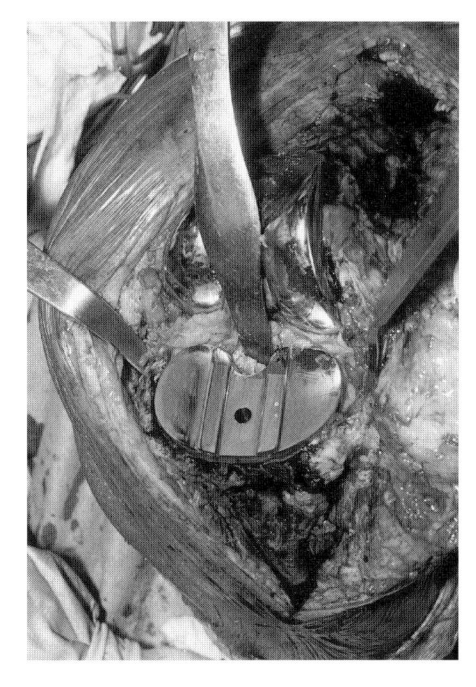

Figure 50.11. Circumferential exposure of the proximal tibia is required to visualize interfaces.

this situation mobilizing the interfaces as described is the first step in removal. When the stem is smooth, disimpaction can be undertaken with confidence that the stem will disengage its mantle without damage to surrounding bone. Difficulties have been encountered in the removal of components with porous coating and that are well fixed with cement.[8] In this situation the stem cannot be disengaged from the stem by use of extraction punches and to attempt to do so risks major damage to the bone. The cement-prosthesis interface must be accessed in order to achieve controlled removal of the stem in this scenario. Options available include windowing the anterior femoral cortex to obtain access to the stem, disrupting the cement mantle under direct vision, then removing the component in its entirety. Alternatively, the component may be transected using a high-speed cutting burr at the base of the stem. The condylar portion of the component can be removed, allowing access to the stem, which can then be removed in a manner similar to that used in extraction of femoral components in total hip arthroplasty.

REMOVAL OF THE TIBIAL COMPONENT

Once the femoral component has been removed, the exposure of the tibial component may be accomplished more readily. The proximal tibia is subluxed anterolaterally through the use of a carefully placed posterior retractor levering forward, with care taken not to damage the bone of the distal femur by using undue force. Once again, the insertion of the patellar tendon is carefully protected in exposing the proximal tibia. If this insertion is at all at risk, despite using additional measures of exposure such as a quadriceps snip or turndown, an unthreaded pin can be driven into the site of insertion to further reinforce it. As is the case in removal of the femoral component, the entire circumference of the component is displayed in order to view the whole implant-bone or cement-bone interface (Fig. 50.11). This measure allows removal of the component with greatest control and hence least potential damage to the patient's bone.

If the tibial component is a metal-backed modular design, the polyethylene liner is removed. A number of implant systems have customized instruments for removal of their respective polyethylene components, and these should be used if possible because they allow the simplest and least traumatic means of removal of that component. If such instruments are not available, most polyethylene liners can be removed by driving an osteotome or similar tool between the polyethylene and the metal baseplate or by transecting the insert (Fig. 50.12).

If the tibial component, whether all-polyethylene or metal-backed has a smooth stem, the situation is relatively straightforward. The interface is carefully taken down under direct vision to minimize damage to bone stock. One can use osteotomes or power instruments as described above for the femoral component to disrupt the component-cement or component-bone interface (Fig. 50.13).

Once the proximal interface has been mobilized sufficiently, an extraction force can be applied to remove the component so the stem, being smooth, will disengage without damage to bone stock. The use here of the technique of stacked osteotomes to progressively extract the component is very effective. Alternatively, an ex-

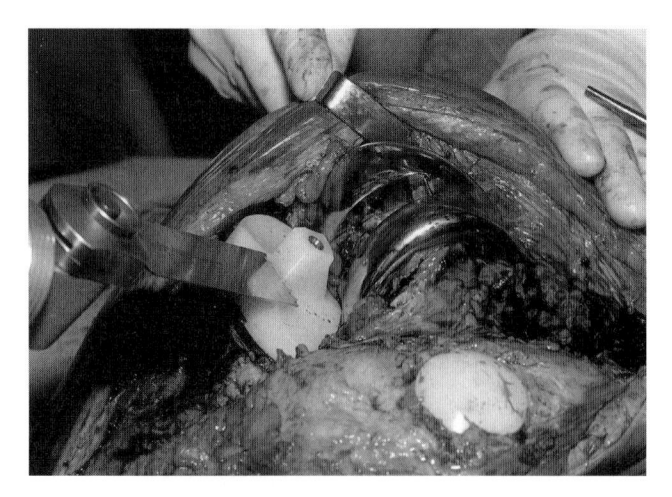

Figure 50.12. Transection of the posterior-stabilizing polyethylene component enables easy removal of the locking pin and then removal of the spacer.

traction device can be attached to the component and a slap hammer used to remove the component (Fig. 50.14).

Following removal of the components the cement is then removed. Cement removal from around stems is similar to that in total hip arthroplasty revision. Cement removal instruments are indispensable when removing cement from the depths of the femoral or tibial canals.

The situation is rendered more complex in the situation in which the tibial component has a stem cemented that is not smooth, or an uncemented distally porous-coated (or similar) stem that is well fixed distally. Here, the application of an extraction force despite having satisfactorily mobilized the proximal interface may seriously damage the bone through either fracture of the shaft or a segment of the plateau, or through avulsion of a segment of central metaphysis, leaving a large cavitatory defect. In these scenarios, one must access the in-

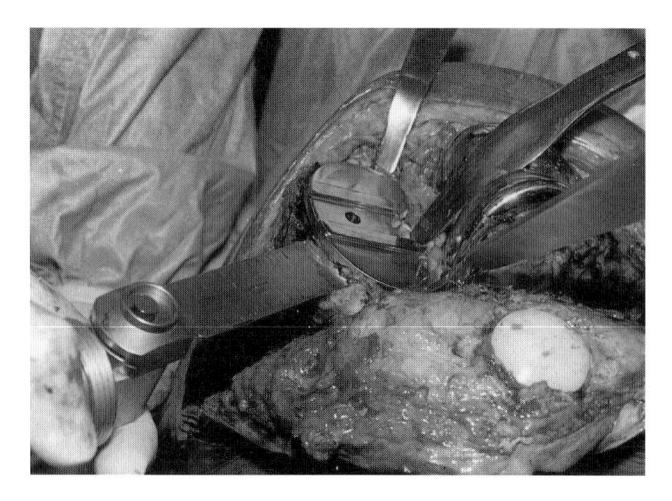

Figure 50.13. A power saw used to take down the tibial component interface.

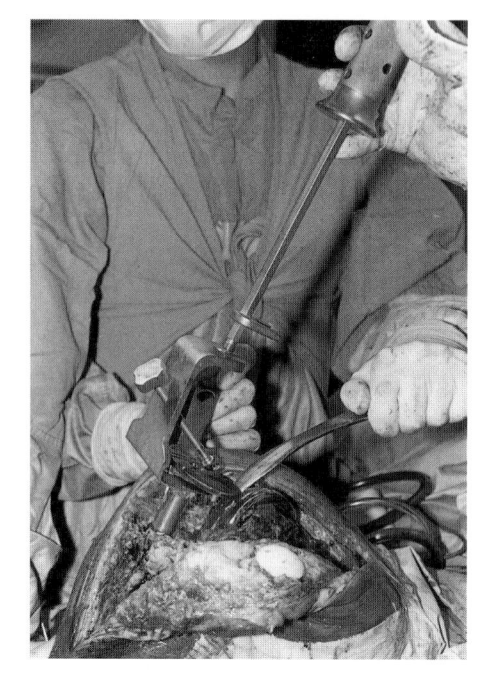

Figure 50.14. An extraction device such as this one allows well-directed and controlled force for removal of the component.

terface at the stem to enable controlled removal of the component. Several strategies can be employed to achieve this. The use of a tibial tubercle osteotomy, as described by Whiteside,[2] allows good access to the stem in such a case. Creating a window in the tibia has the attraction of providing good access to the stem while not disturbing the tibial tubercle, thus avoiding potential problems with obtaining union of the tibial tubercle in the case of an osteotomy.

Alternatively, access to the well-fixed stem can be achieved by transecting the tibial tray at the junction between tray and stem using a diamond-coated cutting wheel. The tray can then be removed independently, allowing free access to the stem. The stem can then be mobilized using a combination of high-speed burrs and osteotomes and then removed. Cement remaining is likewise extracted using cement removal instruments.

EXTRACTION OF THE PATELLAR COMPONENT

In the revision situation the decision to revise the patellar component is often vexed. If the component is well fixed and in good condition, it is often advisable to leave the component in situ even though it may not be an optimal match for the revision system planned, because removal of such a well-fixed component may leave such poor bone stock that reimplantation is difficult. Extraction of the patellar component begins with adequate visualization. The patella should be well mobilized to enable its inversion without placing the quadriceps insertion at risk. The additional exposure measures of tibial tubercle osteotomy and quadriceps snip or turndown all facilitate patellar exposure. The patella is stabilized by the assistant using two large, sharp towel clips placed at either end of the patella. The circumference of the component is exposed using cutting diathermy and rongeurs to expose the component-bone or component-cement interface.

In the case of all-polyethylene patellar components, the patellar button can be removed by first cutting across the stem or lugs with a power instrument (Fig. 50.15). The remaining stem or lugs can then be removed by use of a high-speed burr or a tube saw may be passed over the stem or lug.

Removal of metal-backed patellar components is more difficult to achieve without damaging the patella. In this situation the interface is taken down using either thin osteotomes or power instruments. Once the interface has been fully mobilized, careful levering with an osteotome may well be sufficient to pry the component loose. If this is not sufficient, the technique of stacked osteotomes can be used to extract the component (Fig. 50.16). This is somewhat more difficult in the patella because the component is small and stacking osteotomes around the periphery of the component is rather a balancing act. Very rarely is it necessary to transect a metal-backed component using cutting instruments in order to access well-fixed stems or lugs.

SUMMARY

Removal of the componentry from a failed total knee arthroplasty is only one of the initial steps in what is often a difficult surgical undertaking. The following points are central to successful component removal.

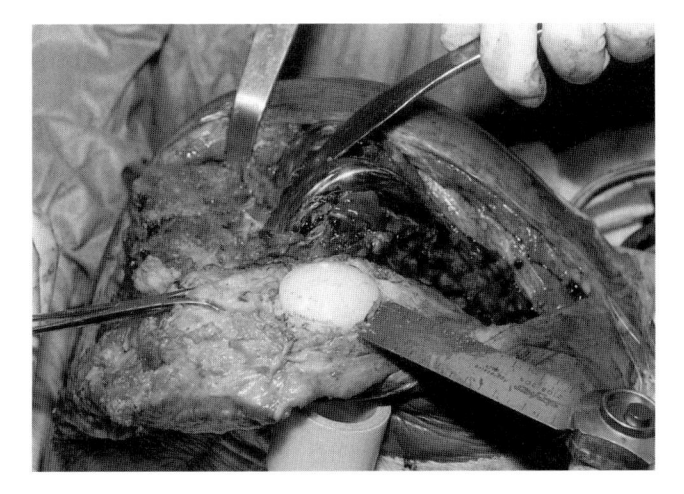

Figure 50.15. The patellar component is circumferentially exposed and the patella stabilized by an assistant. A power saw in this case is being used to transect the component.

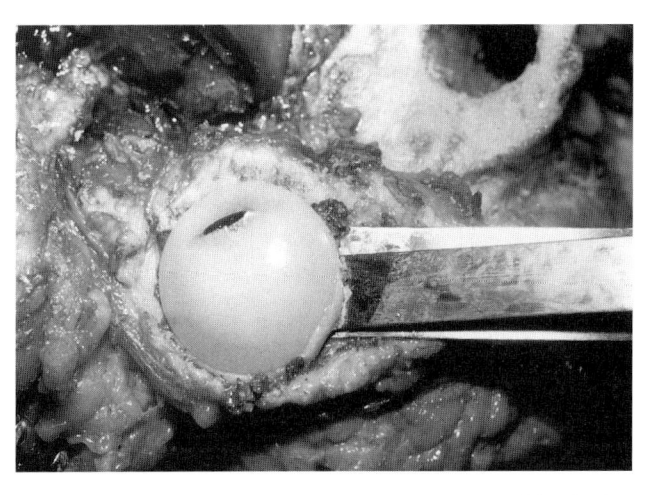

Figure 50.16. Stacking of osteotomes about a metal-backed patellar component.

1. Always plan your removal strategy from the skin incision onward.
2. Do not hesitate to use one of the described extensile exposure measures because you must be able to see all interfaces without struggling for view.
3. Take all the time you need to break down interfaces as described. Time taken here will ensure removal of components with as little damage to bone stock as possible. Haste or undue force can only lead to disaster and an even more difficult revision scenario.

References

1. Insall JN. Revision of aseptic failed total knee arthroplasty. In: *Surgery of the Knee*. 2nd ed. New York: Churchill Livingstone; 1993:935–957.
2. Whiteside LA, Ohl MD. Tibial tubercle osteotomy for exposure of the difficult total knee arthroplasty. *Clin Orthop*. 1990; 260:6–9.
3. Dolin MG. Osteotomy of the tibial tubercle in total knee replacement. A technical note. *J Bone Joint Surg*. 1983; 65A: 704–706.
4. Wolff AM, Hungerford DS, Krakow KA, Jacobs MS. Osteotomy of the tibial tubercle during total knee replacement. *J Bone Joint Surg*. 1989; 71A:848–852.
5. Garvin KL, Scuderi G, Insall JN. Evolution of the quadriceps snip. *Clin Orthop*. 1995; 321:131–137.
6. Coonse K, Adams JD. A new operative approach to the knee joint. *Surg Gynaecol Obstet*. 1943; 77:344–347.
7. Trousdale RT, Hanssen AD, Rand JA, Cahalan TD. V-Y quadricepsplasty in total knee arthroplasty. *Clin Orthop*. 1993; 286:48–55.
8. Windsor RE, Scuderi GR, Insall JN. Revision of well-fixed cemented, porous coated total knee arthroplasty. Report of six cases. *J Arthroplasty* 1988; (Suppl 3):87–94.

CHAPTER 51
Three-Step Technique for Revision Total Knee Arthroplasty

Kelly G. Vince and Daniel A. Oakes

INTRODUCTION

Revision knee arthroplasty surgery requires that order be restored to the chaos of failure. Once the failed components, cement, and useless weak bone have been removed from the knee, a gaping hole confronts the surgeon. The problems of stability, mobility, fixation, and the reconstruction of bone defects as well as restoration of an anatomic joint line all cry out for attention at once. There are undoubtedly a variety of approaches to the revision knee surgery. One thing is certain—an organized approach is essential or the reconstruction is doomed to failure (Fig. 51.1).

This chapter proposes three steps to the reconstruction of any knee regardless of the original cause of failure. The surgeon must (1) reestablish the tibial platform, (2) stabilize the knee in flexion, and (3) stabilize the knee in extension. These steps have been described previously[1–3] and are based upon the principles of knee arthroplasty surgery that were developed for the total condylar knee prosthesis by John Insall, Chit Ranawat, and Peter Walker at The Hospital for Special Surgery in New York in the early 1970s.[4,5] We have applied these concepts to revision knee surgery, expanding them to address the rigors of the failed knee and establishing an appropriate sequence. Faithful adherence to the proposed sequence of steps, building one stage upon the other leads to a successful revision knee arthroplasty (Table 51.1).

Although contemporary instruments have enabled every surgeon to produce good primary knee arthroplasties, they rely on bone for reference. This bone simply does not exist in the failed knee. Consequently, instrument systems have not been reliable for revision surgery. Missing bone, however, is not the greatest challenge facing the surgeon. More problematic are the soft tissues. Working with strong concepts and trial components, the surgeon will be able to understand the vagaries of lost, plastically deformed, overly tight, and unreleased ligaments.

This chapter does not deal with the diagnosis of a failed knee arthroplasty nor with the techniques for the removal of components from a failed knee. It must be emphasized, however, that no revision surgery should be attempted until an accurate mechanical explanation for the failure has been established. Revision of the inexplicably painful knee arthroplasty will yield miserable results.

Step 1   Establish Tibial Platform (Figure 51.2)

The tibia is a platform on which to rebuild the knee. The tibial articular surface is involved with knee function, irrespective of joint position. Whereas the distal femur bears load only in full extension and the posterior femur only in flexion, the tibia is constantly part of the articulation. The phrase tibial "platform" is chosen purposefully. Do not be concerned about the articular surface at this stage, that will come later.

The proximal tibia will have suffered any amount of insult from the failed joint. Although good-quality host bone is respected, any tibial cutting guide can be used to "square up" the surface by removing obviously weak and dispensable tissue. Defects are identified at this point, not eliminated. Any bone cut made now must not sacrifice good bone in an effort to eliminate a bone defect.

In many revision knee arthroplasties, medullary fixation will be required to enhance fixation. If so, open the medullary canal and confirm the measurements of endosteal diameter made on preoperative radiographs, using hand reamers. Bone should not be removed from the tibial canal, which has a relatively thin cortex. A suitable trial rod is selected and attached to a trial tibial component. Once seated in the medullary canal, the tibial trial defines the defective bone that will require re-

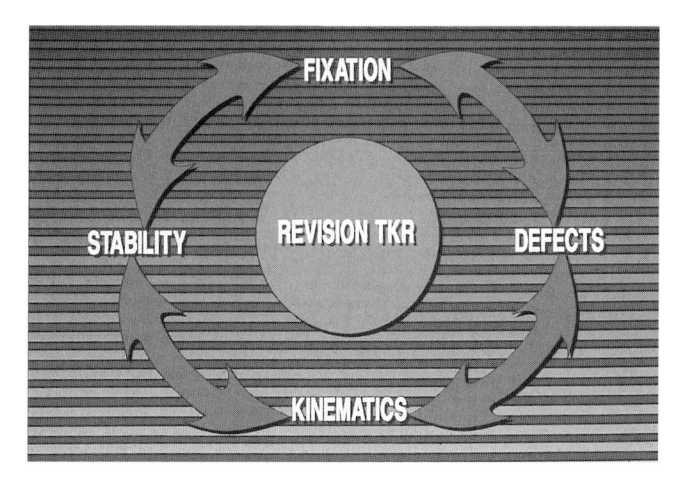

Figure 51.1. Diagram of problems of revision surgery from slides.

construction. If the intramedullary rod, fitted into the canal, is not parallel to the long axis of the tibia, the rod may be too wide for the asymmetric canal and either a narrower rod or one that is offset may be required.

There are several complex classification systems for describing bone defects at revision knee surgery. The simplest approach, in the course of a demanding surgery, will be the most helpful. Defects that are contained and have a rim of bone to hold bone graft, can be filled with particulate graft, be it autograft from the knee, ground up fresh-frozen bone, or freeze-dried allograft bone chips. Noncontained defects, as seen when a tibial component has subsided into varus, will most easily be dealt with by modular wedges or blocks. Combined contained and noncontained defects exist and respond well to a combined approach—the contained area is filled with graft and the noncontained area is reconstructed with an augment on top of the graft (Table 51.2).

Massive defects that offer virtually no host bone on which to seat any of the component will usually require reconstruction with structural allograft. These unusual situations should still be reconstructed following the three steps that are described here.

Tibial defects can be reconstructed at this stage and the tibial component even cemented into place to save time. This is because the tibial platform does not affect how we reestablish alignment, stability, and motion in the knee. We build the knee upon the tibia. Tension and laxity in flexion and extension are manipulated with the femoral component. Nonetheless, in the interest of keeping most of our options open, it is best to leave the trial tibia in place, noting the type of bone defect if any and how we plan to reconstruct it when we implant the final components.

Step 2 Stabilize Knee in Flexion (Figure 51.3)

(A) Choose the Size of the Femoral Component That Stabilizes the Knee in Flexion

Choose the size of the femoral component that stabilizes the knee in flexion. It is a common and deadly error to measure existing bone and simply fit the corresponding femoral component to it. In almost every case, this will lead to the selection of a femoral component that is too small and an arthroplasty that is unstable in flexion or one in which excessive distal femoral bone must be resected to accommodate an unduly thick articular polyethylene. Undue resection of distal femur results in an unacceptable proximal migration of the joint line.

Ignore the residual bone on the distal femur in this step and visualize the normal bone that was present before any surgery had been performed. Use the size of the failed component, and lateral radiographs of the contralateral knee, if unoperated, to estimate the size of the revision femoral component. The final choice of revision femoral component size will depend upon the an-

Table 51.1. Three-step revision knee arthroplasty

Step	Goal	Key
1	Establish tibial platform	Tibia is common to flexion and extension gaps. It is a foundation to build on.
2	Stabilize knee in flexion	Femoral component size and position stabilize the knee in flexion.
2(A)	Sizing the femoral component	Do not simply fit component to the residual bone.
2(B)	Femoral component rotation	The component must not be internally rotated. Feel the residual posterior condylar bone as a guide. Use posterior lateral augments to correct internal rotation.
2(C)	Joint line	In general, a smaller femoral component leads to a higher joint line.
Decision 1	Gap mismatch	Flexion gap is so large due to soft tissue failure that the knee cannot be stabilized in flexion by the size of the femoral component. Need constrained component or ligament reconstruction.
3	Stabilize knee in extension	Seat the femoral component more proximally or distally to create an extension gap that equals the flexion gap.
Decision 2	Varus-valgus instability	The collateral ligaments are incompetent and either a constrained component or a ligament reconstruction will be required.

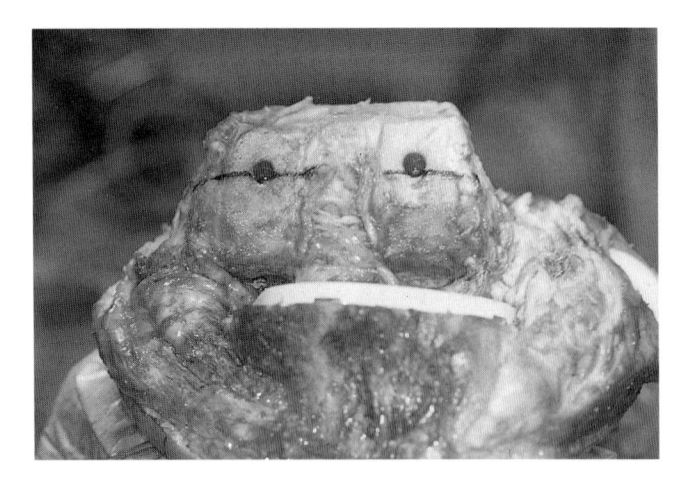

Figure 51.2. The tibial platform is reestablished.

teroposterior dimension that is necessary to stabilize the knee in flexion. The revision femoral component size will be determined not by residual bone, so much as by the soft tissues, specifically the collateral ligaments.

Stability in flexion is determined not only by the size, but also by the anteroposterior location of the femoral component. Unless the original component was oversized, leaving good posterior condyles for the revision component, fixation will be compromised because bone has been lost from the posterior condyles as a result of the failed knee or the removal of components. That is the purpose of posterior femoral augments. They exist to fill in bone defects and consequently to stabilize the knee in flexion by enabling the surgeon to select an appropriately large femoral component. Without them, we would be forced to use components that were too small.

In the presence of defective bone, due either to defects or soft quality, enhance fixation with medullary stems. These will influence the position of the femoral component and accordingly the stability of the knee in flexion. Stems can create problems. If large canal filling stems are selected, there will be little latitude for adjustment of the component position.[6] The component may be positioned in greater varus or valgus, flexion or extension or translated anteriorly or posteriorly, depending on the morphology of the femur. The position of smaller stems that are cemented in the canal (despite the undesirability of methacrylate in the canal) can be manipulated, anterior and posterior to affect the size of the flexion gap.

One situation that may arise when trying to determine the size of the femoral component is a gap mismatch. This important (and unusual) circumstance must be identified in any revision. Simply stated, a knee with an irreconcilable gap mismatch has a capacious flexion gap that, because of soft tissue failure, cannot be balanced to the likely dimensions of the extension gap with conventional releases or selection of the correct femoral component size. When the collateral ligaments, in particular the medial collateral, have stretched, it seems that we cannot find a femoral component large enough to stabilize the knee in flexion without an unacceptably thick polyethylene. The necessary femoral component may be so large that it no longer fits the medial to lateral dimensions of the bone. We have a knee that cannot be stabilized in flexion simply by recreating the anteroposterior dimensions of the femur.

Table 51.2. A simple approach to bone defects

Bone defect	Solution
Contained	Particulate bone graft
Noncontained	Modular wedge or block
Massive	Structural allograft

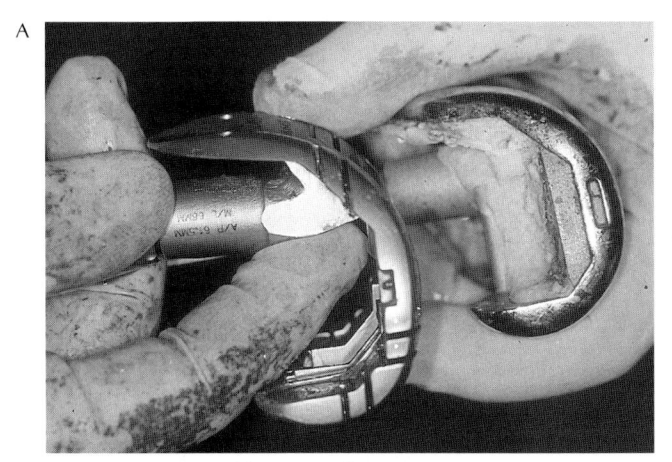

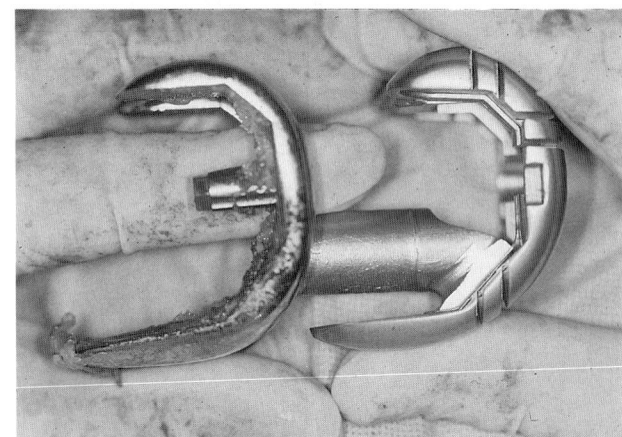

Figure 51.3. The femoral component is sized against the one removed. (A) If the knee was loose in flexion, a large femoral component is selected; or (B) if the original implant was sized correctly, a comparable revision femoral component is chosen.

The gap mismatch marks a decision point in the revision requiring a choice between accepting the laxity in flexion and protecting the patient with a constrained component or advancing the collateral ligament on the femur.[7] Our preference has been to avoid linked, constrained devices (hinges) in all cases, and to even reconstruct ligaments *and* use a nonlinked constrained device. With this decision noted, the femoral component size and position established and the tibial insert selected, the difficult work of the arthroplasty is complete.

(B) Seat the Femoral Component in External Rotation

The femoral component must be correctly rotated in the femoral canal. Internal rotation leads to patellar maltracking and a host of extensor mechanism problems. What landmarks exist for the correct rotation of the revision femur? There are two: the epicondylar axis and the height of residual posterior condylar bone.

The epicondylar axis, an imaginary line joining the medial and lateral epicondyles (where the collateral ligaments attach to the femur) lies in variable amounts of external rotation. It defines the attachment of the collateral ligaments and accordingly their functional length. The residual posterior condylar bone, hidden in the back of the knee, is another reliable guide. Though not visible, it is palpable. With the knee flexed to 90 degrees, one can feel the residual bone above the posterior condyles, by running a finger up onto the posterior femoral cortex (Fig. 51.4). If there is much more bone left on the medial side as compared to the lateral side, we know that the failed femoral component had been implanted in internal rotation. The converse implies external rotation.

Again, do not be fooled by the residual bone and seat a revision femoral component in internal rotation. Defective bone should be reconstructed with augments. Use posterior augments preferentially on the lateral side to correct internal rotation.

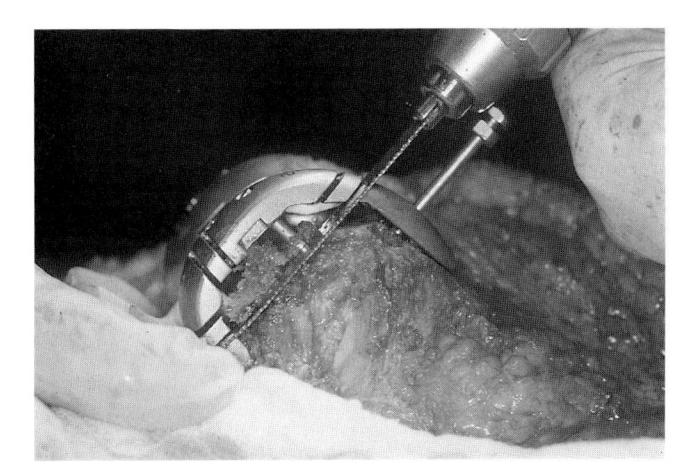

Figure 51.4. Rotational position of the femoral component can be determined by palpation of the posterior femoral condyles.

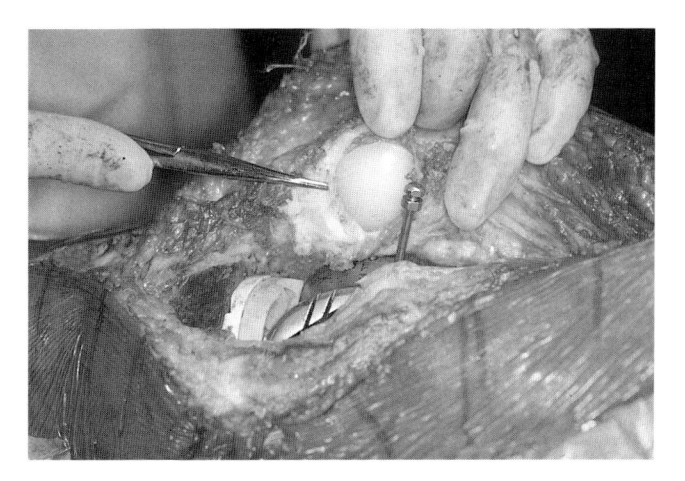

Figure 51.5. The point at which the femoral component meets the tibial articular surface is the joint line. The patella height is then noted.

(C) Reestablish the Joint Line

We have seen that stability in flexion is determined by the revision femoral component size and position. To fully stabilize the knee requires a polyethylene tibial insert so that the combined height of the posterior condyles of the femoral component and the tibial insert match the dimensions of the flexion gap. The point at which the femoral component meets the tibial polyethylene is the joint line. Where then does the patella lie? (Fig. 51.5)

The challenge for the surgeon is to match the prosthetic joint line height as closely as possible to the anatomic joint line. What is the best remaining landmark for approximating the anatomic joint line? The location of the inferior pole of the patella, when the knee is flexed to 90 degrees is an easily identified and reliable indicator of desired joint line. Ideally, the joint line should lie distal to the inferior pole of the patella. In choosing between two femoral component sizes, both of which stabilize the knee in flexion, but each of which requires different thicknesses of tibial polyethylene, select the combination that gives the best patellar height.

Step 3 Seat Femoral Component to Stabilize Knee in Extension (Figure 51.6)

This part is easy. The femoral component must be seated on the distal femur so that there is neither recurvatum nor a flexion contracture. If the trial components result in recurvatum, the femoral component may be seated more distally by using distal femoral augments. This will be the case in the majority of revisions in which bone is missing as a result of failed primary. Selecting a thicker polyethylene tibial insert instead of a distal

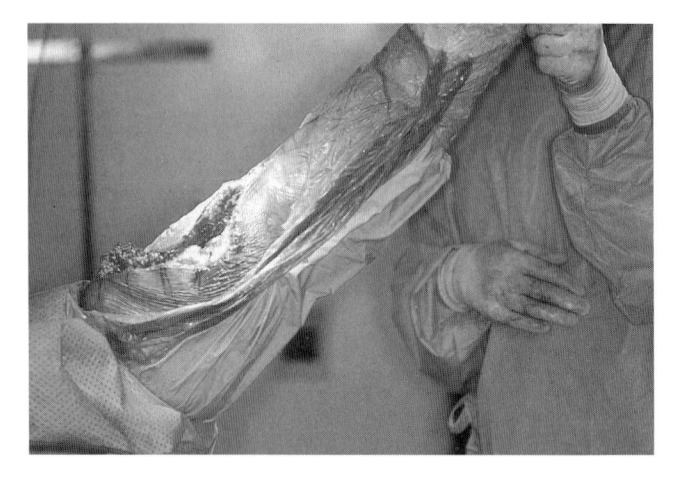

Figure 51.6. With the provisional components in place the knee is brought to full extension.

femoral augment will unbalance the stability that had been achieved in Step 2, in which the knee was stabilized in flexion.

Rarely, the surgeon may resect additional distal femur to stabilize the knee in extension. This may occur for the knee that had failed with a fixed flexion contracture, especially if the joint line had been *lowered* during the primary arthroplasty. When distal femoral resection is contemplated, check that it is not for the purpose of accommodating an inordinately thick tibial insert that is going to result in proximal joint line migration. This could be a gap mismatch.

DECISION POINT: SOFT TISSUE BALANCE IMPOSSIBLE?

In trying to stabilize the knee in extension it may become apparent that one or both of the collateral ligaments is deficient. A failed medial collateral, producing valgus instability, is the most disabling. When the medial collateral has suffered true plastic failure, it will not be possible to stabilize the knee by releasing the lateral side. Despite extensive lateral collateral releases, the medial ligament remains lax. All further releases simply lengthen the lateral side, and increasingly thick articular polyethylene creates a flexion contracture because the posterior structures are intact.[8] This is a decision point. The revision cannot be left without a functional MCL and either a constrained implant or a ligament reconstruction (or both) will be required.

CONCLUSION

Having (1) reestablished the tibial platform, (2) stabilized the knee in flexion, and (3) stabilized the knee in extension, the revision arthroplasty is effectively complete. The trial components can be removed and the bone prepared for implantation of the permanent components. The three steps lend themselves to what-

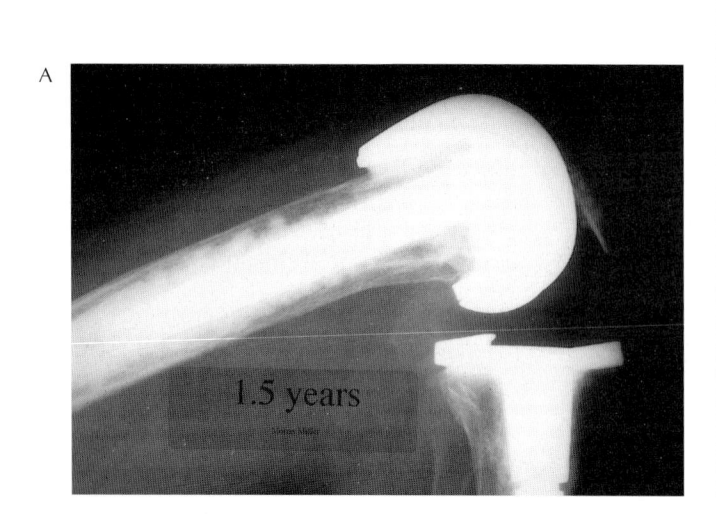

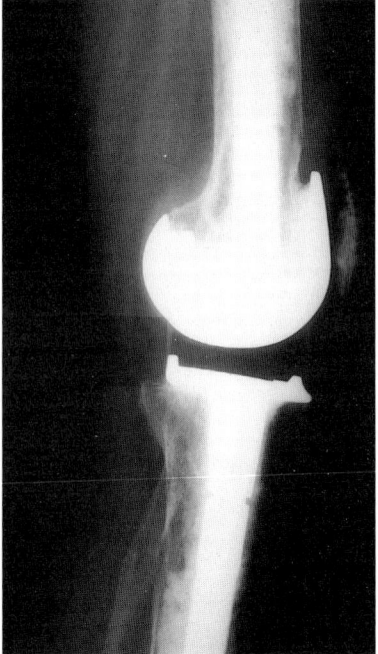

Figure 51.7. The revision arthroplasty should be stable in (A) flexion and (B) extension.

ever implant is planned for the revision. Although posterior-stabilized implants generally provide a higher degree of stability for the revision, these steps can lead to a sound reconstruction when cruciate-retaining implants are selected. As has been indicated by the "decision points," circumstances arise when the pathology of the deformity dictates the best choice of implant.

The three steps to revision knee arthroplasty presented here provide the surgeon with an orderly approach based on sound surgical principles. Meticulous preoperative planning and adherence to the steps should allow the knee surgeon to overcome the daunting challenge of the revision knee arthroplasty (Fig. 51.7).

References

1. Vince KG. Revision Knee Arthroplasty Instructional Course Lectures of the AAOS. Mosby; 1992.
2. Vince K. Revision knee arthroplasty. In: Chapman, ed. *Operative Orthopedics*. Philadelphia: JB Lippincott; 1993:1981–2010.
3. Vince K. Planning revision total knee arthroplasty. *Seminars in Arthroplasty*; 1996.
4. Insall JN. Total knee replacement. In: Insall JN, ed. *Surgery of the Knee*. New York: Churchill Livingstone; 1984:587–696.
5. Vince KG, Insall JN. The total condylar knee arthroplasty. In: Laskin, ed. *Total Knee Arthroplasty*. New York: Springer Verlag; 1991.
6. Vince KG, Long W. Revision knee arthroplasty. The limits of press fit medullary fixation. *Clin Orthop*. August 1995;(317):172–177.
7. Vince K, Berkowitz R, Spitzer A. Ligament Reconstructions in Difficult Primary and Revision TKR. Accepted for presentation at the Annual Meeting of the Knee Society. San Francisco, California, February 1997.
8. Vince KG. Limb length discrepancy after revision total knee arthroplasty. *Techniques in Orthop*. 1988; 3:35–43.

SECTION 15
Management of Bone Loss in Revision Arthroplasty

CHAPTER 52
General Concepts

Emil H. Schemitsch and Thomas S. Thornhill

Bone loss in total knee arthroplasty is a common and difficult problem. Bone defects are seen in both revision and primary total knee arthroplasty. Management of these defects remains controversial. Failure to adequately address bone loss compromises the stability and longevity of newly inserted implants. The current review outlines the various options available and provides a rational approach to management.

ETIOLOGY OF BONE STOCK DEFICIENCY

The etiology of bone loss after total knee arthroplasty is multifactorial. Bone stock deficiency may occur as a result of bone remodeling, osteolysis, implant loosening, and implant removal.[1] Stress shielding of the proximal tibia and distal femur following total knee arthroplasty may cause clinically significant osteopenia.[1–3] Osteolysis is a biologic response to particulate wear debris following total knee arthroplasty so that destruction of bone stock occurs.[4–7] Implant loosening results in pathologic motion between implant and bone that causes increased wear debris and the formation of a biologically active membrane.[1] Removal of a firmly fixed prosthesis, even if performed with an excellent technique, results in removal of some bone with the implant. The loss of bone after total knee arthroplasty is in addition to that normally taken at the time of the original procedure.

CLASSIFICATION OF BONE STOCK DEFICIENCY

An appropriate classification system is necessary to evaluate the various management techniques for bone stock deficiency. Defects are classified by the bone involved (femur or tibia), the location within the bone and by the size and symmetry of the defect.[8] The defect location may be classified as contained, peripheral, or a combination of the two. A contained defect is a cavity surrounded by host cortical or corticocancellous bone that is intact. A peripheral defect is a deficiency of the cortical rim that normally would support an implant and if grafted requires fixation for stability. Both contained and peripheral defects may or may not be load bearing. A symmetric defect results in equal bone loss on either side of the femur or tibia. An asymmetric defect results in unequal bone loss on either side of the femur or tibia. The size of the defect may be classified as grade 1 (less than 1 cm), grade 2 (1 to 2 cm), grade 3 (greater than 2 cm).

MANAGEMENT OPTIONS FOR BONE STOCK DEFICIENCY

The goals of management of bone loss in total knee arthroplasty are to maintain the joint line, to obtain satisfactory alignment, to preserve ligament balance and remaining bone stock, and to create an optimal mechanical environment for support of the prosthesis. Optimal implant stability may be obtained by preserving strong viable remaining host bone and repairing bone defects. Bone defects in primary and revision total knee arthroplasty can be managed by several different methods. Treatment options are limited by the size of the defect. Smaller defects (less than 1 cm) can be managed by resecting the femur or tibia at a higher or lower level, filling the defect with cement, or by shifting the component off of the defect.[9] These methods, however, are less satisfactory for larger defects of bone stock.[9] For larger defects, one can consider the use of cement alone, cement with screw augmentation, modular metallic wedges affixed to the undersurface of the prosthesis, bone grafting (autograft or allograft), and custom prostheses. The choice of method of defect management is based on preoperative planning with intraoperative assessment of defects, as well as availability of bone graft materials and prostheses.

PLANNING FOR BONE STOCK DEFICIENCY

Preoperative planning includes assessment of the size of the original components, if performing a revision total knee arthroplasty, and measuring the opposite knee if normal.[10] This allows for an accurate representation of the true dimensions of the femur and tibia and the amount of femoral and tibial bone loss. Intraoperative estimation of the extent of bone deficiency is made after the initial femoral and tibial resections have been performed.[8] Spacers can be used to estimate the amount of bone loss from the femur and tibia.[10] One must determine the amount of bone stock deficiency that requires restoration, by aiming for a normal joint line and symmetrical flexion and extension gaps. Landmarks that can be used include the femoral epicondyles, the posterior femoral condyles, the tibial tubercle, the insertion of the collateral ligaments, the fibular head, and the patellar position.[10] The tibial bone loss contribution will be the same in both flexion and extension whereas the femoral contribution is posterior in flexion and distal in extension.[10]

TIBIAL DEFECTS—PERIPHERAL

Prior to choosing a method of tibial defect management, one must have an accurate and reliable method of radiographic assessment of defect size. This radiographic measurement technique has been previously described.[9] A point is chosen on the side of the joint contralateral to the defined defect. This point is chosen in the midpoint of the cartilage space. A line perpendicular to the long axis of the tibia is then constructed across the joint surface. A line perpendicular to this is then drawn to the deepest portion of the defect. The defect measured using this technique exceeds the defect encountered during surgery because it incorporates the remaining cartilage and proximal tibia prior to the tibial resection.

Intraoperative evaluation is also critical in defect assessment. Difficulty with tibial preparation occurs when a defect is still present after 1 cm of lateral tibial resection. If tilting of the tibial trial into the defect can be accomplished manually or with trial reduction, then stability of the prosthetic components is compromised.[11] A defect that usually results in compromise of stability of the tibial component is one that extends over an area of half of the tibial condyle and is 5 mm deep.[11] If a defect is present that results in instability of the tibial baseplate, one can consider the use of cement alone, cement with screw augmentation, modular metallic wedges affixed to the undersurface of the prosthesis, bone grafting (autograft or allograft), and custom prostheses. The choice of method of defect management is based both on preoperative planning and intraoperative assessment of defects.

Increased Bone Resection

The most common defect encountered in total knee arthroplasty is the posterior medial defect of the tibia in varus knee deformities.[8,12] This defect is usually grade 1 or less than 1 cm, so that it can effectively be managed by resecting more bone. This allows the component to rest on a flat surface. The safe level of proximal tibial resection is controversial. The level of tibial resection should usually not exceed 1 cm laterally to avoid compromising the durability of the implant.[8,13,14] The mechanical strength of the proximal tibia decreases with increasing depth of tibial resection.[14–17] Increased tibial resection is preferred in elderly patients, if the joint line is not altered more than 2 mm. Recent work suggests that the level of proximal tibial resection may not affect the long-term results of a knee arthroplasty and therefore can be performed deep enough to ensure adequate polyethylene thickness and retention of the original joint line.[18]

Component Translation

Increased tibial resection can also be combined with shifting the component,[19] particularly if small shifts preclude grafting or make it non-load bearing. The concern regarding this technique relates to the use of a smaller tibial component, which does not cap the tibial surface and may result in increased loading of the proximal tibia, inadequate support of the prosthesis, and component subsidence.[8,9]

Cement Fill

Cement fill of defects has been advocated in the past.[20] In biomechanical testing this method of defect management has been found to be inferior.[21] Clinically, the development of a radiolucent line under a defect filled by cement is often seen and clinical results are inferior.[11,12,22,23] The use of cement to fill defects of the tibia should therefore be limited to small peripheral defects that cause no compromise in the support of the tibial component. Cement fill is advantageous for very small defects, because cement conforms to the shape of very small defects. Cement fill is problematic because the cement cannot be pressurized, a large volume of cement may result in thermal necrosis, there is increased susceptibility to infection, formation of a fibrous membrane may occur at the cement-bone interface, and the folds or laminations associated with a large volume of cement may result in fatigue failure.[21,24–26] If cement is used, one should drill the sclerotic bone that is present to improve penetration, and to ensure that the cement does not run out of the defect.

Cement Fill Reinforced with Screws

Some authors have advocated the use of screws within cement to improve the performance of cement as a filler for peripheral defects of the tibia.[27] In biomechanical testing this method of defect management has once again been found to be inferior.[21] Despite this, Ritter and associates followed 47 patients who had a total knee arthroplasty in which cement and screws were used to fill a tibial defect, for an average 6.1 years.[27] There was no evidence of loosening and no components were revised. The screw head supports the undersurface of the tibial component and the addition of cement results in a more stable construct. This technique may have a role for peripheral defects that cause minor instability of the tibial component. Major defects should be managed with either bone grating or metal wedge augmentation.

Metallic Wedge Augmentation

The wedge augmentation technique has been previously described.[9] A tibial alignment or cutting guide is applied in neutral rotation and set for 8 to 10 mm of resection from the normal lateral plateau. The tibial plateau is resected with optional preservation of the posterior cruciate ligament. The tibia is then sized and the appropriate trial tibial tray is placed with a trial insert and articulated with a trial femoral component. The knee is extended, final ligament balance procedures are performed, and the proper rotatory alignment of the tibial component on the femoral component is determined and marked.

The size of the wedge needed is determined by measuring the distance between the bottom of the tray and the base of the defect. A wedge cutting block, if available, is positioned properly to fashion the defect to conform to the wedge slope and height. The bone resection is accomplished with a narrow oscillating sawblade. If a wedge cutting block is unavailable, an approximation of the necessary wedge is made and a trial implant is temporarily fixed to the undersurface of the trial tibial tray with bone wax. The bone defect is then contoured to receive the trial wedge by use of a high-speed burr. The wedge may be secured to the undersurface of the tibial tray by cement, snaps, or screws and the most optimum method is still unknown. If cement is used, one-half package of cement is mixed, and the wedge is permanently cemented to the underside of the tibial tray. A clamp holds the wedge and tray in position as the cement polymerizes. After the cement has polymerized and any extruded cement removed, routine implantation of the tibial and femoral components can proceed.

Any residual sclerotic bone is drilled to promote cement penetration. If screws or snaps are used, cementing is performed in one stage.

Metallic wedge augmentation is attractive because of the ease and simplicity of intraoperative fabrication of a custom implant to match a tibial defect. In biomechanical testing, a modular metal wedge provided superior loading to all other constructs except a custom component.[21] The wedge offers potential load transfer from the implant to the bone.[28] Most total knee systems offer a wide selection of blocks or half and full wedges to deal with most defects. Different shaped wedges (triangular versus rectangular) are mechanically similar,[29] although the load transfer across a large defect is better managed with a rectangular block than an angled wedge.[30] Triangular wedges are usually limited to 15 degrees in magnitude since the shear stresses at the cemented interface are significant.[31] Rectangular wedges avoid shear stresses but may require the removal of healthy bone to insert the wedge. The use of a longer stemmed tibial component has been shown to be biomechanically advantageous when used with a wedge,[29] but this has not been proven clinically.

Further clinical data has come to light to support the concept that a metal wedge affixed to the undersurface of a tibial tray can be successfully employed to augment tibial bone stock.[32–34] At midterm or average 5- to 6-year follow-up, no progressive radiolucencies in association with a tibial metal wedge have been detected.[18,33,34] This suggests that modular metallic wedges are a viable option to manage peripheral tibial defects and are an excellent alternative to standard techniques such as cement, cement and screws, and custom prostheses. Metal wedges do not require incorporation by the host and there is no risk of nonunion or collapse. Donor site morbidity is not a problem. The major concern has been the durability of the wedge-cement-prosthesis interface. Concern of a thin cement layer between implants is not warranted at midterm follow-up.[34] The use of a thin cement layer between implants avoids the concern of corrosion or metal debris. The use of screws between the wedge and tibial baseplate may improve the durability of the wedge-prosthesis interface and reduces operating time. The most optimal method of attachment of the wedge to the undersurface of the tibial baseplate has not been determined.

Cemented wedge fixation appears durable and avoids concerns of bone graft incorporation. The wedge system is appropriate for defects of 20 to 25 mm or smaller, as measured by the technique described previously and assuming a maximal tibial resection of 10 mm.[9] Larger defects will exceed the size of the largest wedge, requiring a significant cement mantle to support the component. In these cases, bone graft or a custom prosthesis should be employed.

The use of a modular wedge system is simple to use, adds minimal operating time, adds little to required inventory, and is versatile, providing the surgeon with the option of customizing a standard tibial tray.[9] The key to the long-term success of this system is proper alignment in the axial plane as well as proper component positioning.[9] The modular wedge system is an acceptable solution to managing severe defects in the elderly, low-demand population.[9] The younger, high-demand patient should be managed with bone graft, to restore bone stock for the future, because the defect remains at the time of future surgery.[8,9,12]

Bone Grafting

Bone grafting is the only management technique which allows for permanent restoration of bone stock.[12,22,25,26,35–42] It is also advantageous because it preserves subchondral bone and provides a uniform cement thickness.[26] There is also no additional implant cost, particularly related to custom components. Disadvantages of bone grafting include the need to find a donor source, difficulty in obtaining a stable fit of the graft into a bone defect and the unpredictable incorporation of the graft.[8] The choice of graft includes both autograft and allograft (cancellous morselized and structural). The use of autograft is usually limited to primary total knee replacement, because local bone is usually nonexistent in revision knee arthroplasty. Indications for autografting include peripheral defects greater than 5 mm in depth and/or greater than 50% of the involved tibial plateau.[8,22] Autografting is advantageous because the graft has osteogenic potential and disease transmission is avoided.

Local bone graft may be obtained from the proximal tibia, femoral condyles, or intercondylar cutout in posterior-stabilized knee arthroplasties. The graft should be prepared resulting in cancellous to cancellous interfaces, should ideally be stabilized with screws, and should have its interface with the host tibial plateau protected so that no cement violates the graft-host junction. Graft success is improved by satisfactory mechanical stability of the graft and an adequate bed for the graft with viable host cancellous bone. Autograft is not usually locally available in revision arthroplasty and, if chosen, one must consider the use of distant iliac crest graft.

There have been a number of techniques described for bone grafting.[22,26,43] These include the use of a self-locking dowel,[26] the use of oblique planar resection with placement of resected bone from the femoral condyles and fixation with perpendicular screws[26] and the creation of a horizontal ledge using a high-speed burr.[22] All techniques rely on exposure of bleeding cancellous bone, precise interference fitting of the graft into the bony defect, rigid fixation of the graft, component coverage of the graft, and correct component and limb alignment.[12] Clinical results have been variable with standard techniques of autografting with concerns related to nonunion, fragmentation and dissolution of the graft.[22,44,45] Failures usually occur due to limb malalignment with overload of the graft and poor graft fit in a sclerotic bony bed.[8,13,22]

Structural bone allografts are usually required in revision knee arthroplasty for uncontained defects that are more than 3 cm long.[46] Bulk allografts are advantageous because they provide for bone stock restoration, have potential for ligamentous attachment, are versatile, avoid unnecessary removal of host bone, and may be cost-effective. Disadvantages of bulk allografts include the potential for bone resorption with poor incorporation, fracture, nonunion, infection, disease transmission, the need for protected weight-bearing, and the uncertain long-term durability.

Various allograft donor locations exist including distal femur, proximal tibia, or femoral head. Biomechanical and structural superiority is offered by the use of femoral head allograft if possible.[47] Allograft preparation includes removal of soft tissue and marrow elements to decrease the immunologic response and orientation in the correct trabecular direction.[1,41] Screw holes or perforations in the graft should be avoided because they increase the potential for early revascularization, resorption, and graft collapse.[1] The allograft should be chosen and prepared to allow a stable interference fit into host bone.

Use of bulk allografts requires adequate fixation of the allograft to host bone, exposure of bleeding well-vascularized host bone and component coverage of the graft.[8] Failure of the allograft is associated with poor mechanical alignment, poor host bed preparation with sclerotic bone, residual cement debris, and membranous tissue and poor graft fit or fixation.[8,22] Any residual bone contributing to ligament origin or insertion should be preserved.[46] A long press-fit tibial stem should be used to protect and off-load a load-bearing structural allograft during its incorporation.[48] Cement should only be used for the condylar surface and not for the stem of the prosthesis. Cement that has access to the allograft host interface may prevent union and graft incorporation. A constrained implant may be required because of ligamentous insufficiency. The long-term outcome of allografts in revision total knee arthroplasty is unknown because most series average less than 5-years follow-up.[37,39–41,46,49] Even with such short follow-up, there is a significant incidence of complications including sepsis, graft collapse, nonunion, and revision.[39]

Bulk allografts can be in the form of smaller wedges or wafers or may be massive in the form of an entire proximal tibia or distal femur. The massive allograft-prosthesis composite technique has been described by

Mnaymneh and colleagues.[39] When there is major loss of cancellous bone from the metaphysis leaving a funnel-shaped cortical tube, an undersized allograft is invaginated and telescoped into the residual tibial empty cortical tube.[39] The allograft is secured tightly in place and rigidly fixed to the bone. When the end of the bone is virtually absent or the cortex is too attenuated to provide any structural support, it is transversely osteotomized leaving a good bony surface with an intact cortex.[39] A size-matched segmental proximal tibial allograft is inserted to replace the resected end of the bone and is rigidly fixed to the patient's bone.[39]

Massive proximal tibial defects can also be reconstructed using morselized cancellous allograft and a rigidly fixed tibial component, stabilized with screw fixation. This technique has been used with peripheral rim defects constituting three-fourths of the tibial circumference with good results.[50] It avoids the disadvantages of bulk allografts including bone resorption with poor incorporation, fracture, and nonunion. Although the experience with this technique is limited, it provides an additional option for reconstruction of deficient tibial bone stock.

Custom Components

Custom components have a limited role in management of bone loss. Their use should be considered for severe bone loss in grade-3 defects that cannot be managed by another technique. Although biomechanically advantageous, allowing excellent force transmission between the implant and the bone, custom components are expensive, often do not allow for a precise fit to the host bone at the time of surgery, require added time for manufacture, and do not allow for reconstitution of bone stock.[8,9,21]

Implant Fixation

Options for implant fixation in the presence of tibial bone loss include cemented, uncemented, and hybrid fixation. A long-stemmed tibial component is required if there is a need to stress shield the proximal tibia or if there is an unstable tibial baseplate. Tibial stems longer than 70 mm can relieve stress on either tibial plateau and bear approximately 30% of the weight-bearing load.[21,51] Although long-stemmed tibial components relieve stress in deficient bone, the effect may be so great as to cause significant stress shielding beyond that intended.[8] The most optimal method of implant fixation if a stem is required includes the use of cement for the condylar surface and the avoidance of cement for the stem.[52] An uncemented press-fit stem is not routinely required when using tibial wedge augmentation. Uncemented stems can engage the isthmus of the tibia with tip fit or enter the isthmus with side fit. Uncemented press fit stems are advantageous because they reduce the incidence of proximal stress shielding and allow for easier removal if revision is required.

TIBIAL DEFECTS—CENTRAL

Small central cavitary tibial defects may be managed with cement or morselized graft. If a rim of tibia remains that can support the tibial component, the durability of the tibial component will not be compromised by either of these methods.[11] If a cavitary defect is so large that it involves almost all the cancellous bone of the condyle, and only a peripheral rim of tibia remains, a structural graft is preferable so that more physiological support of the component is present for long-term durability.[11]

Large central tibial defects are filled with solid graft that is sculpted to press fit into the defect.[39] A long central stem on the tibial tray may be required to unload the graft in this situation by bypassing the graft. A sculpted bulk allograft should be used whenever the tibial component with a stem is not stable or the defect is large. If stability is present, a morselized graft may heal and accomplish long-term support without being in jeopardy of being overloaded during the early healing period.[11] If instability is present, a morselized graft should be avoided.

FEMORAL DEFECTS

Femoral defects are usually seen in revision total knee arthroplasty. A significant defect is one that results in instability of the femoral component on the distal femur.[11] Defects of the distal femur in primary and revision total knee arthroplasty can be managed by several different methods. As in the tibia, treatment options are limited by the size of the defect. Smaller defects can be managed by resecting the distal femur at a more proximal level or by filling the defect, if cavitary, with cement or morselized bone.[9,11] These methods, however, are unsatisfactory for larger defects of femoral bone stock, associated with instability of the femoral component.[9]

One must determine the amount of bone stock deficiency that requires restoration, by aiming for a normal joint line and symmetrical flexion and extension gaps. Landmarks that can be used are the fact that the normal joint line is 25 mm distal to a line drawn through the medial and lateral epicondyles, 20 mm superior from the midpoint of the tibial tubercle, and 14 to 16 mm from the origin of the posterior cruciate ligament.[11] The inferior pole of the patella should also be above the joint line.

Larger defects of femoral bone stock are usually seen only in revision arthroplasty. Bone loss may be anterior, distal, posterior, or combined and may be peripheral or cavitary. As in the tibia, options for filling severe distal femoral defects include the use of cement alone, cement with screw augmentation, modular metallic wedges affixed to the undersurface of the femoral component, bone grafting, and custom prostheses.[9] As in the tibia, the most optimal methods for management of significant femoral bone loss are femoral augmentation, bone grafting and custom prostheses.

Metallic Augmentation

Recent clinical data at early follow-up suggests that a metal augment affixed to the undersurface of a femoral component can be successfully employed to augment femoral bone stock, particularly if condylar loss is incomplete and asymmetrical.[53] Augmentation can be anterior, distal, posterior, medial, lateral, or combined. The augment restores alignment, improves the fit of the femoral component, and prevents subsidence or tilting of the femoral component.[11] There have been no cases of loosening and no revisions using this technique at average 4-year follow-up.[53] The rate of nonprogressive radiolucencies in this study was significant but was not associated with clinical failures. The technique is effective in restoration of the femoral joint line and has minimal morbidity. One must determine the amount of bone stock deficiency that requires restoration, by aiming for symmetrical flexion and extension gaps, in addition to a normal joint line. The femoral bone loss contribution is posterior in flexion and distal in extension.[10] Relative instability in flexion can be managed with posterior augmentation, whereas relative instability in extension can be managed with distal augmentation.

A modular femoral wedge can successfully correct moderate noncontained femoral defects in revision total knee replacement and avoids the unpredictable incorporation of bone grafts. Femoral augmentation is simple to use, adds minimal operating time, adds little to required inventory, and is versatile, providing the surgeon with the option of customizing a standard femoral component.

Bone Grafting

A cavitary defect of the distal femur without instability may be packed with morselized bone. In an elderly patient, a small cavitary defect may be filled with cement. With either cement or morselized graft, a press-fit stem should be used that bypasses the defect, if significant. If a femoral component is unstable, then management should be directed toward obtaining stability of the component. If instability exists, the defect must be managed with either bone graft or metal augmentation.

If distal femoral bone loss is severe, the only treatment options are a custom component or a massive allograft-prosthesis composite.[39,54] If an allograft is used, residual autogenous bone graft is maintained, with retention of a soft tissue sleeve containing the collateral ligaments, to eventually wrap around the allograft-host bone junctions as a vascularized graft.[46] A massive allograft-prosthesis composite is then created using the appropriate cutting jigs and cementing the prosthesis into the allograft.[54] Press-fit stem extensions are employed, obtaining a press fit into the host diaphysis and cemented fixation within the allograft.[54] Further stability is obtained by the use of a step cut at the host-allograft junction and if necessary, the addition of supplementary autograft or allograft struts or cirlage wires. Prolonged rigid fixation is necessary to obtain satisfactory union of the allograft to the host.[19,25,41,49] Fixation of the collateral ligaments is then performed. Protected weight-bearing is required until graft union occurs.

Complications following massive bulk allografts are frequent and include sepsis, nonunion, graft fragmentation, and collateral ligament failure. A reduced risk of allograft failure is obtained by the use of long-stem intramedullary fixation to obtain initial stability, achieving stability at the graft-host junction, satisfactory reattachment of host medial collateral ligaments to the allograft, use of increasing prosthetic constraint to achieve ligamentous stability, liberal use of supplementary autograft and the use of protected weight-bearing until host-allograft union has occurred.[54]

Implant Fixation

Options for implant fixation in the presence of femoral bone loss include cemented, uncemented, and hybrid fixation. The most optimal method includes the use of cement for the condylar surface and the avoidance of cement for the stem. A long-stemmed femoral component is required if there is significant anterior or posterior bone loss, significant anterior notching, or an unstable femoral component.

SUMMARY

Bone defects in primary and revision total knee arthroplasty can be managed by several different methods. Treatment options are limited by the size of the defect. Smaller defects can be managed by altering the resection level, filling the defect with cement, or by shifting the component off of the defect. These methods, however, are unsatisfactory for larger defects of bone stock.

Options for filling severe bone defects include modular metallic wedges affixed to the undersurface of the component, bone grafting, and custom prostheses. Bone grafting is the most physiologic alternative and is recommended for the younger patient. It does, however, have disadvantages including nonunion as well as the possibility of collapse and resorption of the graft. Modular metallic wedges are also a viable option to manage peripheral defects. Wedge fixation appears durable and avoids concerns of bone graft incorporation. The use of a modular wedge system is simple to use, adds minimal operating time, adds little to required inventory, and is versatile, providing the surgeon with the option of customizing standard components. The key to the long-term success of this system is proper alignment in the axial plane as well as proper component positioning. The modular wedge system is an acceptable solution to managing severe defects in the elderly, low-demand population. The younger, high-demand patient should be managed with bone graft to restore bone stock for the future.

References

1. Engh GA, Parks NL. The management of bone defects in revision total knee arthroplasty. In: Springfield DS, ed. *AAOS Instructional Course Lectures*. Vol. 46. Rosemont, Illinois: American Academy of Orthopaedic Surgeons; 1997.
2. Cameron HU, Cameron G. Stress-relief osteoporosis of the anterior femoral condyles in total knee replacement: A study of 185 patients. *Orthop Rev*. 1988; 16:394–495.
3. Mintzer CM, Robertson DD, Rackemann S, et al. Bone loss in the distal anterior femur after total knee arthroplasty. *Clin Orthop*. 1990; 260:135–143.
4. Cadambi A, Engh GA, Dwyer KA, et al. Osteolysis of the distal femur after total knee arthroplasty. *J Arthroplasty*. 1994; 9:579–594.
5. Dannenmaier WC, Haynes DW, Nelson CL. Granulomatous reaction and cystic bony destruction associated with high wear rate in a total knee prosthesis. *Clin Orthop*. 1985; 198:224–230.
6. Nolan JF, Bucknill TM. Aggressive granulomatosis from polyethylene failure in an uncemented knee replacement. *J Bone Joint Surg*. 1992; 74B:23–24.
7. Peters PC Jr, Engh GA, Dweyer KA, et al. Osteolysis after total knee arthroplasty without cement. *J Bone Joint Surg*. 1992; 74A:864–876.
8. Rand JA. Bone deficiency in total knee arthroplasty. Use of metal wedge augmentation. *Clin Orthop*. 1991; 271:63–71.
9. Brand MG, Daley RJ, Ewald FC, Scott RD. Tibial tray augmentation with modular metal wedges for tibial bone stock deficiency. *Clin Orthop*. 1989; 248:71–79.
10. Insall JN. Revision of aseptic failed total knee arthroplasty. In: Insall JN, ed. *Surgery of the Knee*. New York: Churchill Livingstone; 1994.
11. Dorr LD. Management of bone defects. In: Rand JA, ed. *Total Knee Arthroplasty*. New York: Raven Press, Ltd; 1993: 309–317.
12. Dorr LD. Bone grafts for bone loss with total knee replacement. *Orthop Clin North Am*. 1989; 20:179–187.
13. Dorr LD, Conaty JP, Schreiber R, Mehne DK, Hull D. Technical factors that influence mechanical loosening of total knee arthroplasty. In: Dorr LD, ed. *The Knee*. Baltimore: University Park Press; 1985: 121–135.
14. Hvid I. Trabecular bone strength at the knee. *Clin Orthop*. 1988; 227:210–221.
15. Behrens JC, Walker PS, Shoji H. Variation in strength and structure of cancellous bone at the knee. *J Biomechanics*. 1974; 7:201–209.
16. Harada Y, Wevers HW, Cooke TD. Distribution of bone strength in the proximal tibia. *J Arthroplasty* 1988; 3:167–175.
17. Sneppen O, Christensen P, Larsen H, Vang PS. Mechanical testing of trabecular bone in knee replacement. *Int Orthop*. 1981; 5:251.
18. Montgomery TJ, Ritter MA, Keating EM, Faris PM, Meding JB. The clinical significance of proximal tibial resection level in total knee arthroplasty. *Trans Knee Soc*. 1995; 31:32.
19. Lotke P. Tibial component translation for bone defects. *Orthop Trans*. 1985; 9:425 (abstract).
20. Lotke PA, Wong R, Ecker M. The use of methylmethacrylate in primary total knee replacements with large tibial defects. *Clin Orthop*. 1991; 270:288–294.
21. Brooks PJ, Walker PS, Scott RD. Tibial component fixation in deficient tibial bone stock. *Clin Orthop*. 1984; 184:302–308.
22. Dorr LD, Ranawatt CS, Sculco TA, McKaskill B, Orisek B. Bone graft for tibial defects in total knee arthroplasty. *Clin Orthop*. 1986; 205:153–165.
23. Insall JN, Lachiewicz PF, Burstein AH. The posterior stabilized condylar prosthesis: A modification of the total condylar design. *J Bone Joint Surg*. 1982; 64A:1317–1323.
24. Bartel DL, Burstein AH, Santavicca EA, Insall JN. Performance of the tibial component in total knee replacement. Conventional and revision designs. *J Bone Joint Surg*. 1982; 64A:1026–1033.
25. Wilde AH, Schickendantz MS, Stulberg BN, Go RT. The incorporation of tibial allografts in total knee arthroplasty. *J Bone Joint Surg*. 1990; 72A:815–824.
26. Windsor RE, Insall JN, Sculco TP. Bone grafting of tibial defects in primary and revision total knee arthroplasty. *Clin Orthop*. 1986; 205:132–137.
27. Ritter MA, Keating EM, Faris PM. Screw and cement fixation of large defects in total knee arthroplasty: a sequel. *J Arthroplasty*. 1993; 8:63–65.
28. Laskin RS. Management of fixed varus deformity. In: Hungerford DS, Krakow K, Kenna RV, eds. *Total Knee Arthroplasty. A Comprehensive Approach*. Baltimore: Williams & Wilkins; 1994.
29. Touchi H, Loch DA, Genuino VS, Bechtold JE, Gustilo RB. The effect of metal wedges on the strain distribution in the proximal tibia following total knee arthroplasty. *Trans Orthop Res Soc*. 1996; 42:731 (abstract).
30. Fehring TK, Peindl RD, Humble RS, Harrow RS. Modular tibial augmentations in total knee arthroplasty. *Clin Orthop*. 1996; 327:207–217.
31. Chen F, Krackow KA. Management of tibial defects in total knee arthroplasty. A biomechanical study. *Clin Orthop*. 1994; 305:249–257.
32. Jeffery RS, Orton MA, Denham RA. Wedged tibial components for total knee arthroplasty. *J Arthroplasty*. 1994; 9(4):381–387.
33. Pagnano MW, Trousdale RT, Rand JA. Tibial wedge aug-

mentation for bone deficiency in primary total knee arthroplasty. A follow-up study. *Trans Knee Soc.* 1995; 32–33.

34. Schemitsch EH, Scott RD, Ewald FC, Thornhill TS. Tibial tray augmentation with modular wedges for tibial bone stock deficiency. *J Bone Joint Surg.* (Supp) 1995; 77B:79 (abstract).

35. Borja FJ, Mnaymneh W. Bone allografts in salvage of difficult hip arthroplasties. *Clin Orthop.* 1985; 197:123–130.

36. Dennis DA. Structural allografting in revision total knee arthroplasty. *Orthopaedics* 1994; 17(9):849–851.

37. Harris A, Poddar S, Gitelis S, Sheinkop M, Rosenberg A. Arthroplasty with a composite of an allograft and a prosthesis for knees with severe deficiency of bone. *J Bone Joint Surg.* 1995; 77A:373–385.

38. Kraay MJ, Goldberg VM, Figgie MP, Figgie HE III. Distal femoral replacement with allograft/prosthetic reconstruction for treatment of supracondylar fractures in patients with total knee arthroplasty. *J Arthroplasty.* 1992; 7:7–16.

39. Mnaymneh W, Emerson RH, Borja F, Head W, Malinin T. Massive allografts in salvage revisions of failed total knee arthroplasties. *Clin Orthop.* 1990; 260:144–153.

40. Samuelson KM. Bone grafting and noncemented revision arthroplasty of the knee. *Clin Orthop.* 1988; 226:93–101.

41. Tsahakis P, Beaver W, Brick G. Technique and results of allograft reconstruction in revision total knee arthroplasty. *Clin Orthop.* 1994; 303:86–94.

42. Whiteside LA. Cementless revision total knee arthroplasty. *Clin Orthop.* 1993; 286:160–167.

43. Scuderi GR, Insall JN, Haas SB, Becker-Fluegel MW, Windsor RE. Inlay autogenic bone grafting of tibial defects in primary total knee arthroplasty. *Clin Orthop.* 1989; 248:93–97.

44. Altchek D, Sculco TP, Reulin B. Autogenous bone grafting for severe angular deformity in total knee arthroplasty. *J Arthroplasty.* 1989; 4:151–155.

45. Laskin RS. Total knee arthroplasty in the presence of large bony defects of the tibia and marked knee instability. *Clin Orthop.* 1989; 248:66–70.

46. Ghazavi MT, Stockley I, Yee G, Davis A, Gross AE. Reconstruction of massive bone defects with allograft in revision total knee arthroplasty. *J Bone Joint Surg.* 1997; 79-A(1):17–25.

47. Pelker R, Friedlander G. Biomechanical aspects of bone autografts and allografts. *Orthop Clin North Am.* 1987; 18:235–239.

48. Whiteside LA. Bone grafting in revision cementless total knee arthroplasty. *Tech Orthop.* 1992; 7:39–46.

49. Stockley I, McAuley JP, Gross AE. Allograft reconstruction in total knee arthroplasty. *J Bone Joint Surg.* 1992; 74B:393–397.

50. Whiteside LA. Cementless reconstruction of massive tibial bone loss in revision total knee arthroplasty. *Clin Orthop.* 1989; 248:80–86.

51. Reilly D, Walker PS, Ben-Dov M, Ewald FC. Effects of tibial components on load transfer in the upper tibia. *Clin Orthop.* 1982; 165:273–282.

52. Elia EA, Lotke PA. Results of revision total knee arthroplasty associated with significant bone loss. *Clin Orthop.* 1992; 271:114–121.

53. Schemitsch EH, Scott RD, Brick GW, Thornhill TS. Femoral augmentation with modular wedges for femoral bone stock deficiency. *Orthop Trans.* 1995; 19:499 (abstract).

54. Paprosky WG. Use of distal femoral allografts in revision total knee arthroplasty. In: Insall JN, Scott WN, Scuderi GR, eds. *Current Concepts in Primary and Revision Total Knee Arthroplasty.* Philadelphia: Lippincott-Raven Publishers; 1996.

55. Engh GA. Bone defect classification. In: Engh GA, Rorabeck CH, eds. *Revision Total Knee Arthroplasty.* Baltimore: Williams & Wilkins; 1997.

56. Pagnano MW, Trousdale RT, Rand JA. Tibial wedge augmentation for bone deficiency in primary total knee arthroplasty. *Clin Orthop.* 1995; 321:151–155.

CHAPTER 53
Classification of Bone Defects
Femur and Tibia

Gerard A. Engh

An easy-to-use classification system that pinpoints the extent and location of bone damage helps surgeons plan efficiently for revision total knee surgery. Preoperative radiographs should be used to classify such bone defects into categories of comparable difficulty. Once surgeons determine the severity of bone loss, they can make well-informed decisions regarding the type of prosthesis to be used, the need for bone graft, and any special equipment the procedure may require.

When preparing for revision arthroplasty, the surgeon should anticipate the worst-case scenario. Revisions involving severe bone loss require skill, experience, and extra preparation, which may include practice on laboratory sawbone models. Appropriate classification followed by careful preparation and specialized treatment to repair bone damage should improve clinical results. When outcome studies are performed on these cases, the additional expense of modular revision systems would be warranted. In addition, a case mix based on bone defects can justify an implant comparison and validate clinical results.

HISTORICAL REVIEW OF BONE DEFECT CLASSIFICATION SCHEMES

Several attempts have been made to establish a classification of bone deficiencies for both primary and revision knee replacement surgery. In general, these schemes try to either categorize defects with similarities into a small number of defect types, or separate defects into a larger number of more specific groups.

Dorr's classification[1] is the most straightforward; defects are defined as either central or peripheral and cases are separated as primary or revision procedures. No attempt is made to define the size and location of the defect.

Insall[2] uses similar terminology in primary cases of central and peripheral bone defects. His classification is based on how to treat the defect: cement alone (stage 1); cement or augmentation plus a stemmed component (stage 2); or massive defects that require block augmentation and stem extension (stage 3).

In revision surgery, Insall's classification is primarily a visual description of bone defects that describes patterns of bone loss in both the femur and tibia. Femoral defects are categorized as symmetrical and asymmetrical distal loss, central and medial or lateral peg hole defects, distal ice cream cone, and asymmetrical ice cream cone deficiencies. Tibial deficiencies are categorized as proximal loss, asymmetrical loss, full slope, ice cream cone, asymmetrical ice cream cone, and contained defects.

Rand's classification is also based solely on the appearance of the defect at surgery. Rand's classification[3] differentiates three types of defects based on a combination of the depth of the defect and the percentage of the condyle involved. The most severe cavitary defect is further subdivided according to the integrity of the peripheral rim.

A comprehensive classification of bone deficiencies, which covers any and all defects of the femur, tibia, or patella, has been proposed by Bargar and Gross.[4] Four types of defects are defined for the femur and tibia and three types for the patella. Segmental, cavitary, and discontinuity defects can occur in any of the three locations, with intercalary defects as a fourth category for the tibia and femur. This scheme is similar to a classification system recommended by the Hip Society for defects adjacent to failed total hip implants. The large number of defects makes this classification cumbersome and somewhat impractical.

PREREQUISITES FOR A BONE DEFECT CLASSIFICATION

No bone defect classification has been accepted by orthopedic surgeons. Therefore, when the Anderson Orthopaedic Research Institute (AORI) bone defect classification was developed,[5] the goal was to make the system easy to understand and apply. The following criteria were the basis of the AORI classification:

1. The same terminology was employed for femoral and tibial defects because of the similarities in the metaphyseal segments of the femur and tibia.
2. The commonly used definitions in most classifications of bone defects, as central or peripheral, cortical or cancellous, contained or uncontained, were eliminated because of the absence of cortical bone in the metaphyseal segments of the distal femur and proximal tibia (Fig. 53.1).
3. Clear and precise definitions were established that minimize ambiguity when bone defects are categorized.
4. A minimal number of defect types was established to permit clinical investigators to accumulate enough cases to allow meaningful statistical comparisons.
5. This classification was designed to allow retrospective categorization of cases through intraoperative information and postoperative radiographs.

X-RAY TECHNIQUE

It is important to have quality X-rays when classifying a bone defect. A true lateral view is essential to evaluate the location and extent of osteolysis that may be obscured by the prosthesis on an oblique radiograph. To obtain a "true" lateral view of the knee, the radiograph should be taken in 90 degrees of flexion, placing the entire leg, including the knee and ankle, flat on the radiograph table. If a true lateral view is not obtained, repeat radiographs should be performed after rotating the knee either internally or externally or moving the patient a few inches proximal or distal from the center of the beam.

AORI BONE DEFECT CLASSIFICATION

In this system, a defect is only classified when a component has been removed. If both the femoral and tibial components are removed, the femur and the tibia are each assigned a defect classification. Defects are classified from preoperative radiographs for anticipated bone deficiency and then the classification is either confirmed or changed intraoperatively. The femoral epicondyles, the posterior femoral condyles, and location of the patella relative to the joint line may be used as landmarks to differentiate complex femoral defects. The fibular head and the tibial tubercle should be used as landmarks for tibial defects that are difficult to classify.

Occasionally there is the need to classify a bone defect from postrevision radiographs. The metaphyseal segments of the femur and tibia have a distinct profile (Fig. 53.1). The main criterion to look for is a reduction in this profile and the dimensions of the metaphyseal segments of the femoral condyles and/or the tibial plateaus. The distance from the epicondyle to the end of the femur varies according to an individual's bone structure and size, but this distance is proportional to all other dimensions of the bone. A bone defect, however, alters this relationship. For example, a shortened distance from the epicondyle and metaphyseal flare to the end of the femoral component will be visible if a distal bone defect has not been repaired with a bone graft or an augment to restore a normal joint line. If the bone defects were reconstructed with cement, augments, or grafts and the joint line restored, this will be evident on postrevision radiographs and also in the patient's operative note. On the radiograph, the metaphyseal bone segment should appear as a shortened segment, with an augmented component or bone graft filling the deficient area.

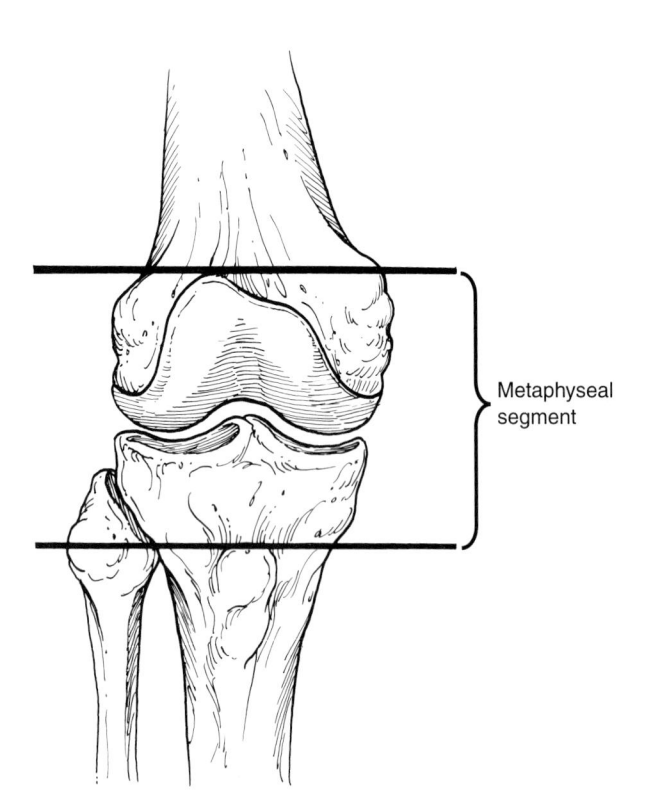

Figure 53.1. Metaphyseal region of the femur and tibia.

Therefore, the following definitions are the foundation of this classification:

Type 1 Defect (INTACT metaphyseal bone): Minor bone defects that do not compromise the stability of the component.

Type 2 Defect (DAMAGED metaphyseal bone): Loss of cancellous bone that necessitates an area of cement fill, augments, or bone graft to restore a reasonable joint line level. Type 2 bone defects can occur in one-femoral condyle or tibial plateau (2A), or in both condyles or plateaus (2B).

Type 3 Defect (DEFICIENT metaphyseal segment): Bone loss that compromises a major portion of either condyle or plateau. These defects are occasionally associated with collateral or patellar ligament detachment and usually require bone grafts or custom implants.

In any classification scheme, some cases will fall on the borderline. To classify these cases, it is necessary to evaluate the postoperative radiographs and the surgical treatment mode. For example, if a primary component was used, no bone defect was addressed in the operative note, and the postoperative radiographs demonstrate joint line restoration, an F3/T3 defect would not apply. If a structural bone graft, major cement fill, or a hinged component with condylar resection was used in the revision, we would conclude that the patient had a significant F2/T2 or F3/T3 bone defect.

Bone defects also occur in the patella but are not classified in the AORI bone defect classification. Patellar defects were excluded because they do not affect management decisions with revision surgery. In these cases, bone grafting is not an option and revision components to address such defects are not available, except for the biconvex patellar design of the Genesis Knee (Smith & Nephew, Memphis, TN). In most instances patellar bone defects are managed simply by not resurfacing the damaged patellar bone.

FEMORAL BONE DEFECT

F1 DEFECTS (Figure 53.2)

The preoperative radiographs of the Type 1 femur demonstrate a correctly aligned component with no evidence of femoral osteolysis. They also show no significant component migration, and a normal joint line level is indicated by patellar height and epicondyle to implant distance. On an anteroposterior radiograph, the quality of bone appears to be strong enough in the metaphyseal segment of the femur to support a component without a stem. The dimensions of the posterior femoral condyles are full, allowing substitution of an implant of the same size with normal condylar dimensions. An augmented component or a modular wedge is not

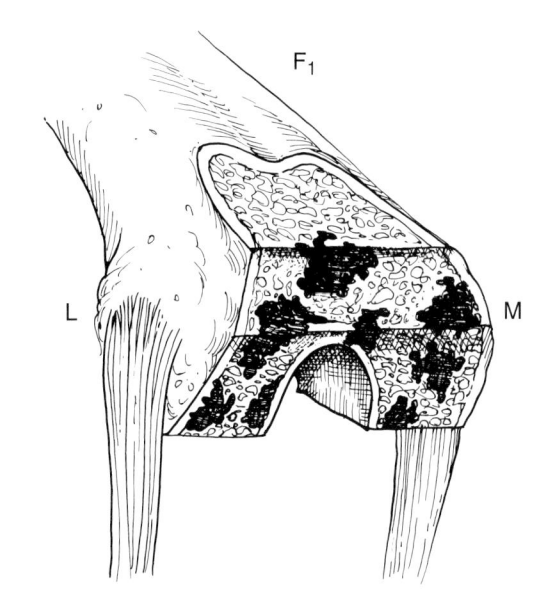

Figure 53.2. F1 Defect

needed to restore joint line level. Minor surface irregularities from cement plugs are managed with particulate bone graft or cement. Table 53.1 summarizes the features and treatment modalities of an F1 defect.

The postoperative radiographs of a Type 1 femur show a relatively normal joint line level with the patella about 1 cm proximal to the tibial plateau. The femoral condyles appear full on the anteroposterior radiograph; the posterior condylar offset created by preserving the posterior condylar bone is evident on the lateral radiograph. The proximal tip of the component's posterior condyle should match the proximal end of the patient's posterior femoral condyle.

F2 DEFECTS

The F2 femoral bone defect is characterized by osteolysis or significant proximal migration of the femoral component. Radiographs may reveal subsidence of the implant with a circumferential radiolucency. Also, the loss of distance from the epicondyles to the end of the implant will be apparent on the anteroposterior radiograph. Femoral osteolysis should not extend above the epicondyles.

In some F2 defects, the normal relationship of the femoral component to the shaft of the femur (6 degrees valgus) is altered. The implant subsides with angular migration into an incorrect varus or valgus posture relative to the anatomic axis of the femur. The F2A defect often demonstrates an increased varus or valgus orientation of the femoral component (from the normal 6 degrees). In an F2A defect, bone of the uninvolved condyle is present at a normal joint line level. See Table 53.1 for a summary of bone defects.

Table 53.1. Guideline for classifying defects

Defect type	Identifying features	Treatment
F1/T1	no component subsidence or osteolysis; no cancellous defects in the peripheral rim; cancellous bone that will support an implant; defects can be filled by small amounts of particulate bone graft or cement; a normal joint line is present	no augments (>4 mm), structural grafts, or cement fill (>1 cm); no stemmed components necessary
	femur—full condylar profile *tibia*—component above the fibular head and a full metaphyseal segment	
F2/T2	cancellous bone inadequate to support the implant; cancellous defects may require bone grafts; the component used requires augmentation to restore the joint line; osteolysis may be more extensive than radiographs indicate	joint line restored with an augmented component (>4 mm), particulate autograft or allograft, or cement fill (>1 cm); stemmed components should be used
	femur—reduced condylar profile *tibia*—component is at or below the tip of the fibular head and the tibial flare is reduced	
F3/T3	marked component migration; knee instability; deficient metaphyseal segment	structural graft, augment or cement, or a hinged component used to reconstruct the condyle or plateau; stemmed components required
	femur—loss of collateral ligament attachments from one or both condyles; severe condylar bone loss from osteolysis or a comminuted supracondylar fracture	

F2A Defects: One Condyle (Figure 53.3)

A Type 2A femur can involve either condyle. The cancellous bone of the involved condyle may have been damaged by osteolysis or iatrogenically if an incorrect angular resection of the distal femur was made at the time of the primary arthroplasty. The bone of the opposite femoral condyle is relatively intact near a normal joint line level.

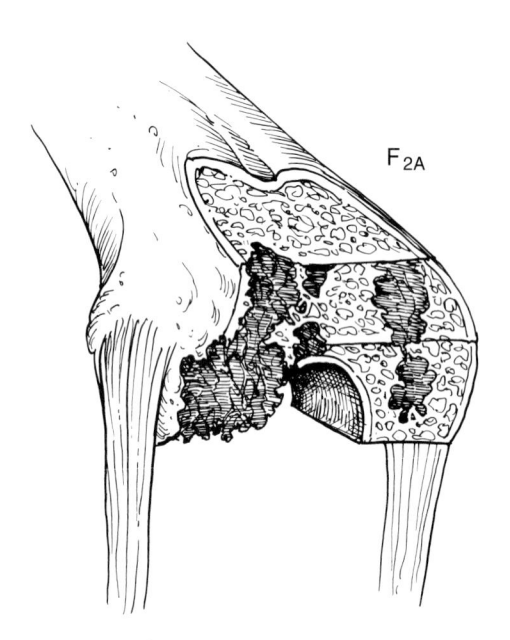

Figure 53.3. F2A Defect

The radiographic criterion for a Type 2A femur is the presence of unilateral elevation of the joint line with adequate bone in the opposite condyle for component fixation. The presence of minor bone defects in the opposite condyle does not alter the classification of a Type 2A defect as long as the opposite condyle maintains a relatively normal joint line level.

Reconstruction of an F2A defect with a primary implant is rarely indicated. In most instances, the damaged condyle should be repaired with a modular augment to restore a normal joint line. In some circumstances, an F2A defect should be treated with incomplete joint line restoration. This may be necessary to correct a large preoperative flexion contracture. An F2A defect is converted to an F2B defect when the opposite condyle is resected at a more proximal level. When the joint line is elevated, a smaller femoral component is needed to restore flexion-extension balance.

Postoperative radiographs of a correctly reconstructed F2A defect should show the augmented or repaired condyle. The anteroposterior radiograph may demonstrate the more proximal resection level of the condyle. However, an augment is not always visible on the lateral radiograph if it is hidden by the box of a posterior-stabilized or more constrained implant.

F2B Defect: Both Condyles (Figure 53.4)

The defect in a Type 2B femur is identical to the Type 2A defect except that it involves both femoral condyles. The damaged metaphyseal bone requires reconstruction

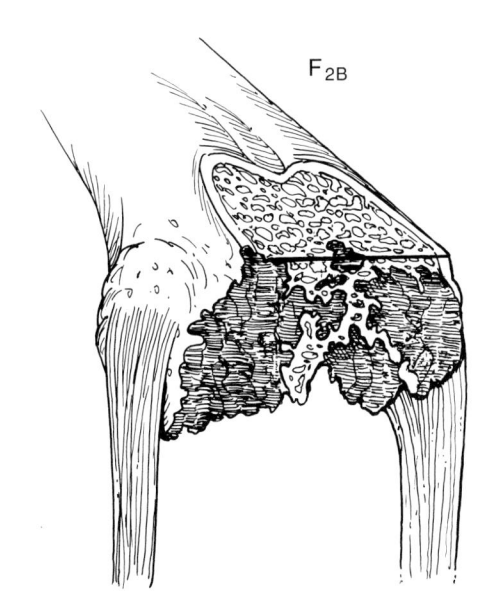

Figure 53.4. F2B Defect

of both condyles with bone, cement, or augments to restore an acceptable joint line level. Cases of multiple revisions and failure of stemmed femoral components often create Type 2B defects.

On the anteroposterior radiograph of a subsided femoral component, the distance from the distal end of the component to the epicondyles appears to have decreased. If the epicondyles are flared by component migration, the defect is extensive and indicative of an F3 defect. On an anteroposterior radiograph, osteolysis may be visible in the bone between the component and the metaphyseal edge of the bone. Also, patella baja may be present on the lateral radiograph. With proximal migration of the prosthetic joint line, the posterior condyle of the component may have migrated to a position above the patient's remaining posterior femoral condyle. Extensive cement fill proximal to a femoral component usually results in an F2B classification.

It is often necessary to augment both femoral condyles distally and posteriorly by using modular wedges to restore joint line level. Cement fill, sometimes reinforced with cancellous bone screws at the base of the defect, may be used to replace lost bone when the interface is not good for cement bonding. An F2B defect should always be revised with a stemmed component.

Some F2B defects require joint line elevation to restore adequate knee motion. This is true in a stiff knee with a flexion contracture greater than 20 degrees. If a release of the contracted posterior capsule proves inadequate, joint line elevation without augmentation may be needed to correct the patient's flexion contracture. A stemmed revision component should be used.

The postoperative radiographs of an F2B defect demonstrate either joint line elevation without repair of a major bone defect, or a joint line that has been restored with augments, bone graft, or a thick mantle of cement beneath the component. The metaphyseal segment of bone will appear shortened and replaced by the increased thickness of the femoral component. Bone grafts may be difficult to see if the graft is in close apposition to host bone and if the host bone has been sufficiently reamed to a cancellous bed. The patella may be at or below the top of the tibial component, thereby indicating joint line elevation.

F3 DEFECT (Figure 53.5)

Type 3 femoral defects have extensive structural bone loss, involving a major portion of one or both femoral condyles. See Table 53.1 for identifying features of F3 defects.

The preoperative radiographs of F3 defects demonstrate osteolysis and/or severe component migration to the level of the epicondyles. When the femur migrates, the epicondyles flare away from the component. Although the severity of osteolysis is not always apparent on radiographs, the surgeon should assume that osteolysis is present and may be far more severe than anticipated. Osteolysis usually appears as a defect in the cancellous bone adjacent to the implant. The most common locations are at the margins of the femoral component, and usually appear with a sclerotic and scalloped border. Lytic lesions of osteolysis frequently begin in areas where the femoral component is not bonded to underlying host bone.[6] Although many osteolytic defects demonstrate a sclerotic border, the most aggressive lesions may not have this radiographic feature.

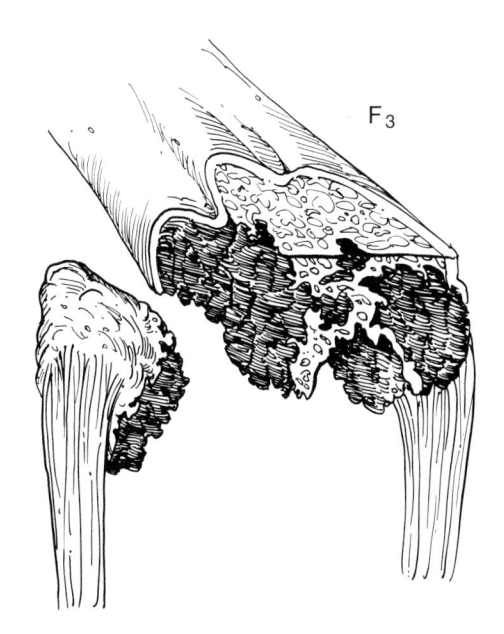

Figure 53.5. F3 Defect

Failure of a hinged, custom, or revision component often results in an F3 defect. These components devices often have stems that migrate in the axis of the femur. A significant amount of bone is lost or sacrificed when these devices are implanted. In these cases, the expanded metaphyseal segment of the femur is shortened.

The surgical reconstruction of an F3 defect is a salvage type procedure requiring a major replacement of metaphyseal bone with either a structural allograft or a custom femoral component. The extensive bone loss may involve one or both condyles. A varus-valgus constrained implant, or preservation and reattachment of one or both collateral ligaments, may be necessary. In this case, a canal-filling stem is required. Rotational stability of the femoral component may require fully cementing the stem or step cutting the allograft and host bone.

The postoperative radiographs of Type 3 femurs demonstrate the reconstruction of a segment of the distal femoral metaphysis and in some instances, diaphysis. Hinged devices are classified as F3 defects because they replace the metaphyseal segment and are recognized by the linkage joining the two components. Demarcation of the allograft from adjacent host bone is often evident because of the differing density of bone and the slower bridging and remodeling that occur if the graft involves the diaphyseal region. The ideal reconstruction of an F3 defect includes restoring the normal joint line using a polyethylene insert of normal thickness.

TIBIAL BONE DEFECT

The same principles used in classifying femoral defects apply to tibial bone deficiencies. Component loosening is more common in tibial implants. Frequently, the tibial prosthesis subsides into varus, creating a bone defect in the medial tibial plateau. Canal-filling stems should be used in cases of large bone defects and whenever increased prosthetic constraint is required for knee stability.

T1 DEFECT (Figure 53.6)

The Type 1 tibia has the same identifying features as the F1 femoral defect (see Table 53.1). Preoperative radiographs reveal a correctly aligned tibial component without significant implant subsidence or tibial osteolysis. There is a full flare to the proximal tibia and the bone is present above the patellar ligament and the fibular head. A standard tibial component is recommended for T1 defects because there is adequate cancellous host bone.

Postoperative radiographs confirm that bone has been preserved above the fibular head and that the fullness and contour of the tibial metaphysis have been maintained. Usually a standard component was used with a combined polyethylene and metal thickness of less than 20 mm.

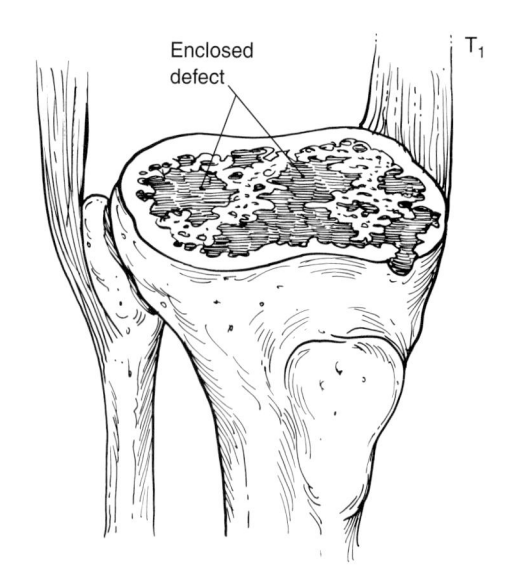

Figure 53.6. T1 Defect

T2 DEFECT

The T2 defect is often caused by component loosening and secondary subsidence of the tibia, commonly into a varus orientation. A circumferential radiolucency develops between the cement and bone as the component subsides. The distance between the top of the fibula and the component is diminished. The lateral radiograph is useful in measuring this distance. Osteolysis may present as cavitary defects beneath the component. See Table 53.1 for a summary of tibial defects.

T2A Defect: One Plateau (Figure 53.7)

The Type 2A defect is usually the result of tibial component loosening and subsiding into varus. The tibia rarely subsides into a valgus orientation, even in knees with valgus alignment. On preoperative radiographs, a widening radiolucency is frequently seen beneath the tibial component. Bone in the opposite tibial plateau is present at a relatively normal joint line level. T2A defects can also occur with aseptic loosening of a unicondylar tibial component.

The surgical management of a T2A defect includes the use of a stemmed implant along with a small bulk autograft, allograft, or a wedged tibial component. The augment can be a horizontal step wedge, a half wedge, or a whole wedge. It is important to avoid converting a T2A defect into a T2B defect by resecting the tibial plateau at a more distal level. When a T2B defect is created iatrogenically, a thicker tibial component is required.

CHAPTER 54
Bone Defects

Tibial Modularity

Russell E. Windsor

Total knee replacement is a successful operation for the treatment of pain due to advanced arthritis, regardless of cause. With the large number of patients that have undergone this operation, there will come a time when revision arthroplasty will probably be needed. Although the longevity and survival of total knee replacements remain high at greater than 94%, it is inevitable that revision surgery will be needed provided the patient survives long enough.

The use of modularity in total knee replacement is confined to the treatment of bone loss. In the primary situation, severe bone destruction will be seen, usually on the posteromedial tibial plateau, in cases of advanced osteoarthritis with varus deformity (Fig. 54.1). Bone loss may also appear in the lateral tibial plateau, in cases of severe valgus deformity in which there is not only severe bone destruction on the femoral side, but also on the tibial plateau. However, it should be noted that femoral bone loss is more characteristically found with severe valgus deformity (Fig. 54.2). Most cases of mild bone erosion are handled easily with the routine proximal tibial resection.

During revision surgery, there is usually bone loss in all regions, with some having severe bone destruction and osteolysis. Particularly in infections, the bone loss after removal of the implants and subsequent reimplantation of a new prosthesis after 6 weeks can be quite severe. In general, it should always be assumed in revision surgery that severe bone loss exists, not only due to the bone loss caused by the initial bone resections during primary total knee replacement, but also the secondary bone loss caused by the failed implant (Fig. 54.3).

PRIMARY TOTAL KNEE REPLACEMENT

During primary total knee replacement, most defects that comprise less than 50% of the tibial condyle may be treated with cement alone or with bone grafting and cementing of the prosthesis. There are numerous techniques for bone grafting and every effort should be made to utilize the bone that is available during primary total knee replacement to build up the tibial plateau. There are, however, cases in which greater than 50% of the condyle is affected. Metal augmentation of the tibial baseplate can be utilized to handle this problem. Bartel[1] and Brooks[2] have shown that a tibial baseplate with a stem is the most secure construct in the proximal tibia. Brooks[2] showed that a metal augment attached to the tibial baseplate yielded the greatest strength of fixation and showed minimal deflection of the prosthesis during mechanical testing in the region of bone loss. A unitized augment is best, but requires custom manufacture, a process that is entirely too expensive for normal use. Thus, most systems utilize modular augments.

Modularity Types

On the tibial side, there are a variety of asymmetrical augments. The modular attachments in some replacement systems consist of half-wedges, which extend from the central portion of the baseplate to the medial or lateral edge of the prosthesis (Fig. 54.4). There are also full wedges that extend from one side of the baseplate to the other. The wedge angles vary in size from 8 to 22 degrees, and they are configured in such a way depending on the region needing buildup to allow augmenting the medial or lateral plateau by simply flipping it. The half-wedges are inherently more stable and have less shear force transmitted across them than the full wedges. When full wedges are used, intramedullary stem extensions should be utilized. The stems themselves are modular and are placed into a Morse-taper. Fixation screws or clips reinforce the connection be-

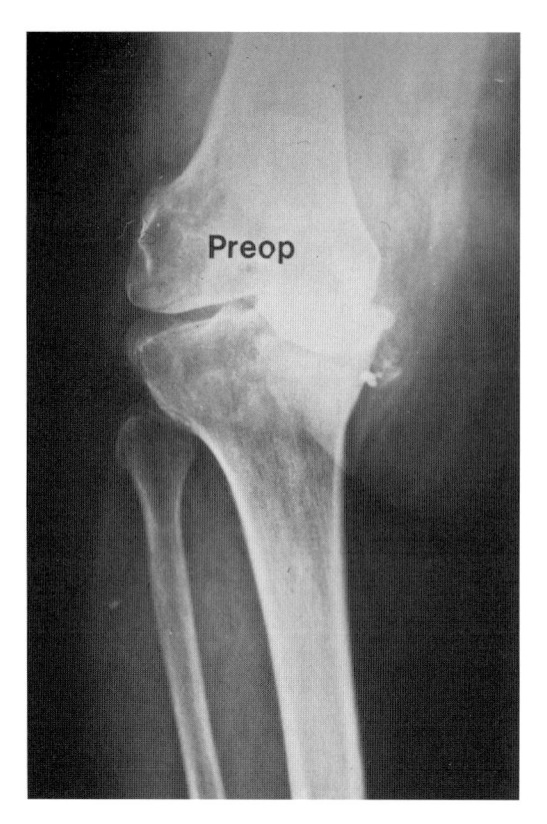

Figure 54.1. Severe varus deformity characteristically is accompanied by tibial bone loss on the medial or posteromedial portion of the plateau.

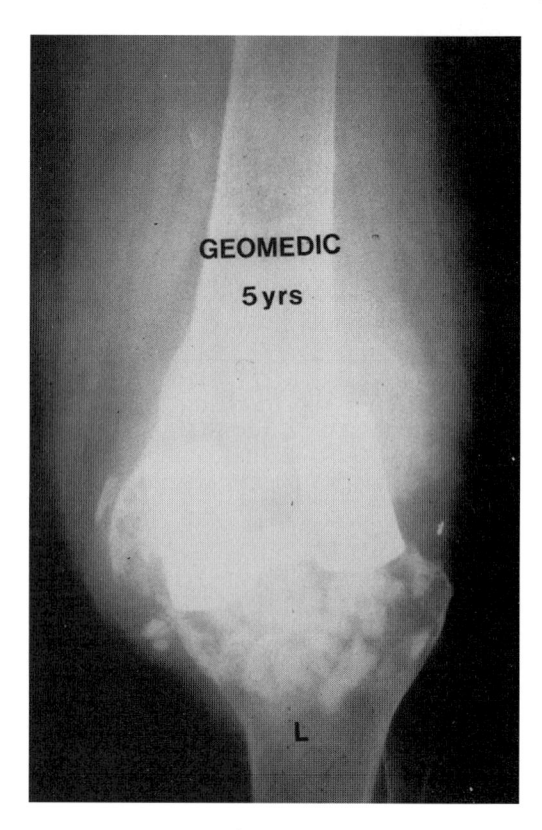

Figure 54.3. Severe aseptic loosening with failure will create substantial bone loss in addition to that which occurred after the routine resections that were made during the initial total knee replacement.

tween the stem and the tibial peg (Fig. 54.5). The stems come in routine lengths of 75 mm and longer lengths at 25-mm increments. The initial stem thickness is 10 mm and increases up to 25, or even 30 mm. When half-wedges are deemed necessary, a stem extension should be attached to the tibial component, especially when a 22-degree wedge is necessary. Otherwise, the normal length of the tibial component peg may suffice for the

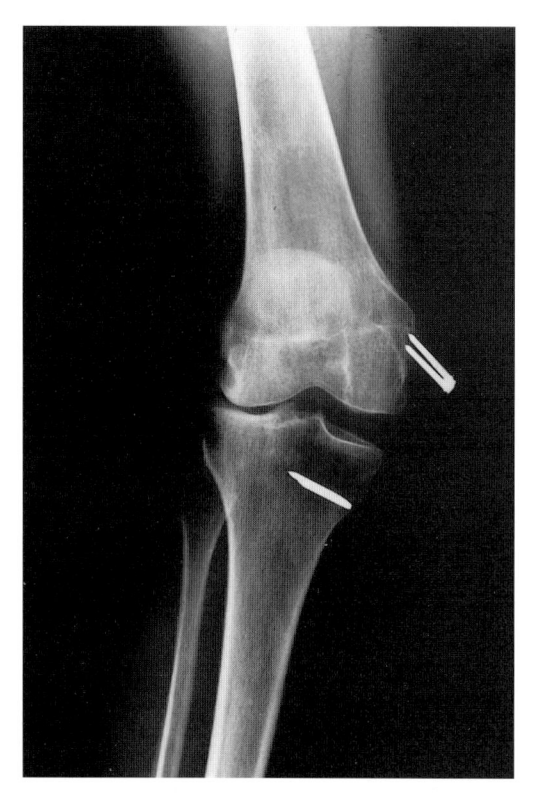

Figure 54.2. Severe valgus deformity characteristically is accompanied by femoral bone loss, although lateral tibial condyle bone loss is seen in the most advanced cases.

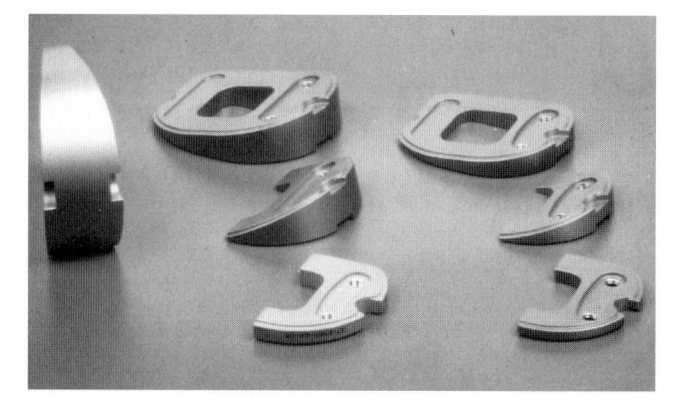

Figure 54.4. Full-wedge and half-wedge augments are available for placement beneath the tibial baseplate. Some manufacturers also have flat metal augments that are affixed beneath the medial or lateral portion of the baseplate.

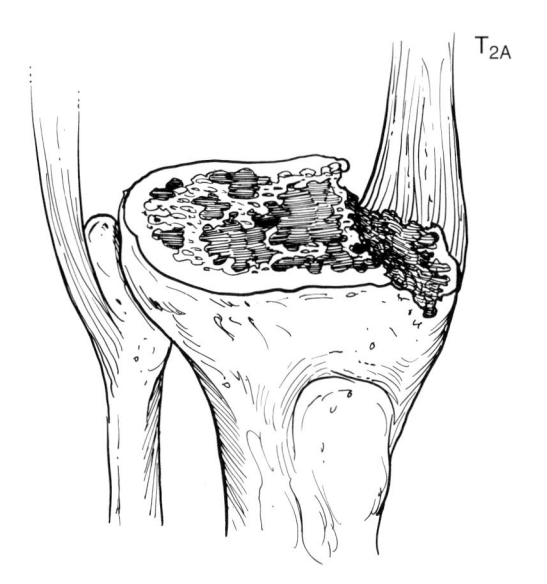

Figure 53.7. T2A Defect

T2B Defect: Both Plateaus (Figure 53.8)

The Type 2B defect (Fig. 53.8) involves both plateaus. Radiographs of T2B defects demonstrate damage to the metaphyseal segment of the tibia by either component subsidence, osteolysis, or both. The damage may extend to the level of the fibular head, but should not include extensive destruction of bone below this level. The metaphyseal flare of the tibia should be reduced but still present. Osteolytic lesions should have a well-defined border with some cancellous bone present for cement interdigitation at the time of the reconstruction.

The surgical management of a T2B defect usually includes the use of a long-stemmed tibial component and reconstruction of the tibial plateaus by bone graft, augments, or an extra thick tibial component. A wedge-shaped component is appropriate for the T2B defect if the bone loss is significant in both plateaus, but greater in one plateau. A canal-filling stem is preferable, particularly if a structural bone graft has been used.

Occasionally, cement fill is used for T2B defect reconstructions. Reinforcement with cancellous screws may provide a stronger construct than cement alone. The most difficult but perhaps the most important aspect of Type 2 and Type 3 tibial reconstructions is achieving cement interdigitation with the graft. An advantage to using allograft bone is recreating a cancellous bone bed for cement interdigitation with host bone. Union of an allograft to host bone is not a problem.[7] In fact, the durability of major structural allografts in revision knee surgery appears to be satisfactory.

Postoperative radiographs of T2B repairs reveal a tibial component augment, cement fill, or allograft to restore joint line level. The augment may be an extra thick tibial baseplate, a step wedge, or an angular wedge beneath the component. There may be a bone graft in addition to the augment. If the defect has not been repaired to restore joint line level, the tibial baseplate is at or below the level of the fibular head. In some instances, the tibial baseplate may be close to the fibular head, with extensive cement penetration below the level of the fibular head.

T3 DEFECT (Figure 53.9)

The Type 3 tibial defect usually results from severe tibial component instability caused by aseptic loosening and implant migration. Osteolysis or an underlying

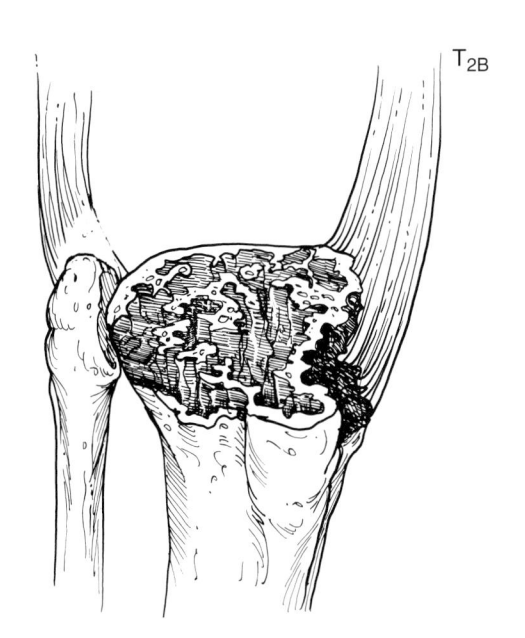

Figure 53.8. T2B Defect

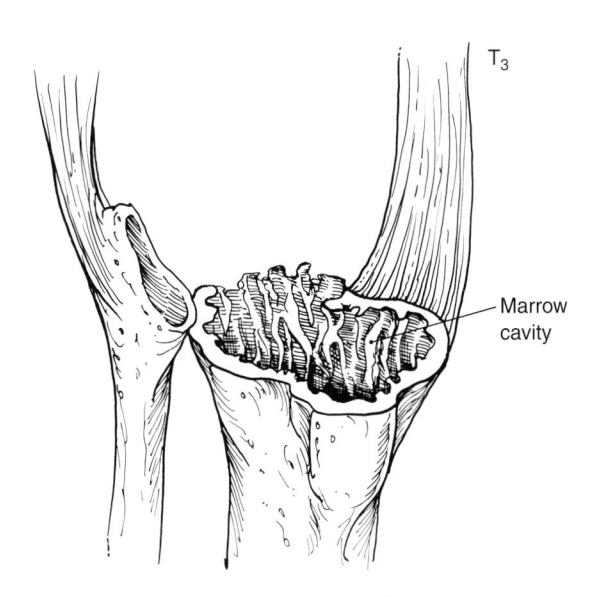

Figure 53.9. T3 Defect

bone fracture may contribute to the development of T3 defects. The T3 tibial defect has extensively damaged cancellous bone of the proximal tibia. The fibular head may be retained, leaving it higher than the proximal tibia. A canal-filling stem must be used to support the component. In severe cases, the metaphyseal flare of the tibia is completely absent. This situation requires a major structural allograft to repair the proximal tibial segment for joint line restoration and component fixation.

Preoperative radiographs of a T3 defect reveal either severe tibial component migration and instability or destruction of a major segment of the proximal tibial metaphysis. Bone loss is severe, so that the patellar tendon insertion or collateral ligament attachment on one or both sides is often compromised. Patella alta may be present with extensor mechanism failure.

To reconstruct a T3 defect, the surgeon must replace a major portion of the proximal tibia with a large structural allograft or a custom tibial component. A canal-filling stem is essential and may need to be fully cemented to achieve rotational stability. A step cut of the allograft in conjunction with cerclage wires provides additional rotational stability. When reconstructing a T3 defect, a varus-valgus constrained implant, reattachment of collateral ligaments, and reconstruction of the extensor mechanism may be needed.

Postoperative radiographs demonstrate the reconstructed metaphyseal segment of the proximal tibia. Femoral head bone grafts may be difficult to identify on postoperative radiographs if the interface with host bone has been adequately prepared for intimate contact with the allograft.

USING A BONE DEFECT CLASSIFICATION SYSTEM

Learning to use a bone defect classification system requires discipline. Preoperative radiographs and intraoperative information should be used to classify the defects. In borderline situations, refer to postoperative radiographs and surgical reconstructive techniques. Generally, an F1-T1 classification is indicated when cancellous bone is present at a normal joint line level, permitting the use of standard nonstemmed implants. F2-T2 categories have damaged cancellous bone that requires augmentation, small structural grafts, or thick cement fill to restore joint line level and knee stability. The F3-T3 category should be reserved primarily for those severe cases in which the damaged metaphyseal segment of bone must be repaired with a salvage hinged implant or with major bone grafts to support the component.

Orthopedic surgeons should examine the complexity of cases included in any study of revision knee arthroplasty. The clinical results of a surgical technique or implant type are valid when a study compares cases according to the severity of bone damage. If the bone defect classification is used correctly, the method of reconstruction used should be appropriate for cases in each category.

References

1. Dorr L. Bone grafts for bone loss with total knee replacement. *Orthop Clin North Am.* 1989; 20(2):179–187.
2. Insall J. Revision of aseptic failed total knee arthroplasty. In: Insall JN, ed. *Surgery of the Knee.* 2nd ed. New York: Churchill Livingstone; 1993: 935–957.
3. Rand J. Bone deficiency in total knee arthroplasty. Use of metal wedge augmentation. *Clin Orthop.* 1991; 271:63–71.
4. Bargar WL, Gross TP. A classification of bone defects in revision total knee arthroplasty. Presented at the Knee Society Interim Meeting. Philadelphia, Pensylvania, 1992.
5. Engh G. A classification of bone defects. In: Engh G, Rorabeck C, eds. *Revision Knee Arthroplasty.* Baltimore: Williams & Wilkins; 1997; 63–120.
6. Engh G. Failure of the polyethylene bearing surface of a total knee replacement within four years: A case report. *J Bone Joint Surg Am.* 1988; 70-A:1093–1096.
7. McAuley J, Engh G. Allografts in Revision Surgery In: Engh G, Rorabeck C, eds. *Revision Knee Arthroplasty.* Baltimore: Williams & Wilkins; 1997; 252–274.

54. Bone Defects: Tibial Modularity

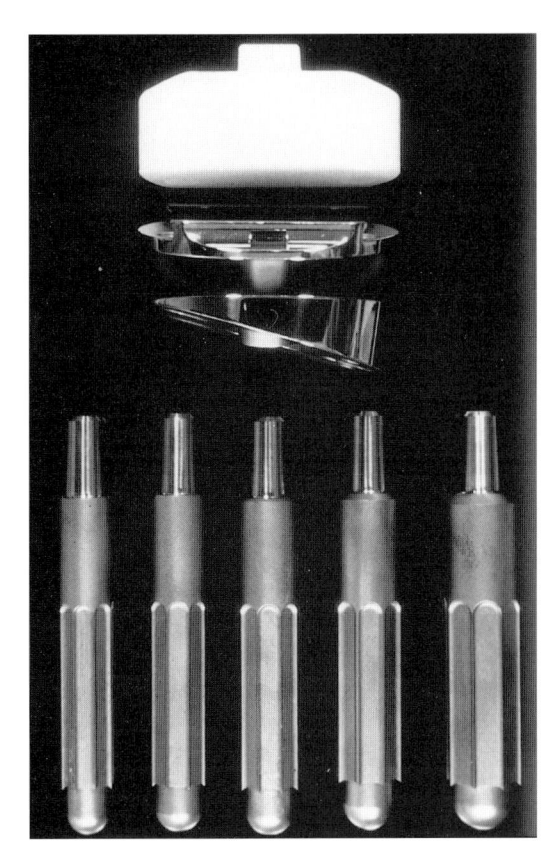

Figure 54.5. The stems are modular and are available in different lengths and thicknesses. They are affixed either by a Morse-taper fitting or by other locking mechanisms.

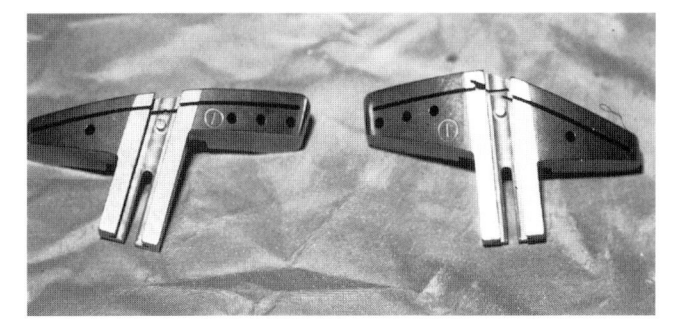

Figure 54.6. Guides are available to permit proper tibial-finishing resections to make a better fit for the tibial augments.

smaller angled half-wedges. These wedges are usually attached to the underside region of the baseplate by screws.

Other systems utilize a series of blocks that are attached beneath the medial or lateral side of the tibial baseplate with cement or small screws. There are also mini-wedges that only modify the posterior aspect of the tibial tray. These are attached usually with a separate batch of acrylic cement. Stems are also recommended when large blocks are needed to make up severe asymmetric bone loss.

In the primary situation, if an augment is going to be used, instrument systems are available to assist making the proper tibial resection to fit the angled wedges with a thin amount of cement. There are guides for both full wedges and half-wedges (Fig. 54.6). When blocks are used, the proximal tibial resection guide can be used to create a separate transverse bone resection that will provide proper placement of the block. After the resection is made, a metal block with an attached alignment rod should be placed on the transversely cut portion of the tibia to check that the resection is perpendicular to the mechanical axis. A novice surgeon may make the mistake of following the region of bone loss and make a resection that is in too much varus. Due to the presence of the patellar tendon, it is difficult to place the component into too much valgus alignment, but clinically there is little risk to the construct. However, excessive varus position of the component will possibly create an early failure of fixation. The stem extensions may also assist the surgeon in obtaining proper tibial mechanical alignment, as good intramedullary fill of the tibial canal by the stem extension is somewhat self-aligning.

Later in the operation, during trial reduction of the prosthesis, the prosthetic fit can be assessed. However, the augmented implant itself can be put together and the fit can be modified slightly by using the implant as a final guide enabling further finishing cuts to assure the best fit (Fig. 54.7). In primary total knee replacement, the bone stock elsewhere on the tibia may be quite good, which allows the stress to be uniformly distributed across the tibial proximal surface.

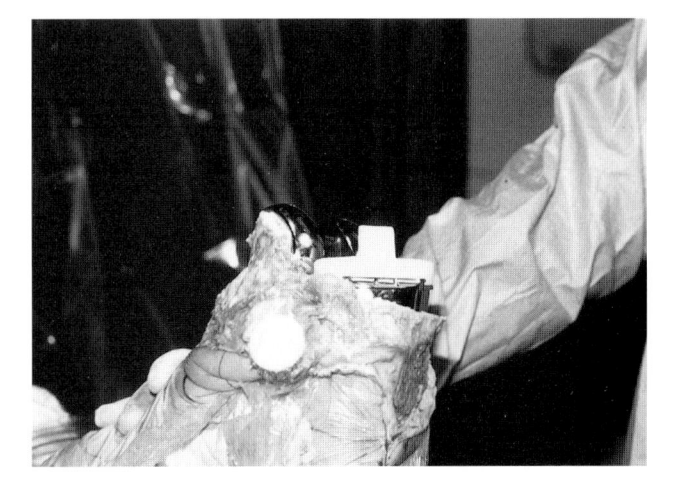

Figure 54.7. The intramedullary stem extension will help self-align the prosthesis that has a metal wedge on it. However, the surgeon should also check the alignment with a separate block and alignment guide as a backup check.

REVISION TOTAL KNEE REPLACEMENT

Bone loss is always a problem the surgeon must address in revision arthroplasty. The mere fact that another implant was placed on the bone means that bone was resected. It is helpful to check the dimensions of the implants that were removed so that proper assessment of the joint line and component sizing can be accomplished.[3]

In grossly loose implants, there will be adjacent bone loss that may be somewhat uniformly distributed around the prosthesis. The bone loss in cases of osteolysis or infection, however, may be quite severe and asymmetric. Cystic cavities may be encountered (Fig. 54.8). Choices for bone augments remain the same as for the primary arthroplasty situation. There are full wedges and half-wedges and blocks. Most systems do not have a thicker baseplate or solid full augment underneath it, because change in the tibial polyethylene insert will provide the proper needed dimension to stabilize the knee. The surgeon must assess the dimension of this bone loss and add to it the dimension of the implant itself. This action will assist the surgeon in preserving the joint line and proper mechanics of the knee replacement.

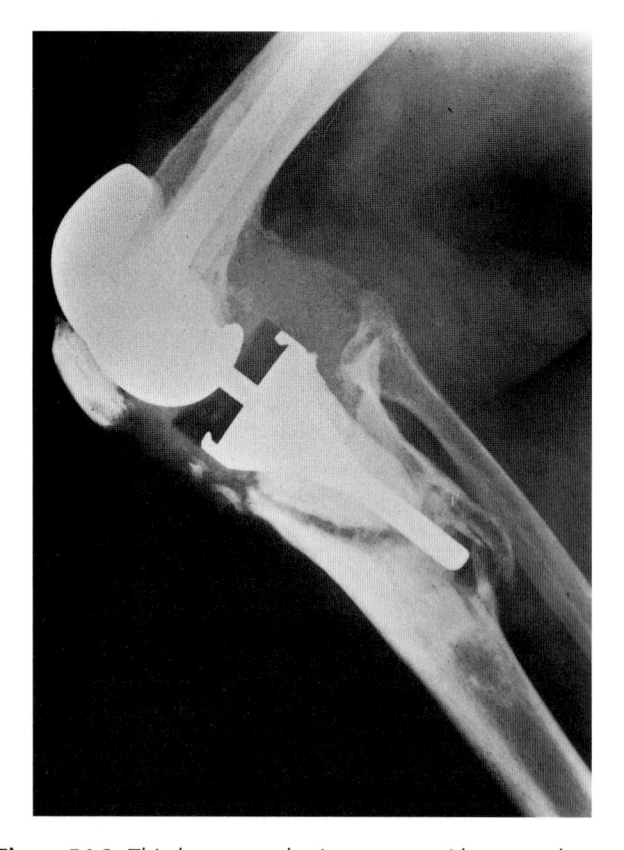

Figure 54.8. This loose prosthesis, as seen with a complete radiolucency, will leave a large cavitary defect in the tibia upon removal.

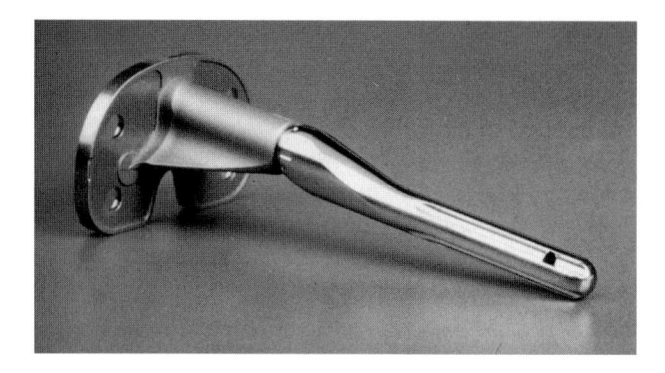

Figure 54.9. Longer stems may be necessary to maintain secure two-point fixation of the tibial prosthesis. Longer lengths usually provide a more secure intramedullary fit, and may be needed in extreme cases of bone loss. This stem has a small offset to allow the surgeon to make up for bone loss by shifting the tibial baseplate through this metal offset.

The revision situation brings with it uncertain stability of component fixation, because the medullary canal has significant bone loss associated sometimes with the removal of a failed stemmed implant. Other implant designs that make use of peripheral pegs for cementless fixation may not have a central stem. However, there may be considerable irregular bone loss in the region of these pegs. The revision prosthesis should have stem extensions available to increase the firmness of fixation of the augmented tibial component. In general, 75-mm stem lengths are utilized for most situations. However, in cases of severe bone loss, it may be necessary to use longer stems from 100 to 200 mm to distribute the force away from the proximal tibia (Fig. 54.9). In cases in which a large 22-degree full wedge is needed, these longer rod lengths should be considered, because even the 75-mm length may not be sufficient enough to provide enough stability (Fig. 54.10).

Just before final implantation, the entire prosthesis should be put together and a trial reduction should be done. Stem attachments will assist the surgeon in placing the tibial component into proper anatomic alignment. The prosthetic trial components or the final implant itself should be placed in the bone and the alignment should be checked with a separate metal block and alignment guide to make certain the implant will be properly aligned. Final resections of bone can be done at this time, using the implant as a guide. The parts should be put together firmly and all screws should be tightened securely. These areas should be checked prior to final cementing of the knee into place. Advocates of cementless fixation in revision arthroplasty may choose to add further bone-grafting techniques to the surface of the tibia. Regardless of the fixation that is used, the implant should be inserted with excellent stability.

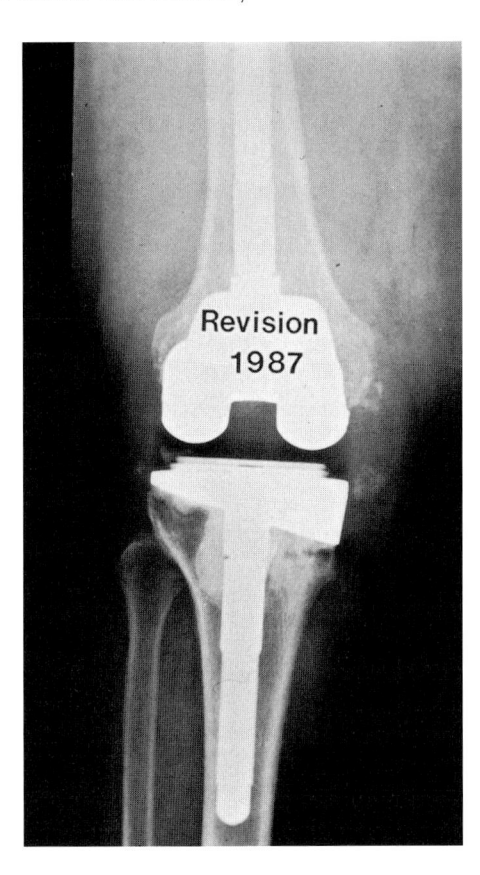

Figure 54.10. With the use of large angled tibial wedge augments, longer stem lengths usually are required.

MODULARITY AND THIRD-BODY WEAR

Because modular components are affixed to the tibial prosthesis by screws or other fixation devices, there is the concern of third-body wear, metal debris, and local osteolysis. There are few reports that provide information regarding this issue. However, the hip replacement literature has shown that osteolysis occurs in situations that seem quite stable, with probable cause being polyethylene wear and third-body wear debris.[4] The cost-benefit ratio of modularity, so far, outweighs the potential disadvantage of third-body wear and osteolysis. Care must be taken to assure firm, rigid attachment of the augments to the underside of the tibial baseplate. Some systems have made use of applying the augments to the baseplate with a separate batch of acrylic cement. Whatever method is used, the component should be put together securely and each fixation point should be checked just prior to final implantation. With secure metal-on-metal fixation, cement may add some structural benefit to the overall construct and alleviate stress that may be repetitively applied to the fixation points by the cyclic loading of the prosthesis during gait.

Engh reported on osteolysis that was observed in a variety of implant designs, which may lead to the manufacture of prosthetic modular augments that will have better fixation.[5] Cementing the prosthesis may decrease the wear somewhat, but the stems should be press fit into the intramedullary canal. Cement should go from the junction of the stem to the proximal portion of the tibial baseplate. Even with cement and metal fixation and a Morse taper, there have been cases in which the rod dissociates in clinically unstable situations due to cyclic loading of the implant. These dissociations have occurred rarely and are seen in the most severely unstable and deficient bony situations.

There has also been concern about rod migration in clinically unstable situations. The intramedullary canal should only be reamed to a mild chatter, leaving as much healthy bone surrounding the prosthesis as possible. If a shorter rod appears to result in little stability, then a longer rod should be used. Thus, modularity allows the surgeon to intraoperatively change the prosthetic design to fit best the needs of the clinical problem at hand. Vince[6] reported on some stem migration in some of his severely compromised revision cases, prompting him to consider cementing the entire prosthesis. In general, however, there is little need to do this. Wolff and associates[7] reported on the use of stems that had no migrations. Cementing the entire prosthesis including the stem would be necessary in only the most severely unstable case in which, perhaps, a longer rod could not be utilized, such as a knee revision beneath an ipsilateral total hip replacement. If something went wrong in the future, however, revision of this fully cemented prosthesis would be daunting.

The benefits of modularity on the tibial side are considerable and most systems today give the surgeon many options to augment the deficient bone frequently encountered in primary and revision replacement situations. Long-term follow-up is still needed to assess the possible third-body wear that may be taking place in these prostheses.

References

1. Bartel DL, Burstein AH, Santavicca EA, Insall JN. Performance of the tibial component in total knee replacement. Conventional and revision designs. *J Bone Joint Surg.* 1982; 64-A:1026–1033.
2. Brooks PJ, Walker PS, Scott RD. Tibial component fixation in deficient tibial bone stock. *Clin Orthop.* 1984; 184:302–308.
3. Berry DJ, Wold LE, Rand JA. Extensive osteolysis around an aseptic, stable, uncemented total knee replacement. *Clin Orthop.* 1993; 293:204–207.
4. Maloney WJ, Smith RL. Instructional course lectures, The

American Academy of Orthopaedic Surgeons. Periprosthetic osteolysis in total hip arthroplasty: the role of particulate wear debris. *J Bone Joint Surg*. 1995; 77-A:1448–1461.
5. Peters PC, Engh GA, Dwyer KA, Vinh TN. Osteolysis after the knee arthroplasty without cement. *J Bone Joint Surg*. 1992; 74-A:864–876.
6. Vince KDG, Long W. Revision knee arthroplasty. The limits of press fit medullary fixation. *Clin Orthop*. 1995; 317:172–177.
7. Wolff DA, Windsor RE, Westrich G. The use of the CCK prosthesis in primary and revision total knee replacements. Proceedings of the Knee Society, 1997.

CHAPTER 55
Bone Defects

Tibial Allograft

Bernard N. Stulberg

INTRODUCTION

Bone loss of the proximal tibia at total knee arthroplasty is frequently encountered in revision total knee arthroplasty (TKA). Loss of bone stock at the tibial surface in revision TKA may be due to a number of factors. These would include over-resection at primary arthroplasty, bone resorption associated with wear debris generation from failed components (metallic, ultra-high molecular weight polyethylene (UHMWPE), carbon-reinforced polyethylene (CRPE), bone cement, or more commonly combinations of these materials), stress fracturing of markedly weakened bone from the above processes, or from loss of bone associated with the removal of components. Local bone graft is infrequently available for these sources of bone loss. Other means of addressing bone deficiency are therefore needed for such cases. As devices using modularity become more sophisticated, the use of bone-grafting approaches may diminish. However, indications remain for the use of bone grafting in the revision situation that can be predictably addressed through the use of bulk or particulate allograft.

The two most important distinctions in the use of allograft techniques relate to the characterization of the defects that exist. For purposes of this discussion, contained defects refer to those areas of bone deficiency that do not compromise the structural shell of the proximal tibia (the cortical shell is intact); uncontained defects extend to the periphery of the shell and involve defects of the cortex. Combined defects, with both cortical and cancellous bone loss, are seen frequently. The published literature on this subject may refer to these types of bone loss in slightly different terms—(1) peripheral versus central and (2) cavitary versus segmental, for example—but conceptually are referring to the same phenomena of bone loss. Contained defects are commonly encountered in revision TKA, and are managed with small particulate graft, whereas uncontained defects can compromise the structural integrity of the proximal tibia and require structural grafting approaches. Combined defects will include a range of defects from minimal to major degrees of cortical bone deficiency. The techniques used to address them are most frequently determined by the degree to which support of the tibial component can be achieved with host bone alone. Cortical and cancellous grafting techniques may be needed in the more severe cases.

Central to the use of bone-grafting techniques is the concept of combined biological and mechanical reconstruction of the proximal tibia. When properly used, bone grafts are used to restore bone stock to the proximal tibial surface.[3,4] To do so requires that they exist in an appropriate mechanical environment for load sharing.[2–6] Proper mechanical restoration requires attention to the devices used for revision arthroplasty (stemmed and/or augmented tibial components) and appropriate fixation methods of the graft itself. Major concerns with the use of allograft reconstruction techniques in other joints (particularly the hip joint) have raised concern regarding the long-term ability of allograft to provide structural support for the implant.[7] It is best therefore to plan to use allograft as part of the reconstruction to provide restoration of bone stock, and to select an appropriate method of implant fixation that will address the stability of the implant itself.[2,5] For contained defects, stabilization of the component may be sufficient to stabilize the grafting material, whereas for uncontained defects, the graft itself will require supplemental fixation to ensure its stability. It is unwise to rely entirely upon a structural allograft for short-term and long-term fixations of a tibial component.[2,4–6,8]

INDICATIONS

Allografting of the proximal tibia in revision total knee arthroplasty (TKA) is indicated in the following circumstances:

1. Any contained bone defects of 2 mm or greater of either medial or lateral tibial plateau (particulate graft).
2. Any remaining contained defects following treatment of combined defects by either grafting or modular implant approaches (particulate graft).
3. Large uncontained defects that are poorly addressed by modular implants (often greater than 3 cm) and might otherwise require custom implants (structural graft).
4. Replacement of massive segmental loss of the proximal tibia in which customized components would be required (structural graft).

CONTRAINDICATIONS

Active or acute periprosthetic infection.

CLASSIFICATION

1. Contained defects (loss of metaphyseal or cancellous bone).
2. Uncontained defects (significant loss of the cortical shell of the proximal tibia).
3. Combined defects (loss of cortical and cancellous bone of the proximal tibia).

MEASUREMENT OF SUCCESS

It is important to remember when gauging success in revision TKA that one is trying to address a number of features of failure, not simply the loss of bone and its restoration. When authors report success rates for approaches to revision TKA that use allografting techniques, they are addressing the role of these techniques in the composite reconstruction. No device or graft will succeed if the basic components of a successful reconstruction are not met.[4] Although it is important that authors report clinical and radiographic success rates of revision arthroplasty, the success of a revision procedure using allograft techniques must also indicate what aspects of success are specifically due to the allograft and what aspects are due to the success of the concept and application of the reconstruction. It is this author's belief that one should consider an allograft technique successful if it restores bone stock by obtaining healing of the allograft to host bone, and if it achieves incorporation of the graft over a long term. This allows the reader to understand why seemingly widely different approaches to revision TKA (such as that of Whiteside's using particulate graft with uncemented techniques[9,10] and Stockley and colleagues using inlay-grafting techniques with cement[11]) can work. It has long been known that graft and implant stability are critical to the short-term success of a reconstruction. It also appears likely that the long-term success of a reconstruction requires allograft incorporation with restoration of bone stock in an environment that reflects proper loading of implant and bone.[2-6] Structural and particulate-grafting approaches will each have value for bone restoration in revision TKA, but will be dependent on differing aspects of the biological performance of the graft.[17]

If the major criteria of the success of the graft are healing and incorporation, the means of measurement most applicable to the follow-up of these patients will be the standardized radiograph. Graft healing is noted when the graft-host junction becomes indistinct and trabeculations can be seen across this junction. Graft incorporation is evident when bone remodeling can be visualized, or when trabecular orientation and density is uniform throughout the graft and host bone in the region. For tibial allografting techniques, evidence of successful healing is usually seen by 11 months, whereas remodeling may occur over a substantially prolonged interval (as in large structural allografts).

The most sophisticated technique reported to date for the assessment of allograft incorporation has been the SPECT scan (single photon emission computerized-tomography scan).[5,12] This is a nuclear imaging study that uses technetium 99m-labeled methylene diphosphonate, as in a planar bone scan, but scans the bone using a rotating tomographic gamma camera generating exposures throughout a 360-degree arc. The data acquired in this fashion can create images in coronal, sagittal, and transverse planes to allow for three-dimensional analysis of the graft. As reported by Wilde and associates,[2] its value has been in the ability to determine the viability of the entire graft, and to identify focal deficiencies in the graft-host junction. They reported that a decrease in activity of greater than 10% suggested nonincorporation of the graft, whereas uniform uptake throughout the allograft suggested continuing incorporation and viability. SPECT may prove an important tool for the understanding of allograft incorporation, and may prove useful in assessing the painful TKA in which allograft has been used, but it is unlikely to prove useful for routine follow-up analysis.

TECHNIQUES

Contained Defects

The technique for the use of allograft for contained defects is usually straightforward.[3,8] Each revision TKA presents its own challenge, and the steps to address the causes of failure must be addressed in a planned and thoughtful manner. The revision of the tibial component is thus not done in isolation, but only after consideration suggests that it is part of what has been problematic for the existing arthroplasty. The decision to use allograft comes after one has made the decision to remove the component, and has determined that sufficient bone is missing and that restoring bone stock to the proximal tibia is an appropriate step in the revision. These steps are evaluated for all components to be revised. The defects in the tibia are thoroughly debrided, and the extent of the defect is determined. Once all bony surfaces are debrided, revision arthroplasty proceeds with preparation of the bone ends and intramedullary canal for placement of revision components. The author prefers intramedullary instrumentation for alignment, and will frequently plan to use components with intramedullary stems as part of the revision. Once resection of the bone surfaces is completed, trial components are used to aid in judgments regarding sizing of components and the degree of constraint required to achieve alignment and stability. If the tibial bone deficiency is small, a standard length stem device may be used. Preparation and trial placement is performed prior to determining the need for grafting. Defined defects are then judged for the appropriate grafting technique. For relatively clearly demarcated defects that are contained, one can use graft material that is either a small block of cancellous bone fashioned to fit the defect, or particulate graft tightly impacted into the defect (see Case 1). For small defects, the nature in which the graft has been rendered particulate may not be important. Freeze-dried and fresh-frozen allografts may be equally effective. For larger defects, there may be advantages to using more uniform particulate graft material and sizes. Fresh-frozen allografts obtained from respected sources (such as the American Red Cross Tissue Banks or Musculoskeletal Tissue Banks)[7,8,13] are shaped either by hand or through the use of available milling devices. Once in place, the trial component is again positioned to be certain that the graft does not interfere with complete seating of the device. Once confirmed as appropriate, the component is then cemented into place. My preference is to place cement on the tibial surface but not around the stem. This is most predictably accomplished by placing "doughy" cement on the component itself, avoiding contact with the stem. This technique can only be used for those component stems designed for use without cement, either short stems with rotational constraint (for example, "fins") or stems designed for intramedullary contact. This technique is *not* appropriate for all-UHMWPE stems or stems *not* designed for uncemented use, in which the entire stem should be cemented. If one chooses uncemented fixation of the tibial component baseplate, then one should supplement this fixation by the use of a long intramedullary stem.[9,10]

There has been recent interest in using an impaction grafting approach to the proximal tibia for extensive defects.[14,15] This represents an approach similar to that described for the hip by Gie and colleagues.[16] This is a useful alternative for those situations in which the deficient cancellous bone of the proximal tibia is extensive. Tools useful to ensure that the graft is firmly impacted and does not interfere with seating of the tibial implant are likely to be developed, and will be useful adjuncts. With this technique, trial reduction should be performed before final fixation is performed to be certain that the graft does not compromise the seating of the component. Cement is used in a viscous state, as for the technique at the hip.[14,15]

As the biological response to cancellous particulate graft appears more rapid than that seen with the more structural forms of allograft,[9,10,17] the author's preference is to attempt to use particulate graft in most cases, including those combined defects in which less than 25% of the cortical shell has been compromised (see Case 2). For any grafting procedure to be successful, the host-graft interface should be prepared to optimize stability and the potential for the graft to heal to the host bone. Thus, if the base of the defect is sclerotic, a small drill is used to make multiple perforations to allow for more intimate interdigitation of host and allograft bone. In addition, one must be careful to avoid cement penetration between host and donor bone. Some authors use host bone to seal a host-donor interface to speed incorporation and minimize cement intrusion. This might be important for the large structural grafts.[2,11,18]

Both conceptually and in practice, it appears that incorporation of the graft is not dependent upon the method of fixation used for the tibial component itself. Uncemented and cemented approaches can be used. If an uncemented approach is used, rigidity of fixation must be achieved and there should not be expectations of bone ingrowth into the prosthesis.[2,9,10] Restoration of bone stock is dependent upon suitable stability of the graft as part of the reconstruction, and the biological process of repair and remodeling of the graft. In cemented approaches using allografting of contained defects the concerns are both the rigidity of fixation of the reconstruction and the need to avoid cement penetration into the bone graft-host interface. In both cemented and uncemented approaches, deficiencies requiring substantive grafting of the proximal tibia will most likely require stemmed implants that provide stabilization and stress transfer to a more distal portion of the tibia.[4,5,8,10,18]

Uncontained Defects or Combined Defects

The revision TKA situations requiring structural allografting are not straightforward, and involve preoperative planning and intraoperative decision making that is complex.[4,6,8,11,18] Although this chapter deals only with the use of allografts on the tibial side, it should be apparent to the reader that these types of cases may involve significant deficiencies of tibial, femoral, and patellar bone stock. It is likely that more constrained components with intramedullary stems will be needed to accomplish the goals of stability and alignment. It is particularly important in these situations that the implant and the structural allograft each be stable independent of the other, in order to achieve success of the reconstruction over the long term.[4,5,8]

The removal of components and debridement of remaining bone stock proceeds the same way as for the uncontained defects noted above. Once all debridement is complete, the resection of the remaining host bone is performed using appropriate alignment and resection guides. Sizing and implant constraint decisions are made as appropriate to achieve the goals of the reconstruction. Once the trial implants, including the size and length of stems, for the tibial component have been determined, the degree of cortical bone support missing can be determined. For smaller cortical defects, the edges of the remaining cortex are trimmed at a right angle to allow for geometric interdigitation of allograft and host. If more substantial bone is missing, a resection guide may be used to make a right angle resection to the mechanical axis to allow for broad contact at the allograft-host junction. Fresh-frozen allografts are used for these defects. If the defects are very large (greater than 5 cm), then proximal tibial allografts are preferred. Medium-sized defects (3 to 5 cm) may also be appropriately addressed using femoral head allografts. The graft is fashioned to approximate the defect and is fixed to the host bone using appropriate internal fixation. Either screws through the graft, or support of the graft with a buttress plate (see Case 3) may be required to achieve stability of the graft. Once the graft is firmly fixed to the host bone, resection of the excess graft material is performed by using resection guides to assure proper alignment. The trial components are then reinserted. Fit and stability are assessed. Once implants have been selected, the host-graft interface is grafted with remaining autograft (if available) and all remaining defects are filled with particulate graft material. The components are cemented in place using a hybrid technique, with cement for the tibial surface and press-fit application of a long intramedullary stem.

Important technical considerations when using structural allografting techniques are the following:

1. Surgical approach for soft tissues—Clear visualization of all surfaces will be required, and extensive soft tissue dissection or release is often required. Patellar tendon avulsion and collateral ligament compromise can occur easily in these circumstances. The surgeon may wish to augment a surgical approach to minimize this potential. In addition, the presence of long-standing deformities and multiple prior operations could make the host soft tissue bed poorly adaptable and make wound closure difficult after reconstruction. The surgeon should make judgments about the suitability of the tissue bed preoperatively.
2. Allograft availability—Major failure situations often involve substantially greater bone loss than one might anticipate by preoperative radiograph. Careful preoperative assessment with implant templating and size matching may be needed to ensure that suitable allograft material is available.
3. Operative timing—The demands of a significant revision arthroplasty could make these operations particularly time consuming. Plans should be made to minimize intraoperative time for fashioning and fixing the allograft, two steps that can add significant time to the length of the arthroplasty.
4. Perioperative infection—The use of structural allograft may require longer operations on patients whose host bed is compromised through multiple operations. Both surgeon and patient should recognize that infections can occur more frequently in this setting, and all steps necessary to minimize the likelihood of this complication should be taken.
5. Postoperative rehabilitation—Because of the more extensive nature of the surgical trauma and the healing needs of the structural allograft reconstruction, the rehabilitation process may be delayed. Large structural grafts may require protection from weight-bearing stress for 6 to 12 weeks, and supplemental bracing may be needed. The surgeon and patient should be aware of this possibility preoperatively.

RESULTS

Several recent reviews address the technical aspects of achieving successful tibial revision with allograft, and discuss the features of the reconstruction that can lead to predictable results. In general, however, the reader will recognize that the published experiences involve small numbers of patients followed for short periods of time. This does not invalidate the findings, but suggests that the massive defects requiring major structural allograft are fortunately not common, whereas the small defects that benefit from morselized grafting may be so common that they do not require reporting. Thus the reader should understand the principles of what is to be accomplished in restoring alignment, stability, and bone stock to a failed TKA, and become familiar with the different techniques that can achieve these goals.

Wilde and associates[5] reported on 12 knees in which allograft was used for large proximal tibial defects. Contained defects were addressed in 5 knees, and uncontained defects in 7 knees. Five of these 7 knees required supplemental internal fixation. Grafts incorporated in 11 of 12 knees with average graft incorporation occurring at 23 months. The authors studied SPECT scans in 5 knees, with 4 knees showing uniform activity consistent with incorporation. All tibial components were fully cemented.

Tsahakis and colleagues[6] reported their experience using allograft for uncontained defects of both femur and tibia. Of the 19 allografts used, 13 were used for the distal femur and 6 for the proximal tibia. They had no failures of the femoral head allografts over the course of their study period (1989 to 1992). They recommend that stems be used for most cases, and advocate the hybrid fixation technique of cementing to the allograft with press-fit fixation of the stem.

Mow and Wiedel[2] reviewed their experience with major structural allografting from 1985 to 1991. They followed 15 allografts, 10 of which were of the proximal tibia. They had one patient with a late failure (3 years) due to allograft failure. At revision, they found evidence for graft incorporation but loss of component support, leading to implant fracture. They felt that all 15 allografts healed to the host bone, with 13 showing evidence of incorporation. Most of their components were fixed without cement.

Ghazavi[18] and Stockley[11] have reported on patients undergoing revision TKA with allografting from The Mount Sinai Hospital, Toronto. In the first report,[11] they examined the results of 32 allograft reconstructions in 20 knees. They used deep-frozen irradiated allografts, and included bulk grafts, cortical strut grafts, and morselized bone grafts. In this group, 16 patients had grafting of the tibia, with 11 having structural grafts. Several different methods of securing graft to tibia and implant were used. For the entire group, three knees suffered infection, and two bulk allografts fractured (one tibial, one femoral). One reconstruction with morselized graft failed due to inadequate implant stabilization at the time of arthroplasty. Their second report[18] focused only on the patients undergoing structural allografting for massive defects. There were 30 knees in 28 patients followed an average of 4.2 years. Their success was 77%, with the causes of failure being infection (three knees), loosening of the tibial component (two), fracture of the graft (one), and nonunion at the allograft-host junction (one). These authors prefer an inlay technique if possible, and try to avoid the use of plates. Using their techniques graft healing and incorporation appear more predictable on the tibial side. They advocate stemmed implants, with the "hybrid" approach to composite fixation.

Whiteside[9] reports a large series of revision TKA in which he has used morselized grafting techniques around uncemented femoral and tibial components. He performed 56 revision TKAs in 56 patients. The characterization of bone loss was not consistent with other reports, making it difficult to determine if the techniques were used mostly for contained or uncontained-combined defects. Grafting was performed on all tibial surfaces, and long stems were used on all tibial components. Screw fixation with a tibial plate was used for 28 knees. Tibial seating was circumferential in 12 knees, 75% in 20 knees, 50% in 14 knees, and 25% in 10 knees. One tibial component has loosened, and two were revised because of recurrent knee dislocations. Other complications included patellar dislocations, patellar tendon avulsion, and patellar fracture. Three patients had biopsies of the grafted area demonstrating viable bone with evidence for remodeling.

CASE STUDIES

The delineation of defects as contained, uncontained, and combined covers a wide variety of situations that would be difficult to account for within the confines of this chapter. The basics of the techniques to be used in such situations are discussed in the case examples that follow.

Case 1

Cancellous grafting of contained defects using cemented devices.

Problem

Bicondylar defects of the proximal tibia related to failed geometric prosthesis with extensive medial and lateral bone defects.

Radiographs

A healed stress fracture of the medial tibial condyle can be seen around a failed geometric prosthesis with an all ultra-high molecular weight polyethylene (UHMWPE) bicondylar tibial component (Fig. 55.1). Osteolysis of bone related to extensive wear debris is apparent.

Technique

The knee is exposed using a standard median parapatellar approach. An extensive medial soft tissue release is performed. The anterior and posterior cruciate ligaments are excised. After component removal, the tibial resection guide is used to resect the proximal tibia perpendicular to the mechanical axis. Because of extensive and deep bone loss, every attempt is made to resect minimal additional tibial bone and to preserve the tibial cortical shell. Sizing of the component is followed by fashioning of the seating hole for the tibial stem. Femoral and patellar resections proceed as needed and the trial components are positioned. Once component

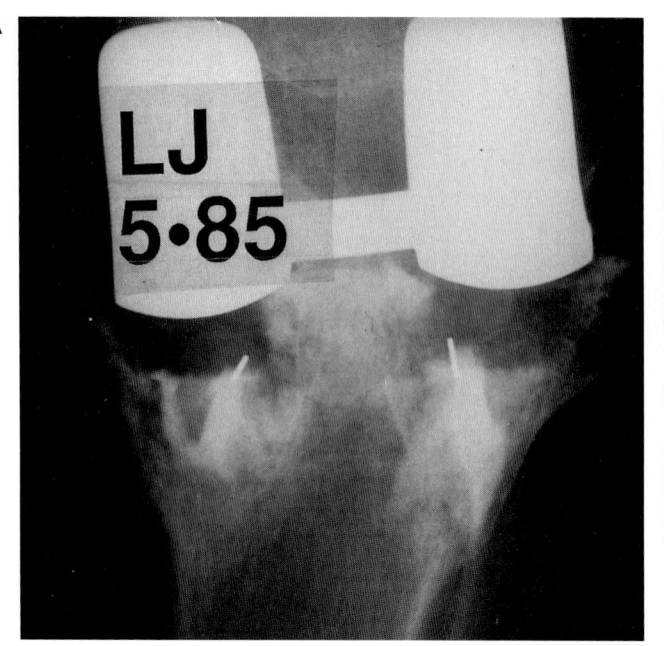

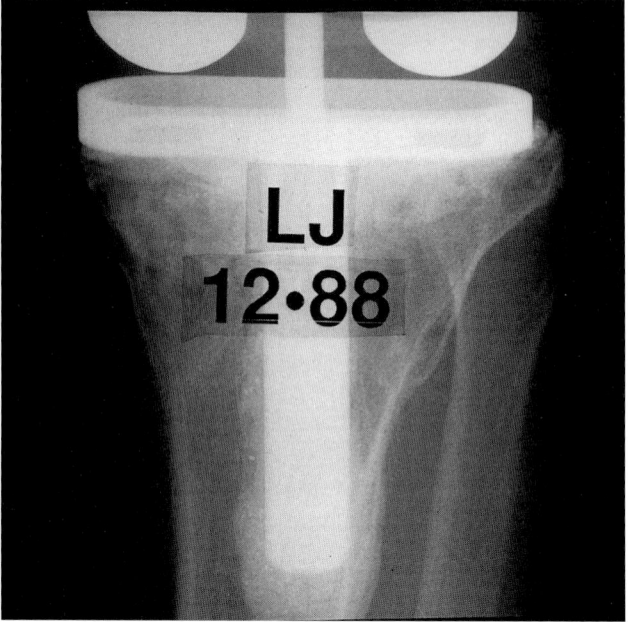

Figure 55.1. Case 1—contained defect. (Courtesy Dr. AH Wilde) (A) Loosening, osteolysis, and medial tibial condylar stress fracture in patient with failed bicondylar geometric prosthesis. (B) Radiograph of proximal tibia 3 years following revision to constrained arthroplasty with a cemented tibial component with fixed long stem. Cancellous block allograft has healed and incorporated. Medial condylar remodeling is apparent.

selection is determined, the extent of bone loss remaining can be adequately judged. In this case, the removal of components left large cavitary but contained defects of the medial and lateral tibial plateaux. Bulk cancellous allograft was fashioned to fit the defects and was impacted into the tibia. A long-stem cemented component was used to permit stress transfer beyond the areas of bone deficiencies. Forty-three months later the grafts are found to be fully incorporated into the proximal tibia. There is evidence of stress transfer distal and laterally about the cemented tibial stem.

Case 2

Cancellous grafting using morselized graft around a modular tibial component.

Problem

Extensive osteolysis around screws of an uncemented tibial component. The femoral and patellar components were well fixed.

Radiographs

Preoperative radiographs demonstrate substantial osteolysis around the medial anterior and posterior screws, and suggest moderate osteolysis around the anterior lateral screw (Fig. 55.2). Component fixation appears stable around the stem and under the plateau. There is no wear apparent of the tibial articular surface.

Technique

After exposure of the knee including an extensive medial soft tissue release, the tibial component is removed and the tibia debrided. The extent of the defect is determined. Femoral and patellar components are evaluated for fixation and evidence of wear. An allograft femoral head is morselized. The proximal tibia is then evaluated for appropriate alignment and depth of resection using revision instrumentation. The remaining tibial surface is resected to allow for placement of the tibial plate perpendicular to axis of the tibia. In this case, a long-stemmed component (150 mm) is to be used. After minimal resection of the remaining tibia (1 mm), the trial component plate is positioned to determine the ability to achieve an even seating of the implant. This step may be performed either before or after the tibial canal is reamed to determine the appropriate diameter and length of the stem. Before grafting, however, it is important to confirm that the implant and modular stemmed trial can be seated fully, and remains stable without the graft. Once this step is completed, the full extent of the contained defect to be grafted can be determined. The cancellous bone graft is then impacted into the defects, using the modular stem trial (and baseplate as needed) to allow for configuration of the graft around the planned implant. Trial reduction is performed with the appropriate insert positioned on the

55. Bone Defects: Tibial Allograft

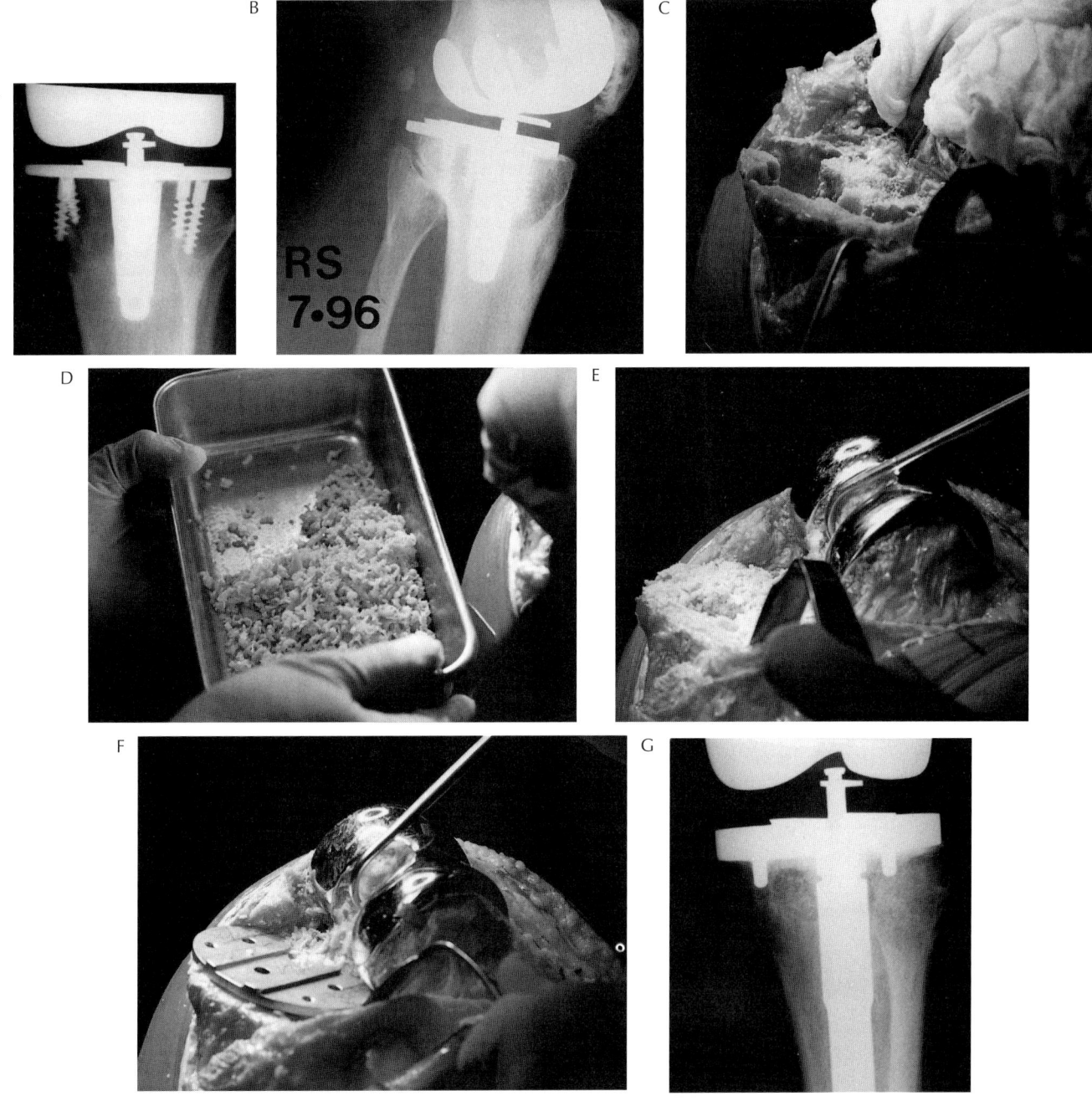

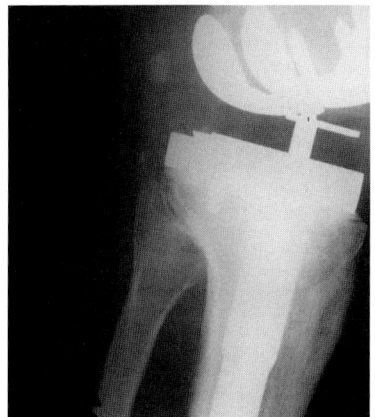

Figure 55.2. Case 2–combined defect. (A,B) Preoperative radiographs demonstrating marked osteolysis around an uncemented tibial component. Significant osteolysis can be seen around the medial and lateral screws, particularly anteriorly. (C) Intraoperative view of proximal tibia after removal of the tibial component and vigorous debridement of the membrane. This view shows extensive medial and lateral contained defects, with a small cortical rim defect medially. Although this would be classified as a combined contained or uncontained defect, it was surgically treated as primarily a contained defect. (D) Fresh-frozen femoral head allograft was morselized using a standardized milling device. (E) Illustration of the proximal tibial surface after extensive grafting. Note that the femoral component was well fixed and was not revised. (F) Illustration of the trial tibial baseplate and stem in position for trial reduction. (G,H) Postoperative radiographs at 6 weeks demonstrating satisfactory stability of the implant. The condylar surface has been fixed with cement whereas the modular long stem has been press fit.

Figure 55.3. Case 3—uncontained defect. (Courtesy Dr. AH Wilde) (A) Radiograph demonstrating failed unicompartmental replacement. Extensive tibial component subsidence is associated with stress-fracture and remodeling of the proximal medial tibia with extensive cortical bone loss. (B) Postoperative radiograph at 2 years demonstrating healing of proximal medial tibial block corticocancellous allograft. A long-stemmed constrained condylar device has been used and alignment has been restored. The graft was supported by the use of supplemental fixation, including the use of a buttress plate.

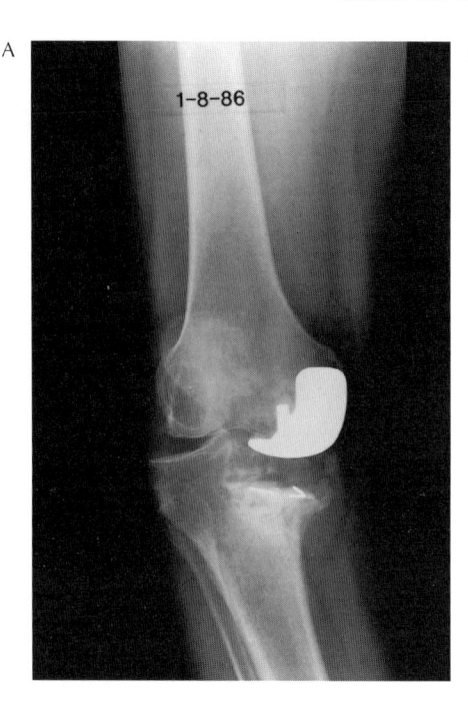

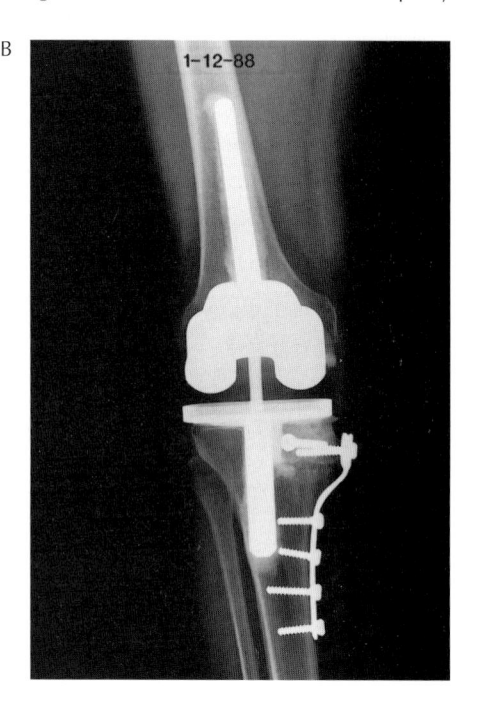

tibial tray prior to placing the graft, but should also be performed after grafting has been completed. The author prefers to use a combined fixation approach cementing the tibial surface but leaving the stem uncemented, with contact distally. To achieve this, cement is placed only on the plateau portion of the tibial component prior to insertion.

Case 3

Structural allografting for massive bone loss associated with failed cemented unicompartmental replacement.

Problem

Uncontained cortical defect along the medial side of the knee with substantial asymmetric bone loss of the proximal tibia, potentially compromising ligament stability.

Radiographs

These radiographs demonstrate failure of a unicompartmental replacement with extensive subsidence of the tibial component with recurrence of advanced varus deformity (Fig. 55.3). A healed tibial stress fracture is visible and persists to the level of the diaphysis. Lateral tibial bone stock is preserved, as is femoral bone stock.

Technique

After routine approach to the knee joint, an extensive soft tissue release is performed to the level of the diaphysis with release of the medial soft tissue structures. After removal of components, resection of the tibial and femoral surfaces is performed as for primary total knee arthroplasty. The tibial cortical shell is trimmed medially and the bony surfaces visualized. A corticocancellous allograft (a proximal tibial graft would be most suitable, but distal femoral, femoral head, or other graft sources could be used) is obtained and contoured so as to mate with the host bone. In this patient it was elected to lay a flat graft onto a flattened tibial bed. This graft requires supplemental stabilization of the graft itself because the component itself will not provide stability. A buttress plate is used to firmly anchor the graft to the host bone. The stabilized graft is then resected flush to the tibial surface to provide a uniformly flat surface for the tibial plate. After sizing, the seating hole for the tibial stem is fashioned. Any remaining areas of contained defects are packed with morselized graft (as in Cases 1 and 2 above) prior to seating of the final components. As an extensive soft tissue release was required to provide proper balancing of the knee, more constrained component geometries were used (Fig. 55.3B).

References

1. Hill RA, Phillips H. Bone grafting in primary uncemented total knee arthroplasty. *J Arthroplasty*. 1992; 7:25–30.
2. Mow CS, Wiedel JD. Structural allografting in revision total knee arthroplasty. *J Arthroplasty*. 1996; 11:235–241.
3. Scott RD. Bone loss: Prosthetic and augmentation methods. *Orthopaedics*. 1995; 18(9):923–926.
4. Harris AI, Poddar S, Gitelis S, et al. Arthroplasty with a composite of an allograft and a prosthesis for knees with severe deficiency of bone. *J Bone Joint Surg*. 1995; 77-A: 373–386.
5. Wilde AH, Shickendantz MS, Stulberg BN, et al. The incorporation of tibial allografts in total knee arthroplasty. *J Bone Joint Surg*. 1990; 72-A:815–824.

6. Tsahakis PJ, Beaver WB, Buick GW. Technique and results of allograft reconstruction in revision total knee arthroplasty. *Clin Orthop*. 1994; 303:86–94.
7. Shinar AA, Harris WH. Bulk structural autogenous grafts and allografts for reconstruction of the acetabulum in total hip arthroplasty. *J Bone Joint Surg*. 1997; 79-A:159–168.
8. Dennis DA. Structural allografting in revision total knee arthroplasty. *Orthopaedics*. 1994; 17(9):849–851.
9. Whiteside LA. Cementless revision total knee arthroplasty. *Clin Orthop*. 1993; 286:160–167.
10. Whiteside LA. Bone grafting in revision cementless total knee arthroplasty. *Instructional Course Lectures*. 1993;42:397–403.
11. Stockley I, McAuley JP, Gross AE. Allograft reconstruction in total knee arthroplasty. *J Bone Joint Surg*. 1992; 74-B: 393–397.
12. Trancik TM, Stulberg BN, Wilde AH, et al. Allograft reconstruction of the acetabulum during revision total hip arthroplasty. Clinical, radiographic and scintigraphic assessment of the results. *J Bone Joint Surg*. 1986; 68-A: 527–533.
13. Czitrom AA. Principles and techniques of tissue banking. *Instructional Course Lectures*. 1993; 42:359–362.
14. Ullmark G, Hovelius L. Impacted morselized allograft and cement for revision total knee arthroplasty. *Acta Orthop Scand*. 1996; 67(1):10–12.
15. de Wall Malefijt MC, van Kampen A, Sloof TJ. Bone grafting in cemented knee replacement. *Acta Orthop Scand*. 1995; 66(4):325–328.
16. Gie GA, Linder L, Ling RSM, Sion JP, et al. Impacted cancellous allografts and cement for revision total hip arthroplasty. *J Bone Joint Surg*. 1993; 75-B:14–21.
17. Burchardt H. The biology of bone graft repair. *Clin Orthop*. 1983; 174:28–42.
18. Ghazavi MT, Stockley I, Yee G, et al. Reconstruction of massive bone defects with allograft in revision total knee arthroplasty. *J Bone Joint Surg*. 1997; 79-A:17–25.

CHAPTER 56
Bone Defects

Femoral Allograft

Douglas A. Dennis

As the number of primary total knee arthroplasties (TKA) performed has steadily increased over the last two decades, the need for revision TKA has similarly increased. Numerous modes of failure have been recognized, including aseptic loosening, ligamentous instability, component malposition and mechanical failure, polyethylene wear, infection, fracture, arthrofibrosis, reflex sympathetic dystrophy, and patellar instability.[1-3] Some degree of bone loss is typically encountered in all cases of revision TKA. Bone defects may be classified as contained (defects with an intact peripheral cortex) or noncontained (defects without a peripheral bony rim).[3] Techniques available to substitute for bone loss include use of polymethylmethacrylate (with or without screws),[4-5] augmented or custom components,[6-9] autogenous bone graft,[10-15] and allograft bone.[3,16-21]

In patients with modest cavitary bone defects, grafting with morselized cancellous autograft or allograft provides favorable results.[22] In cases of revision TKA associated with massive femoral bone loss, multiple surgical options are available, including arthrodesis, amputation, custom TKA, or structural bone allografting. Structural bone allografts offer numerous advantages, including biocompatibility, bone stock restoration, and the potential for ligamentous reattachment,[17-19] particularly if performed utilizing bone block reattachment techniques. Bone allografts provide versatility, allowing the surgeon to shape the allograft to fit the patient's bone deficit and avoid unnecessary removal of host bone. Last, allografts are relatively cost-effective when compared to the high cost of custom-designed TKA.

Disadvantages of using structural allografts include late resorption possibly secondary to immune reaction,[23] fracture or nonunion,[17-19,23,24] and the risk of disease transmission. Buck and associates[24] reported an incidence of HIV transmission from bone transplantation to be less than one in one million cases. This risk may be further minimized through utilization of irradiation sterilization methods.[25,26] This chapter discusses the indications, surgical technique, and results of reconstruction of distal femoral bone defects with structural allograft.

INDICATIONS

Bone loss from the distal femur can occur from the anterior, posterior, or inferior surfaces. Anterior bone loss is commonly found in revision TKA due to stress relief osteoporosis from the anterior flange of the previously implanted femoral component.[27] In the author's experience, bone grafting of anterior femoral defects has not been beneficial due to progressive disappearance of the graft resulting from the same stress shielding phenomenon. Filling of anterior femoral defects with polymethylmethacrylate usually provides satisfactory results if both femoral condyles are intact and femoral intramedullary fixation is utilized.[28]

Bone loss from the distal and posterior femur often occurs in combination. Failure to recognize distal femoral bone loss results in elevation of the joint line and patellar baja, often associated with patellofemoral pain or crepitus and reduction in knee flexion. Ignoring posterior femoral bone loss—by inserting a smaller size of femoral component—risks flexion instability.

Structural allografting of the distal or posterior femur is indicated for osseous defects greater in thickness than the dimensions of available distal or posterior prosthetic femoral augmentations. Common clinical conditions requiring femoral allografting include knees with severe preoperative angular deformity (particularly valgus), TKA with multiple revisions, advanced periprosthetic osteolysis, distal femoral tumor resection, and comminuted supracondylar periprosthetic fractures.

Contraindications to structural allografting of the femur are similar to those of routine TKA, i.e., chronic infection, disruption of the extensor mechanism, and neuropathic arthropathy. Additional contraindications include medical conditions unfavorable to allograft incorporation, such as metabolic bone disorders, severe immunosuppression, and radiation necrosis of adjacent host bone and soft tissues.

PREOPERATIVE PLANNING

Surgical reconstructions requiring structural allografts are often complex, and extensive preoperative planning is essential. Typically, patients requiring structural allografting have undergone multiple previous surgical procedures and thorough testing to rule out preoperative infection is mandatory, including hematologic evaluation (white blood cell count, erythrocyte sedimentation rate, etc.), preoperative aspirations for culture, and nuclear scanning in indicated cases.

The structural allograft must be carefully chosen. Distal femoral, proximal tibial, or femoral head allografts are most commonly used. Attempts are made to utilize an allograft specimen from an anatomically matched site when possible, which will allow trabecular orientation along the line of applied forces.[3] When small defects are encountered, femoral head allografts are typically chosen due to their demonstrated biomechanical superiority over distal femoral allografts.[29] Fresh-frozen processed specimens are presently favored due to superior structural strength.[25] Preoperative sizing of the allograft is critical to ensure sufficient filling of the osseous defect. Oversized allografts may create difficulties with wound closure.[18]

A wide range of prosthetic components should be available at the time of operation. Knees with massive osseous defects are often associated with global ligamentous instability and implants with increased prosthetic constraint are sometimes necessary. Use of intramedullary femoral stems, with lengths sufficient to engage diaphyseal bone, are frequently required to avoid excessive loads on the structural allograft during its incorporation.

SURGICAL TECHNIQUE

In order to achieve optimum results, cases of revision TKA using structural allografts require careful adherence to certain principles of surgical technique. Frequently, due to multiple previous surgical procedures, extensor mechanism fibrosis and contracture are present, creating difficulties with surgical exposure. Surgeons performing these procedures must be skilled in extensile exposure techniques of the knee, including proximal quadricepsplasty[30,31] and tibial tubercle osteotomy.[32]

Initially, the host osseous defect must be meticulously prepared to create a healthy bleeding bed of bone through removal of intervening soft tissue. Efforts are made to maximize prosthetic contact with remaining host bone, thereby lessening load transmission to the structural allograft. To obtain this, a minimal amount of bone (1 to 2 mm) is resected from the most prominent femoral condyle. The structural allograft is then precisely contoured to obtain maximal surface contact and mechanical interlock with the deficient host bone. In some cases, the host defect is contoured to create a more geometric shape that improves allograft-host contact and encourages the intrinsic stability of the allograft. All remaining peripheral cortical bone is maintained for additional allograft support.

Alternatively, the distal femoral defect may be reamed with small acetabular reamers to create a hemispherical defect. A femoral head allograft is then contoured with a female hemispherical reamer of similar dimension to fit into the previously prepared host defect[33] (Fig. 56.1A–D).

Unicondylar femoral defects are typically reconstructed with a femoral head allograft (Fig. 56.2A–E). Bicondylar femoral defects can be managed with either a large femoral head allograft or an undersized distal femoral allograft fit within the remaining cortical contours of the distal femur (Fig. 56.3A–D). In cases in which the entire host distal femur is deficient, reconstruction with a matched-size distal femoral allograft is indicated.

Allograft fixation is temporarily obtained with small K-wires or bone clamps. Permanent fixation is then obtained with the use of axially aligned bone screws and intramedullary stems that extend into diaphyseal bone. In those cases in which satisfactory mechanical interlock is obtained through precise contouring of the allograft, the use of axially aligned bone screws is not required. In some cases, particularly those in which the entire distal femur is reconstructed with structural allograft, an additional unicortical plate may be utilized to ensure rotational stability (Fig. 56.4A–D). Numerous reports have demonstrated the importance of prolonged rigid fixation in obtaining satisfactory union of structural allograft to the host.[16–21,34]

Histologic studies have demonstrated that extended periods are required for allograft incorporation.[35,36] During the process of incorporation, allograft strength is transiently reduced, increasing the risk of allograft fracture and collapse. Long intramedullary stems that engage diaphyseal bone have been shown to reduce proximal tibial cancellous loads by approximately 30%.[37] These load-sharing intramedullary stems are therefore recommended to

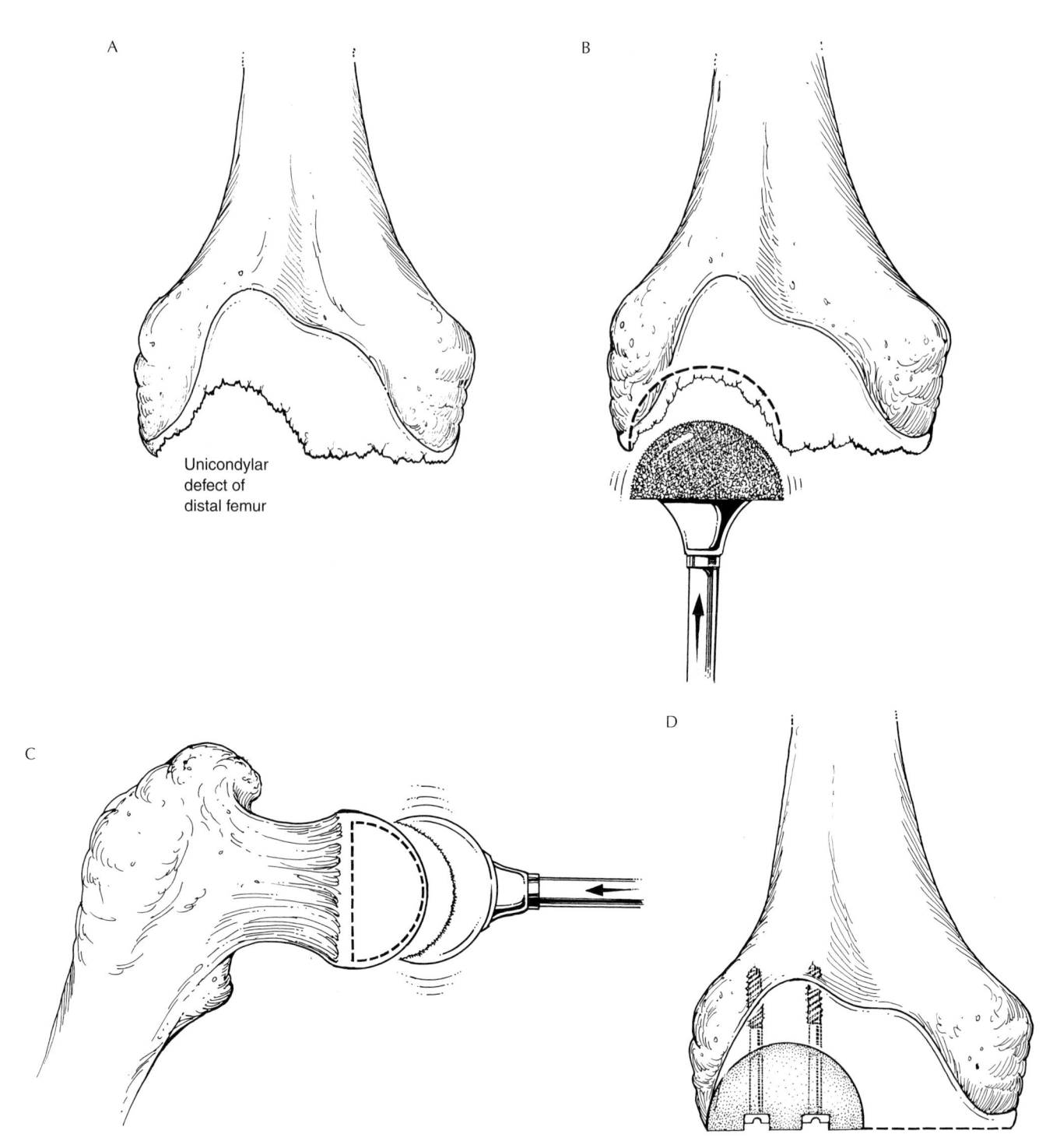

Figure 56.1. Schematic diagrams demonstrating structural allografting using acetabular reamers for defect preparation and reconstruction with a femoral head allograft to fill the osseous defect. (A) Large unicondylar femoral defect. (B) Defect preparation utilizing small acetabular reamers. (C) Femoral head allograft being contoured with a concave reamer to accurately fit previously prepared host femoral condylar defect. (D) Reconstruction with femoral head allograft and screw fixation.

Figure 56.2. (A) Early postoperative lateral view of primary total knee arthroplasty. (B) Postoperative lateral radiograph (5 years) demonstrating osteolytic distal femoral defect (histologically proven polyethylene wear debris induced). (C) Intraoperative photograph demonstrating osteolytic defect of the lateral femoral condyle. (D) Intraoperative photograph following reconstruction with a femoral head allograft. (E) Lateral radiograph 2 years post-reconstruction and suggestive of structural allograft incorporation.

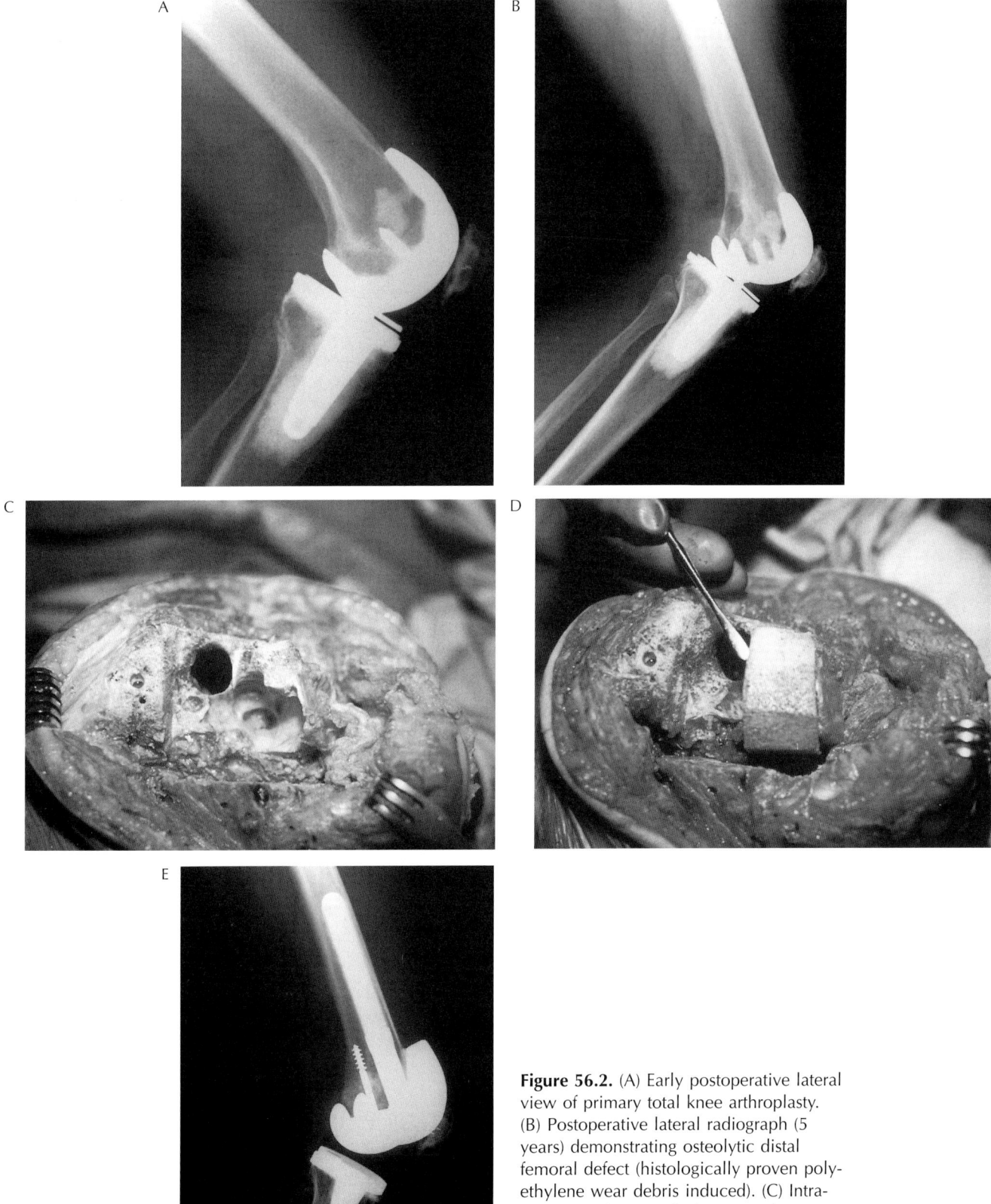

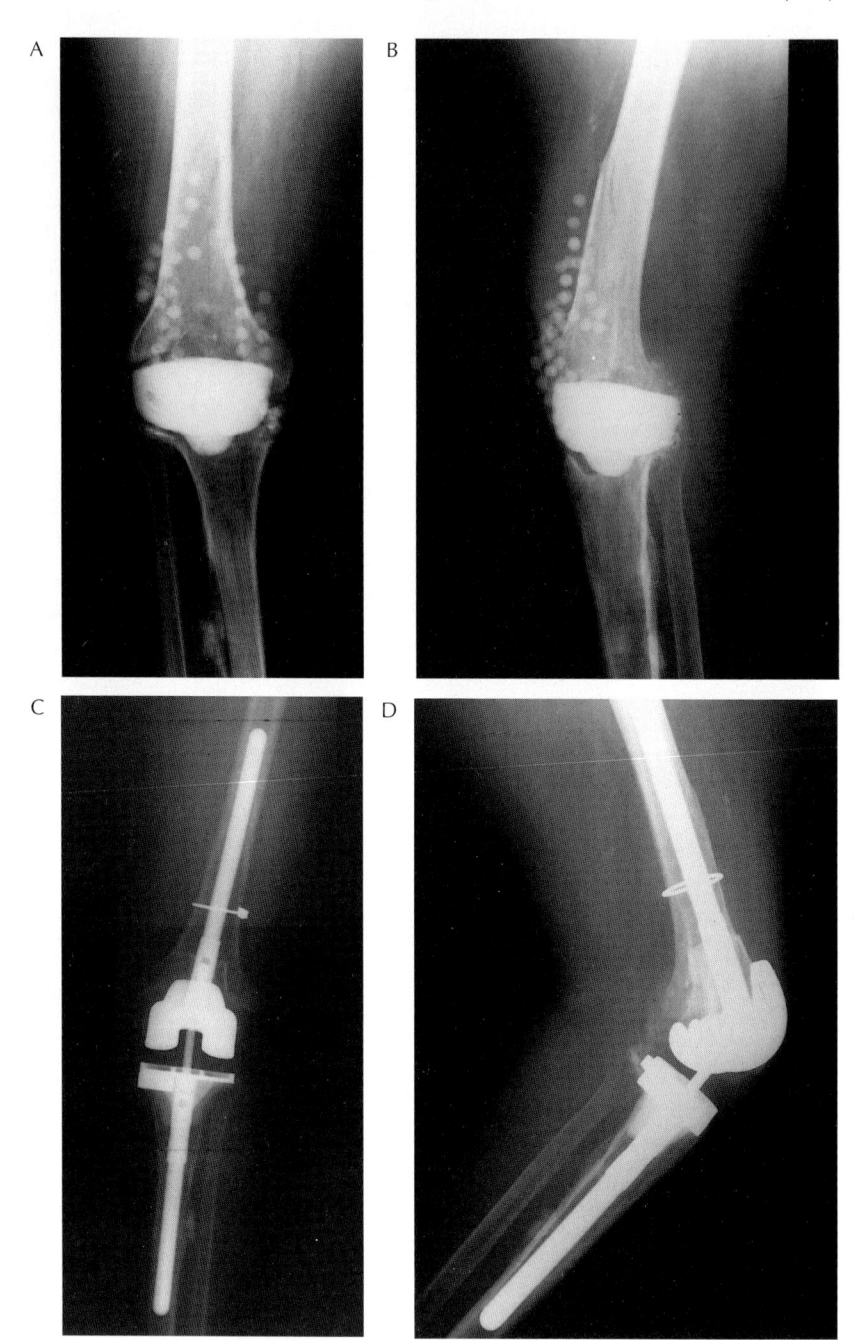

Figure 56.3. (A) Preoperative anteroposterior and (B) lateral radiographs demonstrating a large bicondylar femoral defect following cemented long-stem prosthesis removal and insertion of antibiotic impregnated polymethylmethacrylate spacer for an infected revision TKA. (C) Postoperative anteroposterior and (D) lateral radiographs following reconstruction of large bicondylar femoral defect with a distal femoral allograft invaginated within the remaining distal femur.

protect and off-load the structural allograft during its incorporation.

Fixation of prosthetic components may be achieved using either cemented or cementless methods. The author favors cementation of condylar surfaces and the allograft while press-fitting the longer intramedullary stems into host diaphyseal bone. Porous surfaces adjacent to avascular allograft offer little chance of osseous ingrowth. Montgomery and colleagues[38] demonstrated that when longer intramedullary stems were required in revision TKA, superior results were obtained with press-fit stems, compared to cemented stems, when either a posterior-stabilized or constrained articulation was used.

When necessary, ligamentous reattachment to large structural allografts is most successfully accomplished using bone-to-bone reattachment methods. Although allograft bone can serve as a collagen scaffold for collateral ligamentous reattachment,[17,19] simple ligamentous suturing to allograft bone or its attached soft tissues, in conjunction with prosthetic implantation, often heals with insufficient ligamentous tension.[18] In cases of mas-

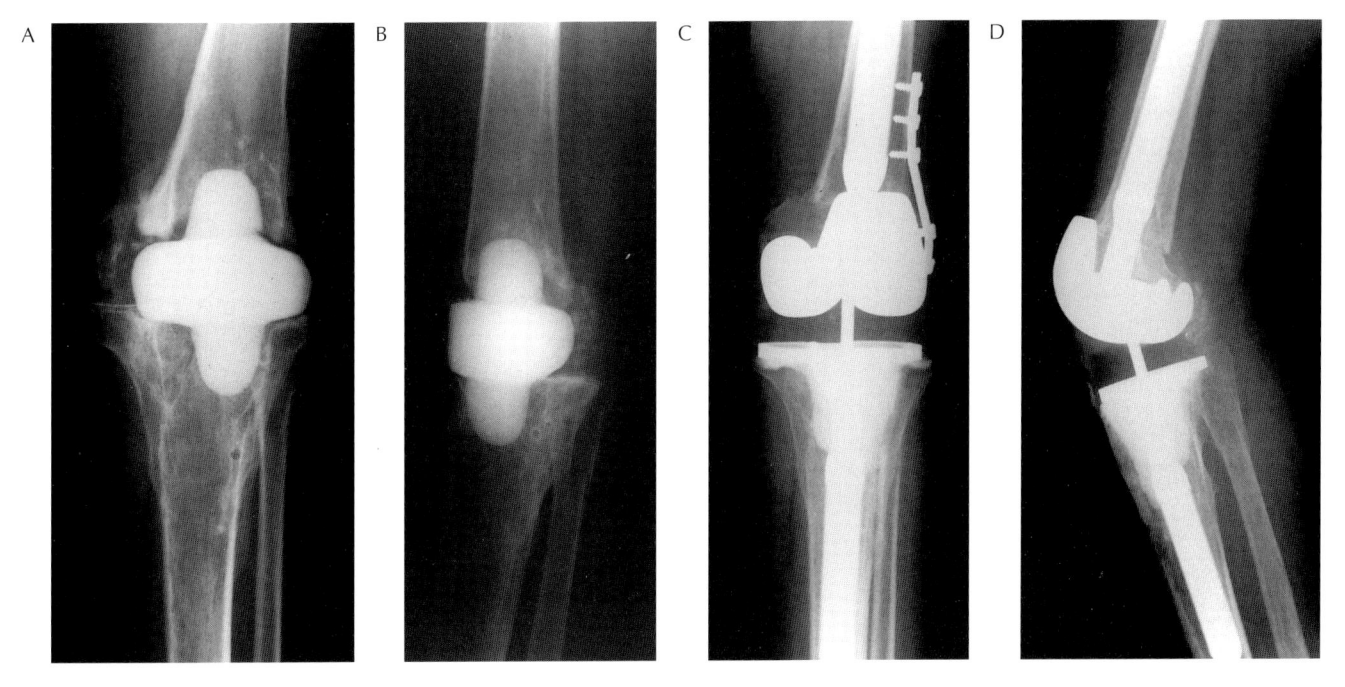

Figure 56.4. (A) Preoperative anteroposterior and (B) lateral radiographs demonstrating a large bicondylar distal femoral osseous defect following removal of an infected, long-stem cemented hinge TKA with insertion of antibiotic impregnated polymethylmethacrylate spacer. (C) Postoperative anteroposterior and (D) lateral radiographs following distal femoral allograft reconstruction with additional unicortical plate fixation.

sive femoral bone loss, efforts to maintain the medial and lateral epicondyles with their respective collateral ligamentous attachments are favored. The epicondyles can then be securely reattached to the distal femoral allograft with screw fixation (Fig. 56.5A–B).

Wound closure without excessive tension, especially in the region of the proximal tibia, may occasionally be difficult if large segmental allografts have been implanted.[18] The use of relaxing skin incisions or rotational myocutaneous flaps are occasionally required to avoid tight skin closure.

Protected weight-bearing by the patient postoperatively is important for allograft incorporation.[19,35,40] In cases in which the majority of the prosthesis is supported by allograft, protected weight-bearing is continued until radiographic signs of allograft union are observed. In those patients requiring allograft reconstruction of the entire distal femur so that little inherent collateral ligamentous stability is present at the time of surgery, postoperative bracing is utilized until allograft-host union is obtained to avoid excessive loads at the allograft-host junction.

CLINICAL RESULTS

Results of structural allografting of the distal femur are few and follow-up is limited. Some reports combine data of allografting of both the proximal tibia and distal femur and do not isolate the results from femoral allografting alone. Mnaymneh and associates[18] reviewed 12 patients in which 14 structural allografts were used to reconstruct either the distal femur or proximal tibia at a mean follow-up of 40 months. Of the seven cases involving structural allografting of the distal femur, nonunion of the allograft occurred in two cases (28.6%) and one tibiofemoral dislocation occurred.

Harris and colleagues[41] reported on 14 cases of revision TKA requiring structural allografts for noncontained osseous defects at a mean follow-up duration of 43 months. Eight of these cases involved allografting of the distal femur. Good or excellent results were obtained in seven of these eight cases (87.5%) with one failure due to nonunion and recurrent infection.

Results of structural allografting of 13 large, noncontained femoral defects were reported by Tsahakis and associates.[3] At a mean follow-up of period of 2.1 years, allograft-host union occurred in all cases with no allograft collapse or reoperations required.

A series of nine cases of complex TKA requiring reconstruction of the entire distal femur with structural allograft was reported by Paprosky.[42] An unlinked, constrained condylar prosthetic design with press-fit diaphyseal engaging stems was utilized in each case. Seven of nine cases (77.8%) were judged good or excellent and union of the allograft occurred in 100% of cases. Com-

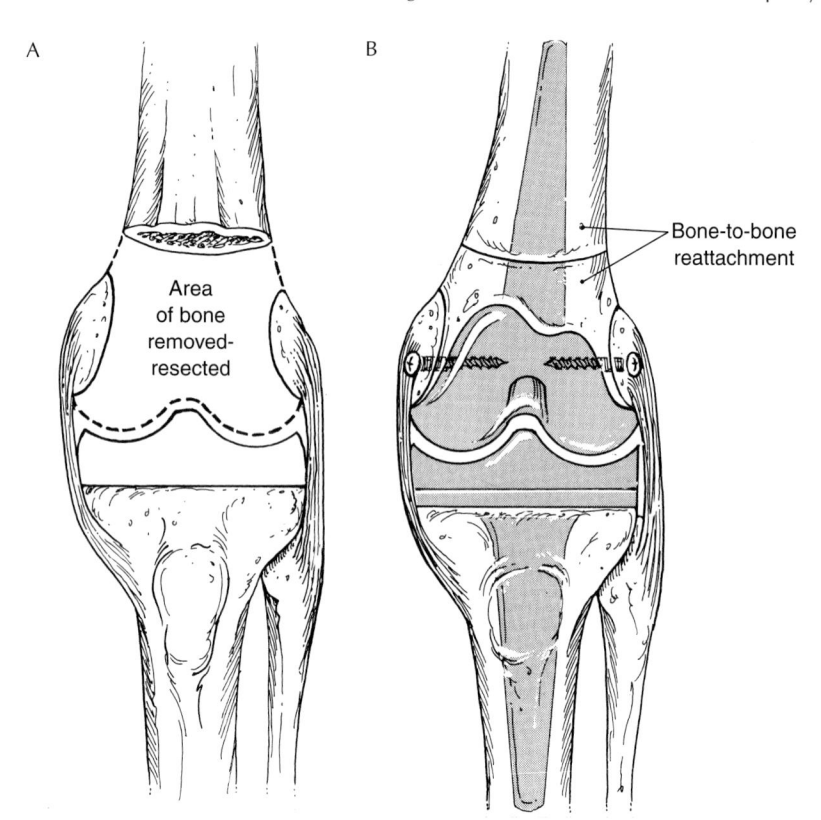

Figure 56.5. (A) Diagram of massive distal femoral defect with maintenance of medial and lateral epicondylar attachments of the collateral ligaments. (B) Diagram demonstrating distal femoral allograft reconstruction with collateral ligamentous reconstruction utilizing epicondylar bone-to-bone reattachment technique.

plications included one case of hyperextension instability requiring bracing and one case of lateral patellar subluxation, which did not necessitate further treatment.

Kraay and colleagues[39] have reviewed a series of seven patients treated with structural allografting of the entire distal femur following complex supracondylar femur fractures and ipsilateral TKA. Three patients had died prior to 2-year follow-up, but had satisfactory pain relief with allograft incorporation. Three of the four remaining patients had satisfactory results at a mean follow-up of 44 months without clinical or radiographic mechanical failure.

SUMMARY

While morselized cancellous autograft or allograft has been shown to be highly successful for management of smaller cavitary defects in revision TKA, structural allografts are often required for large contained or noncontained osseous defects. Early clinical results of revision TKA utilizing structural allografts have been encouraging with high allograft-host union rates, as long as adequate allograft fixation is obtained. The use of intramedullary stems with sufficient length to engage diaphyseal bone is recommended to lessen load transmission to the structural allograft and reduce the risk of late allograft collapse or fracture. Extensive preoperative planning, meticulous operative technique, and an extended period of postoperative rehabilitation are required for optimal results.

References

1. Insall JN. Revision of total knee replacement. *Instr Course Lect.* 1986; 35:290–296.
2. Rand JA, Bryan RS. Results of revision total knee arthroplasties using condylar prostheses. A review of fifty knees. *J Bone Joint Surg.* 1988; 70A:738–745.
3. Tsahakis PJ, Beaver WB, Brick GW. Technique and results of allograft reconstruction in revision total knee arthroplasty. *Clin Orthop.* 1994; 303:86–94.
4. Elia EA, Lotke PA. Results of revision total knee arthroplasty associated with significant bone loss. *Clin Orthop.* 1991; 271:114–121.
5. Ritter MA. Screw and cement fixation of large defects in total knee arthroplasty. *J Arthroplasty.* 1986; 1:125–129.
6. Bartel DL, Burstein AH, Santavicca EA, Insall JN. Performance of the tibial component in total knee replacement. *J Bone Joint Surg.* 1982; 64A:1026–1033.
7. Brand MG, Daley RJ, Ewald FC, Scott RD. Tibial tray augmentation with modular metal wedges for tibial bone stock deficiency. *Clin Orthop.* 1989; 248:71–79.
8. Pagnano MW, Trousdale RT, Rand JA. Tibial wedge augmentation for bone deficiency in total knee arthroplasty. A follow-up study. *Clin Orthop.* 1995; 321:151–155.
9. Rand JA. Bone deficiency in total knee arthroplasty. Use of metal wedge augmentation. *Clin Orthop.* 1991; 271:63–71.
10. Aglietti P, Buzzi R, Scrobe F. Autologous bone grafting for

medial tibial defects in total knee arthroplasty. *J Arthroplasty.* 1991; 6:287–294.
11. Altchek D, Sculco TP, Rawlins B. Autogenous bone grafting for severe angular deformity in total knee arthroplasty. *J Arthroplasty.* 1989; 4:151–155.
12. Dorr LD, Ranawat CS, Sculco TA, McKaskill B, Orisek BS. Bone graft for tibial defects in total knee arthroplasty. *Clin Orthop.* 1986; 205:153–165.
13. Laskin RS. Total knee arthroplasty in the presence of large bony defects of the tibia and marked knee instability. *Clin Orthop.* 1989; 248:66–70.
14. Scuderi GR, Insall JN, Haas SB, Becker-Fluegel MW, Windsor RE. Inlay autogeneic bone grafting of tibial defects in primary total knee arthroplasty. *Clin Orthop.* 1989; 248: 93–97.
15. Windsor RE, Insall JN, Sculco TP. Bone grafting of tibial defects in primary and revision total knee arthroplasty. *Clin Orthop.* 1986; 205:132–137.
16. Harris AI, Gitelis S, Rosenberg A, Rivero D, Sheinkop MB. Structural allografts in revision total knee arthroplasty. Proceedings of the American Academy of Orthopaedic Surgeons 58th Annual Meeting. Anaheim, California, March 11, 1991.
17. Mankin HJ, Doppelt S, Tomford W. Clinical experience with allograft implantation. The first ten years. *Clin Orthop.* 1983; 174:69–86.
18. Mnaymneh W, Emerson RH, Borja F, Head WC, Malinin TI. Massive allografts in salvage revisions of failed total knee arthroplasties. *Clin Orthop.* 1990; 260:144–153.
19. Mnaymneh W, Malinin TI, Makley JT, Dick HM. Massive osteoarticular allografts in the reconstruction of extremities following resection of tumors not requiring chemotherapy and radiation. *Clin Orthop.* 1985; 197:76–87.
20. Stockley I, McAuley JP, Gross AE. Allograft reconstruction in total knee arthroplasty. *J Bone Joint Surg.* 1992; 74B:393–397.
21. Wilde AH, Schickendantz MS, Stulberg BN, Go RT. The incorporation of tibial allografts in total knee arthroplasty. *J Bone Joint Surg.* 1990; 72A:815–824.
22. Whiteside LA. Bone grafting in revision cementless total knee arthroplasty. *Instr Course Lect.* 1993; 42:397–403.
23. Berrey BH Jr, Lord CF, Gebhardt MC, Mankin HF. Fractures of allografts. Frequency, treatment, and end-results. *J Bone Joint Surg.* 1990; 72A:825–833.
24. Buck BE, Malinin TI, Brown MD. Bone transplantation and human immunodeficiency virus. An estimate of risk of acquired immunodeficiency syndrome (AIDS). *Clin Orthop.* 1989; 240:129–136.
25. Pelker RR, Friedlaender GE. Biomechanical properties of bone autografts and allografts. *Orthop Clin North Am.* 1987; 18:235–239.
26. Spire B, Dormont D, Barre-Sinoussi F, Montagnier L, Chermann JC. Inactivation of lymphadenopathy-associated virus by heat, gamma rays and ultraviolet light. *Lancet.* 1985; 1(8422):188–189.
27. Cameron HU, Cameron G. Stress-relief osteoporosis of the anterior femoral condyles in total knee replacement. A study of 185 patients. *Orthop Rev.* 1987; 16:449–456.
28. Vince KG. Revision knee arthroplasty. In: Chapman MW, ed. *Operative Orthopaedics.* 2nd ed. Philadelphia: J.B. Lippincott Co, 1993; 1981–2010.
29. Frick S, Tsahakis PJ, Peindl RD, Barr S, Brick GW. Distal femoral allografts for the reconstruction of structural acetabular deficiencies in revision total hip arthroplasty: A biomechanical study with clinical correlation. Proceedings of the American Academy of Orthopaedic Surgeons 61st Annual Meeting. New Orleans, Louisiana, February 24–March 1, 1994.
30. Scott RD, Siliski JM. The use of a modified V-Y quadricepsplasty during total knee replacement to gain exposure and improve flexion in the ankylosed knee. *Orthopedics.* 1985; 8:45–48.
31. Trousdale RT, Hanssen AD, Rand JA, Cahalan TD. V-Y quadricepsplasty in total knee arthroplasty. *Clin Orthop.* 1993; 286:48–55.
32. Whiteside LA, Ohl MD. Tibial tubercle osteotomy for exposure of the difficult total knee arthroplasty. *Clin Orthop.* 1990; 260:6–9.
33. Herzwurm PJ, Engh GA, Parks NL. Use of bulk allografts and stemmed components for major bone defects in total knee arthroplasty. *Orthop Trans.* 1996; 20(1):32.
34. Tsahakis PJ, Brick GW, Ewald FC, Reilly DT, Sledge CB, Poss R. Use of bulk allografts for uncontained defects in revision total knee arthroplasty. Proceedings of the American Academy of Orthopaedic Surgeons 59th Annual Meeting. Washington, DC, February 22, 1992.
35. Burchardt H. The biology of bone graft repair. *Clin Orthop.* 1983; 174:28–42.
36. Goldberg VM, Lance EM. Revascularization and accretion in transplantation. Quantitative studies of the role of the allograft barrier. *J Bone Joint Surg.* 1972; 54A:807–816.
37. Reilly D, Walker PS, Ben-Dov M, Ewald FC. Effects of tibial components on load transfer in the upper tibia. *Clin Orthop.* 1982; 165:273–282.
38. Montgomery WH III, Becker MS, Haas SB, Insall JN, Windsor RE. The evolution of revision total knee arthroplasty for aseptic failure using metal-backed and custom components. Proceedings of the American Academy of Orthopaedic Surgeons 59th Annual Meeting. Washington, DC, February 22, 1992.
39. Kraay MJ, Goldberg VM, Figgie MP, Figgie HE III. Distal femoral replacement with allograft/prosthetic reconstruction for treatment of supracondylar fractures in patients with total knee arthroplasty. *J Arthroplasty.* 1992; 7:7–16.
40. McGann W, Mankin HJ, Harris WH. Massive allografting for severe failed total hip replacement. *J Bone Joint Surg.* 1986; 68A:4–12.
41. Harris AI, Poddar S, Gitelis S, Sheinkop MB, Rosenberg AG. Arthroplasty with a composite of an allograft and a prosthesis for knees with severe deficiency of bone. *J Bone Joint Surg.* 1995; 77A:373–386.
42. Paprosky WG. Use of distal femoral allografts in revision total knee arthroplasty. In: Insall JN, Scott WN, Scuderi GR, eds. *Current Concepts in Primary and Revision Total Knee Arthroplasty.* Philadelphia: Lippincott-Raven Publishers; 1996: 217–26.

SECTION 16
Fixation Techniques in Revision Knee Arthroplasty

CHAPTER 57
Cemented Revision Knee Arthroplasty

William J. Maloney

INTRODUCTION

Total knee arthroplasty has become a more frequent surgical procedure as the number of primary replacements increases. Interpretation of the results of revision total knee arthroplasty is difficult because reports in the literature on revision knee replacement usually contain a mixture of several different implant types with varying case complexity. As a result, the reported success rates of revision total knee replacement vary tremendously. Success rates as low as 30% at 5 years[1] and as high as 90% at 6 years[2] have been reported. In order to understand this variability, one must understand the factors that have an impact on success. The time period in which the revision surgery was performed is important. In general, older studies report higher failure rates. This is likely related to limited prosthetic selection and a poorer understanding of the importance of ligament balance and implant constraint at the time these surgeries were performed. The complexity of the revision operation has an obvious impact on success. Cases involving severe bone loss and ligamentous instability are technically more challenging with higher complication rates and poorer results. Similarly, the more constrained the implant required to perform a revision surgery, the higher the failure rate. Finally, one has to be aware that there is no single set of criteria that is widely used to define success or failure. Failure may be defined by the need for revision surgery, by radiographic evidence of loosening, or by poor clinical results. Thus, when reviewing reports on the results of revision total knee arthroplasty the reader must determine the time period in which the surgery was performed, the complexity of the cases involved, the implants used as well as the definition of failure to more fully appreciate the significance of these reports. This chapter will focus on the results of cemented fixation in knee revision surgery discussing primarily those cases in which bone loss and instability are problematic.

SURGICAL TECHNIQUE

Although this chapter will focus on the results of cemented fixation in revision knee replacement, some comments concerning the preoperative evaluation are appropriate. It is important when evaluating a failed total knee arthroplasty to try to determine the cause of the failure because this will aid in developing an operative plan. If instability is present, it is generally the result of inadequate balancing during the initial knee implantation. Instability can also result from a malaligned prosthesis. Additionally, instability can occur as a result of the loosening process. When planning a revision procedure, determining the underlying cause of instability will aid the surgeon in planning how to correct it. In some cases, collateral ligament balance is possible at the time of revision surgery, while in other cases, the incompetent ligaments must be substituted for using an appropriate implant. Preoperative radiographs will aid in determining the degree of bone loss. This will aid the surgeon in having the necessary implants and graft material present at the time of surgery.

The individual steps in revision total knee arthroplasty are described in detail in several chapters in this text. The sequence of steps is briefly outlined below. In revision surgery, exposure of the knee is often difficult. Contracture of the extensor mechanism and scarring of the lateral gutter and suprapatellar pouch can make it difficult to evert the patella and flex the knee. Care is required in these cases to avoid patellar tendon rupture or avulsion. Scar tissue in the peripatellar region should be excised and the lateral gutter debrided lysing adhesions and removing dense scar. At this point, the mobility of the quadriceps mechanism in terms of the ease of patellar eversion is assessed. If the patella cannot be everted and the knee flexed without undo stress on the patellar tendon, the surgeon must use another approach. Several techniques have been described to aid in exposure of the tight knee and include lateral retinacular release, quadriceps snip (Chapter 19), V-Y turndown (Chapter 20), and tibial tubercle osteotomy (Chapter 21).

Once the knee has been adequately exposed, the next step is to remove the implant to be revised. Often, at least one of the implants may still be well fixed but will require removal. The goal in implant removal is to avoid further compromise to bone stock (Chapter 50). Next, the soft tissue membrane must be completely debrided exposing host bone. This permits accurate assessment and management of the bony defects (Chapter 53). Finally, the surgeon must balance the ligaments using an implant of appropriate size and design (Chapter 51) to aid in this goal and insert the implants in proper alignment using good cement technique.

In order to optimize cement fixation, all loose cement and soft tissue membrane should be removed. The use of pulsed lavage aids in debridement and helps to identify scar tissue. Scar tissue and hypertrophic synovium should be removed preserving collateral ligaments. The posterior capsule is usually thickened and should be thinned to avoid impairment of joint motion.

IMPLANT SELECTION

In the absence of significant bone loss or ligamentous instability, the choice of implant is not as critical as when there is compromised bone and ligamentous laxity. The majority of patients undergoing revision of a surface type replacement can usually be revised with a total condylar design or a posterior-stabilized total condylar design. The posterior cruciate ligament is often compromised during the aseptic loosening process or damaged during implant removal. It is the opinion of the author that a cruciate-substituting implant should be used if there is compromise of the posterior cruciate ligament.

The more severely damaged the knee, the more constraint required from the implant to substitute for damaged ligaments (Fig. 57.1). With increased constraint, less force on the joint is taken up by soft tissue and more is transferred through the implant to the implant bone interface. When using an implant with more constraint than a standard posterior-stabilized condylar design, extension rods should be used. The advantage of using extension rods in these cases include improved initial implant stability and an increase in the cement–bone interface surface area over which load can be transferred.

RESULTS

In the 1980s, the Mayo clinic revision total knee experience was reported by Bryan and Rand.[3,4] Success was graded based on specific criteria that included no or mild pain, knee flexion to at least 90 degrees, and mild or no instability. Using these criteria, success correlated with whether it was the first or subsequent revision operation. If it was the patient's first revision, the success rate was 66%. In contrast, the success rate dropped to 61% for the second revision and 57% for the third revision. There was no significant difference in survival rates when comparing the older semiconstrained devices (geometric and polycentric designs) with the older more constrained devices (Guepar, Tavernetti, and Walldius designs). However, the newer less-constrained devices of that time period (anametric, total condylar, kinematic condylar designs) demonstrated significantly longer survival than the newer more-constrained implants (kinematic-stabilizer, kinematic rotating-hinge, total condylar III designs) (Fig. 57.1).

During the same time period as the report by Bryan and Rand, Insall and Dethmers[2] reported that when they used a posterior-stabilized implant for revision of aseptic failures, 89% of the results were satisfactory after an average of 2 years following their revision operation. In a subsequent study, Rand and Bryan reported on 50 revision total knee replacements using a condylar prosthesis.[5] This study group represented a selected group of revisions (out of 261) done during 1980 and 1981. None of the cases in this series had more than mild bone loss. Both the femoral and tibial components were seated on an intact rim of bone with central defects less than 1 cm in depth. In addition, all of the patients had intact collateral ligaments. Seventy-six percent of the patients were graded as having either excellent or good results an average of 4.8 years after surgery. Three knees subsequently loosened, two of which were revised.

Donaldson and associates[6] reported on the use of the total condylar III prosthesis (TC-III). The TC-III prosthesis provides increased constraint compared to the original total condylar design, but is less constrained than a hinge. This implant was chosen because of bone loss or collateral ligament instability or both. This implant has a large central eminence to provide increased anteroposterior and mediolateral stability. The implant also has fixed extended tibial and femoral stems. In their study, both primary and revision cases were included. The primary group consisting of 17 patients had good or excellent results. In contrast, only 50% of the 14 revision cases had good or excellent results. Overall, 36% of the revision cases were reported as failures. Three failed secondary to infection and two failed as a result of aseptic loosening.

Rosenberg and colleagues[7] reported on 36 patients (36 knees) using the same prosthesis (total condylar III). The patients were followed for a mean of 45 months (24 to 84 months). The reason for revision was loosening in 19, sepsis in 15, and pain and instability in 2. Sixty-nine percent of the patients were graded as having excellent or good results. Extension lag was common postopera-

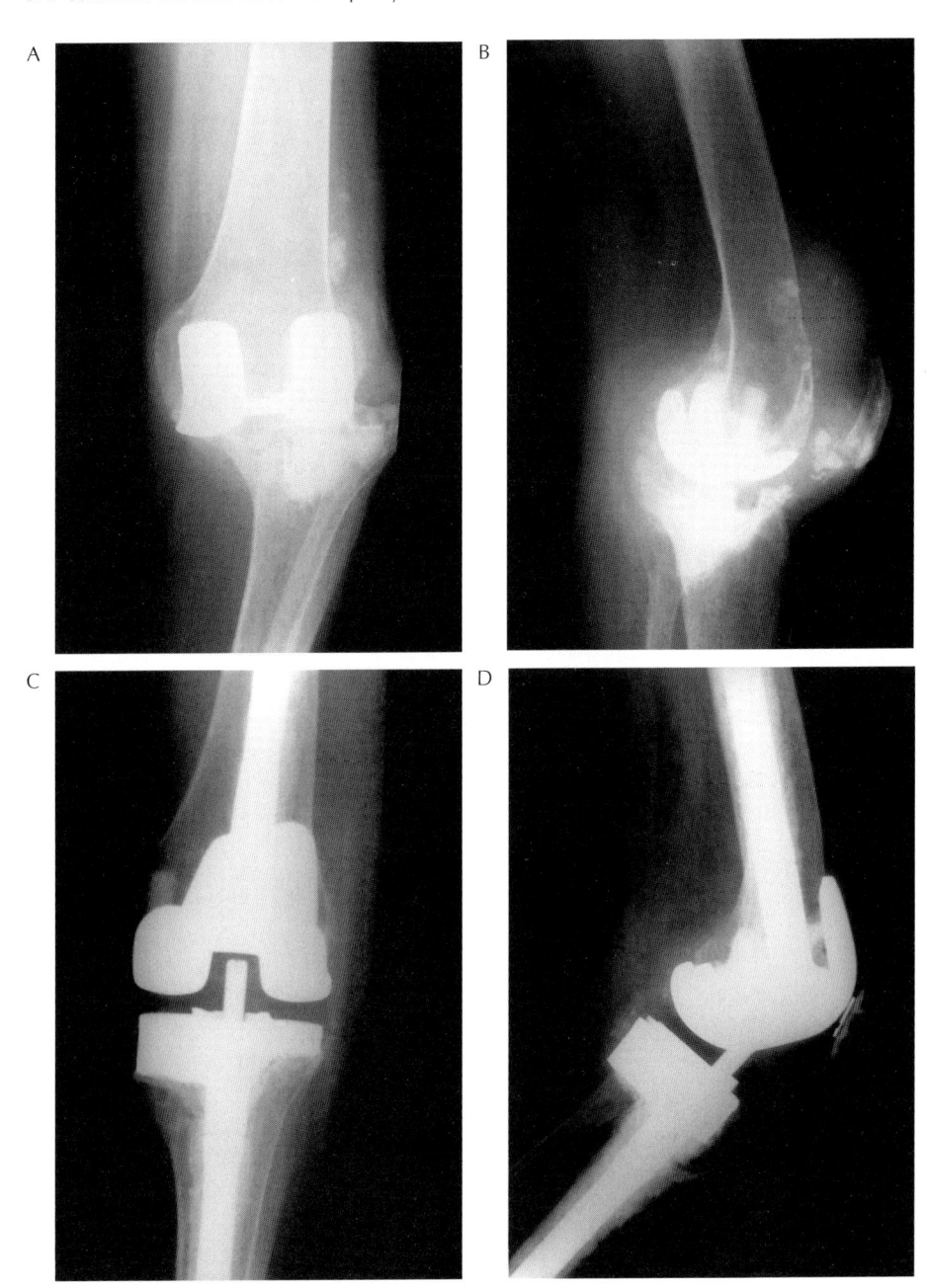

Figure 57.1. (A) AP and (B) lateral radiographs of a failed cemented total knee arthroplasty demonstrating severe bone loss in association with gross ligamentous instability. (C) Postoperative AP and (D) lateral radiographs demonstrating revision total knee arthroplasty performed with cemented components utilizing a constrained insert and a medial tibial augmentation block with extension rods in both the femoral and tibial sides.

tively occurring in 13 patients. One superficial and no deep infections were reported. Two patients required manipulation that resulted in a femoral fracture in one case that was successfully treated in a cast brace. Analysis of the four poor results revealed that three of the patients were minimally ambulatory preoperatively and remained so postoperatively. All four patients continued to have pain with ambulation, but three of four had pain scores of 25 or greater and were satisfied with their results. Only one patient had a poor result and required re-revision for aseptic loosening 28 months after her initial revision operation.

In a more recent review, Rand[8] reviewed 21 knees treated for aseptic loosening of a previous TKA in which the total condylar III prosthesis was used. The patients were evaluated 2 to 7 years after their revision operation (mean 4 years). Using the Knee Society scoring system, the patients improved from a mean of 21 for pain and 11 for function pre-revision to 71 for pain and 56 for function post-revision. The average knee flexion preoperatively was 108 degrees. At the last follow-up visit, the mean flexion was 102 degrees. No radiolucent lines were detected adjacent to 12 of the femoral components and 6 of the tibial components. Seven of the femoral and 11 of the tibial components had radiolucent lines at the cement-bone interface, but only one tibial component had a complete radiolucent line. None of the implants had a detectable change in position. The complication rate in this type of surgery is high. In this series, the overall complication rate was 33%. Complications included two patellar fractures, one patellar tendon rupture, one superficial infection, and one deep infection. In the patient with deep sepsis, amputation was required to control the infection.

The results of modern revision total knee arthroplasty performed with cement reported by other authors are similar. Elia and Lotke[9] studied 40 cases in 38 patients who underwent revision surgery for aseptic failure. At a minimum 2-year follow-up evaluation, they reported 75% good or excellent results, 10% failures, and an overall complication rate of 30%. Friedman and associates[10] reported on 137 revision total knee arthroplasties in 117 patients. Success was defined as having no or mild pain, no or mild instability, and at least 90 degrees of flexion. Using these criteria, a clinical success rate of 63% for a first revision and 50% for subsequent revisions. Goldberg and colleagues[11] reported only 46% good or excellent results in 65 consecutive revision total knee arthroplasties. Forty-two percent had poor results or had failed.

As noted above, the survival rate generally decreases with increasing implant constraint. Rand and associates[12] reported on the first 50 kinematic rotating hinge total knee arthroplasties done at the Mayo Clinic at an average of 50 months after surgery. Thirty-six of the patients in this series were undergoing revision knee arthroplasty. The rotating hinge implant was used because of ligamentous instability or bone loss or both. Forty-two percent of the knees with available radiographs for review demonstrated progressive radiolucent lines at the implant-bone interface. Aseptic loosening requiring revision occurred in 3 knees in 3 patients. Two additional knees were radiographically loose. In addition to aseptic loosening, there was a 16% rate of sepsis, a 22% rate of patellar instability, and a 6% incidence of breakage. They concluded that this implant should only be used in cases of collateral ligament absence that cannot be managed by soft tissue reconstruction.

The optimal fixation mode of tibial and femoral extension rods is unclear. Haas and colleagues[13] reviewed 76 cemented revision total knee replacements performed at the Hospital for Special Surgery in 74 patients. Only patients who had aseptic loosening of the tibial or femoral component or both were included. In this series, cement was applied to the metaphyseal surface of the tibia and femur. Fluted diaphyseal rods were used in all patients and were not cemented. Metal wedges and augments were used to fill bony defects. Eighty-four percent of the patients were rated as having a good or excellent result based on the Hospital for Special Surgery knee rating system. Seven percent of the patients had a fair or poor result. An additional 8% of the patients failed requiring revision. Survivorship at 8 years demonstrated an 83% chance of survival. The most common cause for failure was infection (three cases), followed by aseptic loosening (two cases), and instability (one case). In contrast to the high rate of aseptic loosening reported by Vince and Long[14] following revision with the use of a constrained tibial insert and extension rods inserted without cement, the authors of this study did not have a higher failure rate with constrained inserts compared to posterior-stabilized inserts. Most of the patients who failed in the report by Vince and Long had a history of infection, which may in part explain the higher failure rate in this study.

The radiographic analysis of long-stemmed components inserted without cement frequently demonstrates radiopaque lines adjacent to the intramedullary rods. In the study by Haas and associates,[13] radiopaque lines were noted along 67% of the femoral rods and 69% of the tibial rods. Bertin and colleagues[15] reported 88% of extension rods inserted without cement developed white lines adjacent to the stems. They noted that this radiographic finding had no correlation with pain.

Theoretical concerns about the use of cemented long-stem revision knee implants include stress shielding and difficulty in removal. Murray and associates[16] reported on 35 patients with 40 cemented long-stem kinematic stabilizer revision total knee arthroplasties. In this study, 25 long-stem tibial and 38 long-stem femoral components were implanted. The initial postoperative radiographs showed tibial radiolucencies in 5 knees. An additional 5 knees developed radiolucencies around the tibial component but all were less than 1 mm and incomplete. Two femoral components had cement-bone radiolucencies on the initial postoperative radiographs, one of which demonstrated radiographic loosening that was clinically asymptomatic. With follow-up evaluation, 3 more femoral components developed cement-bone radiolucencies. The authors note the 32% incidence of tibial radiolucencies with cemented long stems in this study was similar to that noted with nonstemmed revision knee replacement using the same implant design.

As noted above, the complication rate in revision total knee arthroplasty is high. Stuart and colleagues[8] reported on the complication requiring reoperation after cemented condylar revision total knee arthroplasties. From a group of 655 condylar revisions, 46 knees without a history of sepsis were identified as requiring 60 reoperations. The most common reason for reoperation was a problem related to the extensor mechanism including the patella. These reoperations accounted for 41% of the cases. Other problems included component loosening (22%), sepsis (20%), wound problems (20%), ligamentous instability (17%), and limited range of motion in four knees (8%). The authors point out that awareness of these failure modes may help to prevent these complications by attention at the time of revision surgery to protection of the patellar tendon and collateral ligaments, balancing of the extensor mechanism, proper component position and sizing, restoration of the mechanical axis, as well as use of more constrained implant designs.

SUMMARY

Successful revision total knee arthroplasty requires careful preoperative planning and attention to surgical technique in order to optimize results. Even in the most experienced hands, complication rates are high. Success in terms of pain relief, function, and survivorship depend on the extent of bone loss, ligamentous compromise, and the degree of constraint inherent in the implant used. In order to interpret the results of cemented revision total knee replacement surgery, the reader must take into account the severity of the cases being performed, the types of implants used, as well as the criteria used to define success or failure.

References

1. Cameron HU, Hunter GA. Failure in total knee arthroplasty: mechanisms, revisions, and results. *Clin Orthop*. 1982; 170:141–146.
2. Insall JN, Dethmers DA. Revision of total knee arthroplasty. *Clin Orthop*. 1982; 170:123–130.
3. Bryan RS, Rand JA. Revision total knee arthroplasty. *Clin Orthop*. 1982; 170:116–122.
4. Rand JA, Bryan RS. Revision after total knee arthroplasty. *Orthop Clin North Am*. 1982; 13:201–212.
5. Rand JA, Bryan RS. Results of revision total knee arthroplasties using condylar prostheses. *J Bone Joint Surg*. 1988; 70A:738–744.
6. Donaldson WF, Sculco TP, Insall JN, Ranawat CS. Total condylar II prosthesis: long-term follow-up study. *Clin Orthop*. 1988; 226:21–28.
7. Rosenberg AG, Verner JJ, Galante JO. Clinical results of total knee revision using the total condylar III prosthesis. *Clin Orthop*. 1991; 273:83–90.
8. Rand JA. Revision total knee arthroplasty using the total condylar III prosthesis. *J Arthroplasty*. 1991; 6:279–284.
9. Elia EA, Lotke PA. Results of revision total knee arthroplasty associated with significant bone loss. *Clin Orthop*. 1991; 271:114–121.
10. Friedman RJ, Hirst P, Poss R, Kelley K, Sledge CB. Results of revision total knee arthroplasty performed for aseptic loosening. *Clin Orthop*. 1990; 255:235–241.
11. Goldberg VM, Figgie MP, Figgie HE, Sobel M. The results of revision total knee arthroplasty. *Clin Orthop*. 1988; 226: 86–92.
12. Rand JA, Chao EYS, Stauffer RN. Kinematic rotating hinge total knee arthroplasty. *J Bone Joint Surg*. 1987; 69A:489–497.
13. Haas SB, Insall JN, Montgomery W, Windsor RE. Revision total knee arthroplasty with the use of modular with stems inserted without cement. *J Bone Joint Surg*. 1995; 77A:1700–1707.
14. Vince KG, Long W. Press fit long stem revision total knee arthroplasty. Read at the Annual Meeting of the Knee Society. New Orleans, Louisiana, February 27, 1994.
15. Bertin KC, Freeman MAR, Samuelson KM, Ratcliffe SS, Todd RC. Stemmed revision arthroplasty for aseptic loosening of total knee replacement. *J Bone Joint Surg*. 1995; 67B:242–248.
16. Murray PB, Rand JA, Hanssen AD. Cemented long-stem revision total knee arthroplasty. *Clin Orthop*. 1994; 309: 116–123.
17. Stuart MJ, Larson JE, Morrey BF. Reoperation after condylar revision total knee arthroplasty. *Clin Orthop*. 1993; 286: 168–173.

CHAPTER 58
Cementless Fixation

Leo A. Whiteside

ABSTRACT

Cementless revision total knee arthroplasty has been used exclusively for 12 years in clean and infected cases. Tight-stem fixation combined with rim seating of the femoral and tibial revision implants left large contained defects that were filled with a combination of morselized cancellous allograft, demineralized allograft bone powder, and local cancellous bone and marrow. These elements produce an effective osteoconductive and osteoinductive material that consistently restores bone stock and produces a durable support structure for the implants.

One-hundred-nineteen clean revision cases followed for 2 to 10 years had a failure rate of 3% due to loosening. The remainder had radiographic evidence of stable fixation. Biopsies of 17 knees showed early, vigorous bone formation and late maturation throughout the grafts. Thirty-three infected knees had revision using this technique 6 to 12 weeks after debridement. Four knees required repeated debridement and revision due to recurrent infection, but currently are functioning well. One had repeated recurrent infection and required amputation.

Cementless reconstruction of severely damaged bone stock using stem fixation, rim seating, and morselized allograft has proven highly effective for difficult revision total knee arthroplasty.

INTRODUCTION

Reconstitution of bone stock is a primary concern at revision surgery for failed total knee arthroplasty (Fig. 58.1). Fixation is often difficult because the cancellous bone has been depleted, so it is tempting to cement the implant to diaphyseal cortical bone. However, revision with cement ultimately destroys more bone stock.

Reprinted with permission from Williams & Wilkins. In: *Total Knee Revision Arthroplasty*, Rorabeck C, Engh G, eds, 1997.

Rather, cementless fixation techniques that use an uncemented stem to engage the isthmus and bone graft to fill the defects can provide adequate fixation as well as the opportunity to reconstruct the bone stock about the knee.[1-3]

The major concerns with massive bone grafting—vascularization and incorporation—remain significant issues in the knee,[4] and bone grafting with allograft still raises the question of immunocompatibility. Bone tissue itself is not highly immunogenic, but the marrow cells incite a vigorous immune response[5] and can create an inflammatory process that blocks ossification and incorporation of the graft.[6]

Early reports of allograft reconstruction in the tibia and cementless fixation of the tibial component have been encouraging,[1,2] and reconstruction of the femur with cementless components has now been well documented in the literature.[7,8] Loss of bone in the distal femur is a major problem after a cemented total knee arthroplasty has failed, and revision surgery with a cemented stem can cause even more bone loss. An effort has been made since 1984 to reconstruct bone defects with morselized allograft bone and to fix the implants to the patient's remaining bone structure without cement. It was initially thought that cementless fixation of the components would be tenuous and that repeat revision would be necessary to achieve durable fixation with the improved bone stock. However, durability of the construct has been surprisingly reliable and repeated revision due to failure of fixation has not been necessary.[3]

In cases of infected total knee arthroplasty, treatment regimens range from debridement and antibiotics to removal and fusion, but the standard treatment has been to remove the implants, treat with antibiotics for 6 weeks, and finally perform revision arthroplasty with antibiotic-impregnated cement.[9-12] However, cementless reconstruction is attractive for these revision cases because further bone destruction is avoided and bone stock can also be restored.[1,2,13,14]

This chapter describes the technique for using bone

58. Cementless Fixation

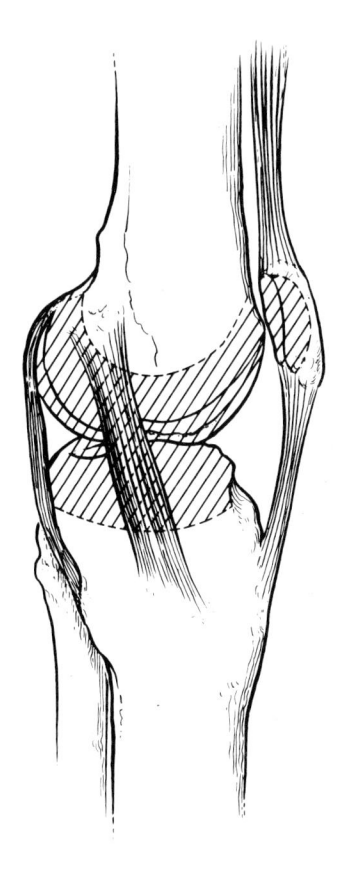

Figure 58.1. Bone loss from the femur, tibia, and patella may be extensive in failed total knee arthroplasty, but the ligaments and capsule are usually competent. Cancellous bone stock is rarely intact. The shaded area represents loss of cortical wall and cancellous structure. The ligaments, capsule, and tendons are usually intact. (From Whiteside,[13] by permission of Lippincott-Raven)

graft to treat massive bone loss in cementless reconstruction of failed total knee arthroplasty, and reports the results of cementless reconstruction since 1984.

BONE PREPARATION TECHNIQUE

Bone loss is one of the major problems in failed total knee arthroplasty, so minimal bone should be resected during preparation to preserve the remaining bone stock (Fig. 58.2). The amount of bone erosion makes complete seating of the component nearly impossible, so that augmented fixation with a stem is almost always necessary to achieve toggle control of the implant. This technique results in substantial, uncontained defects on both the femoral and the tibial sides. Seating the implant on the patient's own bone stock controls axial migration, and the stem prevents the implant from tilting into the defect. Screw and peg fixation can add stability to the construct, thereby allowing the cavitary deficiencies to be filled with morselized bone. This bone-grafting technique promotes rapid healing and reconstitution of bone stock without the technical difficulty and late collapse associated with massive allograft replacement.

Femoral Preparation

When bone destruction is assessed, the medial and lateral condyles are usually found to be at least partially intact. With intramedullary instrumentation as a guide, the distal surface of the femur should be resected just enough to achieve firm seating of the femoral component on one side of the bone. Both sides may be engaged by the implant in some cases, but often only one of the two condyles can afford firm seating for the femoral component without excessive resection of the distal femur (Fig. 58.3). After all the cuts have been made with the saw and all the surfaces are prepared (Fig. 58.4), the femoral component is partially inserted and the morselized allograft is packed into the deficient areas. The implant is then driven until it is fully seated, then more bone graft can be packed tightly into the distal and posterior cavitary defects (Fig. 58.5). Prolonged protection from weight-bearing allows healing of bone into the cavitary defects for mediolateral and anteroposterior support of the implant.

Tibial Preparation

Reconstruction of massive tibial defects also relies upon rim support for axial loading and a stem to stabilize the implant. Screws can be used effectively in the tibial com-

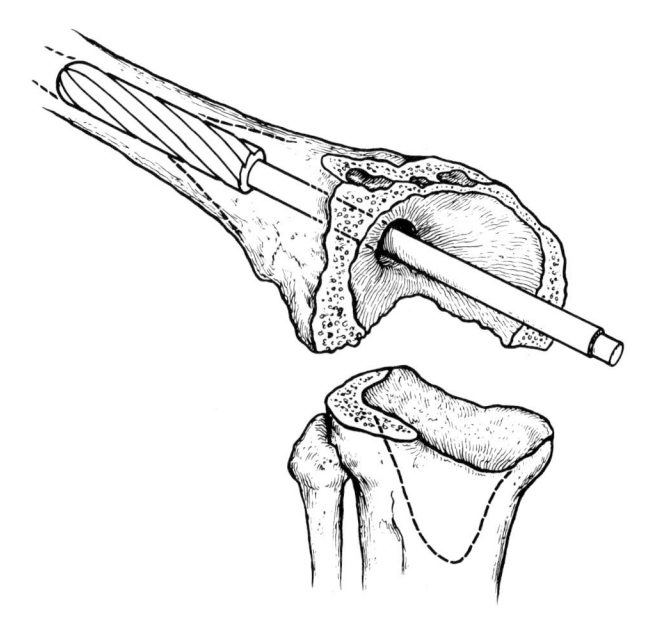

Figure 58.2. Intramedullary alignment provides the only reliable landmarks for minimal resection. Recognizing that severe bone loss has occurred, the surgeon should resect only a small amount of bone to allow firm footing for the implant. (From Whiteside,[23] by permission of Williams & Wilkins)

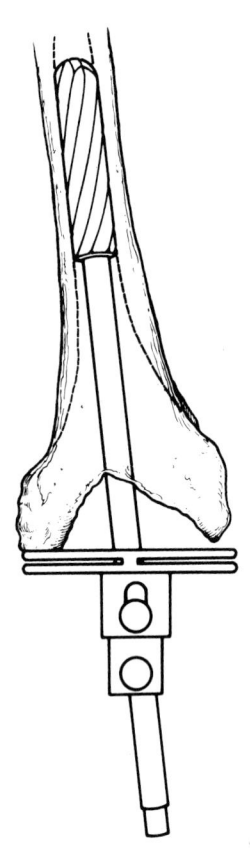

Figure 58.3. Large cavitary and peripheral defects are present with failure of large implants. Intramedullary instruments provide the only reliable landmarks for resection. As little bone as possible is taken from the distal femur. (From Whiteside,[23] by permission of Williams & Wilkins)

and protected until healing and bone formation occur in the grafted area (Fig. 58.7).

GRAFTING TECHNIQUE

Block allografts have traditionally been used for massive bone deficiencies, but their complication rates are high, and the destructive effects of allograft rejection can limit their long-term success.[6,15] Large segments of allograft also heal slowly, are never replaced by new bone, and weaken as the ossification and vascularization front proceeds.[16,17] In contrast, morselized allograft has proven structurally reliable for both small and large defects while supporting new bone formation.[18,19] Morsels that are 1 cm in diameter maintain their integrity long enough to act as a substrate for new bone formation. Morsels less than 0.5 to 1 cm in diameter tend to be resorbed, whereas those larger than 1 cm incorporate slowly, if ever, and tend to collapse.

Rejection can be a major problem with allograft because marrow is immunogenic.[6,15] However, marrow elements can be thoroughly removed from morselized allograft to prevent the inflammatory response and loss of graft and to capitalize on the osteoconductive potential of the allograft. The allograft acts as a scaffolding for new bone growth, and although it is not osteoinductive, demineralized bone, which is mildly osteoinductive, can be added to the allograft to enhance bone formation. The surrounding bone structure supplies most of the osteoinductive activity because metaphyseal

ponent to augment fixation, with nonstructural allograft filling the central and peripheral defects. Massive block allografting is feasible for these defects, but with long-stem and augmented fixation, morselized cancellous allografting can reconstruct the proximal tibial bone with low failure and complication rates.[3]

The lateral tibial cortex is usually relatively well preserved, and the fibular head is almost always present. The fibular head can be used for proximal seating of the tibial component, if the rest of the tibial architecture is severely destroyed (Fig. 58.6). In the worst cases, all cancellous bone is gone, leaving a large cavitary defect and substantial deficiency of the tibial rim. Long-stem fixation is advisable in these cases regardless of whether block allografting or morselized allografting technique is used. When morselized graft is used, the tibial tray should seat on the intact portion of the tibial rim, and the stem should engage the isthmus of the tibia. As with the femoral component, the tightly fit diaphyseal stem maintains stability and prevents tilting of the component, so that massive defects may be filled with allograft

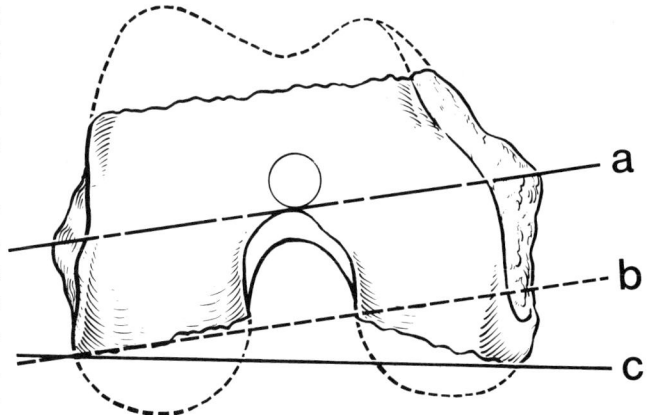

Figure 58.4. A straight line through the medial and lateral femoral epicondyles provides correct rotational alignment. The dotted lines represent the original contours of the distal femur before total knee failure. Line a passes through the epicondyles. Line b represents the proper resection line for the posterior femoral condyles. If line c is followed, severe internal rotation of the femoral component will occur. (From Whiteside,[13] by permission of Lippincott-Raven)

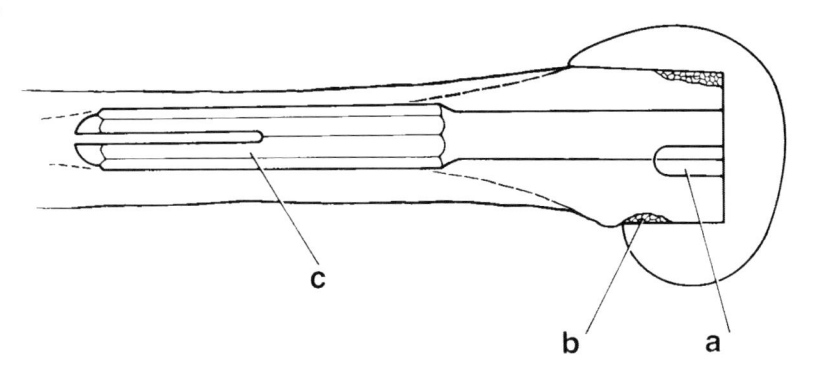

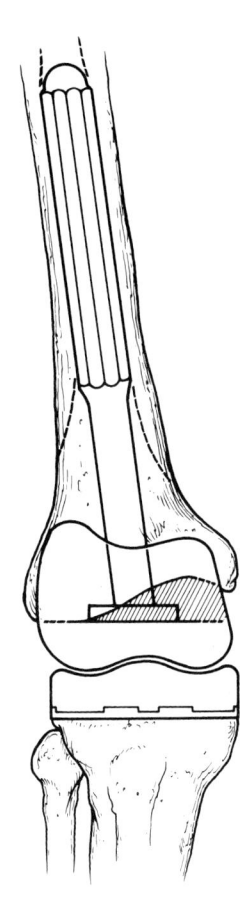

Figure 58.5. (A) Fixation of the femoral component into viable bone is achieved by means of a posterior-stabilizing housing, (a) a peg driven into the distal femoral surface, (b) a thickened posterior surface, and (c) a long stem, which allows soft bone graft to be used. (From Whiteside,[23] by permission of Williams & Wilkins) (B) The stem fixed tightly in the diaphysis in combination with rim seating prevents the implant from migrating proximally and tilting into the defect. (From Whiteside,[23] by permission of Williams & Wilkins)

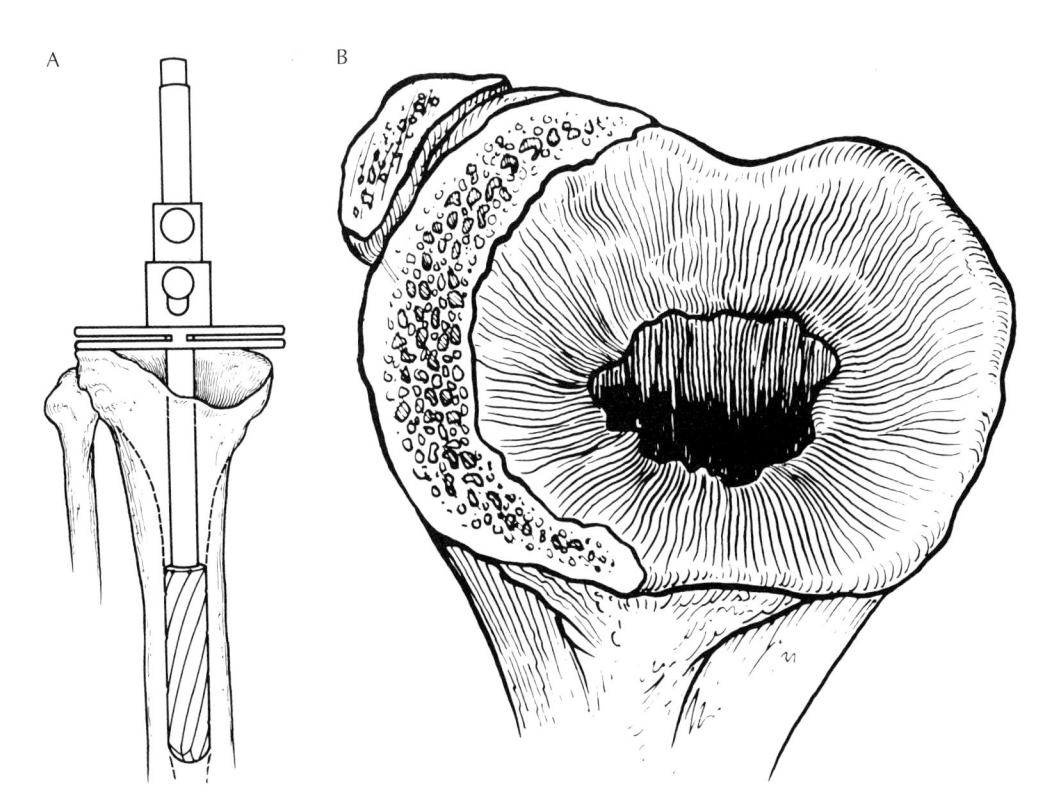

Figure 58.6. (A) Intramedullary instruments allow accurate alignment. Here a planner is used to trim the upper tibial rim. Minimal resection should be done, which may leave large rim defects. (From Whiteside,[23] by permission of Williams & Wilkins) (B) With long-stem support of the tibial component, one-quarter of the rim of the proximal tibia can be used to support the implant. The fibular head may also be used for tibial support. (From Whiteside,[13] by permission of Lippincott-Raven)

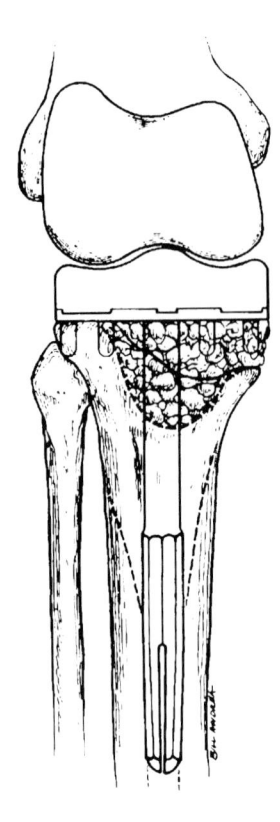

Figure 58.7. Fixation of the tibial component with rim contact on viable bone, screw fixation into the cortical shell, peg fixation into intact bone structure, and stem fixation into the diaphysis allows adequate stabilization until the grafted area can be incorporated. (From Whiteside,[23] by permission of Williams & Wilkins)

bone has a rich blood supply and maintains the capacity to heal even after repeated failed arthroplasty.

Grafting Preparation and Placement

Fresh-frozen cancellous allograft in morsels measuring 0.5 to 1 cm in diameter is soaked for 5 to 10 minutes in normal saline with a concentration of polymixin 500,000 units, bacitracin 50,000 units, and cephazolin 1 g per liter. The fluid is removed and 10 cc of powdered demineralized cancellous bone is added to each 30 cc of the cancellous morsels. Bone fragments and diaphyseal reamings are added to improve the osteoinductive potential. This mixture is packed into the bone defects, then the implants are impacted so as to seat on the remnant of viable bone while compacting the morselized bone graft.

RESULTS SINCE 1984

December 1984–April 1989

Efforts to develop a method for cementless reconstruction in revision total knee arthroplasty began with a tibial-grafting technique developed in 1984. Fifty-six cases of cementless revision total knee arthroplasty in 56 patients were performed using cementless technique, long-stemmed components, and morselized cancellous allograft. Although those in the last year of the study had a similar technique used for the femur, only results from the tibia were reported in this study. Twenty-three patients were men and 33 were women. The mean age was 66 years (range, 34 to 83). Forty-eight patients had osteoarthritis and eight patients had rheumatoid arthritis. Fifty were revised for aseptic loosening, four for unremitting pain and moderate deformity, and two for deformity and instability. All knees had major loss of femoral and tibial bone stock. Bone graft was used on all tibial surfaces and on 39 femoral surfaces. Screws were used to fix the tibial component in 28 knees.

Patients were evaluated postoperatively at 1 month, 3 months, 1 year, and yearly thereafter for pain, range of motion, extensor lag, and stability. Standard radiographs were made at the follow-up visits and were evaluated for evidence of change in bone density, blurring of interfaces within the graft and at the graft-host bone junction, trabeculation in the grafted area, sclerosis around the stem, pedestal at the tip, lucency between the pedestal and tip, migration of the tip of the stem, migration of the tibial tray, and migration of the femoral component. Fusiform enlargement and cortical thickening around the stem tip, and presence of bone atrophy at the articular area also were sought in femoral and tibial radiographs.

In cases of re-revision, a biopsy was taken from the grafted area to assess new bone formation. These specimens were evaluated histologically with hematoxylin and eosin stain and polarized light microscopy.

All patients were able to walk within 3 months postoperative, and 50 discarded their canes before 1 year after surgery. The six who required permanent cane support were restricted by disease in other joints or by general debilitation. Two years after surgery, 30 (54%) of the patients had no pain, 17 (30%) had mild pain, five (9%) had moderate pain, and four (7%) had severe pain. One tibial component migrated into varus and the patient had mild occasional pain, but no other loosening has occurred. Three knees have had occasional recurrent knee dislocation and two of them have had revision of the tibial component for this problem.

The mean valgus angle was 3.8 degrees (range 1 to 8 degrees) at 2 years postoperative. Mean flexion was 104 degrees (range, 65 to 125 degrees) at 2 years after surgery, and increased to 110 degrees (range, 70 to 130 degrees) at 6 years after surgery.

All 56 knees had increasing radiodensity in the grafted areas 1 and 2 years postoperatively as compared with the 1-month radiograph.

Three knees had to be reoperated and a biopsy was

taken from the grafted area of the tibia. One was from a 77-year-old woman 3 months postoperative when she was revised for patellar subluxation. One was from a 68-year-old woman 6 months postoperative when she was surgically treated for persistent valgus laxity, and one was from a 73-year-old woman 18 months postoperative when she was reoperated for recurrent posterior tibial dislocation. All three biopsy specimens contained viable bone in the center of the allograft. New bone trabeculae surrounded by plump osteoblasts was apparent and new bone covered the dead-bone trabeculae in the 3-month specimens. In the 18-month specimen, necrotic trabeculae were still present but were surrounded by varying thicknesses of new bone. New bone trabeculae throughout the specimen appeared viable.

All implants except two achieved stable fixation to bone. Alignment, stability, and comfort of the knee were all improved with this cementless revision technique. Bone stock was reliably reconstructed, and fixation during the short term appeared to be durable. All of the patients with severe persistent pain in this series had well-fixed implants at the time of revision, and were revised for pain only. Although they achieved stable knees with revision, and had no sign of loosening, their pain persisted.

September 1988–January 1993

This group included 63 knees that were grafted with morselized allograft and demineralized bone powder, and all had revision of the femoral and tibial components. Twenty-nine patients were male and 34 were female. Mean age was 71 years (range, 57 to 91 years). Firm seating of the components on a rim of viable bone, and rigid fixation with a medullary stem were achieved in all cases. One knee was lost to follow-up, leaving 62 knees with standard radiographic evaluation at 1 month, 3 months, and 1 year postoperatively. Fourteen patients were reoperated between 1 month and 37 months after revision surgery for loosening, ligamentous laxity, patellar subluxation, patellar tendon rupture, or hardware removal. A biopsy specimen was taken from the central portion of the allograft in each case.

One knee developed a complete radiolucent line around the tibial component and nonprogressive radiolucency behind the anterior femoral flange. Thirty-seven months after the original revision operation, the tibial component was revised. The femoral component was found to be tightly fixed to bone with dense osteointegration along the distal surface. On revision of the loose tibial component, the peripheral tibial rim was found to be complete, and approximately 20 cc of cancellous allograft was needed to fill the tibial defect. One patient developed gross loosening of the femoral component associated with nonunion of an old distal femoral fracture. The femoral component was revised 19 months after the original revision operation, and repeat grafting was done with morselized and strut allografts on the femur. The fracture healed and no further evidence of loosening has occurred.

Table 58.1. Pain score analysis

	Pain score	Type of pain (in %)			
		Severe	Moderate	Mild	None
Preoperative	3.3	90.0	5.0	5.0	0.0
1 month	45.8	0.0	7.7	38.5	53.8
3 months	46.7	1.8	1.8	36.4	60.0
12 months	47.0	0.0	8.7	8.7	82.6

All but one patient in this latest series had significant improvement in their pain score as compared to their preoperative status (Table 58.1). At one year after surgery, the average pain score was 47.0 (on the 50-point Knee Society Clinical Rating System). Although the complication rate was high, all but one knee achieved a successful arthroplasty. The two patients who required revision for loosening had greatly improved bone stock, and new implants were applied with minor additional grafting. The pain decreased to mild in one knee and was eliminated after revision surgery in the other.

Trabeculation and healing were seen in all allografted areas visible on radiograph by one year after surgery with no sign of significant loss of bone graft. Four patients that had subperiosteal extracortical tibial allograft had radiographic signs of incorporation by one year after surgery (Figs. 58.8 and 58.9). Other than the two patients with loosening, none developed progressive widening of radiolucent lines. Mild cortical hypertrophy and partial pedestal formation occurred in all of the stems, but none had full pedestal formation or migration other than those revised for loosening.

All biopsy specimens, including the 3-week specimen (Fig. 58.10), had evidence of active new bone formation in the allografted area. Active bone formation was found within and around the allograft pieces, and new osteoid formed directly on dead allograft trabeculae. The entire graft was permeated with a highly vascular fibrous stroma (Fig. 58.11). Progressive maturation was found in the older biopsy cases, and evidence of osteoclastic activity was absent by 18 months after surgery (Fig. 58.12). From 18 months to 37 months postoperative, the allografted areas showed progressive maturation. By 37 months after surgery, entombed trabeculae were present throughout the biopsied allograft (Fig. 58.13). Mature, viable appearing lamellar bone completely encased all of the visible allograft bone. Few osteoclasts were found

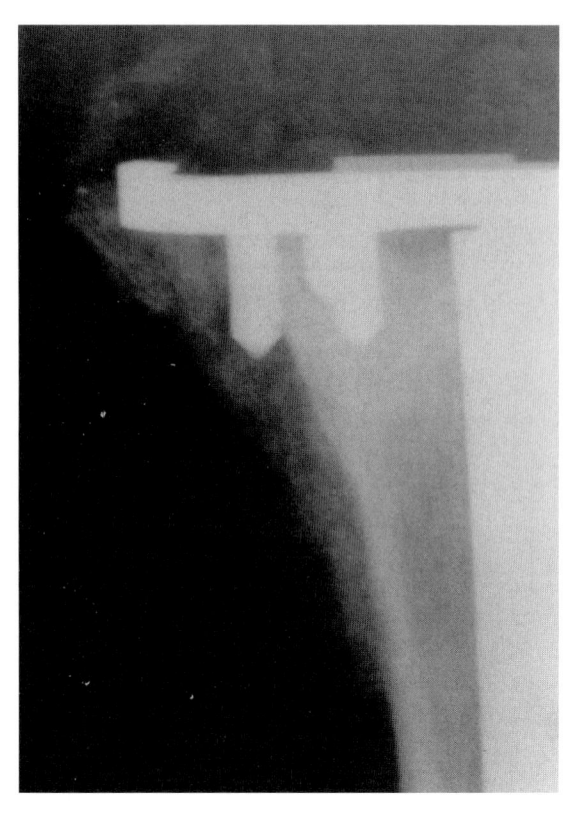

Figure 58.8. Radiograph taken at the 1-month postoperative visit showing the subperiosteal tibial allograft. The allograft is unremodeled, and shows no sign of healing. (From Whiteside,[23] by permission of Williams & Wilkins)

in these sections, and there was minimal evidence of osteoblastic activity.

Infected Total Knee Arthroplasty

Because the morselized allografting method was successful in restoring bone stock in uninfected knees, an effort was made to manage infected knees, after debridement and vigorous antibiotic treatment, with the same technique of bone stock reconstruction and fixation of the implants.[2] A consecutive group of 33 patients (33 knees) with chronically infected total knee arthroplasty was included. Twenty patients were women and 13 were men, and they ranged in age from 35 to 74 years. The original diagnosis was osteoarthrosis in 28 patients and rheumatoid arthritis in five. All knees were treated by implant removal and debridement followed by 6 weeks with antibiotic-impregnated cement beads and spacer and intravenous antibiotics. Cultures of synovial tissue taken at the time of surgery grew *Staphylococcus epidermidis* in 18 knees, *Staphylococcus aureus* in five knees, *Enterococcus* in five knees, *Pseudomonas* in four knees, and mixed gram-negative organisms in one knee. Intravenous antibiotics were given according to the organism grown at the time of surgery.

Six weeks after debridement, the knees were reopened and new components were applied. Morselized cancellous allograft was used to fill all the defects whether they were central or peripheral. The allograft was thoroughly washed by pulsile lavage irrigation solution containing 130,000 units of polymyxin, 17,000 units of bacitracin, and 2 g of ancef per liter. The soft tissue capsule was closed around the defects and the implants to enclose the allograft that filled the peripheral defects. The patients were started on continuous passive motion, and touch-down weight-bearing was allowed. Full weight-bearing was delayed until 3 months after surgery.

A painfree, nondraining wound was achieved with the first incision and drainage in 28 knees, whereas four knees required one or two subsequent procedures to achieve a dry wound and weight-bearing function. Repeat debridement, antibiotic-impregnated cement beads, and bone grafting were necessary in four cases, but they did not lose bone stock with subsequent revisions. One knee continued to drain after repeated attempts at revision and fusion, and amputation above the knee was done at another institution.

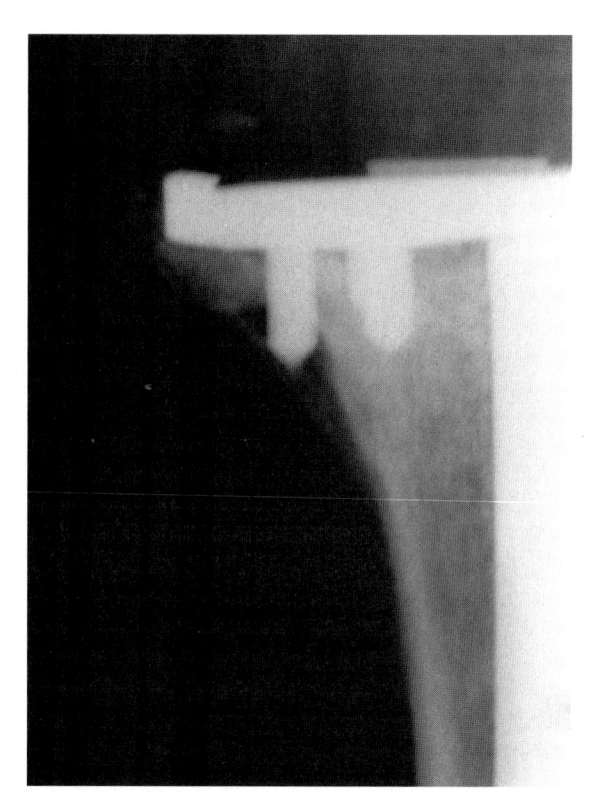

Figure 58.9. Radiograph taken at 1 year postoperative showing the subperiosteal graft. The allograft has healed and has partially remodeled, and now serves as a buttress for the medial edge of the tibial component. (From Whiteside,[23] by permission of Williams & Wilkins)

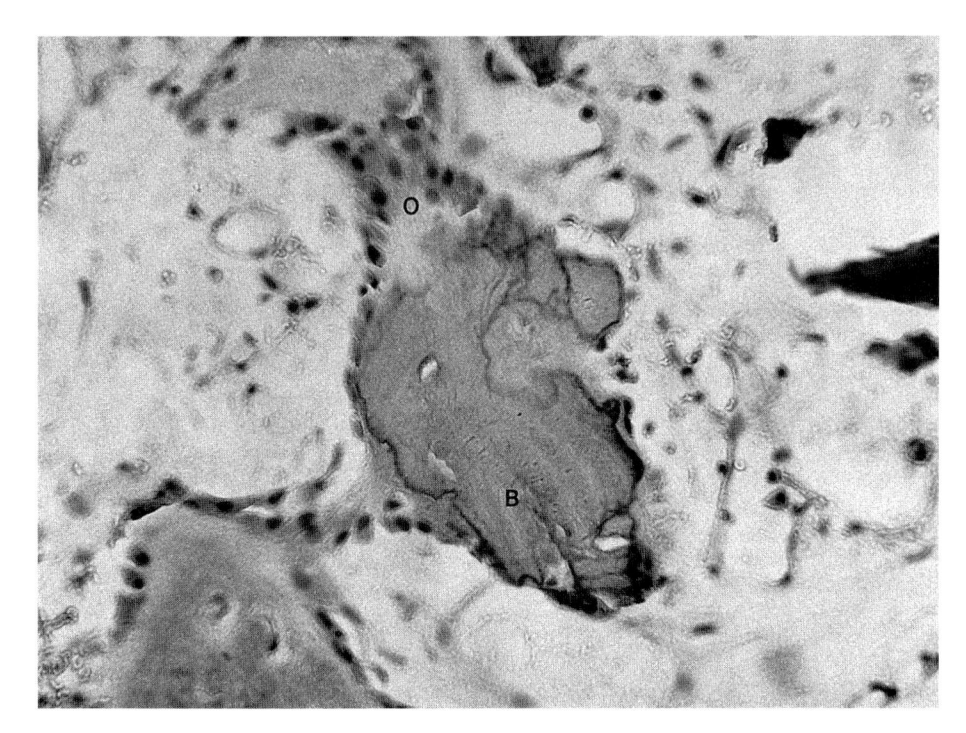

Figure 58.10. Photograph of histological section from the three-week biopsy specimen. Granules of demineralized bone (B) are visible and are surrounded by plump osteoblasts (O) and new osteoid. Vascular stroma is present throughout the allografted area. There is no histological evidence of bone resorption. (From Whiteside,[23] by permission of Williams & Wilkins)

Cementless reconstruction using antibiotic-soaked bone graft and rigidly fixed femoral and tibial components was successful in 32 of 33 knees with intermediate term follow-up. All but one knee have remained free of clinically apparent infection 2 to 8 years after surgery. Two years after surgery 23 patients had no pain in the knee, seven had mild pain, two had moderate pain, and two had severe pain. Mean range of motion was 2 to 100 degrees at the 2-year postoperative evaluation.

None of the knees appeared to have migrated on radiographic evaluation. Partial radiolucent lines appeared under the tibial tray in 11 knees, whereas complete radiolucent lines were apparent under the tibial tray on the anteroposterior and lateral radiographs of two patients. The radiolucency has not progressively

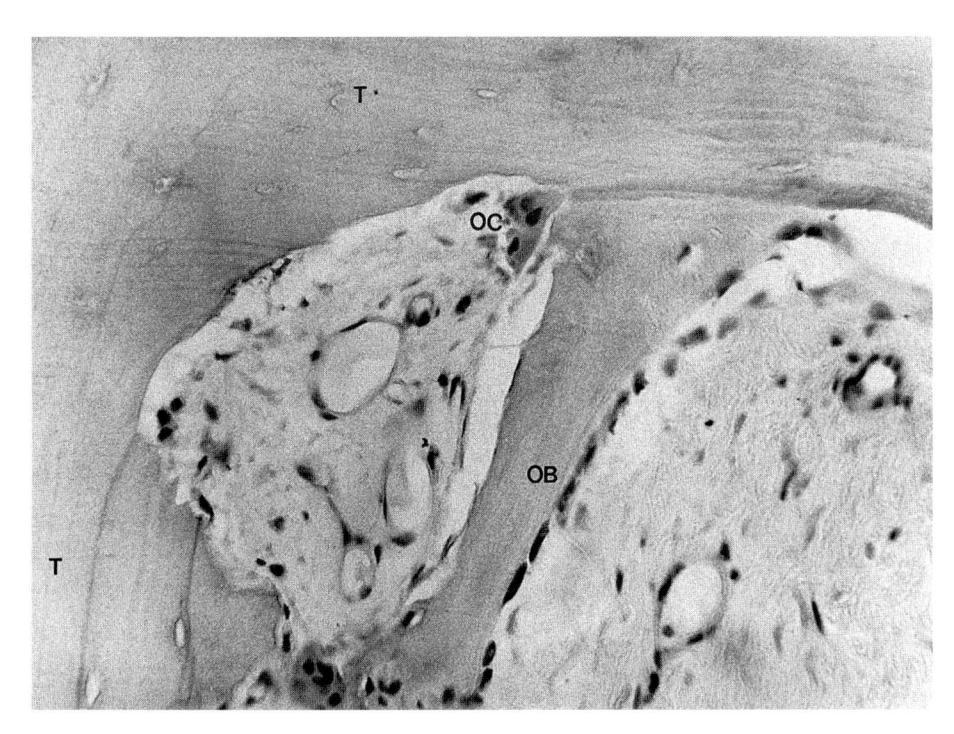

Figure 58.11. Photograph of histological section from the 3-month biopsy specimen. Dead trabeculae (T) are still abundant. Osteoclasts (OC) and new osteoid with osteoblasts (OB) are evident adjacent to the allograft. The allografted area contains multiple sites of bone resorption. New osteoid is often found on one surface of a trabecula and osteoclastic resorption on the opposite surface. Osteoblasts at this time interval are flatter and less numerous than in the 3-week biopsy specimen. (From Whiteside,[23] by permission of Williams & Wilkins)

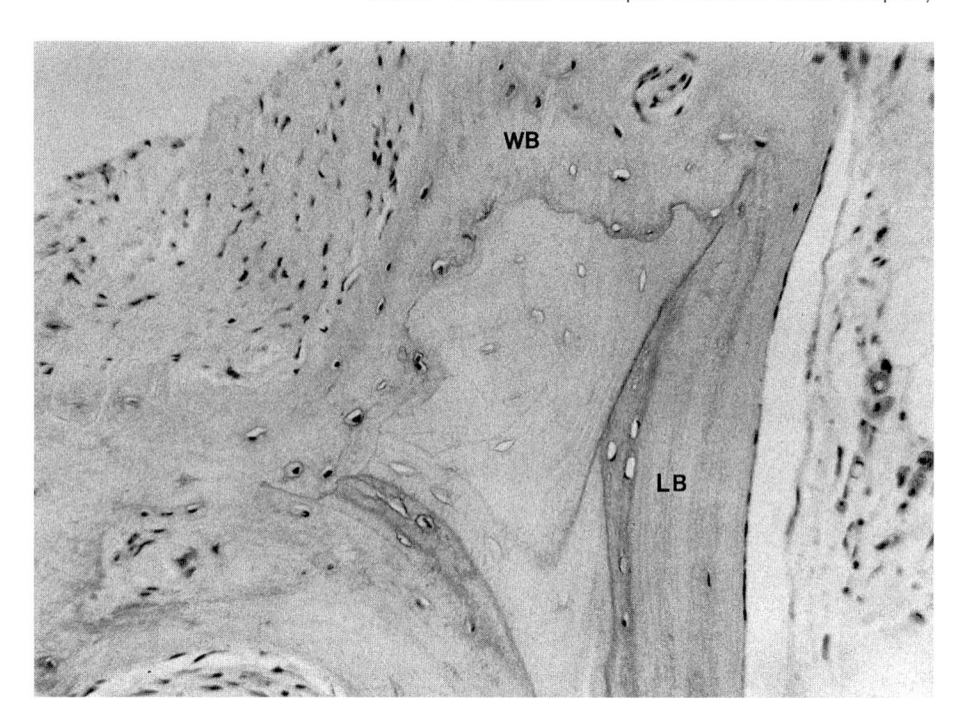

Figure 58.12. Photograph of histological section from the 21-month biopsy specimen. Mature lamellar bone (LB) and disorganized woven bone (WB) surround the allograft. The bone remodeling rate in the allografted area has significantly decreased. Trabecula are now completely entombed by mature or woven bone. Bone remodeling has decreased and osteoblastic or osteoclastic activity is directed toward new bone, not toward allograft. (From Whiteside,[23] by permission of Williams & Wilkins)

widened. Radiographic evidence of healing in regions of massively allografted bone was seen in those knees whose graft was evident on radiograph. The interfaces between graft and host bone were blurred by 6 months postoperative and trabeculation was visible by 2 years postoperative in four cases. All cases had a nonprogressive radiolucency around the smooth tibial stem, and mild lateral cortical hypertrophy was seen around the tibial stem in 15 knees.

In the intermediate term, this method was successful in restoring function, reconstructing bone stock, and eradicating infection.

SUMMARY AND CONCLUSION

Although massive solid allografts can be expected to vascularize and form new bone,[20] variable amounts of replacement as well as collapse and necrosis may

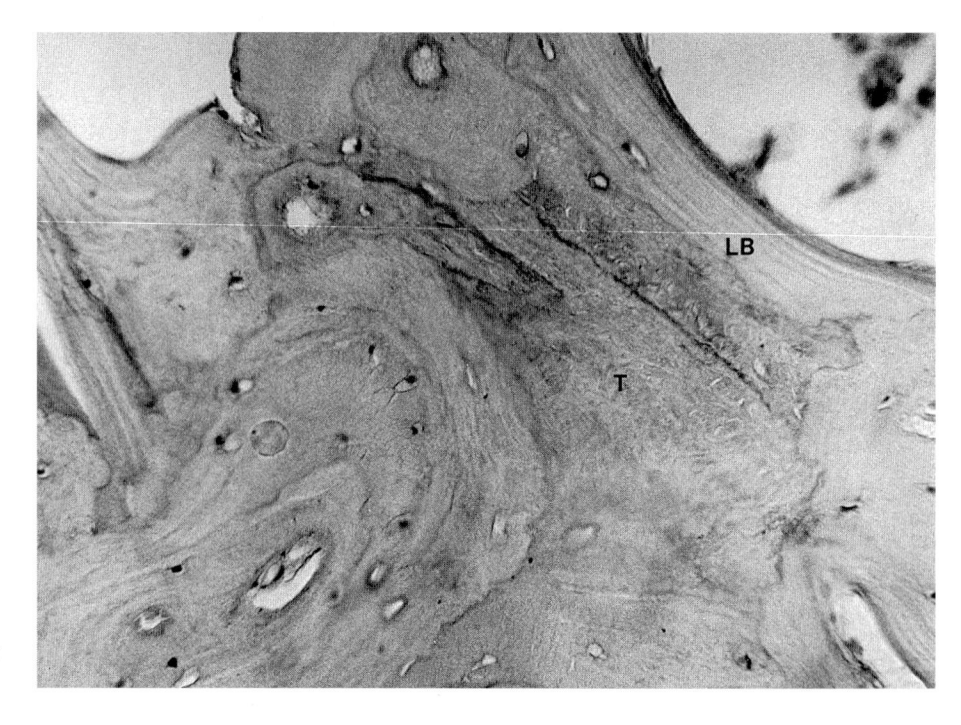

Figure 58.13. Photograph of histological section from the 37-month biopsy specimen. Entombed trabeculae (T) are present throughout the biopsied allograft. The visible allograft is completely encased by mature lamellar bone (LB). Bone remodeling continues at normal levels; few osteoclasts are found, and there is minimal evidence of osteoblastic activity. (From Whiteside,[23] by permission of Williams & Wilkins)

be prominent features of these large block allografts.[16,17]

Immunocompatibility seems to be an important factor in allograft healing and incorporation. Large block allograft of the acetabulum appears to be more likely to succeed if autograft is used.[21] Rejection appears to be a significant factor in survival of large allografts.[6] Although bone itself is not highly immunogenic, the role of marrow elements in the cancellous bone graft may be crucial. When possible, marrow contents should be washed carefully from the interstices of cancellous bone to remove cellular elements that do not contribute to osteoinduction but do produce an inflammatory immune response that can compromise healing and bone formation. Washing and soaking the components in antibiotic solution has the additional benefit of making available a reservoir of antibiotic that is released slowly during the postoperative period.[22]

Morselized cancellous bone rather than finely ground bone, which tends to be destroyed by phagocytosis, is the best available choice for reconstructing large volumes of deficient bone stock. Fixation is completely dependent on the patient's own bone, so that massive defects must be protected until sufficient rigidity develops in the grafted material to allow sharing of weight-bearing loads.

Clinical experience has shown that migration of the tibial component after reconstruction with morselized allograft is rare during the first 2 to 5 years after surgery.[4] These results are surprising in light of reported experience with structural allografts of the acetabulum. Jasty and Harris reported loosening of acetabular components after 4 years in 32% of their cases.[19] The biologic behavior of morselized allograft differs from that of block allograft, however. Vascularization and ossification are rapid, and a permanent, competent load-bearing structure is achieved by filling large deficient areas.[1,2] The biologic response obtained with the correct technique appears to be early and vigorous. It does not seem likely that progressive collapse would occur after remodeling and healing have been established.

Bone graft handling is probably crucial to the success of grafting of the knee. Antibiotic soaking and washing, removal of bone marrow, and adequate support of the implants are all necessary for consistent success of this technique. The results of this salvage procedure have been encouraging. The grafting technique appears to provide long-term support for the implants, so that repeat revision is likely to be uncommon.

ACKNOWLEDGMENT

The author thanks Charles D. Short, MD, and Michael G. Tanner, BS, for histological analysis of bone graft specimens; and Diane J. Morton, BA, for editorial assistance with the manuscript.

References

1. Samuelson K. Bone grafting and noncemented revision arthroplasty of the knee. *Clin Orthop.* 1988; 226:93–101.
2. Whiteside L. Cementless reconstruction of massive tibial bone loss in revision total knee arthroplasty. *Clin Orthop.* 1989; 248:80–86.
3. Whiteside L, Ohl M. Tibial tubercle osteotomy for exposure of the difficult knee arthroplasty. *Clin Orthop.* 1990; 260:6–9.
4. Wilde A, Schickendantz M, Stulberg B, Go R. The incorporation of tibial allografts in total knee arthroplasty. *J Bone Joint Surg.* 1990; 72A:815–824.
5. Goldberg V, Powell A, Shaffer J, et al. Bone grafting: role of histocompatibility in transplantation. *J Orthop Res.* 1985; 3:389–404.
6. Muscolo D, Caletti E, Schajowicz F, et al. Tissue-typing in human massive allografts of frozen bone. *J Bone Joint Surg.* 1987; 69A:583–595.
7. Whiteside L. Treatment of infected total knee arthroplasty. *Clin Orthop.* 1994; 299:169–172.
8. Whiteside L. Radiological and histological analysis of morselized bone grafting in revision total knee replacement. *Orthop Trans.* 1995; 19:448–449 (abstr).
9. Booth Jr R, Lotke P. The results of spacer block technique in revision of infected total knee arthroplasty. *Clin Orthop.* 1989; 248:57–60.
10. Freeman M, Sudlow R, Casewell M, Radcliff S. The management of infected total knee replacements. *J Bone Joint Surg.* 1985; 67B:764–768.
11. Jacobs M, Hungerford D, Krackow K, Lennox D. Revision of septic total knee replacement. *Clin Orthop.* 1989; 238: 159–166.
12. Windsor R, Miller D, Insall J, et al. Two-stage reimplantation for the salvage of total knee arthroplasty complicated by infection. *J Bone Joint Surg.* 1990; 72A:272–278.
13. Whiteside L. Bone grafting in revision cementless total knee arthroplasty. *Techn Orthop.* 1992; 7:39–46.
14. Whiteside L. Cementless revision total knee arthroplasty. *Clin Orthop.* 1990; 286:160–167.
15. Friedlander G. Current concepts review: bone grafts. *J Bone Joint Surg.* 1987; 69A:786–790.
16. Gitelis S, Helgimen D, Quill G, Piasecki P. The use of large allografts for tumor reconstruction and salvage of the failed total hip arthroplasty. *Clin Orthop.* 1988; 231: 62–70.
17. Head W, Malinn T, Berklacich F. Freeze-dried proximal femur allografts in revision total hip arthroplasty. *Clin Orthop.* 1987; 215:109–120.
18. Gerber S, Harris W. Femoral head autografting to augment acetabular deficiency in patients requiring total hip replacement. *J Bone Joint Surg.* 1986; 68A:1241–1248.
19. Jasty M, Harris WH. Salvage total hip reconstruction in patients with major acetabular bone deficiency using structural femoral head allografts. *J Bone Joint Surg.* 1990; 72B:63–67.

20. Kandel R, Gross A, Ganel A, et al. Histopathology of failed osteoarticular shell allographs. *Clin Orthop*. 1985; 197:103–110.
21. Convery F, Meyers M, Minteer-Convery M, Devine S. Acetabular augmentation in primary and revision total hip arthroplasty with cementless prostheses. *Clin Orthop*. 1990; 252:167–175.
22. McLaren A. Antibiotic bone graft: early clinical results. Presented at the 57th annual meeting of the American Academy of Orthopaedic Surgeons. New Orleans, Louisiana, February 8–13, 1990.
23. Whiteside L. Results: cementless. In: Rorabeck CH, Engh GA, eds. *Revision Total Knee Arthroplasty*. Baltimore: Williams and Wilkins; 1997: in press.

CHAPTER 59
Press-Fit Stem Fixation

Wayne G. Paprosky, Todd D. Sekundiak, and John Kronick

In revision total knee arthroplasty, the goal is to recreate a stable joint that is oriented similar to its normal anatomic axis in all planes. Unfortunately, this becomes a more difficult task in the revision setting, where bone and tissue loss has progressed from a combination of factors: primary disease process, infection, osteolysis, aseptic loosening, index procedure, implant removal, and concomitant systemic disease. To recreate the joint, the surgeon is required to use augments of a biological or mechanical nature to compensate for the bony or soft-tissue loss (or must accept the abnormality and place the new components on slightly compromised tissue).

In the normal tibia, the articular cartilage is supported by a thin layer of cortical bone that is in turn supported by cancellous bone. The stiffness of the cancellous bone decreases distally as the stiffness of the cortical shell increases.[1] The joint load is transmitted through the articular cartilage to the thin layer of cortical bone, then to the cancellous bone beneath it, and finally to the cortical shell. In a primary arthroplasty setting, the combination of plastic, metal, and polymethylmethacrylate transmits the load directly to the underlying cancellous and cortical bone. In the revision setting, there is loss of the strongest supporting bone, and transmission of forces to the remaining subsurface bone could lead to early failure.[2]

Revision knee arthroplasty components are commonly stemmed to protect the limited autogenous bone stock remaining. First, this bone may be directly under the component or under cement, metal augments, or bone graft. Second, when using large volumes of morselized contained grafts or structural grafts, the surgeon may want to protect the graft from significant loads and decrease stresses on them.[3] Finally, revision components can place abnormal stresses through even normal bone by their constrained design nature. Joint loads are several times body weight, but a stemmed component can transfer the loads if it is composed of sufficiently strong materials.[4] If the stem fails to transfer the load, then the remaining cancellous bone will experience load beyond its ultimate strength and there will be a loss in fixation.[5]

A stem's purpose, therefore, is to transmit force away from the joint line and, in so doing, lessen the stresses seen at the joint.[6,7] Stems perform this function by being rigid and by being attached to a rigid femoral component or tibial base plate. Brooks has shown that in the varus-deficient proximal tibia the addition of a metal-backed component will decrease stress and allow a more uniform distribution across the proximal tibia.[8] Because these components are more rigid than the remaining cancellous bone, force will be transmitted through them and into the stem or into the remaining cortical rim. Bartel and colleagues have shown by finite element analysis that stresses on the cancellous bone beneath a conventional-design prosthesis can be diminished if a metal tray and a central peg are used.[9] Lewis et al. showed that post designs provided the lowest stresses of all.[10] Once a stem length reaches 70 mm, the axial load at the joint line can be reduced by 23 to 38%.[6–8] The amount of bending moment carried by the stem can be variable, as fixation of the stem occurs distally.[8] However, addition of a central post and stem to the tray will increase the stiffness of the component and, in so doing, decrease the bending moment.[7] The force is then returned to the bone at the metadiaphyseal or diaphyseal area depending on the geometry, size, length, position, and composite of the stem. Bourne and Finlay demonstrated in a fresh cadaveric strain-gauge study that loss of proximal cortical tibial contact resulted in a 33 to 60% decrease in strain values. With stems up to 15 cm in length, marked stress shielding of the proximal tibia cortex and doubling of the strain at the tip occurred.[15]

Two traditional methods of stem insertion have been presented. The cemented stem allows for transmission of load more proximal to the joint line because the stems are shorter and force is transmitted along the bone-cement interface. This is meant to prevent stress shielding.[11] Cement-filling the intramedullary canal can make future revisions more difficult and lead to further bone loss when cement is removed.[12] With cementless stems, forces are transmitted to the tip of the stem where cortical bone contact occurs.[12–14] Concern is sometimes raised as to possible proximal stress shielding, but this is technique dependent.[15] Further, stress shielding may actually be less, because the stem is not anchored in cement.[13] Cementless stem insertion can weaken bone by excessive reaming or can promote early loosening if not sized large enough.[14,16] These arguments are technique-related and should not be indications to avoid cementless stem use. It is essential to realize, however, that stems are not a substitute for optimal component fit; they are an adjunct to relieve a portion of excess stress seen by the components at the joint line. That is, the type and size of stem is irrelevant if the juxtaarticular tissues are not adequately reconstructed. As stresses become greater or tissues more compromised, the approach to stem fixation must also be altered.[16]

Many different geometries of stems are available. Larger-diameter stems lead to increased load transmissions[17] but this is usually negated by the fact that most systems have a set diameter fixation point at the stem component junction. In addition, the bending moment of the base plate will be determined at this junction.[18] Longer stems shield more proximal bone.[7] This factor cannot be assessed in isolation because shorter, wider stems will impinge at their tip secondary to the conical shape of metaphyseal endosteum. Longer, thinner stems prevent tip impingement because the stem can migrate in the sleeve of tubular diaphyseal endosteum. The contact area of the stem within the bone will also determine how the load is transferred to the cortex. In addition, surface preparation of the stem can be altered. Presently, most cementless stems are smooth or blasted but without a porous coating. Flutes have been added to stems to aid in fixation and decrease stem stiffness. Flutes or splines on the stem engage in endosteal bone and are employed to decrease rotational stresses at the joint line. The flutes may also act to decrease the modulus of elasticity of the stems, preventing stress shielding (Fig. 59.1).

PREOPERATIVE PLANNING

Preoperative templating is essential for stem insertion. Full-length anteroposterior and lateral radiographs allow complete assessment of the femur and tibia. Besides determining position of the joint line, alignment of bony cuts, size and placement of components, and need for bone augmentation, the intramedullary canals are assessed to ensure that intramedullary alignment will be accurate to the mechanical axis orientation. Eccentric joint surfaces may require offset stems or tibial housings to ensure alignment of the component while optimizing tibial plateau coverage without overhang (Figs. 59.1, 59.2A,B).

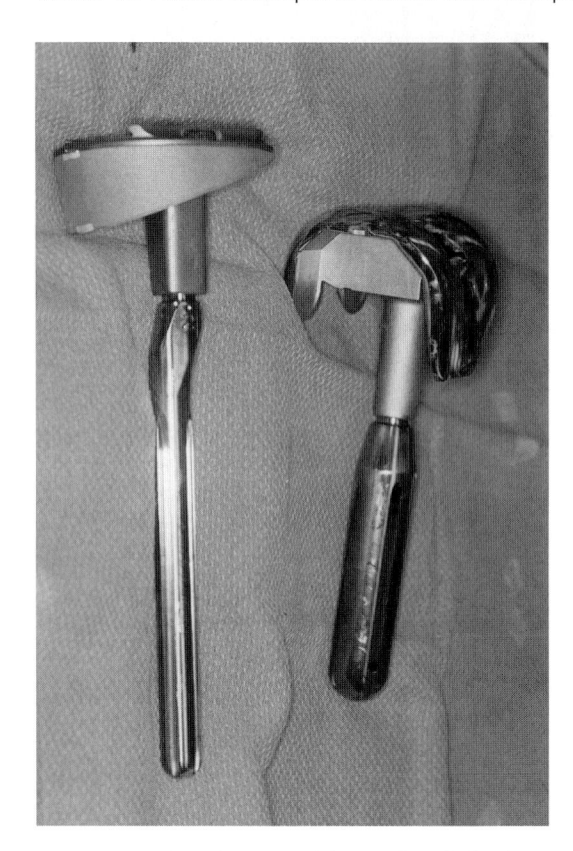

Figure 59.1. Examples of stemmed femoral and tibial components for press-fit use. Stems are fluted to help engage endosteal bone. This allows control of rotational forces. By press fitting the stems, bending forces will also be controlled. The smooth surface allows subsidence to maintain compression forces at the joint line. The tibial stem is offset to compensate for asymmetric joint surfaces. (Courtesy Zimmer, Warsaw, IN)

Canal assessment ensures that straight-stemmed components can be inserted or determines the need of possible osteotomy secondary to the deformity. Estimation of stem length and width is determined to obtain adequate endosteal press fit. Stem length needs to be estimated with the component to account for each component's respective housing. In general, longer stems are used to provide more rigid support because their point of contact extends for a longer length along the endosteal diaphyseal surface. Length and degree of support cannot be assessed in isolation, as the extent of press fit is a significant concomitant factor. Longer stems with tight diaphyseal endosteal cortical press fit are chosen in cases of severe bony deficiencies (Figs. 59.3A,B,C), whereas shorter stems with metaphyseal cancellous contact are used to provide constrained component support in minimal soft-tissue imbalance with normal juxtaarticular bone (Figs. 59.4A,B).

It is useful to template for at least two possible stem lengths with their corresponding different stem widths

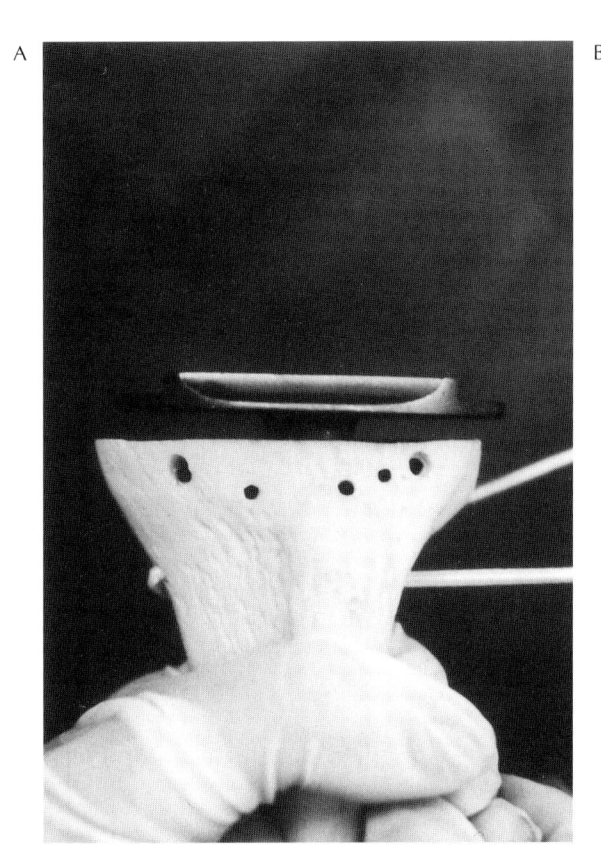

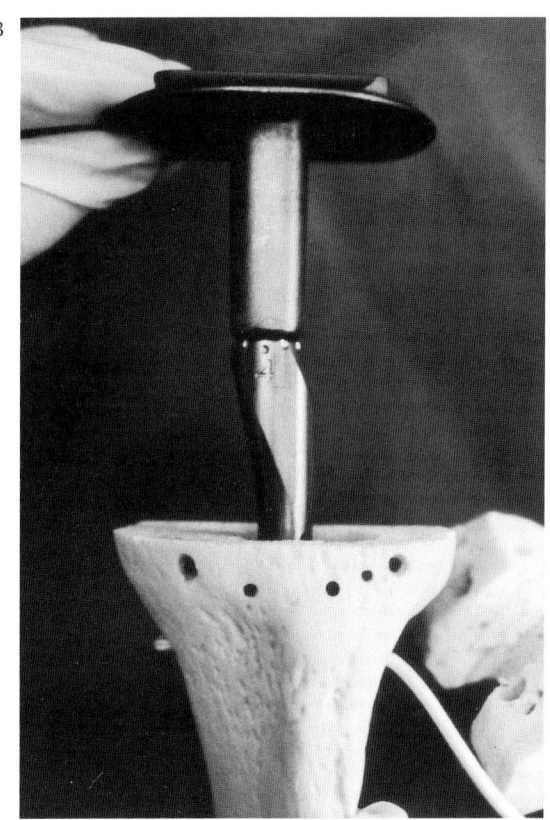

Figure 59.2. (A) A stemmed tibial component with symmetric medial and lateral plates can cause overhang where the intramedullary canal is asymmetrical to the joint surface. This can cause impingement of soft tissues and prevent optimal tibial coverage. (B) An offset stem allows displacement of the tibial base plate in the desired direction to prevent component overhang and allow for optimal coverage. (Courtesy Zimmer, Warsaw, IN)

(Figs. 59.5A,B). Commonly, a stem at one predetermined length may be too loose (from being undersized) or impinge (from being oversized). To attempt at inserting a stem of larger, or smaller, diameter may then cause the reciprocal problem. Usually, the problem of impingement can be avoided by re-reaming more endosteal bone because the impingement occurs at the tip of the stem where the intramedullary canal begins to narrow. If the amount of bone removed is excessive, however, a stress riser can be created at the tip of the stem that can lead to stem tip pain or fracture. An alternative to this problem is to change to a stem of different diameter. Templating will ensure that the stem has been placed to sufficient length that structural bone will be supporting the stem.

Most stems are attached to a fixed point on the arthroplasty component. Estimation of component position in the coronal and sagittal planes is therefore essential. Commonly, the femoral component sizing in the coronal plane will be decided by anatomy because the medial and lateral condyles have relatively symmetric width when related to the intramedullary canal. Placement of the component in the sagittal plane will again be dictated by the stem and, therefore, predetermine the flexion gap. To increase or decrease the flexion gap, the only option is to upsize or downsize the component (Fig. 59.5B). Shifting the component position or adding posterior femoral augments cannot be used to alter flexion gaps because component position has been fixed by the stem. If available, an offset stem or a component with a different housing junction point would be other viable options. On the tibial side, stem positioning tends to be a greater problem in the coronal plane because the medial and lateral tibial plateau are commonly asymmetric. Selection of the component must again correlate to intramedullary alignment to prevent significant overhang of the component.

Newer systems now present with a swivel joint at the component stem junction or an offset stem that allows for adjustment of component positioning (see Fig. 59.1). Curved stems allow for longer support on the femoral side, lessening the possibility of endosteal impingement.

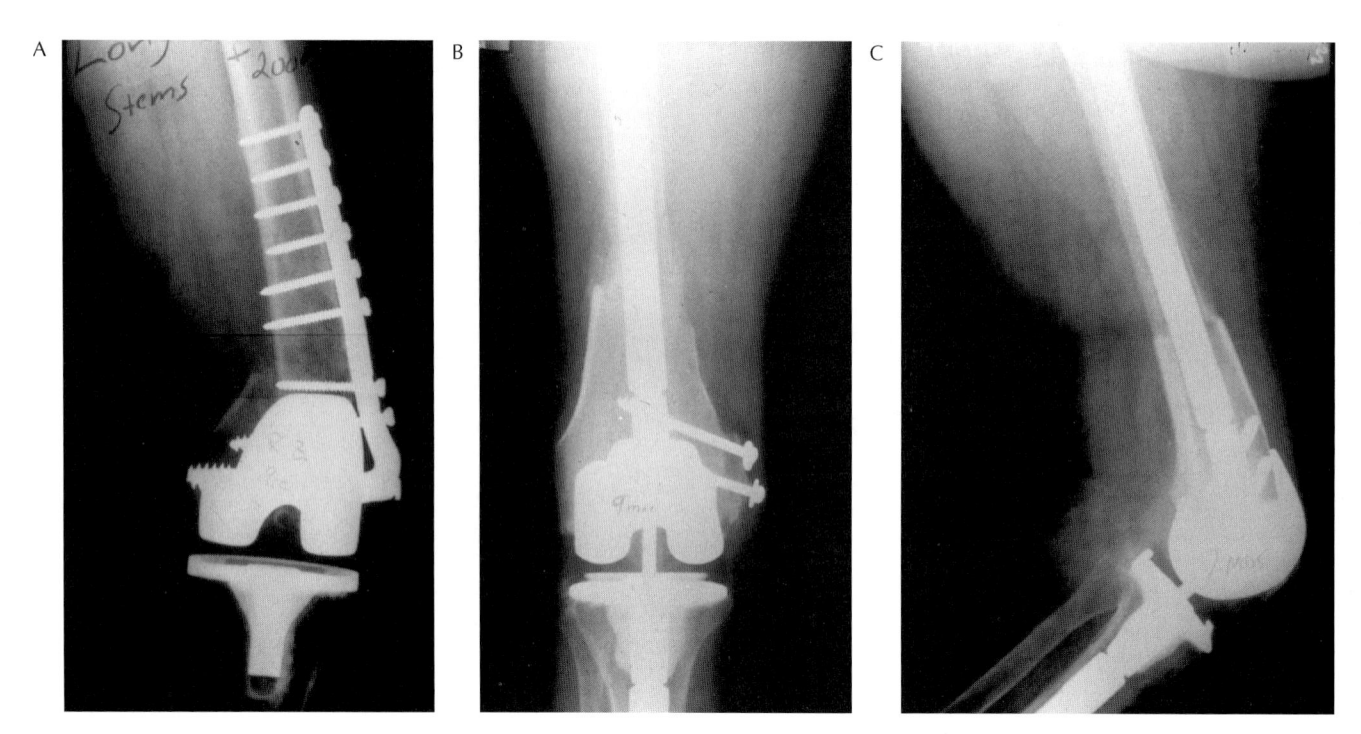

Figure 59.3. Seventy-seven-year-old male who sustained a fall 9 months prior to assessment. Components were stable and correctly oriented prior to trauma. Attempts at open reduction and internal fixation failed to achieve union. (A) Anteroposterior radiograph of severely comminuted nonunion of supracondylar periprosthetic femur fracture following failed internal fixation. Components are malaligned secondary to nonunion with severe osteopenia secondary to disuse. (B) Anteroposterior radiograph 9 months postoperatively showing complete union of host-allograft junction with press fit stemmed components. Medial screw placement reattaches medial collateral complex to aid in joint stability. (C) Lateral radiograph demonstrating graft union and extent of press fit for stable fixation.

Figure 59.4. Fifty-five-year-old female with primary uncemented total knee arthroplasty for degenerative osteoarthritis. Patient was complaining of significant medial knee and lower leg pain. (A) Anteroposterior radiograph of unstable uncemented total knee arthroplasty. Chronological radiographs displayed progressive subsidence of the lateral tibial baseplate. (B) Two-year postoperative AP radiograph of cemented constrained total knee arthroplasty with short press-fit stems to protect bone from increased stresses. Incompetency of the medial collateral ligamentous complex prevented balancing of the joint and therefore required constrained polyethylene to compensate for ligamentous laxity.

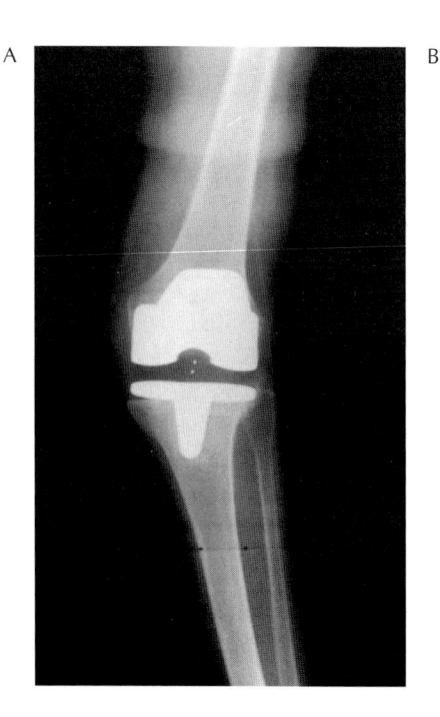

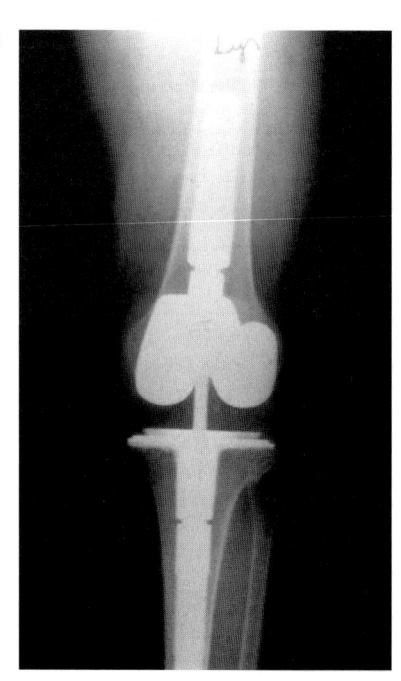

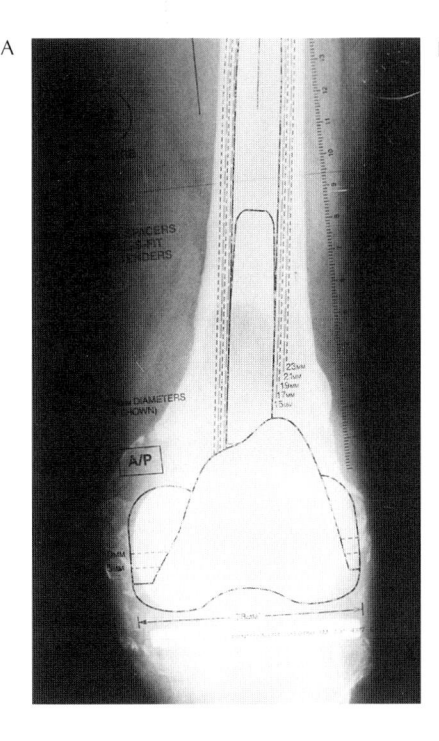

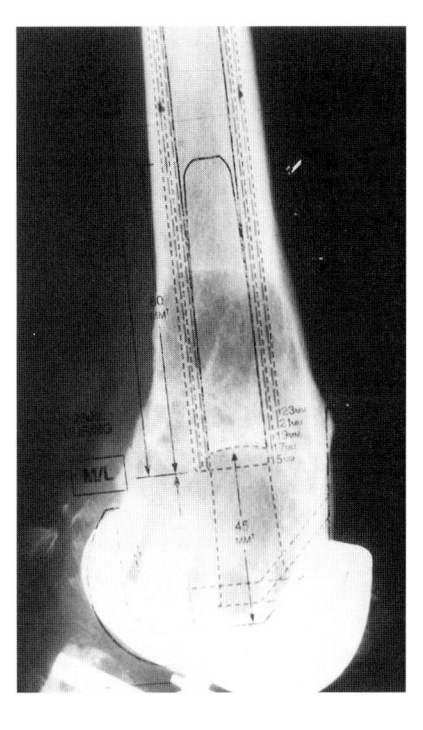

Figure 59.5. Sixty-five-year-old male with severe osteolysis secondary to excessive polyethylene wear from an unrevised scuffed femoral component. The patient previously underwent removal of a metal-backed patella. (A,B) Preoperative AP and lateral radiographs with overlying templates to determine possible lengths and corresponding widths of stems to support compromised bone stock. With severe osteolysis, reconstitution of bone stock with bulk allografting or impaction grafting must be considered.

OPERATIVE TECHNIQUE

Because the stems are of fixed cylindrical geometry with fixed junction points with the components, cutting of the bony surfaces is done with intramedullary alignment. In the primary arthroplasty setting, where a stemmed component may be considered because of severe deformity with significant bone loss or severe ligamentous insufficiency, intramedullary alignment needs to be considered. Conversion to a stemmed component cannot immediately proceed from a regular component if extramedullary alignment has been used. The possibility exists of mismatching the bone cuts to the intramedullary axes, which will cause impingement of the intramedullary stem on the endosteal surface. This can lead to malalignment of components, poor fit of components on the bone surfaces, or iatrogenic bone fractures from attempts at making the component fit through forceful impaction.

Rather than using the narrow intramedullary guide rods that attach to the cutting jigs of most systems, we promote the use of the intramedullary reamers for the cutting-jig guide rod. The initial step is to ream minimally and push the largest-diameter reamer past the isthmus. The initial reamer produces an entry point in the juxtaarticular bone and is rotated to enlarge the entry site. This removes ectatic and sclerotic bone, which can lever the reamers away from the true longitudinal axes of the bones (Fig. 59.6A). Reaming is then continued in millimeter increments until minimal endosteal cortical contact is felt or heard. (As stated earlier, reaming is minimal because the reamers are being used essentially as guide rods for cut alignment and stem position.) Cutting blocks are then attached to this rod and initial cuts are completed (Fig. 59.6B). By using the largest-diameter rod in the canal and ensuring that the rod passes the isthmus, the surgeon can best correlate the bony cuts for the component to the stem orientation and prevent impingement or malpositioning of the component-stem construct. A full-length reamer or a reamer of equal width throughout its length provides the best alignment because there is minimal toggle along its shaft. Note that the reamer is being used under power to open the entry site rather than to ream the intramedullary canal. Once the entry site has been cleared of sclerotic bone, the reamer should be gently pushed up the canal rather than forcibly reamed into the canal. Remember that the reamer is acting as a guide rod at this point.

Balancing the joint stability in the flexion-extension and varus-valgus planes proceeds in a routine manner once the initial cuts have been made. The initial bone cuts required are the proximal tibial cut and distal and posterior femoral cuts. Cuts should resect minimal bone and are performed to assess the flexion and extension spaces adequately. The use of pre-measured spacer blocks or a measurable tensioning device is an essential adjunct at this stage. Joint line positioning will be decided by this assessment and by preoperative templating. The size of the femoral component, the amount of femoral distal buildup and the amount of tibial thickness can then be determined arithmetically. The tibial

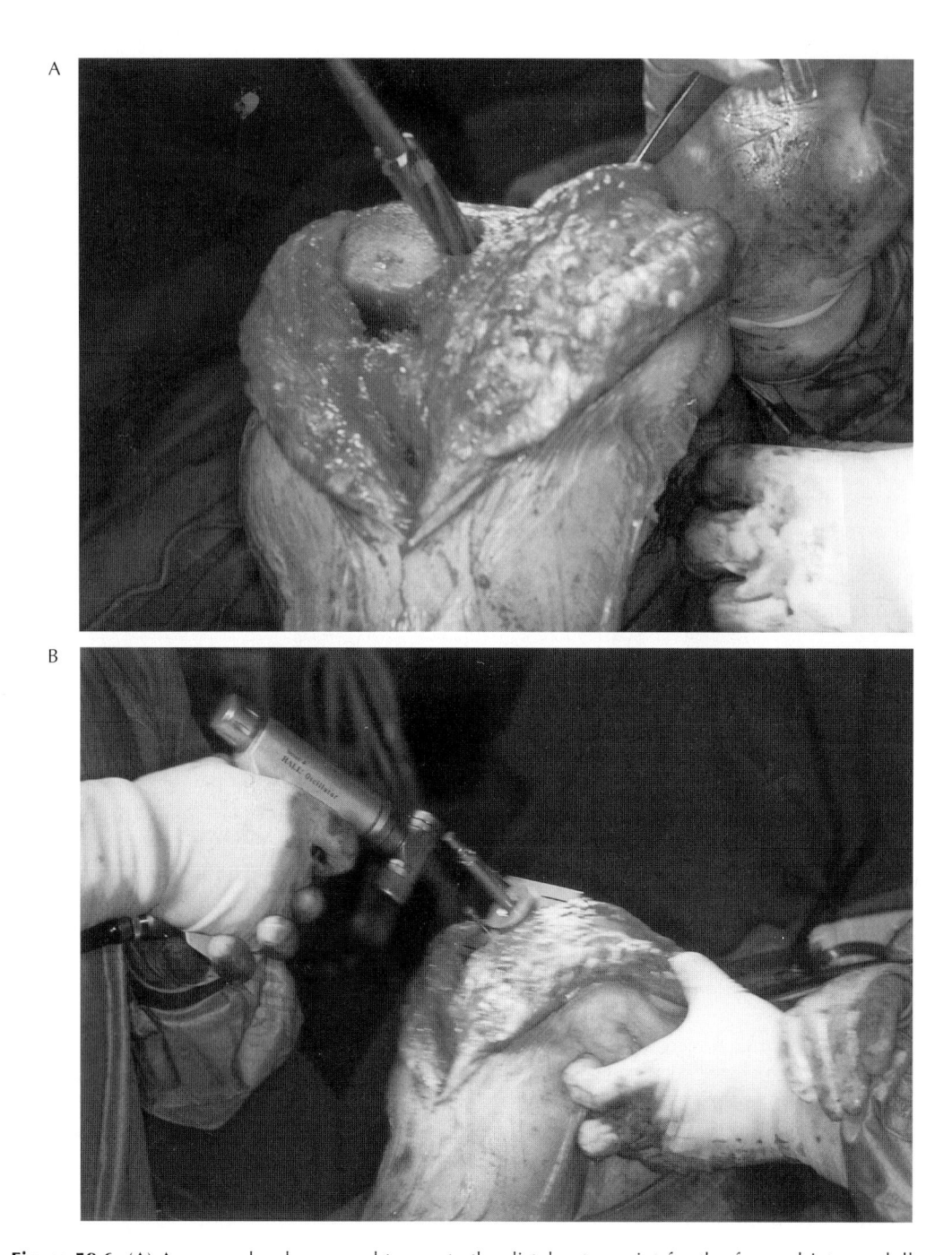

Figure 59.6. (A) A reamer has been used to create the distal entry point for the femoral intramedullary canal. Sequential reamers are then pushed up the femoral canal until endosteal contact is felt. (B) The cutting block is secured to the reamer, which is left within the canal. The bone cuts will then correlate to the intramedullary canal for proper attachment of the component and housing to the stem.

component affects both the flexion and extension gaps. Its thickness is determined by an estimation of the position of the joint line. This measurement can be subtracted from the spacer block measurements of the flexion and extension gaps to determine the size of femoral component required for flexion gap balance and the amount of distal femoral augment for extension gap balance. If the predetermined size of component or augment thickness is unavailable, then a different permutation can be calculated by minimally altering the joint line, synonymous with altering the tibial component thickness.

It is essential to reiterate that the position of the femoral and tibial components is dictated by the position of the press-fit stem. The size of the tibial base plate will determine the amount of coverage and also the amount of overhang on the tibia in the coronal plane. If the canal is eccentric or the tibial plateaus deficient, then a base plate with an offset housing or offset stem will need to be considered to avoid this concern (Fig. 59.7).

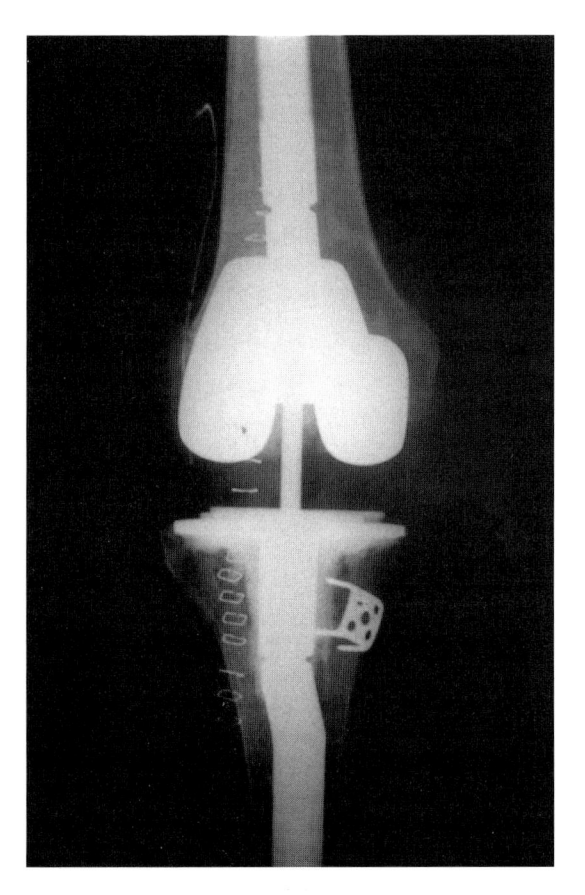

Figure 59.7. A revision total knee arthroplasty requiring a tibial offset stem in a patient who had previously undergone a high tibial osteotomy and was left with a deficient medial tibial plateau. The offset stem allowed for better lateral coverage of the tibial surface with no significant medial overhang of the component.

A similar but less common problem occurs in the sagittal plane.

With the femoral component, there is an additional concern of altering the thickness in the sagittal plane. Changing the femoral sizing will alter the flexion gap thickness by predetermined amounts and is the only way to alter the flexion gap when assessing the femoral component in isolation. The extent that a larger-sized femoral component increases the flexion gap is system specific and must be known. In the same manner, femoral component sizing will determine the degree of fill of the extensor mechanism that will alter patellar tracking. Posterior femoral augments are used as a filler to ensure the posterior aspect of the component is in bony contact and is rotationally stable.

Once the size of femoral component is determined, chamfer cuts and housing resection can be completed. Further resection of tibia, if required, is also performed. Final shaping for augments is completed. All cuts should still be directed by the intramedullary alignment rod.

If bulk allografting is required, sizing of the graft and completion of the graft's shaping and fixation is now performed. Depending on the size of the defect, grafting can be completed prior to gap assessment. If complete structural allografting is required to replace the juxtaarticular bone, length estimates are performed with the previously noted calculations. Completion of bony resection occurs for acceptance of the component and component housing. The cuts are performed on a satellite table with intramedullary alignment. The diameter of intramedullary guide within the graft is determined by the width of reaming required within the host bone to obtain the necessary press fit for stable fixation. Appropriate graft choice is required to ensure that excessive reaming of the graft does not occur and weaken the graft.

Femoral and tibial canals are then sequentially reamed to the appropriate length and width to accept the press fit stem. Both preoperative estimate and the intraoperative assessment are required to determine the extent of press fit required. With a wide variety of stems, different permutations of stem length and width will give adequate press fit in most situations. For more severe defects minimal stem choices exist, which reinforces the need for preoperative templating and ensuring the appropriate availability of stems. Where there is greater structural bone loss with greater soft-tissue imbalance or insufficiency, greater press fit is required. This translates to reaming to greater depths with removal of more endosteal bone to ensure there is a sleeve of cortical endosteal bone supporting the stemmed component.

The width of reaming will be templated preoperatively and will correlate intraoperatively to the point after cortical chatter is felt or heard with the reamer. Assessment of reamings is also of value in determining if endosteal cortical bone is being removed. Traditionally, we ream approximately 1 cm past the tip of the stem to ensure that there is no tip impingement (with the possibility of cortical erosion). Reaming depth must include the stem length and the length of the component housing. If reaming past the tip of the stem will remove excess bone, then a shorter, wider stem is indicated. For routine revisions, reaming should not be overly aggressive and does not need to proceed to the point of significant cortical chatter. Stem insertion and reaming proceeds line-to-line. If the revision requires more support from the stem, then reaming can be more aggressive. It is difficult to quantitate absolutely the extent of reaming for each situation and the surgeon must rely on clinical judgement. It is important to compare the integrity of the bone and soft tissues to the primary arthroplasty setting and then determine the extent of extra support required. For structural bulk allografts, stem fixation along the endosteal bone should have cortical contact and should occur over greater length (Fig. 59.3B,C). Reaming should therefore continue at least a millimeter or two wider after the point that cortical chatter is felt and heard.

Trial reduction of the femoral and tibial components is performed with the required augments but within the stem extensions to assess the accuracy of the bony cuts. Before attempting any recutting, it is important to re-try the components with the stems. Failure to seat components can then be assessed. Failure to seat the components without the stem equates to inaccurate bone cuts that require refinement. Seating of components without the stem, but failing to with the stem, either means that the stem has been incorrectly sized and endosteal impingement is occurring or bony cuts have not correlated to the intramedullary positioning of the stem. If stem impingement is occurring, then re-reaming of the canal or re-sizing of the stem is required. Cortication of the juxtaarticular bone occurs secondary to the osteolytic and loosening process in the revision setting. This bone can deflect the guide rod, reamer, stem, or component housing and lead to malpositioning. Ensuring adequate removal of bone for the component housing will help alignment of the components. Failure to remove this bone or realize this problem will lead to improper cut alignment and component malpositioning. At this stage, the only option is to replace the intramedullary guide rod and recut the femur.

Occasionally, on reassessing the cut surfaces vis à vis the intramedullary alignment guide, cuts will be found to be accurate. However, when upsizing reamers to accept a wider press fit, stem cuts will not correlate to the stemmed component. This occurs secondary to the bowed or noncylindrical nature of the bone with the wider stem seating in a position, in that segment of bone, different from the longitudinal axis as determined by the intramedullary guide. The choice is then to recut the bone, correlating to the wider press-fit stem, or to accept a narrower stem with or without increased length. The latter option better correlates the bone cuts to the longitudinal axis of the bone and, in the majority of cases, the latter is accepted as the risk of malalignment is prevented. Once components are inserted, final assessment of flexion and extension gaps is done.

In many revision situations, bulk allografting is not required for the contained cavitary defects present. Morsellized autogenous or allogeneic bone graft is useful in reconstituting bone stock in these situations. The trial stem with or without the component is inserted into the diaphysis but not fully seated. The stem acts as a mold for the actual component and a stopper to prevent graft from filling the intramedullary canal. Graft is placed around the stem and in the defects, then impacted, which gives it structure and more extensive contact with the host bone. The trial stem is then removed, with the graft maintaining its structural integrity.

Final components are then inserted in a routine manner. If components are cemented, cement should extend to but not include the stem-component junction (Fig. 59.8). If cement extends to a point on the housing where the taper of the component begins increasing in width, as in the junction of the component housing with a wider stem, removal of the component can be extremely difficult. The cement collar will act as an impediment for removal of the stem and can lead to fracturing at re-revision.

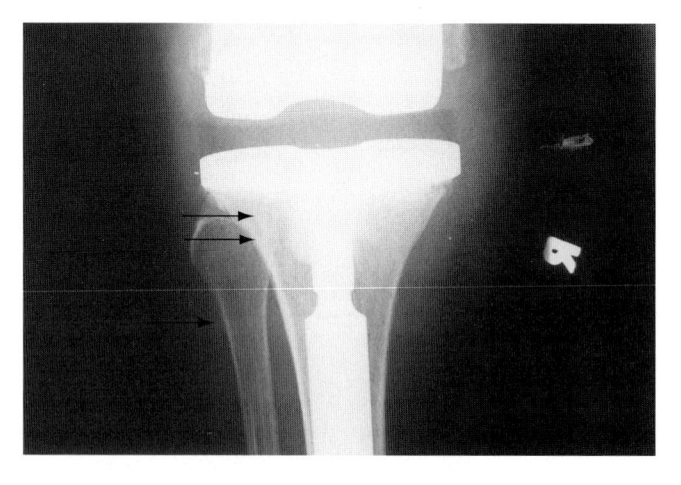

Figure 59.8. A stemmed tibial component with press-fit stem wider than the tibial base plate housing. Cement (double arrow) does not extend to the housing-stem junction (single arrow); the impregnated cement can act as a block to extraction of the component at a later date. If attempts are made to remove the stem with cement extending past this point, fracturing can result. Bone windows or osteotomies are required for controlled removal.

If complete juxtaarticular allografts are being used, attempts at trial reduction without the graft are performed to determine appropriate rotation of the component-allograft composite. Reduction of the joint should be possible because the stemmed component will be stable in the host bone with the press-fit stem. Marking the host bone and graft then allows for reproduction of the appropriate rotation and estimation of stem length. The graft-prosthesis composite is then cemented, with the stem-graft junction being void of cement. The composite is then impacted into the host and final trimming of the junction performed to ensure that host and graft cortical contact is maximized to minimize the stresses through the stem (Fig. 59.9).

RESULTS

The longest follow-up on revision total knee arthroplasties with stemmed components has occurred with cemented stems. Results have been very successful, with a follow-up of 58.2 mon. This is presently the gold standard. Forty stemmed arthroplasty revisions were performed. Only one femoral component was radiographically loose, with three femurs and five tibias developing incomplete progressive lucent lines.[11]

Bertin et al. reported early results of uncemented stems in 53 patients. Stems were of limited sizes and although uncemented were not always press fit. Excluding four knees that had serious postoperative complications, 91% had relief of pain, with 84% having over 90 degrees of motion and 80% being able to walk more than 30 minutes. Eighty-eight percent of the stems were noted to have surrounding radioopaque lines that were unrelated to degree of pain or failure rate.[12]

The Insall group has follow-up with 76 knees at 42 months, with only three failures occurring from loosening and three from infection.[14] Fluted diaphyseal stems were used in all patients. There was a 13% complication rate, with all complications being unrelated to the stems. Overall, 84% of patients had a good or excellent result according to the Hospital for Special Surgery rating scale. Six of the knees failed and required another revision. In 67% of femoral rods and 69% of tibial rods, a 1–2 mm radioopaque line was noted to surround the stems completely or incompletely. These sclerotic lines usually appeared at a few months after the procedure and had no correlation to outcome. In 4% and 6% of the

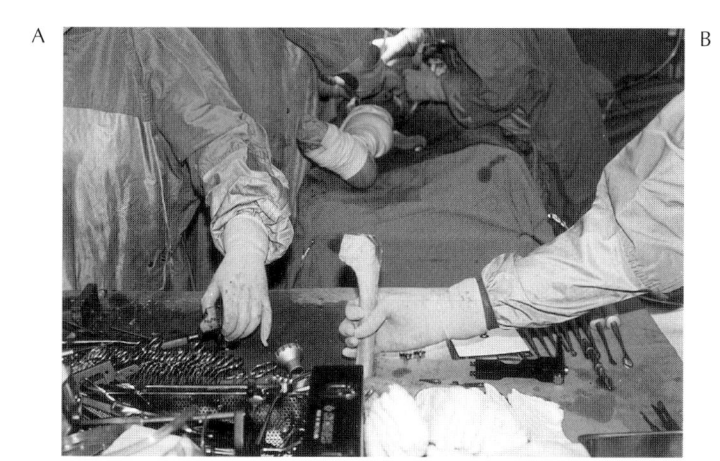

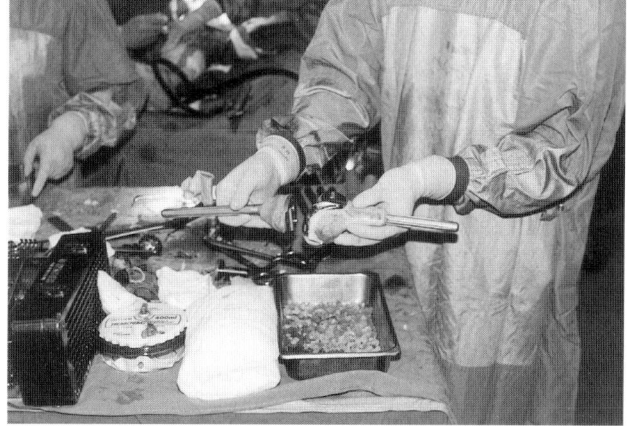

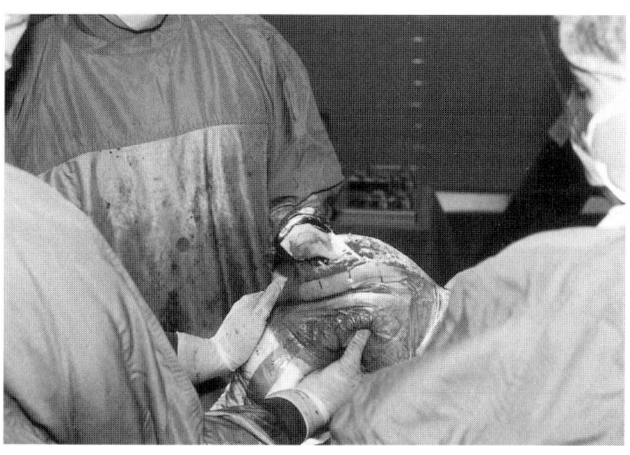

Figure 59.9. Sixty-nine-year-old male requires bulk structural allograft for severe osteolysis and secondary insufficiency fractures. (A) Structural allograft is cut on satellite table with intramedullary rod of equal width to reamer in host endosteal canal. (B) Component-graft composite is cemented, ensuring adequate stem present for press fit into host bone. No cement extends to host-graft junction. (C) Component-graft composite is impacted into host bone with previously determined degree of rotation.

femoral and tibial rods respectively, a >2-mm progressive radioopaque line was present and again had no correlation to outcome.[19] This appearance is markedly different from stems that fail.[16]

Paprosky has reported on a select group of patients where stemmed components were used with distal femoral allografts. This composite was used in periprosthetic femoral fractures, fracture nonunion, and severe distal femoral bone loss. Distinctly absent from this patient population were those with bone tumors. At an average follow-up of 32 months, 7 of the 9 patients had excellent or good results, with the remaining two being fair according to the HSS knee score. Complications were again unrelated to the stems, with soft-tissue balancing being the greatest concern in terms of leading to patellar subluxation or genu recurvatum.[20] Extreme emphasis was placed on protected weight-bearing and bracing till union of the allograft site was evident. Results from Mnaymneh's study have similar results, with union of allograft occurring in 86% of cases and motion averaging 92 degrees; two patients did, however, suffer nonunion and fracture on the femoral side.[21] These procedures were considered salvage procedures.

Vince reported on 44 revision knee arthroplasties using press-fit stems with 2 to 6 year follow-up. Three patients developed clinical or radiographic evidence of loosening despite adequate canal fill. It was concluded that despite adequate canal fill with a press-fit stem, fixation is inadequate in poor-quality bone and that consideration should be given to cementing the stem in position. Significant radiolucencies completely surrounded the stems of those components that failed. In addition to the endosteal lucencies, cortical reaction was evident.[16]

CONCLUSION

As with hip revision arthroplasty, as time progresses the number of revision knee arthroplasties increases. As the number increases, so do the severity of the defects and the complexity of the reconstruction. Use of the press-fit stem on revision components can protect the juxtaarticular bone and transfer the load to stronger diaphyseal bone. The balance between overshielding the juxtaarticular bone and overloading it to failure still needs to be determined. Presently, these stems provide for excellent structural protection of the abnormal bone with no definitive evidence of stress shielding. The stems provide protection from shear, bending, and rotational forces, while still allowing compression of the bone. This necessitates bone of enough structural integrity to support the remaining forces. Medium-term results with these components have provided unparalleled results, leaving these stems as an essential adjunct to the revision arthroplasty procedure. They are not, however, a substitute for ensuring solid juxtaarticular support for the components.

References

1. Behrens JC, et al. Variations in the strength and structure of cancellous bone at the knee. *J Biomechanics*. 1974; 7:201.
2. Albrektsson BEJ, Ryyd L, Carlsson LV, Freeman MAR, Herberts P, Regner L, Selvik G. The effect of a stem on the tibial component of knee arthroplasty. A roentgen stereophotogrammetric study of uncemented tibial components in the Freeman-Samuelson knee arthroplasty. *J Bone Joint Surg (Br)*. 1990; 72:252–58.
3. Dennis DA. Structural allografting in revision total knee arthroplasty. *Orthopedics*. 1994; 17(9):849.
4. Bartel DL, et al. Performance of the tibial component in total knee arthroplasty. *J Bone Joint Surg (Am)*. 1982; 64: 1026–33.
5. Wright T. Biomaterials and prosthesis design in total knee arthroplasty. *Orthopaedic Knowledge Update: Hip and Knee Reconstruction*. Rosemont, IL: AAOS, 1995.
6. Murase K, Crowninshield RD, Pedersen DR, Chang TS. An analysis of tibial component design in total knee arthroplasty. *J Biomechanics*. 1983; 16:13.
7. Reilly D, Walker PS, Ben-Dov M, Ewald FC. Effects of tibial components on load transfer in the upper tibia. *Clin Orthop*. 1982; 170:131.
8. Brooks PJ, Walker PS, Scott RD. Tibial component fixation in deficient tibial bone stock. *Clin Orthop*. 1984; 184:302–308.
9. Bartel DL, Burstein AH, Santavicca EA, Insall JN. Performance of the tibial component in total knee replacement: Conventional and revision designs. *J Bone Joint Surg (Am)*. 1982; 64:1026–33.
10. Lewis JL, Askew MJ, Jaycox DP. A comparative evaluation of tibial component designs of total knee prostheses. *J Bone Joint Surg (Am)*. 1982; 64:129–35.
11. Murray PB, Rand JA, Hanssen AD. Cemented long-stem revision knee arthroplasty. *Clin Orthop*. 1994; 309:116–23.
12. Bertin KC. Freeman MAR, Samuelson KM, Ratcliffe SS, Todd RC. Stemmed revision arthroplasty for aseptic loosening of total knee replacement. *J Bone Joint Surg (Br)*. 1985; 67:242–48.
13. Elia EA, Lotke PA. Results of revision total knee arthroplasty associated with significant bone loss. *Clin Orthop*. 1991; 271:114–21.
14. Haas SB, Insall JN, Montgomery W, Windsor RE. Revision total knee arthroplasty with use of modular components with stems inserted without cement. *J Bone Joint Surg (Am)*. 1995; 77:1700–1777.
15. Bourne RB, Finlay JB. The influence of tibial component intramedullary stems and implant-cortex contact on the strain distribution of the proximal tibia following total knee arthroplasty: An in vitro study. *Clin Orthop*. 1986: 95–99.
16. Vince KG, Long W. Revision knee arthroplasty: The limits of press fit medullary fixation. *Clin Orthop*. 1995; 317:172–77.
17. Donaldson WF, Sculco TP, Insall JN, Ranawat CS. Total

condylar III knee prosthesis: Long-term follow-up study. *Clin Orthop*. 1988; 226:22–28.
18. Askew MJ, Lewis JL, Jaycox DP, Williams JL, Hori RY. Interface stresses in a prosthesis-tibia structure with varying bone properties. *Trans Orthop Res Soc*. 1978; 3:17.
19. Insall JN, Ranawat CS, Aglietti P, Shine J. A comparison of four models of total knee-replacement prostheses. *J Bone Joint Surg (Am)*. 1976; 58:754–65.
20. Paprosky WG. Use of distal femoral allografts in revision total knee arthroplasty. In: *Current Concepts in Primary and Revision Total Knee Arthroplasty*. Philadelphia: Lippincott-Raven 1996:217–26.
21. Mnaymneh W, Emerson RH, Borja F, Head WC, Malinin TI. Massive allografts in salvage revisions of failed total knee arthroplasties. *Clin Orthop*. 1990; 260: 144–53.

SECTION 17
Infection

CHAPTER 60
Single-Stage Revision of Infected Total Knee Replacement

Gareth Scott and Michael A.R. Freeman

Condylar knee replacement commenced at the London Hospital in 1968. At that time joint replacements were undertaken in an operating theater shared with other surgical specialties. There was no modern system of positive-pressure ventilation and an open gulley passed through the operating theater conveying effluent from the neighboring room in which large bowel surgery was conducted.

The incidence of infection at this time was not insignificant. However, the early loosening rate due to a limited understanding of fixation and alignment may well have disguised the true extent of the problem. As the surgical technique became more refined with accompanying improvements in the instrumentation and prosthetic design, a smaller but persistent number of prostheses failed, not through loosening but by sepsis.

It was widely thought in the early days of condylar knee replacement that the only salvage for such an outcome was an arthrodesis of the knee. The surgical preference when infection had been present was to utilize an external fixator such as a Charnley clamp to approximate the femur to the tibia with compression, after the removal of all prosthetic materials and an extensive debridement had been conducted. This method was reported from the London Hospital for 16 cases between 1969 and 1983 with a disappointing functional outcome matched by a fusion rate of only 62%.[1]

This poor outcome and the encouraging reports of one-stage exchange arthroplasty at the hip using antibiotic-laden bone cement produced a change in approach.[2,3] From 1975 onward at the London Hospital a single-stage revision was performed for loose infected prostheses with an arthrodesis reserved for persistent infection after revision. In 1985,[4] the outcome was described in 14 cases, eight of which had loose prostheses that were revised at a one-stage exchange arthroplasty followed by 3 months antibiotics. (The other six who had well-fixed components underwent lavage and drainage.) In all eight cases a staphylococcus species was the infecting organism. None suffered a recurrence of infection (Figs. 1 and 2).

Since the introductory era of joint replacement surgery, supplementary treatment by antibiotic prophylaxis has become effectively mandatory and has led to a decline in the incidence of infection.[5] The confinement of joint replacement surgery to the ultra-filtered laminar flow environment has further reduced the risk.[6] Surgical attire has received attention with recognition that the infecting agents can pass through the weave of cotton fabric. More modern theater clothing blocks the passage of skin squames from the surgical team to the patient while retaining the ability "to breathe" so that the surgical team does not become uncomfortable.[7,8] As a consequence of these improvements, the need for revision surgery for infection has fallen.

In 1992 the results from the London Hospital for the single-stage method were published for 18 consecutive cases operated upon between July 1979 and September 1989, with a mean follow-up of 5 years.[9] There were subsequent infections in two cases. In the first case, who was suffering from rheumatoid arthritis, infection recurred in the revised knee 8 months after the revision. On this occasion the postoperative infection was caused not by the organism found at the single-stage revision but by an organism associated with recurrent episodes of infection in a contralateral knee arthrodesis, itself undertaken for infection in a knee arthroplasty. Lavage and antibiotic treatment resolved the infection in the knee replacement. In the second case, also with rheumatoid arthritis, a new infection occurred 6 years after the single-stage revision. This development arose in association with the formation of an infected ulcer at the ipsilateral ankle. Antibiotics eradicated this infection. Thus it appeared that both infections were "new" and not recurrences of the infection treated by single-stage revision. Encouraged by this outcome, we have

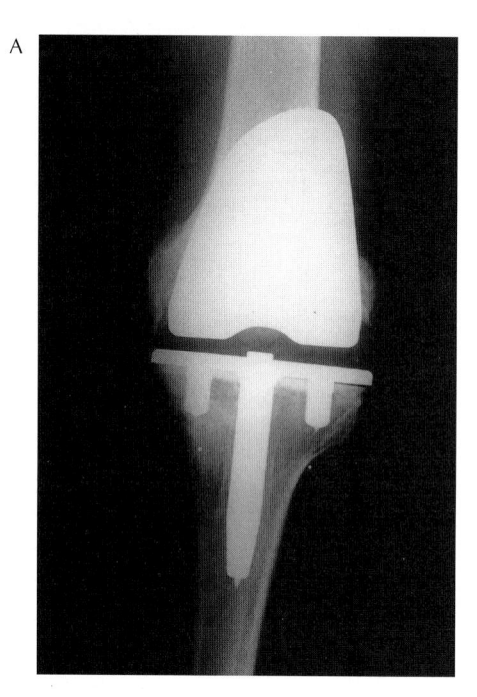

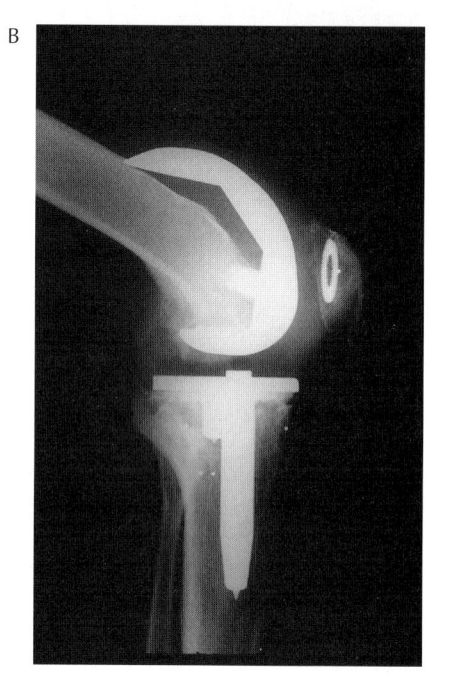

Figure 60.1. (A) Anteroposterior and (B) lateral radiographs of an infected total knee replacement 4 years after the index arthroplasty. Severe bone loss has occurred in relation to the femoral component with subsidence. A radiolucency is present beneath the tibial tray and cement and surrounding the uncemented tibial stem.

maintained the same revision policy from 1989 to the present.

RATIONALE

Both for a single-stage and a two-stage revision procedure the rationale underlying the intervention is first to render the knee joint sterile by a combination of surgery and antibacterial agents and second to implant a new prosthesis covered by antibiotics.

The question at issue when deciding between a so-called "one-stage" and a "two-stage" revision is the length of the interval between these two halves of the procedure. In a two-stage revision the interval is classically about 6 weeks and during this period antibiotics are given parenterally and via an antibiotic-loaded cement spacer in the knee. In a so-called one-stage revision as practiced by the authors, the interval is reduced to half an hour during which the patient remains under anesthesia. As in a two-stage revision antibiotics are

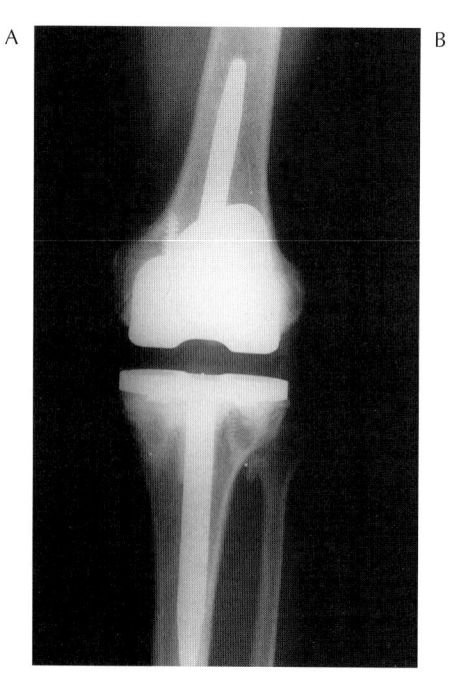

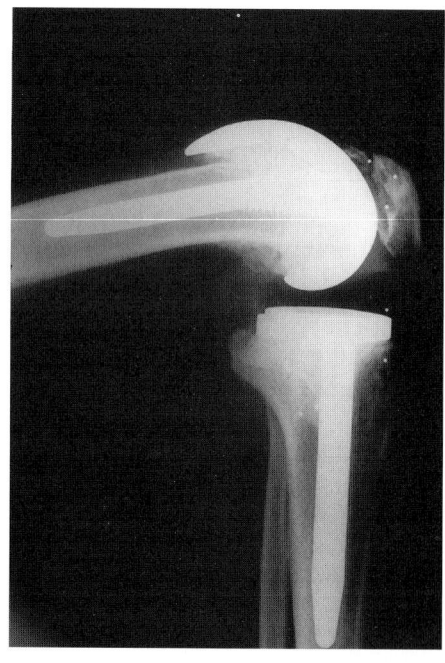

Figure 60.2. (A) Anteroposterior and (B) lateral radiographs following a single-stage revision of the case featured in Figure 60.1.

given intravenously during this time. Instead of an antibiotic-loaded cement spacer the knee is packed with swabs soaked in povidone-iodine. Clearly if the initial debridement has been sufficiently meticulous and if it is followed by a period of exposure to a sterilizing agent sufficient to sterilize a surgical instrument, there is a probability that the tissues will then be sterile. In that event a new prosthesis can be safely implanted at any time thereafter (that is to say immediately or 6 weeks later). However, if the tissues are not sterile at the end of debridement and exposure to a sterilizing agent, a single-stage procedure is almost certain to fail (although the subsequent use of antibiotic-impregnated cement to fix the prosthesis and parenteral antibiotics may, as in the two-stage procedure, kill any remaining bacteria).

The presumption underlying a two-stage operation is that the presence of a foreign body (cement) loaded with antibiotics for 6 weeks in combination with 6 weeks of parenteral antibiotics will offer a better prospect of sterilizing the tissues than would the corresponding situation in a one-stage procedure when the foreign body will consist not only of antibiotic-loaded cement but also for the prosthesis itself. Clearly it is difficult to conceive of an experiment that would allow the efficacy of these two sequences to be accurately compared. In the absence of such an experiment it might be thought wise to rely on the more "conventional and conservative" procedure of two stages. On the other hand, this has the obvious disadvantage of two interventions for the patient and a longer period of time in the hospital.

If a one-stage procedure is to be relied on, the first half of the operation (in which the prosthesis is removed and a debridement is carried out) must be performed with scrupulous attention to detail, perhaps even more so than in the first stage of a two-stage procedure. The knee is then packed with povidine-iodine and the wound closed for 30 minutes while the tourniquet is released and antibiotics are given. Following this, the knee is retoweled and the second half of the operation commences. This sequence results in a long anesthetic time, typically about $3\frac{1}{2}$ hours. It might be thought that prolonged anesthesia would carry risks comparable to two separate anesthetics but in the authors' experience anesthetic complications have been rare.

PREOPERATIVE CONSIDERATIONS

Revision is indicated in all cases in which infection is proven bacteriologically and the prosthesis is loose. The chances of success diminish if there are multiple organisms or if antibiotic sensitivities do not suggest a reliable antibiotic regimen. This is equally true for one-stage and two-stage procedures, but as the prospects of success diminish, it is perhaps wiser to err in the direction of the more conventional two-stage procedure. Similarly the presence of sinuses or difficult scars from previous surgery diminishes the prospects of success for both procedures.

Prior to a one-stage revision and perhaps to a lesser extent prior to the first stage of a two-stage revision it is desirable to reduce edema so far as possible by elevation of the leg for 24 or 48 hours before surgery. If the bacteriology is known for certain preoperatively so that it is not thought necessary to rely solely on additional material at the time of the operation, antibiotics can be given during this preoperative period. However, in general antibiotics preoperatively should be avoided because operative material is the most reliable source of tissue for bacterial identification.

If the prosthesis is well fixed and infection is proven, a combination that for practical purposes only occurs when infection follows immediately after primary procedure, it is worth treating the knee with antibiotics combined with drainage if there is a significant collection in the synovial cavity. This procedure rarely succeeds, but that is not to say that it never does and, if successful, it is obviously a much smaller intervention than revision in one or two stages. It is the authors' preference if the knee is drained to open the knee for lavage and for the insertion of two wide-bore drains (because small diameter drains tend to block). This cannot be done arthroscopically. At the same time the surgeon can determine for certain that the components are well fixed and can biopsy the synovium.

A clinical problem may arise in the early (primary) postoperative period when physical signs strongly suggest an infection but when the absence of a significant intracapsular collection of fluid makes it difficult to know whether the infection is entirely extracapsular (for example, in a subcutaneous hematoma or in tissues infiltrated with blood) or whether it is both intracapsular and extracapsular. In the former event it is unwise to pass a needle through the capsule if the needle in doing so passes through the clinically infected area. This may simply result in producing an intracapsular infection when none previously existed. In these circumstances it may be useful to puncture the skin but not the capsule in the infected area and to send the needle itself for culture because it is not usually possible to aspirate significant quantities of material. A second puncture may be performed through a clinically uninfected area into the synovial cavity itself.

Late infections may present after antibiotics have been in prolonged use. The antibiotics should then be stopped for 2 weeks prior to operation to identify the organism(s) in advance of the definitive procedure by aspiration or open biopsy. Previous antibiotic treatment sometimes prevents identification of the organism, in which case postoperative antibiotic policy has to be planned to be effective against the most probable infecting organism and is guided (post facto) by material taken at revision.

OPERATIVE PROCEDURE

The details of the operative procedure undertaken as a "one-stage revision" are crucial to the outcome. Unfortunately in some reports of the results of "one-stage revision," the exact nature of the operative procedure is not specified. It is not possible therefore to be certain whether the outcome of these (possibly different) procedures can be compared. At the London Hospital the procedure employed is as follows.

No antibiotics are given prior to the operation. The limb is exsanguinated by elevation, never by an Esmark bandage. The incision is made if possible through the previous incision without excision of the skin edges. The prosthesis, all associated cement and all the intracapsular synovial soft tissue including the synovium, the subsynovial tissues and the interface membrane are removed. Specimens from these tissues are sent for culture. The bone surfaces are meticulously freed of soft tissue with a curette and pressure lavage until the bone appears healthy. This stage of the operation may take 90 minutes.

The knee is then packed with swabs (sponges) soaked in povidone-iodine and the wound is temporarily closed. The tourniquet is released and the indicated antibiotics are given. The situation reached at this point in the procedure is essentially equivalent to that at the end of the first stage of a two-stage procedure with the insertion of an antibiotic-laden cement block. In the single-stage procedure as carried out at the London Hospital, there is now a 30-minute interval as distinct from the conventional 6-week interval in a two-stage procedure.

After the 30-minute interval the limb is again prepared for surgery with new towels and new instruments. The temporary sutures and the swabs are removed and the knee thoroughly irrigated. Multiple swabs for culture are taken from the bone and soft tissue surfaces. A new prosthesis is now inserted fixing the implant with antibiotic-laden cement (typically Palacos with gentamicin) confined so far as possible to the bone ends. Intramedullary stems may be used for fixation if required but they should not be cemented so as to facilitate their extraction if infection recurs. Before insertion the stems are dusted with gentamicin powder. Bone defects are filled with cement rather than bone grafts. The knee is drained, the wound closed, and the leg immobilized for 48 hours.

Postoperatively, antibiotics, indicated by the preoperative bacteriology initially and subsequently by the intraoperative bacteriology, are given intravenously for 2 days and then converted to oral antibiotics if this is possible.

If the bacteriological specimens taken at the beginning of the "second" stage of the operation show the presence of bacteria, we would be pessimistic about the outcome but would not alter the postoperative management.

Mobilization of the knee begins as soon as the wound is dry and healing normally. It is not usually difficult to achieve 90 degrees of flexion. The patient walks with the aid of two elbow crutches toward the end of the first week and is typically discharged from hospital at the end of 2 weeks, taking oral antibiotics for an additional 3 months.

At 6 and 12 weeks after operation progress is monitored radiologically and by an ESR, white cell count, and C-reactive protein. It is not established that these investigations are prognostically important but they do form a useful baseline for subsequent evaluation. If at 3 months the knee appears by all criteria to be uninfected, antibiotics cease. The knee is reviewed at 3 monthly intervals to 1 year. If at 1 year there is nothing to suggest infection, our experience suggests that the infection is cured.

CONTRAINDICATIONS

Since 1979, the single-stage method has been applied to 34 consecutive cases of infected total knee replacement regardless of the bacteriology, provided that the patient is not systemically toxic. The operation is a prolonged procedure. If the patient is unfit for such major surgery, simple arthroscopic drainage with lavage would be a safer preliminary option followed by a period of bed rest with elevation of the leg. If this does not produce sufficient improvement to conduct a single-stage definitive revision safely, the prosthetic components should be removed and a staged revision procedure undertaken. The condition of the skin has to be good enough to permit primary wound closure. The presence of marked cellulitis would therefore preclude this method, but again a short period of rest and elevation can quickly transform the quality of the skin. An isolated sinus with noncellulitic margins would not preclude this method providing that excision of the sinus margins would permit primary wound closure without tension at the end of the revision procedure. If the skin is so damaged or infection so far advanced as to have destroyed the stabilizing ligaments, then consideration should be given to arthrodesis of the knee.

In the early report,[9] it was suggested that the operation was appropriate for gram-positive infection but increasing experience has expanded our indications to a broader spectrum of infection that is detailed below.

THE OUTCOME: (1) THE LONDON HOSPITAL

Two postoperative "reinfections" have already been described (see this chapter's Introduction) in our report published in 1992.[9] Since that series, recurrent infection has been confirmed in one additional knee 8 months after a single-stage revision. An arthrodesis was performed.

Of the total series of 34 patients for which a single-stage operation has now been performed, one can therefore be considered a certain failure resulting in an arthrodesis. The rest have functioning total knee replacements, including the two other infected complications discussed earlier. Over the period of this follow-up (i.e., since 1979) six patients have died of unrelated causes with functioning joint replacements. There has been no further case of reinfection. One patient currently has radiographic signs of loosening and is contemplating further revision surgery. Fifty percent of the patients have a continuous uninterrupted walking ability of 30 or more minutes.

In common with the results of Insall and associates[10] the most frequent outcome observed is some weakness in the extensor mechanism. The knee flexion range is generally satisfactory at around 90 degrees but it is not usually as good as in primary joint replacement that has not been complicated in any way.

Initially the single-stage procedure had been considered applicable for gram-positive infections,[9] but as our experience has extended, the spectrum of bacteria encountered has enlarged. This is matched by reports for the two-stage technique.[11]

In our series of 34 patients reported, on only two occasions could no organism be found. However, both patients had loose prostheses with bone loss and a discharging sinus. The majority of infections continue to be caused by gram-positive organisms. In 23 cases a single infecting bacterial species was identified. On eight occasions this was staphylococcus aureus (one case being methicillin resistant); on 13 occasions it was a noncoagulase positive staphylococcus; one case was a streptococcus viridans infection; and on one occasion an infection with proteus mirabilis was found.

On nine occasions mixed infections were found, in eight of these patients one of the staphylococcal species was present in association with one or more other bacteria. In five of these mixed cultures gram-negative organisms were present.

THE OUTCOME: (2) ELSEWHERE

Unfortunately there is little published literature on the single-stage method and such as there is does not permit a general conclusion to be drawn. Most authors have confined themselves to describing the outcome of the two-stage exchange method of reimplantation after various intervals.

Grogan and associates reported one case infected with micrococcus for which reimplantation with a new prosthesis was performed only 5 days after the previous infected implant had been removed. The infection had not recurred at review 97 months later.

In a report[13] from Bristol, United Kingdom, two cases of immediate exchange arthroplasty have been described. Both suffered recurrent infection. The operative technique was not described.

Teeny and colleagues[14] described a series of 24 infected total knee replacements. In the one case for whom a single-stage exchange was performed, the outcome was successful.

Borden and Gearen[15] reported 23 infected total knee replacements. These cases were managed by debridement and retention of the prosthesis or single-stage exchange or two-stage exchange arthroplasty. The infection was eradicated in all three of the cases treated by the single-stage method. All the infections were with gram-positive organisms. Notwithstanding this outcome the authors advocated the two-stage method as their preferred technique.

In the German literature[16] a report from the Endo-Klinik has been published on single-stage revision of 118 infected knee replacements. The outcome of 104 cases was reported at 5 to 15 years follow-up. Seventy-six cases (73%) were cured as a result of the single-stage operation using specific antibiotic-loaded cement. This figure was increased to 84 cases (81%) with a repeated single-stage operation but a third operation did not contribute any further improvement. The preferred prosthesis in this unit was a hinged device, which may have some bearing on the poor outcome. This group of patients was reported again in 1995:[17] survival analysis of 104 cases showed that infection persisted or recurred in 20% of the patients after 2 years and in 30% after 10 years.

Bengston and Knutson[18] published a 6-year follow-up of 357 cases of infected knee arthroplasty. Of these cases 107 underwent exchange arthroplasty, 69 in a single stage and 38 in two stages. This was a retrospective report with the treatment route having been selected by the participating surgeon. No advantage was identified for the two-stage procedure with approximately 75% of the total group of 107 patients cured.

CONCLUSION

Today the "orthodox" treatment for the infected TKR is a two-stage revision. As a consequence there are too few reports of the outcome of the quicker, potentially simpler single-stage revision procedure to permit a balanced view to be taken of its place. However, we believe that as at the hip, successful single-stage revision is certainly possible although technically demanding. Our results have been encouraging and we continue to use this procedure. The literature, such as it is, suggests that the results are no worse than those of a two-stage revision[10,11,13,14] for what remains a challenging complication of TKR.

References

1. Freeman MAR, King JB, O'Riordan SM. The day frame. In: Ackroyd CE, O'Connor BT, De Bruyn PF, eds. *The Severely Injured Limb*. Edinburgh: Churchill Livingstone; 1983: 129–143.
2. Buchholz HW, Engelbrecht E, Röttger J, Siegel A, Lodenkämper H, Elson RA. The management of deep infection involving joint implants. *J Bone Joint Surg Br*. 1979; 61-B:118.
3. Buchholz HW, Elson RA, Engelbrecht E, Lodenkämper H, Röttger J, Siegel A. Management of deep infection of total hip replacement. *J Bone Joint Surg Br*. 1981; 63-B:342–353.
4. Freeman MAR, Sudlow RA, Casewell MW, Radcliff SS. The management of infected total knee replacements. *J Bone Joint Surg Br*. 1985; 67-B:764–768.
5. Aglietti P, Salvati EA, Wilson PD, Kutner LJ. Effect of a surgical horizontal unidirectional filtered air flow unit on wound bacterial contamination and wound healing. *Clin Orthop*. 1974; 101:99–104.
6. Lidwell OM, Lowbury EJL, White W, Blowers R, Stanley SJ, Lowe D. Effect of ultraclean air in operating rooms on deep sepsis in the joint after total hip or knee replacement: a randomized study. *Br Med J*. 1982; 253:10–14.
7. Whyte W, Hodgson R, Bailey PV, Graham S. The reduction of bacteria in the operating room through the use of non-woven clothing. *Br J Surg*. 1978; 65:469–474.
8. Berg M, Bergman BO, Hoborn J. Ultraviolet radiation compared to an ultra-clean air enclosure. *J Bone Joint Surg Br*. 1991; 73-B:811–815.
9. Göksan SB, Freeman MAR. One stage reimplantation for infected total knee arthroplasty. *J Bone Joint Surg Br*. 1992; 74-B:78–82.
10. Insall JN, Thompson FM, Brause BD. Two-stage re-implantation for the salvage of infected total knee arthroplasty. *J Bone Joint Surg Am*. 1983; 65-A:1087–1098.
11. Windsor RE, Insall JN, Urs WK, Miller DV, Brause BD. Two-stage reimplantation for the salvage of total knee arthroplasty complicated by infection. Further follow-up and refinement of indications. *J Bone Joint Surg Am*. 1990; 72-A:272–278.
12. Grogan TJ, Dorey F, Rollins J, Amstutz HC. Deep sepsis following total knee arthroplasty. *J Bone Joint Surg Am*. 1986; 68-A:226–233.
13. Johnson DP, Bannister GC. The outcome of infected arthroplasty of the knee. *J Bone Joint Surg Br*. 1986; 68-B:289–291.
14. Teeny SM, Dorr L, Murata G, Conaty P. Treatment of infected total knee arthroplasty. Irrigation and debridement versus two-stage reimplantation. *J Arthroplasty*. 1990; 5(1):35–39.
15. Borden LS, Gearen TF. Infected total knee arthroplasty. A protocol for management. *J Arthroplasty*. 1987; 2(1):27–32.
16. von Foerster G, Kluber D, Käbler U. Mittel-bis lang fristige Ergebnisse nach Behandlung von 118 periprosthetischen Infektionen nach Kniegelenksersatz durch einzeitige Austauschoperation. *Orthopäde*. 1991; 20, Heft 3:244–252.
17. Nieder E. Results after treatment of 104 periprosthetic infections after knee joint replacement using one-stage revision arthroplasty with a rotating hinge or hinge prosthesis at 5 to 15 years follow-up. *J Bone Joint Surg Br*. 1995; 77-B:S II 128.
18. Bengston S, Knutson K. The infected knee arthroplasty. A six year follow up of 357 cases. *Acta Orthop Scand*. 1991; 62:301–311.
19. Boothe RE, Lotke PA. The results of spacer block technique in revision of infected total knee replacement. *Clin Orthop*. 1989; 248:57–60.

CHAPTER 61
Two-Stage Reimplantation

Giles R. Scuderi and Henry D. Clarke

Two-stage reimplantation of infected total knee arthroplasty has become the treatment of choice for most patients.[1,2,3,4] The treatment protocol is divided into three phases: (1) removal of the prosthesis and all cement with debridement of the soft tissues and bone; (2) six weeks of parental antibiotics; and (3) implantation of a new total knee prosthesis. To have adequate bone stock for the later reimplantation, care should be taken at the time of component removal care. While all attempts to perform a thorough debridement and cement removal are undertaken, overzealous debridement can lead to significant bone loss, complicating the reimplantation.

Following the removal of the infected components, cement spacers are placed between the femoral–tibial and patellofemoral articulations. The use of antibiotic-impregnated cement beads or spacer blocks allows local delivery of high concentrations of antibiotics. While the larger surface area of multiple beads theoretically provides greater allusion of local antibiotics than from a single spacer block, no definite clinical advantage has been proven. However, the spacer block has definite mechanical advantages over the beads. Spacer blocks facilitate ambulation prior to the reimplantation and also allow easier exposure at the time of the later surgery.[5] In most cases a spacer block is fashioned using two to three 40 g batches of polymethylmethacrylate cement mixed with high doses of antibiotics. We typically use 2.4 g of tobramycin and 1 g of vancomycin per pack of cement. When mixing the antibiotics, the lumps in the crystalline vancomycin should not be crushed. Once the cement has reached a doughy consistency it is placed into the femoral tibial space during the final stages of polymerization. Longitudinal distraction is applied to the extremity in an effort to prevent cement interdigitation with the bone; this enables easy removal at the time of reimplantation. If large spacers are used, the heat produced by the exothermic reaction can be significant. Irrigation should be used to cool the cement block, preventing damage to the neurovascular structures that lie only millimeters from the posterior capsule. The cement spacer can be fashioned with short pegs or stems to help provide stability. Extending the spacer anteriorly over the distal femur and into the patellofemoral joint also helps with stability and maintains a plane between the patella and femur. The block should be suitably large to sit on cortical bone and provide stability in extension. If the block is too small and has contact predominantly with cancellous bone or is insufficient to maintain stability, further bone erosion can occur. If the intramedullary canal is opened to remove stemmed components, antibiotic-impregnated cement rods can be placed inside the canals. Use of a cement spacer usually provides enough stability to the knee to allow the patient to walk for short distances in a knee immobilizer, brace, or cast.

During the 1990s, more functional temporary spacers were developed that incorporate small metallic femoral runners and polyethylene inserts into molded polymethylmethacrylate components. One such device, the so-called PROSTALAC (prosthesis of antibiotic loaded acrylic cement) allows joint motion and weight bearing during the period prior to reimplantation.[6] A range of motion up to 75 degrees has been reported with the use of this temporary functional spacer.[6] In a similar manner, some surgeons have sterilized the extracted femoral component and reinserted it temporarily using a small polyethylene insert on a cement block.[7] Again, this can reduce the patient's disability between debridement and staged reimplantation. If an articulating spacer is used, then attention must be paid to equalizing the flexion and extension space or dislocation may occur.

Aspiration prior to reimplantation is considered if there is clinical suspicion of persistent infection. However, in most cases our decision to proceed with reimplantation is determined intraoperatively based upon the appearance of the tissues and an evaluation of histologic frozen section specimens. At the time of reimplantation, adequate surgical exposure must be obtained and use of one of the previously discussed techniques, such as the quadriceps snip, may be required. Although uncemented prostheses with bone graft soaked in antibiotic solution have been used successfully in reimplantation,[8] we favor the use of cemented prostheses. The use of antibiotic-impregnated cement at the time of reimplantation has been shown to be associated with a significantly lower risk of recurrent infection.[9]

Significant bone loss, which requires the use of modular wedges or blocks, is often encountered at the time of reimplantation. Therefore, a prosthesis system, which has a full range of modular augments and stem extensions, should be available at reimplantation. The use of stemmed components does not necessarily require that a fully constrained articulation be implanted. Rather, the use of more constrained designs are reserved for cases with ligamentous insufficiency or instability. In the majority of reimplantations we recurrently use a cemented posterior stabilized prosthesis. We prefer to cement only the core prosthesis and avoid introduction of cement into the canal when stem extensions are used. This facilitates removal of the stems if subsequent prosthesis removal is required. In very rare cases with severe bone loss, custom prostheses or modular tumor prostheses may be required; the need for these devices must be anticipated preoperatively.

The postoperative management of individual patients is dependent on numerous variables, including the status of the soft tissue coverage, the type of exposure required, and whether structural bone grafts were utilized. In general, antibiotics are administered intravenously until final intraoperative culture results and tissue section evaluations have been obtained. If all results are negative for infection, then antibiotics are discontinued.

CLINICAL RESULTS

Insall originally reported on the successful eradication of infected total knee replacements with the two-stage protocol in 1977.[2] Windsor et al later confirmed the success of this technique when they reported on 38 reimplantations with an average follow-up of 4 years.[4] The two-stage protocol successfully eradicated the original deep infection in 37 knees (97.4%) and the reinfection rate was 10.5% (4 of 38 knees). Goldman reported on the largest cohort of two-stage reimplantations for infection.[1] The 64 knees in this study had an average follow-up of 7.5 years. Six knees (9%) became infected after reimplantation. With only two reinfections with the same organism, the infection eradication rate (97%) was identical to the findings of Windsor.[4]

Infection after total knee replacement is a serious and potentially devastating complication. Successful treatment can be obtained with the two-stage protocol. The long-term functional results, reinfection rate, and survivorship are comparable with those of revision total knee replacement.[1]

References

1. Goldman RT, Scuderi GR, Insall JN. Two-stage reimplantation for infected total knee replacement. *Clin Orthop*. 1996; 331:118–124.
2. Insall JN, Thompson FM, Brause BD. Two-stage reimplantation for the salvage of infected total knee arthroplasty. *J Bone Joint Surg*. 1983; 65A:1087–1098.
3. Windsor RE, Bono JV. Infected total knee replacements. *J Am Acad Orthop Surg*. 1994; 2:44–53.
4. Windsor RE, Insall JN, Urs WK, et al. Two-stage reimplantation for the salvage of total knee arthroplasty complicated by infection. Further follow-up and refinement of indications. *J Bone Joint Surg*. 1990; 72A:272–278.
5. Booth RE, Jr, Lotke PA. The results of spacer block technique in revision of infected total knee arthroplasty. *Clin Orthop*. 1989; 248:57–60.
6. Masri BA, Kendall RW, Duncan CP, et al. Two-stage exchange arthroplasty using a functional antibiotic-loaded spacer in the treatment of the infected knee replacement: The Vancouver experience. *Sem. Arthroplasty*. 1994;5(3):122–136.
7. Hofmann AA, Kane KR, Tkach TK, Plaster RL, Camargo MP. Treatment of infected total knee arthroplasty using an articulating spacer. *Clin Orthop*. 1995; 321:45–54.
8. Whiteside LA. Treatment of infected total knee arthroplasty. *Clin Orthop*. 1994; 299:169–172.
9. Hanssen AD, Rand JA, Osmon DR. Treatment of the infected total knee arthroplasty with insertion of another prosthesis: The effect of antibiotic-impregnated bone cement. *Clin Orthop*. 1994; 309:44–55.

CHAPTER 62
Evolution and Design Rationale of the *PROSTALAC* Knee System in the Management of the Infected Total Knee Prosthesis

Bassam A. Masri, Christopher P. Beauchamp and Clive P. Duncan

Since the introduction of the modern total knee replacement,[1] excellent results have been reported with 15-year survivorship up to 94%.[2] Unfortunately an excellent result can quickly become a disaster if a deep infection occurs. In addition to the increased morbidity, infection has a marked socioeconomic effect. Sculco,[3] based on US Medicare data, reviewed the incidence and economic impact of infected total hip and knee arthroplasty. In 1989 in the United States 80,647 total knee replacements were performed on Medicare patients. During the same year, 1795 implants were removed for infection, for an estimated incidence of total knee sepsis of 2.23%. Sculco also estimated the cost of treatment of each infection at $50,000 to $60,000. The overall annual cost for the treatment of infected total knee replacements would therefore be between $90 million and $110 million per year. The majority of the cost of treatment is the expense of the prolonged hospitalization that is often required. Any treatment method that allows earlier discharge from hospital and effective control of infection would be welcomed. An unmeasured burden is the social impact this devastating complication can have. Unfortunately the therapeutic remedies available to patients carry a high morbidity cost.

In this chapter, the authors will outline their preferred method of treating infected total knee replacement. This method is a modification of the well-accepted two-stage exchange arthroplasty, in which the implant is removed and the knee is debrided at the first stage, and following a period of several weeks, a permanent prosthesis is reimplanted. The modification includes the insertion of an antibiotic-loaded facsimile of a total knee replacement prosthesis between stages. In addition to the elution of high levels of antibiotics into the joint, this prosthesis allows ambulation, knee motion permits rehabilitation, and allows for earlier discharge from hospital between stages. The patient is readmitted for the second stage on an elective basis. This temporary functional spacer is now known as the <u>pros</u>thesis of <u>a</u>ntibiotic-<u>l</u>oaded <u>a</u>crylic <u>c</u>ement, or simply the PROSTALAC.[4] The contents of this chapter will therefore be restricted to exchange arthroplasty, particularly as it relates to the use of the PROSTALAC system, and other related articulated spacers.

EVOLUTION OF EXCHANGE ARTHROPLASTY

The most widely accepted treatment for chronically infected total knee arthroplasty is removal of the components, thorough debridement, and a delayed exchange of the components. Historically, the introduction of antibiotic-loaded bone cement by Buchholz and Engelbrecht in 1970,[5] and its use in the successful treatment of infected total hip replacements,[6] stimulated the use of similar techniques in the treatment of the infected knee replacement.

Early reports of successful reimplantation of infected total knee replacements were merely anecdotal. In a 1976 report of GUEPAR hinged knee prostheses, there were nine attempts at reimplantation of infected implants; four subsequently removed for recurrent infection.[7] In 1979, in a series of Attenborough knee arthroplasties, only one infected implant was salvaged by reimplantation using gentamicin-loaded bone cement.[8]

The first report of a successful reimplantation of an infected knee replacement using a two-stage exchange technique with an antibiotic-loaded cement spacer was published in 1979.[9] This was a steroid-dependent 59-year-old patient with rheumatoid arthritis and an infected knee replacement. The infection was treated by removal of the implants and thorough debridement. Gentamicin-loaded bone cement beads were inserted in the joint, and 4 weeks later, the beads were removed and a revision knee replacement fixed with gentamicin-loaded cement was performed. The authors did not comment on the use of oral or intravenous antibiotics between stages. In 1983, Woods and associates[10] reported on the successful salvage in three of three infected knee replacements that were treated with removal of the implants, antibiotic therapy, and reimplantation of another prosthesis 3 to 6 months later.

The first series of reimplantation for salvage of infected total knee replacements were reported in 1983 by Rand and colleagues[11] and Insall and associates.[12] These reports showed good results with two-stage exchange arthroplasty with a delay of at least 6 weeks between stages.[12] When the delay was less than 2 weeks, particularly with more virulent organisms, the results were not as encouraging.[11] In a retrospective review of 14 patients with infected total knee replacements in whom reimplantation was attempted, eventually, six of the 14 patients required either arthrodesis or amputation. Only eight of 14 patients retained well-functioning prostheses at a mean follow-up of 3.3 years after the last revision operation.[11] In this series, however, the treatment protocol was not standardized. Five knees were reimplanted immediately following the removal of the infected implant, and nine were reimplanted no later than 2 weeks following removal of the infected implant. The duration of antibiotic therapy ranged from 4 days to 90 days. Antibiotic-loaded cement was not used either as a spacer or for the fixation of the revision prosthesis.

ONE-STAGE EXCHANGE ARTHROPLASTY

Over the past decade, steadily improving results of reimplantation for treatment of the infected total knee replacement have been reported. In most series, however, successful salvage was achieved using two-stage exchange arthroplasty.

Rand and Bryan[11] reported salvage in only eight of 14 patients who were treated with exchange arthroplasty with a delay of less than 2 weeks between stages. In this series, the patients in whom the infection was caused by low-virulence organisms (*Staphylococcus epidermis*, *Proprionibacterium acnes*, and *Peptococcus*) had a better result with salvage in six of seven knees. In contrast, when the infecting organism was more virulent (*Staphylococcus aureus*, *Escherichia coli*, or *Pseudomonas aerugenosa*), only two of seven knees were salvaged. The definition of virulence in this study, however, was arbitrary, and is not universally accepted. The difference in outcome based on organism virulence is not universally supported in the literature. Bengtson and colleagues[14] were not able to identify a difference in outcome based on organism virulence in a series of 11 one-stage and five two-stage exchange procedures. In Bengtson's study, the knee was salvaged in only seven of 16 knees. Unfortunately, the results were not broken down based on whether a one-stage or a two-stage exchange was performed. The authors concluded, however, that a two-stage exchange arthroplasty with antibiotic-loaded cement beads as spacers between stages, and fixation of the revision implant with antibiotic-loaded cement was a better option.

Borden and Gearen[15] reported no recurrence of infection in three of three patients in whom a one-stage exchange arthroplasty was performed. This is however a small number of patients in whom infection was caused by gram-positive organisms, and these results cannot be used as support for one-stage exchange arthroplasty in all cases.

Freeman and associates[16] were able to control the infection in all eight patients with septic loosening of total knee replacements, who were treated with a one-stage exchange protocol in which gentamicin-loaded Palacos R® (Smith and Nephew Richards, Memphis, Tennessee) cement was used for the fixation of the revision arthroplasty, and oral antibiotics were continued for a minimum of 3 months following surgery. In this series, six knees were infected with *Staphylococcus aureus* and two knees yielded negative cultures because of prior antibiotic therapy. The success of treatment, despite infection with *Staphylococcus aureus*, is in contrast to the results of Rand and Bryan,[11] who characterized *Staphylococcus aureus* as a virulent organism with reference to total knee sepsis. In a later series by Göksan and Freeman,[17] the original infection was controlled in 17 of 18 knees with septic loosening, which were treated using the previously described one-stage exchange technique. All knees in this series were infected with gram-positive organisms. One of these 17 knees subsequently became infected with a different organism, for an overall success rate of 16 of 18 knees (89%). These series by Freeman and colleagues[16,17] are the only ones in the literature in which consistently good results were reported with one-stage exchange arthroplasty. The numbers are small (18 cases), and 17 of 18 knees had at least one loose component at the time of treatment. Moreover, all infections were caused by gram-positive organisms.

In our opinion, one-stage exchange arthroplasty should only be used with great caution, because the findings of Freeman and associates have not been corroborated by other groups. The results may not apply to infections that are caused by gram-negative organisms. Moreover, the presence of draining sinuses, soft tissue deficiency requiring flap coverage, or bony deficiency requiring bone grafting were not addressed. If this technique is to be used, Freeman's protocol should be carefully studied. This includes separate intraoperative preparation and draping for the debridement and reimplantation portions of the procedure. Separate instruments should be used for the implantation portion of the procedure and antibiotic-loaded bone cement should be used for fixation of the implant. Antibiotics should be continued for at least 3 months. It is our opinion after reviewing all the results of treatment options for deep chronic infections that a two-stage exchange arthroplasty is still the treatment of choice of infected total knee replacements.

TWO-STAGE EXCHANGE ARTHROPLASTY

The currently used protocols for the treatment of infected total knee arthroplasties are modifications of the two-stage exchange arthroplasty originally described by Insall and associates.[12] Insall's technique is a two-stage exchange arthroplasty in which the infected implant is removed at the first stage. All infected material and all retained cement are carefully removed. Intravenous antibiotic therapy is then begun and is continued for a 6-week period. Insall advised that serum bactericidal levels be measured using a serial twofold tube-dilution technique, and bactericidal titers are maintained at a dilution level of 1:8 or above. These serum titers are maintained for a full 6-week period, and any days during which the serum titers are not adequate do not count toward the 6-week period. A definitive resurfacing total knee arthroplasty is then reimplanted. Reimplantation should not be delayed by more than 3 months because scarring and contractures preclude good motion following reimplantation, if a spacer is not used between stages.[18] Antibiotic-loaded bone cement is not used. The exposure for the subsequent reimplantation procedure is generally difficult, and skeletonization of the distal femur is often required. The extensor mechanism is often shortened and scarred, frequently requiring a Coonse-Adams[13] quadriceps turndown, or one of its modifications. All antibiotics are discontinued following reimplantation. Using this method, the authors reported no recurrence of the initial infection in a prospective series of 11 infected knee replacements[12] with an average follow-up of 34 months. There was one new infection with a different organism secondary to an infected bunion. Of the 11 knees, five were rated as excellent, four were rated good, and two were rated fair. The most common complication in this series were related to the extensor mechanism. Since Rand and Bryan's[11] and Insall's[12] series, many others have been reported using two-stage exchange arthroplasty (Table 62.1).

In a series of 11 patients treated with a two-stage exchange technique, Borden and Gearen[15] reported control of the infection in 10 cases. The one case that was not controlled was an infected GUEPAR hinged prosthesis. This was treated successfully with a knee arthrodesis. There were three differences between the technique used in this series and that reported by Insall and associates.[12] (1) In eight of 11 cases, antibiotic-loaded cement beads were used as a spacer between stages. (2) In all cases, antibiotic-loaded bone cement was used for the reimplantation. (3) Bactericidal levels of antibiotics were given for 3 weeks, following which, if two separate aspirations revealed no growth of organisms, the second stage was performed. This is in contrast to the 6-week period that was used by Insall and associates.[12] All of the patients in this series had a chronic infection with septic loosening of the implants. In another series,[19] 25 patients with 26 infected total knee replacements were treated with a two-stage exchange arthroplasty, with a duration of 6 weeks (with intravenous antibiotic therapy) between stages. Antibiotic-loaded bone cement was used for reimplantation in all cases. There was no clinical recurrence of infection; how-

Table 62.1. The results of the various series on two-stage exchange arthroplasty are summarized. For the sake of this discussion, any infection following reimplantation is considered a failure of infection cure. The results of the PROSTALAC series are presented later in this chapter

Authors	Year	Number of patients	Number cured	Percent cured
Insall[12]	1983	11	11	100%
Rand[11]	1983	9	5	56%
Borden and Gearen[15]	1987	11	10	91%
Rosenberg[19]	1988	26	23	88%
Wilde and Ruth[59]	1988	15	12	80%
Booth and Lotke[60]	1989	25	24	96%
Windsor[20]	1990	38	34	89%
Teeny[21]	1990	7	7	100%
Scott[62]	1993	7	7	100%
Whiteside[22]	1994	33	32	97%
Hanssen[23]	1994	89	79	89%
Kane[64]	1995	25	25	100%
Cadambi[65]	1995	11	10	91%
PROSTALAC	1995	37	34	92%
Total		344	313	91%

ever, three patients had positive cultures at the second stage. These included one patient with a tuberculous infection that was treated with a long course of antituberculous medication. The other two patients were treated with oral antibiotics for 3 to 6 months following reimplantation. The functional outcome was excellent in 20 of 25 patients (48%), good in six (24%), fair in two (8%), and poor in four (6%).

Windsor and colleagues[20] reported on a larger series with longer follow-up using the technique first described by Insall and associates at the Hospital for Special Surgery.[12] Thirty-eight infected total knee replacements (35 patients) were included in this study. Of these knees, eight had been previously reported by Insall and associates.[12] At a mean follow-up of 4 years (2.5 to 10 years), there was recurrence of the infection in one knee, and reinfection with a different organism in another two knees. One knee was presumed infected; however, no organism could be cultured. This patient was treated with removal of the implant and knee arthrodesis. If successful eradication of infection is defined as prevention of recurrence of the initial infecting organisms, the success rate would be 97%. If all infections and the presumed infection are considered failures, the success rate would be 89%. Similarly, no recurrence of infection was reported by Teeney and colleagues in a series of seven knees that were treated using a two-stage exchange technique following failure of debridement and irrigation.[21]

More recently, Whiteside[22] reported the results of two-stage exchange arthroplasty in 33 infected total knee replacements. In this study, antibiotic-loaded bone cement beads were used between stages, in addition to parenteral antibiotic therapy. In 28 knees, a single debridement was sufficient for control of infection. In four knees, one or two further debridements were required prior to reimplantation in order to control the infection. In one knee, infection could not be controlled, and the patient eventually underwent an above knee amputation. In the 32 knees that were salvaged (97%), reimplantation was delayed by at least 6 weeks following the last debridement, and all revision prostheses were cementless and were implanted with antibiotic-loaded morselized allograft to fill bony defects.

Reimplantation at the second stage is not an easy task. The soft tissues are contracted, and exposure is generally difficult. In order to help preserve length and minimize soft tissue contracture, several techniques have been described. These include methylmethacrylate spacer blocks and articulated spacers, such as the PROSTALAC system. Antibiotic-loaded bone cement has been used in these spacers, as well as for the fixation of the implant at the second stage.

THE ROLE OF ANTIBIOTIC-LOADED BONE CEMENT

Despite the excellent results obtained by Insall and associates[12] and Windsor and colleagues,[20] in which two-stage exchange arthroplasty was performed without antibiotic-loaded bone cement, the current techniques of two-stage exchange arthroplasty include the use of antibiotic-loaded bone cement for fixation of the revision prosthesis at the second stage procedure. In a study of 89 infected total knee replacements,[23] the only factor that was found to correlate with a better result following two-stage exchange arthroplasty was the use of antibiotic-loaded bone cement for the fixation of the definitive prosthesis. The authors used a variety of antibiotics, including tobramycin, gentamicin, erythromycin, vancomycin, and penicillin. The dose of antibiotics used was 1.2 grams of tobramycin or 1.0 gram of the other antibiotics in each 40-gram package of bone cement powder. Of 25 knees in which antibiotic-loaded cement was not used, infection recurred in seven knees (28%). In contrast, infection recurred in only three of 64 knees (4.7%) in which antibiotic-loaded bone cement was used for the fixation of the definitive implant. This was highly statistically significant ($p = 0.0025$).

In a multicenter, randomized, prospective study comparing gentamicin-loaded bead implantation to conventional parenteral antibiotic therapy in infected total hip and knee replacements,[24] antibiotic-loaded bone cement beads seemed to have a protective effect compared with parenteral antibiotic therapy. The study consisted of 22 infected hip and six infected knee replacements. Two-stage exchange arthroplasty was performed, but the group was randomized into two groups. In one group consisting of 13 infected implants, parenteral antibiotics were used between stages, and antibiotic-loaded cement beads were not used. The converse was true for the second group, which consisted of 15 infected implants. Infection recurred in fewer cases in the antibiotic-loaded cement bead group (2 of 15; 15%) than in the parenteral antibiotic group (4 of 13; 30%). Because of the small numbers in this study, this difference was not statistically significant.

Based on this data, we recommend the routine use of antibiotic-loaded bone cement, with a dose of 1.0 to 1.2 grams of antibiotic (usually tobramycin) per 40-gram package of cement. We do not have any experience with cementless revision total knee replacement, and based on results obtained when antibiotic cement is not used for the definitive reconstruction cannot recommend it at the present time. Moreover, our treatment protocol includes the use of antibiotic-loaded bone cement spacers after debridement. The various antibiotic-loaded spacers will be discussed; however, the rational use of antibiotic-loaded bone cement requires an understanding of the properties of this composite material. Therefore, the properties of antibiotic-loaded bone cement will be discussed first.

PROPERTIES OF ANTIBIOTIC-LOADED BONE CEMENT

The properties of antibiotic bone cement have been thoroughly investigated over the past two decades. It is now known, through in vitro[25–38] and in vivo[25–28,30,38–43] studies, that many commonly used antibiotics are released from bone cement in such a way that the local antibiotic levels vastly exceed the minimal inhibitory concentration of most susceptible pathogens, and that these levels are much higher than those achieved with parenteral therapy.[39,44] In our own patients, tobramycin levels as high as 232 mg/L and vancomycin levels as high as 54 mg/L were measured in the suction drainage fluid within 24 hours following insertion of an antibiotic-loaded cement spacer containing tobramycin and vancomycin. These values represent highly therapeutic levels. Different antibiotics have different elution characteristics. For example, when tobramycin is compared to vancomycin (Fig. 62.1), it becomes clear that tobramycin elutes in much higher concentrations early on. Tobramycin elution decays at a much faster rate than vancomycin.[45] The elution of both antibiotics decays with time; however, only a few studies have addressed the long-term elution of antibiotics from bone cement.[28,32,38,40,46]

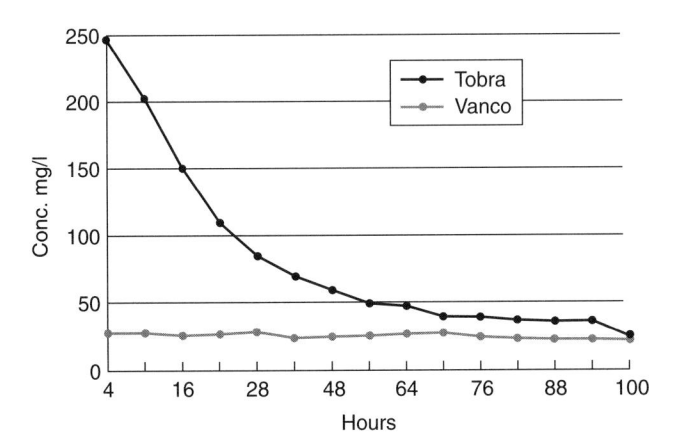

Figure 62.1. The suction drainage fluid was assayed for tobramycin and vancomycin concentrations for the first 5 days following insertion of tobramycin- and vancomycin-loaded PROSTALAC knee spacers. The graph illustrates the better elution of tobramycin from bone cement compared with vancomycin.

In an in vitro assay, clindamycin was found to elute for up to 56 days.[32] In rabbits, antibiotic-loaded cement pellets can elute antibiotics for up to 37 days.[28] In a series of three sheep with gentamicin-loaded bone cement within the femur, gentamicin levels in bone at 18 months following insertion of the antibiotic-loaded cement were 7 to 36 mg/kg.[40]

The in vivo long-term elution of antibiotics in humans has been reported in two series.[38,46] In one study,[38] therapeutic levels of gentamicin were measured in the periprosthetic connective tissue, cancellous, and/or cortical bone in 17 patients several months following total hip arthroplasty with gentamicin-loaded bone cement. In one patient, 5.75 years following surgery, gentamicin concentrations of 5.4 to 6.6 mg/kg of tissue (wet weight) and 6.6 mg/kg were measured from periprosthetic connective tissue and cancellous bone, respectively. Joint fluid, in this study, was not assayed for gentamicin levels. In an investigation by the current authors,[46] long-term antibiotic elution from the PROSTALAC hip[47,48] and knee[4] systems was studied in 49 patients. These results will be discussed later in this chapter.

Not only does antibiotic-loaded bone cement allow the elution of high levels of antibiotics into the periprosthetic milieu, but it has been shown that antibiotics within bone cement implanted within the medullary cavity of a cadaver femur are able to permeate through dead cortical bone.[30] This finding has obvious therapeutic advantages in the case of the severely infected total knee arthroplasty with osteomyelitis and devascularization.

The safety of this antibiotic depot has also been clearly established. In our own patients, who were treated with antibiotic-loaded bone cement for infected hip and knee arthroplasties, we have never been able to measure tobramycin or vancomycin serum levels higher than 3 mg/L. This has also been shown by other investigators in humans and in animal models.[28,30,33,38,41,43,49]

Baker and Greenham,[26] through in vivo and in vitro studies with scanning electron microscopy, described the mechanism of elution of antibiotics from bone cement. The release of antibiotics occurs only from the surface through voids and cracks in the bone cement. They concluded that increasing the concentration of antibiotics within the bone cement would improve the elution characteristics of antibiotics. This was confirmed in human studies by Wahlig and associates[43] who showed that doubling the concentration of gentamicin from 0.5 gms to 1.0 gm per 40 gms of cement allowed doubling of the concentration of gentamicin in wound secretions. Baker and Greenham[26] also concluded that bone cements with a higher porosity would be expected to allow higher antibiotic release than those with a lower porosity. It is then no surprise that Palacos-R® bone cement, which has a higher porosity than other cements, has the best in vitro elution characteristics.[30,33,38,41] Moreover, they also concluded that methods of cement preparation that are designed to minimize porosity (such as vacuum mixing or centrifugation) could have a deleterious effect on antibiotic elution.

The change in mechanical strength of antibiotic-loaded bone cement, when compared with plain cement has also been studied.[50–53] In some studies, the addition of small amounts of antibiotics in the powder form did not seem to significantly weaken bone cement,[52,53] whereas the addition of antibiotics in liquid form to the bone cement caused significant weakening.[52] Other studies have shown that the addition of any amount of antibiotic powder will cause some weakening of the antibiotic-bone cement composite, regardless of the amount of antibiotic added to the cement.[50] The degree of weakening depends on the proportional weight of antibiotics added to the bone cement.[51] Lautenschlager and colleagues[51] showed that mixing more than 4.5 gms of gentamicin sulfate can significantly weaken bone cement to the point that its compressive strength is decreased to below the minimum acceptable standards. This was only when samples were tested in compression. Fatigue testing of the cement is difficult to perform because physiologic cycling would require a very prolonged period of time. Based on the literature, a limit of about 2 gms of antibiotic powder per 40 gms of bone cement appears to be a safe estimate for the maximum allowable concentration of antibiotics in bone cement, particularly when the bone cement is used for the fixation of a permanent revision knee replacement. These limits do not necessarily apply when antibiotics are added to bone cement in temporary spacers, which are removed a few weeks or months following insertion in two-stage exchange arthroplasty.

Another possible advantage to the use of antibiotic-loaded bone cement is its potential role in decreasing bacterial bioadherence. In orthopedic implant infections, bacterial adherence is enhanced by the formation of glycocalyx—a polysaccharide layer that is produced around bacterial colonies and helps to increase bacterial resistance to host defenses.[54,55] In one study,[56] the adherence of *Staphylococcus epidermidis* was reduced when tobramycin was added to bone cement. Another study[57] showed that the use of clindamycin can inhibit glycocalyx production in an experimental streptococcal endocarditis model. Whether such an interaction is applicable in the case of orthopedic implant infections remains to be seen. Also, whether these interactions are as applicable in vivo as they are in vitro is not well documented.

With an understanding of these basic properties of antibiotic-loaded bone cement, the surgeon can take better advantage of this material in the treatment of infected total knee replacements.

METHYLMETHACRYLATE SPACER BLOCKS

In order to preserve a joint cavity following excision arthroplasty in a two-stage exchange protocol, antibiotic-loaded bone cement spacer blocks have been inserted in the joint space. In addition to their ability to elute high levels of antibiotics, these spacer blocks, in contrast to antibiotic-loaded cement beads, decrease the scarring within the joint space and decrease the difficulty of reimplantation. These blocks are handmade in the operating room, and are sized to fit the defect created by removal of the infected prosthesis. Ideally, a small cement stem should be fashioned and added to the spacer block to allow the anchoring of the block to the tibia and to prevent its migration. Moreover, a thin layer of cement between the femur and the patella may prevent the scarring of the extensor mechanism to the distal femur. In most cases, a minimum of two packages of bone cement are required. Despite these efforts, in our experience, the revision procedure is still difficult, and scarring is still substantial, particularly in the lateral and medial gutters. In our opinion, the patient should not be allowed to move the knee with the spacer in place, and full weight-bearing should be discouraged because of the risk of bone erosion with a mobile one-piece spacer, especially in patients with weak bone. These spacers should not be used if further surgery is not possible, and excision arthroplasty will be the definitive method of treatment, because of the risk of dislodgment as well as the risk of this spacer acting as a foreign body following elution of the antibiotics within the surface layer of the spacer.

The use of these spacers was first reported in 1988. Cohen and associates[58] reported on three cases that were treated using this method. Infection was controlled in all three patients, and the authors were able to successfully implant a well-functioning total knee replacement as late as 6 months following excision of the infected implants.

Wilde and Ruth[59] reported a series of 21 infected total knee arthroplasties that were treated using a two-stage exchange technique, but only 15 cases had a longer than 1-year follow-up. A spacer block was used in 10 of these cases. The mean delay between stages was 6 weeks, and the mean duration of intravenous antibiotic therapy was 4.2 weeks. Of these 15 cases, the infection was controlled in 12 (80%), was definitely not controlled in two, and there was a suspicion of continued infection in one. Of the 10 patients with spacers, there were no definite infections, and one patient was presumed to be infected and was revised elsewhere, for an infection control rate of 90%. These numbers are small; however, the presence of a spacer did not seem to have a detrimental effect on infection control.

In a larger series of infected knee replacements treated with two-stage exchange arthroplasty with an interim antibiotic-loaded cement spacer, Booth and Lotke[60] reported one failure of 25 cases with a mean follow-up of 25 months. The delay between stages ranged from 3 weeks to 17 months, and even at 17 months, a successful arthroplasty was achieved with a range of motion of 0 to 105 degrees. The authors felt that the reimplantation was facilitated by the presence of the spacer.

ARTICULATED SPACERS IN TWO-STAGE EXCHANGE ARTHROPLASTY

The majority of the morbidity of two-stage exchange arthroplasty is related to the scarring and lack of motion between stages. As a corollary to the increased ease in reimplantation that was noted by Booth and Lotke,[60] the presence of a spacer that not only allows distraction of the joint space but also motion between stages, would be expected to even further increase the ease of revision, and potentially improve the final functional outcome. Our currently preferred system is the PROSTALAC system, which is primarily made of antibiotic-loaded bone cement, and acts as a functional spacer that preserves mobility and joint stability, while eluting high levels of antibiotics between stages. In our experience, reimplantation is greatly facilitated.

In addition to the PROSTALAC system, which was first reported in 1992,[61] four other articulated space systems have been described.[62,64,66] In 1993, Scott and colleagues[62] described a novel modification of two-stage exchange arthroplasty. In this technique, the infected implant and all cement are removed at first stage. Following a thorough debridement and irrigation, antibiotic-loaded cement beads are threaded on a braided wire, and the beads are inserted within any open medullary canals and also within the joint space. A sterile prosthesis is then loosely cemented with antibiotic-loaded bone cement to act as a spacer and to allow motion. At 6 weeks, a definitive reimplantation using antibiotic-loaded bone cement is performed. The antibiotics that are added to bone cement are chosen according to the sensitivity profile of the infecting organisms. The choice of antibiotic also depends on the criteria outlined by Murray.[63] These include antibiotic safety, thermostability, hypoallergenicity, water-solubility, adequate bactericidal spectrum, and availability in a sterile powder form. These criteria apply to the use of antibiotic-loaded bone cement under any circumstances. In some occasions, where the most appropriate antibiotic is only available in liquid form, the liquid may be lyophilized under sterile conditions and a sterile powder may be obtained, on a custom-basis. However, this requires highly specialized facilities and may not be possible at all centers. The advantages of this articulated spacer include continued mobility, ease of rehabilitation, and ease of reimplantation. The disadvantage would be the increased cost of the prosthesis that is used as a spacer and then discarded at 6 weeks. At first glance, one may wonder why a one-stage exchange is not performed, particularly when a knee replacement prosthesis or facsimile is inserted at the first-stage procedure. The results of one-stage exchange arthroplasty have not been predictable, as already discussed. Moreover, in Scott's series,[62] the authors compared their results using an articulated spacer with a one-stage exchange arthroplasty. Of 10 one-stage exchange procedures, infection persisted in three. On the other hand, all seven knees that were treated using this modified two-stage exchange arthroplasty were free of infection at final review. The other difference between this method and a one-stage exchange is that in this method much higher doses of antibiotic could be added to the bone cement than in a one-stage exchange, in which the surgeon has to limit the dose of antibiotics because of the risk of weakening of the cement. We do not use more than 1.2 grams of antibiotics per 40-gram package of bone cement when antibiotic-loaded bone cement is used for permanent prosthetic fixation, and we strongly discourage the use of more than 2 grams because of the risk of cement weakening. But, in temporary spacers, doses in excess of 5 grams of antibiotics per 40-gram package of bone cement may be used with relative impunity. In cases in which very large amounts of antibiotic are added to bone cement, mixing may be facilitated by the addition of an additional small amount of monomer. Although the numbers are small in this series,[62] they support the safety of this method despite the use of foreign material between stages.

A similar articulated spacer technique was described by Kane and associates.[64] A two-stage exchange technique is used, with a 6-week interval between stages. Following an adequate debridement at the first stage, the removed femoral component is flash sterilized and is reinserted with antibiotic-loaded bone cement, at a late stage in cement polymerization to prevent thorough interdigitation between the cement and bone, and facilitate the removal of the component at the second stage. On the tibial side, a new polyethylene liner of an adequate thickness is likewise fixed loosely with antibiotic-loaded bone cement. Tobramycin was used in bone cement, at a dosage level of 4.8 grams of tobramycin per 40-gram package of Simplex P® (Howmedica, Rutherford, New Jersey) bone cement. Following 6 weeks of intravenous antibiotic therapy, this temporary spacer is removed and a knee replacement is reimplanted using antibiotic-impregnated bone cement. At a mean follow-up of 30 months, with a minimum follow-up of 13 months, there was no infection recurrence or reinfection in 25 infected knee replacements.

Cadambi and associates[65] described another similar technique for the treatment of infected knee and hip replacement. The surgical technique is similar to that described by Scott and colleagues. The only difference is that reimplantation was performed only 2 weeks following the first-stage procedure, and parenteral antibiotic therapy was continued for 6 weeks following reimplantation. Eleven infected knee replacements were treated using this protocol. Infection was controlled in all but one knee. The only failure was in a 72-year-old diabetic with congestive heart failure and peripheral vascular disease. An above knee amputation was required for infection control following recurrence.

McPherson and associates[66] reported on the use of a handmade facsimile of a knee replacement that is inserted between stages in a two-stage exchange protocol. This handmade facsimile is made of antibiotic-loaded bone cement. This allows motion and partial weight-bearing between stages. Because of this crude design, stability was not well maintained, and a knee immobilizer was required for walking.

It is interesting to note that all of these articulated spacer protocols were developed independently over the past few years, at a variety of centers. This possibly reflects the difficulty encountered with reimplantation following a standard excision arthroplasty. It also potentially reflects the dissatisfaction of both the patient and the surgeon with the function between stages, when the patient is left without a functional knee joint. Like others, we have also been dissatisfied with patients' function between stages, hence the development of the Prosthesis of Antibiotic-Loaded Acrylic Cement (PROSTALAC), beginning in 1987. This modified two-stage exchange protocol combines many of the features of the previously discussed articulated spacers. The difference is that it allows intraoperative flexibility, regardless of the intraoperative findings, while using the least possible amount of metal and plastic within the joint.[4]

THE PROSTHESIS OF ANTIBIOTIC-LOADED ACRYLIC CEMENT (PROSTALAC)

The PROSTALAC system is an articulated spacer that is used between stages in a two-stage exchange protocol. Like all other articulated spacers, the purpose of this system is to allow mobility and weight-bearing between stages, while maintaining adequate soft tissue tension and joint stability. It is also intended to simplify the reimplantation procedure. When function is maintained between stages, the patient may be discharged from the hospital, and the cost is reduced.

System Design and Evolution

The PROSTALAC prototype was first implanted in 1987. This was a handmade facsimile of a total knee replacement prosthesis that was made of highly antibiotic-loaded bone cement. Because of the difficulty in fashioning a smooth articular surface using a handmade technique, the first generation PROSTALAC was introduced in early 1991. This was also a facsimile of a knee replacement with a cement-on-cement articulation. The articular surfaces on the femoral and tibial components, however, were smooth. The smooth surfaces were possible because of the use of a flexible polyethylene mold, that allowed molding a perfectly smooth articular surface. Despite the smooth surface, motion was awkward because of the high friction at the articular surfaces. For the most part, motion was painless, and a range of flexion of at least 75 degrees was the norm. However, patients complained that motion was quite noisy, and painless crepitus was easily audible. Because of the high friction, the normal rhythm of gait was disrupted, and gait was awkward. Another problem with the first generation PROSTALAC was knee instability. Because the molds were flexible, it was difficult to adequately control the thickness of the femoral and tibial components, and adequate restoration of the level of joint line, as well as soft tissue balancing, was difficult. Furthermore, this design did not allow substitution of the posterior cruciate ligament function, which is commonly absent in cases of infected total knee replacement. For this reason, posterior instability, as well as mediolateral instability, was not uncommon. The problem with the high-friction articulation was solved by the addition of small stainless-steel femoral runners and polyethylene tibial skids. In order to avoid the use of large amounts of metal and plastic, the design of the tibial skid was quite flat, because a conforming tibial skid would require much thicker polyethylene. This modification allowed us to solve the problem of the high-friction articulation; however, instability persisted. The final modification of the PROSTALAC system is the currently used design. In addition to the low-friction articulation afforded by the stainless steel runners and polyethylene skids, the design was changed to a posterior-stabilized design, with a cement post on the tibial component and a small metal bar connecting the two femoral runners so that a cam mechanism is created. Despite this modification, the amount of metal and plastic within this spacer is still small compared to the much larger amount of antibiotic-loaded bone cement. The other modification is that the flexible polyethylene molds were replaced with more rigid modular molds that not only allow the use of different sizes of components, but within each size, the distal thickness of the femoral component and the thickness of the tibial components could be accurately measured. The thickness of the femoral and tibial components are determined based on intraoperative measurements using any revision total knee system. Specific trial components for the PROSTALAC system are now in production. In the meantime, trial implants from any revision knee system can be adapted and used. With the ability to accurately manufacture the femoral and tibial components intraoperatively, the joint line can be accurately reproduced, and knee kinematics and stability are improved. In the case in which the collateral ligaments are absent, and a constrained knee is required, a hinged knee brace could be used postoperatively so that knee stability is maintained. Motion, however, may be allowed, as may protected weight-bearing depending on bone quality.

Surgical Technique

This is a modified two-stage exchange arthroplasty as described by Insall and associates.[12] At the first stage, the infected implants are removed as is all residual cement. It is controversial whether retained cement affects the outcome of infected total hip arthroplasty, and there is no literature on its effect on the outcome of exchange arthroplasty in infected total knee arthroplasty. Despite the lack of literature regarding retained cement, it is our policy to remove all cement at the first stage. In some cases, an intraoperative radiograph may help to visualize any retained cement.

Excellent exposure is required for removal of the components and a thorough debridement. In many of our cases, a rectus "snip," as described by Insall,[67] or in some cases a modified Coonse-Adams approach may be required.[13]

In infected total knee arthroplasty, one or more components may be loose, or all implants may be rigidly fixed. The removal of loose implants is not difficult. The removal of a rigidly fixed cementless femoral component is greatly facilitated by the use of flexible osteotomes. A Gigli saw may also be passed at the prosthetic interface and facilitate the breakdown of the areas of bone ingrowth. Following loosening of the implant, a variety of extraction devices may be used. For the rigidly cemented femoral component, similar techniques may be used; however, great care has to be taken to remain within the prosthetic-cement interface and not the bone-cement interface. As with any revision surgery, great care has to be taken not to sacrifice bone stock unnecessarily. Similar techniques may be used for the removal of the tibial component, although the Gigli saw is more difficult to apply. Excellent exposure of the tibia is needed for the removal of the tibial component.

Following implant removal, several specimens should be obtained for culture and sensitivity. We generally obtain samples from the capsule, the synovial lining, the membrane at the femoral, tibial, and patellar interfaces, as well as the medullary canals of the tibia and femur if applicable. All antibiotics should be withheld until adequate samples are obtained. These samples should be sent for aerobic and anaerobic cultures, as well as for mycobacterial and fungal cultures. A thorough synovectomy should then be performed. All devitalized tissue and all metal and polyethylene wear debris should be removed. The knee should then be copiously irrigated using several liters of an antibiotic-containing saline solution. At the end of the debridement and irrigation, the appearance of the knee joint should be not unlike that of a knee joint that is being revised for aseptic reasons.

Following the debridement, the knee is prepared for a revision knee replacement and very modest preliminary bone cuts are made removing minimal bone. The flexion and extension spaces are then measured, and the position of the joint line is estimated. A decision is then made on the required thickness of the femoral component and tibial components of the PROSTALAC implants. The minimum thickness of the femoral component is 12.5 mm, and this may be increased distally by 5, 10, or 15 mm. Likewise, the thickness of the tibial component is decided as well. While the knee is being prepared for reimplantation, an assistant then assembles the PROSTALAC molds (Fig. 62.2A,B,C) and manufactures the required implants. Each PROSTALAC component is custom-made, in the operating room, to suit the needs of each individual patient. The antibiotics are selected based on the sensitivity profile of the infecting organism, and on the criteria outlined by Murray.[63] In most cases, however, a combination of tobramycin and vancomycin are adequate. Based on studies on the long-term antibiotic concentrations within the joint following insertion of PROSTALAC implants,[46] we currently recommend the use of 3.6 grams of tobramycin and 1.0 gram of vancomycin. We do not recommend the use of vancomycin alone, because its elution properties, when used alone, are not as reliable as when used in combination with tobramycin. This has been demonstrated in both in vitro[42] and in vivo[46] studies. We also recommend the use of Palacos-R® (Smith and Nephew Richards, Memphis, Tennessee) bone cement because of its more favorable antibiotic elution characteristics.

The femoral component is manufactured as shown in Figure 62.2. The femoral skids are placed within their respective cavities in mold #1. Antibiotic-loaded Papacos-R® cement is then poured into the mold and the appropriate size mold #2 (not shown) is chosen to provide the required distal femoral thickness. Mold #2 is inserted

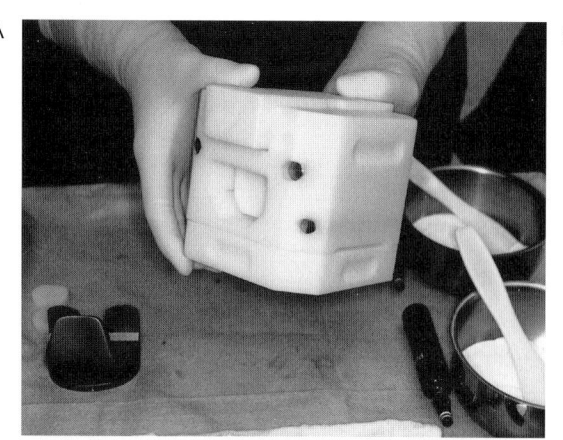

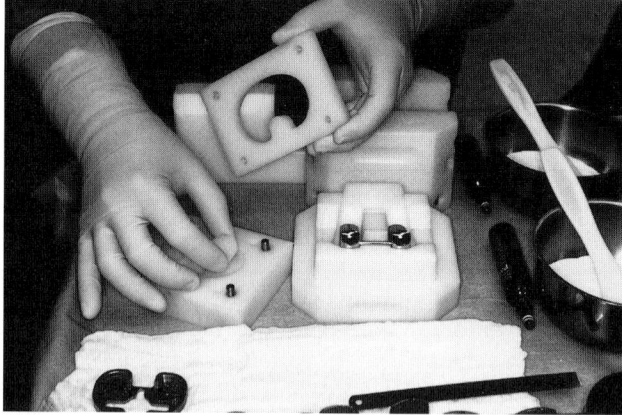

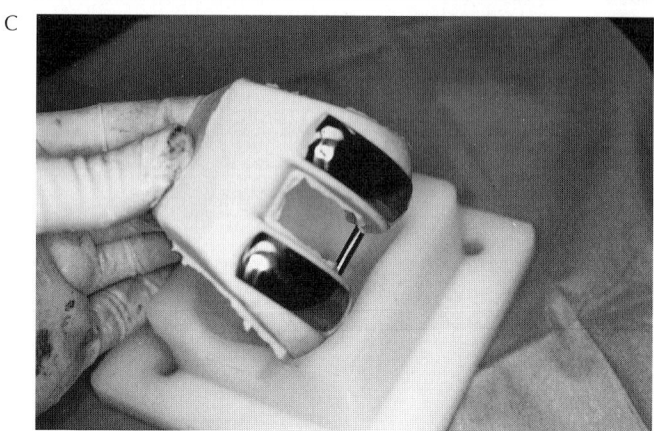

Figure 62.2. Because of the difficulties encountered with obtaining a smooth handmade spacer flexible polyethylene molds were used. Initial experience with a cement-on-cement articulation led to the use of metal runners on plastic skids. The current system uses a series of high-density polyethylene molds resulting in a more accurate facsimile of a knee prosthesis. (A) The femoral mold in its fully assembled state. (B) The tibial mold and femoral mold during the insertion of the metal runners and plastic skids. (C) Note the posterior stabilizer bar on the femoral component. The corresponding post on the tibial component is made of antibiotic-loaded cement. The femoral component is removed from the mold and excess cement is trimmed off.

within mold #1, and its thickness determines the final distal thickness of the PROSTALAC component.

The tibial component is manufactured in the operating room using a similar technique. The tibial skids are placed within their respective cavities within tibial mold #1 and antibiotic-loaded Palacos-R® cement is then poured into the mold. Mold #2 (not shown) is then used to obtain the appropriate thickness of the tibial component. The femoral and tibial components are then cemented to bone with antibiotic-loaded cement, when the cement is at a doughy stage of polymerization, so that fixation is obtained by interference fit and interdigitation without thorough intrusion into bone. This ensures ease of removal at the second-stage procedure without violating valuable bone stock. Bone cement is used to fill any bone defects that are not filled by the PROSTALAC implant. The patella is left unresurfaced; however, great care is taken to ensure appropriate rotation of the femoral and tibial components, and a lateral retinacular release is performed if needed. This minimizes the risk of patellar instability, which was a problem early in our experience with this system (Fig. 62.3).

Postoperatively, the patient is treated with a Jones bandage for 24 to 48 hours, and is then allowed to walk with partial weight-bearing. Free knee motion is allowed, without a brace, unless collateral insufficiency was detected intraoperatively. In this case, a hinged knee brace is used, but the hinges are unlocked to allow free mobility. The patient is then treated with a 3-week course of intravenous antibiotics. It is not our routine to measure minimum bactericidal levels, as suggested by Insall and associates[12] and Windsor and colleagues.[20] The patient is discharged from hospital as soon as possible, and antibiotic therapy is completed at home or at an outside facility. Oral antibiotics are continued for another 3 weeks. Physiotherapy is continued between stages, with an emphasis on range of motion and muscle strengthening.

Three months following the first stage, the patient is readmitted to our hospital for reimplantation. One week prior to reimplantation, the knee is aspirated to ensure negative cultures. In our experience, reimplantation is greatly facilitated by the presence of the PROSTALAC spacer. A rectus "snip"[67] is often required for exposure. A standard revision knee replacement is then performed. Removal of the PROSTALAC is easy and is accomplished in a few minutes. The cement is fractured with the use of an osteotome, and the fragmented components are then removed piecemeal. Following removal of the PROSTALAC, intraoperative cultures are

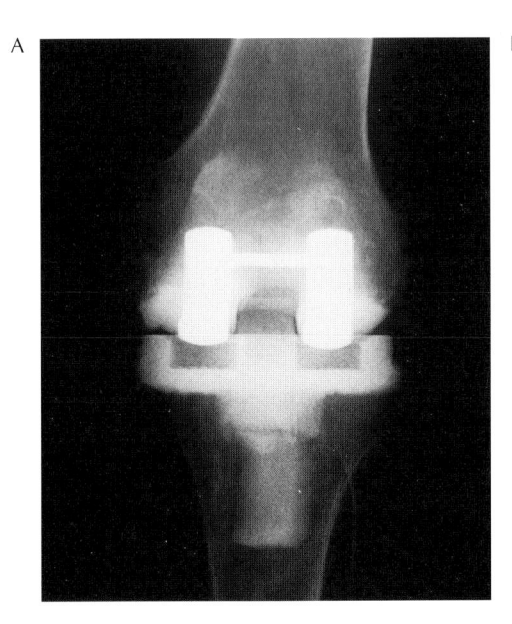

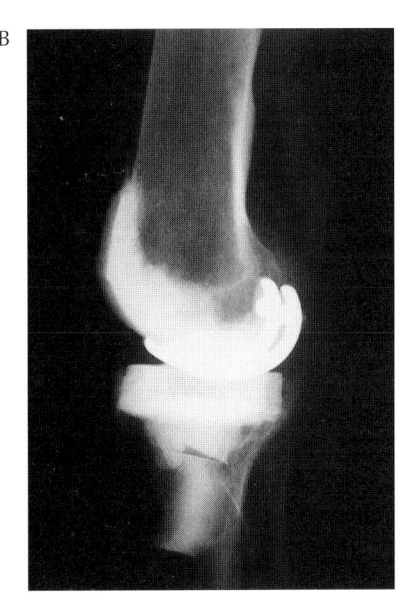

Figure 62.3. (A) The anteroposterior and (B) lateral radiographs illustrate the latest version of the knee PROSTALAC system.

obtained and prophylactic antibiotics are then administered. A thorough debridement and irrigation are performed, and the revision components are implanted. Antibiotic-loaded bone cement is used for the fixation of the components. If tobramycin is an appropriate antibiotic, we use 1.2 grams of tobramycin per package of bone cement. If the infecting organism is not sensitive to tobramycin, another appropriate antibiotic is chosen. Regardless of the type of antibiotic, we prefer not to exceed 1 to 1.2 grams of antibiotic per 40-gram package of bone cement, because of the risk of cement weakening. Intravenous antibiotics are continued for a minimum of 5 days postoperatively, and are discontinued when the final results of intraoperative cultures are reported as negative.

Clinical Results

A total of 44 patients were admitted with a diagnosis of an infected total knee arthroplasty between April 1987 and June 1994. Nine patients were excluded from this series (Table 62.2) for a variety of reasons that made reconstruction using the PROSTALAC system not feasible. An above knee amputation was used in one patient because of severe bone and soft tissue loss, with loss of the extensor mechanism. A knee arthrodesis was performed in two patients in whom knee joint salvage was not technically feasible. One patient had bone and soft tissue loss that was so severe that reconstruction with the first generation PROSTALAC implant was not possible; therefore, a block and bead antibiotic-loaded cement spacer was used between stages. This could likely have been reconstructed with the posterior-stabilized PROSTALAC, but it was not available at that time. Two patients underwent a two-stage exchange procedure using a block and bead antibiotic-loaded cement spacer between stages before the PROSTALAC system became our routine. Another patient underwent an uncomplicated first-stage replacement with the PROSTALAC prosthesis; however, while awaiting reimplantation, the patient died of unrelated causes, and was therefore not included in the final analysis. One patient was a 26-year-old patient with severe juvenile rheumatoid arthritis who had just undergone a revision knee arthroplasty using a custom long-stem femoral component. The femoral component was rigidly fixed, and removal of this prosthesis would have compromised bone stock. We elected to treat this patient with the unusual combination of debridement, retention of the femoral component, and removal of the tibial component and replacement with a highly antibiotic-loaded cement spacer with a thin polyethylene articular surface. This was subsequently revised as a pre-planned second stage procedure. Thus far, 4 years following surgery, there is no evidence of recurrent infection. The last patient who was

Table 62.2. These procedures were used as treatment of the infected knee replacement in eight of the nine patients who were excluded from this series. The ninth patient died between stages and was also excluded.

Procedure	Number of cases
Above knee amputation	1
Knee arthrodesis	2
Two-stage exchange arthroplasty with an antibiotic-loaded cement spacer	3
Debridement and irrigation	1
Two-stage debridement with retention of at least one component	1

not thought to be a candidate for two-stage exchange arthroplasty using the PROSTALAC system was a 76-year-old patient with severe rheumatoid arthritis and a polyarticular deep infection affecting one knee, one hip, and one elbow. Because of frail health and polyarticular involvement, he was treated with debridement, irrigation, and suppressive antibiotics. This patient died 2 years later of unrelated causes.

In addition to the remaining 35 patients with infected knee replacements, one patient with bilateral long-standing deep infections affecting both knee joints was included in this series. This was a 38-year-old with a history of chronic renal failure and previous renal transplantation. He had end-stage osteonecrosis of both femoral condyles and the right femoral head secondary to corticosteroids. He also had multifocal mycoplasma septic arthritis affecting both knees and shoulders. In preparation for an eventual bilateral knee replacements, he was treated with the PROSTALAC knee system as if he had had an infected total knee arthroplasty because of the chronicity of the infection (over 2 years) and because of end-stage degeneration.

A total of 36 patients with 37 infected knees, and a minimum 2-year follow-up are included in this series. There were 17 males and 20 females. Twenty-two left knees and 15 right knees were affected. The mean age was 66.2 (range 26 to 83). All of these patients completed a two-stage exchange knee arthroplasty protocol using the PROSTALAC knee prosthesis as a temporary antibiotic-loaded functional spacer. In seven knees, the PROSTALAC component was a handmade facsimile of a total knee prosthesis with a cement-on-cement articular surface. In three patients a first-generation cement-on-cement molded PROSTALAC implant was used. The first-generation low-friction PROSTALAC prosthesis was used in 14 patients. The second-generation posterior cruciate-substituting PROSTALAC knee design was used in 13 patients in this series. There were no deaths directly related to the procedure; however, two patients (three knees) died of unrelated causes between 2.5 and 7 years following surgery.

The underlying diagnosis was osteoarthritis in 26, rheumatoid arthritis in four, post-traumatic arthritis in two, osteonecrosis in three, hemophilic arthropathy in one, and neuropathic arthropathy in one. Twelve patients (13 knees) were immunocompromised, or at a high risk of infection. Four patients had rheumatoid arthritis, and one of whom was still on corticosteroid therapy, one was treated with chemotherapy for chronic lymphocytic leukemia, one patient (two knees) was on chronic immunosuppressive therapy for a renal transplant, one patient was infected with the human immunodeficiency virus, three were diabetic, one had chronic lymphedema and recurrent cellulitis affecting the ipsilateral lower extremity, and one patient had renal calculi with recurrent urinary tract infections. The mean number of previous procedures was 2.4 (range 0 to 8). One patient (two knees) had undergone no previous procedures. These procedures included nine patients who had already undergone a debridement and irrigation for infection without success. One of these patients had undergone two debridements without success. One patient had undergone excision arthroplasty and insertion of an antibiotic-loaded cement spacer, without resolution of the infection.

Only two patients had an erythrocyte sedimentation rate (ESR) less than 20. The mean ESR was 57 (range 1 to 126). The infecting organisms were known in all but five cases (86%). In each of the five cases in which no organisms were cultured, the patient was on long-term oral antibiotics at the time of presentation, and intraoperative findings at the time of removal of the infected components revealed definite evidence of infection such as gross pus or a draining sinus. There were four cases of mixed infection, and 27 cases (26 patients) of isolated infection. In each of the cases of mixed infection, *Staphylococcus epidermidis* was one of the infecting organisms. Overall, *Staphylococcus epidermidis* was the most common organism, and was isolated in 18 cultures overall. *Staphylococcus aureus* was isolated in eight cases. *Mycoplasma*, *Peptostreptococcus*, and coagulase-negative *Staphylococcus* other than *S. epidermidis* were isolated from two knees each. *Bacillus*, *Streptococcus*, *Serratia*, *Enterococcus*, *Escherichia coli*, and *Mycobacterium tuberculosis* were isolated once each.

Each patient had implanted the prosthesis of antibiotic-loaded acrylic cement (PROSTALAC) during the first stage of a two-stage exchange protocol. In each patient, the antibiotics used in the bone cement were customized based on the sensitivity profile of the infecting organisms. If no organism was isolated, a combination of tobramycin and vancomycin was used. Tobramycin and vancomycin were used in combination in 27 cases, and tobramycin in isolation was used in three. Vancomycin alone was used in four cases. Penicillin G was used in three cases, but never in isolation. In two cases it was combined with tobramycin and in one it was combined with both tobramycin and vancomycin. The amount of antibiotic added to each packet of cement varied between 2.4 and 4.8 grams for tobramycin, 1.0 and 2.0 grams for vancomycin and 5 and 10 million units for penicillin G. Early in our experience, we used Simplex P® bone cement (Howmedica Inc., Rutherford, New Jersey). In the latest nine cases in this series, we used Palacos R® bone cement (Smith and Nephew, Richards, Memphis, Tennessee) because of its better antibiotic elution profile. The mean delay between the two stages was 94 days (range 25 to 234), following which reimplantation was performed. While awaiting reimplantation, each patient was treated with a 3-week course of intravenous antibiotics, followed by oral antibiotics for a minimum of another 3 weeks. All cases were discharged from our hospital prior to the second-stage procedure.

During the course of two-stage exchange arthroplasty, the following additional procedures were required. At first stage, a skin rotation flap and a medial gastrocnemius flap were required for soft tissue coverage in one and two patients, respectively. Repair of a ruptured patellar tendon was required in one patient. At second stage, proximal and distal extensor mechanism realignment was required in one patient and an extensive proximal extensor mechanism realignment was required in nine patients.

Pain Relief

Relief of pain between stages with the use of the PROSTALAC prosthesis was the main advantage of this approach compared with a standard excision arthroplasty. In most cases, there was complete relief of pain following surgery. In the early cases, particularly in those cases in which a low-friction bearing surface was not used, there was mild to moderate residual pain in 5 of 10 knees. This pain was associated with a grating sensation and crepitus with knee movement. Because of this significant incidence of pain, the design of the implant was modified by adding a low-friction articular surface. Only one of the patients who received the modified implant complained of persistent pain. The reason for persistent pain was severe heterotopic ossification in the anteromedial soft tissues (see the section about knee score).

Range of Motion

With the PROSTALAC prosthesis in situ, knee mobility was maintained in the majority of cases. There was no substantial change in range of motion following implantation of PROSTALAC implants when compared with the preoperative range of motion (mean range of motion of 8 to 70 degrees prior to PROSTALAC compared with 8 to 72 degrees following the PROSTALAC). Range of motion following final reimplantation of a definitive total knee replacement prosthesis was improved with a mean gain of 21 degrees in flexion and a 3-degree decrease in flexion deformity. The mean range of motion at final evaluation was 5 to 91 degrees.

Knee Stability

Ligamentous laxity was a common finding in our patients at initial presentation. There was significant ligamentous laxity in 15 of 37 knees. This was due to either failure of the implant with subsequent bone deficiency, or previous excision arthroplasty. Two of these patients had instability so severe that immobilization in a cast was required while the patient was awaiting surgery. Following excision arthroplasty and replacement with the PROSTALAC implant, ligamentous laxity was detected on physical examination in 14 patients; however, this was considered severe in only seven. Instability was marked in only one of the 13 patients who received a posterior-stabilized PROSTALAC. Two of these patients required cast immobilization following implantation of the PROSTALAC prosthesis because of significant tibiofemoral instability. Another patient was immobilized in a cylinder cast prophylactically so that unprotected activity would not cause fragmentation and mechanical failure of the PROSTALAC implant. In this patient, the PROSTALAC implant was used simply as a spacer to maintain the soft tissues out to length and to facilitate revision arthroplasty at the second stage. Another patient required a knee brace between stages because of intraoperative rupture of the extensor mechanism and severe bone loss leading to significant instability. Because of severe bone loss, a hinged implant (Kinematic Rotating Hinge, Howmedica, Rutherford, New Jersey) was used for the final reconstruction at second stage. Postoperatively, he was mobilized with a hinged knee brace. This is the only patient who was using a brace at final review. The only patient with a posterior-stabilized PROSTALAC who required bracing between stages had severe collateral ligament deficiency that could not be controlled with a posterior-stabilized design. A hinged knee brace was used between stages with good success.

Extensor Lag

The mean extensor lag at the time of presentation was 10 degrees (range 0 to 35 degrees). Following excision arthroplasty and replacement with the PROSTALAC prosthesis, the mean extensor lag was unchanged at a mean of 12 degrees (range 0 to 35 degrees). At final review, the mean extensor lag was reduced to 4 degrees (range 0 to 30 degrees), with only one patient with an extensor lag greater than 10 degrees. The one patient with a final extensor lag of 30 degrees was the 62-year-old man with severe rheumatoid arthritis who suffered a rupture of his extensor mechanism at the time of insertion of the PROSTALAC implant. This was the only complication involving disruption of the extensor mechanism. Despite this complication, the final extensor lag was no worse than the preoperative extensor lag of 35 degrees.

Patellar Instability

Maltracking of the patella was encountered in 13 knees in this series (35%). Following insertion of the PROSTALAC prosthesis, there were two complete dislocations of the patella (8%). Patellar dislocation produced a significant decrease in the Hospital for Special Surgery (HSS) knee score following insertion of the PROSTALAC implant (16 points and 18 points in these two patients). This decline in HSS knee score was due to anterior knee pain, quadriceps weakness, and extensor lag. At the second stage, one patient was treated with proximal extensor mechanism realignment with chronic lateral subluxation of the patella and a final HSS knee score of 85, and the other required a tibial tubercle osteotomy and proximal realignment, which resulted in a stable, pain free patella with a final HSS knee score of 89.

There was persistent, yet asymptomatic lateral subluxation of the patella in eight knees (22%) following insertion of the PROSTALAC implant. In all of these patients, the HSS score following implantation of the PROSTALAC prosthesis was improved compared with the preoperative HSS score. At final reconstruction, the patella was stable in all but one of these patients, and all required proximal extensor mechanism realignment. Distal extensor mechanism realignment was not performed in any of these patients. The one patient with persistent subluxation had some anterior knee pain and had an HSS knee score of 76. Patellar instability was not a problem in the patients in whom a posterior-stabilized PROSTALAC design was used.

Knee Score

All patients were evaluated using the Hospital for Special Surgery (HSS) knee score at the time of initial presentation, prior to removal of the PROSTALAC prosthesis, and at final follow-up. The mean HSS knee score at initial presentation was 41 (range 11 to 76). Following excision arthroplasty and replacement with the temporary PROSTALAC spacer, the mean HSS score increased to 55 (range 18 to 87). At final review, the mean HSS knee score was improved to 81 (range 46 to 95). Following insertion of the PROSTALAC prosthesis, there was a significant decline in the HSS knee score in five patients. Two of these patients had a fixed dislocation of the patella, and have already been discussed. Another patient had an 8-point decline in the HSS score following insertion of the PROSTALAC implant. This was the patient who suffered an avulsion of his extensor mechanism at the time of insertion of the PROSTALAC implant. In another patient, there was a 24-point decline in the HSS knee score due to severe heterotopic ossification on the anteromedial aspect of the knee causing significant pain and stiffness. This patient was treated with radiation therapy (single dose of 700 rads) prior to the second-stage procedure. At that time, a lateral parapatellar approach was required because of the severity of the heterotopic ossification within the medial soft tissue structures. At final review, the pain had resolved and the patient achieved a range of motion of 0 to 85 degrees.

His final HSS knee score has improved from 18 to 85. The last patient who had a decline in the HSS knee score following implantation of the PROSTALAC prosthesis had been immobilized in a cylinder cast prophylactically because of severe neuropathic arthropathy.

Summary of Complications

As previously discussed, the following complications were encountered (Table 62.3). *Persistent pain* due to the high-friction articular surface was noted in five patients. This problem was readily corrected by adding a low-friction bearing surface. *Tibiofemoral instability* was seen in 14 patients. However, this was mild and caused no symptoms in the majority of patients (11 of 14) patients. Symptomatic posterior subluxation of the tibia secondary to loss of the posterior cruciate ligament was encountered in two patients. This problem was addressed by modifying the PROSTALAC implant to a more constrained design with a tibial post and a femoral cam as a substitute for the deficient posterior cruciate ligament. *Rupture of the patellar tendon* was seen in one patient. *Patellar instability* was a major complication in this series. Two patients suffered from a fixed lateral dislocation of the patella, which compromised the short-term outcome following insertion of the PROSTALAC implant, although it did not affect the final outcome. One of these two patients had a stable patella at final review, whereas one had an asymptomatic yet chronically subluxed patella at final evaluation. Eight patients suffered from asymptomatic lateral subluxation of the patella following insertion of the PROSTALAC prosthesis. At final review, the patella was stable in all but one of these patients who had persistent, slightly symptomatic subluxation of the patella. The unusual complication of *heterotopic ossification* was encountered in two patients. In one patient, the outcome following insertion of the PROSTALAC was compromised because of pain and stiffness; however, the final outcome was not compromised. This patient was treated with single dose radia-

Table 62.3. These complications were encountered in this series of 36 patients

Complication	Number of patients
Pain with the PROSTALAC in situ	5
Tibiofemoral instability	3
Rupture of the patellar tendon	1
Patellar subluxation with the PROSTALAC in situ	8
Patellar dislocation with the PROSTALAC in situ	2
Patellar instability at final review	2
Heterotopic ossification	2
Intraoperative fracture	1
Recurrent infection	2

tion therapy prior to the second stage. One complication that has not already been mentioned is *an intraoperative fracture of the femur* during removal of the cement from the medullary canal of the femur during the first-stage procedure. The fracture was unicortical in nature, and was stabilized using three 2.0 mm stainless steel cable. The patient was mobilized postoperatively with minimal weight-bearing. The fracture healed without any further complications. The final complication was *failure of the tibial component* in one patient who received a rotating hinge constrained revision total knee replacement prosthesis. He presented 18 months following final reconstruction with dissociation of the tibial component. He underwent a second revision total knee arthroplasty without any complications. At the time of revision surgery, there was no evidence of infection and all intraoperative cultures were negative.

Recurrent Infection

Infection recurred in four patients in this series, for an infection cure rate of 89% at a mean follow-up of 4.1 years. In all patients with recurrence of infection, at least one of the infecting organisms was different from the original infecting organism. In one, the original infection was caused by *Staphylococcus epidermidis*, and the second infection was caused by *Streptococcus agalactiae*. The recurrent infection in the second patient was caused by *Staphylococcus epidermidis* and *Enterococcus sp*. The initial infection was caused by *Staphylococcus epidermidis*. The third recurrence was caused by *Staphylococcus aureus*, whereas the initial infection was caused by *Staphylococcus epidermidis*. The final recurrence was in a patient in whom the initial and recurrent infections were caused by *Staphylococcus epidermidis*. Assuming that the second and fourth patients had a recurrence of the original infection, because *Staphylococcus epidermidis* was cultured on both occasions, the infection recurrence rate would be 5.4%, and the reinfection rate would be 5.4%, for an overall failure rate of 10.8%, which is comparable to the overall failure rate of two-stage exchange arthroplasty as summarized in Table 61.1.

Advantages of the PROSTALAC System

The advantages of mobility between stages are clear. The patient is more functional, can be discharged from hospital, and generally has a better outlook than one treated without a mobile spacer between stages. The reimplantation is much easier because of the presence of the spacer, which stabilizes the soft tissues and preserves the joint cavity. A common criticism of this approach is that it is similar to a one-stage exchange arthroplasty, so why not attempt a one-stage exchange for infected total knee replacements?

The literature to date is clear on the disadvantages of one-stage exchange. This has already been outlined in this and the previous chapters. Moreover, Scott and associates,[62] using an ordinary prosthesis as a spacer and antibiotic-loaded cement beads as an antibiotic depot in a two-stage exchange protocol, clearly showed the advantages of the modified two-stage protocol. The only studies, to date, that have shown favorable results with one-stage exchange arthroplasty have done so only in gram-positive infections.[16,17] For these reasons, one-stage exchange arthroplasty cannot, at the present time, be considered acceptable treatment for all infected total knee replacement.

Another criticism of the PROSTALAC and other articulated spacer techniques is the retention of foreign material within the joint, despite infection. Based on the various reports of articulated spacers, and based on our experience, it is clear that as long as antibiotic-loaded bone cement is used with these articulated spacers, there does not seem to be any adverse effect to the use of small amounts of metal and plastic, in addition to antibiotic-loaded bone cement.

Antibiotic Elution from the PROSTALAC System

One of the advantages of articulated spacers in general, and the PROSTALAC system in particular, is the ability to add large amounts of antibiotic powder to bone cement, without the fear of weakening the cement, because structural integrity of the cement becomes less important when these spacers are used for only a short period of time. This, in theory, should increase the levels and duration of antibiotic elution.

The early elution of antibiotics from bone cement is well documented in the literature, and has already been discussed earlier in this chapter (see section entitled Properties of Antibiotic-Loaded Bone Cement). The long-term elution of antibiotics, however, is not as well documented in the literature. In an effort to address this deficiency, we measured the joint fluid levels of tobramycin and vancomycin in a series of 49 patients in whom the PROSTALAC system was used for the treatment of infected hip and knee replacements.[46] There was no statistically significant difference in the elution profiles of hip and knee PROSTALAC prostheses. The best long-term antibiotic levels were obtained when a combination of at least 3.6 grams of tobramycin and 1.0 gram of vancomycin were added to a 40-gram package of bone cement. At an average delay of 4 months between stages, the mean intra-articular tobramycin concentration was 9.12 mg/L, and the mean intra-articular vancomycin concentration was 2.53 mg/L. We also found that the elution of vancomycin was improved when a higher dose of tobramycin was combined with vancomycin in bone cement. This was also seen in in vitro studies by Penner and colleagues.[42] Based on these results, we recommend the use of at least 3.6 grams of tobramycin in spacers used between stages in the treatment of the infected knee replacement. We also do not recommend the use of vancomycin by itself, instead it should be combined with tobramycin. We have no data on combining vancomycin with other antibiotics; however, the combination of tobramycin and vancomycin should be effective for most periprosthetic infections. Furthermore, based on our long-term antibiotic elution studies, we were unable to detect a statistically significant effect on tobramycin elution by the addition of vancomycin; therefore, tobramycin alone may be used in gram-negative infections, provided a dose of at least 3.6 grams are added to each package of bone cement.

The higher doses of antibiotics that can be added to interim spacers in two-stage exchange arthroplasty are another factor that distinguishes two-stage from one-stage exchange arthroplasty. In one-stage exchange arthroplasty, in which bone cement is used for the permanent fixation of the definitive implant, it is unwise to use such high amounts of antibiotics in the bone cement because of the risk of weakening of the cement.

In conclusion, based on a review of the current literature, the safest approach for the treatment of the chronically infected knee replacement is two-stage exchange arthroplasty. The addition of small amounts of metal and plastic, in addition to antibiotic-loaded bone cement in interim spacers, as in the PROSTALAC system, does not seem to have an adverse effect on infection cure rates, and has the advantage of improved function between stages. Although on the surface it appears that the PROSTALAC system, and other articulated spacers resemble a one-stage exchange, there are vast differences. With the use of the PROSTALAC system, a second debridement is possible at the time of reimplantation, and the amount of antibiotic that is added to bone cement may vastly exceed the safe limits that have to be adhered to in one-stage exchange arthroplasty.

References

1. Gunston FH. Polycentric knee arthroplasty. Prosthetic simulation of normal knee movement. *J Bone Joint Surg Br.* 1971; 53:272.
2. Ranawat CS, Flynn WF, Saddler S, Hansraj KK, Maynard MJ. Long-term results of the total condylar knee arthroplasty. *Clin Orthop.* 1993; 286:94.
3. Sculco TP. The economic impact of infected total joint arthroplasty. In: Heckman JD, ed. *American Academy of Orthopaedic Surgeons, Instr Course Lect Vol. 42.* Rosemont: American Academy of Orthopaedic Surgeons; 1993:349–351.
4. Masri BA, Kendall RW, Duncan CP, Beauchamp CP, McGraw RW. Two-stage exchange arthroplasty using a functional antibiotic-loaded spacer in the treatment of the infected knee replacement: the Vancouver experience. *Sem Arthroplasty.* 1994; 5:122.
5. Buchholz HW, Engelbrecht H. Über die Depotwirkung einiger Antibiotica bei Vermischung mit dem Kunstharz Palacos. *Chirurg* 1970; 41:511.
6. Buchholz HW, Elson RA, Engelbrecht E, Lodenkämper H, Röttger J, Siegel A. Management of deep infection of total hip arthroplasty. *J Bone Joint Surg Br.* 1981; 63:342.
7. Deburge A, GUEPAR. Guepar hinge prosthesis: complications and results with two years' follow-up. *Clin Orthop.* 1976; 120:47.
8. Vanhegan JAD, Dabrowski W, Arden GP. A review of 100 Attenborough stabilised gliding knee prostheses. *J Bone Joint Surg Br.* 1979; 61:445.
9. Hovelius L, Josefsson G. An alternative method for exchange operation of infected arthroplasty. *Acta Orthop Scand.* 1979; 50:93.
10. Woods GW, Lionberger DR, Tullos HS. Failed total knee arthroplasty: revision and arthrodesis for infection and noninfectious complications. *Clin Orthop.* 1983; 173:184.
11. Rand JA, Bryan RS. Reimplantation for the salvage of an infected total knee arthroplasty. *J Bone Joint Surg Am.* 1983; 65:1081.
12. Insall JN, Thompson FM, Brause BD. Two-stage reimplantation for the salvage of infected total knee arthroplasty. *J Bone Joint Surg Am.* 1983; 65:1087.
13. Coonse K, Adams JD. A new operative approach to the knee joint. *Surg Gynecol Obstet.* 1943; 77:344.
14. Bengtson S, Knutson K, Lidgren L. Revision of infected knee arthroplasty. *Acta Orthop Scand.* 1986; 57:489–494.
15. Borden LS, Gearen PF. Infected total knee arthroplasty, a protocol for management. *J Arthroplasty.* 1987; 2:27.
16. Freeman MAR, Sudlow RA, Casewell MW, Radcliff SS. The management of infected total knee replacements. *J Bone Joint Surg Br.* 1985; 67:764.
17. Göksan SB, Freeman MA. One-stage reimplantation for infected total knee arthroplasty. *J Bone Joint Surg Br.* 1992; 74:78.
18. Insall JN. Infection of total knee arthroplasty. In: Anderson LD, ed. *American Academy of Orthopaedic Surgeons, Instr Course Lecture, Vol. 35.* St. Louis: Mosby; 1986:319–324.
19. Rosenberg AG, Haas B, Barden R, Marquez D, Landon GC, Galante JO. Salvage of infected total knee arthroplasty. *Clin Orthop.* 1988; 226:29.
20. Windsor RE, Insall JN, Urs WR, Miller DV, Brause BD. Two-stage reimplantation for the salvage of total knee arthroplasty complicated by infection: further follow-up and refinement of indications. *J Bone Joint Surg Am.* 1990; 72:272.
21. Teeny SM, Dorr L, Murata G, Conaty P. Treatment of infected total knee arthroplasty: irrigation and debridement versus two-stage reimplantation. *J Arthroplasty.* 1990; 5:35.
22. Whiteside L. Treatment of infected total knee arthroplasty. *Clin Orthop.* 1994; 299:169–172.
23. Hanssen AD, Rand JA, Osmon DR. Treatment of the infected total knee arthroplasty with insertion of another prosthesis: the effect of antibiotic-impregnated bone cement. *Clin Orthop.* 1994; 309:44.
24. Nelson CL, Evans RP, Blaha JD, Calhoun J, Henry SL, Patzakis MJ. A comparison of gentamicin-impregnated

polymethylmethacrylate bead implantation to conventional parenteral antibiotic therapy in infected total hip and knee arthroplasty. *Clin Orthop.* 1993; 295:96.
25. Adams KA, Couch L, Cierny G, Calhoun J, Mader MT. In vitro and in vivo evaluation of antibiotic diffusion from antibiotic-impregnated polymethylmethacrylate beads. *Clin Orthop.* 1992; 278:244.
26. Baker AS, Greenham LW. Release of gentamicin from acrylic bone cement. *J Bone Joint Surg Am.* 1988; 70:1551.
27. Bayston R, Milner RDG. The sustained release of antimicrobial drugs from bone cement. *J Bone Joint Surg Br.* 1982; 64:460.
28. Chapman MW, Hadley WK. The effect of polymethylmethacrylate and antibiotic combinations on bacterial viability: an in vitro and preliminary in vivo study. *J Bone Joint Surg Am.* 1976; 58:76.
29. DiMaio FR, O'Halloran JJ, Quale JM. In vitro elution of ciprofloxacin from polymethylmethacrylate cement beads. *J Orthop Res.* 1994; 12:79.
30. Elson RA, Jephcott AE, McGechie DB, Verettas D. Antibiotic-loaded acrylic cement. *J Bone Joint Surg Br.* 1977; 59:200.
31. Goodell JA, Flick AB, Herbert JC, Howe JG. Preparation and release characteristics of tobramycin-impregnated polymethylmethacrylate beads. *Am J Hosp Pharm.* 1986; 43: 1454.
32. Hill J, Klenerman L, Trustey S, Blowers R. Diffusion of antibiotics from acrylic bone-cement in vitro. *J Bone Joint Surg Br.* 1977; 59:197.
33. Hoff SF, Fitzgerald RH Jr, Kelly PJ. The depot administration of penicillin G and gentamicin in acrylic bone cement. *J Bone Joint Surg Am.* 1981; 63:798.
34. Kirkpatrick DK, Trachenberg LS, Mangino PD, Von Fraunhofer JA, Seligson D. In vitro characteristics of tobramycin-PMMA beads, compressive strength and leaching. *Orthopedics.* 1985; 8:1130.
35. Kuechle DK, Landon GC, Musher DM, Noble PC. Elution of vancomycin, daptomycin, and amikacin from acrylic bone cement. *Clin Orthop.* 1991; 264:302.
36. Lawson KJ, Marks KE, Brems J, Rehm S. Vancomycin and tobramycin elution from polymethylmethacrylate: an in vitro study. *Orthopedics.* 1990; 13:521.
37. Seyral P, Zannier A, Argenson JN, Raoult D. The release in vitro of vancomycin and tobramycin from acrylic bone cement. *J Antimicrob Chemotherapy.* 1994; 33:337.
38. Wahlig H, Dingeldein E. Antibiotics and bone cement. *Acta Orthop Scandinavica.* 1980; 5:49.
39. Brien WW, Salvati EA, Klein R, Brause B, Stern S. Antibiotic impregnated bone cement in total hip arthroplasty. An in vivo comparison of the elution properties of tobramycin and vancomycin. *Clin Orthop.* 1993; 296:242.
40. Bunetel L, Segui A, Langlais F, Cormier M. Osseous concentrations of gentamicin after implantation of acrylic bone cement in sheep femora. *Eur J Drug Metab Pharmacokinet.* 1994; 19:99.
41. Marks KE, Nelson CL, Lautenschlager EP. Antibiotic-impregnated acrylic bone cement. *J Bone Joint Surg Am.* 1976; 58:358.
42. Penner MJ, Masri BA, Duncan CP. Elution characteristics of vancomycin and tobramycin combined in acrylic bone cement. Submitted for publication, 1995.
43. Wahlig H, Dingeldein E, Buchholz HW, Buchholz M, Bachmann F. Pharmacokinetic study of gentamicin-loaded cement in total hip replacements: comparative effects of varying dosage. *J Bone Joint Surg Br.* 1984; 66:175.
44. Salvati EA, Callaghan JJ, Brause BD, Klein RF, Small RD. Reimplantation in infection: elution of gentamicin from cement and beads. *Clin Orthop.* 1986; 207:83.
45. Masri BA, Duncan CP, Beauchamp CP, Paris NJ, Arntorp J. Tobramycin and vancomycin elution from bone cement. An in vitro and in vivo study. *Orthop Trans.* 1994; 18:130.
46. Masri B, Duncan CP, Beauchamp CP. Long-term elution of antibiotics from bone cement: an in vivo study using the PROSTALAC system. Presented at the fiftieth annual meeting of the Canadian Orthopaedic Association, Halifax, Nova Scotia, Canada. June 1995.
47. Duncan CP, Beauchamp CP. A temporary antibiotic-loaded joint replacement system for management of complex infections involving the hip. *Orthop Clin North Am.* 1993; 24:751.
48. Kendall RW, Masri BA, Duncan CP, Beauchamp CP, McGraw RW, Bora B. Temporary antibiotic loaded acrylic hip replacement: a novel method for management of the infected THA. *Sem Arthroplasty.* 1994; 5:171.
49. Abendschein W. Arthroplasty Rounds. Salvage of infected total hip replacement: use of antibiotic/PMMA spacer. *Orthopedics.* 1992; 15:228.
50. Bargar WL, Martin RB, deJesus R, Madison MTI. The addition of tobramycin to contrast bone cement. *J Arthroplasty.* 1986; 1:165.
51. Lautenschlager EP, Jacobs JJ, Marshall GW, Meyer PR Jr. Mechanical properties of bone cements containing large doses of antibiotic powder. *J Biomed Mater Res.* 1976; 10:929.
52. Lautenschlager EP, Marshall GW, Marks KE, Schwartz J, Nelson CL. Mechanical strength of acrylic bone cements impregnated with antibiotics. *J Biomed Mater Res.* 1976; 10:837.
53. Davies JP, O'Connor DO, Burke DW, Harris WH. Influence of antibiotic impregnation on the fatigue life of Simplex P and Palacos R acrylic bone cements, with and without centrifugation. *J Biomed Mater Res.* 1989; 23:379.
54. Gristina AG, Costerton JW. Bacterial bioadherence to biomaterials and tissue. The significance of its role in clinical sepsis. *J Bone Joint Surg Am.* 1985; 67:264.
55. Gristina AG, Shibata Y, Giridhar G, Kreger A, Myrvik QN. The glycocalyx, biofilm, microbes, and resistant infection. *Sem Arthroplasty.* 1994; 5:160.
56. Oga M, Arizono T, Sugioka Y. Inhibition of bacterial adhesion by tobramycin-impregnated PMAM bone cement. *Acta Orthop Scand.* 1992; 63:301.
57. Dall L, Keilhofner M, Herndon B, Barnes W, Lane J. Clindamycin effect on glycocalyx production in experimental viridans streptococcal endocarditis. *J Inf Dis.* 1990; 161: 1221.
58. Cohen JC, Hozack WJ, Cuckler JM, Booth RE. Two-stage reimplantation of septic total knee arthroplasty: report of three cases using an antibiotic-PMMA spacer block. *J Arthroplasty.* 1988; 3:369.
59. Wilde AH, Ruth JT. Two-stage reimplantation in infected total knee arthroplasty. *Clin Orthop.* 1988; 236:23.

60. Booth Jr. RE, Lotke P. The results of spacer block technique in revision of infected total knee arthroplasty. *Clin Orthop*. 1989; 248:57.
61. Duncan CP, Beauchamp CP, Masri B, McGraw RW, Paris N, Breault M. The antibiotic loaded joint replacement system, a novel approach to the management of the infected knee replacement. *J Bone Joint Surg Br*. 1992; 74(Suppl III):296.
62. Scott IR, Stockley I, Getty CJM. Exchange arthroplasty for infected knee replacements. A new method. *J Bone Joint Surg Br*. 1993; 74:28.
63. Murray WR. Use of antibiotic-containing bone cement. *Clin Orthop*. 1984; 190:89.
64. Kane K, Plaster R, Tkach T, Camargo M, Hoffmann A. Treatment of Infected total knee replacement arthroplasty using an articulated spacer. *Clin Orthop*. 1995:321:45–54.
65. Cadambi A, Jones RE, Maale GE. A protocol for staged revision of infected total hip and knee arthroplasties: the use of antibiotic-cement-implant composites. *Orthopaedics* (Int. Edition). 1995; 3:133.
66. McPherson EJ, Lewonowski K, Dorr LD. Use of an articulated PMMA spacer in the infected total knee arthroplasty. *J Arthroplasty*. 1995; 10:87.
67. Insall JN. Surgical techniques and instrumentation in total knee arthroplasty. In: Insall JN, Windsor RE, Scott WN, Kelly MA, Aglietti P, eds. *Surgery of the Knee*. 2nd ed. New York: Churchill Livingstone; 1993:739–804.

CHAPTER 63
Alternative Procedures for the Management of an Infected Total Knee

Aaron G. Rosenberg and Richard A. Berger

INTRODUCTION

Many risk factors have been identified that contribute to infection. Deep infection occurs more frequently in patients with rheumatoid arthritis, prior operations, prior knee infection, revision procedures, hinged arthroplasty, and diabetes mellitus. Furthermore, the immune status of the patient, the operating room environment and operative technique, and the use of prophylactic antibiotics all influence the development of infection. However, in spite of the knowledge of risk factors, infection will develop. The prevalence of deep infection has ranged from 0.5% after primary procedures in healthy patients to 16% after hinged arthroplasty. In modern series, the prevalence of deep infection has ranged from 1.2 to 5%.

The prime objective of treatment for an infected total knee replacement is eradication of the infection. Operative debridement is the single most important treatment for an infected knee prosthesis. Eradication of the infection is always the single most important objective. In addition, preservation of the limb and maintenance of a functional extremity are also important. Although every effort should be made to salvage the knee, death from sepsis secondary to an infected arthroplasty can and does occur.

After the infection is treated, reimplantation usually gives the best results. However, reimplantation requires good soft tissue, good bone stock, and a susceptible microorganism. The previous two chapters have covered reimplantation in depth. This chapter explores the options when reimplantation is not possible. In this event five options are available for managing the infected total knee arthroplasty. Antibiotic suppression alone is rarely necessary and is only indicated for patients who are at an extreme risk for surgical intervention. Open debridement with retention of the prostheses is indicated for an acute hematogenous infection (within the time frame of 2 weeks from the onset of sepsis) with a well-fixed implant. Resection arthroplasty is usually reserved for the patient with minimal functional demands and polyarticular disease. Arthrodesis is indicated for the young patient with high-activity demands and single-joint disease or in whom reimplantation is not possible. Finally, amputation is the last resort for patients with life-threatening sepsis or sepsis combined with massive unretrievable tissue loss.

COMPLEX DECISION MAKING

Although advances in soft tissue transfers, bone grafting, and transplantation, and most importantly a better understanding of the pathophysiology of periprosthetic infection, have resulted in a much higher rate of salvage for the failed infected total knee arthroplasty, there are occasions when reimplantation would seem to be a less than reasonable option. Heroic attempts at reconstruction through arthroplasty seem reasonable in some settings, and yet they may be unreasonable in others. Determination of strict indications and hence contraindications for attempts at salvage of a failed infected TKA by reimplantation in all settings are, of course, impossible. The vast number of clinical settings and anatomic variations in which this type of decision must be made renders such decision making complex. The factors involved include an understanding of the limitations of both technology and human physiology. The surgeon (and certainly the patient) facing the consequences of the failed arthroplasty must be cognizant of the potential risks and benefits of intervention.

Multiple factors must be considered in such a decision, including factors unrelated to the knee itself, such as the underlying health and potential longevity of the patient, the willingness to undergo further surgical procedures and the expected outcome, as well as the specific risks of any particular intervention as based on the specific anatomic and pathologic features encountered in the individual patient. Such factors include the conditions of the soft tissues (including the periarticular skin and capsular tissues), the extensor mechanism, the underlying bone stock, and the neurovascular integrity of the limb.

Decision making in these cases can be far from straightforward. Reimplantation may, in some cases, be a technically easier surgical operation than arthrodesis, and in certain cases heroic attempts at infection eradication combined with bone stock and extensor mechanism reconstruction may be warranted. In other cases, the best alternative may be to leave a chronically infected pseudoarthrosis without further surgical intervention.

A basic technique for decision making in these complex settings is a modified form of what is known as expected utility analysis. This technique requires the surgeon to list the potential benefits of any intervention and assign to each benefit both a probability for its occurrence and a specific assignment of numerical ranking to the expected utility or benefit. An important assumption in this method is that utilities (or outcomes) can be expressed using a common scale. This has not been realistically accomplished for many orthopedic utilities. In business decision making, such utilities are mainly economic factors, but in medical decision making, in which factors such as pain and quality of life must be taken into account, these utilities are not as easily described and indeed may be more complex. Nonetheless an approximation of this technique may be quite useful.

For any given procedure each potential benefit of the procedure can be assigned a utility factor. These can then be listed with each utility assigned a probability. One can then sum the product of each utility by its probability, yielding a number representing the expected benefit of a particular intervention. The number derived from a similar sum of risk utilities (in this case, a negative number, indicating a "negative" outcome) multiplied by their individual probabilities can then be subtracted from the number calculated for the potential benefits of the procedure. Thus, for a given procedure with potential benefits listed as 1, 2, 3, ... X, and risks 1, 2, 3 ... Y:

Expected utility = ([Benefit utility 1 × Probability of utility 1] + [Benefit utility 2 × Probability of utility 2]. . . . + [Benefit utility X × Probability of utility X]) − ([Risk utility 1 × Probability of risk 1) + [Risk utility 2 × Probability of risk 2) . . . + [Risk utility Y × Probability of risk Y]).

The resulting number may then be compared to figures generated from similar consideration of alternative procedures.

Of course most of the risk and benefit "utilities" are subjective at this point and there is little hard data on the probabilities of these occurrences in specific unusual or complex settings. Nonetheless, such analysis, even on an informal basis, can assist the surgeon both in complex decision making and in communicating to the patient the potential risks and benefits of intervention involved in complex clinical settings. To make such complex decisions the surgeon must accurately assess multiple patient-related factors as noted above, but must also adequately judge his own skills, experiences, and resources concerning any particular procedure.

As a starting point, the surgeon who treats the failed total knee arthroplasty should be familiar with the prerequisite indications, contraindications, and techniques of reimplantation as well as the alternatives to reimplantation including suppression alone, debridement with retaining the prosthesis, resection arthroplasty, arthrodesis, and amputation.

ANTIBIOTIC SUPPRESSION ALONE

Suppression alone should rarely, if ever, be the treatment for an infected total knee replacement. There are five prerequisites when considering suppression alone. First, the patient must be so medically unstable or compromised that surgical intervention is not possible; this is usually because of a contraindication to anesthesia. Second, the patient must be only locally symptomatic from this infection. If septicemia is present, then surgical decompression of the joint is likely the only way to save the patient's life, even if the patient is a poor surgical risk. Third, only very susceptible organisms such as staphylococcus epidermidis and very susceptible species of streptococcus can even be considered for suppression alone. Fourth, the patient has to have no other prosthesis in place, because without more definite treatment of the infection a hematogenous spread of the initial infection may lead to seeding other joints. Finally, the prosthesis must be well fixed. Because most patients fail to meet at least one of these criteria, antibiotic suppression is rarely indicated.

Even if a patient meets these criteria, suppression alone does not cure the patient and may only delay the inevitable. When indicated, suppression is not without complications. These include development of resistant organisms, septicemia (possibly with a resistant organism), endocarditis, and rapid loosening. Lastly, the long-term effects of antibiotic may be toxic or lead to conditions such as C. Difficile colitis.

There is substantial literature that shows infected knees without a prosthesis can be treated with aspirations and antibiotic treatment alone. However, the literature on suppression of total knee replacements without debridement is less optimistic. Johnson and Bannister reported on antibiotic suppression alone in 25 cases treated for a mean of 15 months. Only two knees (8%) were still in place at final follow-up. In another report, Grogan and associates, reporting on three cases of antibiotic suppression alone, reported that only one knee (33%) was still functioning at 22 months follow-up. Bengtson and colleagues reported on 357 cases of infected knee arthroplasty with a 6-year follow-up. In this multicenter study from Sweden, antibiotic suppression was used in 225 cases and was successful in 47 knees. This success rate of 21% is comparable to the combined results of several series, reported by Rand, in which antibiotic suppression has been successful in 84 of 308 knees (27%).

DEBRIDEMENT WITH ANTIBIOTIC

In chronic infections, the infectious process often extends behind the prosthesis. In the cemented prosthesis, the bone-cement interface is eventually degraded resulting in loosening. This process also occurs at the bone-prosthesis interface in cementless implants, although loosening in this process is slower. Because in chronic infections the implant must be removed to reach the site of infection, debridement, without removal of the prosthesis, is not likely to be successful. Therefore, early operative debridement is indicated for acute hematogenous infection, of less than 2 to 3 weeks duration, occurring around a securely fixed and well-functioning prosthesis. Debridement must be combined with administration of an antibiotic with appropriately selected susceptibility testing. We recommend monitoring of serum levels of antibiotics and administration of antibiotics intravenously for 6 weeks in these cases. Additional oral antibiotics may be indicated but there is little data in the literature to support or guide this process.

The results of debridement are variable. This may be explained by differences in pathogen, the duration of infection to time of treatment, antibiotic management, type of implant fixation, and follow-up interval in several reported studies. Rand and associates report success in six of six infected knees, whereas Morrey and colleagues report success in eight of 10 infected knees treated with debridement. Schoifet and Morrey reported on 31 infected arthroplasties treated with debridement and intravenous administration of antibiotics. The overall success rate for debridement with intravenous antibiotic was 23% at an average of 8.8 years. The average duration of intravenous antibiotics was 4 weeks. Success correlated with the duration of infection prior to debridement: successfully treated knees had averaged 21 days, compared with 36 days in the failures. Failure resulted from this treatment in all gram-negative infections and all hinged prostheses. All the successfully treated knees had a resurfacing implant. *Staphylococcus aureus* was a difficult pathogen to eradicate; it was present in 29% of the salvaged knees compared with 58% of the knees in which debridement failed. Wilson and associates also reported that *Staphylococcus aureus* infections were more difficult to eradicate in their series reporting 12 successes out of a series of 23 debridements.

Many other investigators have found that the results of the treatment of chronic infections compare poorly to acute infections. Johnson and Bannister found no successful results following debridement of 27 chronically infected arthroplasties. Borden and Gearen reported success in five of six acute infections treated with debridement; however, they reported no success in five chronic infections. Using 2 weeks duration as the cutoff between acute and chronic infection, Teeny and colleagues found that debridement was successful in three of five acute infections (60%) but unsuccessful in 13 of 16 chronic infections at 3.5 years follow-up. In a multicenter analysis from Sweden, Bengtson and Knutson reported success in 37 of 154 knees (24%). Rand combined the results of multiple series in the literature. The combined overall success rate in these 377 knees treated with debridement was 110 successes (29%).

In conclusion, debridement is most efficacious in acute hematogenous infection caused by a low-virulence microorganism. The integrity of the prosthesis must be inspected at time of debridement to assure a securely fixed prosthesis.

REIMPLANTATION

Reimplantation or revision TKA is dependent first on the overall health and psychological willingness of the patient. These factors are somewhat subjective and in all cases the surgeon should rely on information provided from an expert in internal medicine with occasional cases requiring input from consultants in psychiatry. Additional concerns regarding multiple joint problems or other barriers to rehabilitation may require additional consultation from neurologists or rehabilitation experts.

Specific surgical prerequisites include the presence of (or when absent, the ability to surgically restore) an aseptic joint space, an adequate soft tissue envelope, extensor mechanism, and bone stock along with the capability to affix the implant to the underlying bone. The absence of any of these dictates alternative treatment. The management of these parameters for the purposes of reimplantation is beyond the scope of this discussion but should be a hallmark of the knowledge base of the surgeon attempting to determine the suitability of reimplantation in these complex settings. This discussion is covered in the last two chapters.

RESECTION ARTHROPLASTY

In the setting in which the limb is salvageable but the requirements for reimplantation cannot be met, the alternatives are arthrodesis or the creation (or maintenance of an already established) resection arthroplasty or pseudoarthrosis. Unfortunately, those cases in which arthrodesis is most difficult due to bone loss are those in which the likelihood of a stable resection arthroplasty is at their lowest.

In resection arthroplasty, the implant is removed with no attempt at reconstruction. The advantage of a resection arthroplasty is that the patient is able to sit more easily than with a straight-legged arthrodesis. However, the disadvantage of resection arthroplasty is that it rarely provides adequate stability and is usually painful during walking. Resection arthroplasty is indicated in a low-demand patient, usually with multiarticular joint involvement, who does not require the increased support and stability of knee arthrodesis and when the lack of knee joint motion of an arthrodesis will hamper mobility and/or excessively stress adjacent joints. Alternatively, in cases in which the patient lacks the prerequisites for reimplantation and/or arthrodesis, and already has a reasonable existing pseudoarthrosis function, the joint should be left alone. An effective pseudoarthrosis provides a compromise between stability and motion with minimal pain. Jones and Wroblewski reported on four knees that had been treated by resection arthroplasty and the use of a cement spacer at 3 years. Three of the four knees were free of infection at follow-up. Unfortunately those series of pseudoarthrosis creation following failed (usually infected) TKA show that clinical results are generally poor. Kaufer reported on 28 patients with knee resection arthroplasty and found that only 50% were functional ambulators. Furthermore, only 17% had joint stability, an additional 17% required further arthrodesis surgery, and average motion was only 40 degrees. All walkers required assistive devices (mainly walkers) for ambulation. Lettin's experience was no better. In 15 patients with knee pseudoarthrosis following removal of constrained TKA, seven were painfree but five had moderate and three severe pain. Seven required long leg bracing for ambulation. The mean range of motion was 52 degrees; however, there was 20 degrees of varus-valgus instability. A conversion of the description of patient function and pain into a Hospital for Special Surgery rating reveals that 12 patients would have had poor results and three only fair.

Rand reviewed multiple series of resection arthroplasty in the literature and combined them. He found that in the 107 knees in these combined studies, a satisfactory result was achieved in 73 (68%). However, although the infections resolved and some motion was achieved, most patients experience some residual pain and instability. Therefore, resection arthroplasty should be reserved for the patient with limited functional demands, most commonly in patients with significant multiarticular involvement such as in rheumatoid disease.

Specific techniques of pseudoarthrosis creation include three steps. First, the knee is debrided of all infected tissues, with removal of the implant and all cement. Second, fixation of the bone ends with pins or sutures to maintain alignment and apposition is done. Finally, cast immobilization is necessary for 6 weeks after joint debridement and the suturing of bone ends. (An alternative technique for stability is filling of the bone gap with an antibiotic-impregnated cement spacer.) Weight-bearing in the cast is permitted as tolerated. The clinical result is dependent on multiple extra-articular factors as well as the specific muscle tone and extensor mechanism function (Fig. 63.1).

ARTHRODESIS

As noted earlier, indications are relative for all procedures in this setting. Arthrodesis is intended to provide a stable and painless knee but does so at the expense of knee motion. In the patient in whom reimplantation is not possible due to loss of bone and/or soft tissue, and/or a functional extensor mechanism (in which the loss is not amenable to reconstruction), or loss of tissue compliancy (which may render any arthroplasty attempt extremely difficult or prone to postoperative ankylosis) or persistent sepsis, arthrodesis will generally provide the best function. Unless a specific indication for resection arthroplasty is present, the bulk of data supports better function and pain relief with arthrodesis.

Contraindications are few and relative: ipsilateral hip or ankle pathology, contralateral knee disease or arthrodesis and sufficient segmental bone loss to prevent arthrodesis. (Even these indications are not absolute; Charnley did report on 11 patients who were satisfied with bilateral knee arthrodesis and segmental bone loss may be handled by both vascularized and nonvascularized bone graft and bone transport techniques.) Of course, additional consideration must be made for the patient's employment and other functional requirements, though these factors are rarely of fundamental importance in the decision making required in these salvage-type situations.

The disabilities and compensations from knee arthrodesis are well documented and include increased energy and oxygen consumption requirements for am-

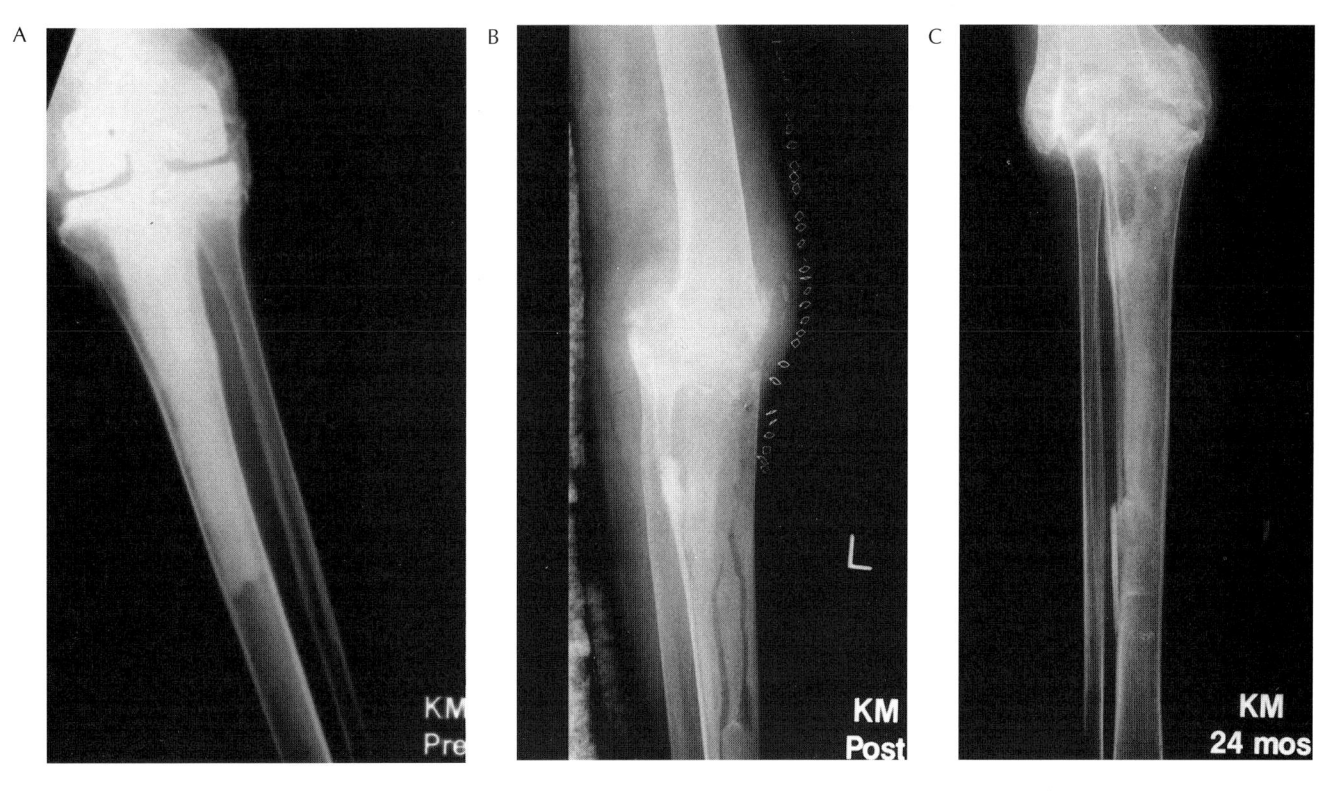

Figure 63.1. Resection arthroplasty: (A) Preoperative radiograph of an infected hinge prosthesis in a patient with rheumatoid arthritis. (B) Initial postoperative radiograph of the resection arthroplasty. (C) Radiograph at 24 months postoperative showing the healed and functional resection arthroplasty.

bulation, hip circumduction for stair climbing and clearing curbs, the difficulties imposed by the stiff limb on seating, and the difficulty using foot controls.

Techniques for arthrodesis are dependent on the amount of bone loss present, the presence or absence of sepsis, and the status of the adjacent bone and joints. The most important principle in arthrodesis is maximizing bone surface contact (interdigitating the bone ends if they are irregular and if this is possible). There should be vascular cancellous bone in apposition. Factors that increase bone loss (hinged implants, stemmed implants, and multiple revisions) decrease the chances of a successful arthrodesis. The success rate of arthrodesis has ranged from 71 to 81% following resurfacing compared with 56% following use of a hinged implant. With bone loss, cancellous bone grafting can improve the chances of success. Furthermore, the bone should be grafted about the periphery of the fusion site, because revascularization usually takes place from the surrounding soft tissues. Bone grafting at the time of arthrodesis resulted in union in 59% of knees, whereas union was achieved in 48% of knees without bone grafting.

Positioning is relatively straightforward. In most cases of salvage arthrodesis bone loss is sufficient so that little or no flexion is required to allow swing through during gait. In primary arthrodesis, in which bone length is not a problem, 10 to 20 degrees of flexion is recommended to allow the foot to clear the ground during the swing phase of gait without circumduction of the hip. Rotation should match the contralateral limb, and sagittal alignment should approximate a neutral mechanical limb axis.

As in all infections, all foreign material must be removed. Retained fragments of cement or metal can harbor residual infection. All devitalized and infected tissue should be excised. A healthy vascularized soft tissue bed should remain. Multiple debridements may be needed. In one study, union occurred in 62% of knees in which infection was controlled compared with 19% in cases with persistent infection. We recommend at least debridement with negative cultures before bone grafting is done.

Surgical exposure is relatively straightforward regardless of the previous status of the knee. Even in the rather severely ankylosed and distorted anatomical situation the hallowed orthopedic exposure principle of going from skin straight down to bone and staying on bone will allow adequate exposure, maintain maximally thick (not undermined) skin flaps, and provide for mobilization of the juxta-articular bone ends.

Fixation choices include external fixation, internal fixation either through plates and/or crossed screws, or intramedullary nailing. All incorporate the concept of compression. Charnley championed the concept of "compression" arthrodesis and noted a 98% success rate with the use of a rather primitive external fixation system for fixation of primary arthrodesis of the knee. External fixation techniques have become considerably more sophisticated since that time, but when the principle is applied to this type of salvage arthrodesis the success rates are considerably lower. Rand at the Mayo Clinic found that success was highly dependent on the parameter of bone loss, which is represented by the type of knee arthroplasty removed with this technique for salvage of infected TKA; finding fusion rates of 56% following removal of hinged TKA, as opposed to fusion rates of 81% following removal of resurfacing TKA. Improved function and arthrodesis success have also been correlated with achieving appropriate alignment and elimination of sepsis by Figgie and Goldberg. Various types of external frame configurations have been reported on from the standpoint of improving rigidity and maintaining compression, which are associated with lowering pin tract infection and pin loosening, the main complications of this method (Fig. 63.2). In addition, the bulky external fixator can be hard for the elderly to manage and makes rehabilitation more difficult than in methods utilizing internal fixation. In addition, improved fusion rates and elimination of the difficulties encountered with this method specific to external fixation are noted in those reports, utilizing internal fixation to achieve fusion. One advantage of external fixation is that it provides immediate stabilization of the knee following debridement of the infected knee. If fusion is successful, no secondary procedure is required. In one study, arthrodesis with the use of biplanar external fixation was successful in 66% of cases, whereas uniplanar fixation was only successful in 33% of cases. In another study, biplanar external fixators resulted in a 71% union rate.

Internal fixation requires the prerequisite of a clean bed, in which case a two-stage procedure is required for management of the infected TKA. Extramedullary internal fixation is best accomplished by dual dynamic compression plating—one placed medially and one placed laterally, both contoured to the knee. A 12-hole plate is recommended. Crossed screws at the fusion site may provide additional compression, but are insufficient fixation in the salvage fusion (Fig. 63.3). One cautionary note: there may be insufficient soft tissue at the knee to cover two plates applied to this relatively subcutaneous location. It also requires rather extensive soft

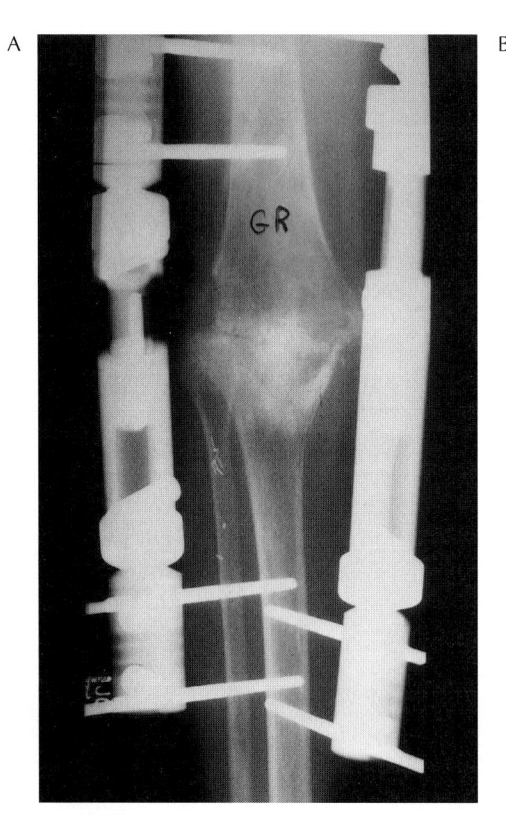

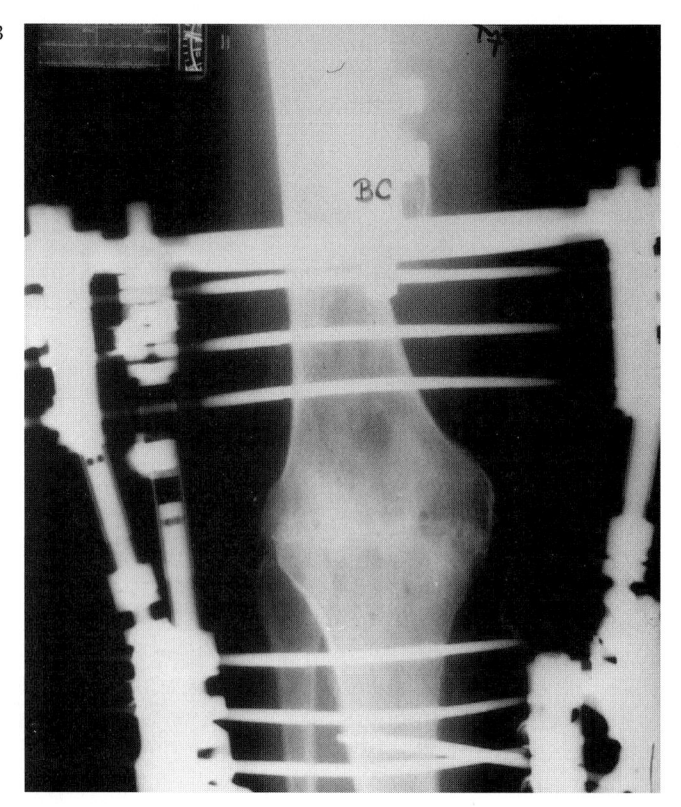

Figure 63.2. Arthrodesis with external fixation: (A) Biplanar external fixation. (B) Biplanar external fixation with compression.

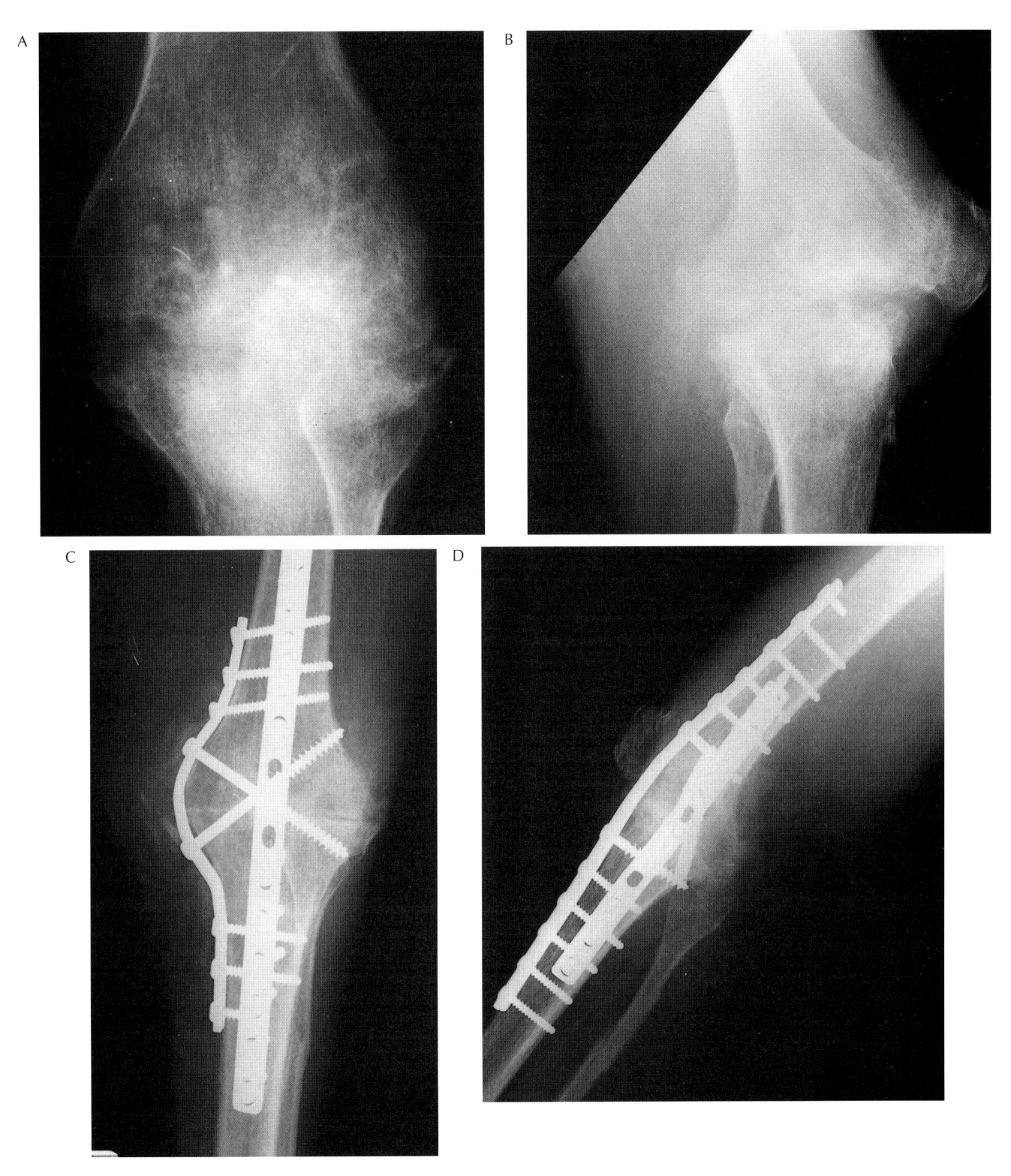

Figure 63.3. Arthrodesis with dual plates: (A) and (B) Preoperative anteroposterior and lateral radiographs after resection of an infected total knee arthroplasty. (C) and (D) Anteroposterior and lateral radiographs of the healed arthrodesis with dual plates 8 months postoperatively.

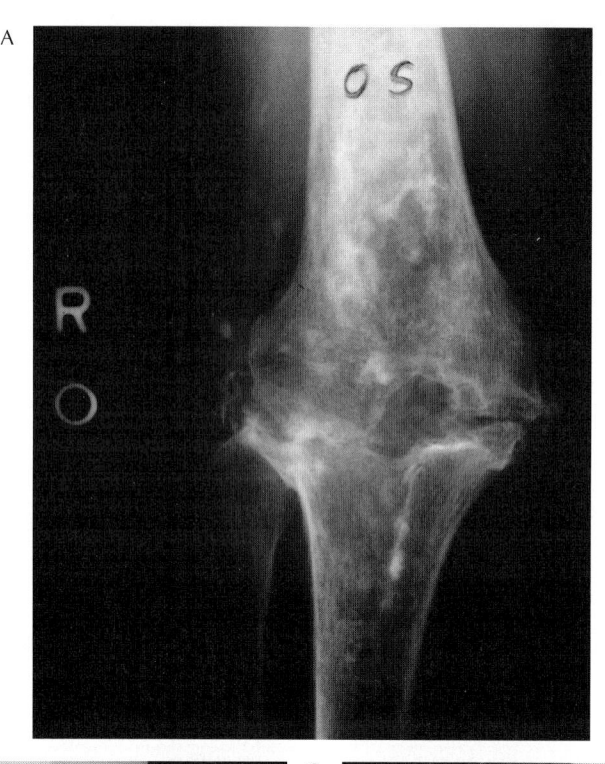

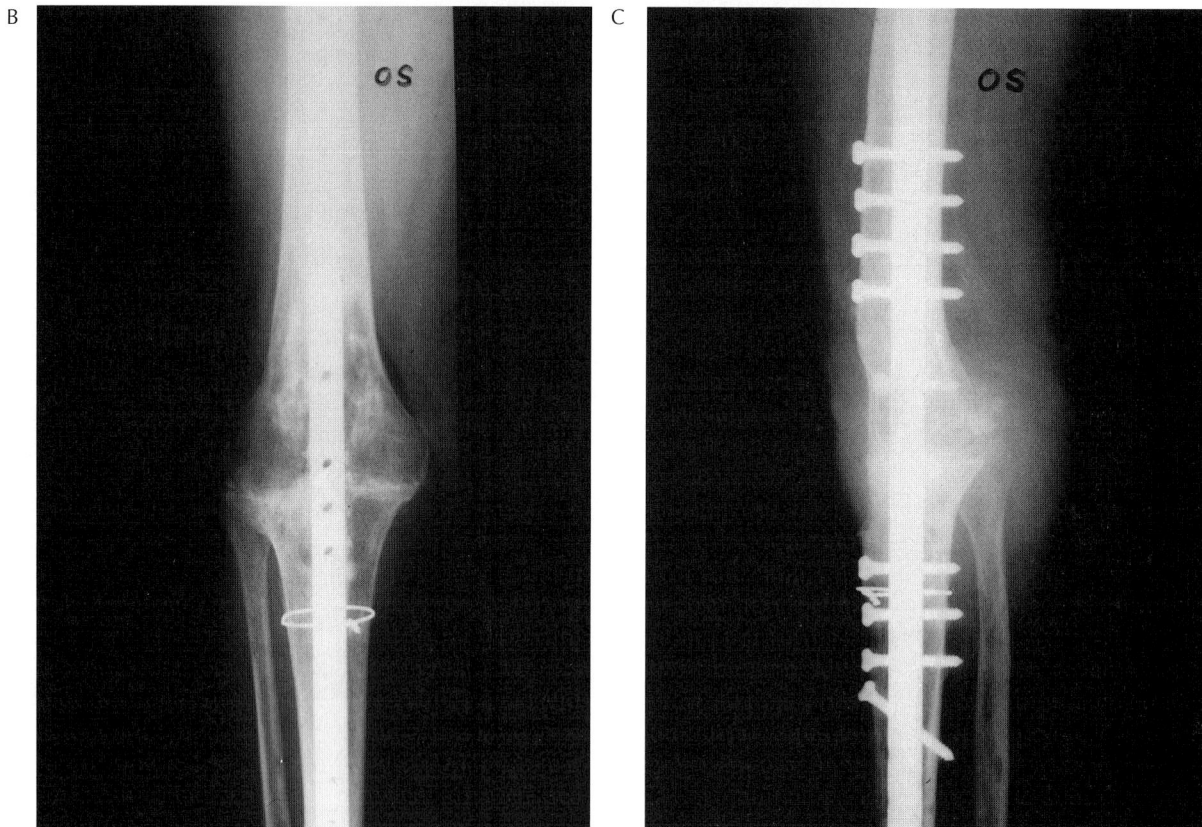

Figure 63.4. Arthrodesis with an intramedullary rod: (A) Preoperative radiograph of a resected total knee arthroplasty done for infection. (B) and (C) Anteroposterior and lateral radiographs of the healed arthrodesis with an intramedullary rod 5 months postoperatively.

tissue stripping from the bone ends. A long leg cast is used, with weight-bearing as tolerated, until radiographs show fusion.

Intramedullary (IM) rod fixation carries with it the need for a clean bed as well with the additional concern that if sepsis is persistent an extensive intramedullary osteomyelitis may be the result of IM nailing. However, this technique, when performed as a second stage following adequate surgical debridement and antimicrobial management of the septic process, has demonstrated the highest fusion rates of any technique when salvaging the failed TKA. Rand reviewed the literature of 13 studies in which IM rod fixation was used. The overall success rate in these combined 98 cases was 91%.

IM rod fixation is particularly useful in cases of severe bone loss. Both vascularized autograft as well as allograft bone segments can be used to bridge extensive defects with this method. It does require relatively straightforward anatomy above and below the knee and the use of special arthrodesis nails. Preoperative planning and templating for nail size is an important part of the procedure. Of course with this technique the tibiofemoral angle is 180 degrees with no knee flexion. We prefer a nail that has locking capabilities proximally and distally to manage the problem of a single diameter nail achieving fixation in canals that may be of widely disparate diameters (Fig. 63.4). In general, the most efficient technique in our hands has been to open and debride the knee region and prepare the bone ends for fusion. The femur is reamed retrograde and the tibia antegrade. A nail that will achieve tight fixation in the tibia is chosen. If the nail achieves sufficient rotational stability in the tibia, there is no need to interlock the nail distally. However, proximally the nail will be undersized for rotational stability. This can be easily managed with the proximal interlock.

AMPUTATION

Amputation is certainly the most difficult alternative for the surgeon to contemplate, yet it may be the easiest to specify definitive indications for the limb that is unsalvageable due to uncorrectable vascular insufficiency, persistent pain unresponsive to efforts at pain relief, progressive life-threatening infection unresponsive to appropriate surgical and medical management, the immunocompromised patient who has uncontrolled systemic sepsis, and in cases of sufficient tissue loss in which tissue restoration is deemed impossible or impractical. The knee in which arthrodesis is unlikely to be successful and another revision procedure is not feasible because of inadequate bone stock may also be a candidate for amputation. Rand reviewed the need for amputation by combining 14 series of attempted knee salvage. The amputation rate in these 14 series, which included 893 knees, was 6%.

Amputation with early prosthetic fitting can allow for rapid rehabilitation. However, most elderly patients are unable to use the above knee prosthesis effectively. They remain limited ambulators or are nonambulatory because of the increased energy expenditure required for walking. Pring reported on 23 patients treated with above-the-knee amputation for failed total knee arthroplasty and fitted with a prosthesis. They found that only seven patients were daily ambulators at 4 years following amputation and 12 were confined to a wheelchair. Furthermore, 20 of the 23 used a wheelchair part of the day.

CONCLUSION

The setting of limb salvage following failure of TKA can be challenging for the surgeon and patient. Best results are achieved when the surgeon has carefully evaluated all the factors influencing the potential success or failure of the various treatment methods available. Although the choice is ultimately the patient's, to be made based on informed consent, it is the job of the surgeon to help guide the patient to an understanding of the situation through the time-honored principles of patient education. This will frequently lead to better understanding on the part of both the surgeon and the patient about the lifestyle and functional requirements involved and allow for individual and customized case management.

References

Bengston S, Knutson K, Lindgren L. Revision of infected TKA. *Acta Orthop Scand*. 1986; 57:489–494.

Bengtson S, Knutson K. The infected knee arthroplasty. A 6-year follow-up of 357 cases. *Acta Orthop Scand*. 1991; 62:301–311.

Bengtson S, Knutson K, Lidgren L. Treatment of infected knee arthroplasty. *Clin Orthop*. 1989; 245:173–178.

Bliss DG, McBride GG. Infected total knee arthroplasties. *Clin Orthop*. 1985; 199:207–214.

Borden LS, Gearen PF. Infected total knee arthroplasty. A protocol for management. *J Arthroplasty*. 1987; 2:27–36.

Broderson MP, Fitzgerald RF, Peterson LFA, Coventry MD, Bryan RS. Arthrodesis of the knee following failed TKA. *J Bone Joint Surg*. 1979; 61A:181–185.

Burton DS, Schurman DJ. Salvage of infected total joint replacements. *Arch Surg*. 1977; 112:574–578.

Chapchall G. Intramedullary pinning for arthrodesis of the knee joint. *J Bone Joint Surg*. 1948; 30A:728–737.

Charnley J, Baker SL. Compression arthrodesis of the knee—A clinical and histological study. *J Bone Joint Surg*. 1952; 34B:187–199.

Charnley J, Lowe HG. A study of end results of compression arthrodesis of the knee. *J Bone Joint Surg*. 1958; 40B:633–635.

Charnley JC. Positive pressure in arthrodesis of the knee. *J Bone Joint Surg.* 1948; 30B:478–486.

England SP, Stern SH, Insall JN, Windsor RE. Total knee arthroplasty in diabetes mellitus. *Clin Orthop.* 1990; 260:130–134.

Fahmy NRM, Barnes KL, Noble J. A technique for difficult arthrodesis of the knee. *J Bone Joint Surg.* 1984; 66B:367–370.

Falahee MH, Matthews LS, Kaufer H. Resection arthroplasty as a salvage procedure for a knee with infection after a total arthroplasty. *J Bone Joint Surg.* September 1987; 69-A:1013–1021.

Fidler MW. Knee arthrodesis following prosthesis removal—Use of the Wagner apparatus. *J Bone Joint Surg.* 1983; 65B:29–31.

Figgie HE, Brody GA, Inglis AE, Sculco TP, Goldberg VM, Figgie MP. Knee arthrodesis following TKA in rheumatoid arthritis. *Clin Orthop.* 1987; 224:237–243.

Freeman MAR, Sudlow RA, Casewell MW, Radcliff SS. The management of infected total knee replacements. *J Bone Joint Surg.* 1985; 67-B(5):764–768.

Goldberg VM, Hardy P. The treatment and outcome of the infected total knee arthroplasty. *Orthop Trans.* 1981; 5:467.

Greind RU. Arthrodesis of the knee with intramedullary fixation. *Clin Orthop.* 1983; 181:146–150.

Grogan TJ, Dorey F, Rollins J, Amstutz HC. Deep sepsis following total knee arthroplasty. Ten-year experience at the University of California at Los Angeles Medical Center. *J Bone Joint Surg.* February 1986; 68-A:226–234.

Hankin F, Louie KW, Mathews LS. The effect of TKA prosthesis design on the K potential for salvage arthrodesis. *Clin Orthop.* 1981; 155:52–58.

Harris CM, Froelich J. Knee fusion with intramedullary rods for failed TKA. *Clin Orthop.* 1985; 197:209–216.

Insall JN, Thompson FM, Brause BD. Two stage re-implantation of salvage of the infected TKA. *J Bone Joint Surg.* 1983; 65A:1087–1098.

Insall JN. Infection in total knee arthroplasty. In: *Instructional Course Lectures. The American Academy of Orthopaedic Surgeons. Vol. 31.* St. Louis: C. V. Mosby; 1982:42–48.

Insall JN, Hood RW, Flawn LB, Sullivan DJ. The total condylar knee prosthesis in gonarthrosis. A five to nine-year follow-up of the first one hundred consecutive replacements. *J Bone Joint Surg.* June 1983; 65-A:619–628.

Jacobs MA, Hungerford DS, Krackow KA, Lennox DW. Revision of septic TKA. *Clin Orthop.* 1989; 238:159–166.

Jacobs MA, Hungerford DS, Krackow KA, Lennox DW. Revision of septic total knee arthroplasty. *Clin Orthop.* 1989; 238:159–166.

Jerry GJ Jr, Rand JA, Ilstrup D. Old sepsis prior to total knee arthroplasty. *Clin Orthop.* 1988; 236:135–140.

Johnson DP, Bannister GC. Outcome of infected arthroplasty of the knee. *J Bone Joint Surg.* 1986; 68-B:289–291.

Jones WA, Wroblewski BM. Salvage of failed total knee arthroplasty: the "beefburger" procedure. *J Bone Joint Surg.* 1989; 71-B(5):856–857.

Kaufer H, Matthews LS. Resection arthroplasty: an alternative to arthrodesis for salvage of the infected total knee arthroplasty. In: *Instructional Course Lectures, The American Academy of Orthopaedic Surgeons. Vol. 35.* Park Ridge, Illinois: American Academy of Orthopaedic Surgeons; 1986:283–289.

Lettin AWF, Neil MJ, Citron ND, August A. Excision arthroplasty for infected constrained total knee replacements. *J Bone Joint Surg.* 1990; 72-B(2):220–224.

Lucas DB, Murray WR. Arthrodesis of the knee by double plating. *J Bone Joint Surg.* 1961; 43A:795–808.

Morrey BF, Westholm F, Schoifet S, Rand JA, Bryan RS. Long-term results of various treatment options for infected total knee arthroplasty. *Clin Orthop.* 1989; 248:120–128.

Morris HD, Mosiman RS. Arthrodesis of the knee: a comparison of the compression method with the non-compression method. *J Bone Joint Surg.* 1951; 33A:982–987.

Petty W, Bryan RS, Coventry MB, Peterson LF. Infection after total knee arthroplasty. *Orthop Clin North Am.* 1975; 6:1005–1014.

Poss R, Thornhill TS, Ewald FC, Thomas WH, Bath NJ, Sledge GB. Factors influencing the incidence and outcome of infection following total joint arthroplasty. *Clin Orthop.* 1984; 182:117–126.

Pring DJ, Marks L, Angel JC. Mobility after amputation for failed knee replacement. *J Bone Joint Surg.* 1988; 70-B(5):770–771.

Rand JA, Bryan RS, Chao EYS. Failed TKA treated by arthrodesis of the knee using the Ace-Fischer apparatus. *J Bone Joint Surg.* 1987; 69A:39–45.

Rand JA, Bryan RS. Reimplantation for salvage of an infected TKA. *J Bone Joint Surg.* 1983; 65A:1081–1086.

Rand JA. Instructional course lectures, the American Academy of Orthopaedic Surgeons. Alternatives to reimplantation for salvage of the total knee arthroplasty complicated by infection. *J Bone Joint Surg.* 1993; 75-A:282–289.

Rand JA, Fitzgerald RH Jr. Diagnosis and management of the infected total knee arthroplasty. *Orthop Clin North Am.* 1989; 20:201–210.

Rand JA, Bryan RS, Morrey BF, Westholm F. Management of infected total knee arthroplasty. *Clin Orthop.* 1986; 205:75–85.

Rand JA, Chao EYS, Stauffer RN. Kinematic rotation-hinge total knee arthroplasty. *J Bone Joint Surg.* April 1987; 69-A:489–497.

Rosenberg AG, Hass B, Barden R, Marquesz DS, Landon GC, Galante JO. Salvage of the infected TKA. *Clin Orthop.* 1988; 226:29–33.

Rud B, Jensen UH. Function after arthrodesis of the knee. *Acta Orthop Scand.* 1985; 56:337–339.

Salvati EA, Robinson RP, Zeno SM, Koslin BL, Brause BD, Wilson PD Jr. Infection rates after 3175 total hip and total knee replacements performed with and without a horizontal unidirectional filtered air-flow system. *J Bone Joint Surg.* April 1982; 64-A:525–535.

Sanders R, O'Neil T. The gastrocnemius myocutaneous flap used as a cover for the exposed knee prosthesis. *J Bone Joint Surg.* 1981; 63B:383–386.

Schoifet SD, Morrey BF. Treatment of infection after total knee arthroplasty by debridement with retention of the components. *J Bone Joint Surg.* October 1990; 72-A:1383–1390.

Schurman DJ. The management of infected total knee replacement. *Orthop Trans.* 1982; 6:477.

Schwartz S, Griffin T. *Medical Thinking. The Psychology of Medical Judgment and Decision Making.* New York: Springer Verlag; 1986.

Teeny SM, Dorr L, Murata G, Conaty P. Treatment of infected total knee arthroplasty. Irrigation and debridement versus two-stage reimplantation. *J Arthroplasty*. 1990; 5:35–39.

Wade PJF, Denham RA. Arthrodesis of the knee after failed TKR. *J Bone Joint Surg*. 1984; 66B:362–366.

Walker RH, Schurman DJ. Management of infected total knee arthroplasties. *Clin Orthop*. 1984; 186:81–89.

Wilson MG, Kelley K, Thornhill TS. Infection as a complication of total knee-replacement arthroplasty. Risk factors and treatment in sixty-seven cases. *J Bone Joint Surg*. July 1990; 72-A:878–883.

Windsor RE, Insall JN, Ors WK, Miller DU, Brause BD. Two stage reimplantation for the salvage of TKA complicated by infection—Further follow up and refinement of indications. *J Bone Joint Surg*. 1990; 72A:272–278.

Woods GW, Lionberger DR, Tullos HS. Failed total knee arthroplasty. Revision and arthrodesis for infected and non-infectious complications. *Clin Orthop*. 1983; 173:184–190.

SECTION 18
Extensor Mechanism Dysfunction

CHAPTER 64
Patellar Fracture

Mark A. Greenfield, Geoffrey H. Westrich, and Steven B. Haas

INTRODUCTION

Patellar fracture following total knee arthroplasty is uncommon, but may cause significant morbidity. Patellar fractures can occur in both resurfaced and unresurfaced patellae. The treatment of these fractures range from a decrease in activity and observation to patellectomy. One must always keep in mind that the treatment and subsequent results of the treatment differ significantly from the non-total knee arthroplasty patient.

INCIDENCE

The incidence of patellar fracture following total knee arthroplasty has been reported in 0 to 21% of cases (Table 64.1), although most recent series report an incidence of less than 6%.[1-16] Most series[2,7] have found a similar incidence of patellar fracture in rheumatoid arthritis and osteoarthritis patients; however, Scott and associates found that patellar fractures were more common in the osteoarthritic patient (3.5%) than the rheumatoid arthritis patient (0.7%).[14] They felt that patients with osteoarthritis have more function and are generating greater force across the patellofemoral joint thereby making them more prone to patellar fracture.

At the time of revision arthroplasty the patellar remnant is generally quite thin and osteoporotic. It is not surprising that these patients have an increased frequency of patella fracture when compared to primary arthroplasty. Although patellar fractures can occur in both resurfaced and unresurfaced patellae, Grace and Sim noted an increased incidence of patellar fractures in the resurfaced patellae (0.33%) compared to unresurfaced patellae (0.05%).[7]

Patellar fractures occur at various times postoperatively.[2,7,8,14-17] They appear to occur most often 1 year following surgery, but can range from the immediate postoperative period to several years following total knee arthroplasty.

ETIOLOGY

Many factors have been implicated about the etiology of patellar fractures following total knee arthroplasty. Those contributing to patellar fractures include vascular, biomechanical, technical, thermal, and traumatic factors. Understanding the vascular anatomy, preservation of bone stock, sound component design, correct component alignment, and attention to detail during surgery are the keys in preventing patellar fractures following total knee arthroplasty.

Compromise of the vascular supply is felt to be a major factor in the development of fractures of the patella following total knee arthroplasty. It is believed that a diminished blood flow will lead to avascular necrosis and predispose the patella to fracture. Lateral retinacular release, medial parapatellar arthrotomy, fat pad excision, cauterization of the prepatellar vessels, and anterolateral capsular release from the tibia have all been reported as contributing to patellar devascularization.

The anatomy of the patellar blood supply can be divided into an intraosseous and extraosseous system. This vascular network is at risk during total knee arthroplasty. A medial parapatellar approach interrupts the medial geniculate circulation, divides the supreme geniculate, superior medial geniculate, and inferior medial geniculate arteries.

Excision of the fat pad, which is done to enhance exposure, may compromise the patellar blood supply.[4,18,19] McMahon and colleagues found that excision of the fat pad did not compromise patellar vascularity.[20] They found that excision of the fat pad, in those knees that were performed with or without a lateral retinacular release, was not associated with an increased incidence of avascular necrosis of the patella.

Stress fractures of the patella have been reported with histologic studies of the bone demonstrating avascular necrosis.[8,10,14,21] Numerous authors regard lateral retinacular releases as having a role in the development of avascular necrosis of the patella following total knee arthroplasty.[2-4,8,10,14-16,18-20,22-25] It interrupts the supe-

Table 64.1. Incidence of patellar fracture following total knee arthroplasty

Author	Year	Incidence
Insall et al.[6]	1979	0%
Thompson et al.[15]	1981	1.75%
Scott et al.[14]	1982	0.7% RA 3.5% OA
Cameron and Fedorkow[3]	1982	21%
Clayton and Thirupathi[4]	1982	5.4%
Dupont and Baker[6]	1982	0.65%
Insall et al.[9]	1982	11%
Levai et al.[11]	1983	4.2%
Lynch et al.[12]	1987	1.8%
Grace and Sim[7]	1988	0.15%
Aglietti et al.[1]	1988	1.3%
Brick and Scott[2]	1988	0.52%
Doolittle and Turner[5]	1988	0.86%
MacCollum and Karpman[13]	1989	6%
Tria et al.[16]	1994	3.6%
Healy et al.[8]	1995	2.4%

rior and inferior geniculate arteries and the anterior tibial recurrent artery. Proper tracking of the patella is nonetheless a greater priority, and a release must be performed when indicated.

In contrast to those who believe the lateral retinacular release is a major factor in the development of patellar fracture, Ritter and Campbell found no increased risk of avascular necrosis in knees that had a lateral retinacular release.[26] They found a higher incidence of stress fractures when a lateral retinacular release was not performed (3.6%) compared to those when a release was performed (1.5%). The former were all noted to have bone lateral to the patellar prosthesis. Therefore, they felt that patellar fractures occurred from an increased lateral tensioning resulting from an intact lateral retinaculum and patellar bone lateral to the patellar prosthesis. The bone fractures as it is pulled away from the prosthesis.

Postoperative technetium bone scans have been used to assess patellar viability following total knee arthroplasty. A decreased perfusion on bone scans after lateral retinacular release has been observed within a few days following total knee arthroplasty.[23,24] Scuderi and associates reported a 56.4% incidence of vascular compromise with sequential bone scans in knees undergoing lateral retinacular release.[23] In those knees that did not have a lateral retinacular release, only 15% were found to have a decrease in the bone scan uptake after surgery. However, the clinical significance was minimal because only 3% developed a patellar fracture, and they responded to nonoperative treatment. Therefore, lateral retinacular release appears to have a causal relationship with patellar viability. It does not seem to be the sole determinant, and implicates other factors that contribute to transient patellar avascularity.

McMahon and colleagues reported an increased likelihood of developing avascular necrosis of the patella with lateral retinacular release.[20] They found that 54.2% of those knees in which a lateral retinacular release was performed compared to 13% in those knees in which a lateral retinacular release was not performed developed cold bone scans postoperatively. However, they felt that patellar revascularization occurred 3 to 10 months postoperatively.

Wetzner and associates reported a decreased bone scan uptake following lateral retinacular release and suggested that lateral retinacular release predisposes to avascular necrosis of the patella.[24] They elected to restrict the activity of those patients and instructed them to avoid certain functions that generate relatively high forces across the knee, such as climbing stairs or arising from a chair without support. They found that uptake improved with time and usually returned to normal by 6 months.

Ritter and colleagues reported no avascular necrosis of the patella associated with lateral release and interruption of the superior lateral geniculate artery.[27] They did recommend that the circumpatellar arteries must be saved along with as many of the contributing vessels as possible from the infrapatellar fat pad and quadriceps tendon. Bone scans returned to normal by 1 year suggesting revascularization.

There are several other surgical considerations that can play a role in the development of patellar fractures following total knee arthroplasty. Excessive bone resection can lead to a thin patella predisposing it to fracture.[3,4,14,22] One should attempt to restore the normal patellar thickness. Reuben and associates recommended not resecting the bony patellar thickness less than 15 mm or the overall patellar thickness should not be less than 25 mm because as the bony patella becomes thinner, the patellar surface strain increases.[28] They suggested that resecting the patella under 15 mm may predispose to patellar fractures. We have not found this to be our experience. We recommend that overall patella thickness should be maintained or thinned 1 to 2 mm, and that the remaining patella should be at least 12 mm thick.

Under-resection of the patella can lead to increased forces across the patella and may predispose to patellar fracture. Increased forces across the patella and patellar implant contribute to increased stress. Increased patellar thickness increases patellar forces at higher flexion angles. And increased patellofemoral forces at higher flexion angles may have implications on the patella and patellar implant. Star and colleagues have shown in a cadaver study that an increased patellar thickness difference of even 10% can significantly alter patello-femoral forces at higher knee flexion angles.[29]

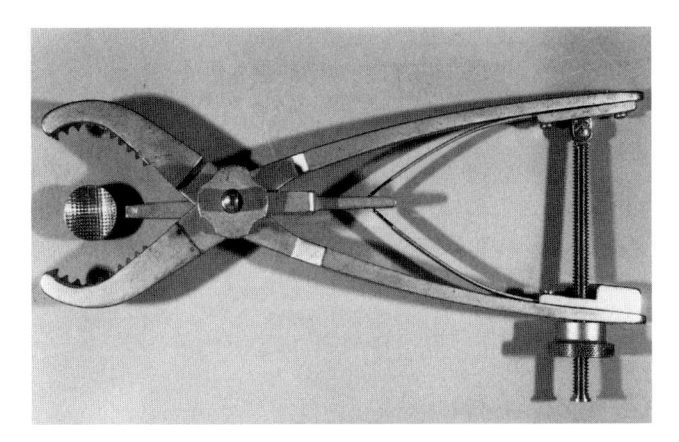

Figure 64.1. Patella resection guide.

Uneven patellar resection may predispose to patellar fractures. A common error in preparation of the patellar osteotomy is to under-resect the medial facet and over-resect the lateral facet. This creates an oblique patellar osteotomy with displacement of the patellar prosthesis too far laterally. Use of a resection guide may prevent tilting of the prosthesis (Fig. 64.1), as well as over-resection or under-resection of the patella.

Removal of peripheral bone has also been implicated in patellar fracture.[15,21] It has been recommended to preserve the peripheral cortex of both the medial and lateral facets.[14,30]

General malalignment of any of the components has been reported to predispose to patellar fracture following total knee arthroplasty.[31] Malalignment causes high patellar strains. Minor malalignment may result in a fracture of the superior or the middle part of the patella, which does not lead to loosening of the component. Major malalignment may be associated with severe fracture and loosening of the component. Figgie and colleagues reported that 15 of 16 knees that had a patellar fracture and minor malalignment had a good or excellent result.[31] In contrast, only three of 20 knees that had a patellar fracture and major malalignment had a good or excellent result. Goldberg and associates stated that those fractures in which major deviations from neutral extremity alignment and implant position had the most severe patellar fractures and the poorest outcomes.[25]

Increased tension in the extensor mechanism due to anterior displacement and increased distance from the tibial tubercle to origin of extensors has been reported as a cause of patellar fracture.[19] This can occur if the anterior femur is under-resected and too large an implant is used.

Weak bone can also lead to patella fracture following total knee arthroplasty. Osteopenia,[2,11,14] steroid therapy,[6] and thermal necrosis from polymethylmethacrylate[4,19] have been reported as contributing to weakened patellar bone.

Patellofemoral component design has been shown to have an influence on the development of patellar fractures. Femoral component design[32] and patellar component design, such as a large, central peg on patella,[4,14,15,19,30] which causes increased patellar strain, and metal-backing of patella,[8] have been linked to patellar fracture following total knee arthroplasty. Patellar components with multiple smaller pegs may reduce the risk of fracture.

Several other factors have been shown to contribute to the development of patellar fracture following total knee arthroplasty—obesity,[6,15] increased general activity level,[5,9,33] and increased range of motion.[1,5,9,14,33] Patients are achieving greater degrees of flexion with newer designs, which increases the patellofemoral compression forces, activity forces, and activity level. Patellofemoral contact stresses are increased with the degree of flexion, and therefore, patellar strains are increased. Reilly and Martins[34] demonstrated that the forces across the patellofemoral joint increase during certain activities. During level gait with the knee flexed to 9 degrees, the force across the patellofemoral joint was 0.5 times body weight. This force increased to 3.3 times body weight with the knee flexed to 60 degrees during stair climbing and increased to 7.8 times body weight during squatting with the knee flexed to 130 degrees.

Fixation failure such as loosening of the patellar component has been linked to the development of patellar fracture after total knee arthroplasty.[15]

Grace and Sim proposed that transverse fractures of the patella may be secondary to abnormally applied forces caused by excessive bone resection or improper button size.[7] Longitudinal fractures may be due to abnormal forces caused by improper soft tissue balance or malposition of the patellar prosthesis.

Care to optimize patellar tracking and thickness and to avoid patellar devascularization may minimize the risk of patellar fracture. The following are recommendations that may reduce the risk of a patellar fracture. A lateral release should not be routinely done unless indicated. The need of performing a lateral release can be minimized by taking care to reproduce or slightly diminish the overall patellar thickness.[35] When it is necessary to improve patellar tracking, it should be done at least 1.5 cm from the patella and preserve the superior geniculate artery. Preserve as much of the fat pad as possible. Avoid cauterizing or stripping of the anterior surface of the patella. Avoid deep saw cuts when removing the articular surface. When performing the patellar osteotomy, the final thickness of the patellar implant and patella should be equal to or slightly less than the original patella.

CLASSIFICATION OF PATELLAR FRACTURES

Classification systems have been described for patellar fractures following total knee arthroplasty.[25,36] Patellar fractures can occur as a result of trauma or fatigue. The majority of these fractures occur as stress, or fatigue, fractures (Fig. 64.2).

Traumatic fractures usually occur as a result of a significant injury, such as a fall. Although the amount of trauma can be minor, the fracture fragments are usually displaced and usually require open repair of the fracture and repair of the retinaculum (Fig. 64.3).

Fatigue fractures occur spontaneously, without significant trauma, and are often asymptomatic. They are often found incidentally on routine follow-up radiographs. In retrospect, the patient may remember a brief period of discomfort that they ignored. Windsor and colleagues further classified fatigue fractures into horizontal or vertical, comminuted and displaced.[36]

Horizontal fractures are usually caused by improper patellar tracking and may be associated with patellar dislocation. Vertical fractures pass through the patellar fixation hole. No specific treatment is required, and these usually heal spontaneously (Fig. 64.4). Comminuted and displaced fractures are a combination of a horizontal or vertical type of fracture. These are usually asymptomatic, and no treatment is required unless the patellar button is loose.[36]

Goldberg and associates classified patellar fractures based on clinical outcome and treatment[25]—type I fractures that had no involvement of the implant-cement composite or quadriceps mechanism; type II fractures that involve the implant-cement composite and/or quadriceps mechanism; type IIIA fractures of the inferior pole of the patella with patellar ligament rupture; type IIIB inferior pole fractures without patellar ligament rupture; type IV fracture-dislocations of the patella.

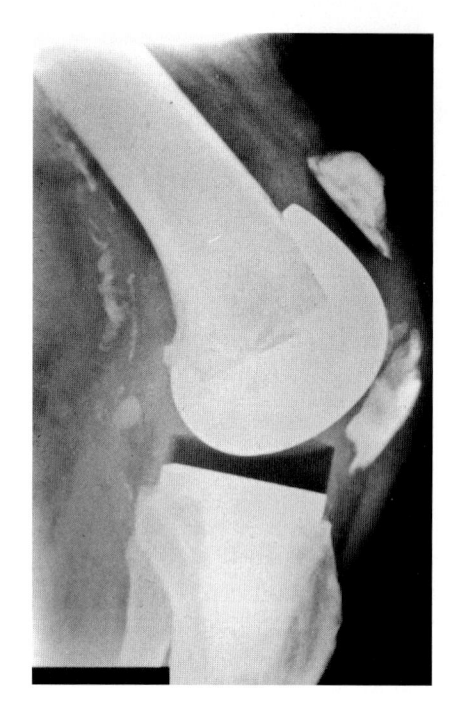

Figure 64.3. Traumatic fracture of the patella with disruption of the extensor mechanism.

DIAGNOSIS

Patients may give a history of trauma; however, the incident might be minor or significant. Many patellar fractures go unrecognized and are only diagnosed retrospectively as part of a routine follow-up examination.

Patients tend to complain about swelling and anterior knee pain, which may be transient. They may recall

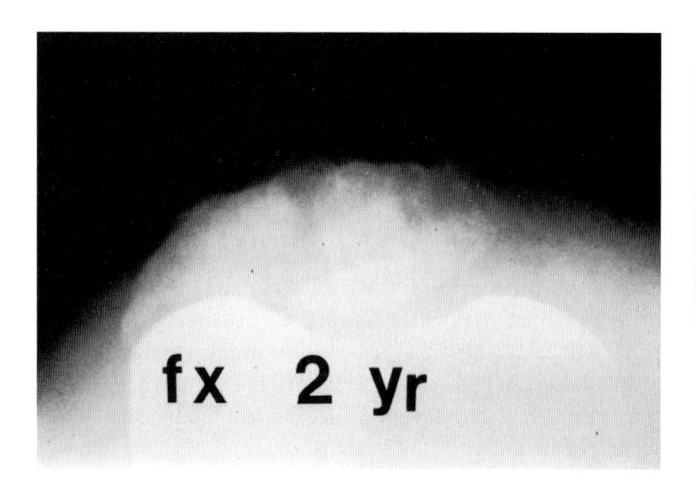

Figure 64.2. Stress fracture of the patella that occurred 2 years post-total knee replacement.

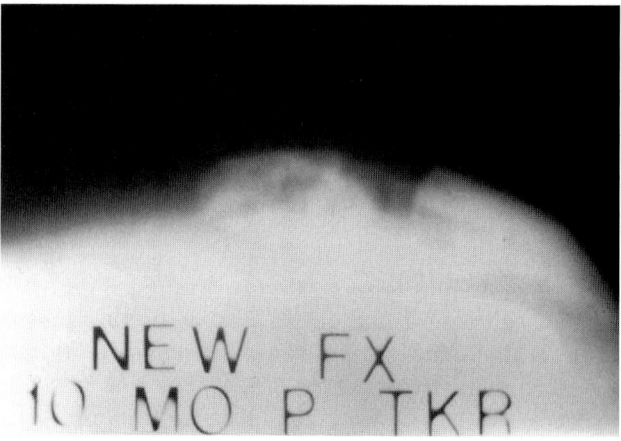

Figure 64.4. Vertical fracture through the fixation hole.

a period of mild discomfort around the knee, primarily with stair climbing.

On examination patients may have patellar tenderness, a palpable gap in the extensor mechanism, ecchymosis, an effusion, and an extensor lag. A complete roentgenographic evaluation is required that should include an anteroposterior, a lateral, and a patellar view such as that described by Merchant.[37]

MANAGEMENT OF PATELLAR FRACTURES

Most patellar fractures following total knee arthroplasty do well without surgery. Insall and colleagues reported that most were found on routine follow-up radiographs and they were usually asymptomatic, required no treatment, and were compatible with an excellent result.[9] Windsor and associates stated that most patellar fractures can be treated with 6 weeks of immobilization, followed by active, assisted exercises and isometric quadriceps strengthening.[36]

For those situations that do require surgical intervention, secure fixation is often difficult and complications are common. And surgical intervention does not guarantee an excellent result. In view of the rather poor results obtained by operative treatment, these fractures should be treated nonoperatively whenever possible. Management of patellar fractures is based on the displacement and location of the fracture; whether the extensor mechanism is disrupted, evidenced by an extensor lag; whether the patellar component is loose as observed on the radiographic studies; and component alignment.

Incidental fractures are asymptomatic and found when radiographs are taken for another reason. No treatment is needed.

Nonoperative treatment is recommended for nondisplaced fractures.[5,7,13,14,25,31,36] If the patellar component is not loose, if the quadriceps mechanism has not been disrupted, if the fracture is comminuted but not displaced, and there is no major implant malalignment, then treatment can be nonoperative. Windsor and colleague recommended for comminuted or vertical fractures, regardless of displacement, 6 weeks of immobilization.[36] Nondisplaced transverse fractures (less than 2 cm of displacement) were treated with immobilization. Small proximal or distal avulsion fractures of the patella were treated by immobilization and active, assisted range-of-motion exercises after discontinuing the immobilization at 3 to 6 weeks.

Grace and Sim treated fractures that were minimally displaced (less than 5 mm), noncomminuted, with an intact patellar prosthesis with immobilization.[7] Fractures with significant displacement (more than 5 mm), excessive comminution, or a loose patellar prosthesis had operative repair.

Scott and associates recommended the initial treatment of a stress fracture of the patella to be nonoperative, with surgery necessary only if the patellar prosthesis became dislodged, or if pain or inadequate active extension persisted.[14]

Goldberg and colleagues analyzed 36 patellar fractures according to the type of fracture and the alignment of the prosthesis.[25] They found that patellar fractures not associated with loosening of the patellar component, disruption of the extensor mechanism (type I or IIIB fractures), and without major malalignment may be treated satisfactorily without surgery. Despite surgery, types II, IIIA, and IV fractures were frequently associated with an unsatisfactory outcome.

Nonoperative treatment of patellar fractures following total knee arthroplasty consists of immobilization in a brace or cast for a period of 4 to 6 weeks in extension. Patients can be partial weight-bearing with crutches, given anti-inflammatory medications, followed by rehabilitation with active range-of-motion and quadriceps-strengthening exercises.

Operative treatment of a patellar fracture is necessary if the fracture is displaced or if there is complete disruption of the extensor mechanism, pole fractures with complete extensor mechanism disruption, loosening of the patellar implant, major component malalignment, or patellar dislocation.

Hozack and associates separated displaced fractures based on the presence or absence of an extensor lag at the time of fracture.[13] They found that displaced fractures without an extensor lag did well with nonoperative treatment. Displaced fractures with an extensor lag had poor results with operative treatment. Even though displacement of the fracture and an extensor lag are compelling indications for operation, these patients did poorly with operative treatment. They recommended that fragment excision should be considered for displaced distal pole fractures with patellar tendon disruption, and patellectomy should be considered for failures of all other treatments.

Brick and Scott recommended surgery for fractures displaced greater than 2 cm, a significant extensor lag causing instability, or a loose, displaced prosthesis.[2] Repeated attempts at fixation should be avoided. If a small fragment of bone is displaced and surgery becomes necessary, a partial patellectomy with quadriceps tendon or patellar tendon repair may be possible. Patellectomy should be considered in comminuted fractures and failed fixation.

Windsor and colleagues felt that displaced transverse fractures (greater than 2 cm) that displayed a significant extension lag and quadriceps weakness required operative treatment.[36] If the patellar component becomes loose, then remove the patellar component and cement. If the patellar bone stock is adequate and the fracture has healed, a new patellar component may be implanted. For severely comminuted fractures with displacement, partial patellectomy, repair of the retinaculum, and removal of the patellar component may be indicated.

A consistent solution to the management of patellar fractures following total knee arthroplasty has not been found. The size, location, and quality of the fractured bone, type of patellar component, and polymethylmethacrylate may limit surgical options. It is often difficult to achieve adequate fixation with conventional tension band wiring, and fixation is rarely successful because of the poor quality of the thin, rather soft avascular bone that remains. Cerclage fixation is often preferred.

Surgical treatment is pragmatic and dependent on circumstance. If the fracture fragments are of adequate size, then consider open reduction and internal fixation with extensor mechanism repair. Tears of the medial and lateral retinaculum should be examined for and repaired. Obtaining apposition of patellar fragments is often not possible. If there is not adequate bone for repair, then consider fragment excision and extensor mechanism repair. If there is an avulsion of the superior or inferior pole of the patella with disruption of the extensor mechanism, then resect the fragment and advance the extensor mechanism. Patella components that have become loose should be removed. If there is sufficient bone stock remaining or if the fracture has healed, then resurfacing may be possible. If the bone remnant is too small for revision, then remove and shape the bone as necessary, remove the patellar component and cement, and perform an extensor mechanism reinforcement. If the fracture is associated with major malalignment, then consider revision arthroplasty.

Windsor and colleagues found that arthroscopic debridement may be beneficial in those cases in which ectopic ossification may develop following a period of healing.[36] This may enable smoother movement of the quadriceps patellar tendon mechanism over the trochlear groove of the femoral component and diminish pain and crepitus.

Patellectomy may be the best treatment alternative if solid fixation and extensor mechanism integrity cannot be restored and maintained.

PARTIAL PATELLECTOMY

The decision to perform a partial patellectomy is dependent upon the type of patella fracture, the integrity of the extensor mechanism, and whether the patella has been resurfaced. In total knee arthroplasty with a nonresurfaced patella, transverse polar fractures that involve retention of one large proximal or distal fragment are amenable to partial patellectomy.[1,38–46] In addition, comminuted displaced patella fractures with a large proximal or distal fragment that remains attached to the extensor mechanism are also managed by partial patellectomy of the comminuted fragments.[1,38–47] Partial patellectomy is always accompanied by reconstruction of the extensor mechanism.

In a total knee arthroplasty patient with a fracture involving a patella that has been resurfaced, every attempt should be made to treat the patient nonoperatively with a period of immobilization. However, in patients with loss of integrity of the extensor mechanism or a loose patellar component, operative intervention is usually necessary. In total knee arthroplasty with a well-fixed patellar component and a displaced polar type fracture, partial patellectomy and reconstruction of the extensor mechanism is indicated. In patients with a loose patellar component, the treatment involves either revision or removal of the patellar prosthesis depending upon the amount of remaining patellar bone stock. Furthermore, in a total knee arthroplasty patient with a vertical patella fracture that involves only a margin of the patella component, one may consider a partial patellectomy of the loose fragment with cementing a smaller component to the remaining patella (Fig. 64.5).

The surgical technique of performing a partial patellectomy involves the complete excision of the small po-

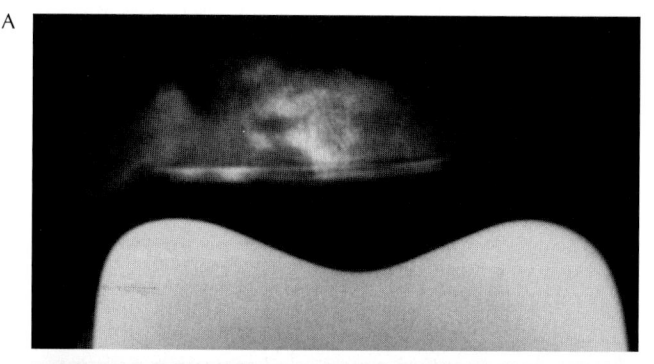

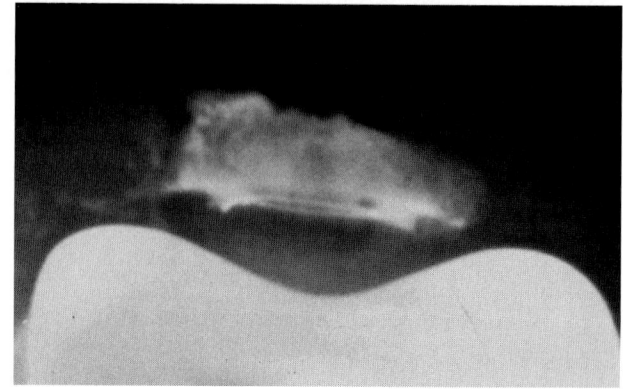

Figure 64.5. (A) Resurfaced patella with displaced vertical fracture and loosening of the component. (B) Excision of fracture fragment and revision with biconvex patella component.

lar fragment or comminuted fragments with repair of the extensor mechanism to the remaining patella. Either the quadriceps tendon proximally or the patellar ligament distally must be repaired with heavy nonabsorbable suture to the remaining fragment close to the articular surface of the patella to avoid tilting of the remaining fragment. At our institution either the Kessler or Krackow stitch is used for this repair.[48,49] In performing a partial patellectomy and extensor mechanism repair, the bone should be imbedded in the tendon or ligament in a layered fashion.[38,50] After suturing the tendon or ligament near the remaining articular surface, to further avoid tilting of the main patella fragment, it is recommended that the aponeurosis of the quadriceps is overlapped and repaired to a denuded surface of the patella.[42,50,51] This is usually accomplished through longitudinal drill tunnels in the patella that begin close to the articular surface at the repair site and exit more superficially at the intact tendon or ligamentous attachment site.

It should be emphasized that the operative treatment of patella fractures in total knee arthroplasty with resurfaced patellae may be difficult secondary to poor bone quality, small remaining patellae for bone tunnels, and patellar components that may interfere with fixation. Therefore, the orthopedic surgeon should utilize extreme caution indicating operative treatment for cases of patella fractures after total knee arthroplasty. If surgery is indicated, however, adequate preoperative planning is essential for a successful outcome.

TOTAL PATELLECTOMY

Total patellectomy is reserved only for the severely comminuted displaced patella fractures that are not amenable to either open reduction internal fixation or partial patellectomy.[42,50–62] Because the results of this technique are controversial, total patellectomy should be performed only when the anatomic restoration of the multiple patellar fragments is unattainable. In patients without a total knee arthroplasty, it should be noted that some authors condemn total patellectomy as the initial procedure and always recommend an attempt at reconstruction of the extensor mechanism with total patellectomy reserved only as a salvage procedure.[63] In total knee arthroplasty patients with a resurfaced patella, total patellectomy should be reserved only for the rare case of patella fracture in which severe comminution, significant extensor lag, and/or loosening of the patellar implant exists so that an attempt at reconstruction is not attainable.

In performing a total patellectomy, the fragments of the fractured patella are carefully excised from the extensor mechanism, and the remaining quadriceps tendon is sutured with heavy nonabsorbable suture to the patella ligament. At our institution either the Kessler or Krackow stitch is utilized for this repair.[48,49] To avoid extensor mechanism laxity and an extensor lag, the tendon to ligament repair is performed end to end. To increase the strength of the reconstruction, a layered repair is recommended with overlapping sutures.

After partial or total patellectomy, the tendon or ligament repair should be protected with immobilization of the knee in extension.[46,50,63] At our institution, a hinged knee brace is utilized for the above postoperative care. Initially, the brace is locked in extension and the patient is allowed to ambulate only partial weight-bearing. Quadriceps isometric exercises are utilized not only to help maintain quadriceps muscle tone, but also to prevent intra-articular adhesions.[46] After a period of immobilization, progressive knee flexion and increased weight-bearing are allowed in the brace. The intraoperative determination of the quality of the repair directs the rate of progression with knee flexion and weight-bearing. Passive stretching of the knee should be avoided, because this may jeopardize the repair.[46,50,63]

In reviewing the results of partial or total patellectomy for patellar fracture in total knee arthroplasty, only a paucity of data currently exists. A few small series exist that report this subset of patients, and the results are far from satisfactory. Hozack and colleagues studied the results of 16 patellar fractures (12 displaced, 4 nondisplaced) that were treated operatively with satisfactory results in only 50% or 8 of the knees. Furthermore, the results were successful for only 50% (2 of 4) of the patients treated with partial patellectomy and 60% (6 of 10) patients treated with total patellectomy.[17] In a study by Brick and associates only one-third (3 of 9) of the patella fractures that were treated operatively had a satisfactory result.[2] However, Grace and colleagues also studied patella fracture after total knee arthroplasty and noted that 72% (5 of 7) patients had a satisfactory result with operative treatment.[7]

At the Hospital for Special Surgery, a retrospective review of 18 cases of patella fracture after total knee arthroplasty were studied.[15] Two open reductions were performed for traumatic fractures, one closed reduction with cast immobilization for a displaced vertical fracture, and one patellectomy with a revision procedure. The results were good in three and fair in one due to persistent quadriceps weakness and an extensor lag. In the remaining 14 knees that were treated nonoperatively, excellent results were attained in 10 patients and good results in four patients. In a subsequent study by Goldberg and associates, 36 patella fractures were evaluated.[25] He noted that fractures not involving the implant or quadriceps mechanism should be treated nonoperatively, although fractures of the patella with disruption of the extensor mechanism or lateral fracture dislocations were treated operatively with six good results and nine poor results. The majority of poor results were attributed to the difficulties obtaining good fixation secondary to avascularity, comminution, and the presence of the patellar implant. Although all of these studies are limited in their interpretation, no single large series exists to adequately report the results of partial or total patellectomy for patella fracture after total knee arthroplasty.

CONCLUSION

The patella is an integral component to the extensor mechanism of the knee and is designed to increase the mechanical advantage of the quadriceps moment arm.[43,50,58,64] Therefore, in patients with a patella fracture after total knee arthroplasty, every effort should be made to retain the patella. The evaluation and management of the patella fracture after total knee arthroplasty with an unresurfaced patella should follow a similar treatment algorithm as a trauma patient without a knee arthroplasty. Nondisplaced fractures should be treated nonoperatively, whereas displaced fractures with disruption of the extensor mechanism should be treated operatively. However, if the extensor mechanism is intact, one can accept a slight amount of displacement, because later operative resurfacing of the patella can be performed.

Because of the poor results that are reported with operative intervention, the initial treatment of a patella fracture after total knee arthroplasty should be nonoperative, as long as the extensor mechanism is intact and the patellar prosthesis is not loose. However, a loose patellar component or disrupted extensor mechanism mandates operative treatment with revision or excision of the patellar prosthesis and restoration of the extensor mechanism. The choice of replacing the patellar prosthesis is dependent not only upon the remaining patellar bone stock, but also the integrity of the extensor mechanism. In this setting, a partial patellectomy with revision to a smaller patellar component may be required. Only in the very rare case of patella fracture with severe comminution and loosening of the prosthesis is total patellectomy with restoration of the extensor mechanism indicated.

References

1. Aglietti P, Buzzi R, Gaudenzi A. Patellofemoral functional results and complications with the posterior stabilized total condylar knee prosthesis. *J Arthroplasty*. 1988; 3:17–25.
2. Brick GW, Scott RD. The patellofemoral component of total knee arthroplasty. *Clin Orthop*. 1988; 231:163–178.
3. Cameron HU, Fedorkow DM. The patella in total knee arthroplasty. *Clin Orthop*. 1982; 165:197–199.
4. Clayton ML, Thirupathi R. Patellar complications after total condylar arthroplasty. *Clin Orthop*. 1982; 170:152–155.
5. Doolittle KH, Turner RH. Patellofemoral problems following total knee arthroplasty. *Ortho Rev*. 1988; 17:696–702.
6. Dupont JA, Baker SA. Complications of patellofemoral resurfacing in total knee arthroplasty. *Orthop Trans*. 1982; 6:369 (abstract).
7. Grace JN, Sim FH. Fracture of the patella after total knee arthroplasty. *Clin Orthop*. 1988; 230:168–175.
8. Healy WL, Wasilewski SA, Takei R, Oberlander M. Patellofemoral complications following total knee arthroplasty. *J Arthroplasty*. 1995; 10:197–201.
9. Insall JN, Lachiewicz PF, Burstein AH. The posterior stabilized condylar prosthesis: a modification of the total condylar design. *J Bone Joint Surg*. 1982; 64A:1317–1323.
10. Insall JN, Scott WN, Ranawat CS. The total condylar knee prosthesis. *J Bone Joint Surg*. 1979; 61A:173–180.
11. Levai JP, McLeod HC, Freeman MA. Why not resurface the patella? *J Bone Joint Surg*. 1983; 65B:448–451.
12. Lynch AF, Rorabeck CH, Bourne RB. Extensor mechanism complications following total knee arthroplasty. *J Arthroplasty*. 1987; 2:135–140.
13. MacCollum MS, Karpman RR. Complications of the PCA anatomic patella. *Orthopedics*. 1989; 12:1423–1428.
14. Scott RD, Turoff N, Ewald FC. Stress fracture of the patella following duopatellar total knee arthroplasty with patellar resurfacing. *Clin Orthop*. 1982; 170:147–151.
15. Thompson FM, Hood RW, Insall JN. Patellar fractures in total knee arthroplasty. *Orthop Trans*. 1981; 5:490–491.
16. Tria AJ, Harwood DA, Alicea JA, Cody RP. Patellar fractures in posterior stabilized knee arthroplasties. *Clin Orthop*. 1994; 299:131–138.
17. Hozack WJ, Goll SR, Lotke PA, Rothman RH, Booth RE. The treatment of patellar fractures after total knee arthroplasty. *Clin Orthop*. 1988; 236:123–127.
18. Kayler DE, Lyttle D. Surgical interruption of patellar blood supply by total knee arthroplasty. *Clin Orthop*. 1988; 229:221–227.
19. Roffman M, Hirsh DM, Mendes D. Fracture of the resurfaced patella in total knee replacement. *Clin Orthop*. 1980; 148:112–116.
20. McMahon MS, Scuderi GR, Glashow JL, Scharf SC, Meltzer LP, Scott WN. Scintigraphic determination of patellar viability after excision of infrapatellar fat pad and/or lateral retinacular release in total knee arthroplasty. *Clin Orthop*. 1990; 260:10–16.
21. Scott RD. Duopatellar total knee replacement: the Brigham experience. *Orthop Clin North Am*. 1982; 13:89–102.
22. Berry DJ, Rand JA. Isolated patellar component revision of total knee arthroplasty. *Clin Orthop*. 1993; 286:110–115.
23. Scuderi G, Scharf SC, Meltzer LP, Scott WN. The relationship of lateral releases to patella viability in total knee arthroplasty. *J Arthroplasty*. 1987; 2:209–214.
24. Wetzner SM, Bezreh JS, Scott RD, Bierbaum BE, Newberg AH. Bone scanning in the assessment of patellar viability following knee replacement. *Clin Orthop*. 1985; 199:215–219.
25. Goldberg VM, Figgie HE, Inglis AE, Figgie MP, Sobel M, Kelly M, Kraay M. Patellar fracture type and prognosis in condylar total knee arthroplasty. *Clin Orthop*. 1988; 236:115–122.
26. Ritter MA, Campbell ED. Postoperative patellar compli-

cations with or without lateral release during total knee arthroplasty. *Clin Orthop.* 1987; 219:163–168.
27. Ritter MA, Keating EM, Faris PM. Clinical, roentgenographic, and scintigraphic results after interruption of the superior lateral genicular artery during total knee arthroplasty. *Clin Orthop.* 1989; 248:145–151.
28. Reuben JD, McDonald CL, Woodard PL, Hennington LJ. Effect of patella thickness on patella strain following total knee arthroplasty. *J Arthroplasty.* 1991; 6:251–258.
29. Star MJ, Kaufman KR, Irby SE, Colwell CW. The effects of patellar thickness on patellofemoral forces after resurfacing. *Clin Orthop.* 1996; 322:279–284.
30. Scott RD, Reilly DT. Pros and cons of patellar resurfacing in total knee replacement. *Orthop Trans.* 1980; 4:328–329.
31. Figgie HE, Goldberg VM, Figgie MP, Inglis AE, Kelly M, Sobel M. The effect of alignment of the implant on fractures of the patella after condylar total knee arthroplasty. *J Bone Joint Surg.* 1989; 71A:1031–1039.
32. Theiss SM, Kitziger KJ, Lotke PS, Lotke PA. Component design affecting patellofemoral complications after total knee arthroplasty. *Clin Orthop.* 1996; 326:183–187.
33. Insall JN, Dethmers DA. Revision of total knee arthroplasty. *Clin Orthop.* 1982; 170:123–130.
34. Reilly D, Martens M. Experimental analysis of the quadriceps muscle force and patellofemoral joint reaction force for various activities. *Acta Orthop Scand.* 1972; 43:126–137.
35. Greenfield MA, Insall JN, Case GC, Kelly MA. Instrumentation of the patellar osteotomy in total knee arthroplasty. *Am J Knee Surg.* 1996; 9:129–132.
36. Windsor RE, Scuderi GR, Insall JN. Patellar fractures in total knee arthroplasty. *J Arthroplasty.* 1989; Supp:S63–S67.
37. Merchant AC, Mercer RL, Jacobsen RH, Cool CR. Roentgenographic analysis of patellofemoral congruence. *J Bone Joint Surg.* 1974; 56:1391–1396.
38. Andrews JR, Hughston JC. Treatment of patellar fractures by partial patellectomy. *South Med J.* 1977; 70:809–813.
39. Bostman A, Kiviluoto O, Nirhamo J. Comminuted displaced fractures of the patella. *Injury.* 1981; 13:196–202.
40. DePalma AF. The management of fractures and dislocations. Philadelphia: W.B. Saunders; 1959.
41. DePalma AF, Flynn JJ. Joint changes following experimental partial and total patellectomy. *J Bone Joint Surg.* 1958; 40:395–413.
42. Johnson EE. Fractures of the patella. In: Rockwood CA Jr, Green DP, Bucholz RW, ed. *Fractures in Adults.* 3rd ed. Philadelphia: J.B. Lippincott; 1991:1762–1766.
43. Maquet PGJ. *Biomechanics of the Knee: with Application to the Pathogenesis and the Surgical Treatment of Osteoarthritis.* Berlin: Springer-Verlag; 1976.
44. Saltzman CL GJ, McClellan RT, et al. Results of treatment of displaced patellar fractures by partial patellectomy. *J Bone Joint Surg.* 1990; 72A:1279–1285.
45. Shorbe HB DC. Patellectomy: repair of the extensor mechanism. *J Bone Joint Surg Am.* 1958; 40:1281–1284.
46. Taylor CJ. Fractures. In: Crenshaw AH, ed. *Campbell's Operative Orthopaedics.* 8th ed. St. Louis: CV Mosby; 1992:841–847.
47. Bostman A, Kiviluoto O, Nirhamo J. Comminuted displaced fractures of the patella. *Injury.* 1981; 13:196–202.
48. Krackow KA, Thomas SC, Jones LC. A new stitch for ligament-tendon fixation. *J Bone Joint Surg.* 1986; 68A:764–766.
49. Wilkinson J. Fracture of the patella treated by total excision. *J Bone Joint Surg.* 1977; 59B:352–354.
50. Aglietti P, Buzzi R, Insall JN. Disorders of the patellofemoral joint. In: Insall JN, Windsor RE, Scott WN, Kelly MA, Aglietti P, eds. *Surgery of the Knee.* 2nd ed. New York: Churchill Livingstone; 1993:1085–1102.
51. Cohn BNE. Total and partial patellectomy. *Surg Gynecol Obstet.* 1944; 79:526–535.
52. Brooke R. The treatment of fractured patella by excision: a study of morphology and function. *Br J Surg.* 1936; 24:733–747.
53. Brooke R. Fractured patella: an analysis of 54 cases treated by excision. *Br Med J.* 1946; 1:231–233.
54. Flinchum D. Patellectomy: when, why, and how. *South Med J.* 1966; 59:897–905.
55. Heineck AP. The modern operative treatment of fracture of the patella: I. Based on the study of other pathological states of this bone. II. An analytical review of over 1,100 cases treated during the last ten years, by open operative method. *Surg Gynecol Obstet.* 1909; 9:177–248.
56. Hohl M, Larson RL. Fractures and dislocations of the knee. In: Rockwood CA J, Green DP, eds. *Fractures.* Philadelphia: JB Lippincott; 1975:1131–1150.
57. Horwitz T, Lambert RG. Patellectomy in the military service. *Surg Gynecol Obstet.* 1946; 82:423.
58. Jensenius H. On the results of excision of the fractured patella. *Acta Chir Scand.* 1951; 102:275–284.
59. Smillie IS. *Injuries of the Knee Joint.* 4th ed. Edinburgh: Churchill Livingstone; 1970.
60. Wass SH, Davies ER. Excision of the patella for fractures with remarks on ossification in the quadriceps tendon following the operation. *Guys Hosp Rep.* 1942; 91:35–45.
61. Watson-Jones R. Excision of the patella (letter). *Br Med J.* 1945; 2:195–196.
62. Wendt PP, Johnson RP. A study of quadriceps excursion, torque and the effect of patellectomy on cadaver knees. *J Bone Joint Surg.* 1985; 67A:726.
63. Kaplan EB. The lateral meniscofemoral ligament of the knee joint. *Bull Hosp Joint Dis.* 1956; 17:176.
64. Weber MJ, Janecki CJ, McLeod P, Nelson CL, Thompson JA. Efficacy of various forms of fixation of transverse fractures of the patella. *J Bone Joint Surg.* 1980; 62A:215–220.

CHAPTER 65
Acute and Chronic Rupture of the Quadriceps Tendon Treated with Direct Repair

Robert E. Booth and Frank P. Femino

Rupture of the quadriceps tendon after total knee arthroplasty is rare and there is scant information in the literature regarding this problem.[1-3] In the nonimplant population, quadriceps tendon rupture is the more common malady in the older patient and patellar tendon rupture in the younger patient.[4-6] The reverse seems to be true after knee replacement despite the older average age of this population.

The causes of quadriceps rupture in the total knee arthroplasty patient are multiple. They include mechanical, systemic, and local factors. Mechanically, the tensile forces generated across the quadriceps tendon are very high, with values approaching 3000 newtons. They are greater than the forces in the patellar tendon at 90 and 120 degrees of flexion but less at 60 degrees of flexion.[7] In the setting of soft tissue compromise and with such large forces being sustained by the extensor mechanism, it is not surprising that rupture of the quadriceps tendon can occur after a total knee arthroplasty. Vascular and soft tissue compromise following surgical procedures such as a lateral retinacular release or a Roux-Goldthwaite procedure can lead to rupture and several cases have also been reported.[2,3]

In a patient with a total knee arthroplasty there is little contraindication to directly repairing the acutely ruptured quadriceps tendon. If there is minimal soft tissue compromise, the techniques used in nonarthroplasty patients are perfectly valid. These techniques are widely described in the literature and include end-to-end repair alone or with supplemental fixation.[4,5,8] The problem arises when, as is often the case in the total knee arthroplasty patient, there is structural compromise of the quadriceps tendon. This can make re-rupture common. Whether the rupture is acute or chronic often makes little difference. Therefore, reinforcement of the repair and augmentation of the soft tissue is advised. Techniques are described using various reinforcement techniques such as a quadriceps turndown flap (Fig. 65.1, Scuderi turndown technique).[6,9] In the chronic situation, the Codivilla technique of quadriceps lengthening may be necessary due to shortening of the extensor mass (Fig. 65.2, Codivilla technique of tendon lengthening and repair).[10]

The results for early repair of acute quadriceps tendon ruptures in nonarthroplasty patients have been excellent.[4,11] The functional outcome in the patient with a total knee arthroplasty has been consistently inferior. Extensor lag and quadriceps weakness are common and may require bracing.[1,2,12] The repair should be protected for several months.[1,3] A series of three repairs reported by Lynch and colleagues resulted in one re-rupture after 6 weeks, leaving a 35-degree permanent extension lag, as well as limited flexion and significant extension lag in the other two.[3] The only exception is a case reported by Fernandez-Baillo and associates[13] in which he repaired a traumatic rupture of the quadriceps tendon occurring over 1 month after a total knee replacement. He used the technique described by Scuderi and reinforced the repair with Dacron tape. The functional result was good after 1 year, with no pain, a range of motion of 0 to 110 degrees, and almost normal quadriceps strength.[13]

It is our recommendation to perform the repair as soon as possible, because acute repair will minimize further quadriceps atrophy and shortening. We prefer the technique as described by Scuderi with the discretionary use of Dacron tape reinforcement, based on intraoperative assessment. Postoperative treatment consists of full weight-bearing in a cylinder cast for 6 weeks. The cast is then removed and gradual flexion is begun in a protective hinged brace. Physical therapy for strengthening is started. Our goal is to reach 90 degrees of flexion at 3 months with minimal extensor lag. Maximum results can be expected between 6 and 12 months.

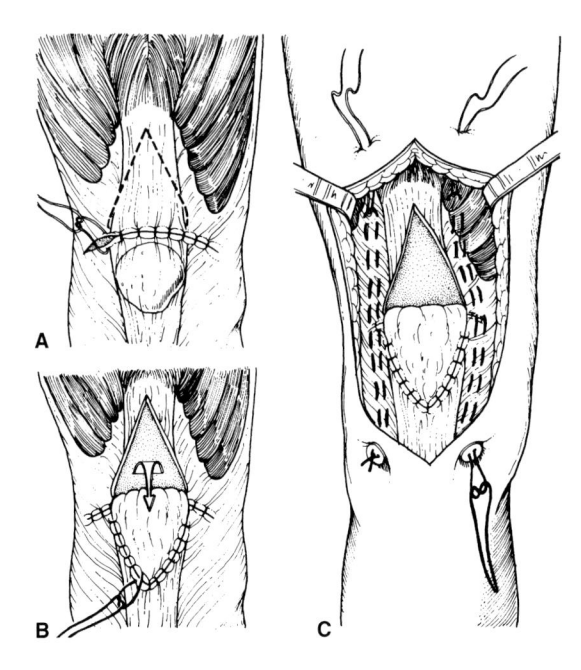

Figure 65.1. The Scuderi technique for repairing acute tears of the quadriceps tendon. (A) The torn edges of the quadriceps tendon are debrided and repaired. (B) A triangular flap of the proximal tendon is developed, folded distally over the rupture, and sutured in place. (C) Pullout sutures are then placed in the medial and lateral retinaculum.

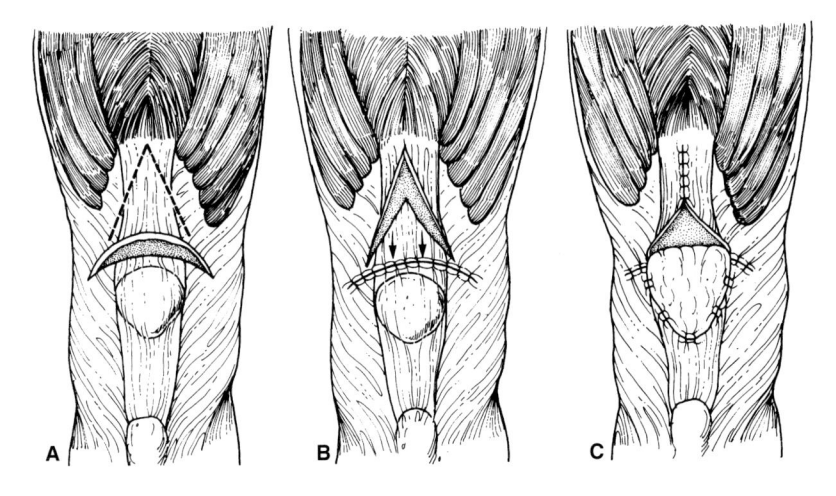

Figure 65.2. The Codvilla quadriceps tendon lengthening and repair for chronic ruptures. (A) The torn tendon edges are debrided and repaired. (B) An inverted V is cut through the proximal tendon. (C) The flap is brought distally and sutured in place. The upper portion on the V defect is then repaired.

References

1. Gustillo RB, Thompson R. Quadriceps and patellar tendon ruptures following total knee arthroplasty. In: Rand JA, Dorr LD, eds. *Total Arthroplasty of the Knee*. Rockville, Maryland: Aspen, 1987:45.
2. Doolittle KH, Turner RH. Patellofemoral problems following total knee arthroplasty. *Orthop Rev*. 1988; 17:696–702.
3. Lynch AF, Rorabeck CH, Bourne RB. Extensor mechanism complications following total knee arthroplasty. *J Arthroplasty*. 1987; 2:135–140.
4. Siwek CW, Rao JO. Ruptures of the extensor mechanism of the knee joint. *J Bone Joint Surg*. 1981; 63A:932–937.
5. Larsen E, Lund PM. Ruptures of the extensor mechanism of the knee joint. *Clin Orthop*. 1986; 213:150–153.
6. Murzic WJ, Hardaker WT, Goldner JL. Surgical repair of extensor mechanism ruptures of the knee. *Complic Orthop*. 1992; 7:276–279.
7. Huberti HH, Hayes WC, Stone JL, Shybut GT. Force ratios in the quadriceps tendon and ligamentum patellae. *J Orthop Res*. 1984; 2:49–54.
8. Walker LG, Glick H. Bilateral spontaneous quadriceps tendon ruptures. *Orthop Rev*. 1989; 18:867–871.
9. Scuderi C. Ruptures of the quadriceps tendon. *Am J Surg*. 1958; 95:626–634.
10. Scuderi C, Schrey EL. Ruptures of quadriceps tendon; study of 14 tendon ruptures. *Arch Surg*. 1950; 61: 42–54.
11. Rasul AT, Fischer DA. Primary repair of quadriceps tendon ruptures. *Clin Orthop*. 1993:205–207.
12. MacCollum MS, Karpman RR. Complications of the PCA anatomic patella. *Orthopedics*. 1989; 12:1423–1428.
13. Fernandez-Baillo N, Garay EG, Ordonez JM. Rupture of the quadriceps tendon after total knee arthroplasty: a case report. *J Arthroplasty*. 1993:331–333.

CHAPTER 66
Reconstruction of the Extensor Mechanism with an Allograft Following Total Knee Arthroplasty

Robert E. Booth and Frank P. Femino

Extensor mechanism disruption after total knee arthroplasty is a dreaded complication that poses a formidable challenge to even the most accomplished knee surgeon. The problem is multifactorial and spans a spectrum of technical difficulty ranging from simple direct repair of the acute rupture to reconstruction of the chronically deficient extensor mechanism. Attrition of the quadriceps and patellar tendons is prone in soft tissue that is already compromised, especially in patients with chronic renal failure, diabetes mellitus, rheumatoid arthritis, and seronegative arthropathies.[1,2] Infection of the TKA and/or mechanical failure of components, causing sharp or abraded surfaces, may hasten soft tissue failure.

One unique solution to the problem of chronic quadriceps tendon rupture or quadriceps deficiency is reconstruction with the use of an extensor mechanism allograft (Fig. 66.1).[3,4] This is used when primary repair or reconstruction with host tissue is not deemed feasible. As described by Emerson and associates, a fresh-frozen or freeze-dried allograft consisting of quadriceps tendon, patella, patellar tendon, and tibial tubercle is used.

The senior author chooses to use fresh-frozen allograft exclusively and, unlike Emerson, does not resurface the patella provided that there is reasonable conformity with the femoral sulcus. Emerson has had two patellar complications related to resurfacing—one fracture in a patella that had been revised from a metal-backed to an all-polyethylene patellar component and loosening of a cemented all-polyethylene component that required excision. These complications have led him to consider eliminating the patellar prosthesis. The senior author's decision not to resurface the patella reflects the belief that any resection of bone will weaken an already-devascularized patella and may predispose the construct to patellar fracture or component loosening. As discussed by Reuben and colleagues, a resurfaced patella has an increased anterior strain across the remaining patellar bone. Furthermore, pain relief is not an issue in a completely denervated structure. The allograft is first debrided of any muscular remnants. This serves the dual purpose of facilitating a secure junction directly to the strong quadriceps tendon and favoring microbiologic factors by eliminating the antigenic muscle fibers.

The graft is first secured distally by wedging the sculpted tibial tubercle bone block on the allograft into the under-cut tibial key hole in the host bone (Fig. 66.2, interlock of the tibial tubercle bone block with the host bone). The senior author prefers fixation using two #18 cerclage wires as described by Whiteside[6] (Fig. 66.3), securing the distal end with cerclage wires around the stem of the tibial component). It is important to properly position the tubercle. Slight medial placement reduces the Q-angle and improves patellar tracking. The proper depth is also important; depressing the tubercle will increase patellar strain and decrease the mechanical advantage, whereas elevating the tubercle could cause excessive skin tension and wound problems.

Proximally, #5 nonabsorbable suture is used to reattach the quadriceps junction using a modified Krackow running-locking stitch (Fig. 66.4, suturing of the proximal end to the quadriceps tendon). The tension of the quadriceps muscle is adjusted at this point to minimize the amount of extensor lag and to ensure horizontal inclination of the graft and smooth tracking in the trochlea. Intraoperative flexion of approximately 60 degrees is adequate; the remaining flexion returns as the

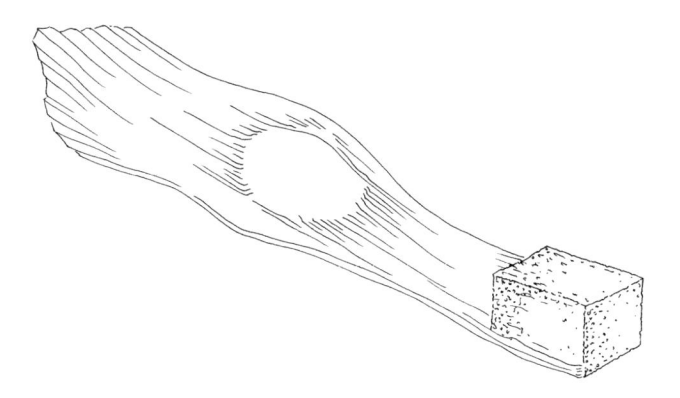

Figure 66.1. The extensor allograft consists of the quadriceps tendon, patella, patella tendon, and tibial tubercle.

retracted quadriceps muscle gradually lengthens over time. It is more critical to prevent extensor lag (measured by the difference between active and passive extension). Minimal debridement of the host soft tissue is performed. This tissue is used to envelope the allograft in an effort to bring vascularity to the donor tissue. This protects the graft from superficial wound healing problems and encourages healing of a strong graft-host interface.

Postoperatively the knee is placed in a well-padded cylinder cast for 6 weeks. Gradually increasing range of motion is then begun in a hinged brace with the goal of 90 degrees at 3 to 6 months. A walking aid is used until adequate quadriceps strength has returned, and the patient is instructed to use the opposite leg for pushing up from a chair and for stair climbing.

Emerson has treated 15 knees out of which nine have greater than 2-year follow-up. Average postop flexion was 106 degrees (80 to 130). There were three

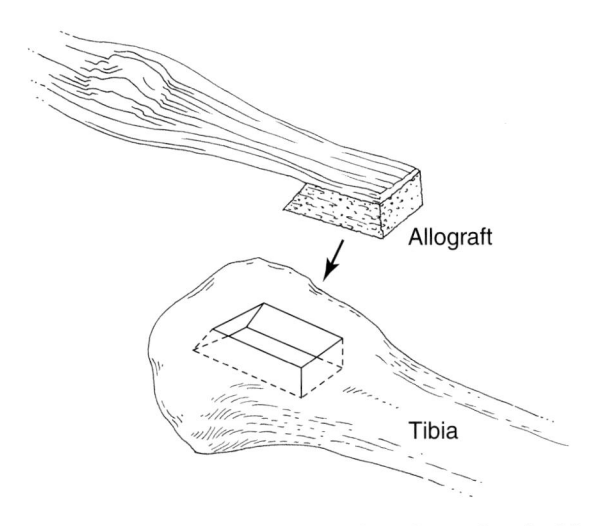

Figure 66.2. The tibial bone block is keyed into the tibial host bone.

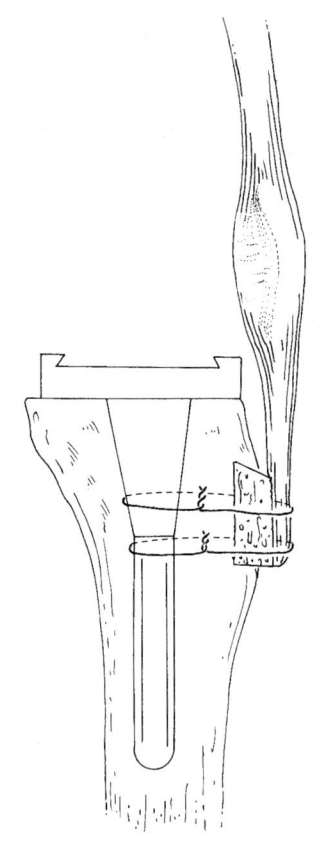

Figure 66.3. The tibial bone block is secured with cerclage wires.

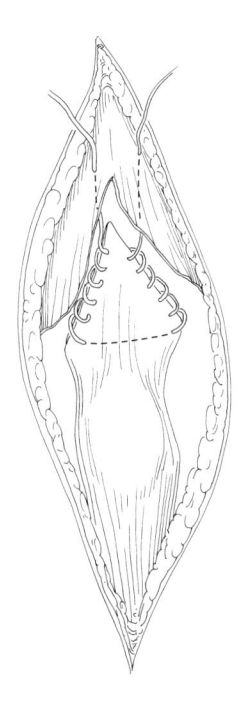

Figure 66.4. The allograft quadriceps tendon is sutured to the myotendinous junction of the host quadriceps tendon with the knee in full extension.

flexion contractures—5, 10, and 20 degrees and three knees with extensor lags: 20, 25, and 40 degrees. The average postoperative knee score was 78 points (60 to 91).

Our results compare favorably with Emerson's. Our group consists of 48 knees, 39 of which have greater than 2-year follow-up. Average postop flexion was 106 degrees (84 to 121). There were 12 flexion contractures at 6 degrees and 44 knees with extensor lags at 8 degrees. The average postoperative knee score was 86 points (74 to 93). There were three recurrent infections, all occurring in previously infected TKAs, which were treated with delayed reimplantation after a spacer block that was treated with irrigation and debridement and suppressive antibiotic therapy. There were no allograft ruptures or dissociations, patellar fractures, or patellar tracking problems.

References

1. Rand JA, Morrey BF, Bryan RS. Patellar tendon rupture following total knee arthroplasty. *Tech Orthop*. 1988; 3:45–48.
2. Walker LG, Glick H. Bilateral spontaneous quadriceps tendon ruptures. *Orthop Rev*. 1989; 18:867–871.
3. Emerson RH, Head WC, Malinin TI. Extensor mechanism reconstruction with an allograft after total knee arthroplasty. *Clin Orthop*. 1990; 303:79–85.
4. Emerson RH, Head WC, Malinin TI. Reconstruction of patellar tendon rupture after total knee arthroplasty with an extensor mechanism allograft. *Clin Orthop*. 1990; 260: 154–161.
5. Reuben JD, McDonald CL, Woodward PL, Hennington LJ. Effect of patella thickness on patella strain following total knee arthroplasty. *J Arthroplasty*. 1991; 6:251–258.
6. Whiteside LA, Ohl MD. Tibial tubercle osteotomy for exposure of the difficult total knee arthroplasty. *Clin Orthop*. 1990; 260:6–9.

CHAPTER 67
Management of Patella Tendon Disruptions in Total Knee Arthroplasty

Giles R. Scuderi and Brian C. De Muth

Extensor mechanism disruptions are an unwelcome complication of primary and especially revision total knee arthroplasty. Management of these disruptions can be extremely challenging, and often fraught with disappointing results. While the previous chapter addressed quadriceps disruptions, this chapter will focus on management of patella tendon disruptions in total knee arthroplasty.

Without question, the optimal method of management for extensor mechanism disruptions in total knee arthroplasty is to avoid them. Even though several types of extensor mechanism repairs will be discussed herein, none can offer results comparable to a repair that is not needed. Therefore, every possible effort should be made to prevent them. This is especially important to bear in mind when planning a TKR for a patient with increased risk for extensor mechanism complications. Those at high risk include patients who are obese, have poor preoperative motion, have had prior surgery about the tibial tubercle or patella tendon, have a connective tissue disorder, or have other metabolic conditions that may compromise their soft tissues.

TIBIAL TUBERCLE AVULSION

Tibial tubercle avulsions are perhaps the most common extensor mechanism disruptions encountered during total knee arthroplasty. Insall has previously described avulsions of the tibial tubercle as *"an intraoperative complication that should be avoided rather than treated."*[1] This point is reinforced by the paucity of documented successes in managing tibial tubercle avulsions once they do occur.[2–5] Therefore, great care should be taken intraoperatively to protect the attachment of the patella tendon to the tibial tubercle.

Three specific preventive measures to avoid this pitfall include:[1]

1. *Protect the tubercle at its insertion site.* Tension from the quadriceps mechanism above can cause the tendon to avulse by tearing across the periosteum, making adequate repair tenuous at best. This can be avoided by bringing the arthrotomy incision for initial exposure medial to the tibial tubercle and then raising a cuff of periosteum up to the tubercle. In tight knees in which exposure is difficult, the reflection of periosteum can be extended laterally with sharp vertical dissection to include up to 40% of the tubercle without significant loss of structural integrity of the extensor mechanism. This creates a "peel" of disection rather than a problematic transverse tear. If the tubercle does begin to avulse, a soft tissue sleeve is preserved that can be later repaired to the medial soft tissue envelope.

2. *Extend proximal exposure when needed.* Several means of enhancing exposure proximally have been described and are reviewed elsewhere in this text. These measures will help to protect the patella tendon attachment distally. The original quadriceps turndown as described by Coonse and Adams[5] has been subsequently modified to become an expansion of a standard medial parapatellar arthrotomy. The proximal apex of the arthrotomy is extended in "inverted-V" fashion by releasing the vastas lateralis distally and laterally until the patella can be adequately everted. The limitation of this exposure approach is the prolonged postoperative rehabilitation that must be observed. The "quadriceps snip" as described by Insall[1] is a more versatile modification that simply extends the quadriceps tendon incision proximally and laterally at an oblique angle. This simple technique is suf-

ficient the majority of the time to allow for adequate exposure. In those instances when the patellar tendon insertion is still under considerable tension, the quadriceps snip can be combined with a lateral retinacular release to afford an even greater exposure. The quadriceps snip release is repaired with the arthrotomy at wound closure. The major advantage of the quadriceps snip is that it allows for immediate motion postoperatively and avoids the problems of extensor lag often seen with the Coonse-Adams release.[1]

3. *Osteotomize the tibial tubercle if necessary.* If all previous measures to enhance exposure still do not afford adequate exposure, traumatic avulsion can still be avoided. It is far better to raise the tibial tubercle with a large wedge of tibial bone to allow for reattachment with wires or screws. Although some authors have reported excellent results with this method,[6,7] others have reported complications at a disappointingly high frequency.[8] Familiarity with the proper technique avoids complication.

RUPTURE OF THE PATELLAR TENDON

Rupture of the patellar tendon after total knee replacement is a rare and typically devastating problem (Fig. 67.1). Unfortunately, the results of several methods of acute repair are almost uniformly poor.[2–4,9]

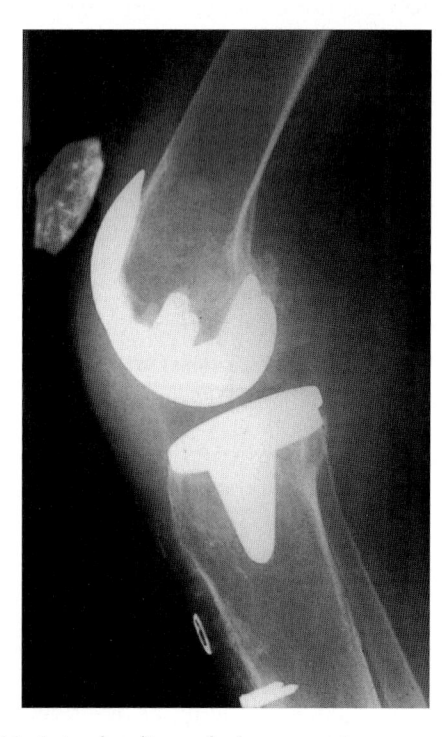

Figure 67.1. Lateral radiograph demonstrating a rupture of the patellar tendon, which is readily identified by the high riding patella.

Numerous theories have been postulated to explain the etiology of late rupture of the patellar tendon following TKA. As mentioned previously, improper surgical technique that malaligns the knee or the position of any single component can play a contributory role. Some authors have found its occurrence more common in knees with limited motion.[10,11] Others have suggested impingement of the prosthesis on the patella tendon to blame.[12] Still others believe that compromise of the vascular supply to the patellar tendon is a critical component of its failure.[12,13]

The time of occurrence of post-arthroplasty patellar tendon rupture has been debated in the literature. In the series reported by Cambi and Engh,[10] six of eight ruptures occurred intraoperatively or soon afterwards. In contrast, Gustillo and Thompson found most of the patellar tendon ruptures in their series to occur later.[4] Regardless of when the disruption occurs, no difference in management has been suggested to be time dependent.

Several repair techniques for patellar tendon disruption have been described. However, because the numbers in all post-arthroplasty case series have been low, no single technique can be considered a gold standard.

Predictably disappointing results have been noted with prolonged cast or brace immobilization alone as the sole means of management. This method of treatment may be adequate for partial tears, but the definitive diagnosis of an incomplete lesion is often difficult and not readily recognized. Therefore, open surgical repair is the preferred treatment. Reconstruction options include direct surgical repair, local autologous graft, distant autologous graft, synthetic graft, or various types of allograft.

Complete acute tendon tears may be managed with direct repair, but will most likely need some method of augmentation. In order to maximize the effectiveness of the repair and minimize ensuing stiffness, the repair should be carried out as soon as possible. If the tear occurs in the mid portion of the tendon, an end-to-end repair technique may be employed. Several means of enhancing the suture fixation during direct repair have been described including a Bunnell suture weave,[7] or a tendon grabbing stitch. The tendon should be repaired with nonabsorbable suture materials and, if present, the paratenon closed with absorbable sutures. Unfortunately, mid-tendon tears are less common than tears near the tendon origin or insertion. These later injuries are far more difficult to treat.

Bony avulsion or patellar tendon tears at the inferior pole of the patella are best managed by a traditional Bunnell-type repair with sutures passed through drill holes at the apex of the patella. It is important to reproduce the original length of the patella tendon when tensioning the sutures. Patella position can be ensured by comparing measurement of tendon length or position on a lateral radiograph with the opposite knee. Patellar baja must be avoided. Many authors also recommend a reinforcing cerclage suture encircling the tibial tubercle and the quadriceps tendon to protect the repair postoperatively. It would be our preference to use a #5 nonabsorbable suture rather than a metallic wire. Postoperative rehabilitation protocols vary. Typically, however, the knee is kept in full extension for 4 to 8 weeks with quadriceps setting exercise begun immediately. After allowing adequate time for soft tissue healing (approximately 6 weeks), the knee is started on a progressive range-of-motion and strengthening program. Unrestricted weight-bearing and flexion activities are permitted at about 12 weeks.

Tendon tears in close proximity to the tibial tubercle insertion pose a far greater repair challenge. A similar scenario occurs when the integrity of the distal remains of the patellar tendon is inadequate for a secure repair. In these clinical settings, the surgeon must choose between one of several reconstructive procedures. Unfortunately, large clinical series that establish the efficacy of any one technique do not exist.

One of the earliest described repair techniques for a patellar tendon-deficient knee was described by Kelikian[14] (Fig. 67.2). He utilized the semitendinosus tendon by harvesting the proximal extent of the tendon up to the musculotendinous junction while leaving the distal insertion site intact. The freed proximal end of the tendon was then routed through holes drilled in the tibial tubercle and the patella before being secured back onto itself near its insertion site. If there is insufficient length, the gracilis tendon can also be harvested, detached, and sutured to the semitendinosis tendon. Ecker and associates[15] described a modification of this technique employing skeletal traction with a Steinmann pin through the superior pole of the patella to regain length of the shortened tendon. However, this technique is not recommended when a total knee replacement is present.

A modification of the Kelikian technique was reported by Cadambi and Engh[10] (Fig. 67.2). In a series of seven patients with a patellar tendon rupture following total knee replacement, the semitendinosus tendon was routed along the border of the remnant of the patellar tendon and then through a transverse hole in the inferior pole of the patella, anterior to the patellar implant-bone interface. In two of their seven patients, the repair was augmented by harvesting the gracilis tendon and passing it through the patella drill hole as well. Postoperatively, weight-bearing was begun within 48 hours in a knee immobilizer or cast. Knee motion was then initiated at 6 weeks and progressed slowly over the next 10 weeks in a hinged knee brace. They reported that quadriceps strength and knee motion was restored in all patients.

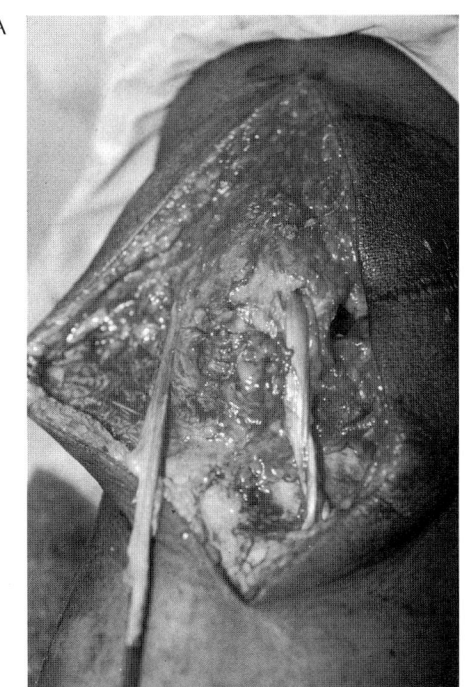

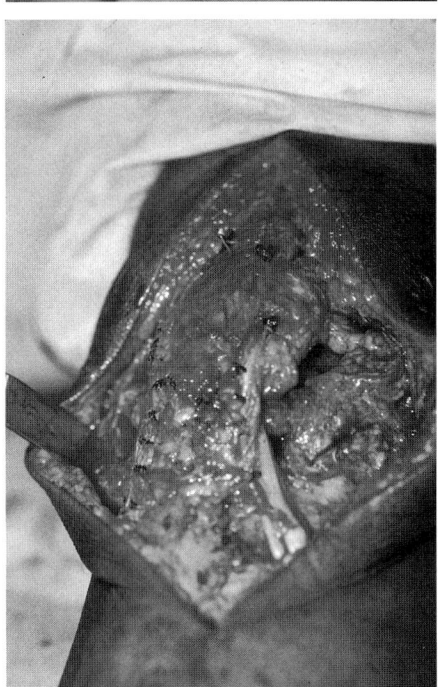

Figure 67.2. The semitendinosis tendon is passed through a transverse drill hole in the patella (A) and is sutured in place along the border of the patellar tendon (B).

Other authors have reported the successful use of allografts to manage disruptions of the extensor mechanism. Emerson and associates[3] have published on the successful use of an extensor mechanism allograft in a series of 15 patients with a rupture of the patella tendon in association with a total knee arthroplasty. The allograft consisted of the tibial tubercle, patellar tendon, patella, and quadriceps tendon that was freeze-dried or fresh-frozen. The graft was secured to the tibia with two screws distally and by nonabsorbable suture attachment to native quadriceps tendon proximally. Motion was begun postoperatively as soon as the wound was sealed limiting flexion to 60 degrees in a hinged knee brace for the first 6 weeks, and progressed to 90 degrees by the end of the second 6 weeks. The authors reported that all but three patients received full active extension, with 66% of patients having no appreciable extensor lag.

More recently, Zanotti and colleagues[16] have reported successful treatment of a patellar tendon-deficient knee in a single patient with the use of a bone-patellar tendon-bone allograft. Their technique employed an irradiated, freeze-dried patellar-patellar tendon-proximal tibial allograft from a fresh cadaver. The host patella was prepared to accept the graft by creating a bone-to-bone interference fit further secured by circumferential sutures. The host tibia was prepared to accept the bone block of the graft, then tibial fixation was secured with a cortical screw. The repair was protected postoperatively in a cast for 3 months, and progressed to ambulation with a KAFO orthosis. They reported the graft to be healed with full active extension at 2-year follow-up.

Our current technique for reconstruction of chronic tears of the patellar tendon utilizes fresh-frozen extensor mechanism allograft that includes the tibial tubercle, patellar tendon, patella, and quadriceps tendon (Fig. 67.3). This is our preference because of the substantial amount of tissue that is available. Because disruptions of the extensor mechanism can lead to flexion instability, it is desirable to use a posterior-stabilized prosthesis. If there is any doubt about stability, then the arthroplasty should be revised to a constrained prosthesis. This may require revision of all the components. Finally, in planning the reconstruction, consideration must be given to the skin and surrounding soft tissues. It is not

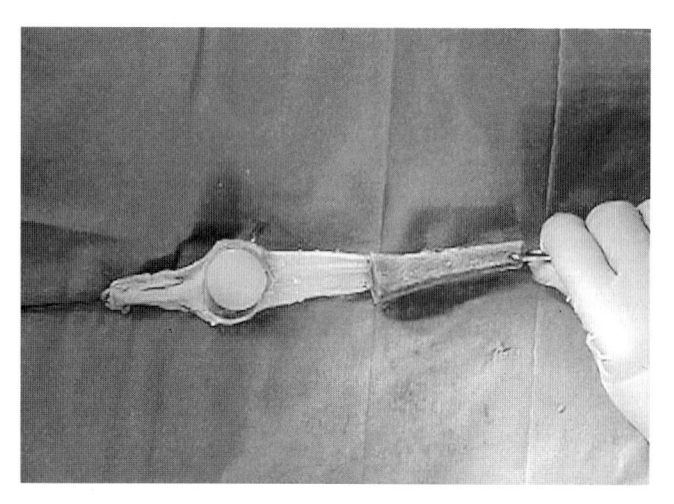

Figure 67.3. The extensor mechanism allograft.

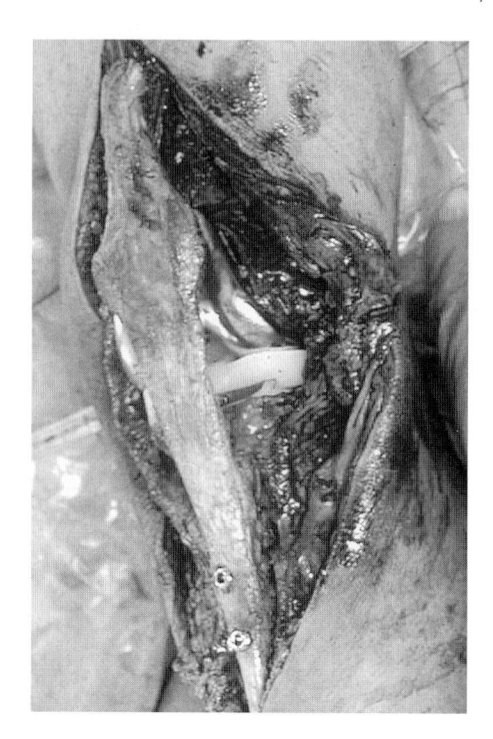

Figure 67.4. The extensor allograft in place.

unusual to be referred a case for allograft reconstruction that has had several prior attempts at repair. Because the skin may be adherent or there may be multiple scars, soft tissue expanders have been shown to be helpful, and should be considered.[12] This is also important because the tibial tubercle allograft does add bulk to the proximal tibia making closure difficult.

TECHNIQUE

Following exposure of the knee, it is preferred to maintain the residual patellar tendon and surrounding fibrous tissue, because this provides a vascular tissue layer for later closure over the allograft. If the femoral and tibial components require revision, it is best to perform this step prior to placement of the allograft. Any hardware about the tibial tubercle should be removed. Whether to resurface the patella allograft remains debatable. It is our current preference not to resurface the patella.

The tibia is prepared by creating a trough about 60 to 80 mm long, which is fashioned along the tibial tubercle and tibial crest. The trough is created by removing the anterior cortex and compressing the underlying cancellous bone. Distally the osteotomy should be oblique in order to reduce the stress riser. Additionally, if possible, a rim of cortical bone should be maintained beneath the tibial component. The allograft then can be "keyed" into place (Fig. 67.4).

At this point, the patella height needs to be determined in order to set the position of the tibial bone graft. With

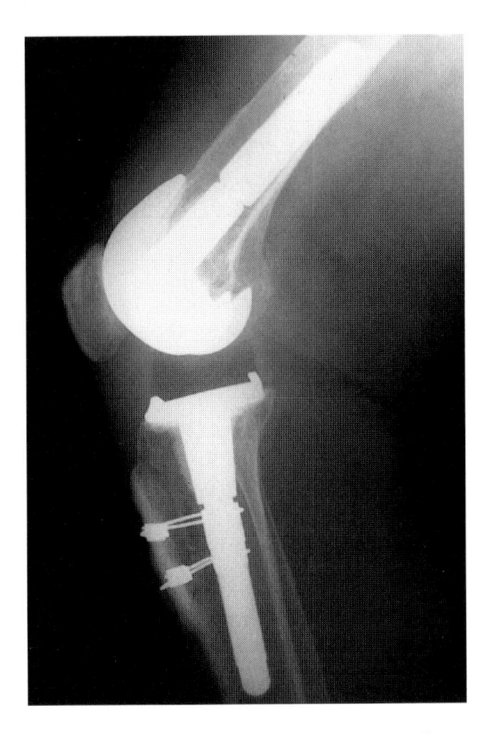

Figure 67.5. Postoperative radiograph showing the extensor allograft in place. Note the double patella.

the knee in full extension, the patella should sit over the anterior flange of the femoral component and the inferior border of the patella approximately 1 cm above the joint line. Once the patella position is selected, the tibial bone graft is secured either with two bicortical screws or two cerclage wires. If the tibial component is being revised, the cerclage wires should be passed through drill holes in the tibial diaphysis and placed posterior to the tibial stem. With a stem extension in place, it may be difficult to set the screws or pass the wires.

The allograft quadriceps tendon is then passed through a transverse slit in the host quadriceps tendon. With the knee in full extension, the quadriceps tendon allograft is secured to the quadriceps expansion with multiple nonabsorbable sutures. The original patella is thinned to a wafer, or cortical shell. A patellectomy is not performed because the residual patella bone facilitates healing and serves as a useful landmark. It usually sits over the patella allograft and makes an interesting postoperative radiograph because two patellae can be seen (Fig. 67.5).

At this point, the range of motion and tension are checked. The range of motion is usually 45 to 60 degrees of flexion, and if properly oriented, the patella tracks centrally without a tilt. While the medial quadriceps retinaculum is sutured to the medial margin of the allograft, the lateral retinacular release is left open. The knee is then closed in a routine fashion and immobilized in extension with a cast or brace for 6 weeks. During this time the patient is allowed to ambulate full weight-bearing and encouraged to practice quadriceps setting exercises. After 6 weeks, the knee is braced and gradual range-of-motion exercises are initiated. The brace is discontinued when there is radiographic evidence that the tibial bone graft is healed, and the quadriceps muscle power is difficult to support the leg.

Our clinical experience with this reconstruction technique includes six cases of extensor mechanism allografts for chronic rupture of the patellar tendon. Although four patients have full active extension, there are two patients who have an extensor lag less than 10 degrees. The average knee flexion is 90 degrees. All six patients are ambulating independently.

References

1. Insall JN, Haas SB. Complications of total knee arthroplasty, In: Insall JN. *Surgery of the Knee*. New York: Churchill Livingstone; 1993: 891–934.
2. Doolittle KH, Turner RH. Patellofemoral problems following total knee arthroplasty. *Orthop Rev*. 1988; 17:696–671.
3. Emerson RH, Head WC, Manlinin TI. Extensor mechanism reconstruction with an allograft after total knee arthroplasty. *Clin Orthop*. 1994; 303:79–85.
4. Gustillo RB, Thompson R. Quadriceps and patellar tendon ruptures following total knee arthroplasty. In: Rand JA, Dorr LD, eds. *Total Arthroplasty of the Knee*. Rockville, Maryland: 1987: 41–47.
5. Coonse K, Adams JD. A new operative approach to the knee joint. *Surg Gynecol Obstet*. 1943; 77:344–347.
6. MacCollum RF, Karpman RR. Complications of the PCA anatomica patella. *Orthopedics*. 1989; 12:1423–1429.
7. Sewik CW, Rao JO. Ruptures of the extensor mechanism of the knee joint. *J Bone Joint Surg*. 1981; 63A:932–937.
8. Whiteside LA, Ohl MD. Tibial tubercle osteotomy for exposure of the difficult total knee arthroplasty. *Clin Orthop*. 1990; 260:6–9.
9. Matava M. Patella tendon ruptures. *J Am Acad Orthop Surg*. 1996; 4:287–296.
10. Cadambi A, Engh GA. Use of a semitendinosus autogenous graft for rupture of the patellar ligament after total knee arthroplasty. *J Bone Joint Surg*. 1992; 74A:974–979.
11. Rand JA, Morrey BF, Bryan RS. Patella tendon ruptures after total knee arthroplasty. *Clin Orthop*. 1989; 224:233.
12. Gold DA, Scott WN. Soft tissue expansion prior to arthroplasty in the multiply-operated knee. A new method of preventing catastrophic skin problems. *J Arthroplasty*. 1996; 11(5):512–21.
13. Laskin RS. Total condylar knee replacement in rheumatoid arthritis. *J Bone Joint Surg*. 1981; 69A:29.
14. Kelikian H, Riashi E, Gleason J. Restoration of quadriceps function in neglected tear of the patella tendon. *Surg Gynecol Obstet*. 1957; 104:200–204.
15. Ecker ML, Lotke PA, Glazer RM. Late reconstruction of the patella tendon. *J Bone Joint Surg*. 1979; 61A:884–886.
16. Zanotti RM, Freidberg AA, Mathews LS. Use of patellar allograft to reconstruct a patellar tendon-deficient knee after total joint arthroplasty. *J Arthroplasty*. 1995; 10(3):271–274.

CHAPTER 68
Revision of Loose Patellar Components

Adolph V. Lombardi, Jr, Thomas H. Mallory, and Stephen M. Herrington

Total knee arthroplasty (TKA) has recently become an extremely reliable and reproducible procedure. Innovations in treatment, application, instrumentation, and materials technology have all contributed to the success of this procedure. Numerous publications have documented excellent long-term results of total knee arthroplasty.[1-6]

The orthopedic community has used the mistakes of the past as a foundation for current improvements in the state of the art of total knee arthroplasty. Historically, concern existed with respect to infection and tibial fixation.[2,4,7-9] Prophylactic antibiotics, clean air operating rooms, and personal isolation suits have all been implemented to reduce the incidence of infection. Experience with numerous arthroplasties has revealed that alignment, coverage of the proximal tibia, implant design, and technique of implantation are all important factors in the success of tibial component fixation. Surgeons in conjunction with engineers continue to seek methods of improving component fixation. With decreasing incidence of infection and tibial loosening, the focus of concern is shifting to the patellofemoral articulation. This shifting of focus to the patellofemoral joint is indicative of a more precise refinement of the total knee arthroplasty technique, rather than a new problem.

PATELLOFEMORAL COMPLICATIONS

A review of the current literature reveals that the patellofemoral articulation is the primary source of complications in total knee arthroplasty.[5,10-14] There are a myriad of complications associated with patellofemoral articulation. These include patellar subluxation,[10,15-17] pain,[18] patellar clunk syndrome,[19-22] patellar fracture,[10,16,23-28] patellar polyethylene wear or dissociation from metal backing,[29-31] fracture of the patellar implant,[11] patellar impingement with the posterior-stabilized tibial eminence,[32] osteonecrosis,[28,33] quadriceps and/or patellar tendon rupture,[16,34] and patellar loosening.[11,24,33,35]

Healy and associates, in an effort to correlate implant design and patient risk factors associated with patellofemoral complications, reviewed the results of 211 total knee arthroplasties. They noted patellofemoral complications in 27 knees (12.8%). Osteoarthritis, obesity, metal-backed patellar implants, and patellar components implanted without cement were associated with increased incidence of patellofemoral complications. Cemented all-polyethylene patellar components demonstrated the lowest rate of patellofemoral complications.[14]

The most common patellofemoral complication is patellar subluxation or dislocation, which can be the result of a number of different factors or combination of factors. These factors include internal rotation of the femoral component, medial displacement of the femoral component,[36] internal rotation of the tibial component,[37] lateral or superior displacement of the patellar component,[19,38] under-resection of the patella,[39] or a contracted lateral retinaculum.[33,40] In addition to these technique-related factors, a number of factors inherent within the femoral, tibial, and patellar components exist. Implant design issues, such as congruency of the patellofemoral articulation, improper transition from the trochlear groove to the condyle or impingement with a posterior-stabilizing eminence on the tibial component can have an adverse effect on patellofemoral tracking.[12,32]

DETERMINING THE NEED FOR SURGICAL INTERVENTION

Correction of the patellofemoral complication may not always require surgical intervention. In the case of periprosthetic patellar fracture, integrity of the extensor mechanism, status of fixation of the patellar component and the degree of displacement of the fracture fragments are all considered in determining the need for surgical management. Patients with intact extensor mechanisms, stable patellar component fixation, and minimal displacement of fracture fragments can be managed nonsurgically.[41] Patellar subluxation or dislocation can initially be managed nonsurgically with physiotherapy in an effort to enhance the strength of the vastus medialis obliquus. If the patient fails conservative management, then surgical intervention is recommended. Certain patellofemoral complications, such as patellar polyethylene wear or dissociation or patellar loosening, cannot be managed conservatively, and therefore, require surgical attention. If surgical intervention is deemed necessary, preoperative planning is imperative because a number of different situations can occur.

PREOPERATIVE PLANNING

Because of the many complications associated with patellofemoral articulation in TKA, a systematic approach to patellar revision is useful. Although the management of extensor mechanism dysfunction is by no means a "cookbook" approach, some general guidelines can be helpful in ensuring a positive outcome. Preoperative planning is extremely critical to the successful performance of patellar revision. Defining the etiological mechanism of the patellofemoral complication is important because it will assist the surgeon in rendering the appropriate treatment.

In planning a patellar revision, an appropriate inventory of patellar components is required. A variety of peg options exist, such as a standard single-peg option, a large single-peg option, and a three-peg option. Additionally, the surgeon must determine whether a "sombrero" versus a dome-shaped, or circular versus ovoid polyethylene component should be utilized. The surgeon should identify the existing components because of the possible congruency issues with the trochlear groove. A femoral component that is designed to articulate with a sombrero patellar implant may not have adequate congruency with a dome patellar component. Differences exist between dome patellar implants from various manufacturers. The radius of the dome may be smaller or larger than the corresponding trochlear groove in the femoral component. This could result in decreased contact area with a concomitant increase in contact stresses, because the contact area would be diminished to either one-point or two-point contact. This should not be interpreted as indicating that at the time of total knee revision arthroplasty, the patella must always be revised. A well-fixed patellar implant with minimal wear may be better left in situ rather than attempting revision of the patellar implant. If the surgeon elects to retain the previously implanted patellar component, close attention should be paid to patellofemoral tracking and specifically the transition from the trochlear groove to the condyles. This area of the patellofemoral track should be checked to ensure that a smooth transition takes place. The detrimental effects of incongruency of the patellofemoral articulation are wear and deformation of the patellar component or possible instability.

At the time of total knee revision arthroplasty, it is the primary author's preference to revise all metal-backed patellar components despite adequate fixation and minimal wear, because historically these components have demonstrated failure secondary to polyethylene wear or dissociation.[29,30,42] Patellar polyethylene wear or dissociation from the metal-backing or polyethylene wear-through generally leads to catastrophic failure of the arthroplasty because abrasion of the femoral component occurs with concomitant debris generation and ultimately osteolysis. Therefore, in the preoperative planning for revision of a patellar component for patellar polyethylene with wear or dissociation, a surgeon should be prepared for a complete total knee revision arthroplasty. A system that incorporates a full array of stems and augments and various degrees of constraint may be required depending on the status of the joint at the time of revision arthroplasty.[43,44]

Preoperative roentgenographs (lateral and merchant views) may be helpful in determining the amount of bone present. According to Reuben and colleagues, patellar strain is significantly increased in patellae with a bony thickness less than 15 mm.[45] Because of this additional concern, the surgeon should advise the patient preoperatively that it may be technically impossible to resurface the patella if sufficient bone stock is not available. It is better to leave the patella unresurfaced if tenuous fixation of the patella is the best that can be accomplished by revision.[46]

SURGICAL APPROACH

Multiple surgical interventions about the knee may compromise the arterial circulation to the skin and subcutaneous tissues. Devascularization of the patella may also occur as a result of interruption of the geniculate arterial circulation by the medial parapatellar approach in conjunction with a lateral retinacular release.[47] As in any revision total knee arthroplasty, the surgeon performing patellar revision must evaluate previous skin incisions about the knee. The surgeon should utilize or incorporate previous skin incisions into the proposed surgical approach.

A formidable challenge in patellofemoral procedures is the stiff knee undergoing patellar revision. Generally, the standard medial parapatellar arthrotomy will accommodate most patellar revisions. However, in the case of contracture of the extensor mechanism, the surgeon may need to consider one of the following approaches—the Coonse-Adams V-Y quadricepsplasty,[48,49] the rectus snip procedure,[50] or the tibial tubercle osteotomy[51] (Fig. 68.1). In revision of the stiff knee total knee arthroplasty, it has been the primary author's preference to begin with a standard medial parapatellar arthrotomy. Exposure is facilitated by extending the incision proximally and tethering slightly the medial insertion of the patellar tendon. Scar excision must be meticulous and thorough. Peripatellar scar, scar within the lateral retinaculum, retropatellar scarring, and scarred fibrous attachment to the proximal lateral resected tibial plateau should be carefully removed and will facilitate mobilization of the extensor mechanism (Fig. 68.2). If exposure continues to be difficult and there is an inability to evert the patella, it is the primary author's preference to use the rectus snip. Occasionally, this must be converted to a V-Y quadricepsplasty. Once the patella is everted, the circumferential border of the patella is identified (Fig. 68.3).

EVALUATION OF EXISTING COMPONENTS

When adequate exposure is attained, the surgeon must begin to evaluate the integrity of all of the total knee components. It is important to note that merely focusing on the patella could be erroneous and lead to recurrent failure of the patellar revision. One does not necessarily have to revise the patellar component in order to correct a patellar tracking problem. In the case of malpositioned tibial or femoral components, patellar revision may not be required, even if slight incongruency exists between the femur and patella.

When evaluating the patella, the thickness, position, and stability of the implant must be assessed. Superior overhang of the patellar component may predispose the patient to patellar clunk syndrome. If patellar clunk syndrome is present, not only will the surgeon need to excise the fibrous nodule, but patellar revision may also be required because of the superior position of the implant.[19] If patellar tilt is evident, the patellar component should be revised. The resection should be corrected to avoid replication of patellar tilt.

When evaluating the femoral component, the anteroposterior and mediolateral positioning of the device

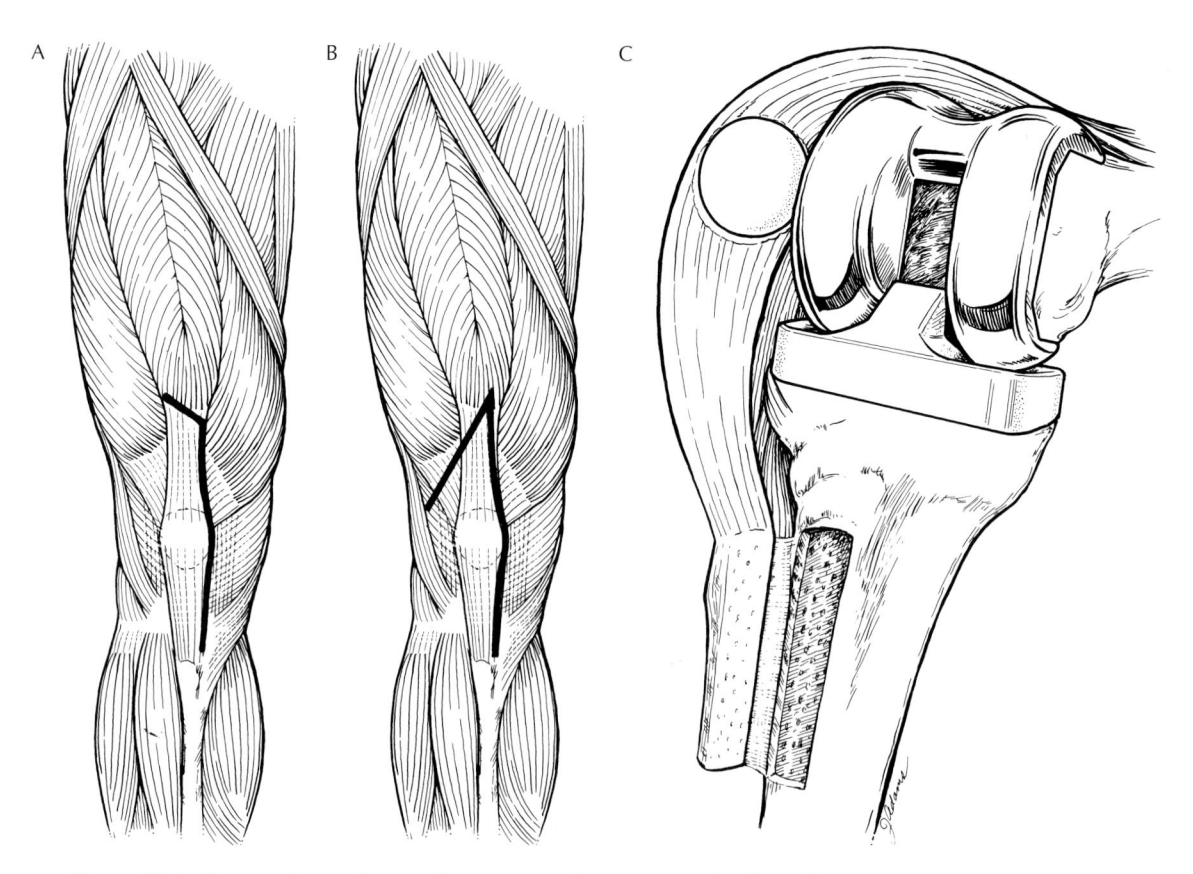

Figure 68.1. Commonly used extensile exposures for revision of stiff total knee arthroplasties. (A) Rectus snip; (B) Coonse-Adams V-Y quadricepsplasty; and (C) tibial tubercle osteotomy.

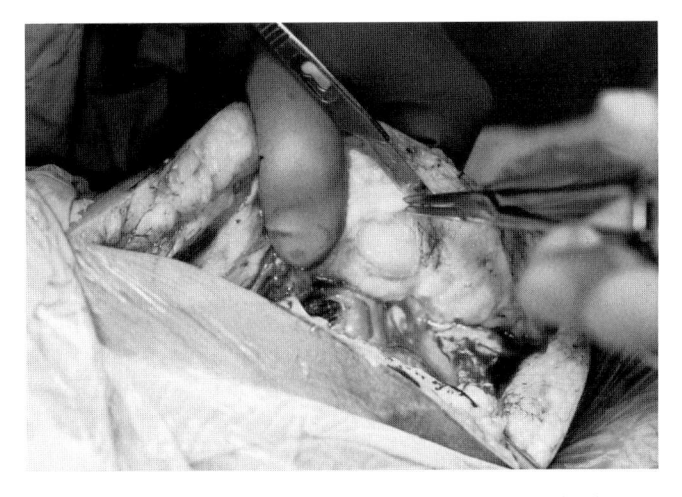

Figure 68.2. Meticulous and complete scar excision facilitates eversion of the patella.

must be considered. If the femoral component is shifted anteriorly, overstuffing of the patellofemoral joint can occur. If the femoral component is shifted too far medially, the patella is forced to move medially, which increases the Q-angle. This increase in the Q-angle predisposes the patellar component to higher stresses on the lateral aspect of the patellar implant, which increases the probability for further patellar complications. Subluxation and/or dislocation could occur if the patella is unable to shift medially. Rotational errors in the placement of the femoral component can also have an effect on the performance of the patellofemoral articulation. If the femoral component is internally rotated, the patella is again shifted medially. The surgeon must therefore be aware that anterior displacement, medial displacement, and internal rotation of the femoral component tend to negatively affect the patellar tracking.[36]

The tibial component must be evaluated for position and rotation. It is especially important to realize the impact of internal rotation of the tibial component on the patellofemoral joint. Internal rotation of the tibial component causes a subsequent external rotation of the tibia, which increases the Q-angle.[37] As stated previously, increases in the Q-angle result in higher stresses on the lateral aspect of the patellar component, which could lead to patellar-tracking problems.

When evaluation of the components individually is complete, the surgeon should evaluate the knee as a system of interacting components and proceed with revision total knee arthroplasty as dictated by this complete evaluation.

REVISION OF THE ALL-POLYETHYLENE PATELLAR COMPONENT

The revision of an all-polyethylene patellar component is straightforward. If the patellar component is grossly loose, removal of the prosthesis can be facilitated with a one-fourth or one-half inch thin osteotome (Fig. 68.4). On the other hand, the reciprocating or oscillating saw can be used to violate the cement-implant interface. The surgeon cuts across the implant-cement interface, without regard for the existing peg or pegs. The primary author has found that the Ultra-Drive thin osteotome (Biomet, Warsaw, Indiana) can also be beneficial to disrupt the cement-implant interface. What remains is a layer of cement on the patella that can easily be removed with an osteotome or oscillating saw. The peg and associated polymethylmethacrylate (PMMA) are removed with a burr.

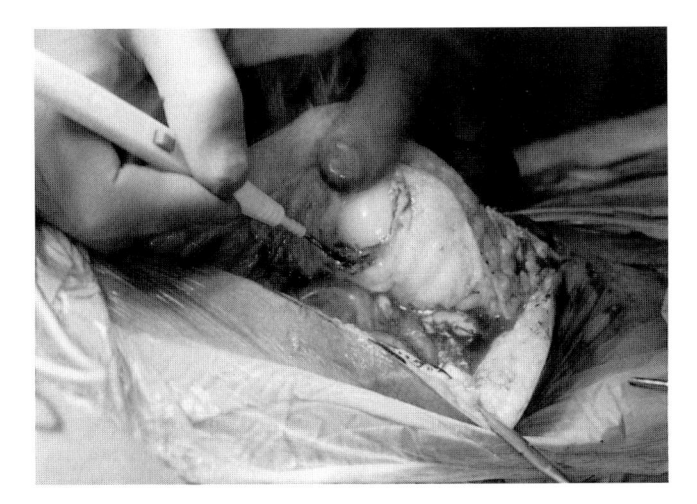

Figure 68.3. Identification of the circumferential border of the patella.

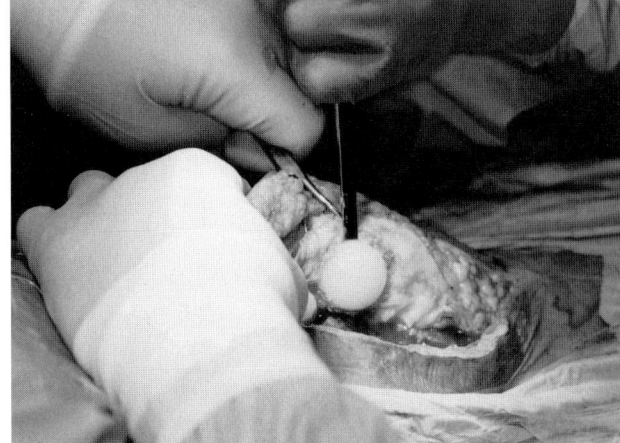

Figure 68.4. Violation of the cement-implant interface with an osteotome.

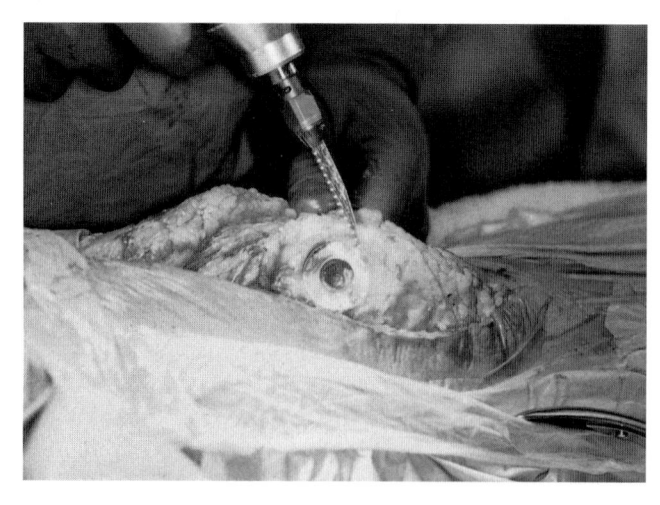

Figure 68.5. Violation of the cement-implant interface with a reciprocating saw.

REVISION OF THE METAL-BACKED PATELLAR IMPLANT

An interesting approach to the revision of metal-backed patellar implants is the approach used by Dennis. A diamond-edged circular saw is used to disrupt the bone-implant interface and the solid pegs from the back of the patellar component. A pencil tip drill is then used to disrupt the peg-bone interface. The procedure is meticulously performed with the use of sponges to prevent the metal debris from entering the joint space. A pulsatile lavage is also used to remove any debris that may have entered into the joint space.^{52}

The primary author has found that a reciprocating saw can be used to revise a metal-backed patellar component. Thin blades can be negotiated around the pegs of the implant to disrupt the cement-implant interface in order to free the patellar implant from the bone (Fig. 68.5).

EVALUATION OF THE REMAINING BONE STOCK

Upon complete removal of the implant and PMMA (if present), the surgeon must assess the patellar bone remaining because this will dictate the type of prosthesis that will be utilized. The thickness of the remaining bone is critical because strains are greatly increased in patellae that are less than 15 mm in overall bony thickness.^{45} It is the primary author's preference not to resurface those patellae that are less than 12 mm thick. If anterior penetration of the patella by the patellar peg is a concern, the implant should be modified by shortening the height of the peg (Fig. 68.6).

Nonresurfacing may be the best option if the existing bone stock cannot support implantation. Use of a single large peg or a three-peg patella will require careful evaluation of the remaining bone in order to minimize the possibility of fracture of the patella. One should always be aware of the placement of the pegs, and their impact

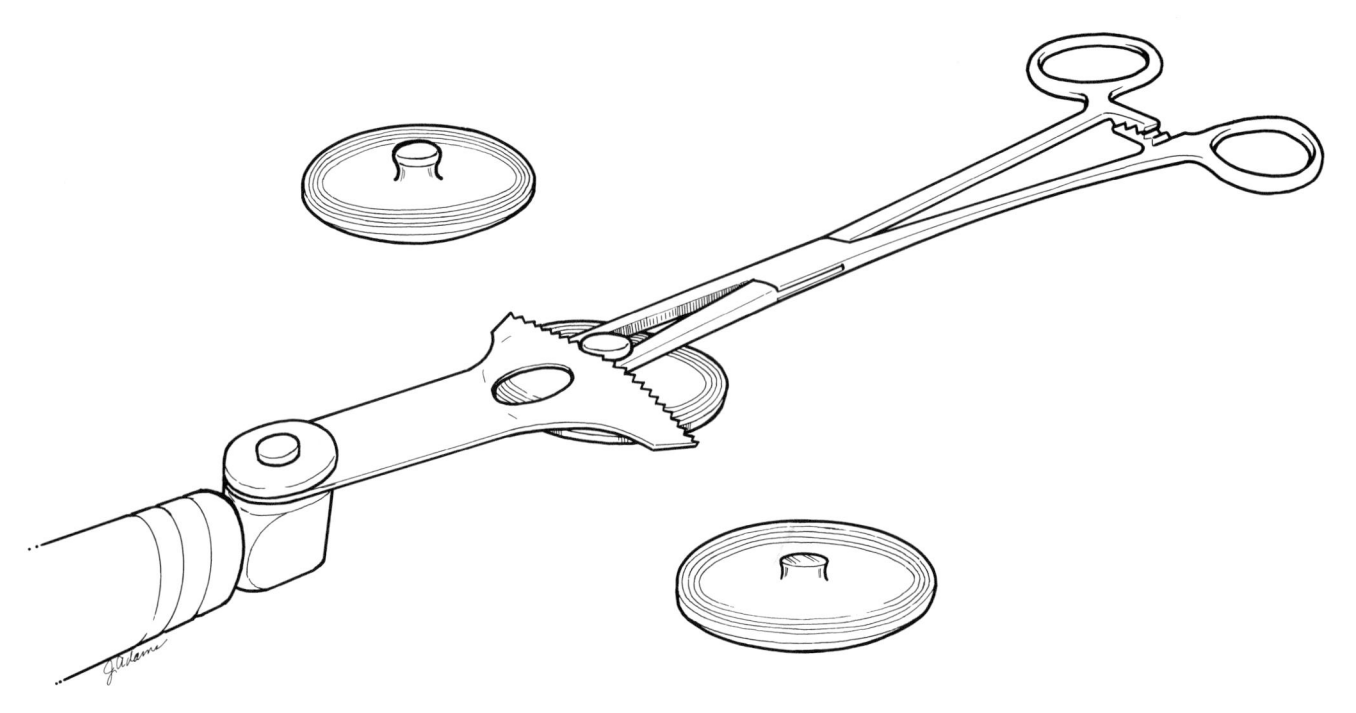

Figure 68.6. Trimming of the patellar peg with a kocher and an oscillating saw.

on the existing bone stock. A three-peg patellar component removes bone closer to the periphery of the patella. The convex shape of the anterior aspect of the patella translates to less patellar thickness at the periphery, which is the location of the pegs in a three-peg patellar component. To avoid disruption of the anterior cortex, a large single-peg patellar component may represent a more appropriate option (Fig. 68.7).

IMPLANTATION

A standard mode of implantation is utilized. Pulsatile lavage is used in conjunction with suction drying to expose the trabecular bony structure. The PMMA is mixed and pressurized into the trabeculae. The component is seated and clamped in place to ensure adequate pressurization of the PMMA. Once cured, the clamp is removed and patellar tracking is evaluated using the "no-thumbs" test.[53] Lateral release and/or proximal realignment of the extensor mechanism, as described by Insall and associates, is used as dictated by the patellofemoral tracking.[15,54]

POSTOPERATIVE TREATMENT

The postoperative regimen is the same as that of a standard primary knee arthroplasty, unless a rectus snip, V-Y quadricepsplasty, or tibial tubercle osteotomy was performed. There is variability among surgeons in the postoperative treatment of patients who have required extensile measures for exposure. Emerson reports that if a tibial tubercle osteotomy is performed, the patient should be fitted with a hinged knee brace with motion allowed up to 60 degrees for the first 6 weeks and increased to 90 degrees during the second 6 weeks.[55] Whiteside suggests that with a tibial tubercle osteotomy, the patient can be treated with a primary postoperative protocol with full range of motion and weight-bearing.[51] It is the preference of the primary author to use either a rectus snip or a V-Y quadricepsplasty, and to immobilize the patient for 2 to 3 weeks immediately postoperatively in full extension. Gentle flexion is commenced following this period of immobilization and gradually increased over the ensuing 6 to 8 weeks.

THE PRIMARY AUTHOR'S CLINICAL EXPERIENCE WITH PATELLOFEMORAL REVISIONS

The primary author follows a systematic approach in dealing with patellar revisions. Figure 68.8 illustrates the algorithm used when evaluating the type of implant that will be utilized to perform the revision. Note that this algorithm is used as a guideline only. The multivariate process of patellar revision can never be sufficiently described by an all-encompassing algorithm.

In a retrospective analysis of 104 total knee revision procedures performed from November 1993 to September 1996, the primary author managed patellar revisions using the previously described algorithm. The implant used most often was the standard single-peg patellar implant. The standard peg patellar implant was used in 38 (36.5%) of the cases. In 29 (27.9%) of the cases, the primary author chose to leave the patella unresurfaced. Three-peg patellar implants were used in 19 (18.3%) of the cases. In 10 (9.6%) of the cases, the existing patellar component was left intact. In the remaining 8 (7.7%) of the cases, a large single-peg patellar implant was used. Reviewing this revision TKA series, 38 patients are 2 years post-op. Of these 38 patients, none have been revised for patellofemoral complications.

CONCLUSIONS

The issues, approach, and technique regarding patellar revision have been presented. Even though patellar complications are a definite clinical problem, many factors causing patellofemoral complications have been determined, which should aid in their reduction. When revising the patellar component, one must be diligent in preoperative planning in order to adequately determine the etiology of the patellofemoral complication. The factors responsible for the specific patellofemoral complication can then be adequately addressed.

A systematic approach to the revision of the patellar component has been described. A system that allows the use of several different types of patellar components can be very beneficial. One must completely understand the total knee arthroplasty that has been used so that an intraoperative determination can be made regarding bone stock, interaction with the femoral component, and overall patellar tracking.

It is hoped that the information presented is used as a guideline, or even as a basis for further discussion.

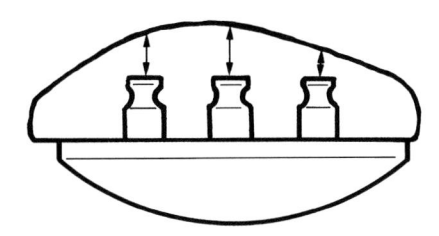

Figure 68.7. Representation of the peripheral placement of pegs in a three-peg patellar implant. Note the peripheral placement of the pegs reduces the distance to the anterior cortex.

A

Patellar Revision Algorithm

```
┌─────────────────────┐  Yes  ┌──────────────────────┐  Yes  ┌────────┐
│ Patellar Component: │─────▶│ Does the patellar    │─────▶│ Retain │
│ Well fixed & aligned│       │ component have       │       └────────┘
│ with minimal wear & │       │ adequate congruency  │
│ deformation?        │       │ with femoral         │
└─────────────────────┘       │ component?           │
          │ No                └──────────────────────┘
          ▼                             │ No
┌─────────────────────┐              ┌──────────────────────────┐
│ Bone Stock          │◀─────────────│ Revise patellar component│
│ Assessment          │              └──────────────────────────┘
└─────────────────────┘
```

Central cavitary deficit < 8mm	Central cavitary deficit 8 to 15 mm	• S/p revision of 3 peg or • Central deficit 15 to 20 mm	• Osteopenic and/or • < 12 mm thickness and/or • Central deficit > 20mm
Standard Single Peg	Large Peg	Three Peg	Do not resurface

B

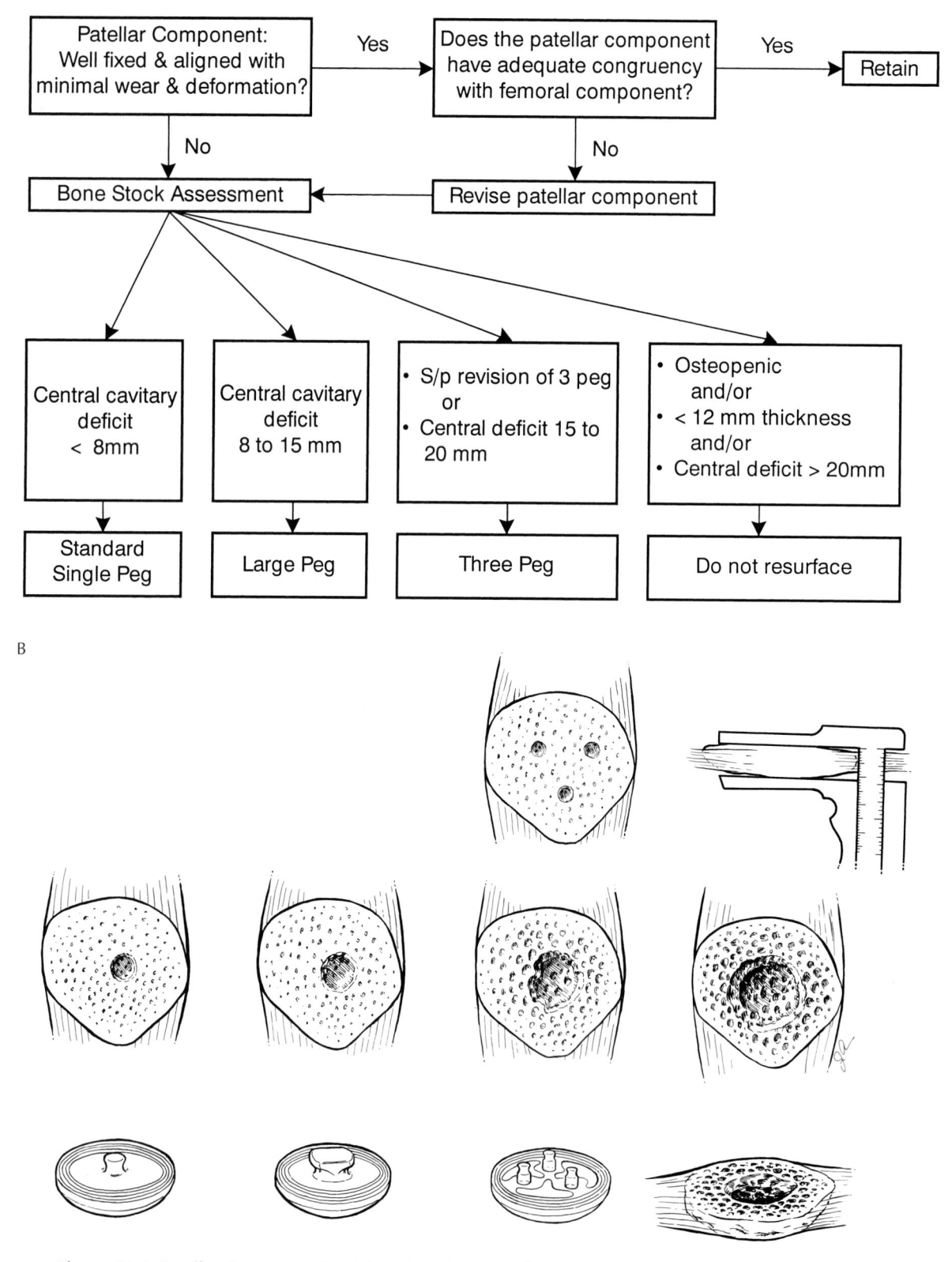

Figure 68.8. Patellar Component Revision Algorithm. (A) Algorithm for revision of patellar components; (B) commonly encountered patellar cavitary deficits and component options. Nonresurfacing may be considered for patellae with less than 12 mm of overall bony thickness or for patellae with very large cavitary deficits.

Further work may be necessary with respect to deficit classification in order to better clarify the cavitary deficits encountered in the patella at the time of patellar revision.

References

1. Scott R, Volatile T. Twelve years' experience with posterior cruciate-retaining total knee arthroplasty. *Clin Orthop.* 1986; 205:100–107.
2. Ritter M, Herbst S, Keating M, Faris P, Meding J. Long-term survival analysis of a posterior cruciate-retaining total condylar total knee arthroplasty. *Clin Orthop.* 1994; 309:136–145.
3. Ranawat C, Flynn W Jr, Saddler S, Hansraj K, Maynard M. Long-term results of the total condylar knee arthroplasty: a 15-year survivorship study. *Clin Orthop.* 1993; 286:94–102.
4. Scuderi G, Insall J, Windsor R, Moran M. Survivorship of cemented knee replacements. *J Bone Joint Surg.* 1989; 71-B:798–803.
5. Cobb A, Ewald F, Wright R, Sledge C. The kinematic knee survivorship analysis of 1,943 knees. Proceedings of the Annual Meeting of the British Orthopaedic Association. *J Bone Joint Surg.* 1990; 72-B:532.
6. Vince K, Insall J, Kelly M. The total condylar prosthesis: 10 to 12 year results of a cemented knee replacement. *J Bone Joint Surg.* 1989; 71-B:793–797.
7. Cameron H, Hunter G. Failure in total knee arthroplasty: mechanisms, revisions and results. *Clin Orthop.* 1982; 170:141–146.
8. Windsor R, Scuderi G, Moran M, Insall J. Mechanisms of failure of the femoral and tibial components in total knee arthroplasty. *Clin Orthop.* 1989; 248:15–20.
9. Moran C, Pinder I, Lees T, Midwinter M. Survivorship analysis of the uncemented porous-coated anatomic knee replacement. *J Bone Joint Surg.* 1991; 73-A:848–857.
10. Clayton M, Thirupathi R. Patellar complications after total condylar arthroplasty. *Clin Orthop.* 1982; 170:152–155.
11. Rosenberg A, Andriacchi T, Barden R, Galante J. Patellar component failure in cementless total knee arthroplasty. *Clin Orthop.* 1988; 236:106–114.
12. Stulberg S. Revision total knee arthroplasty: extensor mechanism complications after total knee arthroplasty. *Orthopedics.* 1995; 18(9):919–920.
13. Campbell D, Mintz A, Stevenson T. Early patellofemoral revision following total knee arthroplasty. *J Arthroplasty.* 1995; 10(3):287–291.
14. Healy W, Wasilewski S, Takei R, Oberlander M. Patellofemoral complications following total knee arthroplasty. *J Arthroplasty.* 1995; 10(2):197–201.
15. Merkow R, Soudry M, Insall J. Patellar dislocation following total knee replacement. *J Bone Joint Surg.* 1985; 67-A:1321–1327.
16. Lynch A, Rorabeck C, Bourne R. Extensor mechanism complications following total knee arthroplasty. *J Arthroplasty.* 1987; 2:135–140.
17. Brick G, Scott R. The patellofemoral component of total knee arthroplasty. *Clin Orthop.* 1988; 231:163–178.
18. Levai J, McCleod H, Freeman H. Why not resurface the patella? *J Bone Joint Surg.* 1983; 65-B:448–451.
19. Hozack W, Rothman R, Booth R, Balderston R. The patellar clunk syndrome: a complication of posterior stabilized total knee arthroplasty. *Clin Orthop.* 1989; 241:203–208.
20. Beight J, Yao B, Hozack W, Hearn S, Booth R Jr. The patellar "clunk" syndrome after posterior stabilized total knee arthroplasty. *Clin Orthop.* 1994; 299:139–142.
21. Shoji H, Shimozaki E. Patellar clunk syndrome in total knee arthroplasty without patellar resurfacing. *J Arthroplasty.* 1996; 11(2):198–201.
22. Figgie H, Goldberg V, Heiple K, Miller H, Gordon N. The influence of tibial-patellofemoral location on function of the knee in patients with posterior stabilized condylar knee prosthesis. *J Bone Joint Surg.* 1986; 68-A:1035–1040.
23. Insall J, Hood R, Flawn L, Sullivan D. The total condylar knee prosthesis in gonarthrosis: a five-to-nine year follow-up of the first 100 consecutive replacements. *J Bone Joint Surg.* 1983; 65-A:619–628.
24. Brick G, Scott R. Blood supply to the patella—significance in total knee arthroplasty. *J Arthroplasty.* 1989; (Suppl):75–79.
25. Cameron H, Fedorkow D. The patella in total knee arthroplasty. *Clin Orthop.* 1982; 165:197–199.
26. Figgie H, Goldberg V, Figgie M, et al. The effect of alignment of the implant on fractures of the patella after condylar total knee arthroplasty. *J Bone Joint Surg.* 1989; 71-A:1031–1039.
27. Roffman M, Hirsh D, Mendes D. Fracture of the resurfaced patella in total knee replacement. *Clin Orthop.* 1980; 148:112–116.
28. Scott R, Turoff N, Ewald F. Stress fracture of the patella following duopatellar total knee arthroplasty with patellar resurfacing. *Clin Orthop.* 1982; 170:147–151.
29. Lombardi A Jr, Engh G, Arlington R, Volz R, Albrigo J, Brainard B. Fracture/dissociation of the polyethylene in metal-backed patellar components in total knee arthroplasty. *J Bone Joint Surg.* 1988; 70-A:675–679.
30. Bayley J, Scott R, Ewald F, Holmes G. Failure of the metal-backed patella component after total knee replacement. *J Bone Joint Surg.* 1988; 70-A:668–674.
31. Wright T, Bartel D. The problem of surface damage in polyethylene total knee components. *Clin Orthop.* 1986; 205:67–74.
32. Grigoris P, Treacy R, McMinn D. Patellotibial impingement in kinemax stabilised total knee arthroplasty. *J Bone Joint Surg.* 1992; 74-B(3):472–473.
33. Ranawat C. The patellofemoral joint in total condylar knee arthroplasty: pros and cons based on five-to-ten year follow-up. *Clin Orthop.* 1986; 205:93–99.
34. Rand J, Morrey B, Bryan R. Patellar tendon rupture after total knee arthroplasty. *Clin Orthop.* 1989; 244:233–238.
35. Landy M, Walker P. Wear of ultra-high molecular-weight polyethylene components of 90 retrieved knee prosthesis. *J Arthroplasty.* 1988; (suppl):S73–S85.
36. Rhoads D, Noble P, Reuben J, Tullos H. The effect of femoral component position on the kinematics of total knee arthroplasty. *Clin Orthop.* 1993; 286:122–129.
37. Nagamine R, Whiteside L. The effect of tibial tray malro-

tation on patellar tracking in total knee arthroplasty. *Trans Orthop Res Soc.* 1992; 38:262–271.
38. Nelissen R, Weidenheim L, Mikhail W. The influence of position of the patellar component on tracking in total knee arthroplasty. *Int Orthop.* 1995; 19(4):224–228.
39. Starr M, Kaufmann K, Irby S, Colwell C Jr. The effects of patellar thickness on patellofemoral forces after resurfacing. *Clin Orthop.* 1996; 322:279–285.
40. Doolittle K, Turner R. Patellofemoral problems following total knee arthroplasty. *Orthop Rev.* 1988; 17:696–702.
41. Scheinberg R, Bucholz R. Fractures of the patella. In: Scott N, ed. *The Knee.* St. Louis: Mosby; 1994; 1393–1403.
42. Peters J, Engh G, Corpe R. The metal-backed patella: an invitation for failure? *J Arthroplasty.* 1991; 6(3):221–228.
43. Lombardi A Jr, Mallory T, Eberle R. Constrained knee arthroplasty. In: Scott N, ed. *The Knee.* St. Louis: Mosby; 1994; 1305–1323.
44. Lombardi A Jr, Mallory T, Eberle R. Constrained knee arthroplasty. In: Fu F, Harner C, Vince K, eds. *Knee Surgery.* Baltimore: Williams & Wilkins; 1994: 1331–1349.
45. Reuben J, McDonald C, Woodard P, Hennington L. Effect of patellar thickness on patellar strain following total knee arthroplasty. *J Arthroplasty.* 1991; 6:251–258.
46. Booth R. Revision technique. In: Fu F, Harner C, Vince K, eds. *Knee Surgery.* Baltimore: Williams & Wilkins; 1994:1573–1585.
47. Scuderi G, Scharf S, Meltzer L, Scott W. The relationship of lateral releases to patella viability in total knee arthroplasty. *J Arthroplasty.* 1987; 2(3):209–214.
48. Coonse K, Adams J. A new operative approach to the knee joint. *Surg Gynecol Obstet.* 1943; 77:344–347.
49. Trousdale R, Hanssen A, Rand J, Cahalan T. V-Y quadricepsplasty in total knee arthroplasty. *Clin Orthop.* 1993; 286:48–55.
50. Vince K. Revision arthroplasty technique. Instructional course lectures. In: Heckman J, ed. *Total Joint Arthroplasty.* Rosemont, IL: American Academy of Orthopaedic Surgeons; 1993: 325–339.
51. Whiteside L, Matthew D. Tibial tubercle osteotomy for exposure of the difficult total knee arthroplasty. *Clin Orthop.* 1990; 260:6–9.
52. Dennis D. Removal of well-fixed cementless metal-backed patellar components. *J Arthroplasty.* 1992; 7(2):217–220.
53. Scott R. Prosthesis replacement of the patellofemoral joint. *Orthop Clin North Am.* 1979; 10(1):129–137.
54. Insall J. Disorders of the patella. In: Insall J, ed. *Surgery of the Knee.* New York: Churchill Livingstone; 1984: 191–260.
55. Emerson R Jr. Extensor mechanism rupture. In: Fu F, Harner C, Vince K, eds. *Knee Surgery.* Baltimore: Williams & Wilkins; 1994: 1483–1490.

CHAPTER 69
Revision of Metal-Backed Patellar Components

Paul F. Lachiewicz

Metal-backed patellar components were introduced in the early to mid 1980s with the goal of eliminating polymethylmethacrylate for fixation of components. A wide variety of metal-backed components were designed and implanted, despite reports showing excellent long-term results with a cemented, all-polyethylene dome patellar prosthesis. Reports of premature failure of metal-backed patellar components began appearing in the late 1980s and prompted redesign and elimination of many of these components.[1] In a study of 132 Miller-Galante porous total knee replacements implanted without cement, Rosenberg and associates[2] reported an 11% rate of reoperation, predominantly for failure of the metal-backed patellar component.[3] Firestone and colleagues reported a 6.1% rate of revision for patellar loosening in a large series of porous-coated anatomic knee arthroplasties.[4] In two knees, metallosis was noted. Others have reported severe polyethylene wear, polyethylene dissociation, and metal failure with these implants.[5,6] Orthopedic surgeons should be aware of the indications and techniques for revision of a wide variety of metal-backed patellar components.

INDICATIONS FOR REVISION OF METAL-BACKED PATELLAR COMPONENTS

There are a wide variety of indications for revision of a metal-backed patellar component (Table 69.1). The most common indication is polyethylene wear (Fig. 69.1). These patients present with synovitis and a complaint of a "squeaking" or "grating" sensation in the knee, which may be most pronounced when arising from a seated position. Radiographs are usually unremarkable and the diagnosis is made on clinical history and examination. Metallosis will eventually occur due to contact between the exposed patellar component baseplate and the femoral component, which becomes burnished. Loosening of metal-backed patellar components was frequently seen with designs that included only two porous-coated pegs for fixation. Bone growth frequently occurs into the porous fiber-metal or beaded fixation peg and not the flat baseplate of the component. Breakage of the metal-backed component may then occur at the junction of the baseplate and fixation peg and also lead to a metallic synovitis. Removal of well-fixed metal-backed patellar components may be required in a variety of situations. In chronic infections or late metastatic infections that do not resolve with drainage and antibiotics, removal of the metal-backed component is mandatory. There are patients with painful subluxation of the patellar component in which the component must be revised or repositioned. There are knees with posterior cruciate or collateral ligament instability, in which the metal-backed patellar prosthesis must be revised because it is incompatible with a more constrained femoral and tibial component. Finally, failure of the metal-backed patellar prosthesis can occur coincidentally with a displaced fracture of the patella.

EVALUATION AND PREOPERATIVE PLANNING

The preoperative evaluation of patients with a metal-backed patellar prosthesis that requires revision includes good lateral and axial (sunrise or Merchant view) radiographs of the patella. This helps in the assessment of the method of fixation of the component (porous-coated or smooth pegs) and the bone structure available for revision. An aspiration of the knee joint in the office is recommended to exclude infection.[7] If the aspirated fluid has a gray or black discoloration, this indicates the presence of metallosis and that the femoral component will also require revision. The surgeon should plan to have specialized equipment available and a variety of

Table 69.1. Indications for revision metal-backed patellar components

1. Infection
2. Polyethylene wear
3. Polyethylene wear and metallosis
4. Implant loosening
5. Implant breakage
6. Painful subluxation
7. Knee instability—metal-backed patellar prosthesis incompatible with revised femoral and tibial components

all-polyethylene patellar components, with both a single, central, large peg and three small pegs for cement fixation.

SURGICAL TECHNIQUES

Problems that may be encountered in revision of a metal-backed patellar prosthesis include difficulties in exposure and extraction of the implant, intraoperative fracture, and excessive bone loss.

Revision should be performed, if possible, in an operating room with vertical laminar air-flow or ultraviolet lights and the members of the surgical team should wear individual body-exhaust suits. Use of a tourniquet is recommended. A generous skin incision, usually incorporating the previous incision, is made to permit adequate exposure. The author prefers an Insall midline approach to the knee,[8] rather than a medial parapatellar arthrotomy. The periosteum of the medial one-third of the patella is elevated sharply in line with the incision of the quadriceps tendon. This approach provides the best exposure of the medial aspect of the patella-prosthesis interface and allows a realignment procedure if required. If necessary for exposure, the patellar tendon may be sharply elevated 25 to 33% from the tibial tubercle, with a cuff of distal tibial periosteum to pre-

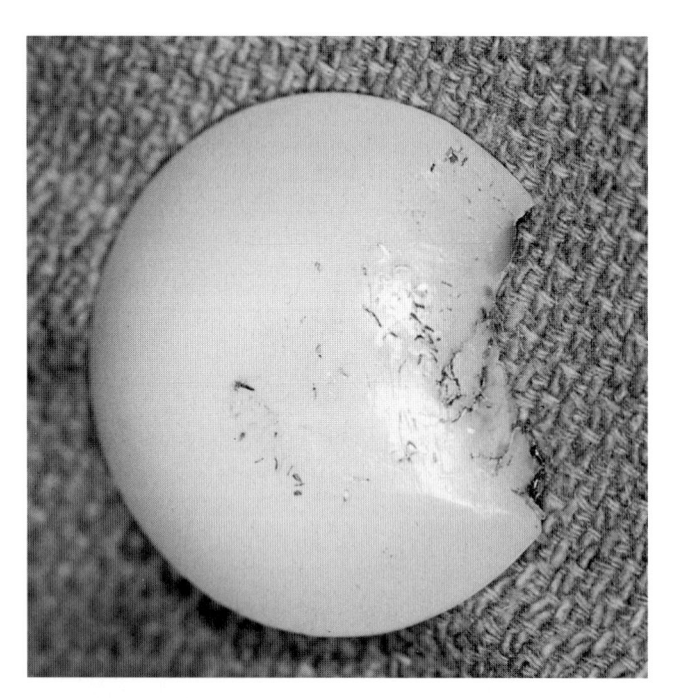

Figure 69.1. Lateral edge of a metal-backed patella component has worn through to the metal plate. Metal debris is imbedded in the remaining polyethylene.

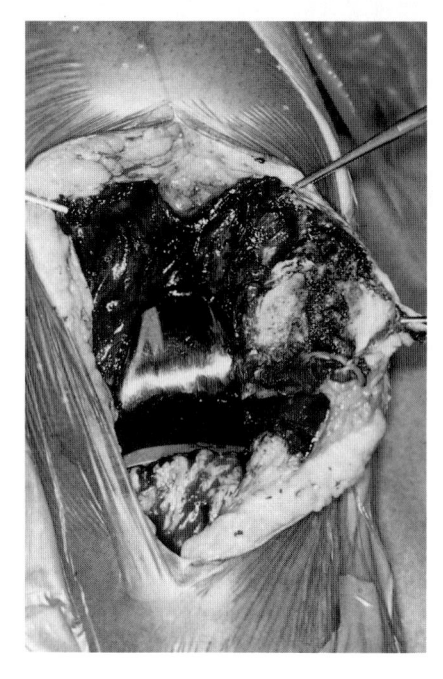

Figure 69.2. Metallosis seen in a knee with worn polyethylene of titanium metal-backed patellar component.

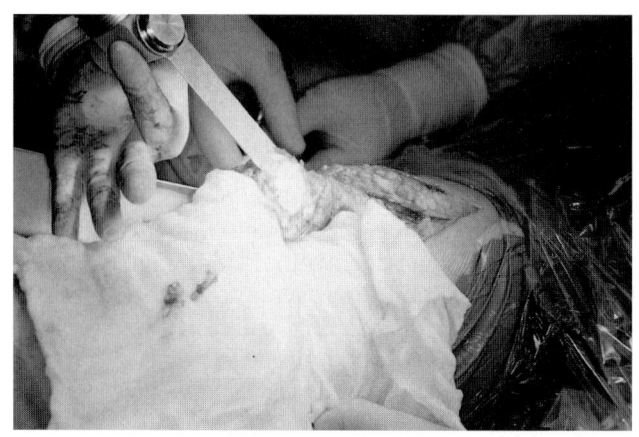

Figure 69.3. Thin, narrow oscillating saw used at periphery of patellar component.

vent avulsion of the tendon. Adequate exposure of the patella in a stiff knee may be facilitated by a lateral retinacular release, a proximal "quadriceps snip," or a combination of the two. Osteotomy of the tibial tubercle or a quadriceps "turndown" has not been necessary for adequate exposure in the author's practice.

Debridement and synovectomy of the anterior, medial, and lateral aspects of the knee, performed using electrocautery, is recommended because of the metal and polyethylene debris that is usually present (Fig. 69.2) and for complete exposure of the patellar prosthesis. Removal of the metal-backed patellar component is performed before revision of the femoral or tibial components to permit the knee to be stabilized by the other components.

The method of removal of the metal-backed patellar prosthesis depends somewhat on the amount of remaining bone and presence or absence of porous-coated fixation pegs (Table 69.2). After complete exposure of the underlying surface of the patella, the polyethylene is usually easily separated from the underlying metal-backed component using a small, thin osteotome. If necessary, the polyethylene may be transected with a high-speed burr. With the everted patella stabilized by two Kocher clamps in the quadriceps tendon, a narrow, thin oscillating power saw is used around the periphery of the implant (Fig. 69.3). If the fixation pegs are smooth, the component may then be removed using a double thin osteotome "wedge-platform" technique or by a gentle "prying" technique. With the "wedge-platform" technique, a wide osteotome is placed at the edge of the metal-bone interface and a small, thin osteotome (placed over the wide one) is then driven into the pegs or spikes. This is continued sequentially around the periphery of the implant. The metal-backed patellar prosthesis can then usually be disimpacted without excessive damage to the underlying bone. With the other technique, two osteotomes are placed on opposite sides of the metal-backed patella (Fig. 69.4). The osteotomes are progressively wedged in alongside the patella until the component is raised sufficiently to be pried free.

If both the baseplate and fixation pegs are porous-coated and well-fixed, removal is somewhat more difficult. Following the use of a narrow, thin oscillating saw

Table 69.2. Methods for removal metal-backed patellar components

---
1. Narrow, thin power sawblade
2. Wedge-platform double osteotome technique
3. Double osteotome-prying technique
4. Diamond-edged wheel saw to disrupt metal-bone interface and cut fixation pegs; then pencil-tip burr to remove porous-coated pegs
---

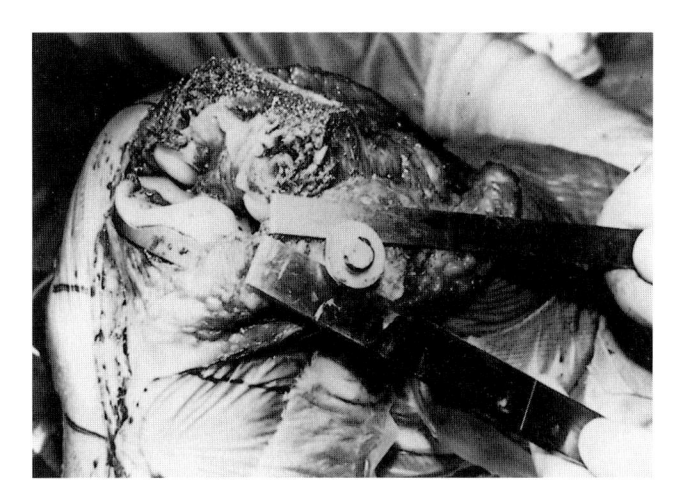

Figure 69.4. With the "prying" technique, two narrow osteotomes are placed on opposite sides of the patella.

at the periphery of the implant, a high-speed pneumatic tool with a thin-wheel diamond-edged saw is used to disrupt the bone-metal interface and separate the porous-coated fixation pegs from the baseplate (Fig. 69.5 A,B). Moist sponges should be placed to isolate the knee from the metallic debris produced with this method. After removal of the baseplate, a pencil-tip cutting device on the high-speed pneumatic tool is used to circumferentially disrupt the interface between the porous peg and the bone (Fig. 69.5C).

A combination of techniques may be necessary to remove some well-fixed metal-backed patellar components. Components fabricated of chrome-cobalt alloy with porous-coated, cruciate-shaped fixation ridges (e.g., LCS patella) are extremely difficult to remove.

Following extraction of the implant, any underlying synovium, fibrous membrane, or cartilage is removed sharply. There is not usually enough bone remaining to permit recutting of the patella. The patella is then prepared for a new polyethylene prosthesis with three fixation pegs (preferably) (Fig. 69.6A,B) or with a single large central peg (Fig. 69.7A,B). If the remaining patella bone structure is inadequate or insufficient to permit fixation of a new prosthesis, the edges should be smoothed, and the knee is left with a resection arthroplasty of the patellofemoral joint. This is preferable to inadequate fixation and possible loosening of a cemented implant.

Dennis described the use of the circular sawblade and pencil-tip drill to remove five well-fixed Miller-Galante porous patellar prostheses without intraoperative or postoperative complications.[3] In the author's series of 19 revisions of porous-coated total knee arthroplasties, the metal-backed patellar prosthesis was well-fixed in all but two, noninfected knees. Seventeen various,

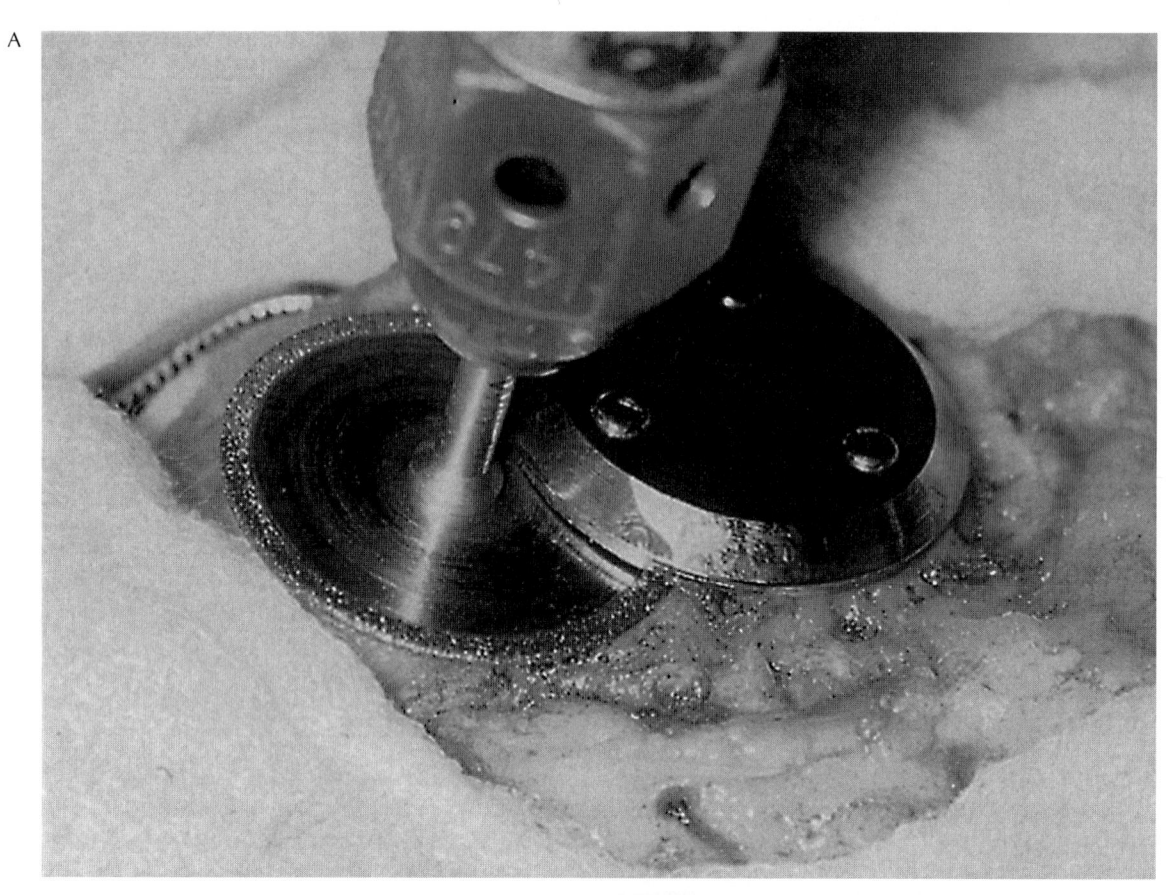

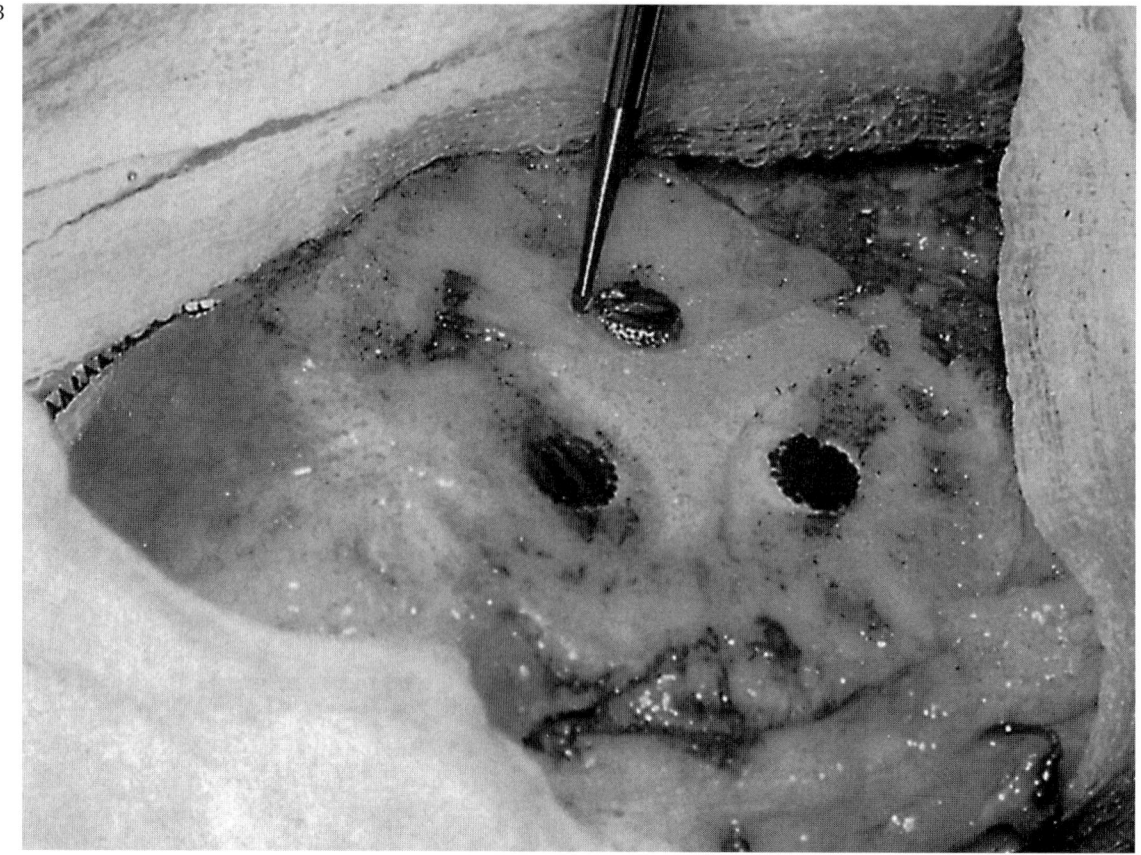

Figure 69.5. (A,B) With patella everted and polyethylene separated from metal backing, a circular saw with a diamond-cutting edge is used to transect the porous-coated pegs at the junction with the metal plate. (B) A thin tip on a high-speed burr then circumferentially disrupts the bone-peg interface.

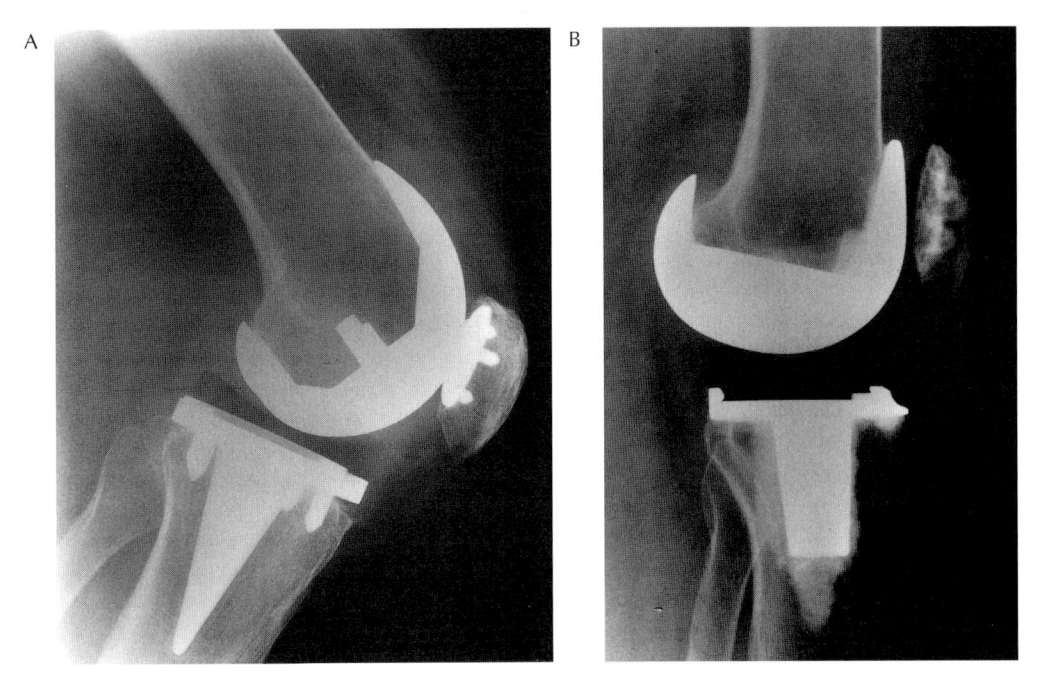

Figure 69.6. (A) This uncemented total knee arthroplasty was revised for pain and chronic synovitis. (B) The metal-backed patella prosthesis was revised using a three-prong all-polyethylene component.

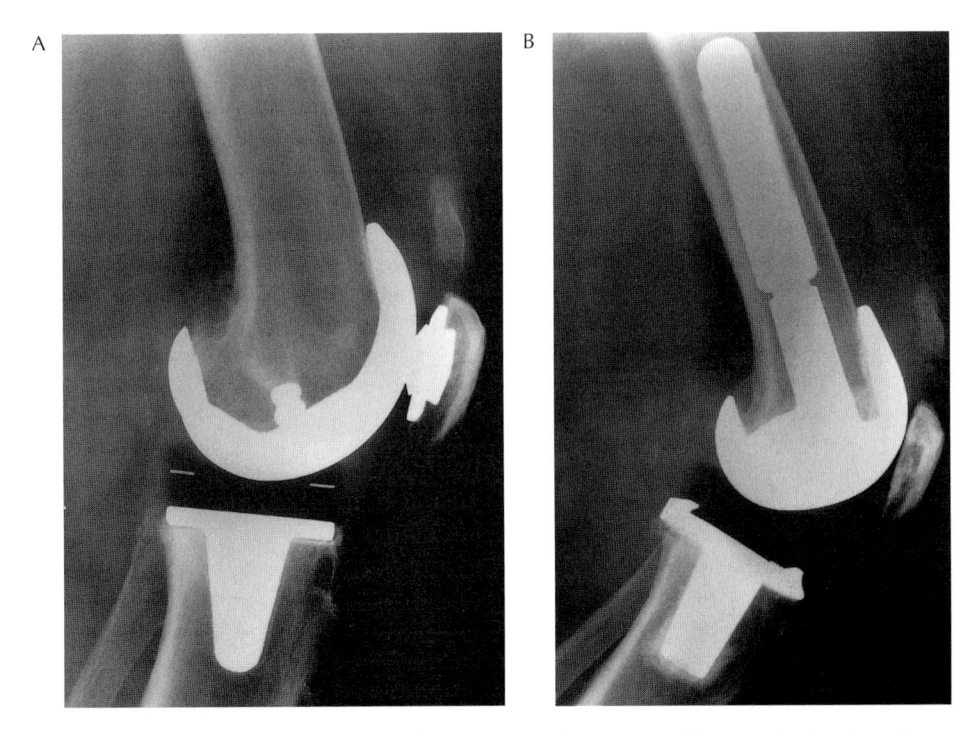

Figure 69.7. (A) This LCS uncemented total knee arthroplasty with metal-backed patellar prosthesis was revised for instability and tibial loosening. (B) The patella was reconstructed with an all-polyethylene component with a single large central peg.

metal-backed patellar components were removed using the techniques described without complication.

References

1. Bayley JC, Scott RD, Ewald FC, Holmes GB. Failure of the metal-backed patellar component after total knee replacement. *J Bone Joint Surg.* 1988; 70A:668–674.
2. Rosenberg AG, Andriacchi TP, Barden R, Galante JO. Patellar component failure in cementless total knee arthroplasty. *Clin Orthop.* 1988; 236:106–114.
3. Dennis DA. Removal of a well-fixed cementless metal-backed patellar component. *J Arthroplasty.* 1992; 7:217–220.
4. Firestone TP, Teeny SM, Krackow KA, Hungerford DS. The clinical and roentgenographic results of cementless porous-coated patellar fixation. *Clin Orthop.* December 1991; 273:184–189.
5. Baech J, Kofoed H. Failure of metal-backed patellar arthroplasty. 47 AGC knees followed for at least 1 year. *Acta Orthop Scand.* April, 1991; 62(2):166–168.
6. Lombardi AV Jr, Engh GA, Volz RG, Albrigo JL, Brainard BJ. Fracture/dissociation of the polyethylene in metal-backed patellar components in total knee arthroplasty. *J Bone Joint Surg.* June 1988; 70A:675–679.
7. Duff GP, Lachiewicz PF, Kelley SS. Aspiration of the knee joint prior to revision arthroplasty. *Clin Orthop.* 1996; 331:132–139.
8. Insall J. A midline approach to the knee. *J Bone Joint Surg.* 1971; 53A:1584.

CHAPTER 70
Patellar Dislocation

Paul F. Lachiewicz

Patellofemoral complications may account for up to 50% of all postoperative complications following total knee arthroplasty.[6] Patellar subluxation or dislocation has been reported to occur from less than 1% to almost 20% in series of total knee arthroplasties. This is usually associated with pain, weakness, and the sensation of instability of the knee. Nonoperative treatment is not successful and a variety of operative procedures have been recommended.

PREDISPOSING FACTORS

Dislocation of the patella following total knee arthroplasty has been reported to occur from 1 to 18 months postoperatively (mean, 5 months). The author has treated one patient with a patellar dislocation 5 years after surgery. Early dislocation may be the result of failure of a medial retinacular suture line or of dehiscence. Trauma (fall or twisting injury) has been associated with patellar dislocation in up to 27% of cases. The prosthetic design has been implicated as a cause of patella dislocations, with a very high incidence reported with the Guepar, variable-axis, and ICLH prostheses. However, the majority of patellar dislocations are likely due to intraoperative technical errors and component malposition (Table 70.1).

It has been shown that patellar tracking after external rotation of the femoral component comes closest to reproducing patellar tracking of the intact knee than any other femoral component position.[1] Thus, internal rotation of the femoral component (relative to the transepicondylar axis) is an important predisposing factor to patellar dislocation. If the tibial component is internally rotated relative to the proximal tibia, the tibial tubercle is laterally displaced, increasing the Q-angle and predisposing the patella to dislocation.[2] The resection level and orientation of the patellar component may also predispose to dislocation.[3] If the patella is insufficiently resected, the patella will be displaced anteriorly, tightening the lateral retinaculum. Similarly, if the patella is incorrectly resected in the coronal plane, with lateral or proximal under-resection, lateral subluxation or dislocation may occur.

EVALUATION AND PREOPERATIVE PLANNING

The diagnosis of patellar subluxation or dislocation after total knee arthroplasty is usually obvious. The patient will complain of pain, weakness, and instability of the knee, particularly when arising from a seated position. The overall femorotibial alignment, range of motion, and varus-valgus stability in full extension should be noted. Good standing anteroposterior, lateral, and axial (sunrise or Merchant) views should be obtained. The clinical diagnosis is confirmed by the axial radiograph (Fig. 70.1). If the femoral or tibial components are loose or malaligned, complete revision of the arthroplasty will be required. The author has performed complete revisions of two knees with subluxed or dislocated patellae because of posterior cruciate or medial collateral ligament instability.

TREATMENT

A variety of operative procedures for patellar dislocation or subluxation have been recommended (Table 70.2). An open or arthroscopic lateral retinacular release of the patella will not usually be successful and is not recommended. A proximal realignment of the patella alone is strongly recommended and is usually successful for the treatment of patellar dislocation or subluxa-

Table 70.1. Patellar dislocation: predisposing factors

1. Preoperative valgus alignment
2. Internal rotation of femoral component
3. Internal rotation of tibial component
4. Tear of medial retinaculum
5. Contracture of lateral retinaculum and iliotibial band

tion.[2] If the components are malaligned, or loose, or the knee is unstable, revision of all components is performed prior to the proximal realignment (Fig. 70.2 A–F).

In the proximal realignment procedure, the quadriceps mechanism and patella are completely exposed through a longitudinal skin incision. Two deep incisions are made, one medial and one lateral (Fig. 70.3A). The surgeon enters the prosthetic knee joint medially by a capsular incision that extends along the musculotendinous junction of the vastus medialis and then distally across the medial third of the anterior surface of the patella and along the medial margin of the patellar ligament. The lateral incision is the lateral release that extends proximally into the fibers of the vastus lateralis. To preserve the continuity of the medial flap, the quadriceps expansion–periosteum overlying the medial third of the patella must be preserved and separated from the underlying bone by sharp dissection (Fig. 70.3B). The realignment is performed by advancing the medial flap over the anterior surface of the patella (Fig. 70.3C). After suturing the edge of the advanced medial flap in place (with nonabsorbable sutures) near the lateral margin of the patella, the suture line should be straight along the front of the patella and the lateral release should be widely opened. The tourniquet should be released prior to closure to check for hemostasis. Although Merkow et al.[2] recommended immobilization in a bulky dressing for 5 to 7 days, the author will allow immediate motion with a CPM machine, but limit flexion to 70–90 degrees for 4 weeks following the procedure.

Merkow et al. reported that a proximal realignment was successful in the treatment of eleven knees with patellar dislocation following total knee arthroplasty.[2]

Table 70.2. Treatment: patellar dislocation

1. Lateral retinacular release
2. Proximal realignment of quadriceps (Insall type)
3. Distal realignment–tibial tubercle transplant
   a. Trillat type
   b. Hungerford type

No patella re-dislocated and there was no radiographic evidence of aseptic necrosis of the patella. Grace and Rand reported four recurrent subluxations in fourteen patients with proximal realignment alone,[4] but this procedure had fewer serious complications than when combined with a distal realignment of the tibial tubercle.

Distal realignment of the patella, with medialization of the tibial tubercle, has been recommended for patellar dislocation following total knee arthroplasty.[3,5] The procedure described by Kirk et al. is a modification of the Trillat procedure.[5] The tibial tubercle is osteotomized and displaced approximately one centimeter medially and fixed with two 4.5-mm AO screws. The knee is immobilized for 4 weeks. The procedure failed in 2 of 15 knees, with a patellar dislocation owing to persistent patellofemoral pain in one knee and a nonunion of the osteotomy in the second knee.[3] Grace and Rand reported two patellar tendon ruptures after a combined proximal and distal realignment, but they medialized only a thin wafer of bone.[4] In the distal realignment described by Briard and Hungerford, the osteotomy of the tibial tubercle extends from behind the patellar tendon to a drill hole 5–6 centimeters distally.[3] The tubercle is rotated medially, leaving the distal periosteum intact and fixed with one or two screws. The medial rotation uncovers cancellous bone laterally, which is then used as a bone graft to fill in the medial overhang. The knee is immobilized for 6 weeks. The author does not recommend tibial tubercle osteotomy and medialization because of the potential for serious complications (nonunion, patellar tendon rupture) and because proximal realignment is technically easier and has a high rate of success.

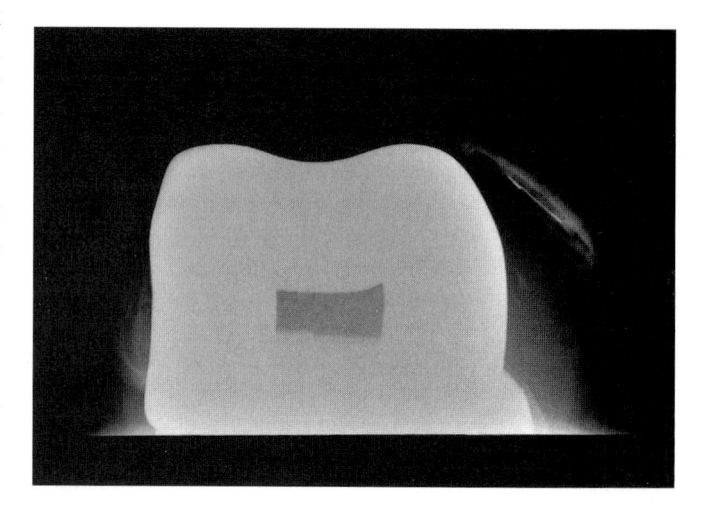

Figure 70.1. Lateral dislocation of patella is easily seen on an axial radiograph.

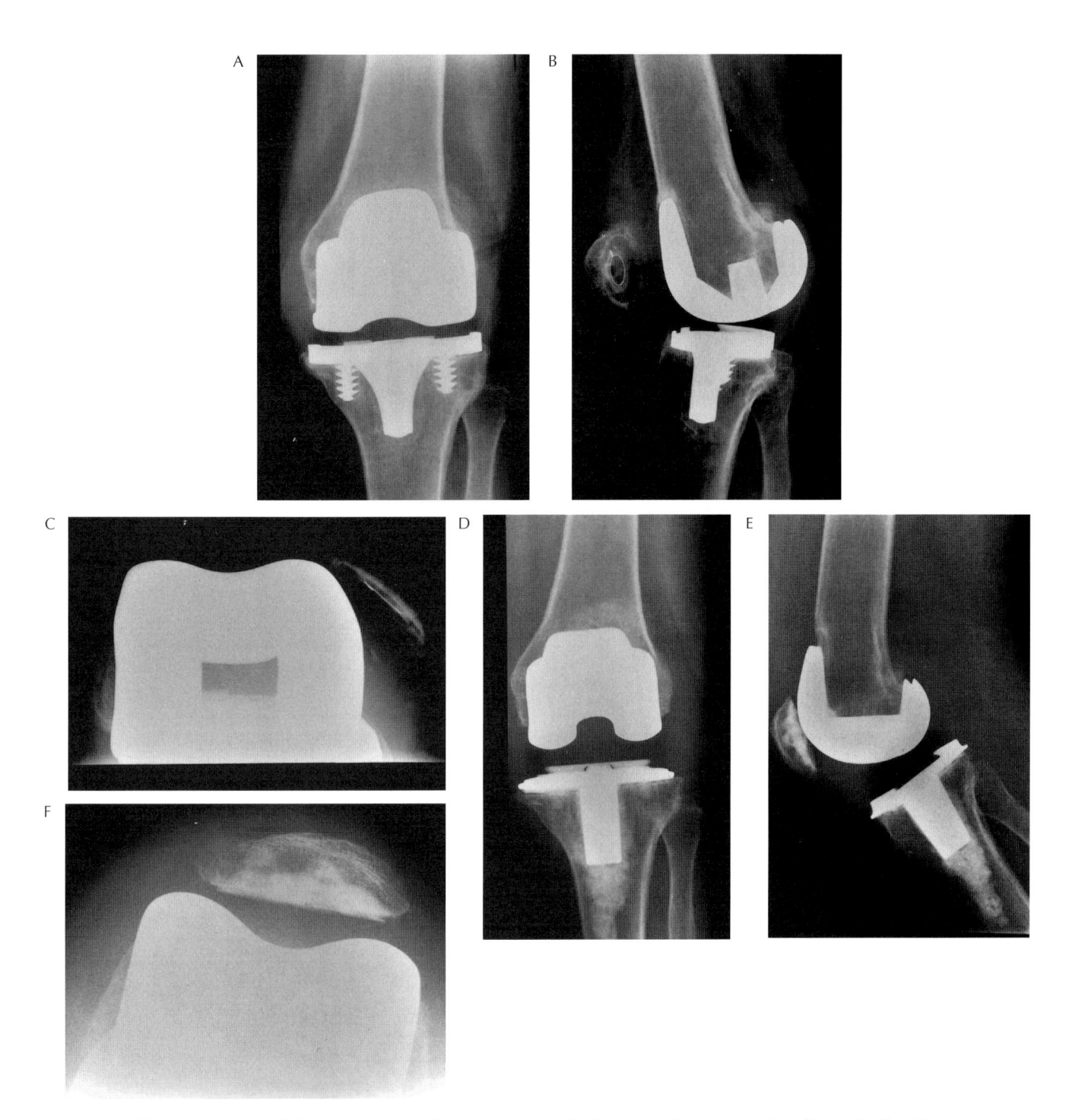

Figure 70.2. (A,B,C) Preoperative standing, anteroposterior lateral, and supine axial radiograph of a 58-year-old woman with a dislocated patella 6 months after uncemented total knee arthroplasty. The knee also had severe posterior instability in flexion. (D,E,F) Postoperative standing anteroposterior, lateral, and supine axial radiographs show that all components were revised to a posterior-stabilized prosthesis. A proximal realignment of the patella was performed.

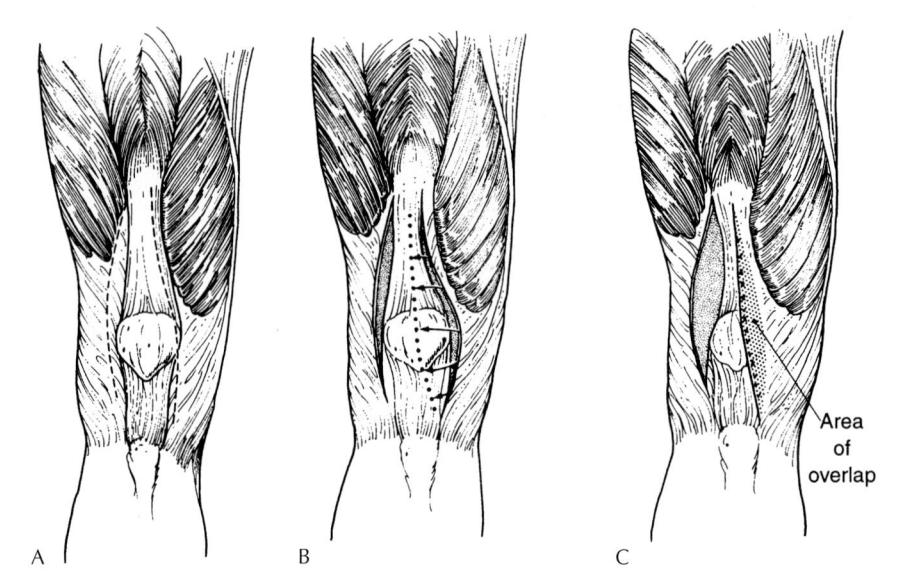

Figure 70.3. (A) With a proximal realignment, two deep incisions are made: one medial (over the medial 1/3 of the patella) and one lateral (1 centimeter lateral to the patella). (B) The quadriceps expansion and periosteum are sharply dissected from the underlying medial patella. (C) The medial flap is advanced over the anterior surface of the patella to its lateral edge.

References

1. Rhoads DD, Noble PC, Reuben JD, Mahoney OM, Tullos HS. The effect of femoral component position on patellar tracking after total knee arthroplasty. *Clin Orthop.* 1990; 260:43–51.
2. Merkow RL, Soudry M, Insall JN. Patellar dislocation following total knee replacement. *J Bone Joint Surg.* 1985; 67A:1321–27.
3. Briard JL, Hungerford DS. Patellofemoral instability in total knee arthroplasty. *J Arthroplasty.* 1989; 4 Supplement: S87–97.
4. Grace JN, Rand JA. Patellar instability after total knee arthroplasty. *Clin Orthop.* 1988; 237:184–89.
5. Kirk P, Rorabeck CH, Bourne RB, Burkart B, Nott L. Management of recurrent dislocation of the patella following total knee arthroplasty. *J Arthroplasty.* 1992; 7:229–33.
6. Brick GW, Scott RD. The patellofemoral component of total knee arthroplasty. [Review] *Clin Orthop.* 1989; 231: 163–78.

SECTION 19
Management of Periprosthetic Fractures

CHAPTER 71
Femoral Periprosthetic Fractures: Nonoperative Treatment

Michael C. Moran

PRESENTATION AND INITIAL EVALUATION

Supracondylar femur fractures above total knee arthroplasty have been associated with osteopenia, notching of the anterior femoral cortex, a diagnosis of rheumatoid arthritis, the presence of neurologic disorders, and the presence of osteolytic bone defects.[1–6] Regardless of the etiology, the initial management of a supracondylar femur fracture after total knee arthroplasty depends upon an accurate initial evaluation of the fracture.

This injury may occur in the early postoperative period, though it is more commonly a late complication, often occurring several years postoperatively. Patients with this injury usually provide a history of minor trauma, such as a fall during ambulation. There is subsequent pain and inability to bear weight. Since these are typically low-energy injuries, they are often not associated with major soft tissue swelling. Unless marked displacement is present, deformity may not be apparent on examination.

Fractures above total knee replacement are considered supracondylar fractures if they extend within 7 centimeters of the prosthetic joint line or if they are within 2 centimeters of the femoral flange.[5,7] Radiographically, nondisplaced or minimally displaced fractures may be obscured by the femoral flange. It is important to identify nondisplaced fractures, since late displacement may occur without appropriate precautions. The diagnostic evaluation must include a direct lateral view (if necessary, obtained with fluoroscopic guidance) of the distal femur in order to guide subsequent treatment. The direct lateral view facilitates assessment of fracture displacement, while also revealing the bone available for fixation devices, the location of femoral lugs of posterior cruciate-retaining components, and the proximal extent of the central femoral recess in cases with posterior stabilized components.

CLASSIFICATION

The most important factors in classifying supracondylar femur fractures above total knee arthroplasty are the status of prosthetic stability and the degree of fracture displacement. Displaced fractures have been described as those with displacement at the fracture site of greater than 5 millimeters or angulation greater than 5 degrees.[5,8–10] The Neer classification system has been used for these injuries in some series, with Neer Type I fractures considered to be nondisplaced or minimally displaced, while Neer Types II and III include displaced fractures.[11] In general, the fractures are considered to be displaced versus nondisplaced, while in each case the prosthesis is judged to be either well-fixed or not well-fixed.

TREATMENT OPTIONS
General Principles

For nondisplaced or minimally displaced fractures with a well-fixed prosthesis, closed treatment is usually successful (Fig. 71.1). Cylinder casts, long leg casts, hinged knee braces, and cast braces have all been employed in this setting.

Significant controversy exists regarding the initial management of displaced fractures with a well-fixed prosthesis. In reported series, displaced fractures with a well-fixed prosthesis represent the most frequent presentation of fractures above total knee arthroplasty. Unfortunately, a majority of reports have included certain variables that made comparison of closed versus open therapy difficult. Problems included: (a) the inclusion of a wide variety of early prosthetic designs or stemmed implants, and (b) the inclusion of a variety of techniques of internal fixation.

Some authors have recommended an initial trial of

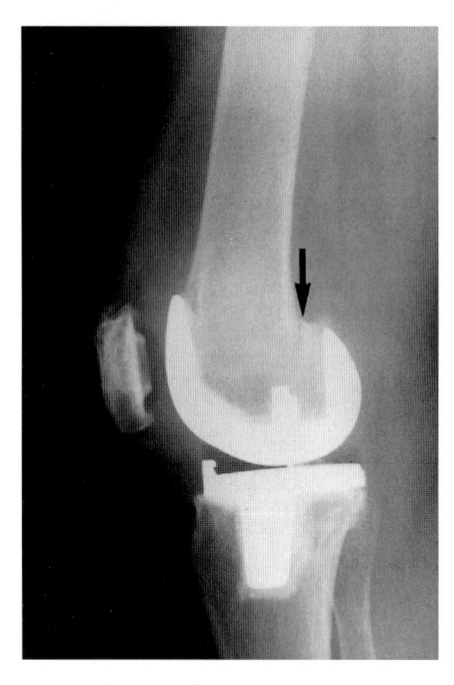

Figure 71.1. Lateral view of a knee with a minimally displaced fracture (arrow) that healed in satisfactory position after treatment in a standard knee immobilizer.

closed treatment for displaced fractures.[2,12–15] Skeletal traction, closed reduction with cylinder casting, and cast wedging have all been employed for the nonoperative management of these injuries.

Malunion has been reported to be common after closed treatment of displaced fractures. Malunion may produce diminished function and limited motion, while potentially compromising prosthetic survival through excessive asymmetric loading of the implant. In addition, malunion complicates any subsequent revision procedure. For these reasons, in recent years a majority of authors have recommended early internal fixation of displaced fractures associated with a well-fixed prosthesis.[5,7,10,16,17] Advocates of internal fixation feel that prompt surgical intervention may preserve motion and avoid malunion.

METHODS OF NONOPERATIVE TREATMENT

The early nonoperative treatment for these injuries falls into two general categories: (1) ambulatory (immediate splinting, casting, or hinged bracing, and (2) nonambulatory (skeletal traction).

Ambulatory Treatment

Nondisplaced or minimally displaced fractures may be managed successfully using one of several immobilization devices. The simplest of the available options is the standard knee immobilizer, which typically consists of a nonhinged splint with multiple straps. Use of this device may be best limited to noncomminuted, nondisplaced fractures that are considered at minimal risk for displacement.

Standard cylinder casts or long leg casts have been the most frequently used devices in reported series of fractures above total knee replacement. Pressure areas should receive special attention during application of these casts in elderly patients in order to prevent pressure ulcers. For displaced fractures, several reports have included cases in which cast wedging was performed in attempts to achieve adequate alignment.[4,5,13]

The "cast brace" has also been frequently reported as an option for fractures above total knee replacement (Fig. 71.2). Popularized by Mooney et al., the cast brace has been successfully used to treat a large series of supracondylar femur fractures that were not associated with prosthetic knees.[18] This report noted that in comparison to previously reported internal fixation techniques, the cast brace appeared promising for the treatment of displaced supracondylar fractures. However, more-recent reports of modern surgical techniques have generally shown internal fixation to be superior to cast brace treatment for displaced fractures in the nonarthroplasty setting.[19,20] In particular, malunion may occur even within a properly applied cast brace (Fig. 71.3).

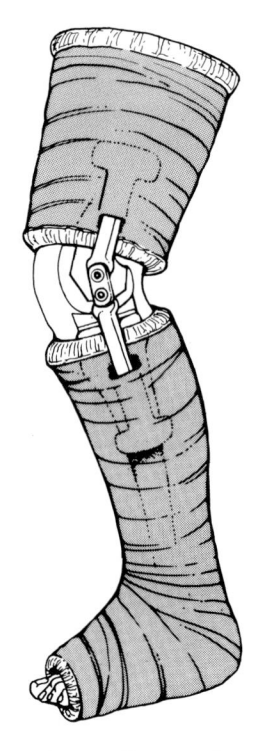

Figure 71.2. The cast brace allows early motion, while partial weight-bearing is theoretically facilitated by transmission of load to the soft tissues of the thigh.

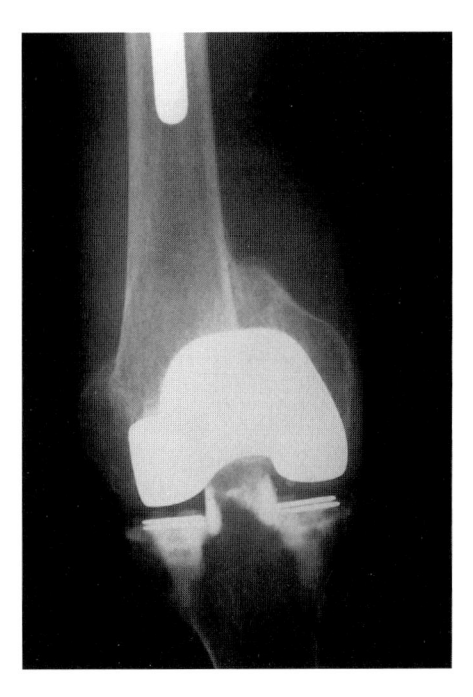

Figure 71.3. Anteroposterior radiograph of a varus malunion after closed treatment of a displaced fracture using a cast brace.

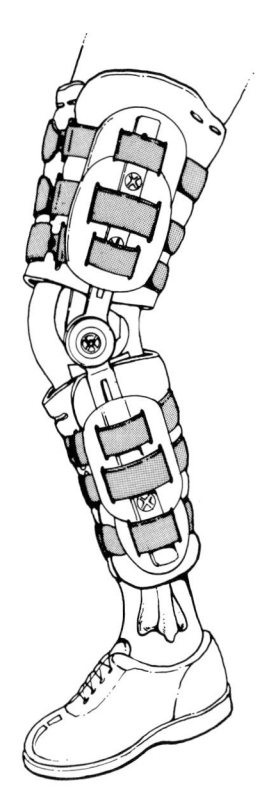

Figure 71.4. A functional hinged brace may be used for nondisplaced or minimally displaced fractures.

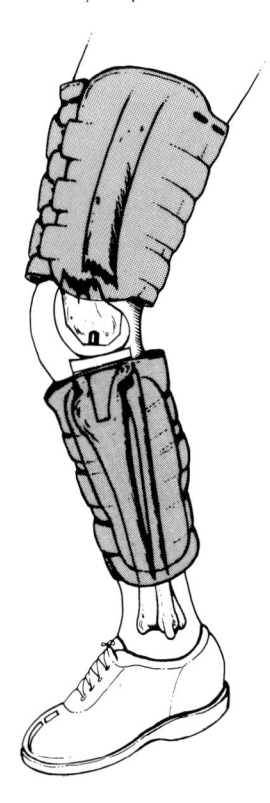

Figure 71.5. One deficiency of hinged knee braces is the difficulty in maintaining the hinge at the center of rotation of the knee. If a fracture is considered at risk for displacement, the hinge is kept locked during the first few weeks of treatment.

The cast brace includes a well-fitting thigh portion made of plaster or fiberglass that is connected by medial and lateral hinges to a short leg cast.[18] The resulting construct may control fractures of the distal femur while allowing knee motion. Weight-bearing loads are theoretically transmitted through the short leg cast portion, the hinges, and the thigh portion to the soft tissue around the thigh. This load transmission through the cast brace continues to the proximal femur and hip, thus partially unloading the knee and distal femur. A device that is similar to the cast brace is the hinged functional fracture orthosis as described by Sarmiento and Latta. This so-called functional brace is lighter and less bulky than the traditional cast brace, using closely fitting, custom-molded thigh and leg portions.[21]

Hinged knee braces with foam padding and multiple straps may also be used for the management of nondisplaced or minimally displaced fractures (Fig. 71.4). During the application of the hinge, strict attention is required to place the center of rotation of the hinge at the center of rotation of the knee. The straps of these braces must remain securely fastened and may require tightening as swelling subsides. Since the brace may shift in position (most commonly, sliding distally) the patient should be carefully instructed about the correct position of the brace (Fig. 71.5). If early motion is allowed, it is imperative to follow frequent radiographs to assure that fracture displacement does not occur (Fig. 71.6). Patient reliability is therefore essential to assure proper readjustment of the brace.

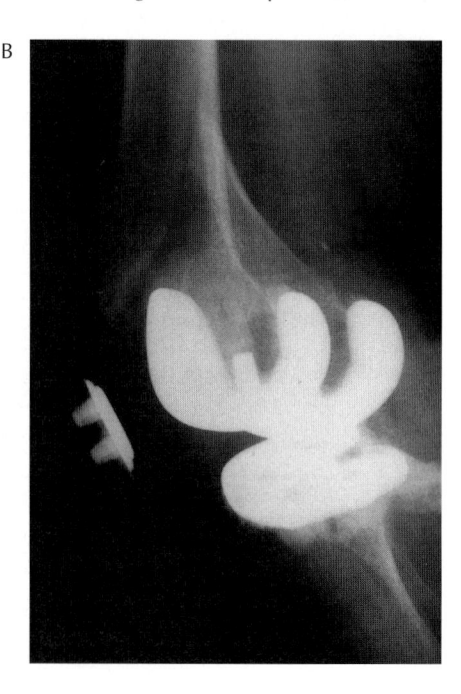

Figure 71.6. Displacement during treatment in a hinged knee brace. (A) Lateral radiograph obtained immediately postinjury of a minimally displaced fracture (arrow). The extremity was placed in a hinged knee brace and motion was initiated at three weeks. (B) Lateral radiograph obtained 6 weeks postinjury demonstrates displacement of the fracture. Surgical intervention was then required.

The surgeon may wish to keep a hinged brace locked in one position—usually in full extension or slight flexion—for the first several weeks to allow early fracture healing prior to the initiation of motion. After serial radiographs demonstrate stability of the fracture and new bone formation, the hinges may be opened to allow motion.

Nonambulatory Treatment

The predominant form of nonambulatory treatment for these injuries is skeletal traction. This treatment modality has been used for displaced fractures that would not be amenable to ambulatory treatment in a cast or brace. If conservative treatment is chosen, fractures that are displaced at initial presentation may require traction to maintain acceptable alignment.

The skeletal traction is used for a variable time period, typically 4 to 6 weeks, followed by a period of ambulatory immobilization using one of the devices (e.g., a cast or brace, as described above). It may be difficult to determine the time at which the fracture is healed enough to allow this conversion to ambulatory treatment. Neer has mentioned resolution of pain and tenderness at the

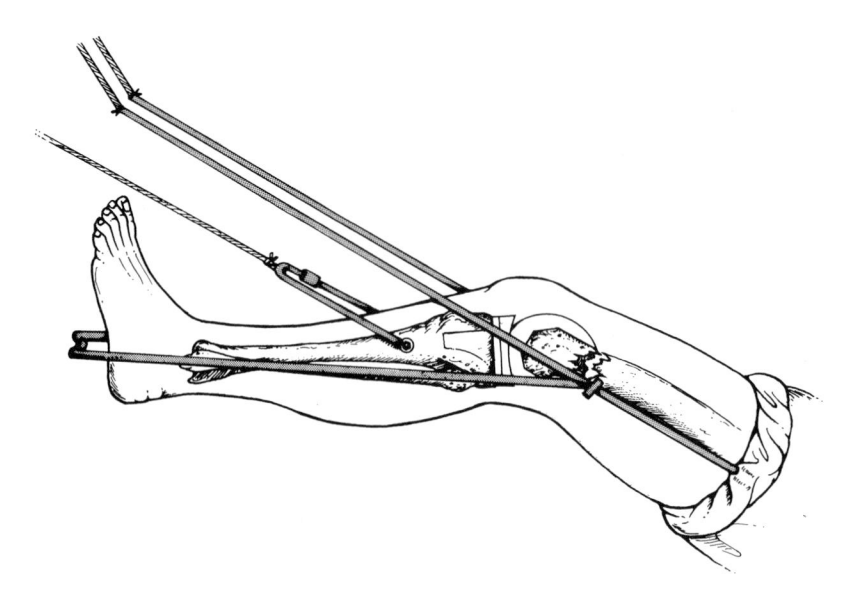

Figure 71.7. Skeletal traction using a tibial pin and balanced suspension has typically been used for fractures too unstable to allow ambulatory treatment.

fracture site as an indicator that early fracture consolidation has occurred, allowing discontinuation of traction and conversion to ambulatory treatment.[11]

The most commonly used skeletal traction type for fractures above total knee replacement is tibial pin traction in balanced suspension (Fig. 71.7). A balanced suspension apparatus may be assembled using described techniques.[22] While placing the tibial traction pin in the presence of a tibial component, it is important to keep the pin sufficiently distal so that the stem of the tibial component is avoided. Pin track infection in such a situation could conceivably jeopardize the arthroplasty.

Tibial pin traction may fail to fully correct varus-valgus deformities. In addition, correction of sagittal plane (flexion-extension) deformities may be impossible despite application of substantial amounts of traction (Figs. 71.8, 71.9). Most importantly, obtaining a satisfactory alignment in traction does not prevent redisplacement after removal of traction, especially in cases of comminution (Fig. 71.10).

RESULTS OF NONOPERATIVE TREATMENT

Due to the relatively small number of cases treated by any one center, it is necessary to perform a meta-analysis of the literature. During such an assessment, attention is restricted to reports that provide adequate information regarding fractures associated with bicompartmental or tricompartmental prostheses that were treated nonoperatively.[2,4,5,8,12–15,23,24] In these reports, the decision whether to relegate a specific fracture to ambulatory immobilization or skeletal traction has probably

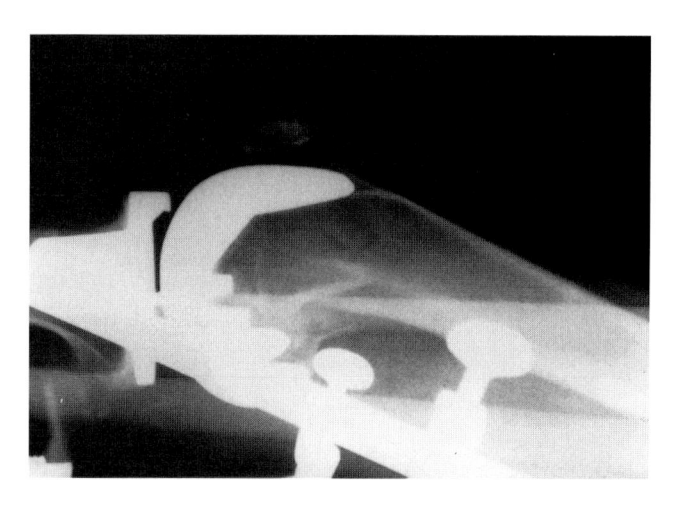

Figure 71.9. Lateral radiograph of another case in balanced suspension with tibial pin traction. The fracture healed with a flexion deformity (anterior angulation at the fracture site), with resultant pain as the patella tracked over the bony prominence proximal to the femoral flange. There was also a 20-degree loss of active knee extension. (Reprinted with permission from Moran MC, et al: Supracondylar femur fracture following total knee arthroplasty. *Clin Orthop* 1996; 324:196–209.)

been influenced by the severity of the fracture. In other words, more severe fractures that could not be controlled in a cast may have been selectively managed with skeletal traction. A fair comparison of simple immobilization versus skeletal traction is therefore difficult to make.

On the basis of this meta-analysis, nonoperative treatment overall is shown to yield satisfactory results in 64%

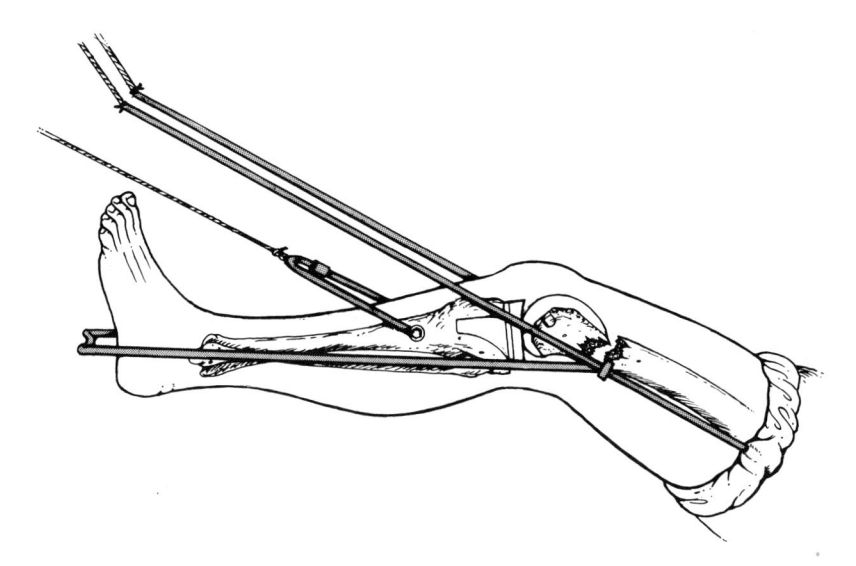

Figure 71.8. Despite using enough weight to distract the fracture, sagittal plane deformities may not be corrected with traction. In this illustration, increasing the traction has failed to correct an extension deformity (posterior angulation at the fracture site). This type of deformity has been attributed to the pull of the gastrocnemius muscles.

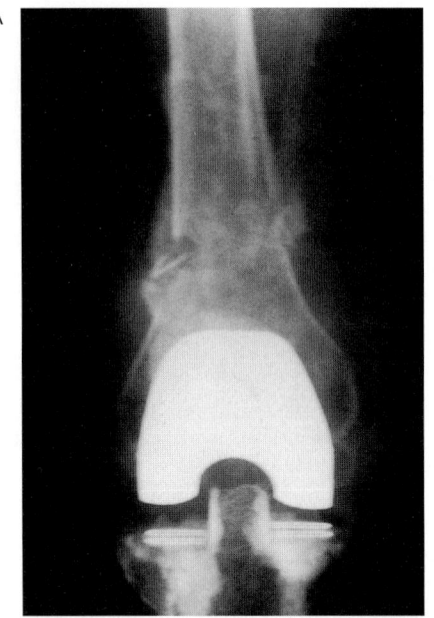

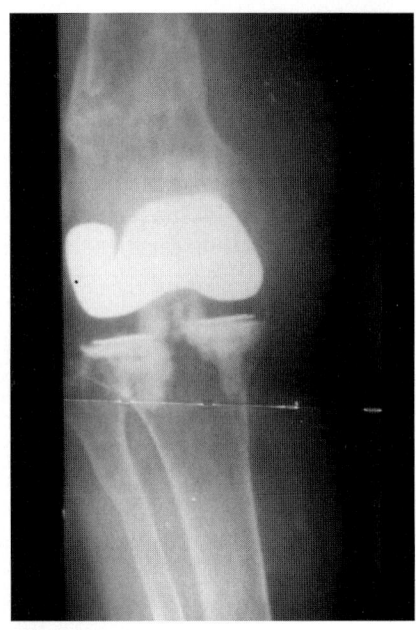

Figure 71.10. An example of redisplacement of a fracture after treatment with skeletal traction. (A,B) Anteroposterior and lateral radiographs with the extremity in balanced suspension with tibial pin traction demonstrates adequate tibiofemoral alignment. The extremity was placed in a cast brace 6 weeks after the fracture. (C) Despite early acceptable alignment in traction, the fracture redisplaced and healed in varus alignment. In addition, the knee had significant decrease in its range of motion.

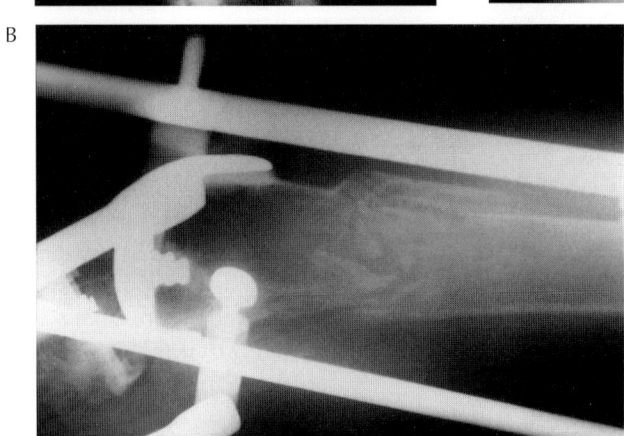

of cases, with malunion as the most common reason for a result to be considered unsatisfactory (Table 71.1). However, when one separates out the nondisplaced fractures from the displaced fractures, it becomes clear that the prognosis is very different for these two categories (Table 71.2). Nondisplaced fractures managed nonoperatively have yielded satisfactory results in 80% of cases, while displaced fractures have yielded satisfactory results in only 32% of cases. This low rate of satisfactory results for displaced fractures is substantially lower than that reported for surgical treatment of displaced fractures.[3]

It is difficult to determine, on the basis of existing reports of displaced fractures, whether ambulatory treatment or skeletal traction is the better of the two options. Two reports specifically noted no significant difference in the results of traction versus immediate ambulatory treatment in the treatment of displaced fractures.[5,13] In these reports, both traction and ambulatory treatment were unsuccessful in controlling displaced fractures.

OTHER COMPLICATIONS OF NONOPERATIVE TREATMENT

Aside from malunion, nonunion, and loss of motion, there are certain other complications that may be more likely with nonoperative treatment than with surgical treatment. The incidence of these complications may be increased with prolonged immobilization or bedrest. Such reported complications include cast ulcers,[5] sacral ulcers, and heel ulcers related to prolonged bedrest,[2,12] thromboembolic events related to prolonged cast immobilization or skeletal traction,[2,4] and gastric outlet obstruction.[5]

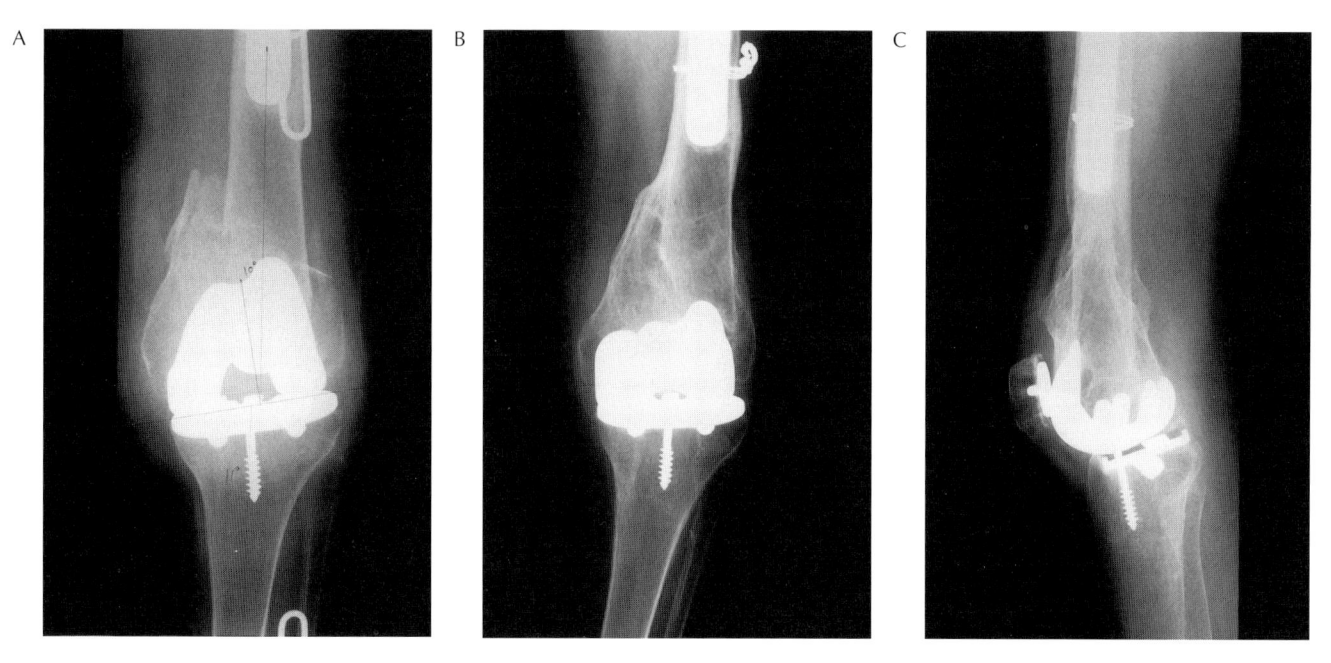

Figure 71.11. A fracture in a minimally ambulatory, debilitated patient with dementia. Prior to fracture, the patient had a subsided, yet asymptomatic, tibial component. (A) Anteroposterior radiograph showing a comminuted fracture with an ipsilateral long-stemmed total hip replacement. The extremity is being treated in a standard knee immobilizer. (B,C) Anteroposterior and lateral views 1 year later demonstrated union of the fracture with no significant change from the prefracture alignment. The patient remained minimally ambulatory and had a decreased range of motion compared to the prefracture status.

THE DEBILITATED, MINIMALLY AMBULATORY PATIENT

A special circumstance arises when this injury occurs in very elderly patients who are minimally ambulatory. This is not a rare occurrence, considering that these are patients with the type of osteopenic bone that may be prone to a supracondylar femur fracture. Often these patients also have severe medical problems. Such patients are best assessed on an individual basis. If a potential surgical procedure is expected to be too major an undertaking considering the patient's medical status, it may be reasonable to manage such cases nonoperatively (Fig. 71.11). Such an approach in displaced fractures must take into account the potential for malunion. Even more important, other potential complications of nonoperative treatment (e.g., pressure sores) may be more likely in the debilitated patient.

SUMMARY

In the setting of a well-fixed prosthesis, closed treatment is indicated for nondisplaced or minimally displaced fractures. Most of these fractures may be managed with ambulatory treatment consisting of one of several techniques.

Some early reports also recommend attempted closed treatment even when the fracture is displaced. These displaced fractures have typically been managed with skeletal traction during the early period of fracture healing. Closed reduction and casting followed by cast wedging have also been attempted, with unpredictable results. Fractures with acceptable early alignment may proceed to malunion, while fractures that heal in good alignment may be complicated by a loss of motion from prolonged immobilization. More recent reports advocate prompt surgical intervention for displaced fractures, which represent the most common reported presentation for supracondylar femur fractures above total knee arthroplasty.

References

1. Aaron RK, Scott RD. Supracondylar fracture of the femur after total knee arthroplasty. *Clin Orthop*. 1987; 219:136–9.
2. Bogoch E, Hastings D, Gross A, et al. Supracondylar fractures of the femur adjacent to resurfacing and MacIntosh arthroplasties of the knee in patients with rheumatoid arthritis. *Clin Orthop*. 1988; 229:213–20.

3. Chmell MJ, Moran MC, Scott RD. Periarticular fractures after total knee arthroplasty: Principles of management. *J Am Acad Orthop Surg*. 1996; 4:109.
4. Culp RW, Schmidt RG, Hanks G, et al. Supracondylar fracture of the femur following prosthetic knee arthroplasty. *Clin Orthop*. 1987; 222:212–22.
5. Moran MC, Brick GW, Sledge CB, et al. Supracondylar femur fracture following total knee arthroplasty. *Clin Orthop*. 1996; 324:196–209.
6. Rand JA. Supracondylar fracture of the femur associated with polyethylene wear after total knee arthroplasty. A case report. *J Bone Joint Surg Am*. 1994; 76:1389–91.
7. McLaren AC, Dupont JA, Schroeber DC. Open reduction internal fixation of supracondylar fractures above total knee arthroplasties using the intramedullary supracondylar rod. *Clin Orthop*. 1994; 302:194–98.
8. Cain PR, Rubash HE, Wissinger HA et al. Periprosthetic femoral fractures following total knee arthroplasty. *Clin Orthop*. 1986; 208:205–214.
9. Degoia AM, Rubash HE. Periprosthetic fractures of the femur after total knee arthroplasty. *Clin Orthop*. 1991; 271:135–42.
10. Zehntner MK, Ganz R. Internal fixation of supracondylar fractures after total knee arthroplasty. *Clin Orthop*. 1993; 293:219–24.
11. Neer CS, Grantham SA, Shelton ML. Supracondylar fracture of the adult femur. *J Bone Joint Surg Am*. 1967; 49:191.
12. Figgie MP, Goldberg VM, Figgie HE, et al. The results of supracondylar fracture above total knee arthroplasty. *J Arthroplasty*. 1990; 5:267–76.
13. Merkel KA, Johnson EW. Supracondylar fracture of femur after total knee arthroplasty. *J Bone Joint Surg Am*. 1986; 68:29–43.
14. Nielson BF, Peterson VS, Vamarken JE. Fracture of the femur after total knee arthroplasty. *Acta Orthop Scand*. 1989; 59:155–57.
15. Sista DJ, Lachiewics PF, Insall JN. Treatment of supracondylar femur fractures following prosthetic arthroplasty of the knee. *Clin Orthop*. 1985; 196:265–72.
16. Ritter MA, Keating EM, Faris PM et al. Rush rod fixation of supracondylar fractures above total knee arthroplasties. *J Arthroplasty*. 1995; 10:213–16.
17. Healy WL, Siliski JM, Incavo SJ. Operative treatment of distal femoral fractures proximal to total knee replacements. *J Bone Joint Surg Am*. 1993; 75:27–34.
18. Mooney V, Mickel VL, Harvey JP, Snelson R. Cast brace treatment for fractures of the distal part of the femur. *J Bone Joint Surg Am*. 1970; 52:1563.
19. Shatzker J, Lambert DC. Supracondylar fractures of the femur. *Clin Orthop*. 1979; 138:77.
20. Sanders R, Regazzoni P, Ruedi TP. Treatment of supracondylar-intercondylar fractures of the femur using the dynamic condylar screw. *J Orthop Trauma*. 1990; 3:214–22.
21. Sarmiento A, Latta LL. Fractures of the femur. In Sarmiento A, Latta LL, *Closed functional treatment of fractures*. Berlin, Springer-Verlag, 1981:297–338.
22. Bucholz RW, Brumback RJ. Fractures of the shaft of the femur. In Rockwood CA, Green DP, Bucholz RW, *Fractures in adults*. New York, 1991, Lippincott, 1653.
23. Hirsch DM, Bhalla S, Roffman M. Supracondylar fracture of the femur following knee replacement. *J Bone Joint Surg Am*. 1981; 63:162–63.
24. Short WH, Hootnick DR, and Murray DG. Ipsilateral supracondylar femur fractures following knee arthroplasty. *Clin Orthop*. 1981; 158:111–16.

CHAPTER 72
Femoral Periprosthetic Fractures: Rush Rods

Jeffrey R. Ginther and Merrill A. Ritter

SUPRACONDYLAR FRACTURES AFTER TOTAL KNEE ARTHROPLASTY

The treatment of supracondylar fractures of the distal femur following total knee arthroplasty has presented a challenge to the orthopedic surgeon both in complexity of the fracture and type of fixation. This is an uncommon injury, with incidence reported as 0.3 to 2.5%.[1,2] The accelerating number of knee replacements being performed will result in an increasing frequency of this injury. Common treatments for this injury include both operative and nonoperative techniques. The common operative choices of treatment include internal fixation with a supracondylar screw or blade plate, revision arthroplasty, and the use of intramedullary fixation (e.g., Rush rod).

We reported a simple treatment using the Rush rod for this fracture in 1985 and because of our success continue to advocate this method of treatment.[3] The limited exposure needed to use a Rush rod gives the advantages of internal fixation without having to make a large dissection. Our results have been satisfactory, with a lower incidence of complications (i.e., infections, loss of motion, nonunions, etc.). All of our fractures have healed within 3 to 4 months and the patients' range of motion was unchanged from before surgery. A treatment that allows for early ROM, early mobilization, and minimal tissue dissection is an ideal choice for this injury.

Previous literature has reviewed both operative and nonoperative treatments for this fracture. Cain reviewed the literature from 1974 to 1983 and reported on 14 fractures. Ten patients had nonoperative treatment and three of these patients had poor results. Four patients were treated by open reduction and internal fixation and three patients had poor results.[4] Healy reviewed the literature between 1981 and 1989, reporting on 173 fractures. Seventy-eight patients were treated operatively and 31% of these had poor results. Ninety-five patients were treated nonoperatively and 32% of these had poor results.[1] The high percentage of poor results led us to our current treatment for supracondylar fractures using the Rush rod.

INDICATIONS FOR USE OF RUSH ROD

Conservative treatment has often yielded poor results. We use Rush rods on almost all adult patients who sustain a supracondylar fracture following a knee replacement (nondisplaced, displaced, angulated, and comminuted). Typically, the patients that sustain this injury are elderly, osteoporotic, and have multiple medical problems. The Rush rod is ideal in this patient population.

We treat nondisplaced fractures with Rush rods, though this may be an aggressive approach (Fig. 72.1A,B,C). Cast immobilization is not a good alternative because casting for greater than 3 weeks is associated with a decrease in the range of motion of the knee and difficulty with ambulation.[5] Culp found that patients immobilized lost 26 degrees of motion and those treated with early motion lost an average of 7 degrees of motion.[6] Skeletal traction is not a good alternative because knee replacement patients are typically older and do not tolerate prolonged bed rest well. These fractures do much better when motion is initiated early.

Patients who have underlying medical diseases that would normally preclude them from an extensive surgical procedure *are* possible considerations for this procedure. These conditions, normally considered contraindications, should instead be considered relative indications. Fixation with Rush rods can be done rapidly with little blood loss. This surgery is little insult to the patient. The alternative of prolonged immobilization and bedrest, in our opinion, has much greater risks of morbidity and mortality for the patient.

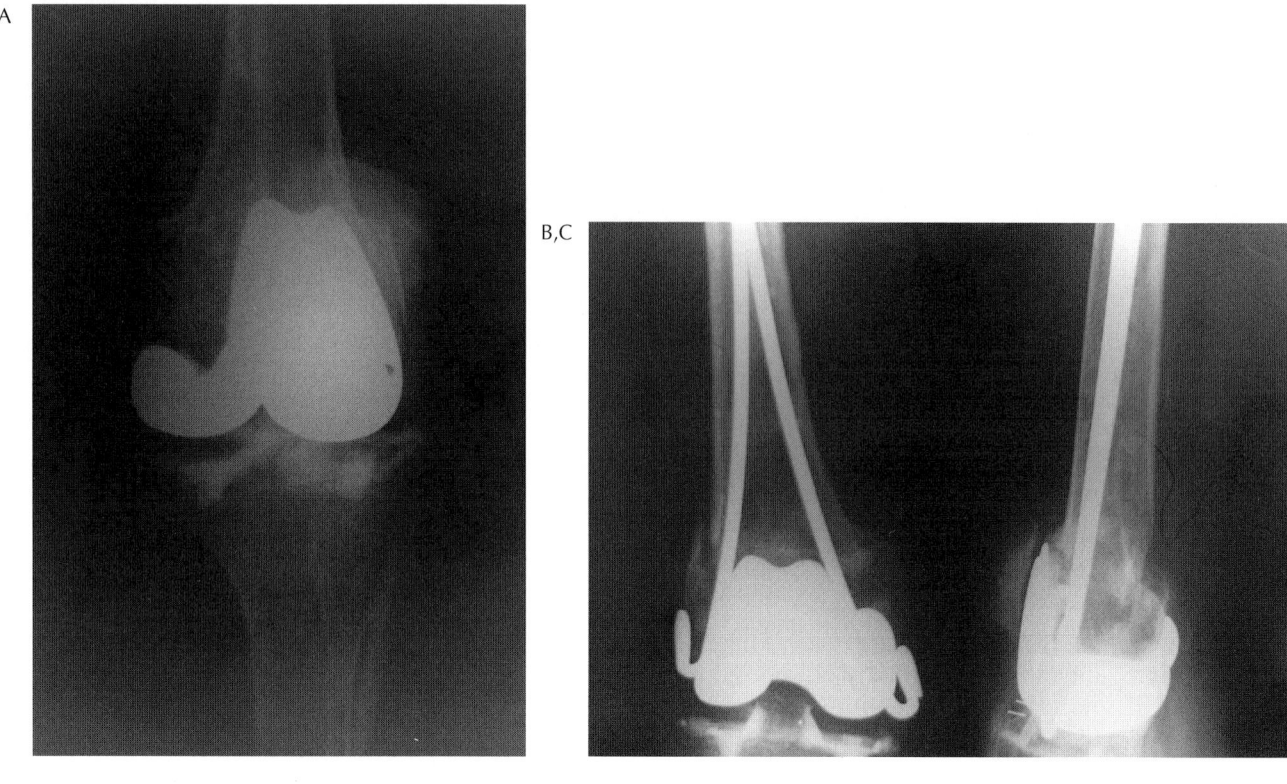

Figure 72.1. (A) Sixty-year-old female who fell and sustained a nondisplaced supracondylar fracture. (B,C) Six weeks postoperative radiographs demonstrating healing of the fracture without displacement. Patient is not tender and ambulates without pain. Alignment and range of motion were preserved.

CONTRAINDICATIONS FOR USE OF RUSH RODS

Component loosening or a nonunion of a previous supracondylar fracture are relative contraindications to treatment with Rush rods. These fractures should be treated with revision arthroplasty with a long-stemmed prosthesis, or possibly plate fixation with bone grafting. The advantages to revision arthroplasty are numerous. The patient can immediately be full weight-bearing and start aggressively working on regaining motion. Concern always exists that the trauma which caused the fracture could have caused some motion at the bone–cement interface and the prosthesis now may be a setup for loosening.[7] If intramedullary fixation was performed and the fracture heals but the prosthesis is loose, the patient will need another surgery. Early revision surgery at the time of the fracture will prevent additional surgery in the future. Additionally, if the components were malaligned after surgical treatment the prosthesis could become loose after ambulation begins. We demonstrated that there is an increased incidence of loosening when the anatomic alignment is in varus.[8] If revision arthroplasty is to be done, care must be taken in prosthesis selection. A femoral component with a large medullary stem that is in 6–8 degrees of valgus should be chosen to follow the anatomic valgus of the knee.[7]

As previously discussed, in the past patients with numerous medical problems were considered contraindicated for surgery. The sentiment now is that these medical problems may give the patient a *relative* indication for surgery with limited operative intervention.

OPERATIVE TECHNIQUE

The patient is positioned on a fracture table such that image intensification can be used to see both the anteroposterior and lateral aspects of the distal femur. The fracture is then reduced and the alignment is checked before inserting any rods. It is critical that the long axis of the femur be positioned in 6–9 degrees of valgus to the distal surface of the femoral component. Fracture reduction before surgery is mandatory because the rods are designed to hold the reduction, not to reduce the fracture. A fracture table with a counter-support posterior to the distal femur will aid in reducing the fracture. After a reduction is achieved, the leg is prepped and draped, maintaining the position of the fracture; this reduction is checked with image intensification (Fig. 72.2).

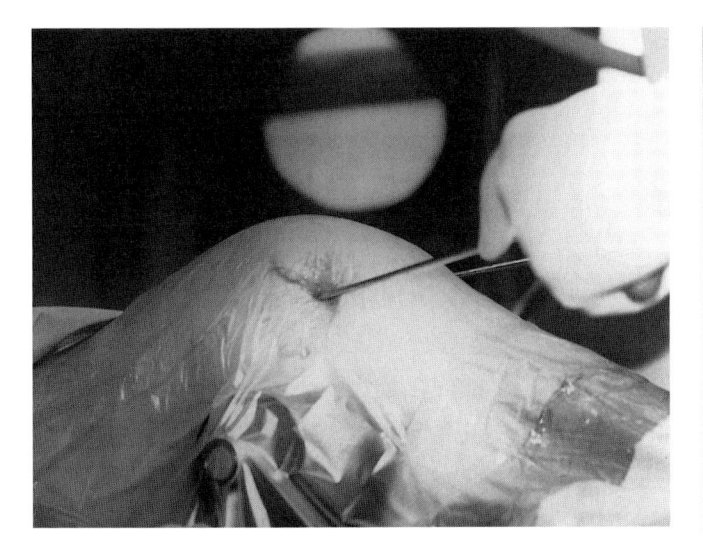

Figure 72.2. Initial positioning of the fracture. The counter support is posterior to the distal femur. Reduction is evaluated with image intensification.

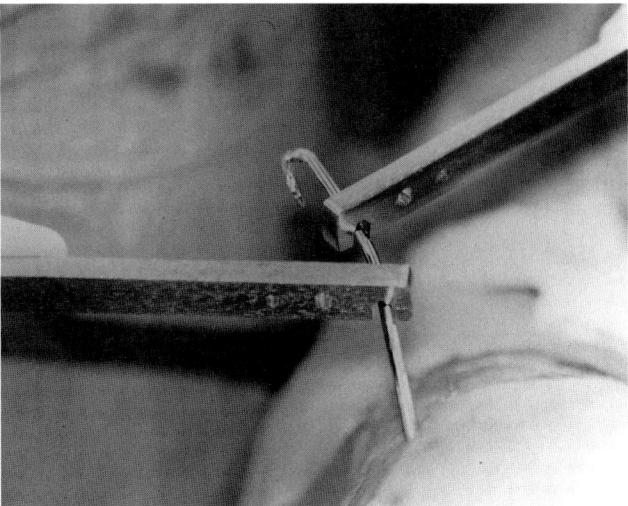

Figure 72.3. Rush rod is being stress relieved (bent) such that the bend will be at the level of the fracture site.

Before making the incision, a transverse mark is made medially and laterally at the level of the distal femur just proximal to the metal component. The incisions are then made extending distally from that line 3–4 cm centering on the epicondyles. The location of the entrance needs to be as close to the prosthesis as possible and centered on the femoral shaft. The bone is hardest in this area and the best purchase of the rods will be obtained. The rods must be in the anterior aspect of the condyles because the shaft of the femur lies anteriorly in relationship to the condyles. The entrance position is checked in both the sagittal and coronal planes prior to entering through the cortical bone. The Rush awl is pushed into the bone initially at a right angle to the femur. The awl is twisted and the femur cut such that it can be brought down until it is almost parallel to the femur. The same technique is repeated on the other side.

The Rush rods are introduced through the awl holes, first laterally, then medially. The beveled aspect of the rods are turned such that they will slide up inside the medullar cavity of the cortical bone. The rods are stress-relieved (bent) on both the medial and lateral sides (Fig. 72.3). Determining the position of the bend is critical. The bend should be at the position of the fracture site when the rods are in place. This can be easily determined by visualization with image intensification. Although the fracture should be fully reduced prior to placement of the Rush rods, the rods can help reduce the fracture if proper stress relief is done. If the fracture has a tendency to go into varus then stress relief should be performed laterally and not medially (or to a lesser degree, medially). If the fracture has a tendency to go into valgus, stress relief should be done medially and less so laterally. This fracture usually results in a valgus deformity because of the pull of the abductor magnus and longus on the proximal fragment.

The rods are now pushed by hand, or tapped gently, across the fracture site and into position (Fig. 72.4). The entire femur is viewed with the image intensifier to ensure that the reduction has been maintained and to

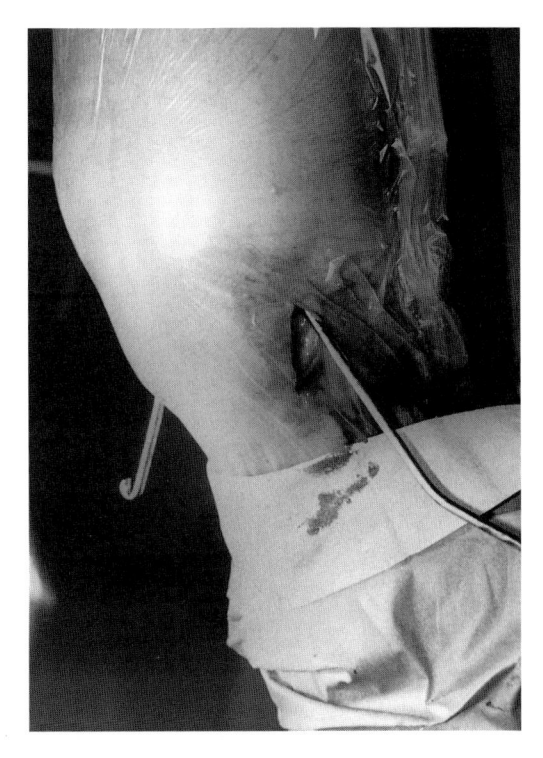

Figure 72.4. Both rods are placed through the awl holes and then pushed by hand or tapped gently across the fracture site. The surgeon should alternate between positioning the medial and lateral Rush rods in order to not lose the reduction.

check that the rods have not penetrated through the femur. It is not necessary for the rods to cross more than once in the intramedullary canal. The knee is taken through a range of motion to assess for any obstruction. The condylar hoops are next buried under soft tissue but superficial to the femur itself; if they are not buried, they will remain prominent and frequently be painful. It is preferable that one use the supracondylar rods rather than the hook rods because they have a larger, flatter surface in the hook area. This allows for better purchase on the cortical bone, which is crucial in osteoporotic patients because the cortical bone is so thin. The knee is now taken through a range of motion to assess for any obstruction to motion.

Postoperatively, the patients are placed in a compression dressing and then a hinged knee brace. Protected ambulation with crutches or a walker begins the first postoperative day. Range of motion exercises are begun immediately and motion is progressed as tolerated. Patients continue with their hinged knee brace and partial weight-bearing with crutches or a walker until the fracture unites, which is usually within 3 to 4 months.[2,9]

RESULTS

We have reported on 22 displaced supracondylar fractures in patients who have had total knee arthroplasties and were treated with Rush rods from various orthopedic surgeons throughout Indiana. The primary diagnosis was osteoarthritis in 15 patients and rheumatoid arthritis in 6 patients. Seven of the patients were on steroids. Eight of the procedures were performed by one of the surgeons at The Center for Hip and Knee Surgery. All of the patients were ambulatory before the fracture. The average flexion prefracture was 102 degrees and all but 2 knees had full extension. One patient had a 5-degree flexion contracture and one patient had a 10-degree contracture. The average flexion postoperatively was 108 degrees. The only knees to have flexion contractures were the same knees that had a contracture preoperatively, and these were both 10 degrees. All other knees achieved full extension.[3]

The average alignment prior to the fracture was 7 degrees of anatomic valgus. At the most recent follow-up evaluation this averaged 10 degrees. The tendency is to place the knees in valgus, which we feel is beneficial. In 1993, we reported to The Knee Society that a TKA in valgus is statistically less likely to fail than one in varus.[8] We therefore have a tendency to place the knee in this position.[10] Cain reviewed 14 cases of supracondylar fractures after knee replacement surgery and found a strong correlation between those fractures that were left in varus angulation and those that were treatment failures.[4] The primary diagnosis was osteoarthritis in 15 patients and rheumatoid arthritis in 6 patients (Fig. 72.5A,B,C).

Between 1981 and 1989, thirteen articles in the English literature reported on the treatment of supracondylar fractures of the femur after total knee arthro-

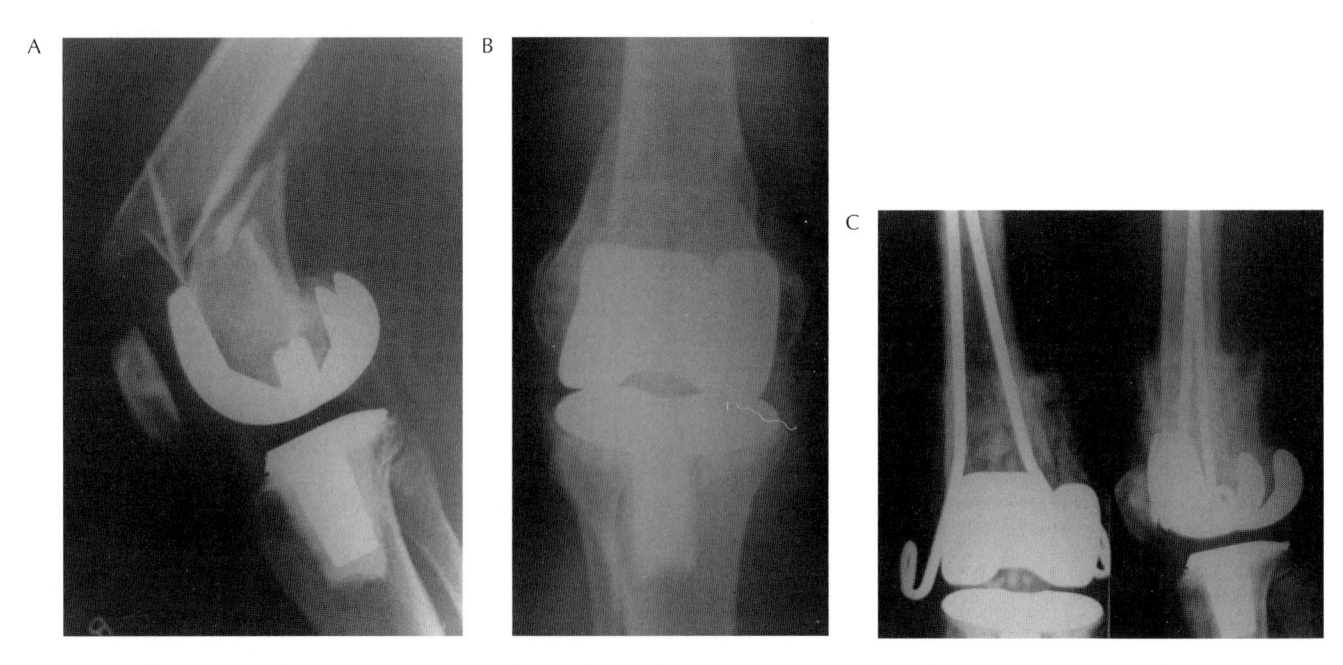

Figure 72.5. Knee replacements in slight valgus fail less than those in varus. The reduction is placed in slightly increased valgus. Stability of this fracture is enhanced by settling of the fracture. The Rush rod allows for controlled collapse such that the load is shared by the fracture and the rods. (A and B) Preoperative radiographs. (C) Healed fracture that demonstrates anatomic valgus and controlled collapse of the fracture.

plasty. The results of these articles were reviewed by Healy. He found good to excellent results in 69% of the patients managed operatively and 68% of the patients managed nonoperatively. Multiple complications—including nonunion, stiffness, deformity, infections, and amputations—have been noted with the treatment of supracondylar fractures. The results of this review in comparison with our results indicate that patients with Rush rods have fewer complications. We experienced none of the complications that are reported so frequently with other methods of treatment.[11–16]

In order to examine if there was a correlation between notching the anterior femoral cortex and sustaining an ipsilateral supracondylar fractures, we reviewed 670 knee replacement surgeries performed between 1975 and 1983 with a 2- to 10-year follow-up period. Only two supracondylar fractures occurred in this series: one in a patient with a 5-mm anterior notch and one in a patient without evidence of notching. In our series, significant notching (i.e., greater than 3 mm) occurred in 20.8% of the total knee arthroplasties performed in our institution. No correlation was found between anterior femoral notching and ipsilateral supracondylar femur fractures. Culp found that a 3-mm anterior notch creates a decrease in torsional stress to fracture of 29% and this has generally been considered to be the standard for significant notching in the literature. These findings did not consider the remodeling capability of bone. In dogs, bone remodeling around screw holes returns the strength of the bone to normal in 8 weeks after screw removal.[6] We feel that remodeling of bone proximal to the prosthesis occurs and that notching of the cortical bone only weakens the bone in the acute setting. The reason the fracture occurs is because of osteoporosis and torsional strain. The fractures in our study occurred between 6 weeks and 16 years following TKA (average, 5 years). In only two cases did the fracture occur earlier than 1 year after total knee arthroplasty.

We concluded that anterior notching of the femur is not a risk factor for sustaining a supracondylar fracture. We feel that the most significant risk factor causing this injury is the increase in activity that elderly patients display after knee replacement. This makes them more prone to slipping and falling, which is consistent with the minor trauma that is typically the mechanism for this type of injury. Other risk factors include steroid use, osteoporosis, revision arthroplasty, rheumatoid arthritis, and neurologic disorders.[4,6]

In conclusion, we believe that the use of Rush rods with this type of fracture is the best solution to this complex problem. Our surgical precept of doing what is easy to make the tough problem simple could never be more applicable. This technique provides the advantage of both open and closed techniques. It also offers enough stability to allow early motion at the knee without the necessity of prolonged bedrest, immobilization, extensive surgical exposure, or the resultant disruption of blood supply. Early knee motion and protective weight-bearing allow the fracture to settle and maintain proper varus-valgus alignment. The muscle contraction during early healing and early partial weight-bearing will work to simulate fracture healing. The minimal dissection will result in a lower infection rate and less scarring. This also makes regaining motion less difficult for the patient. Our results support the use of Rush rods for this fracture and allow the surgeon to have excellent reproducible results.

References

1. Healy W, Siliski J, Incavo S. Operative treatment of distal femoral fractures proximal to total knee replacements. *J Bone and Joint Surg*. 1993; 75A:27–34.
2. Ritter M, Keating M, Faris P, Meding J. Rush rod fixation of supracondylar fractures above total knee arthroplasties. *J Arthroplasty*. 1995; 10:213–16.
3. Ritter M, Stiver P. Supracondylar fracture in a patient with total knee arthroplasty. *Clin Orthop*. 1985; 193:168–70.
4. Cain M, Rubash H, Wissinger H, McClain E. Periprosthetic femoral fractures following total knee arthroplasty. *Clin Orthop*. 1986; 208:205–214.
5. Digiora A, Rubash H. Periprosthetic fractures of the femur after total knee arthroplasty. *Clin Orthop*. 1991; 271:135–42.
6. Culp R, Schmidt R, Hanks G, Mak A, Esterhai J, Heppenstall R. Supracondylar fracture of the femur following prosthetic knee arthroplasty. *Clin Orthop*. 1987; 222:212–22.
7. Cordeiro E, Costa R, Carazzato J, Silva J. Periprosthetic fractures in patients with total knee arthroplasties. *Clin Orthop*. 1990; 252:182–89.
8. Ritter M, Faris P, Keating M, Meding J. Postoperative alignment of total knee replacement. *Clin Orthop*. 1994; 299:153–56.
9. Shelbourne K, Bureckmann F. Rush-pin fixation of supracondylar and intercondylar fractures of the femur. *J Bone and Joint*. 1982; 64A:161–69.
10. Ritter M, Faris P, Keating M. Anterior femoral notching and ipsilateral supracondylar femur fracture in total knee arthroplasty. *J Arthroplasty*. 1988; 3:185–87.
11. Aaron R, Scott R. Supracondylar fracture of the femur after total knee arthroplasty. *Clin Orthop*. 1987; 219:136–39.
12. Hanks G, Mathews H, Routson G, Loughran T. Supracondylar fracture of the femur following total knee arthroplasty. *J Arthroplasty*. 1989; (4):289–92.
13. Kray M, Goldberg V, Figgie M, Figgie H. Distal femoral replacement with allograft/prosthetic reconstruction for treatment of supracondylar fractures in patients with total knee arthroplasty. *J Arthroplasty*. 1992; 7:7–15.
14. Merkel K, Johnson E. Supracondylar fracture of the femur after total knee arthroplasty. *J Bone and Joint Surg*. 1986; 68A:29–43.
15. Moran C, Brick G, Sledge C, Dysart S, Chien E. Supracondylar femoral fracture following total knee arthroplasty. *Clin Orthop*. 1996; 324:196–209.
16. Sisto D, Lachiewicz P, Insall J. Treatment of supracondylar fractures following prosthetic arthroplasty of the knee. *Clin Orthop*. 1985; 196:265–72.

CHAPTER 73
Femoral Periprosthetic Fractures: Retrograde Intramedullary Nail

Lawrence A. Schaper and David Seligson

Supracondylar fractures of the femur after total knee arthroplasties are relatively uncommon, with an incidence from 0.3 to 2.5%. Most agree that nondisplaced fractures can be treated conservatively with bracing or cast-brace immobilization. If the femoral component is loose or unstable, it should be revised to a long-stemmed implant. The treatment of displaced fractures, however, has been somewhat controversial. A comprehensive review of the literature by Chen et al. in 1994 showed that 83% of patients with Neer type 1 (nondisplaced) fractures were satisfied, whereas only 64% of patients with types 2 and 3 (displaced) fractures were satisfied, with no statistical difference between operative or nonoperative treatment.[1] Healy et al. reported on twenty displaced supracondylar fractures above total knee replacements, all treated with open reduction and internal fixation using blade plates, condylar screw-plates, and buttress plates. Eleven patients eventually healed and returned to their previous level of function, although two required a second procedure for delayed union.[2] Intramedullary fixation using a retrograde interlocking nail to yield excellent results in displaced supracondylar and intercondylar fractures has been increasingly reported in the recent literature.[3-8] This technique has several advantages over traditional open reduction with plate fixation. Intramedullary implants are biomechanically superior to laterally placed fixation devices, with larger bending moments. Periosteal stripping, which can lead to compromise of blood supply to the fracture site and increase the risk of nonunion, is not necessary. Plate fixation can be technically demanding and often requires the use of supplemental bone grafting. The retrograde nail can often be placed percutaneously, thereby reducing some of the morbidity associated with exposure and periosteal stripping of the fracture site.

PREOPERATIVE PLANNING

Preparation for fracture treatment should begin with a radiograph of the entire femur in two planes. The fracture pattern, amount of displacement, bone quality, prosthetic stability, and (if possible) model and size of the implant should be assessed. Nails are available in lengths of 15 cm, 20 cm, and 25 cm, with outer diameters of 11 mm, 12 mm, or 13 mm. Two designs are available (Fig. 73.1) and should be selected on the basis of the fracture pattern. Rolston et al. have investigated the intercondylar distances of commonly used prostheses and have published a table with dimensions that can assist in determining whether the nail will fit a given design (Table 73.1).[4]

TECHNIQUE

The patient should be positioned supine on a radiolucent operating table. A U-shaped adhesive drape is useful to isolate the groin and perineum, leaving the entire thigh and leg areas exposed. The knee should be flexed 30 to 40 degrees with a roll under the distal thigh (Fig. 73.2). Rotational alignment can be verified by the iliac crest, patella, and first web space of the foot. In situations with intercondylar extension, fixation can be achieved with percutaneous cannulated screws placed over guidewires prior to insertion of the nail. If there is any question that the fracture might have compromised fixation of the femoral component, a formal arthrotomy should be done and the stability of the femoral component assessed.

After the lower extremity has been prepped and draped, the fluoroscope should be used to check the adequacy of closed reduction. Attention to the amount of flexion and valgus required for proper alignment will

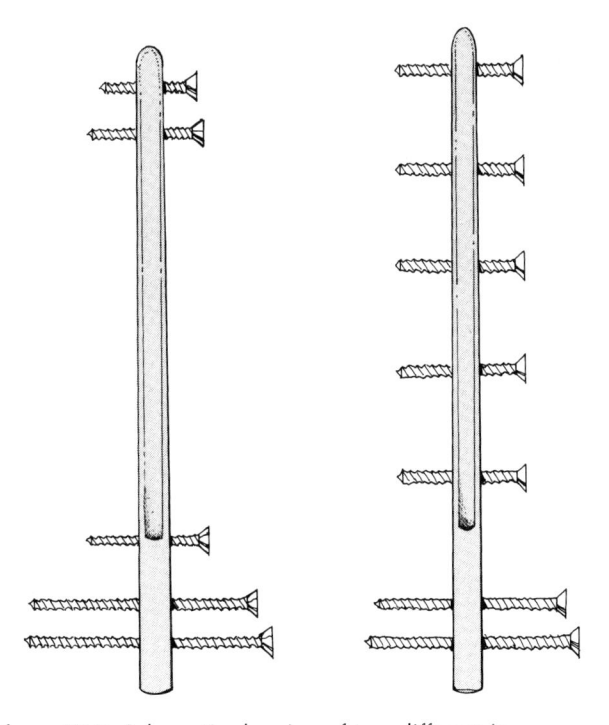

Figure 73.1. Schematic drawing of two different intramedullary supracondylar nails. The IMSC nail (left) is fully cannulated with 7–12 holes for placement of 5.0 mm locking screws. The standard multihole nail (right) has an 8-degree anterior bend for easier insertion.

help later when the nail is inserted. When possible, the nail should be inserted percutaneously. A longitudinal incision is made over the patellar tendon. The fibers are split, allowing access to the intercondylar notch. A curved awl is inserted under direct vision below the anterior flange of the prosthesis (Fig. 73.3). It is extremely important that the fracture is properly aligned in both planes when the awl is inserted because the later reamers will follow this path. A ball-tipped guidewire is inserted past the fracture site and flexible reamers are passed over the guide, beginning with 8 mm and advancing to 1 mm larger than the selected nail. The nail and drill guide are then assembled and the nail is advanced over the guidewire, holding the fracture reduced. The nail can be placed with the apex either anterior or posterior and should be oriented to achieve best reduction. This is done with manual pressure only and a gentle twisting motion. The tip of the nail should be countersunk slightly beneath the bone surface (Fig. 73.4). Interlocking screws are used to hold the nail both in the condylar region and the diaphysis. The screws are placed percutaneously from lateral to medial and should be confirmed with anteroposterior and lateral fluoroscopic images. At least two screws should be placed in the diaphysis and up to three screws may be used in the condylar region. If the bone is osteopenic, locking boulons are available to add strength to the fixation and can add transverse compression to intercondylar fractures.[9]

AFTERCARE

Most fractures will be stable enough to allow early motion with use of a hinged brace during ambulation. Continuous passive motion (CPM) may be started within 24 to 48 hours after surgery and should be supplemented with an isometric quad strengthening program. Touchdown weight-bearing is allowed initially with gradual progression to tolerance over a 6- to 12-week period, guided by radiographic signs of callus formation. The rehabilitation program should be modified based upon the surgeon's assessment of fracture stability. Routine

Table 73.1. Intercondylar distances of commonly used femoral prostheses

Manufacturer	Model	Intercondylar distance (smallest size, in mm)
Biomet (Warsaw, Indiana)	AGC Universal	18
DePuy (Warsaw, Indiana)	AMK	18
Dow Corning Wright (Arlington, Tennessee)	Whitesides modular	20
Howmedica (Rutherford, New Jersey)	PCA	18.5
Intermedics (Austin, Texas)	Natural	14
Johnson and Johnson (New Brunswick, New Jersey)	Press-fit condylar	20
	Insall-Burstein* (Posterior stabilized)	15
Kirschner (Timonium, Maryland)	Performance	14
Zimmer (Warsaw, Indiana)	Insall-Burnsetin I*	16
	Insall-Burnstein II (posterior stabilized* or constrained condylar**)	15
	Miller-Galante I	
	Small/small+[//]	11
	Regular/regular+	12.5
	Large/large+	15
	Large++	18
	Miller-Galante II	13

*The intercondylar box will accommodate the nail. However, it is necessary to countersink the nail to prevent impingement on the tibial spine.
**The prosthesis includes a femoral stem and thus will not accommodate the nail.
[//]The prosthesis will not accommodate even the smaller nail (eleven millimeters).
Source: Rolston L, Christ D, Halpern A, O'Connor P, Ryan T, Uggen W. [4].

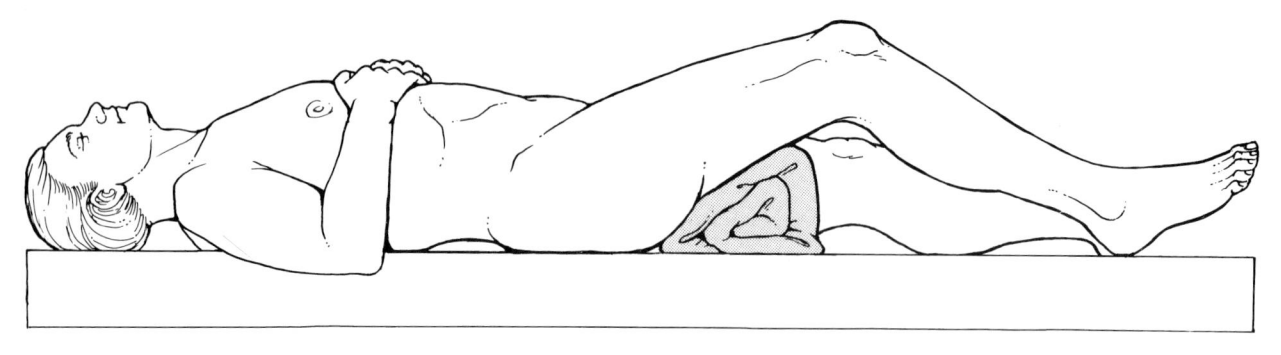

Figure 73.2. Schematic of patient positioning. Note the patient in a supine position on a radiolucent table. Fluoroscopic control should be used in association with a radiolucent extension table. The knee is flexed to 30–40 degrees with a leg roll to provide adequate access for reduction and fixation of the intercondylar fracture. Rotational alignment is achieved by aligning the iliac crest, patella, and first web space of the foot.

prophylaxis against thromboembolic phenomena should be instituted postoperatively.

SUMMARY

Supracondylar fractures of the femur after total knee replacement should be assessed to determine the amount of displacement and whether the femoral prosthesis is stable. Minimally displaced fractures are best treated with immobilization. If the femoral component is unstable, it should be revised with a long-stemmed implant, using supplemental bone graft when significant comminution is present. Displaced fractures with a sta-

Figure 73.3. Schematic of a curved awl. Entry into the intracondular notch is made with a curved awl over a 3.2-mm guide pin.

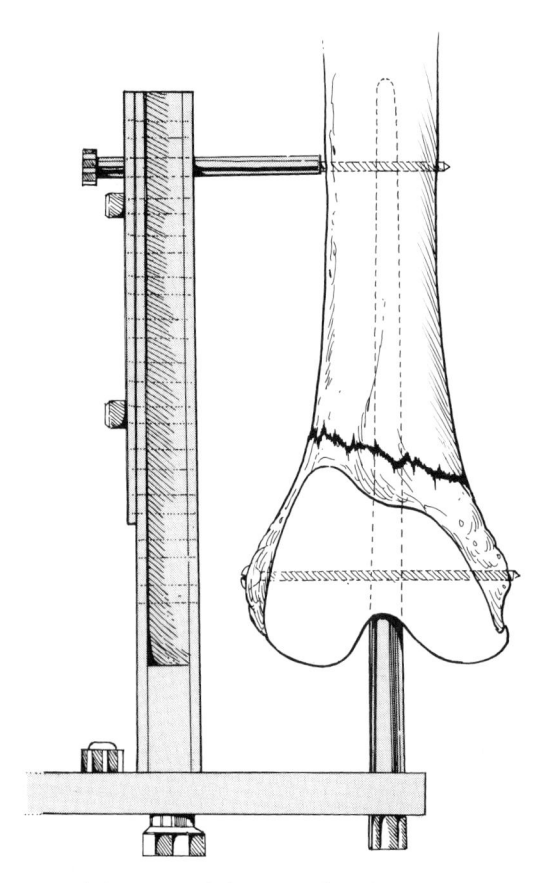

Figure 73.4. Schematic of the procedure for inserting the 5.9-mm locking screws or the step screws. With the leg over a bolster, place the screws percutaneously through the drill guide beginning with the most distal screw and progressing to the most proximal screw.

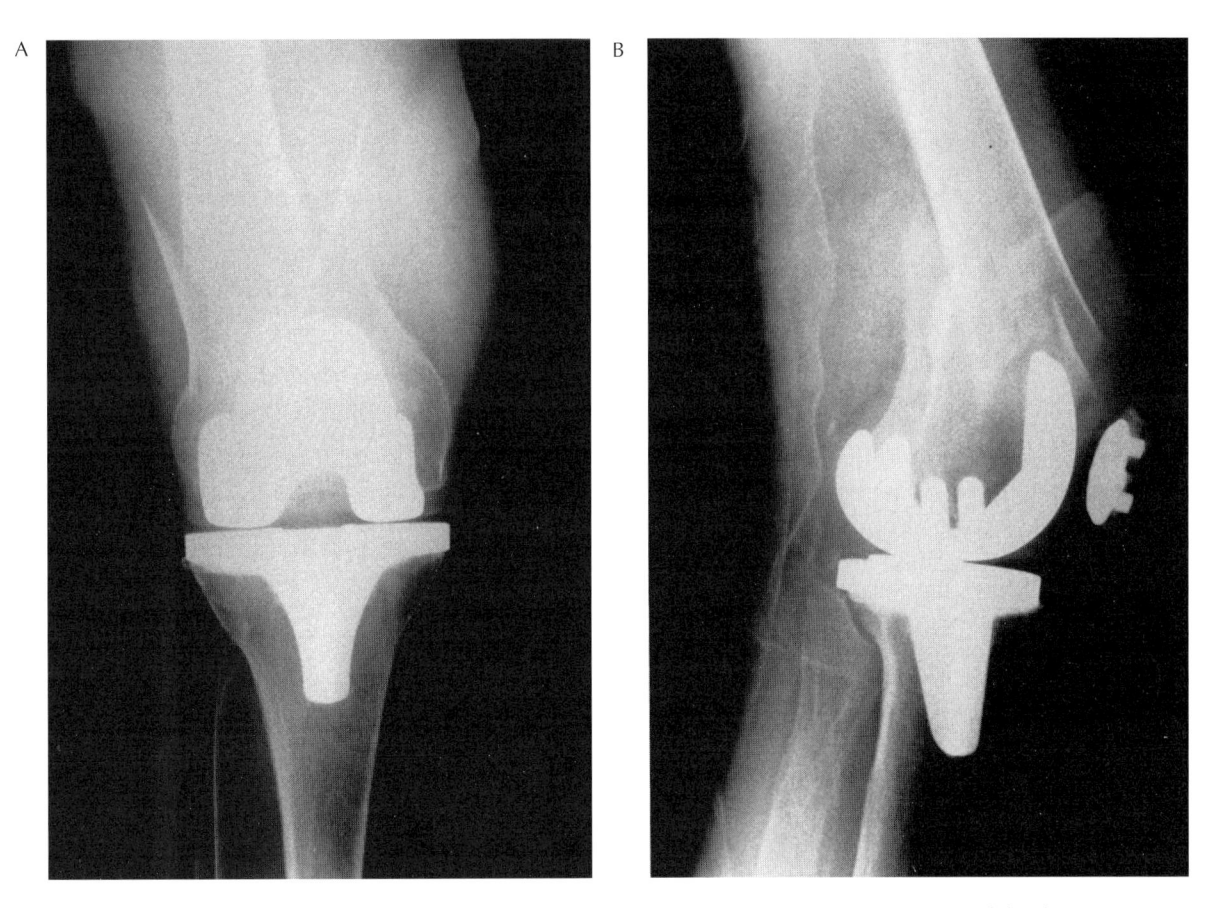

Figure 73.5 A,B. Anteroposterior and lateral preoperative roentgenograms of a supracondylar fracture of the right distal femur above a total knee replacement in a 78-year-old female.

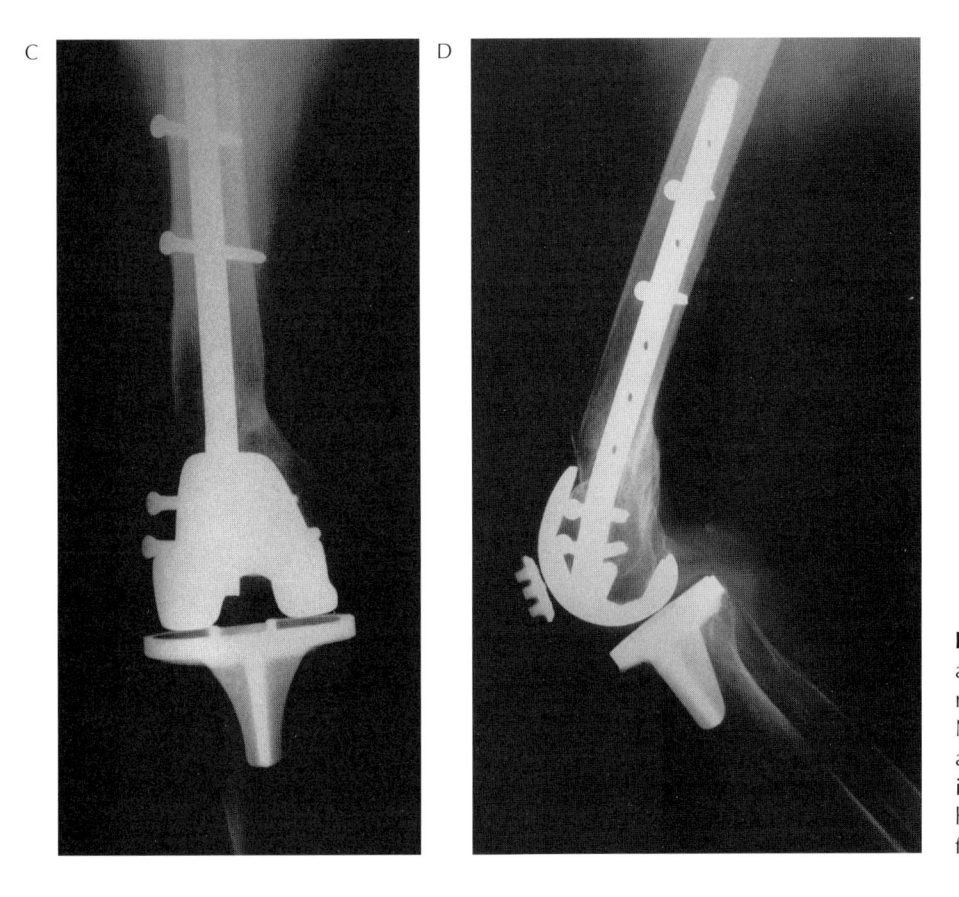

Figure 73.5 C,D. Anteroposterior and lateral 2-year postoperative roentgenograms of the same patient. Note the distal blocking screw appears somewhat angulated and is probably broken. The GS nail, however, is in place and the fracture healed.

ble prosthesis should be managed by reduction and internal fixation. At least one series has shown good results with open reduction and osteosynthesis with blade plates or condylar plates; however, this method is technically demanding and requires direct fracture exposure with increased periosteal stripping (Fig. 73.5A–D). The recent introduction of a specialized retrograde intramedullary nail has greatly simplified the treatment of these historically difficult fractures. Most prosthetic designs are suitable for this technique, although it is extremely important to know the model and size of the implant to ensure that the nail will pass safely. Percutaneous placement is usually possible, thus minimizing disturbance of the fracture site. Good functional and radiographic outcomes using the retrograde intramedullary nail with few complications have been documented in several recent series and suggest that, when indicated, the retrograde intramedullary nail is an excellent method for treatment of supracondylar fractures of the femur after total knee arthroplasty.

References

1. Chen F, Mont M, Bachner R. Management of ipsilateral supracondylar femur fractures following total knee arthroplasty. *J Arthroplasty*. 1994; 9[5]:521–25.
2. Healy W, Siliski J, Incavo S. Operative treatment of distal femoral fractures proximal to total knee replacements. *J Bone and Joint Surg*. 1993; 75A[1]:27–33.
3. Ritter M, Keating M, Faris P, Meding J. Rush rod fixation of supracondylar fractures above total knee arthroplasties. *J Arthroplasty*. 1995; 10[2]:213–16.
4. Rolston L, Christ D, Halpern A, O'Connor P, Ryan T, Uggen W. Treatment of supracondylar fractures of the femur proximal to a total knee arthroplasty. *J Bone Joint Surg*. 1995; 77A[6]:924–31.
5. Jabczenski F, Crawford M. Retrograde intramedullary nailing of supracondylar femur fractures above total knee arthroplasty. *J Arthroplasty*. 1995; 10[1]:95–101.
6. Murrell G, Nunley J. Interlocked supracondylar intramedullary nails for supracondylar fractures after total knee arthroplasty. *J Arthroplasty*. 1995; 10[1]:37–42.
7. McLaren A, Dupone J, Schroeber D. Open reduction internal fixation of supraconcylar fractures above total knee arthroplasties using the intramedullary supracondylar rod. *Clin Orthop*. 1994; 302:194–98.
8. Cole J, Huff W, Blum D. Retrograde femoral nailing of supracondylar, intercondylar, and distal fractures of the femur. *Amer J of Ortho*, supp. 1996; 22–30.
9. Wozasek GE, Seligson D, Durgin R. Distal interlocking screw fixation strength in femoral intramedullary nailing: Influence of bone quality and supplemental buttress nut. *Osteo Int*. 1996; 2:123–27.

CHAPTER 74

Femoral Periprosthetic Fractures: Blade Plates Fixation

Laurence D. Higgins and Mark P. Figgie

Periprosthetic fractures pose a challenging management problem for the orthopedic surgeon. Supracondylar femur fractures above ipsilateral total knee replacements (TKRs) may be the most formidable of all. The principles of fracture management are complicated by prosthetic component location, poor bone quality, the necessity for anatomic alignment, and achieving sufficient stability to allow for early postoperative motion. The goals of management include maintenance of leg alignment and length, conservation of well-fixed components to avoid unnecessary revision TKR with its incumbent morbidity, and restoration of prefracture ambulatory status and motion in a pain-free knee.

HISTORICAL OVERVIEW

The earliest report of supracondylar femur fractures above TKRs appeared in 1977 in the German literature.[1] The first reported series in the English literature was authored by Short et al. in 1981, detailing five cases.[2] Since then, we are aware of 40 articles published in the English literature describing this problem.

The definition of supracondylar femur fractures above TKRs has varied. Several studies define supracondylar femur fracture after TKR as those occurring within 15 cm of the joint line, whereas others have limited inclusion to fractures within 9 cm of the joint line. DeGioia and Rubash have further proposed that any fracture that occurs within 5 cm of the most proximal extent of an intramedullary femoral device should also be included in the definition of supracondylar femur fractures above TKRs.[3] Of note, stress fractures and intraoperative fractures have not routinely been included in published series.

INCIDENCE

Undoubtedly, supracondylar femur fractures after TKRs are rare fractures. The published incidence ranges from 0.3 to 2.5%.[4–8] Despite varying definitions, most articles consist of small case series and only ten articles exist to our knowledge that report on more than ten patients each.[4,6,7,9–15]

RISK FACTORS

Various risk factors have been identified for the development of supracondylar femur fracture after TKR (Table 74.1). Merkel and Johnson[7] published the first large series, with 36 fractures and correlated osteopenia, rheumatoid arthritis, oral steroid use, revision TKR, and anterior femoral notching with increased fracture risk. Subsequently, a variety of other factors were added to this list, including neurologic disorders with gait ataxia, female gender, and occurrence during the seventh decade of life.[4,6,7,9,10] Despite consensus regarding most risk factors, the correlation between anterior femoral notching and supracondylar femur fractures above TKRs is still controversial.

Culp et al.,[10] in the largest series published to date, addressed the issue of anterior femoral notching on both clinical and biomechanical grounds. Using a retrospective analysis of supracondylar femur fracture after TKR treated by the Pennsylvania Orthopaedic Society between 1975 and 1984, Culp documented that 27 of the 61 patients with supracondylar femur fractures above TKRs had anterior femoral notching. This 44% prevalence served as the catalyst to evaluate the biomechanical consequences of such a lesion. By deriving a formula for polar moment of inertia, Culp demonstrated that a 3-mm defect in the anterior

Table 74.1. Risk factors for supracondylar femur fractures

- Osteopenia
- Rheumatoid arthritis
- Steroid use
- Neurologic disorder
- Revision TKR
- Female gender
- Age in seventh decade
- Distal femoral osteolysis
- ± Anterior femoral notching

femoral cortex theoretically diminishes torsional strength by 29.2%.[10]

Ritter et al.[8] subsequently reviewed 670 TKRs performed between 1975 and 1983. The study retrospectively documented 138 of 670 cases with 3 mm or more of anterior femoral notching (20.5%). With a follow up of 2–12 years, only two supracondylar femur fractures after TKR occurred. Furthermore, one of the two fractures occurred in a patient without evidence of anterior femoral notching. Ritter concluded that the remodeling capability of bone remedies torsional strength weakness over time and that notching is only of minimal concern in the early postoperative period (0–6 months).[8] In addition, such fractures were multifactorial in origin and may be attributed to osteopenia, inadequate bone remodeling, stress shielding, or increased use of the extremity after the operation.[8]

In 1994, Rand reported on a single case of a supracondylar femur fracture after TKR associated with polyethylene wear.[42] Massive osteolysis, measuring 7 by 5 by 5 cm, was measured intraoperatively with a fracture extending through the osteolytic region. Soon thereafter, Cadambia et al. documented an 11.1% incidence of femoral osteolysis (30 of 271 primary TKRs with cementless implantation) accompanying two minimally constrained TKR designs.[16] With a mean follow-up of 52 months, polyethylene debris was noted in all revised components. Femoral osteolysis was present more frequently with male gender, younger age, increased weight, presence of concurrent tibial osteolysis, osteoarthritis, and the length of time in situ.[16]

In addition to notching and osteolysis, distal femoral deficits may result from degenerative or rheumatoid cysts.[12,17] Moran et al.[12] recently reported three fractures associated with large anterior femoral cysts filled with polymethylmethacrylate (PMMA) at the time of arthroplasty. Adequate remodeling may be inhibited when these defects are filled with cement. Therefore, current recommendations for such defects include curettage with bone graft packing. The use of a long-stemmed intramedullary femoral component has been advocated to protect this area until adequate remodeling has occurred.[17]

EVALUATION

A thorough history and physical examination are essential in evaluating any periprosthetic fracture. Indepth questioning regarding prefracture ambulatory status, level of pain (if any), and function must be detailed. During physical examination, particular attention should be directed at three areas: (1) a detailed neurovascular exam; (2) evaluation of the soft tissue envelope; and, (3) the location and appearance of previous incisions.

Radiographic evaluation including AP, lateral, and oblique images are necessary. Additionally, long cassettes may provide important information regarding overall leg alignment, which is not adequately assessed on standard x-ray cassettes. The fracture pattern and its relation to the prosthesis, presence of comminution, displacement (including angulation, rotation, and shortening), limb alignment, and quality of the bone must be carefully noted. Furthermore, meticulous attention must be directed at the component itself, seeking evidence of component loosening or failure. Comparison with prefracture radiographs is critical in determining the necessity for revision. Areas of osteolysis or cyst formation, and their treatment (if any), must be noted. Finally, documentation of the exact prosthesis involved, including size, will allow for appropriate preoperative planning of fracture repair.[17]

CLASSIFICATION

Classification of supracondylar femur fractures above TKRs has been problematic. As no specific classification system exists for periprosthetic femur fractures above TKRs, a large number of studies failed to classify fractures, assigning to them either stable or unstable configurations. Furthermore, a variety of generic fracture classification systems have been applied to such fractures in other studies. These classification systems have not been demonstrated to fulfill the criteria for a clinically significant classification system, which must possess the following properties:

(1) Provide accurate documentation of the fracture
(2) Possess high inter- and intra-observer reliability
(3) Possess a logical and simple framework
(4) Provide direction for clinical management
(5) Possess prognostic information

Neer et al. provided a general classification system for supracondylar femur fractures in 1967.[18] This classification system has been most widely employed in the literature and therefore will be reviewed. Briefly, type I fractures are minimally displaced. Type II fractures, demonstrating displacement of the condyles are subdivided into two categories: (1) type IIA, with medial displacement; and (2) type IIB, with lateral displacement. Finally, type III fractures have concomitant supracondylar and shaft fractures.[18]

DiGioia and Rubash[3] modified Neer's classification system in 1991. After detailing a thorough physical and radiographic exam, the authors proposed a three-part classification. Grade I fractures are extraarticular, nondisplaced fractures (defined as less than 5 mm translation or 5 degrees angulation in any plane). Grade II fractures are also extraarticular, but possess displacement of greater than 5 mm or greater than 5 degrees angulation in any plane. Finally, grade III fractures are severely displaced fractures with loss of cortical contact, severe angulation (greater than 10 degrees) and may include intercondylar components. The presence of fracture comminution is separately classified as minimal or severe.[3] Despite the broad application of the Neer and modified-Neer classification systems, a specific clinically significant classification system needs to be developed.

REVIEW OF LITERATURE

To date, only ten articles published on supracondylar femur fractures above TKRs describe series of ten of more patients. The remainder of the reports in the literature document case reports of small numbers of patients, which are accordingly unable to achieve statistical significance. Those publications that include more than ten cases each are reviewed next.

The first large series of supracondylar femur fractures above TKRs was published by Sisto et al.[15] in 1985. Documenting 15 fractures in 15 patients (all within 15 cm of the joint line), the study group comprised nine patients with rheumatoid arthritis and six with osteoarthritis. All fractures occurred after minimal trauma and twelve were classified as displaced. Treatment was divided into three groups. Group I (4 patients) underwent cast immobilization with early weight-bearing. Group II (8 patients) was initially treated with traction followed by cast or cast-brace immobilization. Group III (3 patients), all with displaced fractures, underwent immediate open reduction with internal fixation (ORIF). Using a mean follow-up of 18 months (range, 10 to 48 months) all patients completed the Hospital for Special Surgery (HSS) Knee Rating Scale. In group I, 3 of 4 patients had lower post-injury knee ratings on the HSS score, with one patient requiring a supracondylar osteotomy for a symptomatic nonunion. In group II, 4 of 8 had lower HSS knee scores, and one nonunion required a revision TKR with a fluted femoral rod. In group III patients, all fractures united within 5 months and HSS knee scores were unchanged from prefracture ratings.[15]

The criteria for success included union of the fracture with proper prosthetic alignment, maintenance of fixation of all components, and a minimum of 90 degrees of knee motion. In conclusion, Sisto et al. proposed a treatment protocol that recommended gentle closed reduction with skeletal traction as initial treatment. Early ORIF was recommended for the prosthetic fracture that could not be maintained in acceptable alignment with traction. No specific guidelines were offered to assess the success of closed reduction with traction, nor were details provided regarding the choice of device or technique of fixation.[15]

Merkel and Johnson[7] reported the Mayo Clinic experience in 1986, documenting 36 supracondylar femur fractures above TKRs. Of the 36 fractures, each of which resulted from slight trauma, 11 were classified as nondisplaced and 25 displaced. Using Neer's classification system, the authors divided the treatments into three groups. The first group was "nonoperative" and consisted of traction, cast immobilization, or both. The second group underwent early ORIF, whereas the third group underwent immediate external fixation. Twenty-six fractures (25 patients) were treated in the nonoperative group, all of which were classified as Neer grade I, IIA, or IIB. Seventeen of 26 (65%) healed without a secondary procedure. Nine failed nonoperative treatment with four nonunions, two malunions, two prosthetic loosenings, and one extensor dysfunction that required an above-knee amputation (AKA) for fulminant sepsis following a failed quadricepsplasty. In group II (early ORIF), 3 of 5 had a satisfactory result, all Neer grade II. Of the two failures, one patient died intraoperatively and another underwent AKA for a periprosthetic infection with sepsis. Of the three fractures treated with external fixation, all had either good or excellent results.[7]

The authors recommended nonoperative treatment for initial management. Furthermore, they proposed that leg alignment was critical in predicting clinical success after closed reduction, requiring less than 10 degrees of angulation in both planes for a satisfactory result. Poor outcomes following nonoperative treatment were best treated with revision arthroplasty, which routinely yielded a satisfactory result. Using Neer's classification system, Merkel and Johnson proposed a treatment algorithm. Neer grade I fractures were best treated with immediate cast immobilization, followed by cast bracing at 4 weeks. Neer grade IIA or IIB fractures should undergo gentle closed reduction and skeletal traction. If the alignment is unacceptable, early ORIF was recommended; revision arthroplasty was proposed if ORIF was not technically feasible. Furthermore, allowing the fracture to heal with delayed revision arthroplasty best treated loose components at the time of fracture. Overall, the loss of motion with nonoperative treatment averaged only 10 degrees and, given the higher rates of complication with ORIF, the authors concluded that ORIF was not warranted. The only groups for which ORIF was recommended were those patients who did not have osteopenia, in whom stable fixation could be obtained, who required a highly functioning knee, or in whom adequate reduction could not be maintained.[7]

In 1986, Cain et al.[9] reported on 14 supracondylar femur fractures above TKRs, all of which occurred after minimal trauma. Ten patients were treated nonoperatively, with three unsatisfactory results (two with excessive loss of knee function and one nonunion). Four patients underwent ORIF with a variety of techniques (two rush pins, one rush pin with cancellous screws, and one compression plating). Three of 4 ultimately resulted in poor results, with two nonunions and one ligamentous instability. All of the poor results occurred in patients with displaced fractures with significant comminution. The authors determined that the degree of comminution at the fracture site confers a poor prognosis and should be noted. In addition, the authors correlated translations of more than 5 mm in prosthetic alignment with a poor outcome. In conclusion, Cain et al. proposed a plan for treatment based on their results. Nondisplaced fractures should be casted for 4 to 6 weeks, followed by cast-brace application. Displaced fractures were best treated with closed reduction and skeletal traction. ORIF was indicated only for failed closed-reduction and skeletal traction.[9]

The largest series to date was published by Culp et al.[10] in 1987. Describing 61 fractures in 58 patients (obtained from the Pennsylvania Orthopaedic Society), the authors directly compared the outcome between operative (31 fractures) and nonoperative (30 fractures) treatment. In the operative group, 21 fractures were comminuted and 21 were classified as displaced. A wide assortment of internal fixation devices was utilized, including 20 compression plates and four immediate revision TKRs. In the nonoperative group, 19 of 30 were treated with immediate cast immobilization, 10 patients were treated with traction followed by cast immobilization, and 1 patient managed with bedrest alone. No documentation of fracture displacement or comminution in the nonoperative group was provided.[10]

In the operative group, 25 of 31 fractures showed satisfactory union. Of the remaining six fractures, three malunions and one nonunion occurred; two patients underwent above knee amputations secondary to deep sepsis after surgery. Those operative patients who received postoperative casting lost a mean of 27 degrees of knee motion, whereas only a 7-degree loss of motion occurred when immediate postoperative motion was implemented. Ultimately, five of these patients underwent revision TKRs.

The nonoperative group yielded 17 successful unions, seven malunions and six nonunions. The rate of complications (defined by malunion, nonunion or amputation) was statistically higher in the nonoperative group. Six of the 30 fractures required a secondary procedure and resulted in a substantial loss of motion. Those patients treated with immobilization (casting) lost a mean of 26 degrees of motion; when early motion with traction was initiated, patients only lost a mean of 12 degrees of motion. This was the only study large enough to obtain statistical significance, and the authors concluded that supracondylar femur fractures above TKRs are best treated with rigid internal fixation accompanied by early motion.[10]

In 1988, Bogoch et al.[4] reported on twelve patients with rheumatoid arthritis who had periprosthetic fractures above TKRs (resurfacing or MacIntosh prostheses). Eight of these fractures were treated nonoperatively with splints, casts, and traction. The authors documented that such treatment did not maintain correct alignment and restore leg length in most cases. Eleven fractures healed, with one patient requiring a second operative procedure to obtain union. Only one patient retained prefracture alignment and length; nine axial nonunions occurred, and ten fractures resulted in excessive shortening (mean shortening, 2.8 cm). The authors concluded that neither operative nor nonoperative treatment was ideal. However, given the difficulties of ORIF with severe osteoporosis, nonoperative management was recommended unless rigid, secure internal fixation was possible in the presence of adequate bone stock.[4]

Nielsen et al.[13] published the Scandinavian experience in 1988. Reporting on 16 patients, the authors divided the patients into three groups. The first group consisted of ten patients, all of whom received casting. A second group, totaling four patients, underwent AO plating. The last group, with two patients, was treated with Rush pins after closed reduction. There were no complications in the nonoperative and Rush pinning group, and all patients regained prefracture ambulatory status by 1 year. Three of the patients with AO plating had complications, including a deep infection necessitating arthrodesis, a chronic fistula formation in continuity with the femoral prosthesis, and a failure of fixation with a subsequent nonunion. The authors surmised that stable, nondisplaced fractures, or slightly displaced supracondylar fractures after TKR may be treated conservatively with a cast. Unstable or displaced fractures should be treated with ORIF, with the caveat that the risks are substantial. Finally, Rush pin fixation should be considered for these fractures as an alternative to plate osteosynthesis.[13]

Figgie et al.[6] reported their results of 24 supracondylar femur fractures above TKRs in 22 patients. The treatments were divided into five modalities—namely, traction followed by cast application (10 fractures), ORIF (10 fractures), custom TKR with distal femoral allograft (2 fractures), external fixation (1 fracture), and primary arthrodesis (1 fracture). Fractures were classified using the Neer classification system with Neer Type II fractures comprising 80% of the nonoperative group and 90% of the operative (ORIF) group. Follow-up averaged approximately six years with a range of 3 to 12 years.[6]

In the nonoperative group, 9 of 10 fractures treated conservatively healed primarily, whereas only 5 of 10 in the ORIF group healed primarily. Two of the 5 surgical failures healed with a secondary ORIF and bone grafting, while the remaining three ultimately underwent revision TKR. Twelve of 14 fractures that healed primarily (in both operative and nonoperative groups) resulted in varus orientation of the femoral component. Nine of these 12 fractures developed progressive tibial radiolucency that mandated revision TKR.[6]

The authors proposed guidelines for treatment based upon Neer's classification system. Closed reduction and skeletal traction with subsequent cast bracing was recommended for Neer type I or II fractures. If acceptable alignment is not achieved, then ORIF with medial and lateral buttress plates is recommended, with the caveat that even this may not ensure acceptable alignment. Neer type III fractures and Neer type II fractures with inadequate bone stock or fractures in the presence of a loose prosthesis are best treated with immediate revision TKR to minimize prolonged immobilization. The use of distal femoral allografts was encouraged if bone stock was inadequate for standard revision TKRs.[6]

Healy et al.[11] reported on 20 supracondylar femur fractures above TKRs treated by the New England Trauma Study Group with ORIF. Nineteen of 20 fractures resulted from low-energy trauma and fractures were classified either comminuted, transverse, short oblique, or spiral. No documentation about fracture displacement was provided and at the time of ORIF no components were loose. Furthermore, a variety of fixation devices were utilized, including seven blade plates, seven dynamic compression screw (DCS) plates, and six condylar buttress plates. Uniformity in outcome evaluation was supported by the use of the Knee Society's clinical and radiographic scoring systems.[11]

Fifteen of 20 cases underwent bone grafting at the time of primary ORIF. Of the 20 fractures, 18 healed after the primary procedure at a mean of 16 weeks. Two patients underwent reoperation for delayed union with autogenous bone grafting and revision of hardware where necessary. Postoperative tibiofemoral alignment was unchanged, as were mean knee scores, with no loss of function or range of motion. Specifics regarding operative technique were provided, with the preference for blade plate fixation over both DCS and condylar buttress plates. The authors stated that although DCS plates may be technically easier to insert, the shortcomings with this device, including mandatory removal of bone during insertion, potential motion in the distal fragment with tenuous fixation in osteoporotic bone, and larger volume generate preference to the use of blade plates. The condylar buttress plate, while most flexible for screw placement, provides the least secure fixation. Finally, a straight lateral approach with intraoperative fluoroscopy is preferred for operative technique. The use of PMMA and corticocancellous struts, if necessary, is encouraged.[11]

The authors concluded that while operative management of all supracondylar femur fractures above TKR is not appropriate, it is the procedure of choice for any displaced, unstable, or poorly reduced fracture. The use of bone grafting was stressed to increase the likelihood of union in these challenging fractures. Furthermore, maintenance of 5 to 7 degrees valgus tibiofemoral alignment to prevent early tibial component loosening was emphasized. Rapid mobilization with early motion in the presence of rigid fixation allowed for maintenance of knee scores and range of motion.[11]

Ritter et al.[14] documented 22 displaced supracondylar femur fractures above TKRs treated with Rush rod fixation in 1995. All fractures were classified as displaced and a mean follow-up was 7 years. There were two intraoperative technical errors yielding excessive valgus orientation over 15 degrees. There were no postoperative complications and all fractures healed within 4 months of surgery. Range of motion was unchanged from preoperative values. The authors recommended closed reduction with Rush rod fixation as an alternative to ORIF with a shorter operative time and postoperative convalescence and fewer complications.[14]

Moran et al.[12] recently reported on 29 supracondylar femur fractures above TKRs from the Brigham and Women's Total Joint Registry. All fractures occurring more than 7 cm above the joint line and those fixed with external fixation devices or internal fixation devices not classified as plates were excluded. Each patient completed a Knee Society Clinical Rating System questionnaire and underwent detailed radiographic assessment. A satisfactory result was defined as a fracture that healed within 6 months, loss of range of motion of less than 30 degrees, and healing with less than either 15 degrees of tibiofemoral angulation or 10 degrees of flexion or extension. Using the Muller AO system for classification, the patients were divided into three groups. Group I patients were nondisplaced fractures, totaling five fractures. All fractures were type A1 fractures, and patients underwent nonoperative treatment (application of a cast brace or skeletal traction in the majority). Group II, totaling nine fractures, were displaced fractures treated with closed methods. All were type A fractures, treated with 4 to 6 weeks of skeletal traction in four patients and cast or brace immobilization in the remaining five patients. Group III consisted of 15 displaced fractures (the majority type A fractures), undergoing operative treatment. A variety of fixation devices were employed including nine blade plates. All but one patient in this group began knee range of motion within 48 hours of surgery.

The outcome of nondisplaced fractures (Group I) demonstrated satisfactory results with no nonunions or malunions and healing time of approximately fourteen weeks. Furthermore, there were no complications in this group. Group II patients (displaced fractures treated nonoperatively) yielded no satisfactory outcomes. No fracture healed in acceptable alignment with two requiring revision TKR at the time of publication. The patients with displaced fractures undergoing ORIF (Group III) had 10 of 15 satisfactory results. Of the unsatisfactory results, two malunions were managed conservatively, while two nonunions underwent revision TKR. Three of five of the unsatisfactory results were deemed secondary to technical error or poor implant choice at surgery. Four complications occurred in this group, including an incomplete peroneal nerve palsy, wound necrosis, and exuberant callus formation necessitating resection.[12]

Moran et al.[12] concluded that closed management with immobilization and subsequent partial weight-bearing was the treatment of choice for nondisplaced fractures. However, displaced fractures that were treated closed invariably obtained a poor result. The authors attributed these unsatisfactory results to the inability to obtain and maintain appropriate alignment. Therefore, despite a high complication rate, early open reduction with internal fixation was recommended. Strict adherence to the principles of internal fixation, meticulous preoperative planning, and the careful selection of an appropriate fixed-angle device (i.e., blade plate or DCS) can minimize the risk of failure.

MANAGEMENT

Supracondylar femur fractures above TKRs are complex fractures complicated by prosthetic location, poor bone stock, and the necessity for stable anatomic alignment with early motion to obtain optimal results. A critical analysis of the radiographs, including prefracture films, coupled with a detailed physical exam are mandatory components of the decision-making process.

The decision to attempt ORIF of these fractures is predicated upon two major factors: Is the implant well fixed, and is reduction necessary? (Fig. 74.1) If the prosthesis is loose, closed treatment or ORIF will result in a poor outcome unless revision TKR is a component of treatment. Although the recommended timing of such revision has varied from immediate[6] to delayed,[7] the results of treatment of a loose prosthesis in this setting universally yield unsatisfactory results. Secondarily, if implant fixation is solid, a detailed fracture analysis must be performed to assess the necessity for reduction. While closed treatment of nondisplaced fractures above supracondylar femur fractures has been nearly universally espoused as definitive treatment, the paucity of displaced fractures at any single institution has made definitive criteria for fracture reduction difficult to establish. While Schatzker and Lambert's[19] criteria for acceptable reduction has been applied to supracondylar femur fractures above TKRs, current literature suggests that even those measurements enjoy tolerances that may be too high with the presence of a prosthesis. Figgie et al.[6] documented a greater than 50% radiolucency rate with fractures healing in varus, whereas progressive radiolucencies were not observed with valgus alignment. The tendency for such fractures to fall into a varus alignment has been well documented in both native and periprosthetic supracondylar femur fractures.

Once the need for open reduction with internal fixation has been established, the selection of the appropriate device naturally follows. A wide variety of fixation devices have been employed, including compression plates, standard locked intramedullary nails, flexible

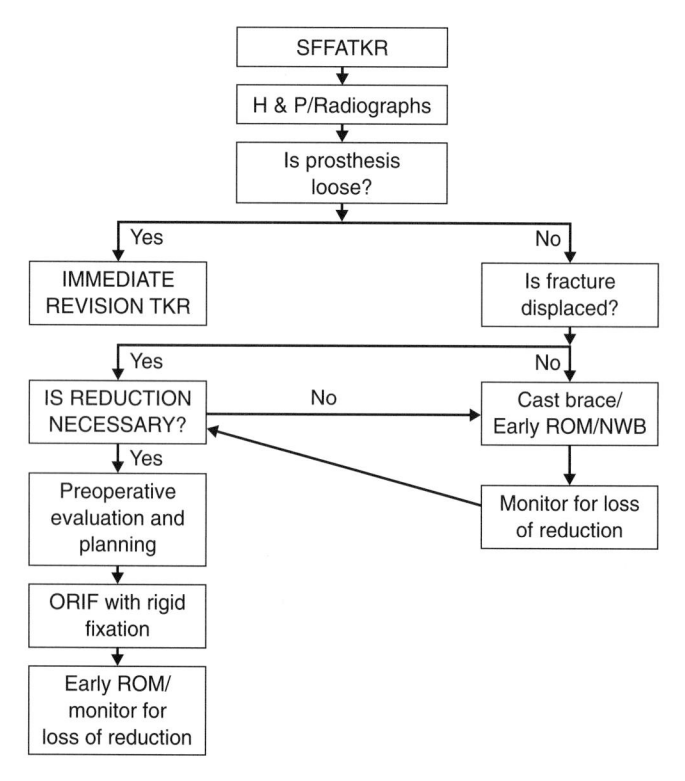

Figure 74.1. Treatment algorithm.

Rush rods, retrograde supracondylar nails, and fixed angle devices.

Initial reports of ORIF for native supracondylar femur fractures provide results that varied whether treatment was rendered in "accordance with the principles" of rigid internal fixation or not. Fracture healing reviewed in Schatzker and Lambert's[19] article that fulfilled the rigid fixation principles resulted in 71% good-to-excellent results. Those patients in whom fixation was not rigid yielded only 21% good-to-excellent results. Early reports of internal fixation in supracondylar femur fractures above TKRs remarked upon tenuous fixation and, not surprisingly, had poor results with this technique.[7,9]

When rigid fixation was obtained, follow-up results often approached prefracture function, range of motion, and pain scores. Culp et al.[10] documented improved ROM with internal fixation versus nonoperative treatment. Furthermore, their experience demonstrated a statistically significant decrease in the number of complications with rigid internal fixation. Healy et al.[11] utilized 14 fixed angle devices in 20 cases in which rigid internal fixation was obtained. Furthermore, prefracture ambulatory status was achieved in all patients without diminished Knee Society clinical scores. In order to attain the best clinical results in supracondylar femur fractures above TKRs, rigid internal fixation is the treatment of choice.

The choice of internal fixation device is critical in obtaining rigid fixation. Analysis of extramedullary fixation demonstrates several advantages of blade plate fixation over simple plate or dynamic condylar screw (DCS) devices. First, the thinness of the blade allows it to be placed close to the femoral component both anteriorly and distally. The large size of the DCS, for example, prohibits such distal fixation and may inhibit rigid stabilization of certain fractures. Second, the blade plate offers the most rigid biomechanical fixation, superior to other fixed-angle devices or plate and screw devices. Third, the DCS often requires removal of bone for insertion, which may be undesirable, particularly in those fractures with poor bone stock. Finally, blade plate purchase may provide increased control of micromotion over the DCS, condylar buttress plate, or simple plate-and-screw fixation.[11]

TECHNIQUE

Ideally the patient should be supine with the iliac crest prepped for autogenous bone graft. Careful positioning upon a radiolucent table for intraoperative fluoroscopy will significantly facilitate blade plate insertion. Furthermore, due to the presence of a prosthetic joint, meticulous sterile technique must be maintained.

A straight lateral approach is recommended for open reduction with internal fixation. Using the anterior approach may be problematic in fractures with proximal extension and complicate blade plate insertion. The lateral approach also permits fracture fixation without an arthrotomy. Maintenance of 7-cm "skin bridges" reduces the likelihood of flap compromise.

Once adequate exposure has been obtained, the blade plate insertion site is critical. The surgical anatomy of the distal femur resembles a trapezoid with 25-degree medial inclination and 10-degree lateral inclination. Furthermore the posterior diameter is longer than the anterior diameter in the coronal plane. Blade plates that appear to be the exact diameter of the femur on an AP x-ray will by definition protrude through the medial cortex and may create pain or restrict movement.

The sagittal alignment is similarly critical. The plate must line up along the shaft of the femur. In native supracondylar femur fractures, the ideal position is at the midpoint of the anterior one-half, approximately 2 cm from the joint surface. However, this guideline is less accurate because the position of the prosthesis may distort the insertion site. Therefore, it is recommended to align the plate along the shaft of the femur and mark the appropriate entrance site, using the midpoint of the anterior one-half as an initial reference point.

If the entrance point of the blade plate is too posterior, both medialization and anterior displacement will occur. This occurs since the posterior condyles are slightly larger. The net result is a nonanatomic reduction and significantly higher failure rates. It is rare that the entrance point will be too anterior, particularly in the presence of a prosthetic joint.

The seating chisel with the guide should be utilized, with particular attention to aligning the guide along the femoral shaft. The blade length typically measures approximately fifteen millimeters less than the AP diameter of the femur due to its rhomboidal geometry. The use of PMMA may enhance screw purchase in the presence of osteoporotic bone. Autogenous bone graft should be used in virtually every case to provide the optimal environment for fracture healing during the initial attempt (Fig. 74.2).

CONCLUSION

Supracondylar femur fractures above TKRs are uncommon fractures complicated by poor bone stock, component location and the necessity for rigid stabilization in an anatomic alignment to obtain satisfactory results. Meticulous preoperative evaluation and planning, in concert with the principles of rigid fixation, must be observed. Displaced fractures with well-fixed components are best treated with rigid internal fixation, and the use of the blade

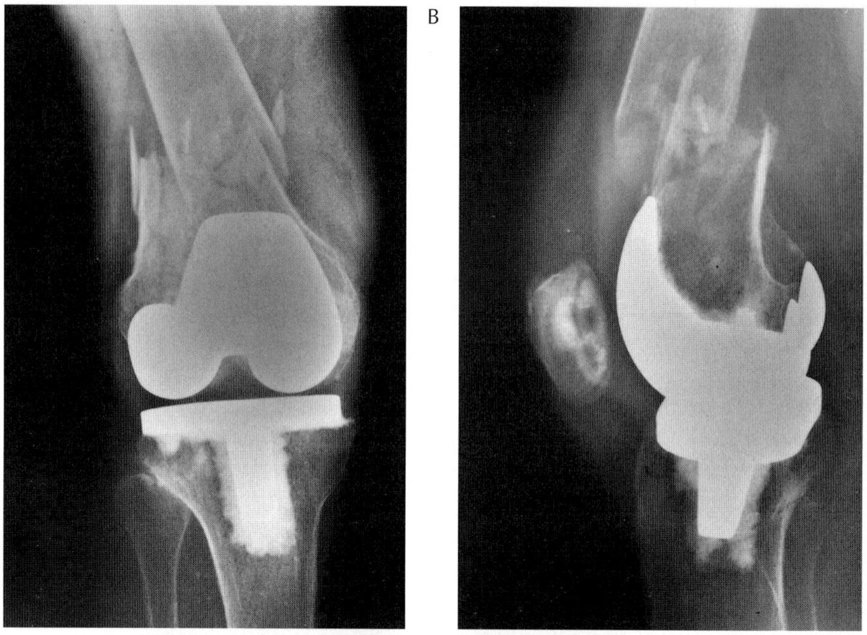

Figure 74.2A,B. (A) Anteroposterior and (B) lateral views of a comminuted supracondylar femur fracture above a TKR with displacement in the presence of a well-fixed prosthesis. Note poor bone stock.

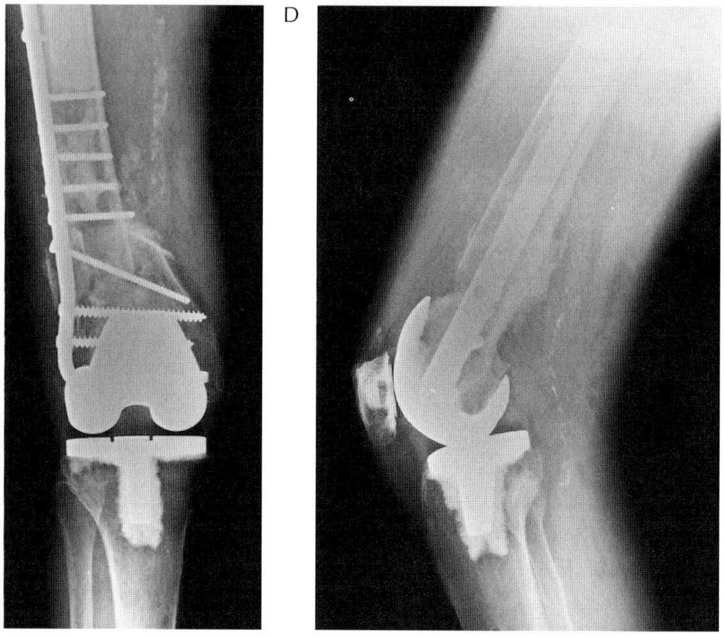

Figure 74.2C. Anteroposterior projection of supracondylar femur fracture above TKR after blade plate fixation. Some shortening was accepted to enhance fracture stability and PMMA was used to increase screw purchase. Note stem of ipsilateral THR. The patient achieved unrestricted ambulation with maintenance of prefracture ROM.

Figure 74.2D. Lateral projection showing appropriate entrance site of blade plate with good sagittal alignment.

plate is advocated. Newer devices (i.e., intramedullary fixation) offer attractive alternatives that merit further study and comparison to blade plate fixation.

References

1. Rinecker H, Haiboeck H. Zur operativen Behandlung periprothetischer Oberschenkelfrakturen nach Kniegelenktotalendoprothesen. *Arch Orthop Unfall.* 1977; 87:23.
2. Short WH, Hootnick DR, Murray DG. Ipsilateral supracondylar femur fractures following knee arthroplasty. *Clin Orthop.* 1981:111–16.
3. Digioia AM III, Rubash HE. Periprosthetic fractures of the femur after total knee arthroplasty. A literature review and treatment algorithm. *Clin Orthop.* 1991:135–42.
4. Bogoch E, Hastings D, Gross A, Gschwend N. Supracondylar fractures of the femur adjacent to resurfacing and MacIntosh arthroplasties of the knee in patients with rheumatoid arthritis. *Clin Orthop.* 1988:213–20.
5. Delport PH, Van Audekercke R, Martens M, Mulier JC. Conservative treatment of ipsilateral supracondylar femoral fracture after total knee arthroplasty. *J Trauma* 1984; 24:846–49.
6. Figgie MP, Goldberg VM, Figgie HE III, Sobel M. The results of treatment of supracondylar fracture above total knee arthroplasty. *J Arthroplasty.* 1990; 5:267–76.

7. Merkel KD, Johnson EW Jr. Supracondylar fracture of the femur after total knee arthroplasty. *J Bone Joint Surg Am*. 1986; 68:29–43.
8. Ritter MA, Faris PM, Keating EM. Anterior femoral notching and ipsilateral supracondylar femur fracture in total knee arthroplasty. *J Arthroplasty*. 1988; 3:185–87.
9. Cain PR, Rubash HE, Wissinger HA, McClain EJ. Periprosthetic femoral fractures following total knee arthroplasty. *Clin Orthop*. 1986:205–214.
10. Culp RW, Schmidt RG, Hanks G, Mak A, Esterhai JL, Jr. Heppenstall RB. Supracondylar fracture of the femur following prosthetic knee arthroplasty. *Clin Orthop*. 1987:212–22.
11. Healy WL, Siliski JM, and Incavo SJ. Operative treatment of distal femoral fractures proximal to total knee replacements. *J Bone Joint Surg Am*. 1993; 75:27–34.
12. Moran MC, Brick GW, Sledge CB, Dysart SH, Chien EP. Supracondylar femoral fracture following total knee arthroplasty. *Clin Orthop*. 1996:196–209.
13. Nielsen BF, Petersen VS, Varmarken JE. Fracture of the femur after knee arthroplasty. *Acta Orthop Scand*. 1988; 59:155–57.
14. Ritter MA, Keating EM, Faris PM, Meding JB. Rush rod fixation of supracondylar fractures above total knee arthroplasties. *J Arthroplasty*. 1995; 10:213–16.
15. Sisto DJ, Lachiewicz PF, Insall JN. Treatment of supracondylar fractures following prosthetic arthroplasty of the knee. *Clin Orthop*. 1985:265–72.
16. Cadambi A, Engh GA, Dwyer KA, Vinh TN. Osteolysis of the distal femur after total knee arthroplasty. *J Arthroplasty*. 1994; 9:579–94.
17. Chmell MJ, Moran MC, Scott RD. Periarticular fracture after total knee arthroplasty: principles of management. *J Amer Acad Orthop Surg*. 1996; 4:109–116.
18. Neer CS II, Grantham SA, Shelton ML. Supracondylar fracture of the adult femur. *J Bone Joint Surg*. 1967; 49A:591–613.
19. Schatzker J, Lambert DC. Supracondylar fractures of the femur. *Clin Orthop*. 1979:77–83.

Bibliography

Aaron RK, Scott R. Supracondylar fracture of the femur after total knee arthroplasty. *Clin Orthop*. 1987:136–39.

Anderson SP, Matthews LS, Kaufer H. Treatment of juxtaarticular nonunion fractures at the knee with long-stem total knee arthroplasty. *Clin Orthop*. 1990:104–109.

Biswas SP, Kurer MH, MacKenney RP. External fixation for femoral shaft fracture after Stanmore total knee replacement. *J Bone Joint Surg Br*. 1992; 74:313–14.

Booth RE Jr. Management of periprosthetic fractures. *Orthopedics*. 1994; 17:845–47.

Booth RE Jr. Supracondylar fractures: All or nothing. *Orthopedics*. 1995; 18:921–22.

Chen F, Mont MA, Bachner RS. Management of ipsilateral supracondylar femur fractures following total knee arthroplasty. *J Arthroplasty*. 1994; 9:521–26.

Cordeiro EN, Costa RC, Carazzato JG, Silva JDS. Periprosthetic fractures in patients with total knee arthroplasties. *Clin Orthop*. 1990:182–89.

Courpied JP, Watin-Augouard L, and Postel M. [Femoral fractures in subjects with total prostheses of the hip or knee]. *Int Orthop*. 1987; 11:109–115.

Dave DJ, Koka SR, James SE. Mennen plate fixation for fracture of the femoral shaft with ipsilateral total hip and knee arthroplasties. *J Arthroplasty*. 1995; 10:113–15.

Fitzek JG, Wessinghage D. [Intramedullary nailing of periprosthetic fractures following total knee joint replacement]. *Aktuelle Traumatol*. 1990; 20:248–53.

Freund KG. [Bilateral supracondylar fracture of the femur following total knee replacement (letter)]. *Ugeskr. Laeger*. 1989; 151:1333.

Garnavos C, Rafiq M, Henry AP. Treatment of femoral fracture above a knee prosthesis. Eighteen cases followed 0.5–14 years. *Acta Orthop. Scand*. 1994; 65:610–14.

Goodman SB. Supracondylar fractures above a total knee arthroplasty: A novel use of the Huckstepp nail [letter; comment]. *J Arthroplasty*. 1995; 10:255.

Grob D, Gschwend N. [Periprosthetic fractures after total replacement of knee joint (author's transl)]. *Orthopade*. 1982; 11:109–117.

Hanks GA, Mathews HH, Routson GW, Loughran TP. Supracondylar fracture of the femur following total knee arthroplasty. *J Arthroplasty*. 1989; 4:289–92.

Harlow ML, Hofmann AA. Periprosthetic Fractures. In Anonymous 1996.

Heisel J. [Intra- and postoperative fractures in alloarthroplastic knee replacement]. *Aktuelle Traumatol*. 1988; 18:76–83.

Hirsh DM, Bhalla S, Roffman M. Supracondylar fracture of the femur following total knee replacement. Report of four cases. *J Bone Joint Surg Am*. 1981; 63:162–63.

Jabczenski FF, Crawford M. Retrograde intramedullary nailing of supracondylar femur fractures above total knee arthroplasty. A preliminary report of four cases. *J Arthroplasty*. 1995; 10:95–101.

Jahn K, Siegling CW. [Fractures of the femur following prosthetic replacement of the hip and knee joint (author's transl)]. *Zentralbl Chir*. 1981; 106:463–68.

Kraay MJ, Goldberg VM, Figgie MP, Figgie HE, III. Distal femoral replacement with allograft/prosthetic reconstruction for treatment of supracondylar fractures in patients with total knee arthroplasty. *J Arthroplasty*. 1992; 7:7–16.

Kress KJ, Scuderi GR, Windsor RE, Insall JN. Treatment of nonunions about the knee utilizing custom total knee arthroplasty with press-fit intramedullary stems. *J Arthroplasty*. 1993; 8:49–55.

Maceachern AG, Ling RS. Ununited supracondylar fracture of the femur following Attenborough stabilized gliding knee arthroplasty treated by distal femoral replacement [letter]. *Injury*. 1983; 15:214–16.

McLaren AC, Dupont JA, Schroeber DC. Open reduction internal fixation of supracondylar fractures above total knee arthroplasties using the intramedullary supracondylar rod. *Clin Orthop*. 1994:194–98.

Murrell GA, Nunley JA. Interlocked supracondylar intramedullary nails for supracondylar fractures after total knee arthroplasty: A new treatment method. *J Arthroplasty*. 1995; 10:37–42.

Nielsen BF, Lind T, Olsen PA. [Supracondylar fracture of the femur following total knee replacement]. *Ugeskr Laeger*. 1989; 151:422–26.

Oni OO. Supracondylar fracture of the femur following Attenborough stabilized gliding knee arthroplasty. *Injury*. 1982; 14:250–51.

Ostermann PA, Hahn MP, Ekkernkamp A, David A, Muhr G. [Treatment of supracondylar femoral fracture proximal to a knee joint endoprosthesis by retrograde interlocking nailing]. *Zentralbl Chir*. 1995; 120:731–33.

Patch DA, Iorio R, Healy WL. Distal femur fracture above a total knee arthroplasty. *Orthopedics*. 1994; 17:371–74.

Rand JA. Supracondylar fracture of the femur associated with polyethylene wear after total knee arthroplasty: A case report. *J Bone Joint Surg Am*. 1994; 76:1389–93.

Rehnberg L, Karlstrom G. Second arthroplasty of the knee combined with medullary nailing for non-union of fracture of the femur: A case report. *Injury*. 1987; 18:211–12.

Ritter MA, Stiver P. Supracondylar fracture in a patient with total knee arthroplasty. A case report. *Clin Orthop*. 1985: 168–70.

Rolston LR, Christ DJ, Halpern A, O'Connor PL, Ryan TG, Uggen WM. Treatment of supracondylar fractures of the femur proximal to a total knee arthroplasty: A report of four cases. *J Bone Joint Surg Am*. 1995; 77:924–31.

Roscoe MW, Goodman SB, Schatzker J. Supracondylar fracture of the femur after Guepar total knee arthroplasty: A new treatment method. *Clin Orthop*. 1989:221–23.

Scott RD. Anterior femoral notching and ipsilateral supracondylar femur fracture in total knee arthroplasty [letter]. *J Arthroplasty*. 1988; 3:381.

Sekel R, Newman AS. Supracondylar fractures above a total knee arthroplasty: A novel use of the Huckstepp nail [see comments]. *J Arthroplasty*. 1994; 9:445–47.

Shepperd JA, Franklin A. Supracondylar fracture of the femur following Attenborough stabilized knee arthroplasty treated by a long-stem prosthesis plus internal fixation [letter]. *Injury*. 1984; 16:65–66.

Stulberg SD, Dorr LD, Hungerford DS, Insall JN, Scott RD, Whiteside LA. Knee challenges: What would you do? *Orthopedics*. 1995; 18:941–47.

Zehntner MK, Ganz R. Internal fixation of supracondylar fractures after condylar total knee arthroplasty. *Clin Orthop*. 1993:219–24.

CHAPTER 75
Revision of Periprosthetic Femur Fractures

Robert E. Booth and David G. Nazarian

Distal femoral fractures associated with a total knee arthroplasty are mercifully rare, as they are arguably among the most difficult osseous infractions to treat. Fractures occurring *outside* the "no-man's land" between the femoral epicondyles and the femoral diaphysis (some 12 cm proximal) are less problematic. Femoral diaphyseal fractures have good bone, less comminution, and sufficient distance from the joint to be minimally affected by the arthroplasty itself. Fractures distal to the femoral epicondyles do not involve the collateral ligaments of the knee, and they can be treated with simple revisional augmentations.

Periprosthetic total knee fractures within 3 to 15 mm of the joint line, however, hold several distinct hazards. First, they can occur with surprisingly little trauma to the limb yet with severe bony comminution. In fact, as a general rule, the less the trauma, the worse the fracture. This is explained by the second point, which is that the supracondylar area of the femur is extremely osteoporotic in these patients, with thin cortices and practically no intramedullary cancellous bone. Once the "eggshell" of the distal femur has cracked, reconstructive efforts will be frustrated by the simple lack of substance proximal to the arthroplasty.

Third, it is rarely appreciated that one of the contributing factors to the fracture is the unsatisfactory nature of the original arthroplasty. This is particularly true of stiff total knees, most commonly the result of a tight posterior cruciate ligament or oversized components. The stress that this stiff arthroplasty places on the femoral bone not only predisposes to fracture, but also confounds attempts at stable fixation. While one would prefer to treat either the fracture or the failed total joint individually, it is often necessary to address these problems simultaneously, since they are so interrelated.

For biologic as well as sociologic reasons, conservative treatment of supracondylar femoral fractures is almost impossible today, and open intervention of some variety is usually necessary. Many techniques of internal fixation are available, but all share significant technical difficulties as well as a surprisingly high incidence of nonunion and malunion. The medial mechanical axis of the lower limb, the concerted action of the posterior knee musculature, and the sagittal plane of motion of the joint itself all conspire to destabilize even the most rigid internal fixation. This is compounded by the effects of bony comminution, severe femoral osteopenia, and a stiff knee arthroplasty. It is not surprising, therefore, that many fractures develop nonunions or go on to a tardy malunion with the typical deformity of adduction, flexion, and internal rotation of the distal femoral fragment.

Rush rod fixation, as espoused by Ritter[1] is economical and expeditious, but in most cases has provided insufficient stabilization. Better results have been found with distal condylar plate and screw devices,[2] although even good surgical results will often deteriorate into nonunion or malunion and the bone available for distal screw fixation is often compromised by the intercondylar design of the femoral prosthetic component. New plating systems with abundant supracondylar screw options may improve this situation, but the biologic issues of bone quality and joint dynamics will remain.

The competing principles of fracture immobilization in the face of joint mobility require ever more rigid fixation. The use of intramedullary rods, introduced through the intercondylar notch of most prostheses, is an attractive option that requires minimal disturbance of the arthroplasty. Excellent results have been reported with this technique,[3] although several important technical issues should be considered. First, the precise design of the prosthetic femoral component must be known, so that a rod of sufficient diameter to achieve intramedullary stabilization of the fracture can be introduced through the open box of the femoral component. The diameters of these components are well known (Table 75.1). There have been apocryphal reports of the need for a "prosthetic notch plasty" using a Midas Rex burr to enlarge the metallic intercondylar space, although this is clearly not to be recommended.

Second, one should be prepared for the necessity to open the fracture site above the femoral prosthesis and place an intercalary allograft—sculpted from a distal femur—to surround the intramedullary rod, fill the metaphyseal void, maintain femoral limb length, and provide support for the comminuted host cortical bone, which can be wired about the graft. Without this graft material, the rod alone may be insufficient to maintain length and promote healing of the fracture. Finally, one may enhance the function of the stiff arthroplasty after stabilization of the fracture by sectioning an excessively tight posterior cruciate ligament or downsizing an excessively thick patellar button.

All too frequently, none of these options will suffice. The total knee arthroplasty may be too bad to salvage, compromising the fracture healing and yielding a dysfunctional limb even if union should occur. The "personality" of the fracture may be unattractive, with such problems as profound comminution, insufficient distal bone for screw or rod fixation, periprosthetic bone loss secondary to prefracture osteolysis, or intercondylar fragmentation and compromise of collateral support. In these and other severe situations, simultaneous revision of the arthroplasty and stabilization of the fracture must be considered. This can be a heroic endeavor, to be undertaken only by those with a full array of revisional prostheses and tools, an adequate supply of allograft material, and extensive total knee revisional experience.

In the operating room, one must be prepared for an extended surgical procedure, with sufficient anesthetic to last several hours. Some thighs will be too short to permit a proper tourniquet, although a sterile tourniquet can be used to maintain hemostasis through much of the procedure. The preferred incision is an extension of the knee arthrotomy midline incision well up into the proximal thigh. This approach will even allow the removal of prior failed fixation devices from the medial or lateral side of the femur without the use of parallel skin incisions. All prior prosthetic materials must be removed, and it is generally preferable to address the previous fracture materials before removing the femoral component of the total knee. This will protect the fragile distal femoral bone as long as possible during the surgery.

The optimal stabilization of the fracture usually involves a long intramedullary rod, extending several inches at least above the fracture site. This must be compatible with the new total knee arthroplasty and systems such as the constrained condylar knee remain the industry standard. Curved rods may be necessary to match the femoral bow, and they have the additional advantage of conferring some rotational stability upon the ultimate construct. Rods of 150 to 200 mm of length are most helpful. Offset rods may additionally allow for accommodation of previous fracture malunions.

The mechanism of failure of the index arthroplasty must be clearly understood and reversed. Most frequently this involves conversion from a cruciate retaining to a cruciate substituting design, downsizing of prosthetic components, and correction of internal rotational malalignment of the femoral and tibial components. Extra hands are often needed during surgery even to place trial components, since the distal femoral fragment in particular will be difficult to control, tending to flex and internally rotate in response to muscle influences about the knee.

Once a prosthetic device has been selected and trials implanted, the fracture can be addressed. Particular attention should be paid to the proper rotation of the limb, often using palpation of the posterior linea aspera to confirm position. Whether fresh fracture, malunion, or nonunion, the interface between the proximal and femoral and distal femoral fragments may need to be simplified and freshened. This is preferably performed in an oblique fashion, avoiding butt or step cuts. An oblique osteotomy provides greater bone surface for healing, partial correction of flexion deformities, and significant stability against rotation. Occasionally, supplemental cortical plating of the fracture may be necessary, although only unicortical screw fixation will be available if the intramedullary rod is of appropriate substance.

Extensive grafting of the fracture may be required. At the very least, small bone fragments or *paste* will be helpful at the termination of the procedure to enhance healing in an area of extreme osteopenia. An *intercalary graft*, fashioned to surround the intramedullary rod but pro-

Table 75.1. Intercondylar distances of commonly used total knee implants*

Implant	Intercondylar distance (mm)
Miller-Galante (Zimmer, Warsaw, IN)	12
Insall-Burstein (Zimmer)	14–19
Biomet (Warsaw, IN)	22
Intermedics (Austin, TX)	18
AMK (DePuy, Warsaw, IN)	14–17
Osteonics (Allendale, NJ)	19
PFC (Johnson & Johnson, New Brunswick, NJ)	20
Kirschner wires (Timonium, MD)	20
Genesis (Smith & Nephew Richards, Memphis, TN)	20
Duracon (Howmedica, Rutherford, NJ)	12–16

*Reproduced, with modification, from: Engh and Ammen[4]

vide bulk and fill for the supracondylar area may be extremely helpful, as previously described in the retrograde rodding technique. Occasionally, the distal bone is of such poor quality that an entire distal *femoral allograft* may be needed. An arthroplasty of the graft can be performed on a back table, then mated with the host femur within the operative field. The junction of the massive allograft can be accomplished either by invagination of the graft within the residual femoral canal or—as described previously—by an oblique osteotomy. In either situation, the graft surmounting the intramedullary rod should be made intentionally too long, then whittled to proper limb length once the arthroplasty has been balanced in flexion. This allows the secondary adjustment of proper extension balance in the same way that one would balance a simple revisional arthroplasty using prosthetic augments.

If an intercondylar fracture should occur during the procedure, the bony fragments should be preserved with their attached collateral ligaments. These can be cemented at the time of fracture reduction within the "pockets" of the femoral component, secured with methylmethacrylate and held temporarily by a bone clamp, potentially reinforced with mersilene tape. The medial collateral ligament is, of course, of the highest priority, since even a constrained condylar knee system will display rotational instability in its absence. Onlay cortical plates or struts may be wired about the host/graft junction to augment bone stock, contain residual cortical fragments, and confer further rotational stability. The late incorporation of these grafts is quite good, much as has been observed in proximal femoral hip reconstructions.

Finally, it is the obligation of the surgeon to confer stability upon both the fracture and the arthroplasty at the time of surgery. Occasionally, this may require cementation of the intramedullary stem. This should be done with caution because of potential future revisional difficulties as well as possible sequestration of some of the fracture fragments. Intramedullary rods appropriate for cementation should be used, as well as cement restrictors. Internal stabilization of these fractures is far preferable to subsequent external bracing, although this adjunctive therapy may be helpful in the early mobilization of some reconstructions. Protected weightbearing is at the discretion of the surgeon, influenced by the extent of the allograft, the stability of the reconstruction, the need for postoperative motion, and patient compliance.

When successful, simultaneous revision of an unsatisfactory knee arthroplasty and fixation of the fracture it precipitated can be an extremely satisfying and cost-effective procedure.

References

1. Ritter MA, Keating EM, Faris PM, Meding JB. Rush rod fixation of supracondylar fractures above total knee arthroplasties. *J Arthroplasty*. 1995; 10:213–216.
2. Healy WL, Siliski JM, Incavo SJ. Operative treatment of distal femoral fractures proximal to total knee replacements. *J Bone Joint Surg*. 1993; 75-A:27–34.
3. Henry SL, Booth RE. Management of supracondylar fractures proximal to total knee arthroplasty with GSH supracondylar nail. *Contemp Orthop*. 1995; 31:231–238.
4. Engh GA, Ammeen DJ. Periprosthetic fractures adjacent to total knee implants. *J Bone Joint Surg*. 1997; 79-A:1100–1113.

CHAPTER 76
Classification of Periprosthetic Tibial Fractures

Arlen D. Hanssen, Michael J. Stuart, and Nancy A. Felix

INTRODUCTION

Contrary to the extensive literature detailing periprosthetic femur fractures associated with total knee arthroplasty, there is little information available regarding periprosthetic tibial fractures. Between 1970 and 1992, there were 32 cases of tibial fractures located below a total knee arthroplasty that were mentioned in nine different reports.[1] The largest report described 15 stress fractures of the tibia following Geomedic and Polycentric knee arthroplasty.[2] This fracture pattern was associated with axial malalignment and improper component orientation and all knees eventually required revision arthroplasty. Since 1992, several authors have reported tibial fractures in association with a tibial tubercle osteotomy.[4,5] Two different fracture patterns were described in these reports, which included five tibial shaft fractures and two minimally displaced tibial tubercle fractures.

We recently reviewed 102 periprosthetic tibial fractures that were diagnosed and treated at our clinic between 1970 and 1995 and concluded that classification and treatment of these fractures could be based on three primary factors: (1) the anatomic location of the fracture, (2) the timing of the fracture's being in either the intraoperative or postoperative periods, and (3) the radiographic determination of prosthesis fixation as being well-fixed or loose at the time of the fracture.[3] Accordingly, we suggest the following fracture classification and treatment recommendations for periprosthetic tibial fractures associated with total knee arthroplasty.

CLASSIFICATION

Initially, fractures are classified into 1 of 4 major anatomic fracture patterns (Fig. 76.1). Type I fractures involve the tibial plateau and extend to the interface of the prosthesis and the tibial plateau. Type II fractures typically occur in the metaphyseal-diaphyseal region adjacent to the tibial stem. Type III fractures occur distal to the tibial prosthesis and the Type IV fracture involves the tibial tubercle. These four major fracture patterns are then further categorized into three subtypes:

1. Prosthesis appears radiographically well-fixed
2. Prosthesis appears radiographically loose
3. The fracture occurred intraoperatively

The major fracture pattern and appropriate subtype are combined to describe a specific fracture group (Fig. 76.2). For example, if the tibial plateau is fractured during the surgical procedure, this is described as a Type I C fracture. If a tibial shaft fracture occurs distal to the prosthesis postoperatively and the prosthesis appears well-fixed, the fracture is designated as a Type III A fracture. There were 62 Type I, 22 Type II, 16 Type III, and 2 Type IV fractures. The specific fracture categories are listed in Table 76.1. For purposes of description and treatment it is easier to consider separately the intraoperative and postoperative fractures.

POSTOPERATIVE FRACTURES

Type I

Type I fractures in the postoperative period have invariably occurred in association with a loose prosthesis (Table 76.1). Many of these fractures were associated with first-generation knee prostheses such as the Geomedic or Polycentric designs, but they also happened with modern condylar knee designs (Figs. 76.3, 76.4). Of 51 Type IB fractures, it was elected to initially treat the fracture and allow consolidation of the fracture fragments in 23 knees. Twenty knees (83%) required revision arthroplasty at a mean duration after fracture of 17

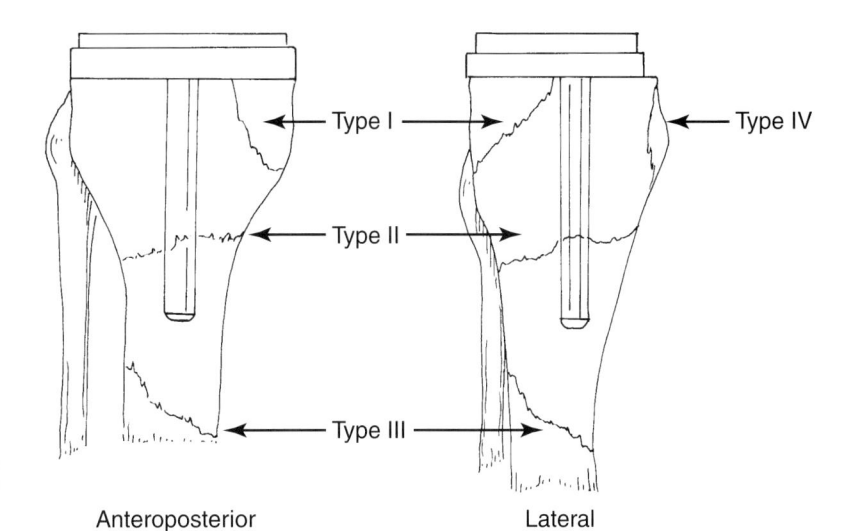

Figure 76.1. Anteroposterior and lateral illustrations of four-part Mayo fracture classification of periprosthetic tibial fractures.

months. Twenty-eight knees with fracture underwent immediate revision surgery and at a mean of 92 months after revision surgery; only one knee required additional surgery. In the presence of a loose prosthesis, early surgery to treat the loose prosthesis and stabilize the fracture simultaneously provides the benefit of earlier treatment resolution for the patient, and isolated treatment of the fracture only delays the inevitable need for revision surgery.

The Type IB fracture typically occurs in the medial plateau with a bone deficiency characterized as a combined cavitary and segmental defect of the tibial plateau (Fig. 76.5). At revision surgery, this type of bone defect can be managed with a variety of treatment modalities including: (a) cement fill, (b) bone graft, (c) modular metal augments, or (d) a custom prosthesis. It is advisable to bypass the bone defect with the use of a stemmed tibial component utilizing either cemented or press-fit stems (Fig. 76.6). Our preferred treatment method has been structural graft or metal augments in combination with a stemmed tibial component.

Type II

These fractures may occur in association with well-fixed or loose prostheses (see Table 76.1). Type IIA fractures usually occur as a result of a defined traumatic episode such as a fall or a motor vehicle accident and are most often associated with modern condylar knee designs (Fig. 76.7). To date, all of these fractures, treated with rigid immobilization until fracture healing is complete, have successfully healed without untoward effect on knee function. None have required revision surgery at a mean follow-up of 59 months.

Type IIB fractures typically occur adjacent to loose-stemmed knee arthroplasties, often a hinged knee design, and in the presence of extensive osteolysis (Fig. 76.8). The resultant bone defect is an extensive cavitary defect of the proximal tibia often combined with severe ectasia distally and segmental deficiencies in the metaphyseal-diaphyseal region (Fig. 76.9). These bone defects are extremely difficult to manage and often require structural or morseled

Major Anatomic Pattern

I: Tibial Plateau
II: Adjacent to Stem
III: Distal to Prosthesis
IV: Tibial Tubercle

+

Subcategory

A: Prosthesis well-fixed
B: Loose prosthesis
C: Intraoperative

→ Fracture Type

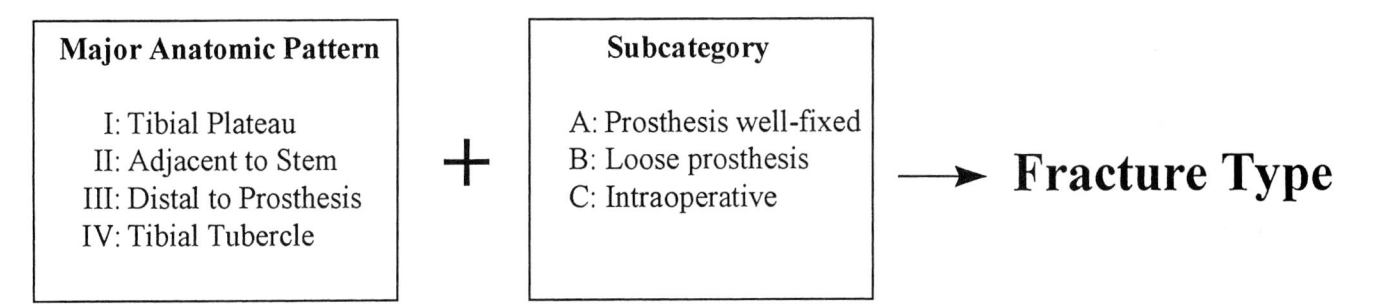

Figure 76.2. The specific fracture type is obtained by combining one of the four major fracture patterns with one of the three subtypes.

Table 76.1. 102 periprosthetic tibial fractures

I	B	51
	C	11
II	A	5
	B	10
	C	7
III	A	14
	B	1
	C	1
IV	A	2

bone grafting with long-stemmed tibial components (Fig. 76.10).

Type III

This fracture pattern, a tibial shaft fracture that occurs below a knee prosthesis, transpires from one of three mechanisms: (1) a definitive traumatic event, (2) a stress fracture resulting from limb malalignment or improper component orientation, or (3) a fracture in association with a tibial tubercle osteotomy.[4,5] In our recent review, all but 1 of 15 fractures occurred in association with a prosthesis that was radiographically well-fixed (Type IIIA) (Fig. 76.11A,B). All traumatic fractures were treated with cast immobilization while the stress fractures were managed with immobilization and limitation of weight-bearing followed by gradual return to activities when fracture healing was complete. Two of the knees with

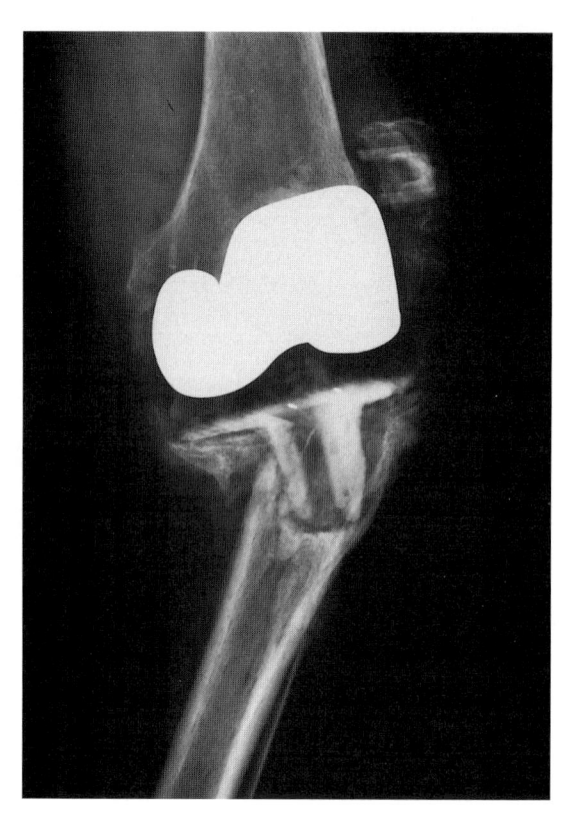

Figure 76.4. Anteroposterior radiograph of a cemented condylar knee replacement in association with a Type IB fracture.

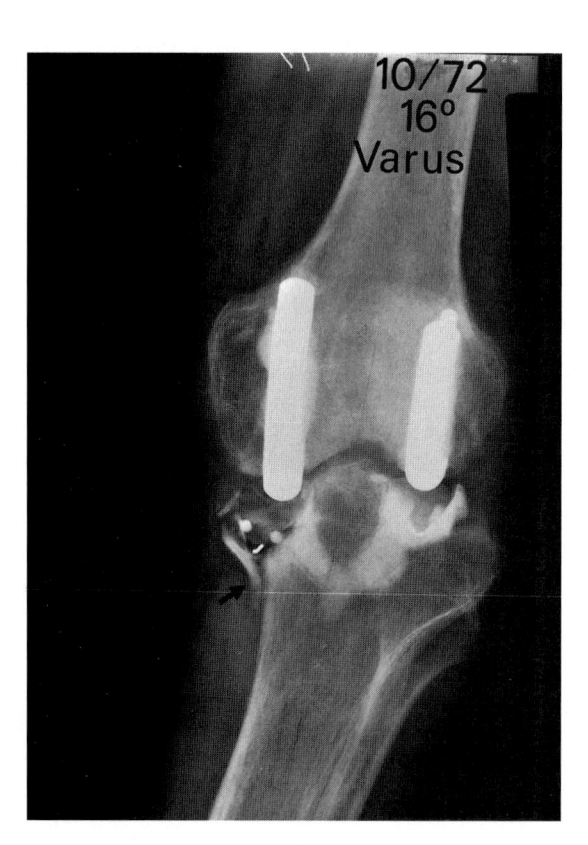

Figure 76.3. Anteroposterior radiograph of a polycentric knee arthroplasty with a Type IB fracture.

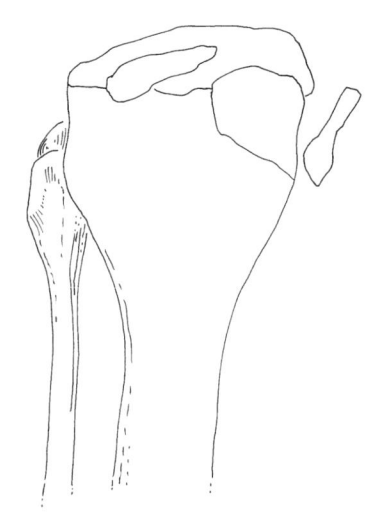

Figure 76.5. Illustration of a typical bone defect associated with a Type IB fracture.

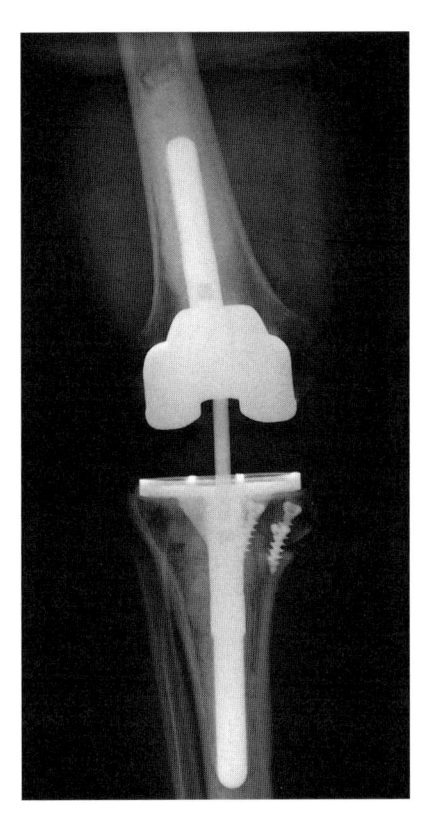

Figure 76.6. Anteroposterior radiograph of revision knee arthroplasty using structural bone graft and cemented stem bypass for the treatment of a Type IB fracture.

stress fractures and limb malalignment eventually required revision surgery for aseptic loosening (13 and 84 months following fracture treatment). The one Type IIIB fracture, also treated with immobilization, underwent revision surgery 27 months later.

For Type IIIA fractures, we recommend that treatment proceed in accordance with the usual principles of tibial shaft fractures emphasizing proper limb alignment and maintenance of knee function. Treatment of Type IIIB fractures need to be individualized and, although the only fracture we treated was done by sequential staging of fracture immobilization and revision surgery, it is possible that certain variations of this fracture pattern could potentially be managed with revision of the loose tibial component and stabilization of the fracture site with a long-stemmed tibial component.

Type IV

Fractures of the tibial tubercle signify extensor mechanism disruption and are potentially a catastrophic event. Both Type IV fractures in our recent review occurred after a fall and were observed in association with well-fixed components (Type IVA). The minimally displaced fracture was successfully treated with extension immobilization, whereas the displaced Type IVA fracture was successfully treated with open reduction and internal fixation with a tension-band wiring technique. Recently we have treated two additional Type IV fractures, one

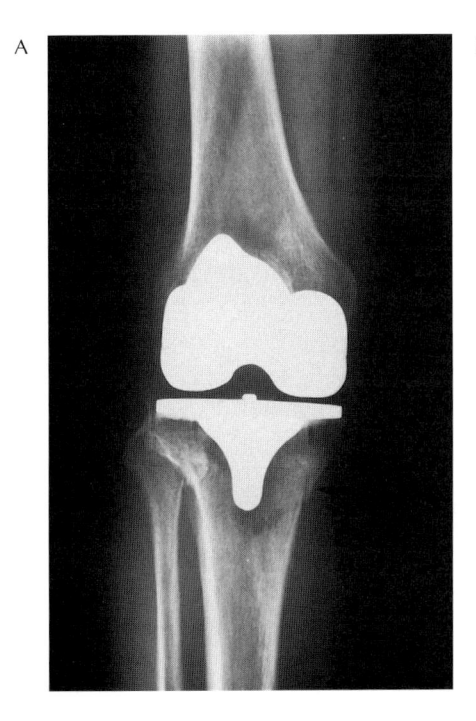

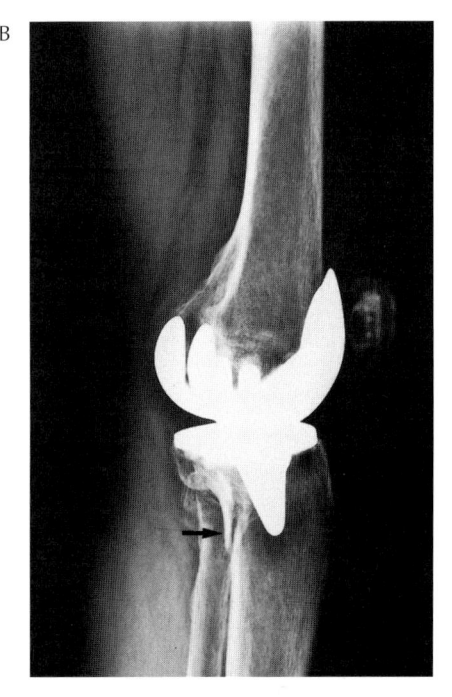

Figure 76.7. (A) Anteroposterior and (B) lateral radiographs of a cemented condylar knee arthroplasty associated with a Type IIA fracture.

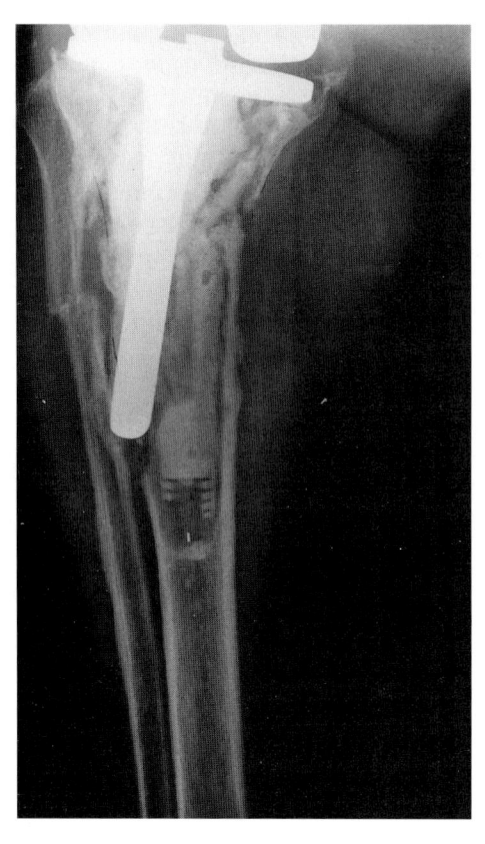

Figure 76.8. Anteroposterior radiograph of a stemmed cemented total knee arthroplasty associated with a Type IIB fracture.

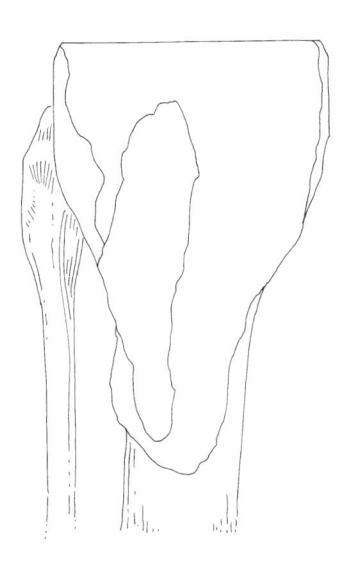

Figure 76.9. Illustration of a typical bone defect associated with the Type IIB fracture.

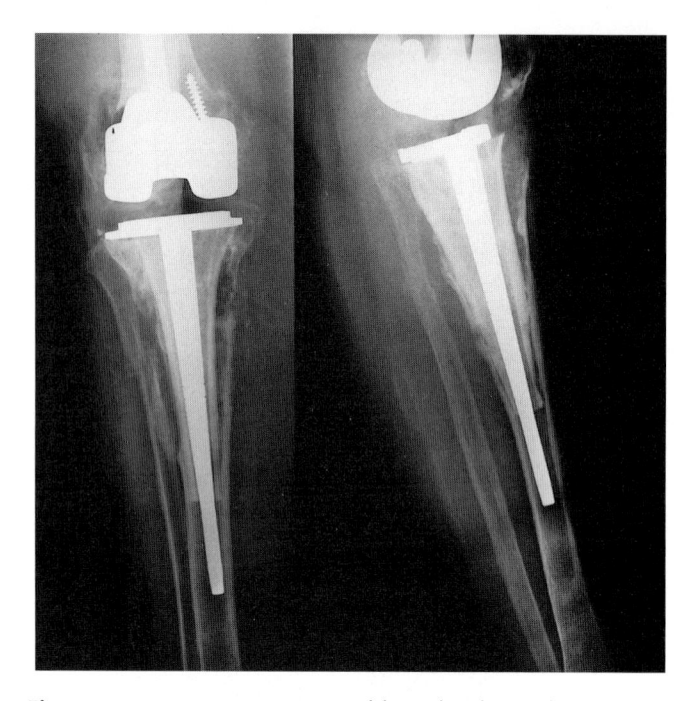

Figure 76.10. Anteroposterior and lateral radiographs of a Type IIB fracture treated with large structural allograft inset within the patulous bone defect and bypassed with a long-stemmed tibial component.

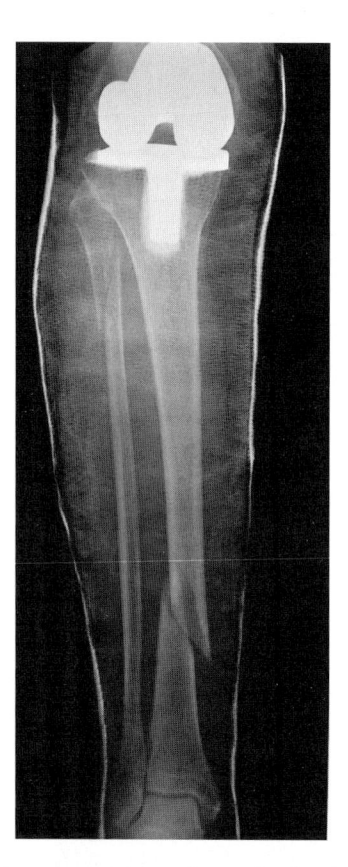

Figure 76.11. Anteroposterior radiograph of a Type IIIC fracture treated with cast immobilization.

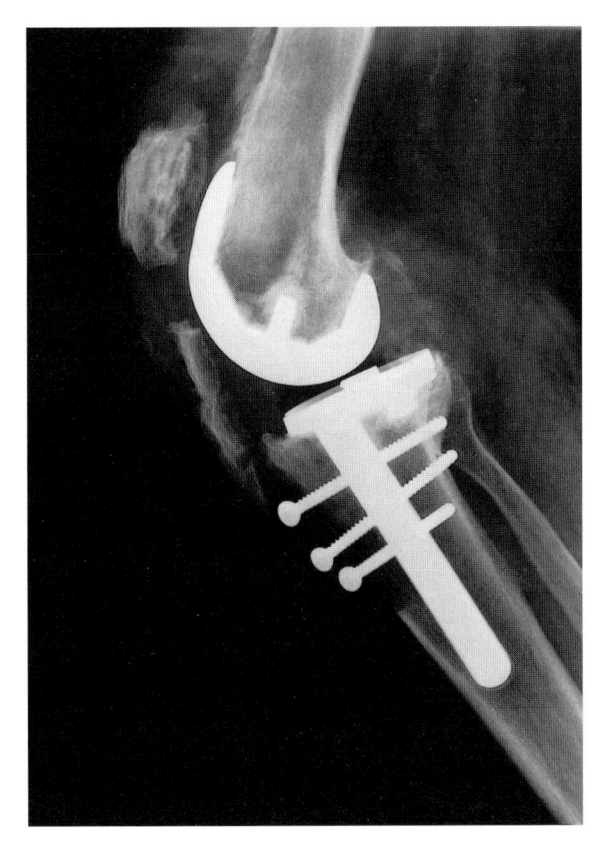

Figure 76.12. Lateral radiograph of Type IVB fracture that occurred after tibial tubercle osteotomy.

being a Type IVB fracture that occurred after a tibial tubercle osteotomy and was treated with extensor mechanism repair utilizing Marlex augmentation and revision knee surgery (Fig. 76.12). The other Type IV fracture was an intraoperative fracture (Type IVC) and is discussed later.

INTRAOPERATIVE FRACTURES

Tibial fractures occurring during knee arthroplasty are created by a variety of mechanisms including: (a) fracture of the plateau or diaphysis with an osteotomy during cement or prosthesis removal, (b) split of the tibial plateau during trial reduction, (c) retraction on bone, (d) preparation of the medullary canal for tibial stems, (e) tibial stem–cortex conflict during insertion of a stemmed tibial component, and (f) torsional stress applied to the limb during the knee arthroplasty.

Type I

These tibial plateau fractures were most commonly caused by the use of an osteotome during cement removal or when the trial reduction was being performed. Fractures are usually minimally displaced, and in several instances have been discovered only on review of the immediate postoperative films. When discovered during surgery, the treatment of choice has been to use cancellous screw fixation prior to insertion of the real component (Fig. 76.13A). A long-stemmed cemented tibial component was usually used in addition to the screw fixation to bypass the fracture site (Figs. 76.13B, 76.14).

Type II

These fractures all occurred in association with the removal, preparation, or insertion of a long-stemmed tibial component. In the four primary total knee arthroplasties, the intraoperative fracture occurred as a result of tibial stem–lateral tibial cortex conflict during insertion of the real tibial component (Fig. 76.15). The mechanisms causing this fracture in three revision surgeries included cement removal, trial reduction, and preparation of the medullary canal.

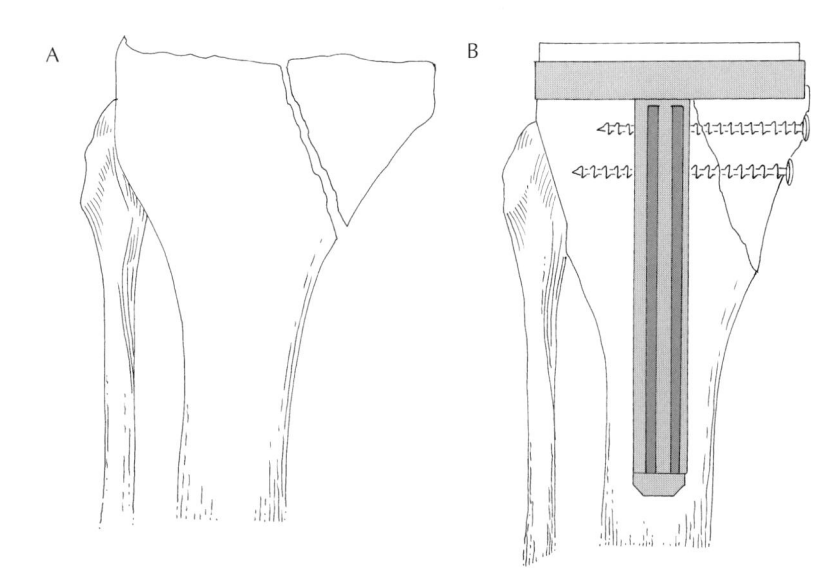

Figure 76.13. (A) Illustration of the Type IC fracture. (B) Fixation of the Type IC fracture with stem bypass and transverse cancellous screw fixation.

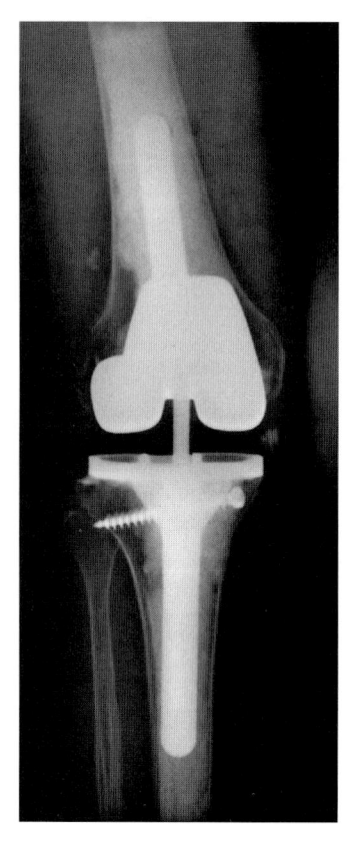

Figure 76.14. Anteroposterior radiograph of a Type IC fracture, which occurred during revision total knee arthroplasty, treated with screw fixation and stem bypass.

Four fractures were discovered on initial postoperative radiographs and treatment consisted of external immobilization with bracing and limitation of weight-bearing for 6 weeks. Of the three fractures discovered intraoperatively, two were treated with bone grafting and stem bypass whereas the other fracture was treated with stem bypass only. One of the fractures treated with bone grafting loosened by 3 years and revision surgery has been recommended.

Type III

In our initial review, there was only one of these fractures in a patient with rheumatoid arthritis and severe osteopenia. This distal tibial fracture was treated by casting and nonweight-bearing for 7 weeks. Since then, we have observed an additional Type III C fracture, which was discovered on intraoperative films after cementing a long-stemmed custom tibial prosthesis. The tibia was fractured just distal to the tip of the prosthesis and was detected by the presence of extruded cement at the fracture site. Through a separate incision, the extruded cement was removed and the tibia was fixed with plate and screws and supplemental bone graft.

Type IV

One of these intraoperative tibial tubercle fractures recently occurred during removal of a chronically infected knee prosthesis in a patient with severe osteoporosis. The tibial tubercle was reapproximated with monofilament absorbable suture after insertion of an antibiotic-loaded cement spacer and the patient is currently being treated in a long leg cast. If the tibial tubercle is satisfactorily healed in several months, reinsertion of another prosthesis is planned.

SUMMARY

We propose a classification for periprosthetic tibial fractures based on the anatomic location of the fracture, timing of the fracture (postoperative or intraoperative), and the radiographic appearance of prosthesis fixation. Based on this classification and a review of our experience, the following treatment algorithm

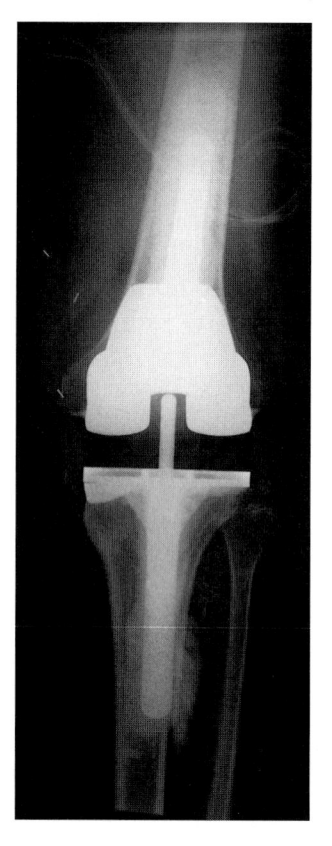

Figure 76.15. Anteroposterior radiograph of a Type IIC fracture discovered on postoperative radiographs.

Periprosthetic Tibial Fracture Treatment Algorithm

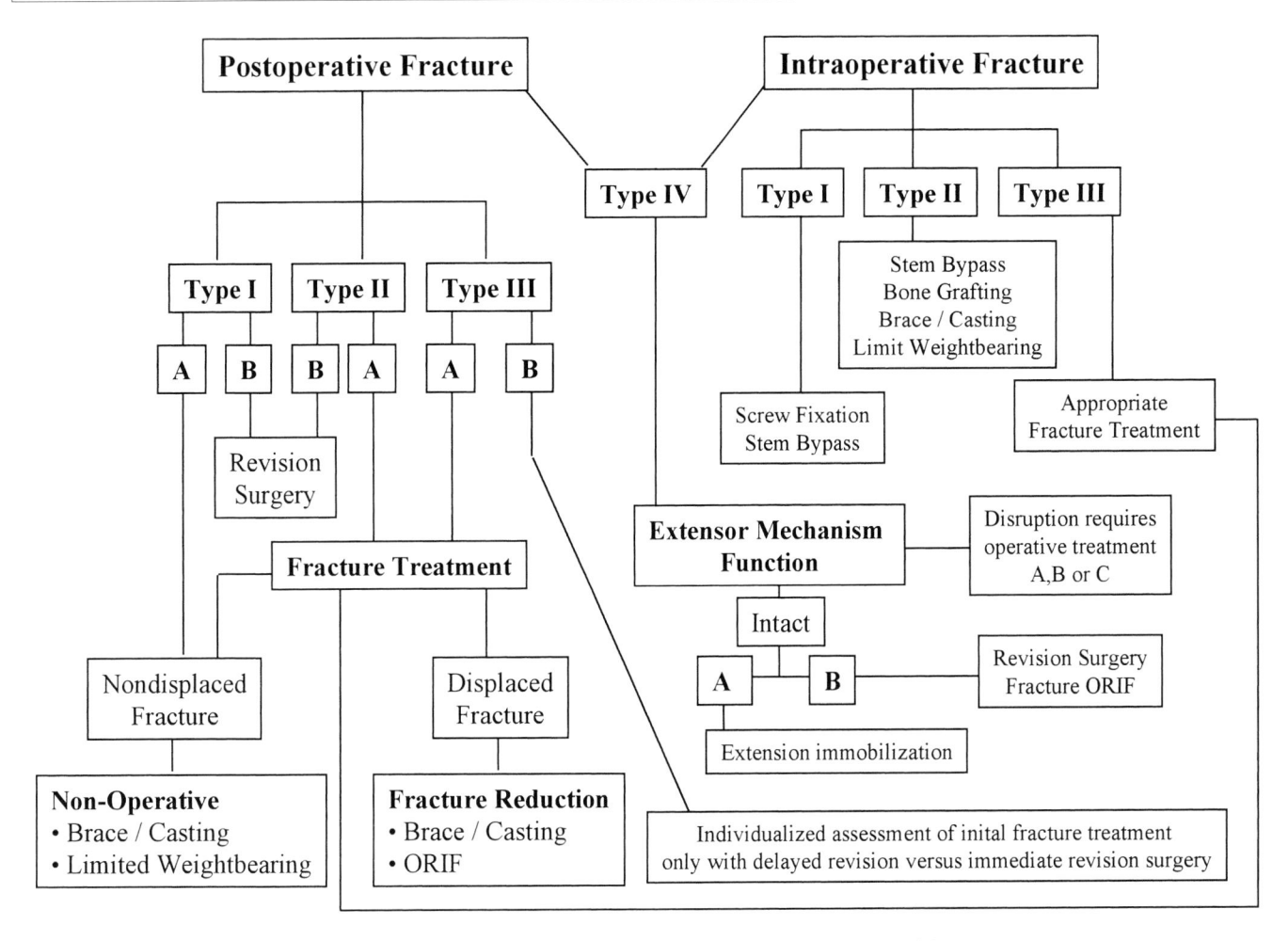

Figure 76.16. A proposed treatment algorithm of periprosthetic tibial fractures.

is suggested (Fig. 76.16). In general, for fractures occurring postoperatively, those that happen in association with a loose prosthesis are managed best by early revision surgery with appropriate fracture fixation and bone grafting, which may often be accomplished by the use of stemmed revision prostheses. These same principles may be used for fractures discovered intraoperatively. For fractures associated with a well-fixed prosthesis, closed reduction and casting until fracture healing is achieved is usually adequate; however, careful attention to maintenance of appropriate limb alignment is important. If extensor mechanism function is intact, extension immobilization of nondisplaced tibial tubercle fractures may be reasonable; however, internal fixation of displaced tibial tubercle fractures seems advisable.

References

1. Healy WL. Tibia fractures below total knee arthroplasty. In: Insall JN, Scott WN, Scuderi GR, eds. *Current concepts in primary and revision total knee arthroplasty.* Philadelphia: Lippincott-Raven Publishers; 1996:163–67.
2. Rand JA, Coventry. Stress fractures after total knee arthroplasty. *J Bone Joint Surg.* 1980; 62A:226–33.
3. Felix NA, Stuart MJ, Hanssen AD. Periprosthetic fractures associated with total knee arthroplasty. Presented at the Annual Meeting of the Knee Society, San Francisco, February 1997.
4. Ritter MA, Carr K, Keating EM, Faris PM, Meding JB. Tibial shaft fracture following tibial tubercle osteotomy. *J Arthroplasty.* 1996; 11:117–19.
5. Whiteside LA. Exposure in difficult total knee arthroplasty using tibial tubercle osteotomy. *Clin Orthop.* 1995; 321:32–35.

CHAPTER 77
Tibial Periprosthetic Fractures: Nonoperative Treatment

Philip M. Faris

Periprosthetic tibial fractures involving TKR may be categorized into traumatic and nontraumatic (atraumatic) types. Atraumatic fractures predominate. They occur almost exclusively in the medial plateau, beneath the tibial prosthesis in standard tibial components. In articles by Rand et al.,[1] Skolnick et al.,[2] Lotke et al.,[3] Bryan et al.,[4] and Cordeiro et al.,[5] these fracture patterns are similar and are related to varus malalignment and inadequate subprosthetic bone. Bony collapse and fragmentation, along with prosthetic loosening and subsidence, are seen on x-ray. Faris et al.[6] has described similar stress-related tibial fractures beneath the medial plateau in well-aligned, all-polyethylene tibial components in a flat-on-flat total knee replacement design. Stress-related fractures may also result from inadequate stress distribution in well-aligned arthroplasties (Fig. 77.1).

Although these fractures were often treated initially with limited nonweight-bearing and/or cylinder casts, the results of conservative treatment appear to be universally unacceptable, with progressive deformity, pain, and prosthetic subsidence. Revision arthroplasty is the treatment of choice.

Traumatic types of fractures theoretically could occur just as they do in normal knees; however, the stress required to fracture a tibial shaft or to create a periprosthetic tibial plateau fracture must be considerably greater than the forces that create a periprosthetic supracondylar femur fracture because supracondylar femoral fractures are much more common. In reviewing our

Figure 77.1. (A) Two-month follow-up x-ray, left total knee replacement, showing satisfactory axial alignment with a well-cemented all-polyethylene tibial component. (B) Two-year follow-up x-ray revealing stress fracture and bone failure beneath the medial tibial plateau, apparently related to excessive stress transfer to the medial compartment.

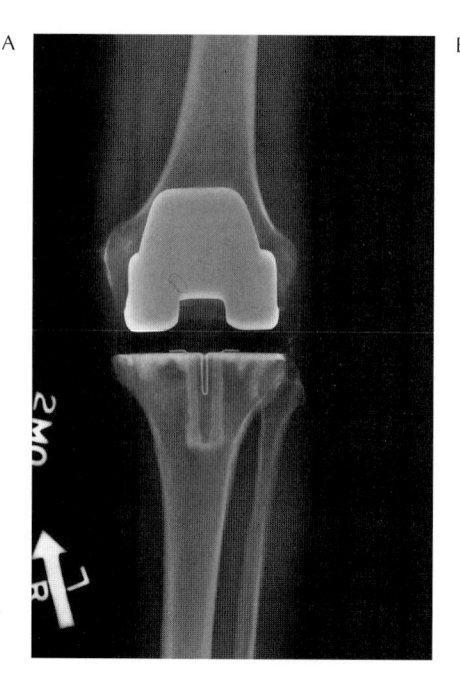

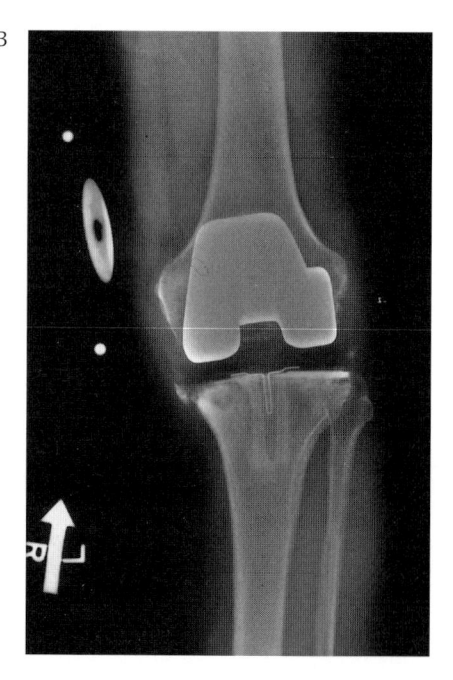

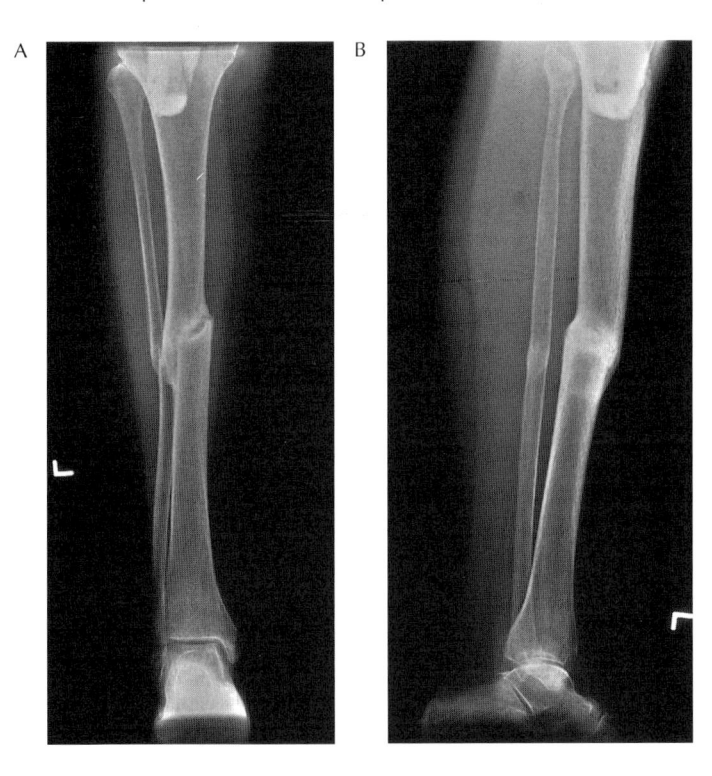

77. Tibial Periprosthetic Fractures: Nonoperative Treatment

Figure 77.2. Anterior/posterior and lateral views of a healed left mid-shaft tibial fracture that occurred traumatically below a cemented left total knee replacement.

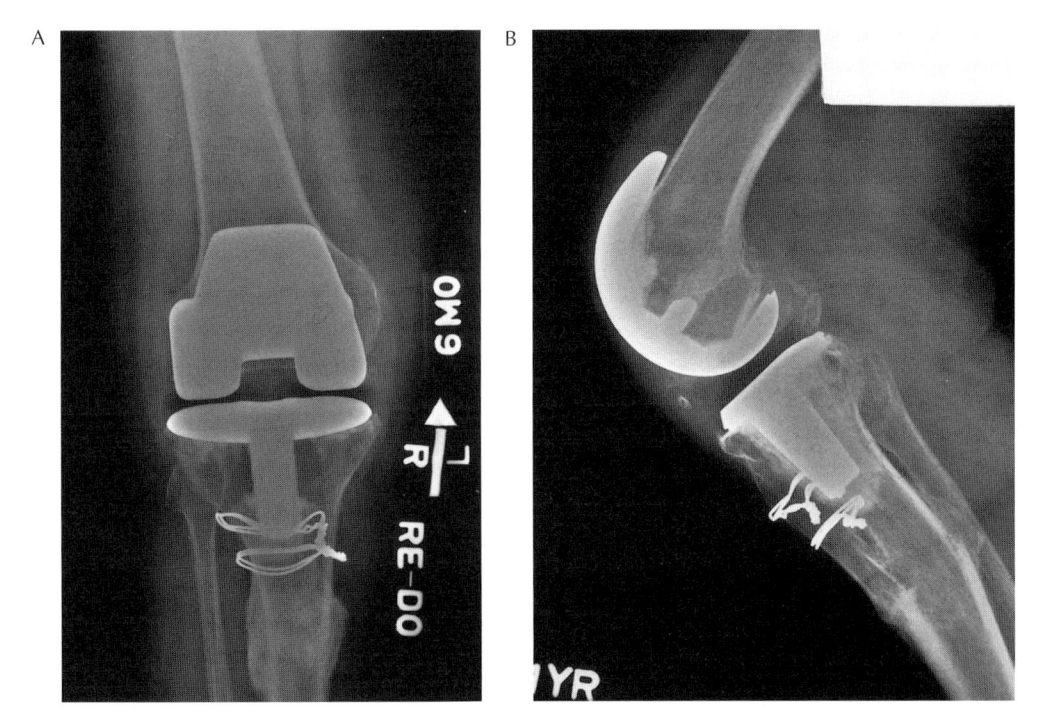

Figure 77.3. Healed fracture through a tibial tubercle osteotomy at the distal extent of the osteotomy. Acceptable alignment was obtained in a cast, the fracture healed, and the patient is doing well.

databank of over 3000 total knee replacements, I found only two traumatic tibial fractures that were treated conservatively, including one tibial shaft fracture (Fig. 77.2) and one fracture that occurred through a tibial tubercle osteotomy screw hole (Fig. 77.3). Both fractures were treated with casting and had satisfactory outcomes. There was reocurrence of two other fractures through tibial tubercle osteotomy. One required revision of the tibial component with long intramedullary extensions. The other was initially treated with cast immobilization and healed in malalignment, requiring revision. A review of the literature reveals no other reports of conservatively treated periprosthetic tibial fractures.

CONCLUSION

Periprosthetic tibial fractures are generally related to bone stress overload in varus-aligned total knee replacements or knees with prostheses that inadequately distribute load. Traumatic fractures are rare and conservative treatment of these fractures is reserved only for fractures in which adequate alignment can be maintained with cast immobilization.

References

1. Rand JA, Coventry MB. Stress fractures after total knee arthroplasty. *J Bone Joint Surg Am*. 1980; 62:226–233.
2. Skolnick MD, Brian RS, Peterson LFA, Combs JJ, Ilstrup DM. Polycentric total knee arthroplasty: A two year follow-up study. *J Bone Joint Surg Am*. 1976; 58:743–48.
3. Lotke PA, Ecker ML. Influence of positioning of prosthesis in total knee replacement. *J Bone Joint Surg Am*. 1977; 59: 77–79.
4. Bryan RS, Peterson LFA, Combs JJ. Polycentric knee arthroplasty: A preliminary report of postoperative complications in 450 knees. *Clin Orthop*. 1973; 94:148–52.
5. Cordeiro EN, Costa RC, Carazzato JG, Silva Jdoss. Periprosthetic fractures in patients with total knee arthroplasties. *Clin Orthop*. 1990; 252:182–89.
6. Faris et al. Three- to 5-year follow-up of all polytibial component; in preparation for publication.

CHAPTER 78
Tibial Periprosthetic Fractures: Open Reduction Internal Fixation

William L. Healy

Periprosthetic fractures of the tibia below knee replacements are uncommon and infrequently reported. Between 1970 and 1992, 32 of these fractures were reported in nine articles published in the English language orthopedic literature. Rand and Coventry[1] reported 12 periprosthetic tibia fractures below 705 knee replacements after a 4-year follow-up of the knee replacement surgery. This study from 1980, which reports on knee replacements performed in the 1970s, notes a 1.7% incidence of periprosthetic tibia fractures below knee replacements.

Although the reported incidence of periprosthetic tibia fractures distal to knee replacements is small, this number might be expected to increase in the future. In 1995, 243,919 total knee operations were performed in the United States. This represents a 5.9% increase from 1994. The prevalence of knee replacement operations is increasing faster than hip replacement operations.[2] As knee replacement operations are performed more frequently, and as knee replacement patients become more active following TKA surgery, the incidence and prevalence of periprosthetic tibial fractures below knee replacements may increase.

Periprosthetic fractures of the tibia below knee replacements are most commonly stress or fatigue fractures associated with minimal or low-velocity trauma. However, minimal trauma can cause significant problems for patients in terms of pain and disability. Factors predisposing to these fractures include: osteopenia from disuse, medications or systemic illness, limb malalignment, implant malposition, and loosening of the tibial implant.

Periprosthetic tibia fractures below knee replacements can be classified according to the integrity of the bone-cement-implant interface. When this interface is disrupted and a tibial implant is loose, ultimate treatment of the fracture will require revision knee replacement surgery. Depending on the displacement of the fracture, revision of the tibial implant can be associated with nonoperative treatment of the tibia fracture or open reduction internal fixation of the tibia fracture. When the bone-cement-implant interface is not disrupted, the tibial implant can be left intact and the fractured tibia can be treated with nonoperative or operative treatment.

Periprosthetic fractures of the tibia below knee replacements can also be classified according to anatomic location and function. Surgeons at Mayo Clinic have proposed a four-part classification for these fractures, based on the location of the fracture, the integrity of the tibial implant, and the integrity of the extensor mechanism of the knee.[3] The four types of periprosthetic tibia fractures in the Mayo classification are: Type I, tibial plateau fractures; Type II, fractures adjacent to the tibial implant; Type III, fractures distal to the tibial implant; Type IV, fractures involving the extensor mechanism/anterior tibial tubercle. The Mayo classification subclassifies these fractures into: an A group when the tibial implant is well fixed; a B group when the tibial implant is loose; and a C group for intraoperative fractures.

The Mayo group reviewed 102 periprosthetic tibia fractures below knee replacements that were treated between 1970 and 1995. The distribution of their fractures included: 62 Type I (51 IB, 11 IC); 22 Type II (5 IIA, 10 IIB, 7 IIC); 16 Type III (14 IIIA, 1 IIIB, 1 IIIC); and 2 Type IV (2 IVA). Successful outcome following treatment of these fractures was associated with restoration of skeletal integrity around a well-fixed implant in a stable mobile knee.

Treatment of periprosthetic tibia fractures below knee replacements must restore limb alignment, limb rotation, knee stability, and knee mobility. Functional fracture treatment may achieve these goals by nonoperative treatment of the fracture or operative treatment of the

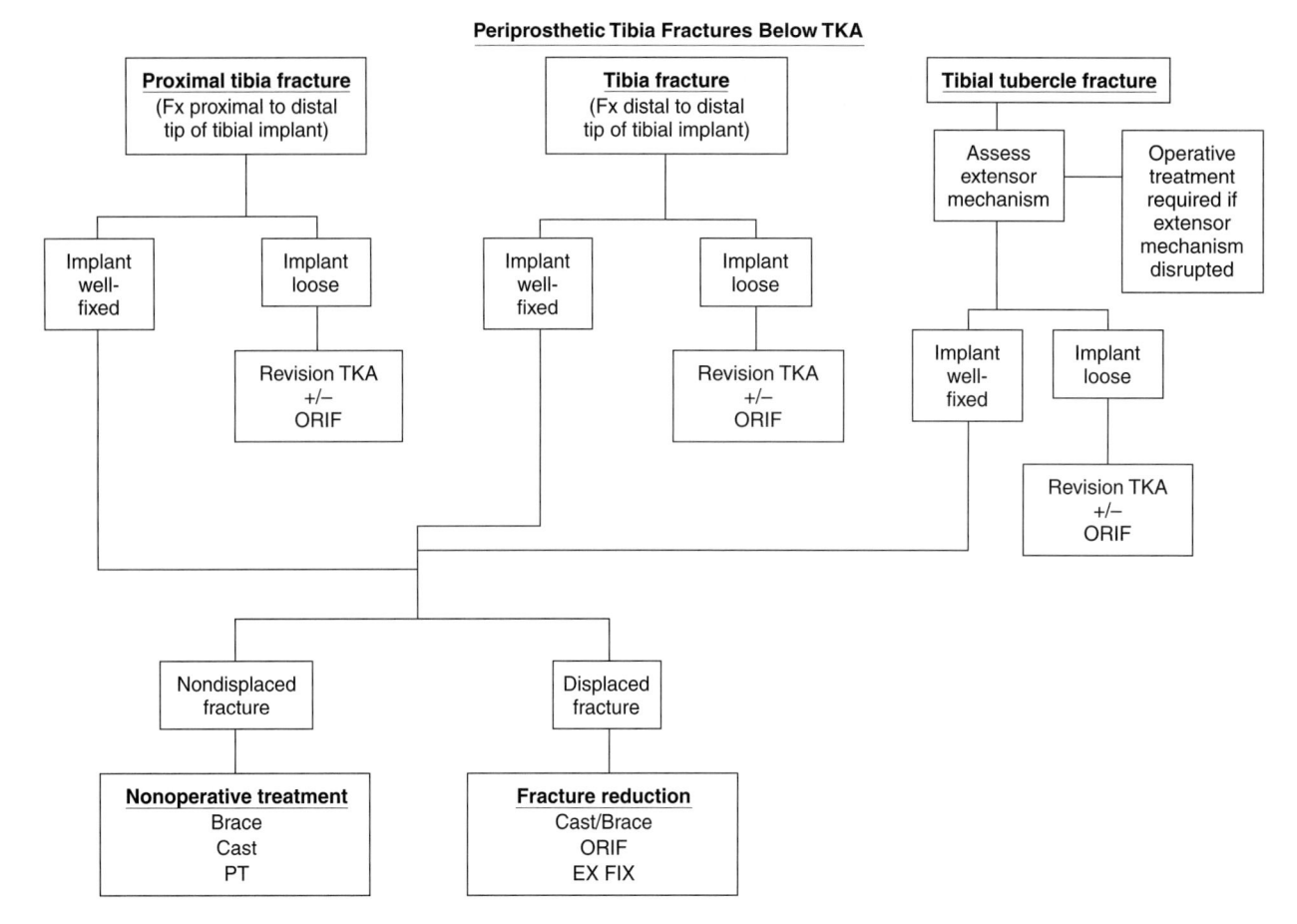

Figure 78.1. Treatment algorithm for periprosthetic tibia fractures below knee replacements.

fracture. Nonoperative fracture treatment usually involves cast or brace immobilization followed by physical therapy. Operative treatment may include ORIF and revision knee replacement surgery. Rand and Coventry[1] stated that early revision surgery at the time of fracture did not adversely affect fracture healing. Five of their knees were revised within 2 days and ten knees were revised between 3 and 24 weeks following fracture.

An algorithm for treatment of periprosthetic tibia fractures below knee replacements is presented in Figure 78.1. Three fracture patterns, based on location, are described: (1) proximal tibia fractures, which are proximal to the distal tip of the tibial implants; (2) tibia fractures, which are distal to the distal tip of the tibial implant; and (3) tibial tubercle fractures, which involve the tibial attachment of the patella ligament and the extensor mechanism. When choosing a treatment method, it is also important to determine whether the tibial implant fixation is satisfactory.

For fractures in which the implant is well-fixed, a decision as to nonoperative or operative treatment depends on fracture displacement and potential for function. For fractures in which the tibial implant is loose, revision knee replacement is suggested with or without open-reduction internal fixation of the fracture. In tibial tubercle fractures, the extensor mechanism must be assessed and treated surgically if the extensor mechanism is disrupted.

Nondisplaced tibia fractures below well-fixed tibial implants can be treated nonoperatively with a pre-

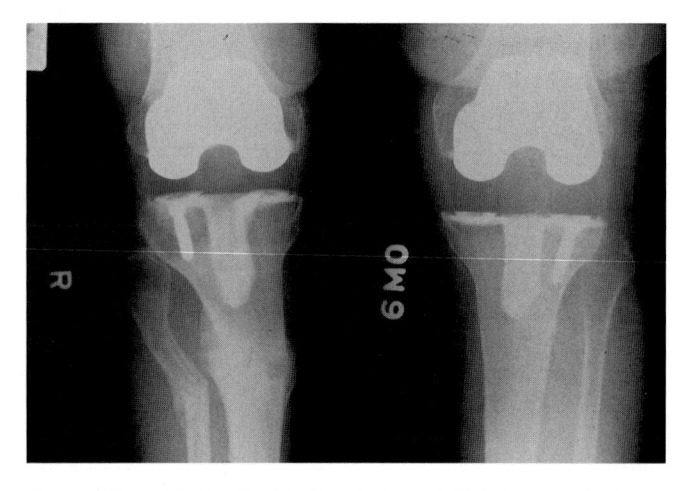

Figure 78.2. Minimally displaced Type II tibia fracture below a well-fixed right knee replacement. Nonoperative treatment achieved fracture union and a functional knee.

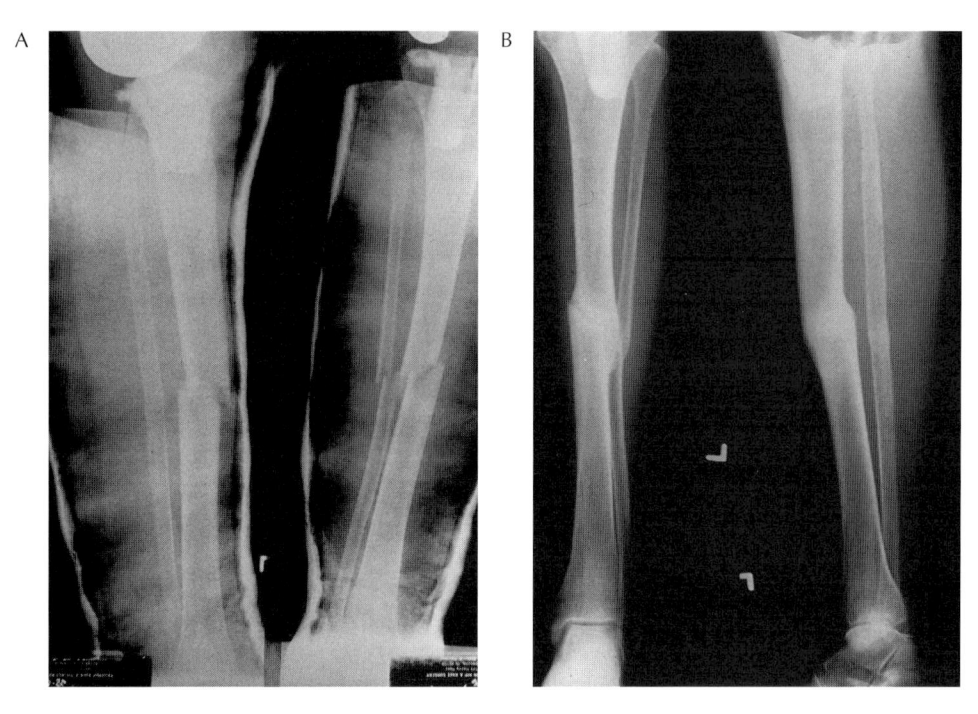

Figure 78.3. (A) This 65-year-old patient experienced a Type IIA mid-shaft tibial fracture distal to a knee replacement. The patient was treated with cast immobilization. (B) The fracture healed with full function of the knee and limb.

dictably successful outcome (Figs. 78.2 and 78.3). Immobilization can be achieved with a cast or a fracture brace. Motion can be added to a fracture brace as clinically indicated. When sufficient bony union is achieved, the knee can be rehabilitated with physical therapy. Displaced tibia fractures below knee replacements require surgical treatment when: (a) proximal tibial bone is disrupted such that the tibial implant will not have sufficient support; (b) the fracture has caused a loss of skeletal integrity (alignment, rotation) inconsistent with satisfactory knee function; or (c) loss of extensor mechanism integrity. Whenever the anterior tibial tubercle and its attachment at the patella ligament is disrupted from the proximal tibia, it must be repaired. Extensor

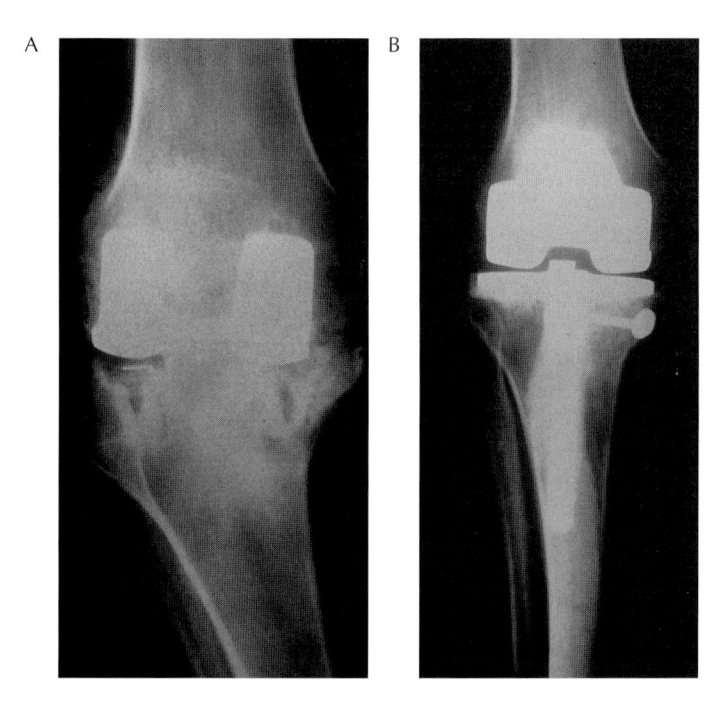

Figure 78.4. (A) This 70-year-old woman experienced a Type IB tibial plateau fracture associated with a loose tibial implant. This fatigue/stress fracture occurred following minimal trauma. (B) Treatment of this fracture required revision knee replacement. A femoral head allograft was used for bone augmentation of the medial tibial plateau. The allograft was fixed in place with a medial buttress screw and washer. The fracture and bone graft were bypassed with a cemented long-stemmed tibial implant.

mechanism insufficiency is disabling, and this clinical condition is not compatible with a satisfactory outcome following these fractures.

Technical considerations for operative treatment of these fractures include bone stock, fracture fixation technique, fracture fixation implant, and choice of tibial knee implant. Frequently, tibia fractures below knee replacements are associated with osteopenia, and augmentation of bone stock may be required. Methods for proximal tibial bone augmentation include allograft bone, wedges or blocks for attachment to the tibial knee implant, and custom tibial implants (Fig. 78.4).

Fracture fixation techniques must sufficiently buttress the proximal tibia to support the tibial implant. Buttress plates should be applied medially or laterally to the proximal tibia, depending on the location of the fracture. Bicondylar proximal tibia fractures may require medial and lateral plates. Small-wire external fixation techniques and hybrid external fixators may be useful for severely comminuted fractures. Fixators may span the knee if necessary. Fracture fixation must also address disruptions of skeletal integrity between the proximal tibia and the tibia diaphysis. If lag screw fixation is used to reduce and compress oblique fractures in the metaphysis and the diaphysis, these reduced fractures should be neutralized with plates that extend from the proximal tibia into the tibial diaphysis, or with external fixation. When revision surgery is required in association with open-reduction internal fixation, the position of bone screws should take into account the need for placement of an intramedullary stem from the tibial base plate into the intramedullary space. Long tibial stems provide increased stability for the tibial implant, provide increased stability for the fracture reconstruction, and can reduce the stress applied to proximal tibial bone grafts used for augmentation (Fig. 78.5).

Successful surgical treatment of tibia fractures below knee replacements requires an understanding of principles and techniques of operative fracture fixation and revision knee replacement surgery. Open-reduction internal fixation and revision knee replacement surgery are indicated when tibial implants are loose, malposi-

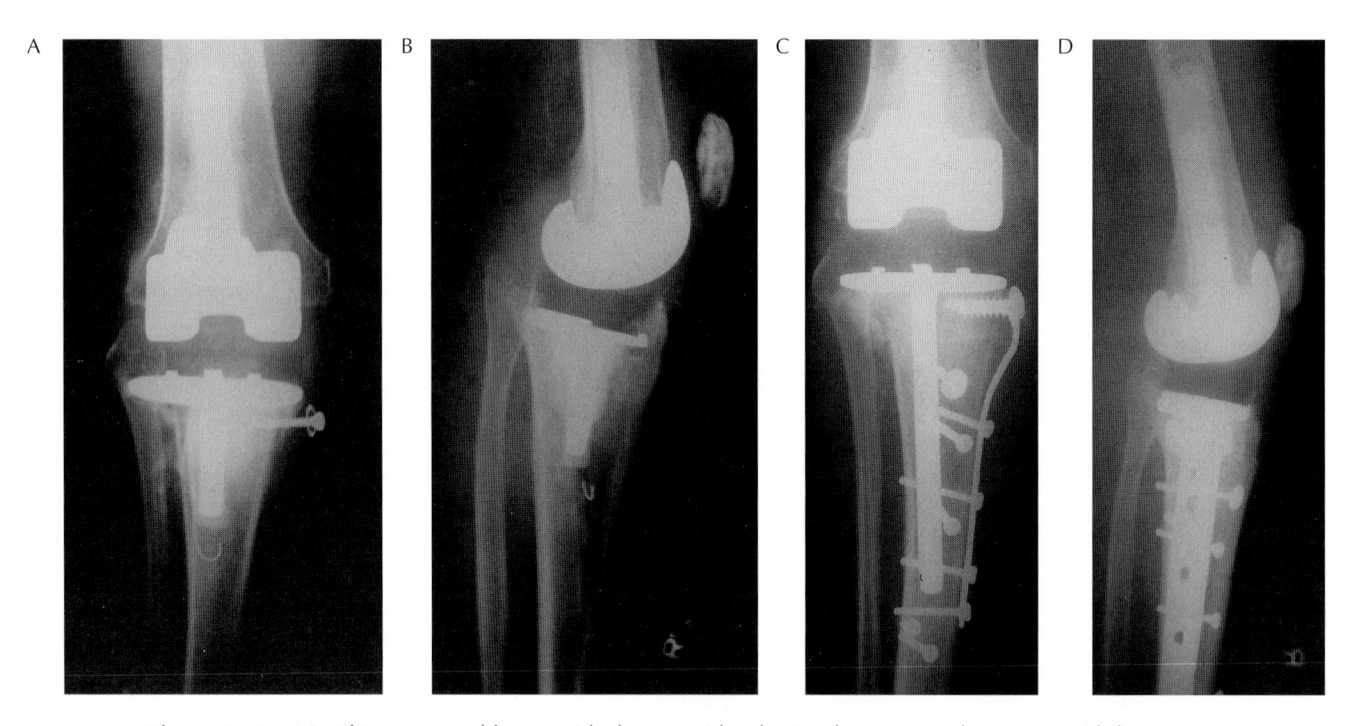

Figure 78.5. (A,B) This 68-year-old man with rheumatoid arthritis who was on chronic steroid therapy had previously had two revision knee replacement operations for aseptic loosening. Following minimal trauma, the patient experienced a Type IIB fracture of the proximal tibia extending from the tibial implant bone cement interface into the tibial diaphysis. The tibial component was imploded into the proximal tibia. (C,D) Treatment of this fracture required open-reduction internal fixation of the tibia and revision knee replacement. The medial tibial plateau required bone augmentation with a femoral head allograft. The long oblique fracture was fixed with interfragmentary lag screws. A plate was used to buttress the metaphysis of the proximal tibia and neutralize the lag screw fixation in the tibial diaphysis. A long-stemmed tibial implant provided intramedullary support of the fracture and bypassed the allograft, stabilizing the tibial implant.

tioned, malrotated, or malaligned, or when the tibia is displaced to the point where functional treatment of the fracture is not possible. Clinical results of operative treatment of these fractures depend on patient selection and choice of operative technique and, ultimately, on a surgeon's skill in achieving a reconstruction that can restore prefracture function.[4]

ACKNOWLEDGMENTS

The author acknowledges the contribution of clinical cases to this chapter by Merrill A. Ritter and Steven A. Wasilewski. The author also acknowledges the contribution of the Mayo Clinic classification for tibia fractures below knee replacements, which was provided by Arlen D. Hanssen.

References

1. Rand JA, Coventry MB. Stress fractures after total knee arthroplasty. *J Bone Joint Surg Am*. 1980; 62:226–233.
2. Mendenhall S, ed. Editorial. *Orthopaedic Network News*. July 1996; 7:3,1.
3. Felix NA, Stuart MJ, Hanssen AD. Periprosthetic fractures of the tibia associated with total knee arthroplasty. *Clinical Orthopaedics*. 1997; 345:113–124.
4. Healy WL. Tibia fractures below total knee arthroplasty. In: Insall JN, Scott WN, Scuderi GR, eds. *Current concepts in primary and revision total knee arthroplasty*. Philadelphia: Lippincott-Raven Publishers, 1996:163–167.

CHAPTER 79
Revision Arthroplasty for Tibial Periprosthetic Fractures

Wayne G. Paprosky, Todd D. Sekundiak, and John Kronick

Despite the increasing number of total knee arthroplasties being performed,[1] the rate of periprosthetic tibial fractures has remained low. Healy performed a retrospective review of the English-language literature from 1970 to 1992 and found 32 reported cases in nine published articles.[2-11] These fractures are much less common than supracondylar femoral fractures with Cordeiro and associates reporting a relative ratio of nine to one.[4] Treatment options for these fractures have included a host of different operative and nonoperative techniques with revision arthroplasty being indicated in a select group.

No complete series of periprosthetic tibial fractures has been reported in the literature. The 15 tibial plateau fractures reported by Rand and Coventry[8] only included fractures that they felt were stress related from component malalignment or improper component rotation. It excluded fractures that occurred intraoperatively, secondary to trauma, or component failure. All fractures involved the medial plateau and were attributable to excessive medial displacement and varus positioning of the tibial component. This increased eccentric loading of the medial tibial plateau, in bone of poor quality and with a component that does not distribute force, led to resultant fracture.[12,13] These stress fractures had concomitant component loosening and required revision arthroplasty ultimately. Other authors have also correlated these stress fractures to component loosening and malalignment.[3,6,9,11]

These stress fractures have to be differentiated from fractures that occur from definitive trauma. As the prevalence of total knee arthroplasties increases in a younger more active population, periprosthetic tibial fracture from associated trauma will also increase. Treatment modalities will need to consider a host of variables, as with fracture management in general, to determine the most judicious approach. Traumatic injuries must be differentiated further by the amount of energy when determining treatment. High-energy fractures may preclude certain treatments secondary to the degree of bone and soft tissue loss, the higher risk of infection, the possibility of multiple or bilateral fractures, and the concern of multisystem injuries.

INCIDENCE

The incidence of periprosthetic tibial fractures has been reported at 1.7%.[8] This may actually be higher than that which exists because this rate has iatrogenic influence secondary to component malpositioning and selection. In Weidel's review of 800 total knee arthroplasties, no traumatic periprosthetic tibial fractures were found.[12] Bryan reported on 450 patients and reported a rate of 1%.[3] No difference has been found between control and fracture groups when body weight, duration of disease, disease of the contralateral lower extremity, or steroid use was compared.[8] Surprisingly, most series and case reports of periprosthetic tibial fractures occur from minimal trauma.[3-11] The most common presenting symptom is pain that can be present from 1 day to a year.[8] The delay in diagnosis is most commonly from the patient delaying medical advice.

TREATMENT OPTIONS

The goals with periprosthetic tibial fractures are similar to any particular fracture—to obtain fracture union with satisfactory limb alignment while maintaining ligamentous and tendinous tissue attachments and function. Chen and associates have proposed an algorithm for supracondylar femoral periprosthetic fractures that can be applied to tibial periprosthetic fractures.[15] Rand has also considered five factors in assessing the fracture character that determines an algorithm for treatment options. These are timing, location, and extent of the fracture, presence or absence of union, and the effect of the fracture on limb alignment as well as fracture alignment.[16] These then must be combined with host factors such as age, activity level, and concomitant systemic disease to determine treatment. Finally, consideration is given to the premorbid joint replacement that provides us with the following algorithm.

Most authors agree that with well-fixed, painless total knee arthroplasties, that union of a nondisplaced, stable fracture can be obtained with nonoperative measures secondary to the low-energy nature of these fractures.[17] Motion is preserved in a knee that has previously functioned well and has been casted for a short period to obtain union.[17]

For fractures that are displaced or unstable but occurring with a component that is well fixed and previously functioning well, there is controversy whether these should be treated open or closed—and if opened, if revision or internal fixation should proceed. Closed treatment should only be considered when reduction can be obtained and maintained. When closed treatment is not an option for a fracture because of the patient's inability to tolerate prolonged immobility or the surgeon's inability to reduce the fracture or maintain the alignment, open reduction and internal fixation is the next option.

Significant bone loss can occur with removal of previously well-fixed components, making revision arthroplasty indicated only when the soft tissue coverage, the previous implant and stem, or the fracture pattern precludes internal fixation. It is critical to summate the amount of bone loss that will occur from removal of the components, combined with the fracture pattern itself. Removal of components can extend the degree of comminution and must be considered with the patient's overall bone quality, to determine the type of prosthesis, stem, augmentation, and bone graft required. Further, it must be determined if it is technically feasible to reconstruct the joint immediately. It may be prudent to initially accept a malunion that allows bone stock and soft tissue coverage to improve with healing. Revision arthroplasty or osteotomy may then be easier and more effective than undertaking an immediate massive initial reconstruction that requires extensive resources to reconstruct an extremity with deficient bone and soft tissues.

The assessment of bone loss is even more critical when assessing a fracture with a component that is well-fixed but malpositioned. Because of the malpositioning of the component, one may feel obliged to revise the joint immediately. Ultimately all tibial periprosthetic stress fractures will require revision when they have occurred in the presence of a malpositioned component.[8]

However, the revision procedure can be technically demanding and may be easier achieved once union has initially been obtained. If, however, stable fixation can be obtained with a revision arthroplasty without compromising significant host bone or soft tissues, then revision should be considered as the immediate definitive treatment.

In cases in which the component is loose, irrespective of the fracture being displaced or nondisplaced, revision arthroplasty is indicated. Some authors still initially seek union by closed treatment or internal fixation because reconstruction is fraught with hazards in the presence of a fresh fracture.[17] As stated previously, the technical demands of the reconstruction and the resources required will determine the timing of the reconstruction. Further caveats to this approach would be for patients unable to tolerate an operative procedure or where infection would be at high risk.

Nonunions, malunions, or delayed unions of tibial fractures can also be treated with a stemmed tibial revision component (Fig. 79.1). An established delayed or nonunion of the femur can be treated with internal fixation and bone grafting.[18] The periprosthetic tibia fracture, however, may have a tenuous soft tissue envelope that may lead to skin slough if one were to open the

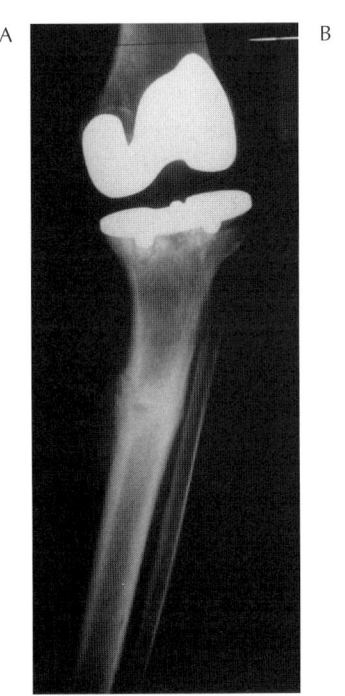

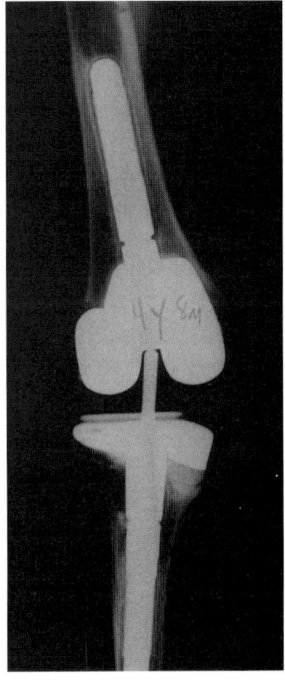

Figure 79.1. (A) Tibial nonunion with malpositioned uncemented components. (B) Revision arthroplasty at 4½ years. Nonunion has healed with stem bridging nonunion site. Joint deformity required metal augmentation to reconstruct joint line. Sclerotic halo around femoral stem is not indicative of failed component.

fracture site, graft, and obtain osteosynthesis. Open reduction and internal fixation of these fractures with plate osteosynthesis may also preclude future revision by encroachment of screws in the intramedullary canal. Placement of a stemmed component and use of intramedullary bone graft, for metaphyseal or diaphyseal fractures, can be used with great success as the fracture site is stabilized. Deformity is corrected. Motion of the joint can be maintained and the fracture site can be loaded (Fig. 79.1B).[19-21]

PREOPERATIVE PLANNING

The objectives in revision of total knee arthroplasty for ipsilateral periprosthetic tibial fractures are the same as for the principles of total knee arthroplasty. If revision arthroplasty is to be considered, preoperative planning must consider bone and soft tissue losses from traumatic and atraumatic causes—and the degree of deformity. Preoperative assessment includes full-length standing anteroposterior and lateral radiographs with magnification markers of the lower extremity. This provides accurate assessment of defect size, deformity angle, as well as component size, augment or stem length and width, and the need for an osteotomy. Treatment choices will be tempered not only by the noted anatomical deficits of the injury but also by the functional limitations or expectations of the patient. A custom long-stemmed tumor prosthesis can easily substitute for a comminuted metaphyseal fracture in an elderly debilitated patient, whereas a short-stemmed minimally constrained arthroplasty with limited internal fixation may function better for a younger active patient.

Removal of components, osteolysis, and osteopenia, in addition to the comminuted fracture fragments can significantly increase the amount of bone loss. This can necessitate the use of cement, bone graft, or augments in the revision procedure to fill defects. In instances in which severe bone loss or comminution exists, bulk structural allografting must be considered. Length and width of graft are measured, as well as the possible need for ligament and tendinous reconstruction (Fig. 79.2).

In the late setting of nonunions or malunions, angular deformities can be corrected in the metaphyseal region by bone resection or augmentation at the time of arthroplasty as long as the collateral ligaments or extensor mechanism is not compromised. Knowledge of ligamentous and tendinous insertions is essential and must be correlated to bony resection to determine if insertions will be compromised. For translational tibial deformities, offset tibial stems or baseplates with eccentric housing connections are useful for obtaining better tibial coverage without needing an osteotomy. Deformities that exist in the diaphyseal area of the tibia with greater than 10 to 15 degrees of angulation in the coronal plane or 20 degrees in the sagittal plane may require osteotomy and correction to perform a satisfactory arthroplasty.[16] To restore a normal mechanical axis, tracing paper outlining the deformity and resultant operative correction is used in deciding the method of correction.

Surgical exposure must be planned to include these adjunctive procedures of fracture fragment reduction, removal of old components or fixation devices, as well as new component insertion. If possible, exposure should include previous operative incisions to prevent the possibility of skin ischemia and resultant slough.

Stemmed components have been indispensable adjuncts to these revision procedures. The use of stems in the revision setting has been discussed elsewhere. Most systems now have an array of fluted press-fit stems. Cemented stems have previously been used with great success but run the risk of nonunion by the presence of cement into the fracture site. For fractures that occur in the metaphyseal or diaphyseal region, the stem can be used like an intramedullary rod to bridge the fracture site and obtain rotational and bending stability (Fig. 79.1). For epiphyseal fractures, the stem can be used as an unloader to transmit force away from the joint and prevent collapse or migration of bony fragments after limited fixation, grafting, or removal of fragments has been performed (Fig. 79.3). The need for a constrained or nonconstrained component is also determined. The compatibility of the stem to the type of component must also be considered because bridging a fracture with an intramedullary rod does not obligate the use of a constrained component.[19] Compatibility of the revision tibial stem and baseplate with the in situ femoral component must also be considered to determine the need and technical difficulty of its removal.

OPERATIVE TECHNIQUE

Revision knee arthroplasty for tibial periprosthetic fractures begins with an incision that must be extensile to allow adequate access to the knee for removal of components and for the possibility of exposure of fracture fragments. Tissues are compromised from previous operative procedures, but now also have the acute traumatic insult. Previous operative incisions must be incorporated as discussed elsewhere. Osteotomes or sliver osteotomes are routinely used for removal of well-fixed components. One needs to be cognizant of the force imparted on the arthroplasty interfaces because the force can be transmitted to the bone and lead to propagation of the fracture or fracture fragmentation. The use of a power saw or burr may remove some extra bone at the interface being debonded but avoids the peak forces that a mallet and osteotome may impart. This leads to a re-

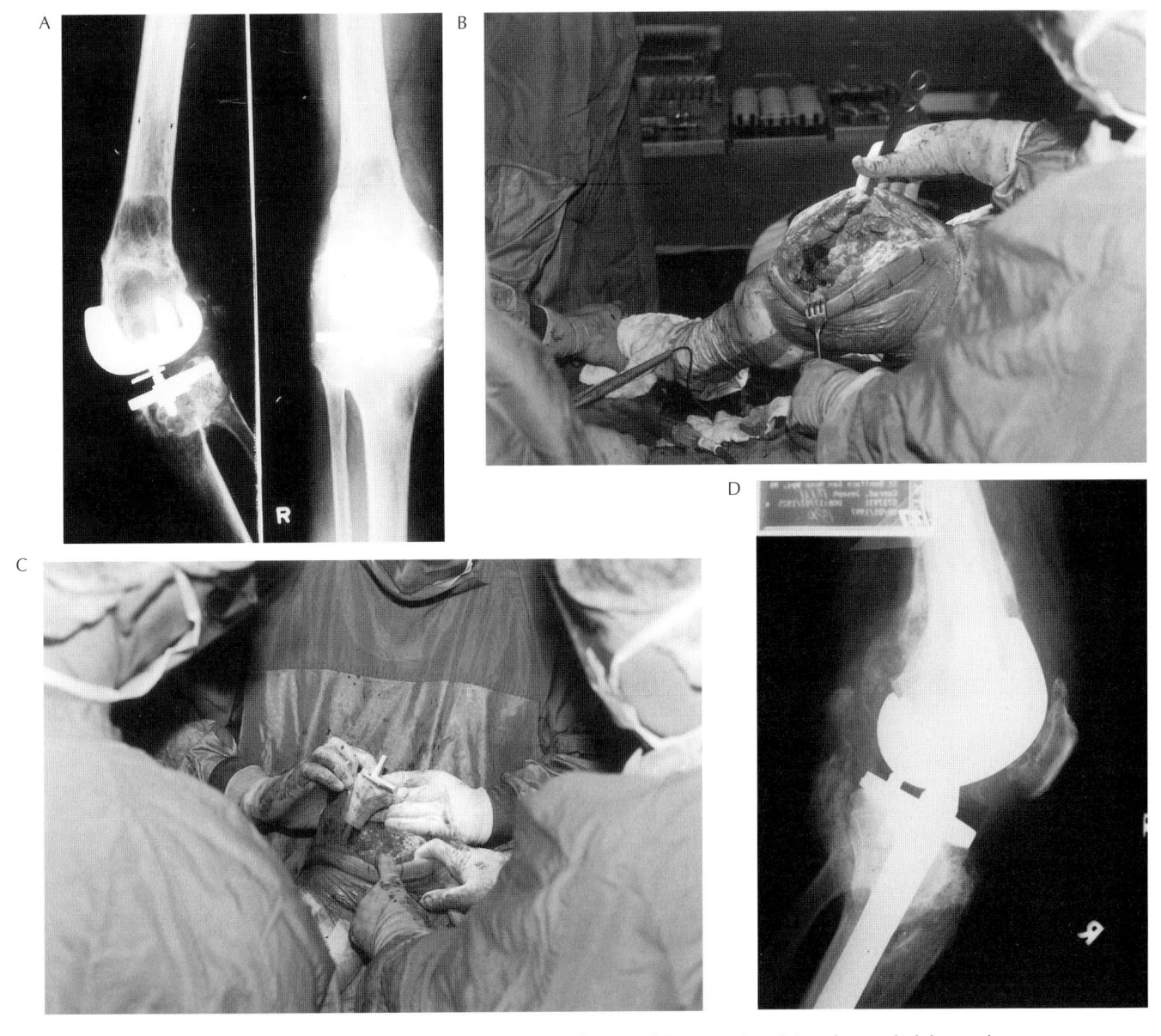

Figure 79.2. A 69-year-old male with severe osteolysis and fractures involving the medial femoral condyle and lateral tibial plateau. (A) Preoperative radiographs. (B) Tibial defect demonstrating severe loss of bone but integrity of tibial tubercle and extensor mechanism. (C) Cemented tibial component and allograft press-fit in host bone. (D) Postoperative radiograph demonstrating graft invaginated in host bone with maintenance of host extensor mechanism.

sultant increase in final bone stock integrity. Removal of components can proceed in a host of different ways but patience must be employed. Once component interfaces have been debonded, the components should be digitally pulled off the bone surfaces without the use of a mallet to expedite the removal.

With the components removed, the bone is curretted and cleansed to assess the bone defects present. In nearly all cases in which tibial component revision is the treatment for a periprosthetic fracture, a tibial intramedullary stem will be used to augment the component. This requires intramedullary alignment for the proximal tibial cut. The method of alignment is described elsewhere. Initially a minimal amount of proximal tibia is resected. "Clean-up" cuts are also performed on the femur, which then allows flexion and extension gaps to be assessed.

The presence of the fracture may prevent adequate assessment of the gaps at this time. If the fracture is metaphyseal or epiphyseal, then initial internal fixation should proceed. This will provide bony stability and then allow for assessment of ligamentous stability and

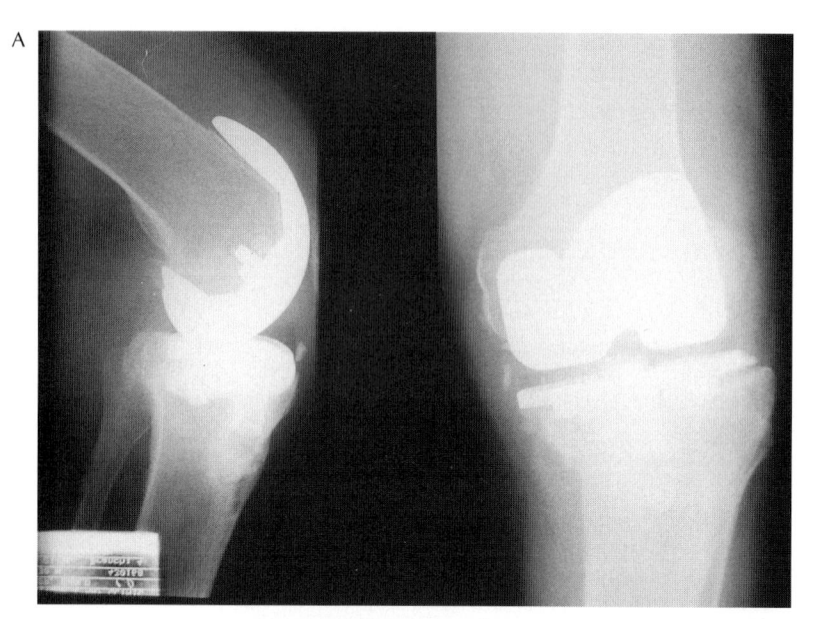

Figure 79.3. A 70-year-old male with two previous knee arthroplasties in two consecutive years. Patient began complaining of significant medial knee pain and sudden increasing deformity. (A) Preoperative radiograph demonstrating varus positioning of the tibial component with subsidence and fracturing of the medial tibial plateau. (B) Intraoperative photograph demonstrating lag screw fixation of medial tibial plateau fracture with stemmed component and augment then being positioned. (C) Postoperative radiograph of stemmed components. An offset stem was used to increase load on the intact lateral tibial plateau.

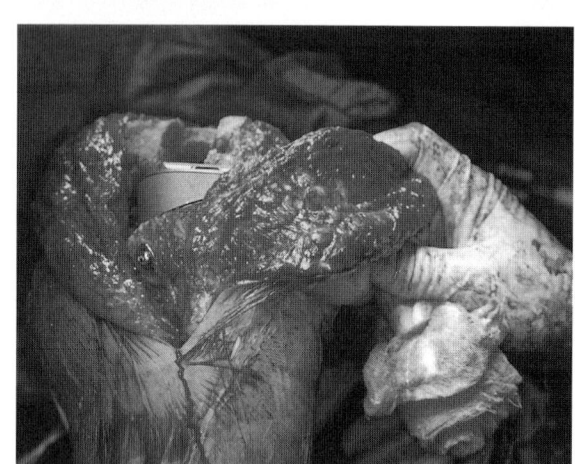

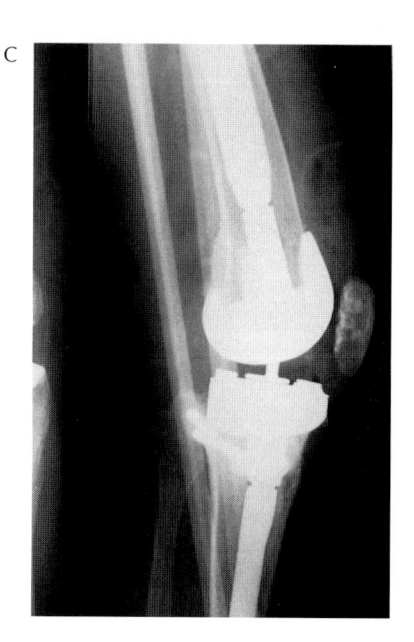

flexion-extension gap balance. If fractures are metadiaphyseal or diaphyseal, fractures can be splinted with an intramedullary trial stem or guide rod that then allows the surgeon to place the appropriate strains to assess balance. Final cuts are then determined and made. Intramedullary reaming continues to accept the appropriate width and length of stem. Trial components are then placed and the joint reduced and moved through a range of motion. Final adjustments are made to accept the actual components.

Epiphyseal fractures or metaphyseal extensions of plateau fractures should be reduced and fixed to maintain as much host bone as possible and to help support the prosthesis. Screw or screw-and-plate fixation can be used as described by Schatzker with screw placement occurring to avoid possible impingement with an intramedullary revision stem or extension[22] (Fig. 79.3). Fixation should be stable but limited to avoid complications of the "dead bone sandwich." With revision arthroplasty being considered, stability will be augmented with stemmed components. If fracturing is limited to a small compression or split component, then metal base tray augmentation or small bulk allografting fixed with screws can be used to substitute for the defect.

The revision procedures for periprosthetic metaphyseal or diaphyseal tibial fractures, in which significant bone loss or comminution does not exist, proceed in a manner as previously described for revision knee arthroplasty but with a few modifications. If the fracture is metaphyseal, cementing the housing of the baseplate will provide stability to the proximal fracture fragment. A stem extension can then be press-fit into the diaphyseal bone to bridge the fracture and maintain alignment (Fig. 79.1). If the rod is being used to bridge the diaphyseal fracture site and not simply to protect epiphyseal fractured bone, intramedullary fixation occurs to a point approximately two to two-and-one-half diameters of the tibial shaft past the fracture site to allow for stability. Press-fitting of the rod occurs with reaming line-to-line. Reaming is slightly more aggressive than in routine revision with the aim of removing some endosteal cortical bone. This ensures cortical contact of the rod along a farther length of the endosteal cortical bone that gives stability to the fracture site in the bending and rotational planes.

Grafting of the fracture site to obtain union is indicated as for other fractures. Bone resected from the cut surfaces can occasionally be used as a structural graft but is indispensible in its morselized form for its osteoinductive potential. Its employment at the fracture site will also obviate the potential morbidity from another donor site. To improve stability and bone stock, morselized allogenic or autogenous bone can be impacted around the stem at the metaphyseal flare as previously described.[23] This grafting helps to control motion of the fracture site if it occurs at or proximal to the metaphyseal flare. Grafting will also support the tibial tray and provide a smoother transmission of joint forces to the host bone. When cementing the component in place, only the surface and housing of the component are cemented, ensuring that no cement intrudes at the fracture site.

Where proximal bone loss is significant or if the fracture is epiphyseal with significant comminution, use of a bulk structural allograft can be considered (Fig. 79.2). No series exists for periprosthetic fractures but has been described for salvage revisions or periarticular tumors.[24-26] A custom metaphyseal-replacing prosthesis can also be considered but cost and longevity of the system need to be realized. The allograft can replace the proximal bone that is missing or damaged. If loss extends past the tibial tubercle, then extensor mechanism reconstruction is required. Ligamentous replacement or possible reconstruction must also be considered with the use of constrained components. Alternatively a hinged prosthesis must be evaluated. The allograft can be sculpted to invaginate into the remaining host bone that may obviate the need for reconstruction of the soft tissues (Fig. 79.2B). Augmentation of the soft tissues can occur with screw or wire fixation from the host bone into the allograft.

The tibial component is sized to the allograft and cemented into the prepared allograft with an attached press-fit stem. Size of the stem is determined by reaming into the distal tibial intramedullary canal until adequate cortical chatter is felt and heard. With the use of fluted stems, fixation is usually stable in the bending and rotational planes so that no augmentation of fixation is required (Fig. 79.2B). Alternatively, a step cut at the host-graft junction can improve rotational stability. A transverse host-graft junction allows for final fine-tuning length adjustments while the stem is being impacted into the host. A transverse saw cut can also be trimmed for optimal contact at the host-graft interface.

Plate fixation for rotational control is unnecessary and causes undo soft tissue stripping and furthers the risk of nonunion or soft tissue slough.

Tibial nonunions, delayed unions, or malunions are managed differently depending on the location of deformity. As discussed earlier, if the deformity is metaphyseal, then deformity can be corrected by performing the arthroplasty bone resections and augmenting further defects with metal or a small bulk allograft fixed with screws. The use of an offset stem or eccentric housing on a tibial baseplate allows for tibial coverage while maintaining mechanical alignment for those deformities that may be translational. Diaphyseal deformities require exposure of the site and debridement of the pseudoarthrosis or osteotomy of the malunion. Use of a guide rod and cannulated reamers passed across the deformity under fluoroscopy ensures that reaming is symmetric and that the deformity will be corrected with stem insertion.

Postoperative protocols include continuous passive motion for all patients with weight-bearing being dependent on the fracture configuration and stability of the implant. Stemmed tibial revisions that substitute for bone loss with metal augments or small bulk allografts can begin immediate weight-bearing as tolerated. Touch weight-bearing and bracing is used for a period of 3 to 6 months when bulk allografts are used. Weight-bearing is increased once graft union is seen.

RESULTS

Results and complications can be variable and dependent on the energy to cause the fractures and the type of reconstruction required. With the number of periprosthetic tibial fractures being small and with revision arthroplasty being reserved for a select group of patients, the success and complication rates for revision arthroplasty can only be estimated by extrapolation. For fractures with minimal bone loss and low energy, complication rates likely parallel other revision series. When fracturing is comminuted with severe bone loss, rates will likely parallel rates for complex allograft revisions for salvage procedures or tumor resection.[24] Overall, success of revision can be expected to be approximately 90% with 4- to 5-year follow-up if the fracture is uncomplicated.[15,20] Kress and associates reported on four tibial nonunions treated with knee arthroplasty and intramedullary rod fixation. All patients achieved union with 90 degrees of painfree motion.[20] However, if the fracture pattern necessitates structural allografting with the use of the revision component, complications vary from 36 to 85%[24-27] with results only being short term. Complications include infection, component dislocation, component loosening, refracturing, nonunion, muscle weakness, and tissue loss.[26] Union of the graft to the host will occur in 92 to 100% of the cases and satisfactory results averaging 90%.[27,28]

CONCLUSION

With the incidence of total knee arthroplasty increasing annually, the prevalence of active mobile patients will also increase. The low-energy stress fractures of the past will then be supplanted by high-energy complex fractures. This in addition to the fact that components are being implanted for ever-increasing durations will demand sound surgical algorithms to obtain optimal fracture treatment results. As with any long bone fracture, the first aim is to obtain fracture union with normal extremity alignment. The character of the fracture, with the functional and medical level of the patient, is combined with the status of the total knee arthroplasty to determine successful management. If this is not possible by closed or open means or not possible without significant morbidity to the patient, then revision arthroplasty for tibial periprosthetic fractures should be considered as a viable option.

References

1. Mendenhall S. Hip and knee implant review. *Orthopedic Network News*. 1995; 6:1–6.
2. Healy WL. Tibial fractures below total knee arthroplasty. In: *Current Concepts in Primary and Revision Total Knee Arthroplasty*. Lippincott-Raven; 1996:163–167.
3. Bryan RS, Peterson LFA, Combs JJ. Polycentric knee arthroplasty: a preliminary report of postoperative complications in 450 knees. *Clin Orthop*. 1973; 94:148–152.
4. Cordeiro EN, Costa RC, Carazzato JG, Silva J. Periprosthetic fractures in patients with total knee arthroplasties. *Clin Orthop*. 1990; 252:182–189.
5. Kjaersgaard-Andersen P, Juhl M. Ipsilateral traumatic supracondylar femoral and proximal tibial fractures following total knee replacement: a case report. *J Trauma*. 1989; 29:398–400.
6. Lotke PA, Ecker ML. Influence of positioning of prosthesis in total knee replacement. *J Bone Joint Surg Am*. 1977; 59:77–79.
7. Makela EA. Capacitively coupled electrical field in the treatment of a leg fracture after total knee replacement. *J Orthop Trauma*. 1992; 6:237–240.
8. Rand JA, Coventry MB. Stress fractures after total knee arthroplasty. *J Bone Joint Surg Am*. 1980; 62:226–233.
9. Skolnick MD, Brian RS, Peterson LFA, Combs JJ, Ilstrup DM. Polycentric total knee arthroplasty: a two year follow-up study. *J Bone Joint Surg Am*. 1976; 58:743–748.
10. Tietjens BR, Cullen JC. Early experience with total knee replacement. *NZ Med J*. 1975; 82:42–45.
11. Wilson FC, Venters GC. Results of knee replacement with the Walldius prosthesis: an interim report. *Clin Orthop*. 1976; 120:39–46.
12. Wiedel JD. Management of fractures around total knee replacement. In: *Total Knee Arthroplasty: A Comprehensive Approach*. Williams & Wilkins; 1984:258–267.
13. Haemmerle J, Bartel D, Chao E. Mechanical analysis of polycentric tibial tract loosening. Read at the Joint Applied Mechanics, Fluids Engineering and Bioengineering Conference. New Haven, Connecticut, June 15–17, 1977.
14. Nogi J, Caldwell JW, Kauzlarich JJ, Thompson RC. Load testing of geometric and polycentric total knee replacements. *Clin Orthop*. 1976; 114:235–242.
15. Chen F, Mont MA, Bachner RS. Management of ipsilateral supracondylar femur fractures following total knee arthroplasty. *J Arthroplasty*. 1994; 9:521–526.
16. Rand JA, Franco MG. Revision considerations for fractures about the knee. In: *Controversies of Total Knee Arthroplasty*. Raven Press; 1991:234–247.
17. Stulberg SD, et al. Case challenges in hip and knee surgery. Knee challenges: what would you do? *Orthopedics*. 1995; 18:941–947.
18. ZumBrunnen C, Brindley H. Nonunion of long bones: analysis of 144 cases. *JAMA*. 1967; 203:637.
19. Cameron HU. Double stress fracture of the tibia in the presence of arthritis of the knee. *Can J Surg*. 1993; 36:307–310.
20. Kress KJ, Scuderi GI, Windsor RE, Insall JN. Treatment of nonunions about the knee utilizing custom total knee arthroplasty with press-fit intramedullary stems. *J Arthroplasty*. 1993; 8:49–55.
21. Wilkes RA, Thomas WG, Ruddle A. Fracture and nonunion of the proximal tibia below an osteoarthritic knee: treatment by long stemmed total knee replacement. *J Trauma*. 1994; 36:356–357.
22. Schatzker J, McBroom R, Bruce D. The tibial plateau fracture: the Toronto experience 1968–1975. *Clin Orthop*. 1979; 138:94.
23. Whiteside LA. Cementless revision total knee arthroplasty. *Clin Orthop*. 1993; 286:160–167.
24. Brien EW, Terek RM, Healey JH, Lane JM. Allograft reconstruction after proximal tibial resection for bone tumours. *Clin Orthop*. 1994; 303:116–127.
25. Dennis DA. Structural allografting in revision total knee arthroplasty. *Orthopedics*. 1994; 17:849–851.
26. Mnaymneh W, Emerson RH, Borja F, Head WC, Malinin TI. Massive allografts in salvage revisions of failed total knee arthroplasties. *Clin Orthop*. 1990; 260:144–153.
27. Tsahakis PJ, Beaver WB, Brick GW. Technique and results of allograft reconstruction in revision total knee arthroplasty. *Clin Orthop*. 1994; 303:86–94.
28. Wilde AH, Schickendantz MS, Stulberg BN, Go RT. The incorporation of tibial allografts in total knee arthroplasty. *J Bone Joint Surg Br*. 1992; 74:815–824.

SECTION 20
Special Situations

CHAPTER 80
Total Knee Arthroplasty Following High Tibial Osteotomy

Charles L. Nelson and Russell E. Windsor

INDICATIONS AND CONTRAINDICATIONS

Evaluation of patients with knee pain following high tibial osteotomy begins with a thorough history and physical evaluation. Key points to be addressed include the character and duration of the patient's pain. A history of instability or mechanical symptoms must be ruled out. Whether a traumatic injury preceeded the onset of pain must be established.

Knee history prior to the high tibial osteotomy should be characterized, including a history of prior knee surgeries or infections. How did the patient's symptoms respond to the high tibial osteotomy? Was there a pain-free interval and, if so, of what duration? Before considering interventions to address intraarticular sources of pain, extraarticular sources of knee pain such as tendonitis and bursitis need to be ruled out. The history should examine whether there are clues suggesting referred pain from the hip or lower back. Groin pain radiating into the anterior thigh or knee is suggestive of hip pathology. Buttock pain radiating below the knee with associated neurologic symptoms suggests referred or radicular pain from the lower back.

The social history should include whether the patient is currently working and if the patient returned to gainful employment following the previous surgery. Are there Workers' Compensation or other issues involving litigation? A previous study identified five factors associated with poor outcomes in total knee arthroplasties following high tibial osteotomies.[1] These five factors were: (1) a Workers' Compensation patient; (2) a patient diagnosed with reflex sympathetic dystrophy following the total knee arthroplasty; (3) a patient in which there was less than 1 year of pain relief following the high tibial osteotomy procedure; (4) a patient who had undergone multiple surgical procedures prior to the high tibial osteotomy; and (5) a patient employed as a laborer (independent of Workers' Compensation patients).[1]

The physical examination begins with evaluation of the patient's gait, paying particular attention to the presence of an antalgic gait or lateral thrust. A Trendelenberg or coxalgic gait suggesting hip pathology should be noted. A list suggestive of spinal pathology must also be ruled out. The physical examination should rule out extraarticular and referred sources of knee pain. Examination of the knee notes the alignment while standing. Identification of the condition of the soft tissues is essential. Note the presence of sinus tracts suggestive of infection or signs that the wound healing may be compromised. Identification of previous scars allows planning future incisions at the time of arthroplasty. The presence of an effusion is strongly suggestive of intraarticular knee pathology. A careful examination of ligamentous stability assists in determining the likelihood of requiring a knee design with more constraint if arthroplasty is entertained. Occasionally, an intraarticular injection of local anesthetic can assist in determining if perceived knee pain is from an intraarticular source or an extraarticular (or referred) source in cases that are not straightforward. Atrophic skin changes, decreased skin temperature, increased skin moisture, or skin hypersensitivity should be noted. These findings associated with pain out of proportion to physical findings should raise suspicion of reflex sympathetic dystrophy.[2] However, patients with a successfully performed high tibial osteotomy will nevertheless experience further arthritic degeneration to a level that may require conversion to a total knee arthroplasty.

The history and physical examination should be followed by a radiographic series consisting of, at a minimum, a standing anteroposterior (AP) radiograph on a long casette, a lateral view, and a Merchant or other tangential patellar view. Ideally, previous radiographs will be available for comparison. Radiographs should be evaluated for the presence of a nonunion at the osteotomy site, or fracture or stress fracture at another site. The AP radiograph should be evaluated for tibiofemoral alignment. Was there excessive overcorrection or undercorrection? Evidence of progressive degenerative changes should be noted. Do the radiographic findings explain the patient's complaints? The presence and type of hardware should be noted. The amount of resection of the medial and lateral plateaus should be planned. Normally, the resected medial plateau is thicker than the resected lateral plateau for total knee arthroplasties following high tibial osteotomies.[3] The relationship of the tibial intramedullary canal to the templated resection should be determined during preoperative planning, as the component may need to be shifted medially, or a tibial tray with an offset stem may be required.[3] This occurs because the medial periosteal hinge maintains the correct relationship on the medial side at the osteotomy site, but the resected wedge at the flare of the proximal tibial metaphysis results in a step-off laterally and in medial displacement of the tibial shaft relative to the articular surface. The lateral radiograph should be evaluated specifically for the presence of patella infera and the slope of the proximal tibia. There is a higher incidence of patella infera following high tibial osteotomies.[3,4] Often there is a decreased posterior slope or even an anterior slope (Fig. 80.1) of the tibial articular surface following high tibial osteotomy.[3] The patellar tangential view should be evaluated to detect evidence for lateral subluxation or tilt.

Occasionally, additional radiographic or other radiological studies may be needed. Nuclear medicine scintigraphy may be necessary to rule out active infection or occult neoplasm. Magnetic resonance imaging (MRI) may be helpful in evaluating intraarticular pathology treatable by conservative or minimally invasive means. Additional radiographs, tomograms, or CT scans may assist in the diagnosis of a nonunion.

Conservative management of the patient's symptoms is reasonable in cases where the etiology of the patient's pain remains obscure following a comprehensive history, physical examination, and radiographic evaluation. Surgical arthroscopy should be considered when the patient has a history of mechanical symptoms and physical findings and/or radiological findings consistent with intraarticular pathology that can be managed arthroscopically. When conservative measures have been exhausted, and the patient's pain is determined to be secondary to advanced degenerative changes and not likely to benefit from minimally invasive procedures, consideration for total knee arthroplasty is appropriate.

Total knee arthroplasty is obviously inappropriate when the patient is unlikely to benefit from the procedure, or is likely to be made worse. Once reflex sympathetic dystrophy or additional sources of pain unlikely to respond to total knee arthroplasty have been effectively screened, additional relative contraindications for total knee arthroplasty following high tibial osteotomy include active infection, Charcot arthropathy, medical comorbidities that predispose to unacceptable risk, and soft-tissue coverage problems that are not reconstructable or where reconstruction is inappropriate. The patient needs to understand the occupational and recreational restrictions imposed by a total knee arthroplasty prior to the surgical procedure.

TECHNIQUES

Preoperative planning is critical once there is a decision to proceed with total knee arthroplasty in a patient with a previous high tibial osteotomy. The history, physical examination, and radiographic studies should be reviewed for evidence of severe overcorrection or excessively unstable knees. Both may be associated with a poorer prognosis and may require special surgical techniques or more constrained implants. The hardware used to stabilize the earlier high tibial osteotomy may also dictate the type of prosthesis required. For example, following removal of a plate, using a tibial tray with a stem augment may be necessary to bypass old screw tracts and avoid creation of stress risers (Figs. 80.2, 80.3). Whenever possible, hardware should be removed.

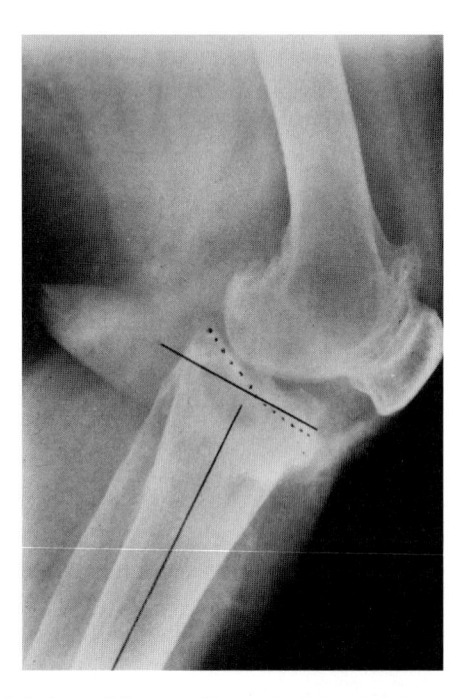

Figure 80.1. Lateral knee radiograph demonstrating anterior slope of the articular surface (dotted line) following high tibial osteotomy.

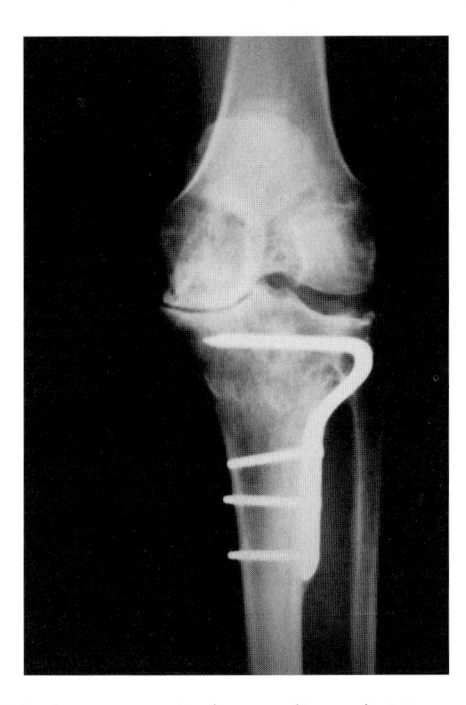

Figure 80.2. Anteroposterior knee radiograph 10 years following a high tibial osteotomy fixed with a lateral blade plate. The patient did well initially following the osteotomy procedure, but subsequently developed gradually advancing arthritic disease, which ultimately required conversion to a total knee replacement.

The condition of the soft tissues is critical to preoperative planning. In one series that reported a higher complication rate for total knee arthroplasty following high tibial osteotomy than for total knee arthroplasty following failed unicompartmental arthroplasty the higher complication rate was secondary exclusively to wound problems, or infections directly related to wound problems.[5]

Previous transverse incisions can be ignored, and a standard anterior midline incision made.[3] If staples were utilized for fixation, they can be left in place so long as they do not preclude resection of the tibia at a suitable level to create a stable platform (Fig. 80.4). If necessary, staples can be bent or burred down to allow passage of the tibial stem or keel. When removal of staples is necessary (Figs. 80.5A,B), this can generally be performed through the anterior midline incision by raising a full-thickness flap laterally without major risk of wound compromise as long as the flap is developed below the deep fascia (Fig. 80.6).

Following lateral longitudinal incisions, three options exist. A more medial than normal anterior midline longitudinal incision can be utilized, leaving as large a skin bridge as possible. Previous experience with tibial pilon fractures and skin flaps suggests maintaining a skin bridge of at least 7 cm.[6,7] This option may not provide sufficient exposure for removal of lateral hardware, particularly in cases involving internal fixation with blade plates or L-plates. In this case, we recommend remov-

Figure 80.3. Postoperative anteroposterior radiograph of the patient in Figure 80.2, demonstrating use of a tibial stem augment to bypass screw holes at the time of conversion to total knee arthroplasty.

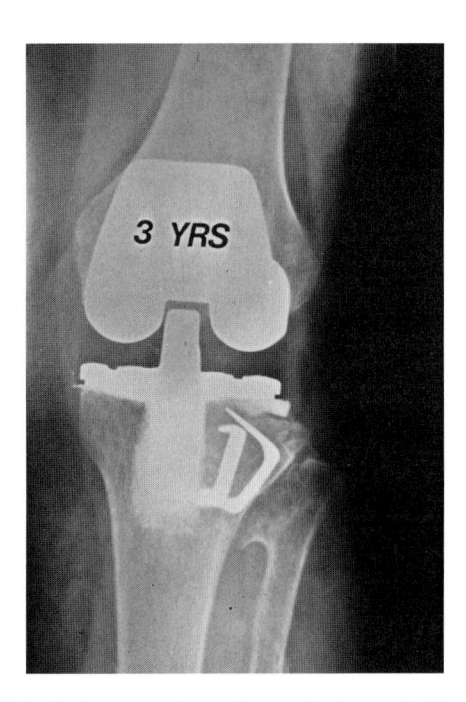

Figure 80.4. Anteroposterior radiograph demonstrating successful conversion of a high tibial osteotomy to a total knee arthroplasty without the need for staple removal.

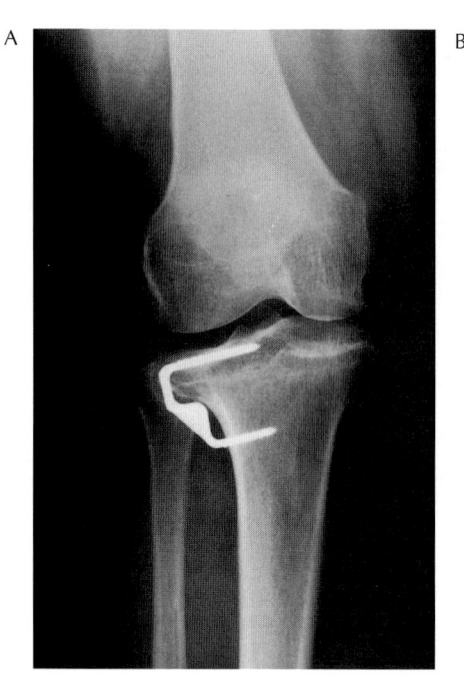

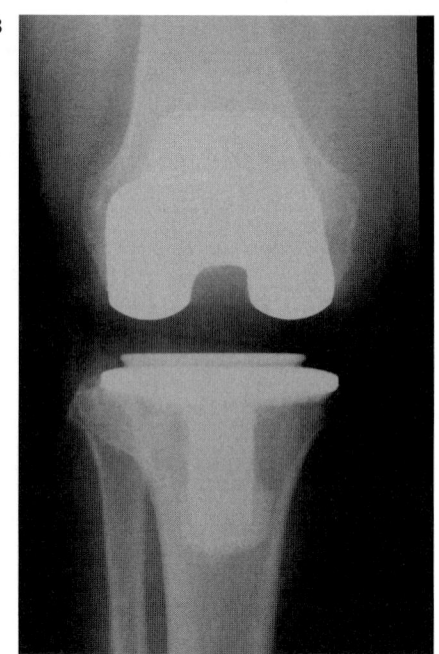

Figures 80.5. A,B. Preoperative and postoperative knee radiographs. In this case, staple removal was required in order to create a stable platform perpendicular to the long axis of the tibia.

ing the hardware prior to the total knee arthroplasty, allowing wound healing, and performing the arthroplasty as a second stage. Alternatively, the lateral longitudinal incision can be utilized, allowing removal of the implant and exposure of the knee through a lateral parapatellar arthrotomy.[8,9] This approach requires a tibial tubercle osteotomy in order to evert the patella and expose the knee adequately. The third option involves utilizing the distal aspect of the lateral longitudinal incision, and extending the incision obliquely in a medial direction at the patella (Fig. 80.7). Plate removal can be performed from the distal aspect of the incision. The fascia over the tibialis anterior is incised along the tibial flare just dis-

tal to Gerdy's tubercle, leaving a small cuff for repair. The muscle is then stripped in a subperiosteal fashion, being careful not to injure the anterior tibial artery as it enters the anterior compartment. Following plate removal (Fig. 80.8), a flap is developed deep to the deep fascia and superficial to the patellar tendon and tibial tubercle, allowing a standard medial parapatellar arthrotomy to be performed through this incision. We recommend that the angle between the proximal aspect of the lateral longitudinal incision and the oblique inci-

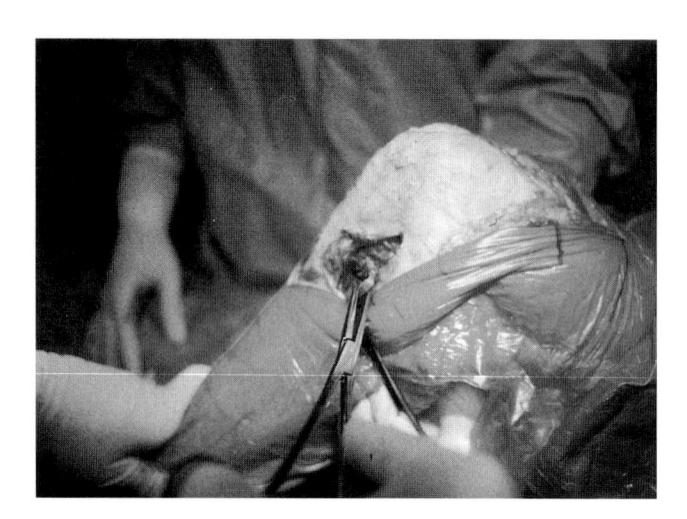

Figure 80.6. Photograph demonstrating staple removal through a lateral window from within a standard midline longitudinal incision.

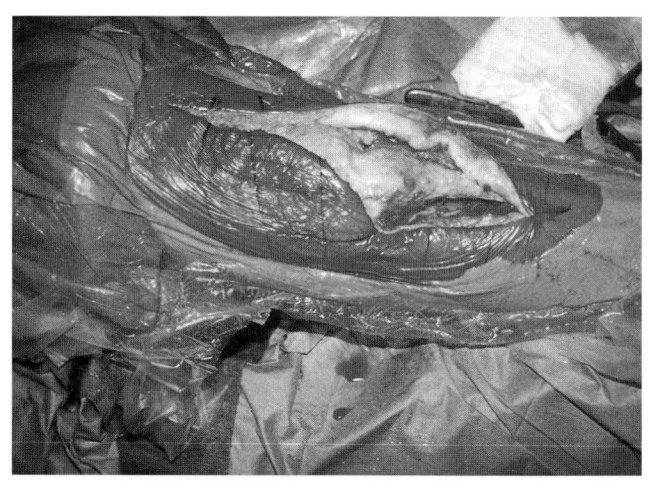

Figure 80.7. Photograph demonstrating oblique medial extension of a prior lateral longitudinal incision. Note the oblique medial extension begins at approximately the inferior pole of the patella. Note the 60-degree angle between the proximal aspect of the previous lateral longitudinal incision and the oblique medial incision.

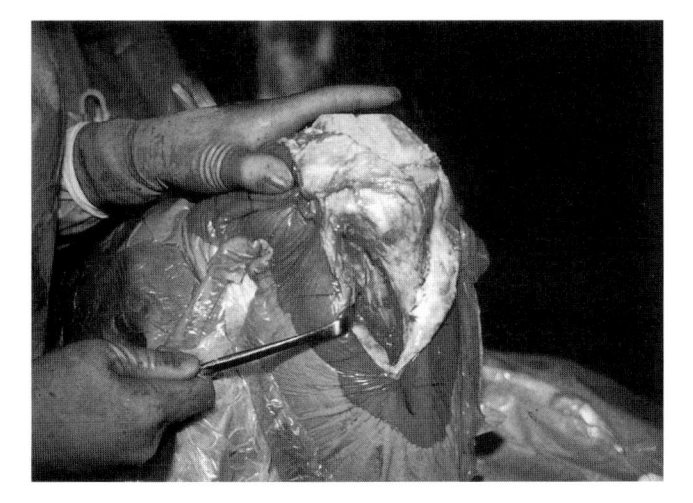

Figure 80.8. Photograph following lateral blade plate removal and preparation of bony surfaces for conversion to a total knee replacement. Note the incision through fascia overlying tibialis anterior followed by subperiosteal posterior reflection of anterior compartment muscles, which allowed removal of lateral blade plate. Note the full-thickness medial flap over tibial tubercle and patellar tendon, which allowed the medial parapatellar arthrotomy to be performed through this approach.

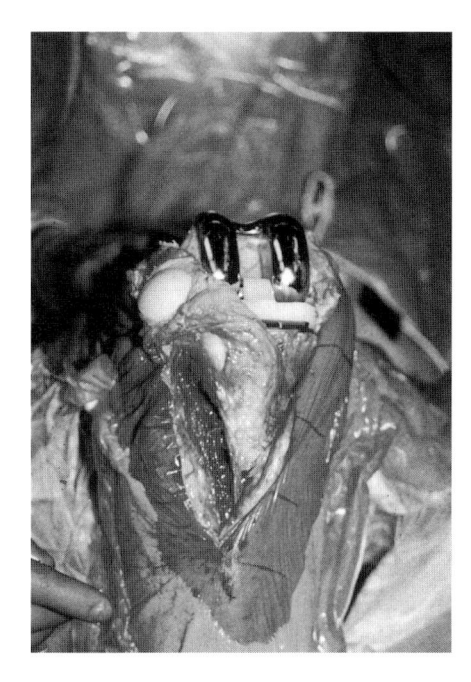

Figure 80.9. Photograph following blade plate removal and implantation of total knee arthroplasty components.

sion be between 45 and 60 degrees to minimize the risks of wound healing.[10] This approach allows successful removal of lateral L-shaped or blade plates and performance of a medial arthrotomy as a single stage following prior lateral longitudinal incisions without subsequent wound healing problems (Fig. 80.9).

Inverted L-shaped incisions allow anterior midline incisions by utilizing the longitudinal limb of the prior incision as the inferior aspect of the longitudinal incision and extending the incision in a proximal direction.[3] The result is an incision similar to the anterior midline incision utilized with a prior transverse incision, with the exception that in some cases the incision may end more laterally secondary to placement of the longitudinal limb of the previous inverted L-shaped incision. In this case a small full-thickness medial flap may be raised to allow medial parapatellar arthrotomy.

We strongly recommend templating the radiographs preoperatively, as in some cases where the medullary canal is excessively offset medially a custom-made component with an offset stem may be required (Figs. 80.10, 80.11). Preoperative templating can reveal whether hardware must be removed. Removal as a separate procedure prior to total knee arthroplasty may decrease risks of wound problems later. The presence of patella infera can be determined from the lateral radiograph, as described by Insall and Salvati.[11] Patella infera results in more difficult exposure and increases the risk of avulsion of the patellar tendon insertion during surgery.[3,12] The inclination of the tibial plateau can also be deter-

mined from the lateral radiograph. Anterior slope of the tibia may result in excessive posterior bone removal during tibial resection.[3] The medial and lateral thicknesses of the resected specimen can be templated and compared to the resected specimen at the time of sur-

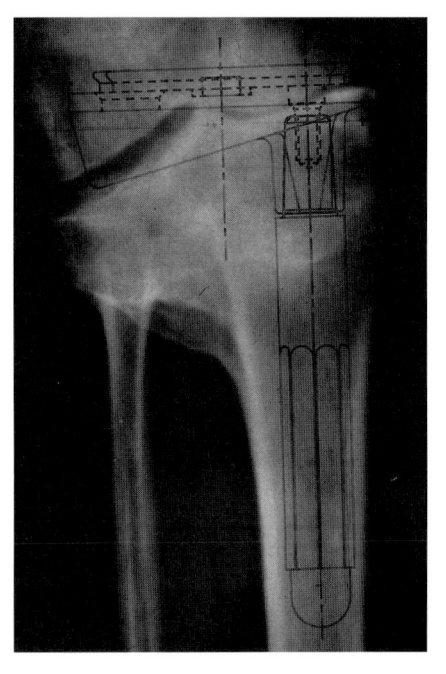

Figure 80.10. Preoperative radiograph in a patient with a failed previous high tibial osteotomy, demonstrating need for a custom-made prosthesis with a medially offset stem and a full lateral wedge.

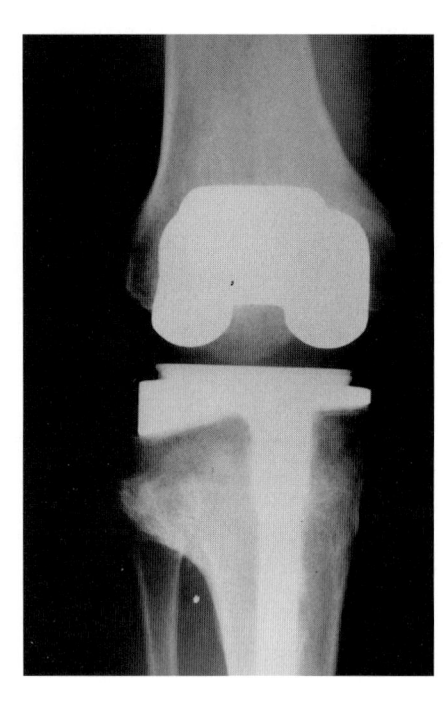

Figure 80.11. Postoperative radiograph of the knee in Figure 80.10 following conversion to a total knee arthroplasty utilizing the custom-made tibial component.

gery, providing an additional clue to alignment. In some cases, bone grafting or augments may be required to replace bone loss secondary to overcorrected tibial osteotomies.

Administration of antibiotics, induction of anesthesia, and prep and drape of the lower extremity are performed in standard fashion. The total knee arthroplasty procedure can be performed with or without tourniquet control, although we typically utilize a tourniquet. The incision is chosen as described earlier based on prior incisions about the knee. When creation of skin flaps is necessary for exposure, it is critical that the plane be developed below the deep fascia to maximize perfusion to the overlying skin. We prefer to expose the knee through a medial parapatellar arthrotomy. Surgeons interested in performing lateral parapatellar arthrotomies with concurrent tibial tubercle osteotomies are referred to the approach described by Buechell.[8] We prefer to make the distal aspect of our arthrotomy 1 cm medial to the patellar tendon. The resulting cuff of tissue adds support to the patellar tendon, decreasing the chance of avulsion, and facilitates closure of the arthrotomy at the completion of the case.[3] A medial subperiosteal sleeve is developed with a scalpel, while being careful to protect the medial collateral ligament. Elevation of the scarred patellar tendon from the proximal tibia may be necessary to allow eversion; however, care must be exercised so as not to disrupt the patellar tendon insertion into the tibial tubercle. The fat pad is released from the lateral meniscus. In many cases (particularly cases with patella infera) there may be difficulty with patellar eversion. Tight lateral structures need to be released. In some cases, a formal lateral retinacular release may be necessary prior to patellar eversion to prevent excessive tension on the patellar tendon insertion. In a series cited earlier, this was required in 21 out of 45 patients.[3] A pin through the patellar tendon and tibial tubercle helps protect against avulsion of the patellar tendon insertion. If patellar eversion cannot be performed safely at this stage, a quadriceps snip, quadriceps V-Y plasty, or tibial tubercle osteotomy may be required, although in our experience this is seldom necessary. It was necessary in 2 out of 45 in the previous series.[3] Following eversion of the patella, the knee is flexed with the foot externally rotated to protect the patellar tendon insertion. Generous release of the patellofemoral ligaments facilitates exposure of the lateral tibial plateau without undue tension on the patellar tendon insertion.

Exposure of the knee is completed with incision of the anterior cruciate ligament and anterior subluxation of the tibia. The tibia is resected using an extramedullary or intramedullary guide, at the discretion of the operating surgeon. Caution should be exercised with intramedullary guides because the medullary canal may be displaced medially secondary to the previous osteotomy procedure. The tibial resection should remove minimal bone laterally to create a stable platform perpendicular to the long axis of the tibia. Usually this results in a greater thickness of resected bone medially. If an anterior slope of the tibial articular surface was noted on the preoperative lateral radiograph, resection of the tibia should be done with a minimal posterior slope to avoid creating an excessively large flexion gap in comparison to the extension gap. If the knee is subsequently noted to be tight in flexion, a second tibial resection creating a normal posterior slope can be performed. The resected specimen should be compared to the anticipated resection from the preoperative template. The tibial alignment is checked using an alignment block and rod. In cases of marked bone loss or severely overcorrected high tibial osteotomies, bone grafting or augments may be required for deficiencies of the lateral tibial plateau.

Following tibial resection, the femur is prepared at the discretion of the operating surgeon using standard cutting or milling techniques. With a laminar spreader in the opposite compartment, the menisci are resected, leaving a small rim adjacent to the medial meniscus to avoid injury to the medial collateral ligament. Posterior osteophytes require curved osteotomes and can be removed using angled curettes. We prefer to resect the posterior cruciate ligament and use a posterior stabilized prosthesis. If use of a posterior cruciate–preserving prosthesis is entertained, advancement of the posterior cruciate ligament may be necessary for appropriate balance.[13]

We check flexion and extension gaps with both rectangular blocks and laminar spreaders. The surgeon may observe a larger flexion than extension gap, particularly following conversion of high tibial osteotomies associated with anterior tibial slopes and resection of a significant amount of posterior bone. This problem is best minimized by resecting the tibia with minimal posterior slope. Increased distal femoral resection and use of a thicker polyethylene equalizes flexion and extension gaps in this setting at the expense of joint-line elevation and increased relative patella infera. Another option is to upsize the femoral component, if necessary, utilizing posterior augments.

Flexion and extension gaps are also checked for medial and lateral balance. Appropriate ligament releases are performed as necessary. When necessary, we perform a medial subperiosteal release from the tibia as a continuous sleeve, as described by Insall.[14] When the lateral side is tight in extension, we prefer to perform the lateral release initially in extension, with a laminar spreader, releasing the posterolateral capsule with a multipuncture technique as modified by Insall from his previous description.[14] If necessary, we release the iliotibial band at the resected surface of the tibia, also with the knee in extension. In cases where the flexion space is trapezoidal with a tight lateral side, release of the lateral collateral ligament and/or popliteus from the femur is performed with the knee in flexion. In cases of marked ligamentous imbalance, a more constrained implant may be required.[14] When an excessive lateral release is necessary, predisposing to peroneal nerve palsy or lateral flexion instability, we prefer to perform a more conservative release, accepting some imbalance and use of a constrained condylar style prosthesis. Alternatively, an advancement of the lax medial collateral ligament, medial hamstring tendons, and posterior cruciate ligament can be performed as described by Krackow.[13] This technique is demanding, requires a more protected postoperative rehabilitation, and should be done only by an experienced knee surgeon.

The trial components are inserted. The knee is taken through a range of motion when patellar tracking, ligament balancing, and stability are checked. We do not perform posterior cruciate ligament–retaining total knee arthroplasty following high tibial osteotomy because of the unpredictable function of the posterior cruciate ligament in this setting. However, if use of a posterior cruciate–retaining prosthesis is entertained, a careful assessment of anterior-posterior stability must be performed because the posterior cruciate ligament may not be functional in these patients.[13] We recommend balancing the posterior cruciate ligament utilizing the techniques described by Ritter[15] and by Swany and Scott.[16]

The posterior cruciate ligament should be assessed with the patella reduced and tracking appropriately in the trochlear grove.[16] Lift-off of the anterior portion of the tibial tray with flexion indicates an excessively tight posterior cruciate ligament.[15,16] The knee should be stable to anteroposterior displacement at 90 degrees of flexion, and the posterior cruciate ligament should deflect only 1 to 2 mm with firm digital pressure in this position.[16] In cases of patella infera, care must be taken to ensure that the patellar component does not impinge on the tibial tray in extension. If this occurs, our preference is to utilize a smaller patellar polyethylene, and place it more superiorly on the patella. The inferior aspect of the patella, which is not supporting the component, can then be thinned with a burr, taking care not to damage the patellar tendon. We prefer to avoid moving the joint line distally with distal augments in this setting. Once satisfactory patellar tracking, ligamentous balance, and stability are demonstrated, the components are implanted in standard fashion.

Postoperative rehabilitation must be individualized based on the particular procedure performed. Most total knee arthroplasties following high tibial osteotomies can be rehabilitated as if they had a primary total knee arthroplasty. In settings at substantial risk for wound complications secondary to the need to raise large flaps or have parallel incisions, we prefer to keep the knee immobilized until the first postoperative day and start continuous passive motion at 0–30 degrees at that time. We increase range of motion more slowly in these patients. In cases of severely overcorrected high tibial osteotomies or significant bone loss requiring either bone grafting or augments, postoperative rehabilitation mimics that following revision total knee arthroplasty.

RESULTS

The results of total knee arthroplasty following high tibial osteotomy have varied in the literature, with some reports describing results comparable to primary total knee arthroplasty[17–19] and others describing results approaching those of revision total knee arthroplasty.[1,3,12] The discrepancy between these series is most likely secondary to the fact that knees requiring knee replacement following high tibial osteotomy represent a heterogeneous group, with varying degrees of coronal and sagital-plane deformity, bone loss, ligament imbalance, patella infera, and soft tissue compromise. Conversion of a high tibial osteotomy without significant preoperative deformity, without patella infera, and without a compromised soft-tissue envelope probably is similar to a primary total knee arthroplasty, both in terms of technical difficulty and results. On the other hand, converting a severely overcorrected high tibial osteotomy with marked lateral soft-tissue scarring, medial and posteromedial ligamentous laxity, and significant patella infera, probably approaches a revision total knee arthroplasty in terms of technical difficulty, need for more constrained prostheses, and anticipated results.

Review of the series where the results of total knee arthroplasty were not compromised by a previous high tibial osteotomy[17-19] demonstrates that these series had a lower percentage of knees with significant preoperative deformity and a lower percentage of patella infera compared with series in which total knee arthroplasty was noted to be compromised by previous high tibial osteotomy.[1,3,12] This has led some surgeons to hypothesize that patella infera and significant coronal-plane deformity lead to a more difficult total knee arthroplasty with less satisfactory results following high tibial osteotomy.[3,13] Our experience is consistent with this hypothesis. However, in the only series where the authors made an attempt to stratify the results of total knee arthroplasty following high tibial osteotomy and evaluate poor prognostic factors, the coronal-plane deformity and Insall-Salvati index were not shown to influence their results.[1] There was insufficient documentation in the article to determine whether this failure was secondary to a beta error or a true finding. Five poor prognostic factors in patients undergoing knee replacement following high tibial osteotomy were identified in this series. These included a Workers' Compensation patient, a diagnosis of reflex sympathetic dystrophy following total knee arthroplasty, less than 1 year pain relief following the high tibial osteotomy, multiple knee surgeries prior to the high tibial osteotomy, and an occupation as a laborer.

Although a prior high tibial osteotomy did not compromise the results of total knee arthroplasty in a few series with regard to knee scores or pain, one of these series demonstrated a decrease in knee range of motion of 14 degrees (101-degree arc versus 115-degree arc) at follow-up in these patients compared with primary total knee arthroplasties done at the same institution.[17] Another series noted a trend toward decreasing range of motion in the postosteotomy group, but this difference was not significant.[18] The other series did not specifically address range of motion.[19] There were several limitations of this latter study.[19] One hundred of the 135 knees enrolled in the study were excluded. Seventy-one of these were excluded because prosthetic designs were used that were not part of the inclusion criteria of this retrospective study. Of these, at least six were excluded because of requirement of a more constrained prosthesis secondary to either excessive valgus deformity preoperatively (five cases) or because of nonunion of the high tibial osteotomy (one case). Therefore, this series actually evaluated the results of selective patients with less deformity than other series showing less satisfactory results.

One series attempted to evaluate the results of conversion of a high tibial osteotomy to a total knee arthroplasty, and compare this with the results following conversion of a unicompartmental arthroplasty to a total knee arthroplasty.[5] This study demonstrated similar results in terms of knee scores and range of motion at follow-up. The knees, having undergone a prior high tibial osteotomy, had a higher rate of wound problems and infection. These problems were attributed to the prior high tibial osteotomy incision. The prior series at our institution also noted a higher incidence of infection in these patients compared with primary total knee arthroplasty.[3] These findings were not statistically significant.

Our experience has been that conversion of a high tibial osteotomy to total knee arthroplasty is in many cases technically more challenging than primary total knee arthroplasty. Windsor et al. published results on conversion of total knee arthroplasty to high tibial osteotomy at the Hospital For Special Surgery with intermediate follow-up.[3] The results were evaluated using the Hospital For Special Surgery Knee Score[20] and Lund Score.[21] Fifty-one percent of patients had an excellent result, 29 percent a good result, 4 percent a fair result, and 16 percent a poor result at minimum 2-year follow-up (mean, 4.6 years). Four of the 45 knees in this series required revision, two for aseptic loosening and two for infection. These results are similar to published results of revision total knee arthroplasty.[22]

References

1. Mont MA, et al. Total knee arthroplasty after high tibial osteotomy. *Clin Orthop Rel Research*. 1994; 299:125–30.
2. Cooper DE, DeLee JC, Ramamurthy S. Reflex sympathetic dystrophy of the knee: Treatment using continuous epidural anesthesia. *J Bone Joint Surg*. 1989; 71-A:365–69.
3. Windsor RE, Insall JN, Vince KG. Technical considerations of total knee arthroplasty after proximal tibial osteotomy. *J Bone Joint Surg*. 1988; 70-A:547–55.
4. Scuderi GR, Windsor RE, Insall JN. Observations of patellar height after proximal tibial osteotomy. *J Bone Joint Surg*. 1989; 71-A:245–48.
5. Jackson, M., Sarangi PP, Newman JH. Revision total knee arthroplasty. *J Arthroplasty*. 1994; 9(5):539–42.
6. Mast J. Fractures of the tibial pilon. *Clin Orthop Rel Research*. 1988; 230:68–82.
7. Craig SM. Soft tissue considerations in the failed total knee arthroplasty. In: Scott WN, ed. *The knee*. St. Louis: Mosby-Year Book; 1994:1279–95.
8. Buechel FF. A sequential three step lateral release for correcting fixed valgus knee deformities during total knee arthroplasty. *Clin Orthop Rel Research*. 1990; 260:170.
9. Keblish PA. Valgus deformity in total knee replacement. *Orthop Trans*. 1985; 9(1):28–29.

10. Wright PE. Basic surgical technique and after care. In: Crenshaw AH, ed. *Campbell's Operative Orthopaedics*. St. Louis: Mosby–Year Book; 1992:2976.
11. Insall JN, Salvati E. Patella position in the normal knee joint. *Radiology*. 1971; 101:101.
12. Katz MM, et al. Results of total knee arthroplasty after failed proximal tibial osteotomy for osteoarthritis. *J Bone Joint Surg*. 1987; 69-A:225–33.
13. Krackow KA, Holtgrewe JL. Experience with a new technique for managing severely overcorrected valgus high tibial osteotomy at total knee arthroplasty. *Clin Orthop Rel Research*. 1990; 258:213–24.
14. Insall JN. Surgical techniques and instrumentation in total knee arthroplasty. In: Insall et al., eds. *Surgery of the knee*. New York: Churchill Livingston; 1993: 779–84.
15. Ritter MA. Posterior cruciate ligament balancing during total knee arthroplasty. *J Arthroplasty*. 1988; 3:323–26.
16. Swany MR, Scott RD. Posterior polyethylene wear in posterior cruciate ligament–retaining total knee arthroplasty. *J Arthroplasty*. 1993; 8:439–45.
17. Amendola A et al. Total knee arthroplasty following high tibial osteotomy for osteoarthritis. *J Arthroplasty*. 1989; S12: S11–17.
18. Bergenudd H, Sahlstrom A, Sanzen L. Total knee arthroplasty after failed proximal tibial valgus osteotomy. *J Arthroplasty*. 1997; 12(6):635–38.
19. Staeheli JW, Cass JR, Morrey BF. Condylar total knee arthroplasty after failed proximal tibial osteotomy. *J Bone Joint Surg*. 1987; 69-A:28–31.
20. Insall JN, et al. Comparison of four models of total knee replacement prosthesis. *J Bone Joint Surg*. 1976; 58-A:754–65.
21. Tjornstrand BAE, Niels E, Hagstedt BV. High tibial osteotomy: A seven-year clinical and radiographic follow-up. *Clin Orthop Rel Research*. 1981; 160:124–36.
22. Haas SB, et al. Revision total knee arthroplasty with use of modular components with stems inserted without cement. *J Bone Joint Surg*. 1995; 77-A(11):1700–1707.

CHAPTER 81
Total Knee Arthroplasty after Supracondylar Femoral Osteotomy

Giles R. Scuderi, John N. Insall, and Alberto Bolanos

Though performed less frequently than proximal tibial osteotomy for a varus deformity, supracondylar femoral osteotomy (SCFO) is indicated for patients with lateral compartment arthritis and a valgus deformity. While in the adult this is usually associated with posttraumatic arthritis, osteoarthritis, or osteonecrosis, a valgus deformity in the young patient may be recased to a metabolic bone disorder or growth plate injury. Supracondylar femoral osteotomy is then considered a joint sparing procedure in an attempt to correct the limb malalignment.[1-10] The question then is, What is the natural history of SCFO? and What are implications when the knee is converted to a TKA? Let us then look at each of these questions individually.

Jackson and Waugh[9] in 1958 were the first to report on the results of SCFO. It was their thesis that this procedure to correct limb malalignment would restore the normal loads across the knee joint, thereby reducing the progression of the generative process. This was later supported by Coventry.[7] Most reports in the literature tend to have short follow-up with a limited number of patients. While Johnson[11] reported 41% satisfactory results in 53 knees at an average follow-up of 44 months, McDermott[12] demonstrated 92% satisfactory results at an average follow-up of 4 years. The longest follow-up of SCFO was published by Finkelstein and coworkers[5] who reported in their survivorship analysis a cumulative success rate of 64% at 10 years. This demonstrates that while the initial results of the procedure may be beneficial the results tend to deteriorate with time. This is especially the case in young patients with metabolic bone disorders; Nercessian has documented a 100% recurrence of the angular deformity following SCFO.[13] As a consequence to the deterioration of the clinical results, progression of the degenerative arthritis, or recurrence of the deformity, SCFO appears to be only a temporizing procedure. Further surgery may then be needed and in some cases this may include total knee arthroplasty (TKA).

The incidence of failed SCFO necessitating conversion to TKA varies among reports. While Beaver[14] reported 5 of 42 osteotomies requiring conversion to TKA at an average follow-up of 3.6 years, McDermott[12] reported only one conversion to TKA in a group of 24 SCFO at an average follow-up of 4 years. With an average follow-up of 11 years, Finkelstein noted that one-third (7/21) of the SCFO were converted to TKA.[5] In our own series of 13 osteotomies, six were converted to TKA at an average of 10.7 years after the SCFO (range, 4.8 to 17.5 years).

TKA following a SCFO needs to be approached like a revision arthroplasty, taking into account prior skin incisions, joint exposure, previous hardware, limb alignment, and component position. The SCFO creates an extraarticular deformity in close proximity to the knee joint.

When planning a conversion, it is our preference to remove all previous hardware as the first procedure. The TKA is staged about 3 to 6 months later when there is radiographic evidence that the screw holes have filled in with bone, since they tend to act as a stress riser. If the medial displacement of the distal femur is not excessive, we might consider removing the hardware at the time of the arthroplasty and using a stemmed femoral prosthesis (Fig. 81.1); placement of the stem may be difficult if the displacement is too medial. When in doubt, the procedure should be staged. Beyer reporting on 17 conversions, retained the hardware in six knees and removed it from nine.[15] Though he did not clearly define his indications for retention of the hardware, there were no reported complications.

The surgical approach in most cases should be performed through the prior skin incision to minimize the

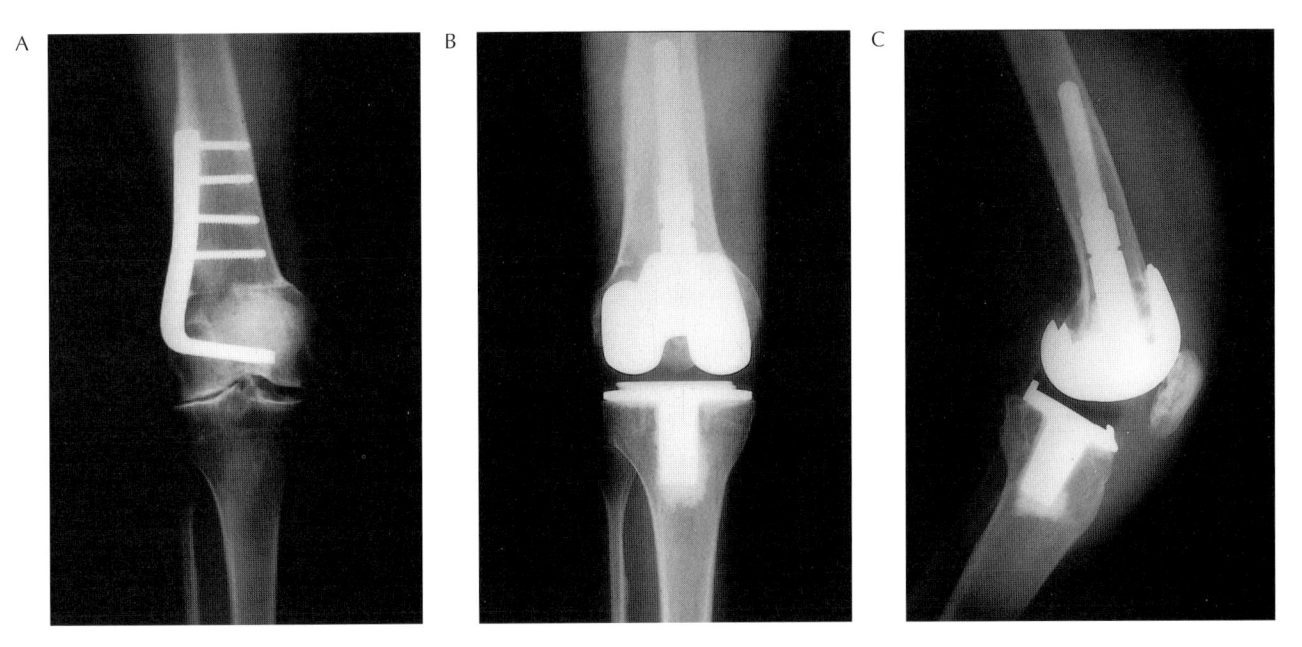

Figure 81.1. The preoperative anteroposterior radiograph (A) shows the alignment of the knee and the position of the hardware following a supracondylar femoral osteotomy. The postoperative anteroposterior (B) and lateral (C) radiographs reveal the position of the posterior stabilized prosthesis and the use of a femoral stem extension.

risk of skin necrosis. If the prior incision is too lateral for routine exposure, then a standard midline skin incision could be utilized, as long as care is taken to maintain an adequate bridge of skin. In cases where there are multiple skin incisions, soft-tissue expansion or a sham incision may be considered.

Our standard arthrotomy is through a medial parapatellar incision because this can easily be converted to a quadriceps snip if there is any difficulty with exposure. In fact, there may be scarring of the quadriceps musculature following SCFO, and for this reason we would hesitate to recommend a subvastus or midvastus approach. Difficulty in exposing the knee following SCFO was noted by Beyer, who recommends a tibial tubercle osteotomy.[15]

The SCFO creates an extraarticular deformity with medial displacement of the distal femur. When using an intramedullary femoral alignment guide, the femoral entry hole should be placed more lateral than usual to ensure that the intramedullary rod is placed centrally within the femoral canal. The angle of distal femoral resection should be templated from the preoperative long films and confirmed with an extramedullary guide prior to resection. If the hardware remains in situ an extramedullary femoral guide needs to be utilized. As we have previously reported, the rotation of the femoral component is set along the epicondylar axis and appropriate ligament balancing must be performed to ensure equal flexion and extension spaces.

CLINICAL RESULTS

Results of TKA after failed proximal tibial osteotomies have been well documented.[16–18] In the best-case scenario, the results have been equal to those of primary TKA, whereas in the worse-case scenario, they have been comparable to revision TKA.

The literature has few reports on TKA after SCFO, but clinical results appear favorable. Beyer followed 12 TKA with a cemented condylar prosthesis following SCFO.[15] At an average follow-up of 75 months, he noted a difference between patients with osteoarthritis and rheumatoid arthritis. Six of eight knees with osteoarthritis had an excellent result and the remaining two knees had a good result compared with one excellent and three good in the rheumatoid group. Cameron and Park reported in eight conversion arthroplasties with an average follow-up of 4 years.[19] The Hospital for Special Surgery score was excellent in five and good in three knees. These investigations noted that, despite the fact that the distal femur was medially offset, the alignment and clinical results were uniformly excellent and SCFO does not adversely affect subsequent TKA. In our own series of 16 conversion arthroplasties, the outcome has been good or excellent with no problems related to the prior SCFO.

References

1. Aglietti P, Stringa G, Buzzi R, Pisaneschi A, Windsor RE. Correction of valgus knee deformity with a supracondylar V osteotomy. *Clin Orthop*. 1987; 217:214–20.

2. Briggs LC. Surgical treatment of unicompartmental arthritis of the knee. *Resident Reporter.* 1996; 1:6–10.
3. Coventry MB. Current concepts review. Upper tibial osteotomy for osteoarthritis. *J Bone Joint Surg.* 1985; 67-A:1136–40.
4. Coventry MB. Osteotomy about the knee for degenerative and rheumatoid arthritis. *J Bone Joint Surg.* 1973;55-A:23–48.
5. Finkelstein JA, Gross AE, Davis A. Varus osteotomy of the distal part of the femur. *J Bone Joint Surg.* 1996; 78-A:1348–52.
6. Goutallier D, Hernigou P, Lenoble E. Debeyre intercondylar femoral osteotomy for severe lateral compartment osteoarthritis of the knee with laxity. *Fr J Orthop Surg.* 1988; 2:573–83.
7. Healy WL, Barber TC. The role of osteotomy in the treatment of osteoarthritis of the knee. *Am J Knee Surg.* 1990; 3:97–109.
8. Healy WL, Wilk RM. Osteotomy in treatment of the arthritic knee. In: Scott WN, ed. *The knee*, vol 2. St. Louis. Mosby–Year Book; 1994.
9. Jackson JP, Waugh W. Osteotomy for osteoarthritis of the knee. In: *Proceedings of the Sheffield Regional Orthopaedic Club. J Bone Joint Surg.* 1958; 40-B:826.
10. Learmonth ID. A simple technique for varus supracondylar osteotomy in genu valgum. *J Bone Joint Surg.* 1990; 72-B:235–37.
11. Johnson EW, Bodell LS. Corrective supracondylar osteotomy for painful genu valgum. *Mayo Clin Proc.* 1981; 56:87–92.
12. McDermott AGP, Finkelstein JA, Farine I, Boynton EL, Macintosh DL, Gross A. Distal femoral varus osteotomy for valgus deformity of the knee. *J Bone Joint Surg.* 1988; 70-A:110–16.
13. Nercessian OA, Roye DP, Bini SA, Dick HM. Supracondylar femoral osteotomies for the correction of angular deformity about the knee in children. *Am J Knee Surg.* 1995; 8:48–51.
14. Beaver RL, Yu J, Sekyi-Otu A, Gross AE. Distal femoral varus osteotomy for genu valgum. *Am J Knee Surg.* 1991;4:9–17.
15. Beyer CA, Lewallen DG, Hanssen AD. Total knee arthroplasty following prior osteotomy of the distal femur. *Am J Knee Surg.* 1994; 7:25–30.
16. Katz MM, Hungerford DS, Krackow KA, Lennox DW. Results of total knee arthroplasty after failed proximal tibial osteotomy for osteoarthritis. *J Bone Joint Surg.* 1987; 69-A:225–33.
17. Staeheli JW, Cass JR, Morrey BF. Condylar total knee arthroplasty after failed proximal tibial osteotomy. *J Bone Joint Surg.* 1987; 69-A:28–31.
18. Windsor RE, Insall JN, Vince KG. Technical considerations of total knee arthroplasty after proximal tibial osteotomy. *J Bone Joint Surg.* 1988; 70-A:547–55.
19. Cameron HV, Parks YS. Total knee replacement after supracondylar femoral osteotomy. *Am J Knee Surg.* 1997; 10(2):70–72.

CHAPTER 82
Total Knee Replacement after Maquet Osteotomy

Douglas Padgett

INTRODUCTION

The management of refractory patella pain is an often-perplexing situation for both physician and patient. Patellofemoral pain as a result of patellar arthrosis has been the topic of debate for some time. Unfortunately, the results of patellectomy are not uniformly successful in terms of pain relief and may lead to compromise of extensor mechanism function.[1,2] It is for these reasons that patellectomy has fallen out of favor. The results of patellofemoral arthroplasty, a relatively conservative arthroplasty, have not been routinely successful in alleviating pain, have been associated with high rates of loosening and clinical failure, and unfortunately may compromise later conversion to total knee arthroplasty.[3,4] Thus patellofemoral arthroplasty has been performed with decreasing frequency. Alternatively, some have advocated the performance of total knee arthroplasty in situations where degenerative disease only involves the patellofemoral joint. However, the role of total knee arthroplasty for isolated patellofemoral arthrosis, as well as the results in this well-defined group, are not known.[5]

The role of tubercle osteotomy in the management of refractory patellofemoral disease is fairly well established. Based upon his detailed analysis of joint reaction forces about the knee, Maquet was one of the first to describe the technique of anterior displacement of the tibial tubercle in an attempt to reduce patellofemoral contact forces.[6] While initial clinical results were compromised by technical problems with fixation and wound slough in cases of excessive tubercle elevation, many clinical successes were achieved.[7] Maquet's success was confirmed clinically by the work of Radin[8] and Ferguson[9] and, with subsequent technical modifications, the technique became widely accepted in the orthopedic community.

Currently, the role of tubercle osteotomy for the treatment of isolated patellofemoral arthrosis is well-defined.[10] Whether the technique is of pure anteriorization of the tubercle, as in correction of a prior distal advancement (prior Hauser, Fig. 82.1) or a combination of anteromedialization for correction of malalignment, the results appear to be consistent in obtaining relief of pain. Unfortunately, as with many procedures done for degenerative conditions about the knee, there is often progression of the arthritic process, which ultimately involves bicompartmental or tricompartmental disease. At this stage, the only reasonable treatment option may be total knee arthroplasty. Bessette[11] and Mendez[12] both found that 5 to 10% of their patients undergoing tubercle osteotomy eventually became candidates for knee arthroplasty. Because of the deformity of the proximal tibia caused by the osteotomy, conversion to total knee arthroplasty presents some unique features that can compromise the surgical result. In this chapter, we will attempt to outline the salient features of performing total knee arthroplasty following tubercle osteotomy and propose solutions to the problems the surgeon will encounter.

TUBERCLE OSTEOTOMY: UNIQUE FEATURES

The presence of a prior tibial tubercle osteotomy should alert the surgeon that the upper tibia has been significantly distorted. In general, there are three features that require attention when converting a prior tubercle osteotomy to a total knee arthroplasty. First, whether there has been a classic Maquet operation with 1 to 2 cm of straight anterior elevation (Fig. 82.2) or a combination with some degree of medialization in order to improve patellofemoral tracking, the proximal tibia is distorted.

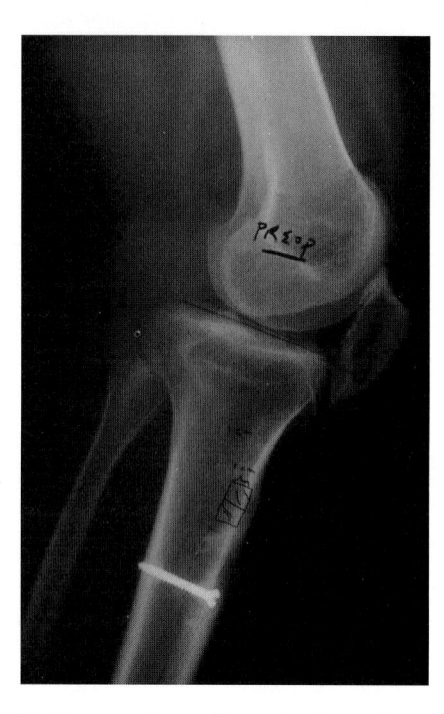

Figure 82.1A. Preoperative radiograph of a patient who had undergone a prior tibial tubercle distal advancement (Hauser procedure) and subsequently developed intractable patellofemoral pain.

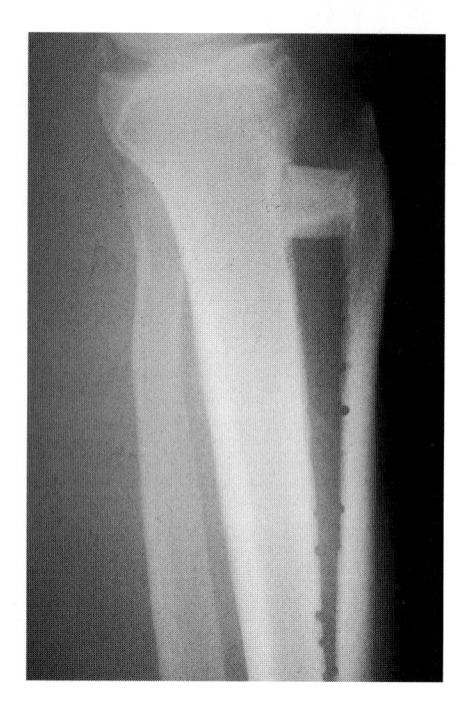

Figure 82.2. Lateral radiograph demonstrating 15-mm bone block elevation of the tibial tubercle. Note that this degree of anterior displacement can compromise soft tissues in front of the knee.

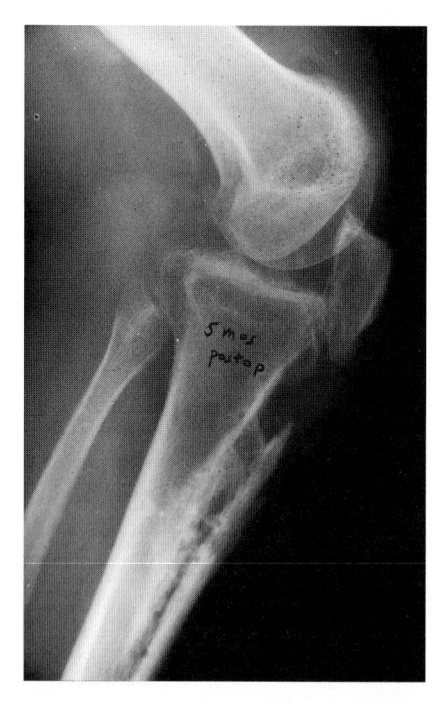

Figure 82.1B. Postoperative radiograph demonstrating anteriorization of the tibial tubercle in attempt to relieve patellofemoral symptoms.

This distortion will have a profound effect upon tibial component orientation. While most surgeons are comfortable using the tibial tubercle as a guide for orientation when placing cutting guides or components onto the proximal tibia, this landmark is no longer valid. Recognizing this from the beginning will reduce the risk of component malposition that leads to a poorly functioning arthroplasty.

Secondly, in addition to distorted position of the tibial tubercle, the proximal tibia is often bulky, with an increased anterior-posterior dimension. The prominence of the proximal tibial bony architecture will affect exposure, soft-tissue balancing, and placement of the external tibial cutting guide. The prominence of the bone will affect the guide's relationship to the upper tibia.

The third effect of prior tibial osteotomy upon the proximal tibia involves the tibial medullary canal. While some tibial tubercle osteotomies do not require any form of internal fixation, many osteotomies will enhance fixation of the tubercle with screw fixation to allow early mobility of the joint. The presence of prior hardware as well as the depth of osteotomy may have disturbed the medullary canal of the tibia. This may either prevent the use of any type of tibial intramedullary alignment device or compromise the placement of such a device. In summary, prior tubercle osteotomy will affect (a) tibial tubercle location, (b) proximal tibial bulk, and (c) proximal tibial medullary canal.

PREOPERATIVE PLANNING
Clinical Evaluation

As with any arthroplasty, a thorough clinical assessment is imperative prior to surgery. Specifically, the surgeon should evaluate the knee for the presence of prior incisions and whether they are sufficient to incorporate into the total knee incision. Preoperative range of motion is important, with particular focus upon the presence and extent of flexion contractures, degree of maximal flexion, and presence of any extension lag. Quadriceps strength should be assessed at this time. The alignment of the limb should be evaluated and assessed as to the extent of fixed coronal plane deformities (i.e., fixed varus or valgus). The degree to which the knee can passively be corrected preoperatively will give an indication as to how much ligament release will be necessary at the time of surgery. An assessment of anteroposterior stability should be performed. Evidence of posterior ligament insufficiency may preclude the use of a posterior cruciate retaining device and appropriate implant decisions should be based upon this. Last, evaluation of the patellofemoral joint must be performed. Clinical assessment of patellar tracking may provide some information as to anticipated patellofemoral stability following arthroplasty. Gross evidence of instability may be problematic at the time of arthroplasty and may require more extensive correction.

Radiographic Evaluation

The standard radiographic Knee Clinic series at The Hospital For Special Surgery consists of (a) standing anteroposterior projection, (b) flexed knee lateral, (c) notch view, and (d) a Merchant view tangential to the patellofemoral joint. In most instances, these views should provide sufficient information prior to total knee arthroplasty. However, due to the deformity of the proximal tibia after Maquet osteotomy or other types of tubercle osteotomies, we will be orienting tibial rotation and alignment to the ankle. For this reason, it is recommended that the preoperative knee series include a standing long alignment film which includes the entire tibia. Any deformity of the distal tibia can be identified and confirmation of tibial alignment can be made. At this time, drawing in the neutral mechanical axis line of the tibia is performed. At the proximal tibia, a line perpendicular to the tibial mechanical axis line is drawn (Fig. 82.3). Performing this on the preoperative radiograph will give the surgeon an idea of the relative resection of the proximal tibia from the medial and lateral tibial plateaus. Resecting equal amounts of medial and lateral tibial plateau at the time of surgery often results in a tibial resection in varus. Preoperative radiographic assessment of bone resection is helpful in anticipating the relative resection amounts.

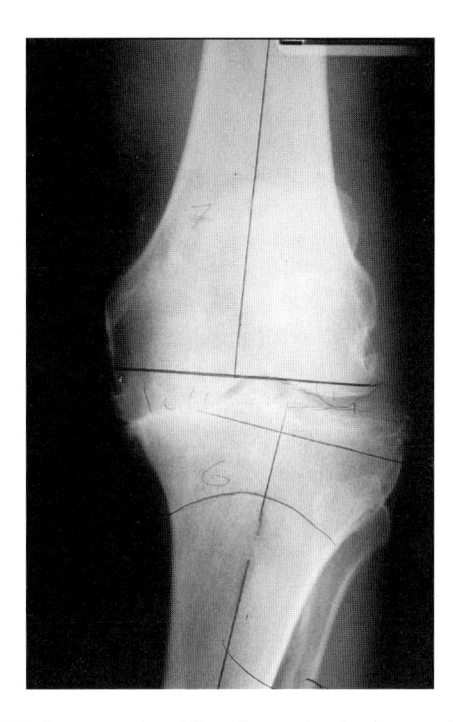

Figure 82.3. Preoperative AP radiograph of a knee with significant varus deformity. In addition to the tibial axis line, a line perpendicular to the tibial axis has been drawn demonstrating the relative resection amounts of medial and lateral tibial plateaus.

SURGICAL TECHNIQUE
Approach

The presence of prior incisions is the most important factor in determining your approach for total knee arthroplasty. Whenever possible, utilize old incisions. If the previous surgical incision will require excessive undermining of skin and subcutaneous tissue in order to perform the arthroplasty, then a second incision should be contemplated. However, the surgeon should never use crossing incisions, especially about the knee because they will dramatically increase the risk of skin slough. Fortunately, most tubercle osteotomies have utilized straight anterior incisions and these are usually extensile enough to incorporate into an anterior knee incision. However, when other incisions are present and are not compatible with exposure for total knee arthroplasty, parallel incisions may be used—but they should have at least 6 to 7 cm between incisions in order to reduce the risk of skin compromise.

Following skin incision and division through the subcutaneous layer, the surgeon removes any previous hardware (i.e., screws, staples). At this time, the parapatellar arthrotomy is performed. The decision to use a medial or lateral parapatellar arthrotomy should be based upon location of skin incision, to some degree upon the site of tight structures (i.e., tight medial in varus, lateral side in valgus) but most important, the surgeon's familiarity with the use of one or the other. Following the arthrotomy, the incision is carried down to the level of the tubercle. The bulk, as well as orientation, of the tubercle can be appreciated at this time. Most commonly, elevation of the periosteum off the medial tibia is performed at the level of the flare of the tibia, raising the superficial medial collateral ligament in a subperiosteal fashion. Following excision of the anterior cruciate ligament, the posterior cruciate ligament in situations where cruciate substitution is performed, and menisci, the tibia is hyperflexed and subluxated anteriorly.

Tibial Resection

It is crucial to realize that, in addition to the amount of tibia resected, resection of the proximal tibial is performed in three planes: anteroposterior, varus/valgus, and, to some degree, internal/external rotation. The advent of more sophisticated cutting and alignment systems has made resection of the tibia more predictable. These include both intramedullary and extramedullary devices. The use of intramedullary tibial devices appears to have fallen out of favor after reports of increase risk of fat embolism[13] and distortions of the tibial canal, which can lead to erroneous tibial resections. In cases of prior tibial tubercle osteotomy, tibial canal sclerosis may preclude the use of an intramedullary tibial alignment guide and the surgeon may be forced to use the extramedullary resection guide. The use of the tibial resection guide is greatly influenced by prior tubercle surgery and how it affects proximal tibial resection, a key element to successful knee arthroplasty.

Anteroposterior Plane

During placement of the external tibial cutting device during routine total knee arthroplasty, the distal end of the device is usually secured to the lower limb with either a clamp or spring and the proximal end is applied against the upper end of the tibia just proximal to the tibial tubercle. The long axis of the cutting device is parallel to the long axis of the tibia. In this situation, the applied cutting guide will allow for the appropriate degree of anteroposterior slope during resection. For most cruciate-substituting designs, this is a 3-degree posterior slope. For cruciate-retaining knee designs, the posterior slope mimics the anatomic slope of approximately 10 degrees (Fig. 82.4A).

Following tibial tubercle osteotomy, especially Maquet osteotomy (which is exclusively an anteriorization of the tibial tubercle), the tubercle is obviously more prominent, more "forward." The net effect of this prominent tubercle is seen during placement of the tibial cutting guide. Following attachment of the guide distally, the proximal end of the guide is placed against the upper tibia but, due to prominence of the tibial tubercle, the guide is *pushed forward*. As the guide is pushed forward, the posterior inclination of the guide is effectively diminished. With the guide in this position, and if resection were to occur, there would be a decrease in the net posterior slope of the tibia (Fig. 82.4B). While minor reductions in posterior slope of the tibia may be of min-

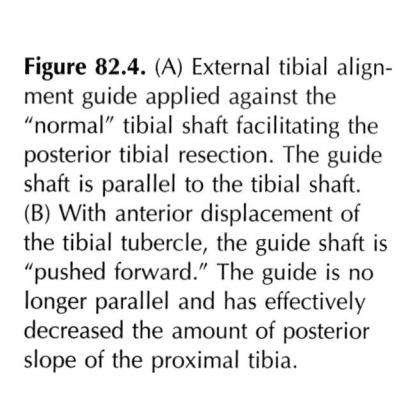

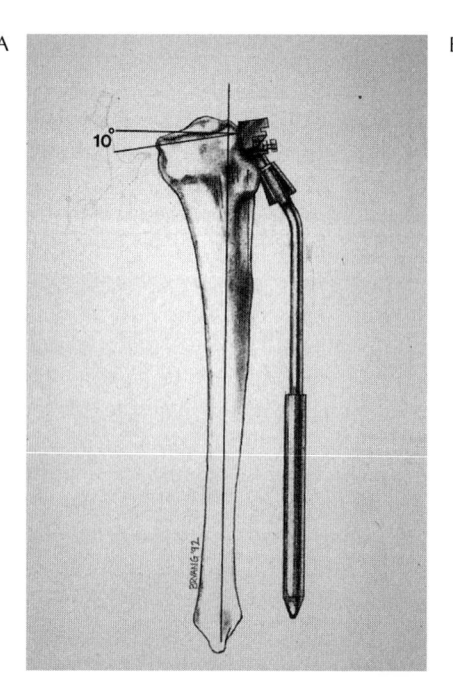

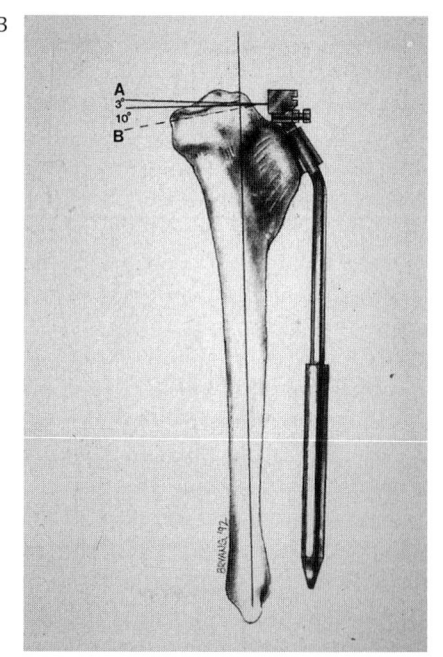

Figure 82.4. (A) External tibial alignment guide applied against the "normal" tibial shaft facilitating the posterior tibial resection. The guide shaft is parallel to the tibial shaft. (B) With anterior displacement of the tibial tubercle, the guide shaft is "pushed forward." The guide is no longer parallel and has effectively decreased the amount of posterior slope of the proximal tibia.

imal significance, reduction in posterior slope of more than 5 to 7 degrees may have a major impact upon function of the arthroplasty. For both cruciate-retaining and cruciate-substituting knee designs, posterior slope is provided to enhance the phenomena of femoral rollback. Proper rollback of any total knee will maximize knee kinematics, especially knee flexion. A reduction in posterior slope, or insufficient posterior slope, especially in cruciate-retaining knee designs, will decrease femoral rollback, lead to "tightening" during flexion, and result in a net decrease in knee motion. Tibial slope is crucial to restoring knee kinematics following total knee arthroplasty.

To avoid the inadvertent reduction of posterior slope during tibial resection, the surgeon must pay particular attention to the relationship of the extramedullary guideshaft to the tibial shaft. Following Maquet osteotomy, the proximal end of the guide becomes divergent due to the prominent tibial tubercle. The key is to keep the guide parallel to the tibial shaft. If the tubercle is 10 to 15 mm prominent, advancing the distal guide attachment anteriorly a distance of 10 to 15 mm will restore the parallel relationship between guide and tibia. This can be achieved with the use of sponges, sterile sheets, or (with some systems) simply sliding the distal guide attachment anterior. Care should be taken not to overdisplace the distal guide anteriorly. Excessive anterior displacement of the distal end of the guide will have the reverse effect, i.e., excess posterior slope, which, while enhancing knee flexion, may make knee extension difficult.

Varus/Valgus Plane

Having noted the effect that prior tubercle osteotomy has upon anteroposterior extramedullary guide placement, proper varus-valgus alignment must now be attained. Unfortunately, prior tubercle surgery makes guide placement difficult because of the bony prominence. This is especially true if there has been both anterior displacement and some degree of medialization. With medial prominence, the medial aspect of the tibial guide can be "pushed" either proximal or distal. It is this sliding of the tibial guide that can lead to inadvertent varus or valgus resection. This coronal plane alignment must be based upon distal landmarks such as the bimalleolar axis or the relationship to the first web space. Referring to the preoperative tibial radiograph will confirm relative resection amounts from the medial or lateral side so as to avoid resultant varus or valgus resection. Unfortunately, provisional pin fixation of the guide is often difficult once varus-valgus alignment has been determined. With the associated anteriorization and medialization of the tubercle, the face of the proximal medial tibia is somewhat oblique. Our experience has shown that during placement of provisional pins, there is a tendency for the pins to "skive" distally, thus yielding varus alignment (Fig. 82.5). It is imperative that the guide not translate during pin insertion. Placement of lateral fixation pins first appears to yield satisfactory fixation and prevents guide displacement during medial pin insertion. Once the appropriate degree to coronal alignment has been determined, all that remains is tibial rotation before proceeding with tibial resection.

Internal/External Rotation

Proper tibial rotational alignment is essential to a functioning arthroplasty. Tibial malrotation can lead to altered femoral-tibial kinematics, resulting in loss of motion, abnormal stresses upon the articulation leading to polyethylene material failure, and abnormal patellofemoral mechanics causing subluxation. In uncomplicated primary total knee arthroplasty, tibial resection and component placement is often described in relation to the tibial tubercle.[14] Unfortunately, this landmark is not present or is distorted and therefore not reliable. It is important to remember that tibial resection guide rotation is just as important as varus/valgus and anterior/posterior alignment. With resection guides set for approximately three to ten degrees of posterior slope, inadvertent malrotation, either internal or external, will cause the resultant tibial resection to be oblique rather than perpendicular to the tibial axis, resulting in varus or valgus alignment.

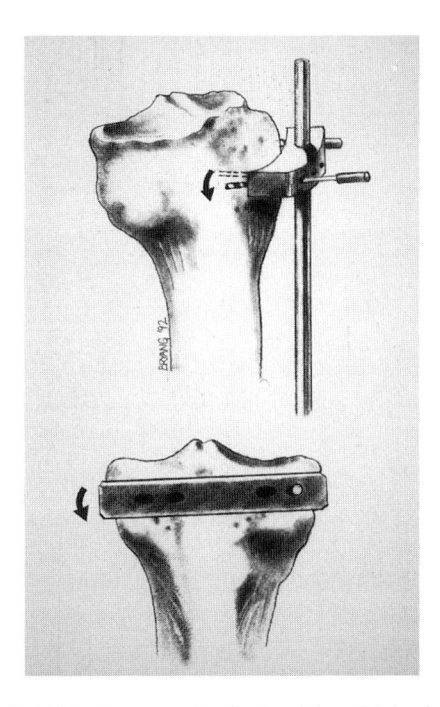

Figure 82.5. With the excessive bulk of the tibial tubercle, guide placement and fixation may be difficult. The tendency for the guide to displace requires careful attention at this stage of the operation.

When major distortion of the tubercle has occurred, landmarks (e.g., the tibial crest, the transmalleolar axis) should be used. Attempting to determine tibial rotation based upon maximal coverage of the resected upper tibia often results in tibial component internal rotation. Proper tibial rotation provides optimal femoral tibial mechanics as well as a stable patellofemoral articulation.

Once the tibial resection guide replacement is fixed, resection of the proximal tibia can proceed. Due to the excessive bulk of the tubercle anteriorly, it is often not possible to complete the tibial osteotomy using the standard-length saw blades (Fig. 82.6). Options include (a) the use of extra-long saw blades, or (b) to provisionally cut the tibia with the guide attached, remove the guide to continue resection as much as the saw blade length will permit, and complete the resection with an osteotome. Following resection, tibial alignment should be checked for: varus/valgus orientation, anterior-posterior slope, and internal/external rotation. If proper alignment has been attained, femoral and patellar preparation may begin. In general, there are no unique problems during femoral or patellar preparation following tubercle osteotomy and therefore preparation is routine.

Tibial Sizing and Fixation

Tibial base plate sizing may be affected by prior tubercle surgery, depending upon the level of proximal tibial resection: the more distal the resection, the larger the proximal tibial surface area. Proper tibial sizing is influenced by ability to obtain rim fit of the implant, avoiding competent oversize or undersize. In addition, some knee systems require matching sizes between femoral component and tibial component, which may dictate which size tibial base plate to utilize. Each surgeon must be familiar with the specifics of the knee system being used. My general tendency is to strive for cortical rim coverage even if some degree of component overhang occurs. Undersizing of tibial implants and failure to obtain rim contact has been shown to be less biomechanically sound.[15]

In performing the final implant positioning, tibial rotation must be assessed. Use of distal landmarks such as first web space and bimalleolar axis should be employed rather than the tibial tubercle. In addition, using the posterior tibial cortical rim as a guide for anterior-posterior placement is advised. Remember that the anterior tibial cortex may be distorted and displaced anteriorly due to the prior tubercle osteotomy. Reliance upon the anterior cortical margins as a landmark for placement may result in unnecessary anterior placement of the tibial component. Anterior displacement of the tibial component may also affect the ability to use any type of stemmed or rodded tibial component. Once tibial preparation is complete, component insertion, either with or without acrylic bone cement, can proceed. As with all knee arthroplasties, final checks of alignment, motion, and stability of both femorotibial and patellofemoral joints are made prior to closure. While patellofemoral mechanics following Maquet osteotomy are often improved, patellar tracking must still be thoroughly evaluated. Following surgery, standard knee arthroplasty rehabilitation can begin without any specific precautions.

RESULTS

There is very little in the literature on the subject of total knee arthroplasty following tibial tubercle osteotomy. In our experience, the major difficulties were all technical in nature, relating specifically to the deformity and distortion of the proximal tibia.[16] As outlined here, attention to detail and understanding the specific consequences of prior tubercle osteotomy upon execution of knee arthroplasty is the key to successful arthroplasty. The short-term follow-up of our patients has shown that there is no untoward effect of prior Maquet osteotomy upon functional recovery following total knee arthroplasty. The use of either a cruciate-retaining or cruciate-substituting knee design did not have any adverse effect; thus the decision to use either knee system is a matter of preference for the surgeon (Fig. 82.7).

SUMMARY

The use of tibial tubercle osteotomy has been shown to be a success in the management of refractory patellofemoral pain due to arthrosis. Despite these successes,

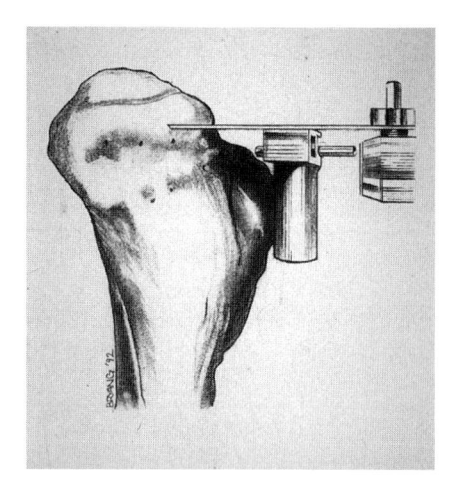

Figure 82.6. Following anterior displacement of the tibial tubercle, the use of standard-length saw blades may be inadequate to resect the proximal tibia. The use of longer saw blades will facilitate resection.

82. Total Knee Replacement after Maquet Osteotomy

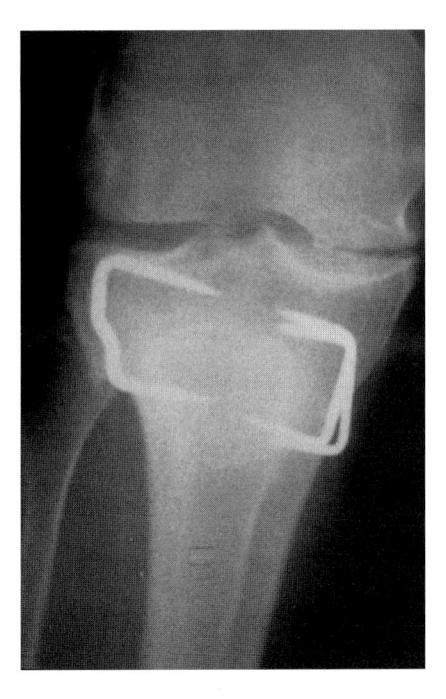

Figure 82.7A. Preoperative AP radiograph of a patient who had previously undergone Maquet osteotomy, who presents now with advanced degenerative disease of the knee.

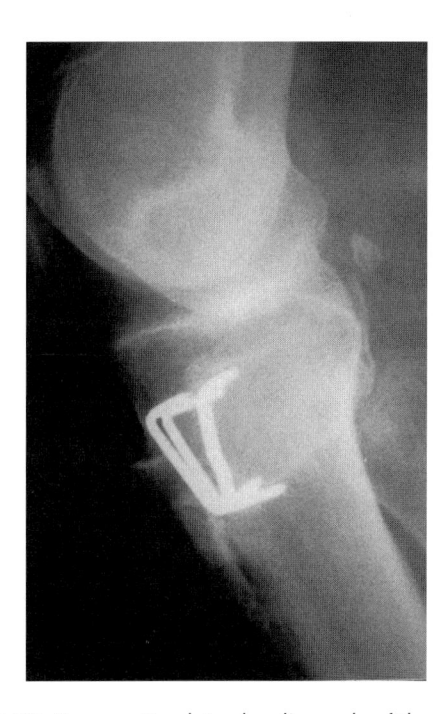

Figure 82.7B. Preoperative lateral radiograph of the same patient.

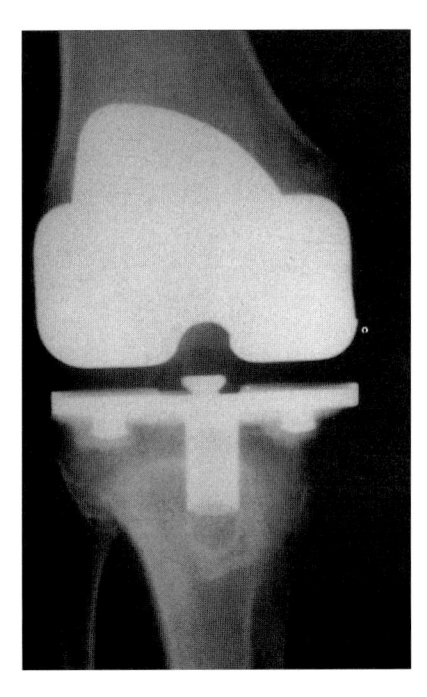

Figure 82.7C. Postoperative AP radiograph following total knee arthroplasty. Note that coronal plane alignment to neutral has been achieved.

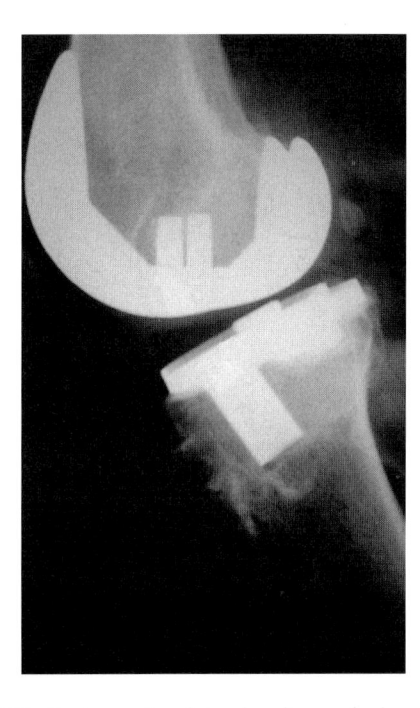

Figure 82.7D. Postoperative lateral radiograph demonstrating 10 degrees of posterior slope of the tibial component. Adequate posterior inclination is essential for knee function, especially in a cruciate-retaining knee like this one.

some patients will inevitably progress, with femorotibial arthrosis eventually requiring total knee arthroplasty. The presence of prior tubercle osteotomy should alert the surgeon to a series of unique potential pitfalls in performing total knee arthroplasty. These pitfalls are specifically due to (a) distortion of the proximal tibia, (b) the bulky nature of the proximal tibia, and (c) the effect of prior osteotomy upon tibial canal. Strict attention to de-

Table 82.1. Common problems encountered during total knee arthroplasty after Maquet osteotomy

Problem	Cause	Solution
AP resection with insufficient posterior slope	Anteriorization of tubercle forces extramedullary guide forward	Tibial resection guide must be parallel to the tibial shaft
Proximal tibial resection in varus alignment	Anterior and/or medial displacement of tubercle can cause resection guide tilt	Pre-resection and post-resection check for varus/valgus alignment
Malrotation of tibial component (excess int/ext rotation)	Loss of tibial tubercle as reference landmark	Check rotation of proximal tibia relative to distal extremity: first web space, transmalleolar axis

tail and an understanding of the effect of prior osteotomy upon execution of total knee replacement is essential in order to attain a successful, well-functioning knee arthroplasty (Table 82.1).

References

1. Ackroyd CE. Polyzoides, Patellectomy for osteoarthritis: A study of 81 patients followed from 2 to 22 years. *J Bone Joint Surg.* 1978; 60B:353–57.
2. Kelly M, Insall JN. Patellectomy. *Orthop Clin North Am.* 1986; 17(2):289–95.
3. Worrell R. Resurfacing of the patella in young patients. *Orthop Clin North Am.* 1986; 17(2):303–309.
4. Harrington KD. Long-term results for the McKeever patellar resurfacing prosthesis used as a salvage procedure for severe chondromalacia patellae. *Clin Orthop.* 1992; 279: 201–213.
5. Fulkerson JP. *Disorders of the patellofemoral joint*, 3rd ed. Baltimore: Williams & Wilkins; 1997.
6. Maquet P. Considerations Biomechaniques sur l'arthrose du genou. Un Traitment biomechanique de l'arthrose femoropatellaire. L'advancenent du tendon rotulien. *Revue Rheumatologie.* 1963; 30:779–90.
7. Maquet P. Advancement of the tibial tuberosity. *Clin Orthop.* 1988; 115:225–29.
8. Radin EL. The Maquet procedure: Anterior displacement of the tibial tubercle. Indications, contraindications and precautions. *Clin Orthop.* 1986; 213:241–48.
9. Ferguson AB, Brown T, Fu FH, Rutkowski R. Relief of patellofemoral contact stress by anterior displacement of the tibial tubercle. *J Bone Joint Surg.* 1979; 61A:159–61.
10. Fulkerson P, Becker G, Meaney J, Miranda M, Folcik M. Anteromedial tibial tubercle transfer without bone graft. *Am J Sports Med.* 1990; 18(5):490–97.
11. Bessette GC, Hunger RE. The Maquet procedure: A retrospective review. *Clin Orthop.* 1988; 232:159–67.
12. Mendez DG, Soudry M, Iusim M. Clinical assessment of Maquet tibial tuberosity advancement. *Clin Orthop.* 1987; 222:228–38.
13. Fahmy NR, Chandler HP, Danylchuk K. Blood-gas and circulatory changes during total knee replacement: Role of the intramedullary rod. *J Bone Joint Surg.* 1990; 72A:19–23.
14. Merkow RL, Soudry M, Insall JN. Patellar dislocation following total knee replacement. *J Bone Joint Surg.* 1985; 67A:1321–27.
15. Bourne RB, Finlay JB. The influence of tibial component intramedullary stems and implant-cortex contact on the strain distribution of the proximal tibia following total knee arthroplasty. *Clin Orthop.* 1986; 208:95–99.
16. O'Brien TJ, Padgett DE, Lyons P. Technical considerations in total knee arthroplasty following the Maquet procedure. *Am J Knee Surg.* 1993; 6(3):108–111.

CHAPTER 83
Total Knee Arthroplasty after Patellectomy

Frankie M. Griffin and Michael A. Kelly

Patellectomy has been used for many years in the treatment of a variety of patellofemoral disorders. The indications for patellectomy have narrowed considerably because the importance of the patella for normal knee function has become apparent.[1–5] This chapter reviews the described techniques of patellectomy and the effects and special considerations of total knee arthroplasty after previous patellectomy.

FUNCTIONAL ANATOMY OF THE PATELLA

The clinical importance of the patella has been debated for years. Early authors believed the patella actually inhibited extensor mechanism function.[6–8] Most current investigators now agree that the patella plays an important role in normal knee function.[1–3,9,10] Recent publications have also substantiated the importance of the patella in total knee arthroplasty.[11–15]

Important functions of the patella include the following:

1. It contributes to the extensor moment arm.[1,4,16,17]
2. It reinforces the anteroposterior stability of the knee.[14]
3. It provides a smooth articulation for the extensor mechanism.[18]
4. It gives the knee a normal cosmetic appearance.
5. It decreases the compressive stress of the patellofemoral articulation.[19]
6. It shields the underlying distal femoral articular cartilage from trauma.

The patella gives the quadriceps muscle a mechanical advantage for extending the knee joint; it increases the moment arm of the quadriceps at the joint by displacing the quadriceps tendon anteriorly. Kaufer[1] found that the patella contributed 10 to 30% of the quadriceps moment arm depending on the amount of knee flexion. By increasing the perpendicular distance between the applied force and the center of rotation of the knee joint, the patella decreases the amount of force required from the quadriceps to generate enough torque to straighten the leg. Investigators have found that patellectomy decreases the amount of torque generated by the quadriceps by 15 to 50%.[3,4,17,20] For patients, the mechanical disadvantage of patellectomy translates into diminished ability to ascend and descend stairs, changes in gait patterns, and decreased ability to run.[3,4]

The patella is important for the anteroposterior stability of the knee. The knee has been described as a four-bar linkage with the patellar tendon parallel to the posterior cruciate ligament and the quadriceps tendon parallel to the anterior cruciate ligament.[2] The posterior cruciate ligament prevents anterior translation of the femur on the tibia during flexion, and the forces directed through the patellar tendon parallel to the PCL reinforce this stabilizing function of the PCL (Fig. 83.1A). After patellectomy, the patellar tendon is no longer parallel to the PCL (Fig. 83.1B), and anteroposterior stability of the knee during flexion is diminished accordingly. This is especially important in the total knee arthroplasty patient and will be discussed later in this chapter.

The patellar provides a smooth articulation for the extensor mechanism. Its presence protects the quadriceps tendon from direct friction and wear.[20] In addition, the hyaline cartilage articular surface allows for efficient near frictionless force transmission across the knee during motion. The hyaline cartilage is adapted to bear high compressive loads and ultimately decrease the compressive stress of the patellofemoral joint.[19]

The patella has some obvious practical functions. The articular cartilage of the femoral condyles and trochlea are protected from direct trauma by the patella. The patella also helps to give the knee a normal cosmetic appearance.

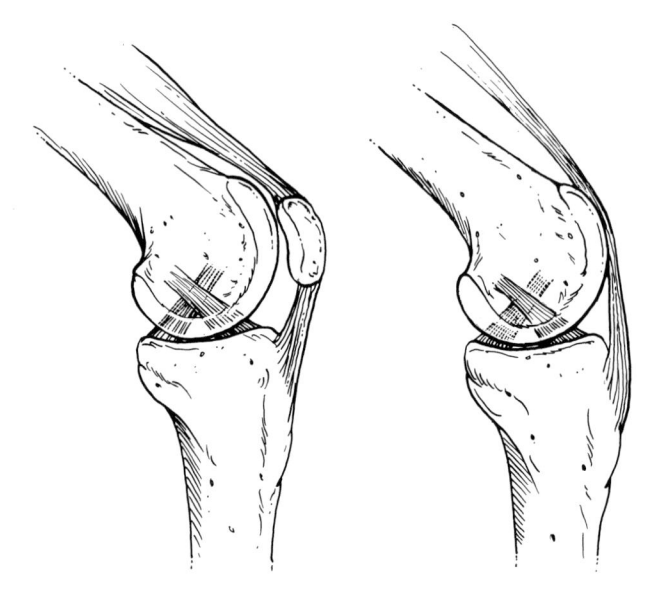

Figure 83.1. Drawing demonstrating the four-bar linkage system of the knee proposed by Sledge and Ewald.[2]

TECHNIQUE OF PATELLECTOMY

One commonly used technique of patellectomy involves simple enucleation of the patella through an incision in the extensor mechanism. The appropriate orientation of the incision and repair is controversial. Kaufer[1] advocated a transverse repair. Based upon biomechanical evaluation of eight fresh human amputation specimens, he reported a 15% reduction in extensor mechanism force when the tendon was repaired transversely after patellectomy, compared to a 30% reduction when the repair was longitudinal in orientation.[1] Fulkerson and Hungerford[21] disputed this conclusion. They believed that the longitudinal repair was performed side-to-side without imbrication and that the quadriceps force was being transmitted to the tibia through the retinaculum rather than through the central tendon. Additionally, they noted that the transverse incision necessitates a longer period of immobilization to protect the repair.[22] Longitudinal techniques similar to that described by Boyd and Hawkins[23] employ a side-to-side or imbricated closure to permit early knee motion with minimal tension on the repair. Fulkerson and Hungerford[21] reported no extensor lag in their patients when an imbricated longitudinal closure was used. Similar results have been reported with cruciate-type repairs.[24]

Several techniques have been described that reinforce the patellar defect. Baker and Hughston[25] reported long-term results using the Miyakawa technique for patellectomy. This procedure realigns the extensor mechanism with proper tension and centralizes the pull of the quadriceps. The vastus lateralis and medialis are advanced with a strip of quadriceps tendon used to fill the patellar defect. Ninety-five percent good-to-excellent results were reported.

Past reports have suggested that calcification in the extensor mechanism following patellectomy can be a source of pain following patellectomy.[26-28] To address this potential problem, Compere and associates[27] described a surgical technique to create a "tube within which any bone regeneration would be contained" (Fig. 83.2). Enucleation of the patella is performed through medial and lateral parapatellar incisions, and the medial border of the quadriceps tendon is brought under-

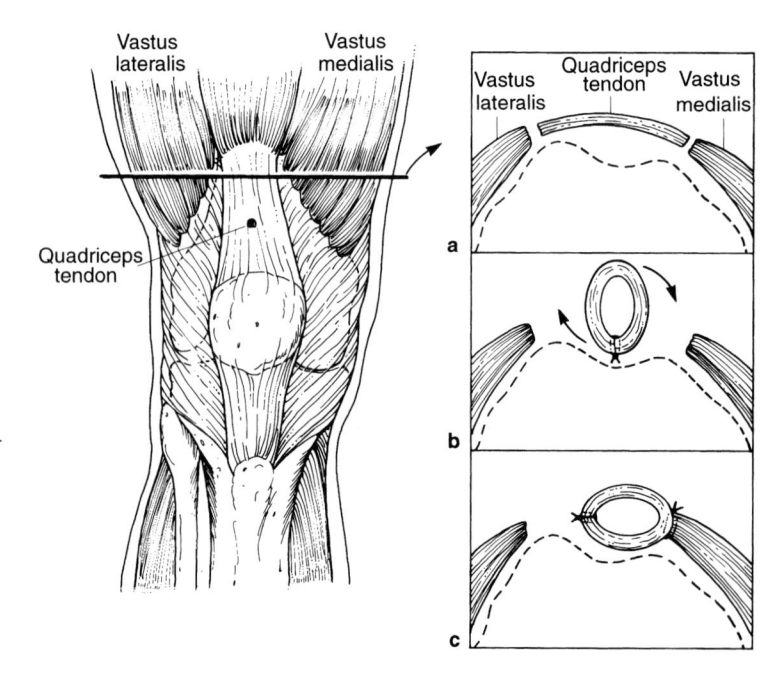

Figure 83.2. Surgical technique of Compere patellectomy. (A) Enucleation of the patella through medial and lateral parapatellar incisions. (B) The medial border is rolled underneath the tendon and sutured to the lateral border to form a tube. (C) The vastus medialis is advanced and sutured to the tube. (Reprinted with permission from *The Patella*, ed. G. Scuderi, M.D.)

neath and sutured to the lateral border of the quadriceps tendon to create a tube (Fig. 83.2). Ninety percent good and excellent results were reported. We have used this technique successfully and have noted improved cosmesis compared to other techniques of patellectomy.

Bandi and Maquet[29,30] proposed increasing the effectiveness of the extensor mechanism by transposing the patellar tendon anteriorly. Anteriorization of the tibial tubercle may be helpful in mitigating some of the adverse effects of patellectomy by lengthening the extensor moment arm. Radin and Leach[31] reported good results in six of nine knees following anteriorization of the tibial tubercle for failed patellectomy.

Regardless of the technique utilized, careful attention to proper tracking of the extensor mechanism is mandatory. Postoperative care varies with the individual surgical technique. Adequate restoration of extensor strength is critical to a satisfactory result.

TOTAL KNEE ARTHROPLASTY AFTER PREVIOUS PATELLECTOMY

In general, the results of total knee arthroplasty after previous patellectomy have been inferior to those reported for similar patients with patellae.[11–15,32–34] However, in properly selected patients, significant improvements in function and reduction of pain have been achieved.[13,14]

Patient Selection

For patients with previous patellectomy, factors that predict a more successful outcome for total knee replacement include severe tibiofemoral arthritis, few previous knee procedures, and excellent quadriceps function.[12] A patient with multiple previous knee procedures and continued pain, with only mild to moderate tibiofemoral arthritis, and with compromised quadriceps function is a poor candidate for total knee arthroplasty after previous patellectomy. Nonoperative treatment or arthrodesis should be considered in the latter population. In addition, Paletta and Laskin[14] found that patients who had undergone patellectomy for fractures of the patella had better outcomes after total knee arthroplasty than those who had undergone patellectomy for chondromalacia or osteoarthritis. Several authors have also found that a longer time interval between patellectomy and total knee arthroplasty correlated with higher postoperative knee scores.[13,14]

Surgical Technique

As previously mentioned, the patella helps to position the quadriceps and patellar tendons so that the knee functions as a four-bar linkage system[2] (Fig. 83.1). Without the patella, the force directed through the patellar tendon is no longer parallel to the PCL and the restraints to anterior translation of the femur on the tibia in flexion are diminished. Some investigators believe that anteroposterior instability is the cause of residual pain in patients with a previous patellectomy.[14,15,32,33]

The correct surgical method to handle this anteroposterior instability is controversial. Several authors have advocated retention of both cruciate ligaments. Sledge and Ewald[2] recommended retention of the cruciate ligaments to maintain the intact portion of the four-bar linkage system of the knee. Bayne and Cameron[32] initially advocated use of unicompartmental prostheses both medially and laterally (bicompartmental unicompartmental TKA) with cruciate retention at all costs. They felt that bicompartmental unicompartmental arthroplasty preserved the cruciates and allowed the patellar tendon to articulate with smooth, articular cartilage anteriorly. However, a later study by Cameron and Jung[35] of 11 patients who underwent total knee arthroplasty after previous patellectomy found that the posterior-stabilized total knee arthroplasty (IB-II) provided a technically simpler procedure and better results than the use of bicompartmental unicompartmental arthroplasty. Marmor[33] also has advocated preservation of both cruciates and recommended use of unicompartmental arthroplasty in patients with unicompartmental disease and a "prosthesis that preserves the cruciate ligaments" in patients with bicompartmental disease. However, Larson and associates[11] noted that 5 of the 10 patients in their study who required revision of total knee arthroplasties after previous patellectomy had Marmor modular knees. Marmor[33] recommended a posterior-stabilized knee arthroplasty in patients with severe arthritis and associated instability. Most surgeons would agree that an intact, competent PCL is a minimal prerequisite to consider use of a PCL-retaining device in this population.

Several authors have found the PCL to be an unreliable source for stability in patients who have undergone patellectomy. Paletta and Laskin[14] suggested that loss of the stabilizing effect of the patella in the four-bar linkage system increases the stresses across the PCL, and over time, the PCL and posterior capsule become stretched. Therefore, they felt that the PCL is not a reliable source for stability. In fact, Larson and colleagues[11] found that in their group of primary total knee patients with previous patellectomy most of the PCLs, although intact, did not appear normal. Therefore, they said "it was impossible to rely on the PCL for anteroposterior stability." Similarly, Lennox and associates[12] noted that 3 of their 11 patients had PCLs that were either absent or had to be sacrificed due to their poor condition.

Two recent clinical studies have supported the use of a posterior-stabilized prosthesis in patients with a previous patellectomy. Paletta and Laskin[14] retrospectively reviewed 22 cases of total knee arthroplasty after previous patellectomy to compare the results of posterior-stabilized prostheses to cruciate-sparing prostheses. Nine patients had posterior-stabilized prostheses and 11 had posterior cruciate-sparing designs. They found that the posterior-stabilized group had results similar to control groups without previous patellectomy. The posterior-stabilized group did significantly better than the cruciate-sparing group with regard to knee scores, pain scores, arc of flexion, extension lag, anteroposterior stability, and stair climbing. They concluded that the posterior cruciate-sparing arthroplasties provided less reliable results than the posterior-stabilized arthroplasties. Martin, Haas, and Insall[13] found that their patients with posterior-stabilized arthroplasties (IB-II) did better than those with the cruciate-sacrificing design (total condylar 1).

The design of the posterior-stabilized prosthesis ensures that the center of rotation moves toward the posterior aspect of the tibial plateau during flexion (rollback) (Fig. 83.3).[20] Femoral rollback results in a greater lever arm and resultant force produced by the quadriceps on contraction, and this biomechanical advantage is especially important for total knee arthroplasties without patellae.

Some authors advocated the use of constrained implants to address the potential anteroposterior instability in total knee arthroplasty after patellectomy. Bayne and Cameron[32] recommended the use of hinged prostheses in knees without adequate cruciates. Multiple other investigators have reported similar results with unconstrained prostheses including cruciate-sparing, cruciate-sacrificing, and posterior-stabilized designs.[11–14,33,35,36] The majority of the literature suggests that if an unconstrained posterior-stabilized prosthesis is performed with appropriate soft tissue balancing so that the implant properly tenses the knee in flexion and extension, there is no need to use a constrained device.[13–15,35] Historically, avoiding increased constraint in prosthetic selection is a sound principle.

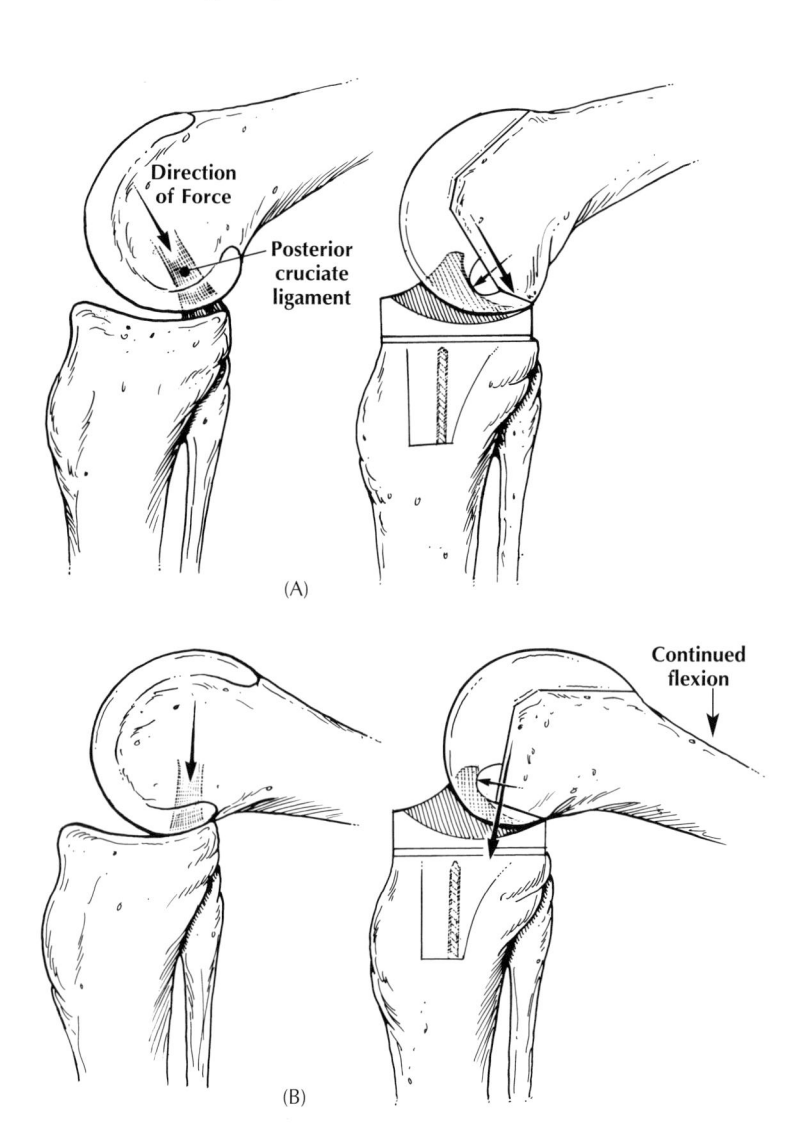

Figure 83.3. Rollback of the femur on the tibia in the posterior-stabilized prosthesis. (Reprinted with permission from Insall.[20])

Results of TKA after Previous Patellectomy

The results of total knee arthroplasty after previous patellectomy have been variable. Because many of the studies include primary and revision arthroplasties and a variety of implant designs, the results reported in the literature are difficult to interpret. Among these reports, classification of results into good or excellent categories was based upon a variety of different factors that make comparisons difficult.

When compared to patients with patella, patients with total knee arthroplasties after previous patellectomy have lower overall knee scores. Postoperative pain, flexion contracture, extension lag and decreased range of motion contribute to the lower knee scores.[11] More chronic pain has been reported after total knee arthroplasty in patellectomized patients than in control groups without patellectomy in several studies.[11,12,14,32,35] Flexion contracture has also been reported. Larson and associates (1990) found that 10 of 22 patellectomized patients had preoperative flexion contractures ranging from 5 to 35 degrees, and half of these patients had flexion contractures (5 to 15 degrees) after total knee arthroplasty. Marmor[33] similarly reported 10 of his 11 patellectomized patients had preoperative flexion contractures up to 40 degrees (7 to 40 degrees), and three had flexion contractures up to 20 degrees (7 to 20 degrees) after TKA. Paletta and Laskin[14] reported flexion contractures averaging 10 degrees in 5 of 13 cruciate-sacrificing TKAs. Additionally, postoperative extensor lags may contribute to poor knee scores. Railton and associates[15] found an extensor lag of 30 degrees in 2 of 7 patients and of 5 degrees in one of the same seven patients; they report that the extensor lags were present preoperatively and were unchanged after TKA. Lennox and colleagues[12] reported an average extensor lag of 9 degrees in their 11 total knee arthroplasties after patellectomy. Martin and associates[13] found that 4 of 22 patients had extensor lags that averaged 11 degrees. Larson and associates (1990) noted that 5 of 14 patients had preoperative extensor lags from 5 to 35 degrees and that only two had postoperative extensor lags (5 and 7 degrees). Decreased arc of knee motion has also been reported. Larson and associates (1990) reported decreased arc of motion compared to total knee replacements with patellae. Paletta and Laskin[14] found the mean arc of flexion for posterior-stabilized knees to be equal to patients with total knee arthroplasty without patellectomy, whereas in the cruciate-retaining group, Paletta found a decreased mean arc of flexion for the patellectomized patients compared to the knees with patellae.

Anteroposterior instability has been reported by several authors in total knee arthroplasty after previous patellectomy and may contribute to postoperative pain. Paletta and Laskin[14] found anteroposterior instability of greater than 1 cm in 12 of 13 patients with cruciate-retaining arthroplasties. Railton and associates[15] found asymptomatic laxity of the knee in flexion in two of the seven patellectomized patients who underwent total knee arthroplasty. Larson and colleagues,[11] however, reported an average anterior drawer of only 3.8 mm in their 22 patients. In addition, recurvatum deformity has been reported in this population. Paletta and Laskin[14] found that 4 of their 13 cruciate-retaining knees had recurvatum deformities of 5 degrees at 5-year follow-up.

Decreased quadriceps torque is an issue in total knee arthroplasties in patellectomized patients and translates to relatively weak quadriceps function for this patient population. As predicted by biomechanical and anatomical models, Lennox and associates[12] reported decreased peak torque of the quadriceps at both high and low speeds in patellectomized patients after total knee replacement. The importance of aggressive postoperative quadriceps rehabilitation should be stressed. Difficulty walking stairs has also been reported when these patients are compared with controls without patellectomy. Szalapski and colleagues[36] found in their cruciate-retaining total knee arthroplasties that patellectomized patients had increased difficulty in walking stairs compared to nonpatellectomized patients. Paletta and Laskin[14] similarly noted increased difficulty climbing stairs in their group of cruciate-retaining total knees, whereas they noted no differences between the patellectomized group and the controls when a posterior-stabilized prosthesis was used.

CONCLUSIONS

Total knee arthroplasty after previous patellectomy can provide significant improvements in function and control of pain in properly selected patients. The ideal patient for total knee replacement after patellectomy has had few other procedures on the knee for pain relief, has gotten several years of satisfactory function from their knee after patellectomy, had the patellectomy for a patellar fracture, has good quadriceps function, and has severe arthritis of the tibiofemoral joint. When compared to nonpatellectomized patients, the patient can expect to have decreased range of motion, decreased quadriceps torque, increased extensor lag, diminished ability to walk stairs, and more pain postoperatively. The surgeon should ensure anteroposterior stability of the knee intraoperatively through proper soft tissue technique so that the implant properly tenses the knee in flexion and extension and through selection of an appropriate prosthesis. Better results are reported when the posterior cruciate-substituting design is used in this population. In addition, postoperative rehabilitation should include aggressive quadriceps rehabilitation to improve function and stability.

References

1. Kaufer H. Mechanical function of the patella. *J Bone Joint Surg*. 1971; 53A(8):1551–1560.
2. Sledge CB, Ewald FC. Total knee arthroplasty: experience at the Robert Breck Brigham Hospital. *Clin Orthop*. 1979; 145:78–84.
3. Sutton FS Jr, Thompson CH, Lipke J, Kettelkamp DB. The effect of patellectomy on knee function. *J Bone Joint Surg*. 1976; 58A(4):537–540.
4. Watkins MP, Harris BA, Wender S, Zarins B, Rowe CR. Effect of patellectomy on the function of the quadriceps and hamstrings. *J Bone Joint Surg*. 1983; 65A:390.
5. West FE. End results of patellectomy. *J Bone Joint Surg*. 1962; 44A:1089–1108.
6. Brooke R. The treatment of fractured patella by excision: A study of morphology and function. *British J Surg*. 1937; 24:733–747.
7. Hey Groves EW. A note on the extension apparatus of the knee joint. *British J Surg*. 1937; 24:747–748.
8. Watson-Jones R. Excision of patella (correspondence). *British Med J*. 1945; 2:195–196.
9. Jakobsen J, Christensen KS, Rasmussen OS. Patellectomy—a 20 year follow-up. *Acta Orthop Scand*. 1985; 56:430–432.
10. Peeples RE, Margo MK. Function after patellectomy. *Clin Orthop*. 1978; 132:180–186.
11. Larson KR, Cracchiolo A III, Dorey FJ, Finerman GA. Total knee arthroplasty in patients after patellectomy. *Clin Orthop*. 1991; 264:243–254.
12. Lennox DW, Hungerford DS, Krackow KA. Total knee arthroplasty following patellectomy. *Clin Orthop*. 1987; 223:220–224.
13. Martin SD, Haas SB, Insall JN. Primary total knee arthroplasty after patellectomy. *J Bone Joint Surg*. 1995; 77A(9):1323–1330.
14. Paletta GA, Laskin RS. Total knee arthroplasty after a previous patellectomy. *J Bone Joint Surg*. 1995; 77A:1708–1712.
15. Railton GT, Levack B, Freeman MAR. Unconstrained knee arthroplasty after patellectomy. *J Arthroplasty*. 1990; 5(3):255–257.
16. Haxton H. The function of the patella and the effects of its excision. *Surg Gynecol Obstet*. 1945; 80:389.
17. Wendt PP, Johnson RP. A study of quadriceps excursion, torque, and the effects of patellectomy on cadaver knees. *J Bone Joint Surg*. 1985; 67A:726–732.
18. Kelly MA, Brittis DA. Patellectomy. *Orthop Clin North Am*. 1992; 23(4):657–663.
19. Mow VC, Proctor CS, Kelly MA. Biomechanics of articular cartilage. In: Nordin M, Frankel V, eds. *Basic Biomechanics of the Musculoskeletal System*. 2nd ed. Philadelphia: Lea and Febiger; 1989:31–58.
20. Insall JN. *Surgery of the Knee*. 2nd ed., New York: Churchill Livingstone, 1993.
21. Fulkerson JP, Hungerford DS. *Disorders of the Patellofemoral Joint*. Baltimore: Williams and Wilkins; 1990.
22. Ficat RP, Hungerford DA. *Disorders of the Patellofemoral Joint*. Baltimore: Williams and Wilkins; 1977.
23. Boyd HB, Hawkins BL. Patellectomy: a simplified technique. *Surg Gynecol Obstet*. 1948; 86:357.
24. Steurer PA Jr, Gradisar IA Jr, Hoyt WA Jr, et al. Patellectomy: a clinical study and biomechanical evaluation. *Clin Orthop*. 1979; 144:84.
25. Baker CL, Hughston JC. Miyakawa patellectomy. *J Bone Joint Surg*. 1988; 70A:1489–1494.
26. Boucher HH. Results of excision of the patella. *J Bone Joint Surg*. 1952; 34(B):516.
27. Compere CL, Hill JA, Lewinnek GE, et al. A new method of patellectomy for patellofemoral arthritis. *J Bone Joint Surg*. 1979; 61(A):714–719.
28. Duthie HL, Hutchinson JR. The results of partial and total excision of the patella. *J Bone Joint Surg*. 1958; 40(B):75.
29. Bandi W. Chondromalacia patellae and femoropatellarre arthrose aetiologie, klinik und therapie. *Helv Chir Acta*. 1972; (suppl 11):1:3.
30. Maquet PCJ. *Biomechanics of the Knee with Application to the Pathogenesis and Surgical Treatment of Osteoarthritis*. Berlin: Springer-Verlag; 1976.
31. Radin E, Leach R. Anterior displacement of tibial tubercle for patellofemoral arthrosis. *Orthop Trans*. 1979; 3:291.
32. Bayne O, Cameron HU. Total knee arthroplasty following patellectomy. *Clin Orthop*. June 1984; 186:112–114.
33. Marmor L. Unicompartmental knee arthroplasty following patellectomy. *Clin Orthop*. 1987; 218:164–166.
34. Joshi AB, Lee CM, Markovic L, Murphy JCM, Hardinge K. Total knee arthroplasty after patellectomy. *J Bone Joint Surg*. 1994; 76(B):926–992.
35. Cameron HU, Jung YB. Prosthetic replacement of the arthritic knee after patellectomy. *Canadian J Surg*. 1990; 33(2):119–121.
36. Szalapski EW Jr, King TV, Siliski J, Ritter MA. Total knee replacement in the patellectomized knee. *Orthop Trans*. 1991; 15:725–726.

CHAPTER 84
Total Knee Arthroplasty for Patients with Prior Knee Arthrodesis

Paul A. Lotke and Elizabeth A. Cook

Patients with an ankylosed or arthrodesed knee find that the inability to bend the joint is disabling. An awkwardness of gait, the inability to have the foot touch the floor while sitting, and the awkwardness of the foot remaining in the extended position for social events and while dining is uncomfortable. Consequently many seek the surgical solution of a knee arthroplasty in order to achieve some motion. This chapter will review the feasibility, indications, and results of reversing an arthrodesed or ankylosed knee and inserting a total knee replacement.

INDICATIONS

The indications for the takedown of an ankylosed or arthrodesed knee have become relatively limited because the long-term results of this procedure have been better defined.[1] Although it is technically possible to complete a knee arthroplasty in an ankylosed knee, the short-term complications and long-term results should be clearly defined for each prospective patient. This significantly narrows the pool of appropriate candidates. At present, it appears to be indicated for low-demand patients with lower extremity malalignment and pain, or ankylosis of both knees. There should be a functional extensor mechanism. Finally, the patient should be willing to accept the possibility of failure, revision, and possible re-arthrodesis (Fig. 84.1).

RESULTS

There have been scattered reports in the literature indicating the feasibility of the conversion of a knee fusion to a total knee arthroplasty.[2–6] The small series with short-term follow-up report satisfactory results.

The longest and largest study in the literature to date presents a more dismal outlook. Naranjan and associates[1] accumulated data on 37 patients from several institutions with ankylosed or arthrodesed knees. The mean age at surgery was 53 years and the average follow-up was 90 months. The results showed that only modest motion was achieved; the average range was 7 to 62 degrees. There were 24% significant short-term complications and 35% major long-term complications, with a 14% infection rate and 14% aseptic loosening. The total complication rate was 57%. A satisfactory result, with no pain and unlimited walking tolerance was achieved in only 29%. The latter patients were younger and had achieved a better than average range of motion, with a mean 87-degree flexion. The authors suggested that careful consideration be given a takedown of a fusion for a total knee. Because they inconsistently obtained adequate motion and there were many short-term and long-term complications, they advised caution.

SURGICAL TECHNIQUE
Prosthetic Choice

The prosthetic choice depends on the etiology of the ankylosis or arthrodesis. Those patients who had spontaneous ankylosis secondary to infection, inflammatory arthritis, or trauma will likely have an intact medial collateral ligament, and therefore some intrinsic ligamentous stability. On the other hand, those patients who had a surgical fusion may or may not have retained the medial collateral ligament, and the length and balance of their collateral ligaments will be difficult to determine. In the former case, with the probability of the medial collateral ligament being intact, the standard total knee or moderate constraints from a total condylar III prosthesis may be appropriate. On the other hand, if there is doubt that the medial collateral ligament is intact or functional, then a more constrained prosthesis such as

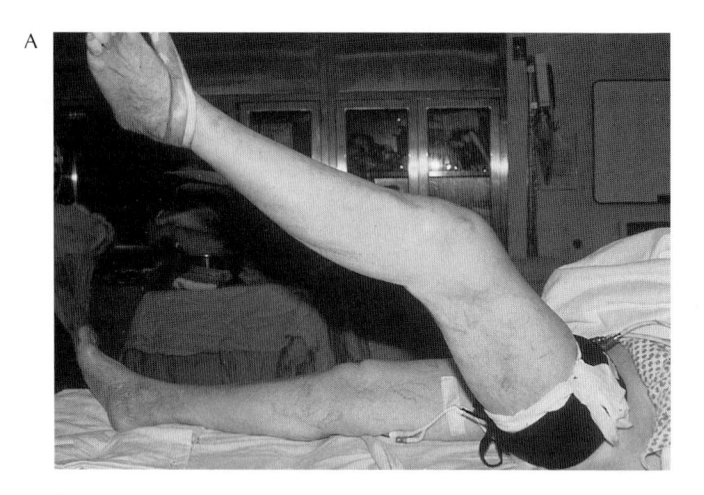

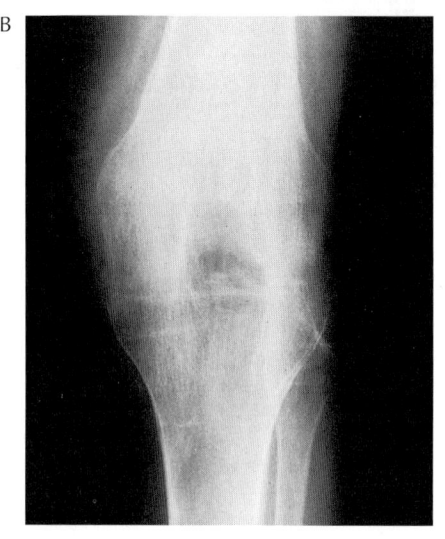

Figure 84.1. Patient with a solid fusion in 25 degrees of flexion (A) and 15 degrees of valgus (B).

a total condylar III or rotating hinged device will be required. Appropriate equipment should be available at the time of surgery for either circumstance.

Incision

The incision will depend on the quality of the skin and the presence of previous incisions. If the skin is very tight or adherent to underlying bone from prior trauma or infection, the use of soft tissue expanders should be considered.[7,8] If prior incisions are present, they should be incorporated into the new incision. This is usually possible with most prior anterior, anteromedial, and anterolateral incisions. If not, then every effort should be made to move as far from the preexisting incisions as possible or to cross them with as wide an angle as practical. Transverse incisions generally do not create wound-healing problems, but parallel incisions place the wound healing at significant risk.

The incision should give good exposure to the anterior aspect of the knee.[8] The quadriceps tendon, patella, and tibial tubercle should be well visualized. In order to obtain flexion of the knee, a tibial tubercle osteotomy is required,[9,10] and therefore the incision should extend more distally than a standard arthroplasty approach. The alternatives for exposure, such as quadriceps turndown with a V-Y plasty, may be considered.[12–15] However, it is not recommended for an ankylosed knee because a manipulation and rigorous postoperative therapy would then be required.

Exposure

It is important to obtain good visualization of the anterior structures of the knee. A medial parapatellar incision is taken through the quadriceps tendon along the border of the patella and the border of the tibial tubercle. The osteotomy is completed as described by Whitesides.[9] The osteotomy of the anterior tibial tubercle is taken 8 to 10 cm distally. It is important to leave the tibial tubercle thick enough to allow screw or wire fixation at the end of the procedure, but not so thick as to create a stress riser and potential for tibial fracture. The osteotomy is taken through both medial and lateral cortexes and rolled laterally on an intact lateral soft tissue sleeve. This preserves the vascular supply to the tubercle, which aids in early healing.

An elevator is placed under the patella, which gently lifts the patella, and osteotomized tibial tubercle, and releases scar and adhesions from under the medial extensor mechanism. Proximally there will be a soft tissue plane under the vastus medialis. This can be dissected with a finger or an elevator to assure that the true anatomic plane is being maintained. With gradual dissection, the medial extensor mechanism is folded laterally. The medial sleeve is similarly elevated from the distal femur, femoral condyle, and medial tibial plateau. There is usually a soft tissue fatty plane, which can be entered and elevated and which serves as a guide to developing the vastus medialis plane over the distal femur. If the medial collateral ligament is intact, care should be taken not to disrupt its origin from the femur.

After full exposure, the contours of the distal femoral condyle and tibial plateau will be appreciated. The medial exposure is taken distally to the insertion of the pes anserinus tendons and medial collateral ligament. Care is taken not to elevate these structures from the proximal medial tibia. This dissection should allow good exposure to the anterior, medial, and lateral aspects of the ankylosed knee. Elevators can be placed posteriorly under the medial and lateral collateral ligaments in order to better define and protect the ligaments.

Osteotomies

When good exposure has been achieved, a preliminary osteotomy is completed. This should be transverse to the long axis of the tibia. It is safest to do this with an osteotome, and not a power saw, in order to protect the posterior neurovascular structures. The osteotomy should take place at the original joint line. In knees that had "spontaneous" ankylosis, the anatomy is normally surprisingly well preserved. In the surgically ankylosed knee, there is marked anatomic distortion and no absolute guidelines can be given for the location of the joint line.

When the osteotomy is completed, an osteotome can help to mobilize the femur from the tibia. The extensor mechanism is displaced laterally and the knee is gradually flexed. This is done slowly. When the knee is flexed, the tibial tubercle is everted, taking the entire quadriceps mechanism laterally. Medially, the soft tissue sleeve should be dissected as necessary in order to allow the vastus medialis to slide posteriorly. The knee can then be flexed to 90 degrees.

After the knee is flexed, good exposure is obtained and the alignment guides can be used to complete the final osteotomies for alignment and ligament balance (Fig. 84.2).

Alignment

Standard alignment guides are utilized for the femur and tibia. Preferences are generally for an intramedullary femoral alignment guide and intramedullary or extramedullary tibial guide. A 5- to 7-degree valgus osteotomy is taken in the distal femur, and a transverse osteotomy is taken in the proximal tibia. The amount of bone resection should be equivalent to the dimensions of the prosthetic thickness. Anterior and posterior cuts and chamfers can then be completed. Preliminary cuts should be made to allow later adjustment for rotation. Once the posterior femoral condyles have been osteotomized, better mobility can be achieved. The remnants of the anterior and posterior cruciates should be cleared from the intercondylar notch. The soft tissue adhesions on the posterior aspects of the tibia are dissected from the proximal portions of the tibia. There should be good exposure circumferentially around the distal femur and tibia, sparing only the collateral ligamentous attachments. Following this soft tissue mobilization, final anterior and posterior bone resections for rotation and size can be accomplished.

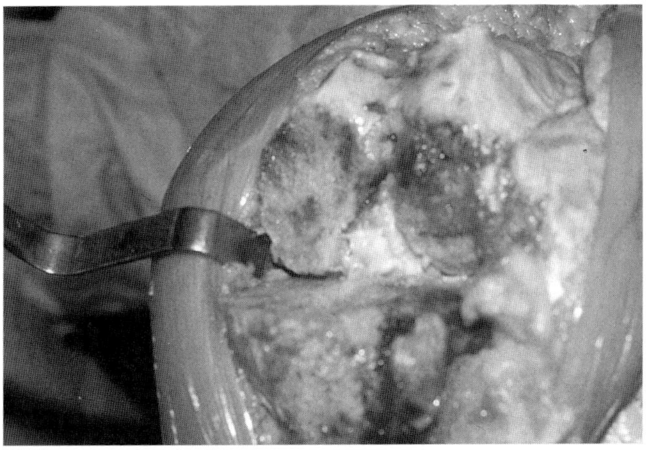

Appropriate rotation of the femoral component can be determined by one or all of three techniques.[3,12,13] The transepicondylar axis gives a reasonable approximation of the rotational axis. If the patellar groove still remains in the femur, a transverse line to the intercondylar notch confirms the transepicondylar axis. If ligaments are present, then equal balance with the knee at 90 degrees of flexion confirms appropriate rotation. It is important to avoid internally rotating the femoral component.

Ligament Stability

Integrity of the medial and lateral collateral ligaments should be evaluated. The most important structure to the knee is the medial collateral ligament and if intact, a semiconstrained device may be selected. As mentioned previously, this could be either a posterior cruciate-substituting device or a *total condylar III* style device with a high central tibial spike. If the medial collateral ligament is absent, then significant constraint must be utilized (Fig. 84.3).

If a constrained prosthesis is chosen, then a stem is required for fixation. This could either be a short cemented or long uncemented stem. Fixation is addressed in other chapters. At this point, the osteotomies for the distal femur, proximal tibia, and rotation on the posterior femoral condyle are complete. Trial reductions can now be initiated.

Trial Reduction

The trial reduction should be completed without constraints in the prosthetic device. In this manner, the soft tissue sleeve can be assessed independently. If the soft tissue sleeve is intact and the knee has good kinematics, less prosthetic constraint is required. On the other hand, if there is marked instability or ligament imbalance, then constraint is required.

After the knee is reduced, the quadriceps mechanism is usually found to be tight and limits flexion. Hope-

Figure 84.2. Osteotomy at the joint line with tibial tubercle folded laterally and knee brought to 90 degrees of flexion.

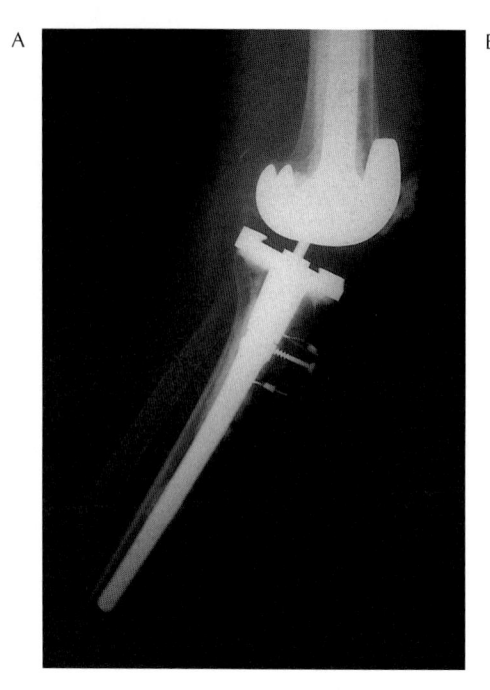

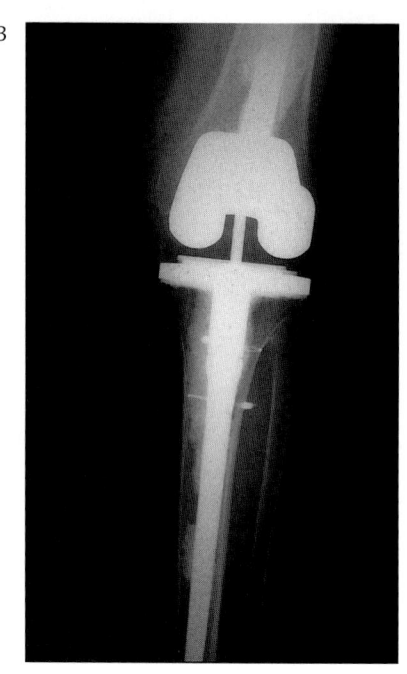

Figure 84.3. (A) and (B) X rays of postoperative total knee after fusion. Prosthetic choice of stems and partial internal constraint.

fully, 90 degrees or more of motion can be achieved. A finger should be slid under the quadriceps mechanism to be sure that no residual adhesions are present along the distal femur or under the vastus medialis and lateralis. The tourniquet makes it difficult to fully assess the mobility of the extensor mechanism. If there is severe restriction in flexion, you can briefly release the tourniquet and reassess flexion.

The prosthetic joint should then be implanted and fixed according to the surgeon's choice. If cement fixation is chosen, the patient can immediately bear weight and be rapidly mobilized.

Reattachment of the tibial tubercle is completed before soft tissue closure. This can be done with either screws or wires. The wiring technique is usually most effective because it obviates the problems with screws abutting a central fixating stem. If wires are chosen, care should be taken to place them well laterally in the tibial tubercle and replace the tubercle into its anatomic position.

The wound is closed in a routine manner, with care to be sure that the patella tracks centrally. The amount of flexion achieved on the operating table is carefully noted because this will be the immediate postoperative flexion goal.

Postoperative Care

The ultimate goal after the total knee arthroplasty is to achieve maximum motion. In the recovery room, continuous passive motion (CPM) is initiated to the maximum flexion achieved at the time of surgery. CPM is maintained while the patient is in bed and/or until the soft tissue inflammation begins to resolve.

Complications

As mentioned previously, there are a variety of complications that are unique to this procedure. Outcome depends on the preoperative deformity, etiology of ankylosis, and age of the patient. There is an increased risk for infection, higher incidence of wound-healing problems, and frequently significant reduction in anticipated range of motion as compared to TKA for osteoarthritis or rheumatoid arthritis. Recognition of the importance of these complications assists the surgeon in the postoperative period in planning follow-up management. The loss of motion is a problem and may require manipulation under anesthesia. This should be done as soon as the loss is recognized and repeated if necessary.

Summary

Total knee arthroplasty after a prior ankylosis or arthrodesis of the knee is feasible and recommended for a carefully selected set of patients. The overall quality of the result is often limited because of only modest gains in motion, high rates of infection, loosening, and revision. The decision to take down an akylosed knee and expectations for outcome should be carefully reviewed. The surgical technique depends on the presence of scar and the ligaments. Good exposure can be achieved with the tibial tubercle osteotomy and careful soft tissue dissection under the vastus medialis and vastus lateralis. Postoperatively the patient should be mobilized as rapidly as possible. The motion that was achieved at the time of surgery should be assiduously protected and maintained. Postoperative management should recognize the increased frequency of problems from wound healing, infection, and loss of motion.

With appropriate selection and surgical techniques, this procedure can have benefit for a limited group of patients.

References

1. Narajan RJ, Lotke PA, Pagnano MW, Hanssen AD, Total knee arthroplasty in a previously arthrodesed knee. *Clin. Orthop.* 1996;331:1–4.
2. Aglietti P, Windsor R, Buzzi R, et al. Arthroplasty for the stiff or ankylosed knee. *Arthroplasty.* 1989; 4:1–5.
3. Berger RA, Rubash HE, Seel MJ, Thompson WH, Crosset LS. Determining the rotational alignment of the femoral component in total knee arthroplasty using the epicondylar axis. *Clin Orthop.* 1993; 286:40–49.
4. Holden D, Jackson D. Considerations in total knee arthroplasty following previous knee fusion. *Clin Orthop.* 1988; 227:223–228.
5. Mullen J. Range of motion following total knee arthroplasty in ankylosed joints. *Clin Orthop.* 1983; 179:200–203.
6. Schurman J, Wilde A. Total knee replacement after spontaneous osseous ankylosis. *J Bone Joint Surg.* 1990; 72A: 455–459.
7. Gold DA, Craig-Scott S, Scott WN. Soft tissue expansion prior to arthroplasty in the multiply operated knee. *J Arthrop.* 1996.
8. Lotke PA. Surgical approach to the knee. In: *Master Techniques of Total Knee Arthroplasty.* Raven Press; 1995.
9. Whitesides LA. Exposure in the difficult total knee arthroplasty using tibial tubercle osteotomy. *Clin Orthop.* 1995; 321:32–35.
10. Wolff A, Hungerford D, Krackow K, et al. Osteotomy of the tibial tubercle during total knee replacement: a report of twenty-six cases. *J Bone Joint Surg.* 1989; 71A: 849–852.
11. Coonse K, Adams J. A new operative approach to the knee joint. *Surg Gynecol Obstet.* 1943; 77:344–347.
12. Insall JN, Tria A, Scott N. The total condylar knee prosthesis. The first five years. *Clin Orthop.* 1979; 145:68–77.
13. Scott RD, Siliski JM. The use of a modified V-Y quadricepsplasty during total knee replacement to gain exposure and improve flexion in the ankylosed knee. *Orthopaedics.* 1985; 8:45–48.
14. Whiteside LA, Arima J. The anteroposterior axis for femoral rotational alignment in valgus total knee arthroplasty. *Clin Orthop.* 1995; 321:168–172.
15. Trousdale RJ, Hanssen AD, Rand JA, Calahan TD. V-Y quadricepsplasty in total knee arthroplasty. *Clin Orthop.* 1993; 286:48–55.

CHAPTER 85
The Effect of Extra-Articular Deformity on the Tibial Component

David S. Hungerford

INTRODUCTION

The fundamental issues involved in extra-articular deformity have been reviewed in considerable detail in the chapter on femoral articular deformity. They are briefly reviewed here in order to allow this chapter to stand more or less on its own. Most deformity confronting the surgeon at total knee arthroplasty is the result of lost substance within the knee caused by the erosive process of inflammatory or osteoarthritis. The loss of intra-articular substance often produces a concomitant instability. The process of total knee arthroplasty restores the lost substance through properly aligned and oriented proximal tibial and distal femoral cuts and the selection of the appropriately sized implants. Thus, both alignment and stability are re-created. Extra-articular deformity is uncommon but not unknown. Perhaps the most common such deformity is a previous high tibial osteotomy, particularly one that has been poorly done. The clinical examples in this chapter will show such cases. Other causes of extra-articular deformity in the tibia include congenital bowing, rickets, and fracture with malunion. Unlike the more common intra-articular deformity, and extra-articular deformity, does not impose or imply any intra-articular instability. In fact, if the surgeon offsets an extra-articular deformity with a compensating proximal tibial resection, ligament instability will be created. When confronted with an extra-articular deformity, the surgeon has two choices. The deformity can be corrected by an extra-articular osteotomy, either prior to proceeding to total knee arthroplasty, or in association with the total knee arthroplasty. Alternatively, the surgeon can correct the extra-articular deformity by an offsetting proximal tibial cut, accepting, or dealing with the resultant instability. The purpose of this chapter is to present the issues to allow the surgeon to make an informed choice.

DETERMINING THE IMPLICATIONS OF EXTRA-ARTICULAR DEFORMITY ON THE TIBIAL COMPONENT

For purposes of this discussion, we are limiting the observation to deformities in the coronal plane (varus, valgus). Deformities may, however, occur in the transverse plane (rotation) or the sagittal plane (flexion, extension). The basic *principles* of the discussion will apply to extra-articular deformity in these other planes.

The accurate orientation of the proximal femoral cut to reestablish lower extremity alignment can be simply determined by creating the proper angular relationship of the distal femoral cut to the mechanical axis (center of the knees to the center of the ankle). This requires a long-standing film in which the knee and the ankle are well visualized with the tibia positioned in neutral rotation. Any extra-articular malalignment will require an offsetting and compensatory malalignment of the proximal tibial cut. The magnitude of this will be influenced by two factors—(1) the absolute magnitude of the axial deformity, and (2) the distance of the deformity from the center of the knee. Although there is a mathematical formula for calculating the angular relationships that would be required, this can be carried out very simply by templating (ref). Templating demonstrates the magnitude of the required compensatory intra-articular cut. This will help the surgeon to determine the magnitude of the ligament imbalance that would be created by the compensatory cut. Figure 85.1 shows the influence of the location of the deformity to the magnitude of the required cut. In this illustration it can be seen that a 20-degree valgus malunion of the supramalleolar fracture has virtually no influence on the orientation of the proximal tibial cut, whereas the same degree of malunion in the proximal tibial metaphyseal region produces the requirement for dramatic over-resection of the medial tib-

85. The Effect of Extra-Articular Deformity on the Tibial Component

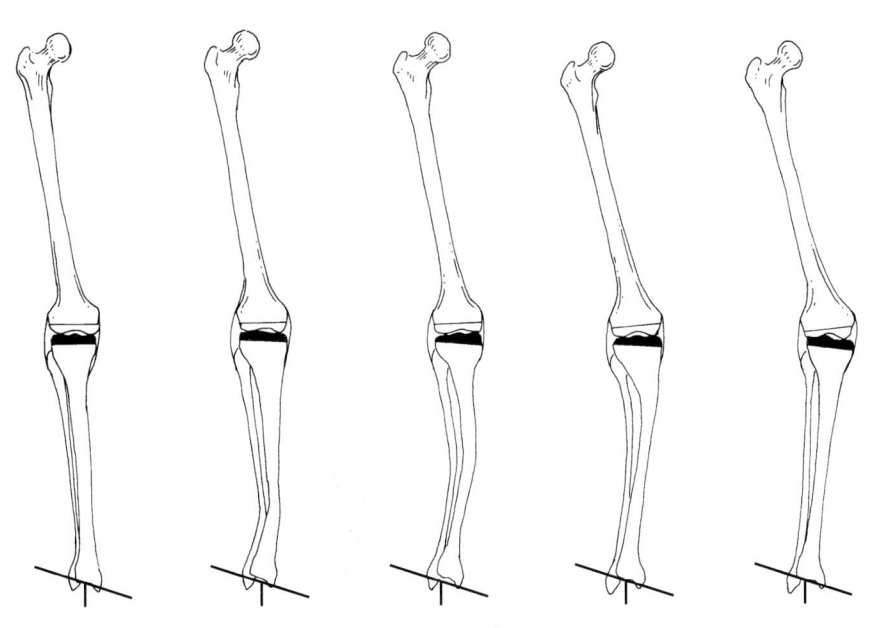

Figure 85.1. Resection level and orientation is shown necessary to correct the malalignment of a 20-degree valgus malunion of the tibia, beginning in the supramaleolar region on the left, proceeding up the tibia to the proximal metaphysis.

ial plateau to achieve alignment of the knee. In this illustration, such a malalignment, solved by intra-articular compensation, will result in severe medial instability, which in turn would require either a complex major ligamentous reconstruction of the use of a highly constrained prosthesis (Fig. 85.2). With this information of the required proximal compensatory cut, the surgeon can estimate the magnitude and complexity of the soft tissue imbalance that such a compensatory cut would create and make the decision whether to resolve the soft tissue issue by ligamentous reconstruction, constrained prosthesis, or extra-articular correction of the deformity. A varus deformity of the tibia will require an overresection of the lateral tibial plateau. This will produce instability throughout the range of motion. Minor degrees of lateral instability are well tolerated because the lateral side of the knee is dynamically stabilized by the iliotibial tract, the biceps tendon, the popliteus, the lateral head of the gastrocnemius muscle, and to a certain extent, by the joint reaction force. Medial compartment instability, however, does not have the same degree of dynamic stabilization because the medial hamstrings are not positioned in a way to provide significant resistance to valgus forces. Therefore, valgus deformities are more likely to require extra-articular correction than a varus deformity of similar magnitude.

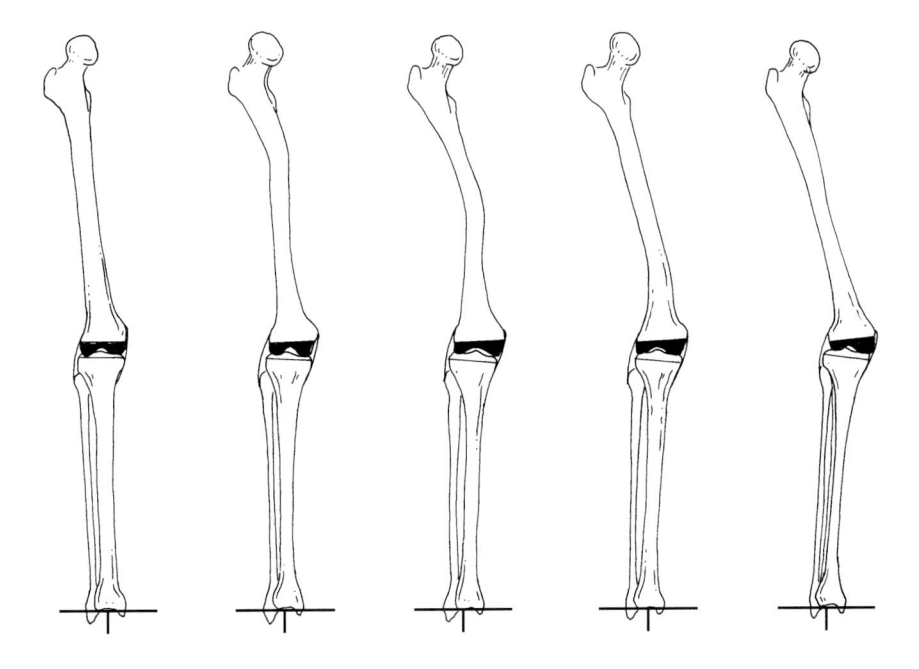

Figure 85.2. Medially based wedge resection has produced extremity alignment and medial ligament laxity. Notice also that the effect of the malalignment in the ankle is incompletely corrected.

In most instances, when a decision is made to carry out an osteotomy to compensate for an extra-articular deformity, this will be carried out at the proximal metaphysis. However, only a correction at the site of the deformity will correct all aspects of the deformity. A tibial deformity produces both implications for the knee and the ankle. For example, from Fig. 85.1, it can be seen that a mid-shaft angular deformity produces a malalignment at the ankle, which would require hindfoot valgus to compensate. A proximal tibial osteotomy would correct the implications at the knee but would leave the implications at the ankle incompletely corrected. A more complex deformity involving flexion and/or rotation would lead toward correction of the deformity at its site rather than at the proximal tibial metaphysis.

There is a major difference between extra-articular tibial deformity and extra-articular femoral deformity. A compensatory intra-articular cut for a tibial deformity will produce instability that is applicable throughout the whole range of motion, whereas a compensatory distal femoral cut will produce instability in extension only. Therefore, extra-articular tibial deformity is somewhat more straightforward to resolve with an intra-articular tibial cut. If the required compensatory cut is moderate, the tight side can be released to equal the loose side, which will restore ligament balance throughout the range of motion. Such loosening is likely to impact tension on the posterior cruciate ligament and the optimal choice of prosthesis in such a case would probably be a posteriorly stabilized component. However, posteriorly stabilized components are likely to be desirable for most extra-articular malalignments in which resolution is chosen to be affected by an offsetting intra-articular cut. Even in more severe degrees of deformity, ligament advancement to stabilize instability of tibial origin is much more straightforward than for the same instability of femoral origin. In the latter, the ligament attachment to the femur would have to be adjusted to find the new isokinetic point. In the case of tibial deformity, the isokinetic point for the femur is unchanged and therefore, only the tibial attachment of the loose ligament would have to be adjusted.

SUMMARY AND CONCLUSION

Extra-articular deformity of the tibia is fundamentally different from deformity caused by loss of intra-articular substance. Correction of the latter restores alignment and also usually stability. Extra-articular deformity can be corrected by compensatory intra-articular resections, but to do so introduces instability. The magnitude of the necessary correction can be assessed by templating from the mechanical axis. Although the magnitude of a deformity is obviously important, the distance from the knee also is a determinant in the magnitude of the necessary correction. Because the lateral side of the knee is dynamically stabilized, varus deformities, requiring a laterally based compensatory wedge (producing lateral laxity) will be better tolerated than intra-articular correction of a valgus deformity. Because a compensatory proximal tibia cut creates equal instability in both extension and flexion, the instability pattern is much less complex than a similar degree of femoral deformity. Therefore, the decision to correct an extra-articular tibial deformity by a compensatory extra-articular osteotomy or correction at the site of the deformity will probably be appropriate only for larger degrees of tibial deformity compared to femoral deformity. Finally, long-standing extra-articular deformity is often the cause of the arthrosis leading to the need for consideration of arthroplasty. In some instances, when the arthrosis is not severe, correction of the extra-articular malalignment will provide sufficient symptomatic relief so that arthroplasty can be deferred or avoided altogether.

CHAPTER 86
Total Knee Replacement with Associated Extra-Articular Angular Deformity of the Femur

John W. Mann III, Giles R. Scuderi, and John N. Insall

INTRODUCTION

Osteoarthritis of the knee with associated extra-articular angular deformity of the femur is an infrequent but challenging problem that must be thoughtfully addressed in patients requiring total knee replacement surgery. Common etiologies of extra-articular deformities are as follows: fracture malunion, failed osteotomies, physeal trauma, osteomyelitis, metabolic bone disease, and Paget's disease.[1] Historically, extra-articular deformities have been approached by corrective osteotomy at the site of the deformity to ensure that the overall alignment of the extremity is corrected prior to total knee arthroplasty.[1–4] Angular correction by osteotomy avoids the need for alteration of the routine joint line resections at the time of knee replacement surgery. This approach is particularly useful when large resections beyond the origins of the collateral ligaments are required to obtain normal alignment.[1,4] An alternative method for handling these difficult deformities has been correction of limb alignment by alteration of the joint line resections.[4,5] Soft tissue releases, including sacrificing the posterior cruciate ligament, are critical when employing this technique.[5] The major advantages of this method are that an additional procedure for osteotomy is not required and there are no concerns regarding healing of the osteotomy site.

PREOPERATIVE PLANNING

Preoperative planning for total knee arthroplasty in cases with associated extra-articular angular deformities must include long-standing radiographs of the lower extremity. Care should be taken when obtaining these radiographs to keep the extremity in neutral rotation because external rotation may accentuate a varus deformity due to the anterior bow of the femur.[6,7] Preoperative templating should be performed to determine the degree of the distal femoral cut. The mechanical axis is drawn from the center of the femoral head to the center of the knee joint and the anatomic axis is drawn from the center of the knee to the center of the intramedullary canal of the femur distal to the deformity.[1,3,8–10] Variations from the standard 6- to 7-degree valgus cut of the distal femur are dependent upon the magnitude of the deformity and its proximity to the knee joint.[1] If the templated distal femoral resection extends above the level of the epicondyles, the level of resection should be moved farther distally to avoid the origin of the collateral ligaments. It is not unusual to only resect bone from one condyle and set the level of resection on the other. For instance, with a severe varus deformity, bone may only be resected from the lateral femoral condyle. If this is still not acceptable, then an osteotomy may need to be considered. Templating is also done to ensure that the femoral components will seat securely because there may be a need for femoral augmentation or bone grafting. If the need for increased constraint arises, there may be some difficulty in seating the intercondylar box of a constrained condylar prosthesis (CCK) (Zimmer USA, Warsaw, Indiana). This is especially noteworthy if there is a need for a stem extension, because the stem may impinge on the medial cortex or, in the most extreme cases, may not be able to be inserted. Offset stem extensions may be of some value in these cases. A custom femoral component (Fig. 86.1) with the appropriate stem angle may have to be prefabricated if the coronal or sagittal plane deformity is outside the capability of a

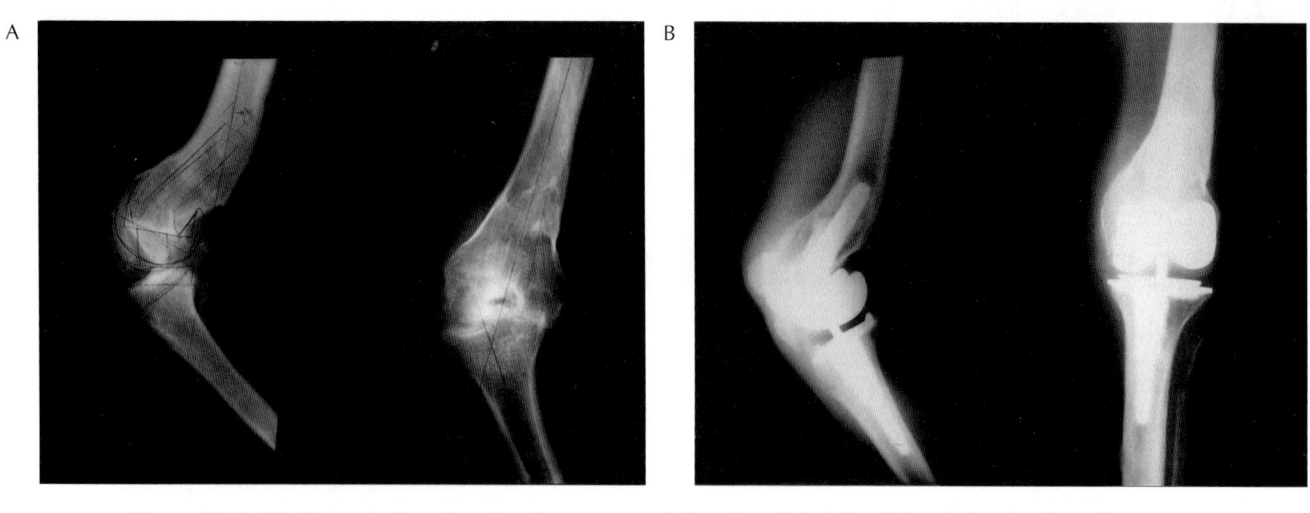

Figure 86.1. (A) Preoperative planning for a severe deformity of the distal femoral metaphyseal region following malunion in a supracondylar osteotomy in a 52-year-old female school teacher with a history of polio in the involved extremity. (B) Ten-year follow-up radiographs of this patient reveals restoration of axial alignment with a custom femoral component.

fixed degree of valgus, which in the case of the standard constrained condylar knee is 5 degrees of valgus. Soft tissue releases should be anticipated and planned accordingly.[7] Because these cases require extensive soft tissue release, it is our belief that the posterior cruciate ligament should be resected and a posterior cruciate-substituting prosthesis be implanted. Finally, if ligamentous stability is not achieved with the posterior-stabilized insert, a more constrained articulation should be available.

SURGICAL TECHNIQUE

The surgical approach is carried out through a standard anterior midline incision unless a prior surgical scar is present.[7] Utilization of previous incisions is recommended whenever feasible to decrease the risk of soft tissue complications. During the exposure limited soft tissue flaps are developed and a medial parapatellar arthrotomy is performed to allow eversion of the patella. When the exposure is limited by tension of the extensor mechanism, a quadriceps snip has been useful in improving exposure. A quadriceps snip is performed by releasing the quadriceps tendon from the apex of the medial arthrotomy laterally in an oblique fashion.[11] A tibial tubercle osteotomy allows wide exposure of the distal femur and proximal tibia in rare cases when the quadriceps snip is not adequate.[12]

Soft tissue releases are performed at this time to achieve provisional soft tissue balance and to enhance surgical exposure. The soft tissue release for a fixed varus deformity should be performed to allow the knee to come to neutral alignment.[7] The medial release has been described previously in this book (chapter 25), but in summary involves subperiosteal release of the deep and superficial collateral ligament as a contiguous soft tissue sleeve along the proximal tibia. The semimembranosis and posterior capsule are also released from the posteromedial corner. This allows excellent exposure and correction of deformity in almost all cases of varus deformity. The medial head of the gastrocnemius may require release in severe cases. Obviously, an extensive medial release should not be performed with valgus deformities. The valgus release may be performed at this time, but it is generally easier following completion of the distal femoral and proximal tibial cuts as described earlier in this book (chapter 26). Complete release of the posterior cruciate ligament facilitates correction of these fixed deformities.

The distal femoral cuts are performed at this time for correction of the mechanical axis in all femoral deformities. Following the preoperative template, the distal femoral cut should be perpendicular to the mechanical axis so as to avoid any joint line obliquity[7,9] (Fig. 86.2). Verification of the resection angle must be made intraoperatively with an extramedullary alignment device prior to performing the definitive resection. The external alignment rod is attached to the distal femoral cutting block and the patient's anterior superior iliac spine is palpated and a point 2 cm medial to this should correspond to the center of the femoral head. A radiographic skin marker whose position has been confirmed preoperatively may also be used. The distal femoral resection should not extend proximally beyond the epicondyles and it should correct the mechanical axis without creating any joint line obliquity. It should be

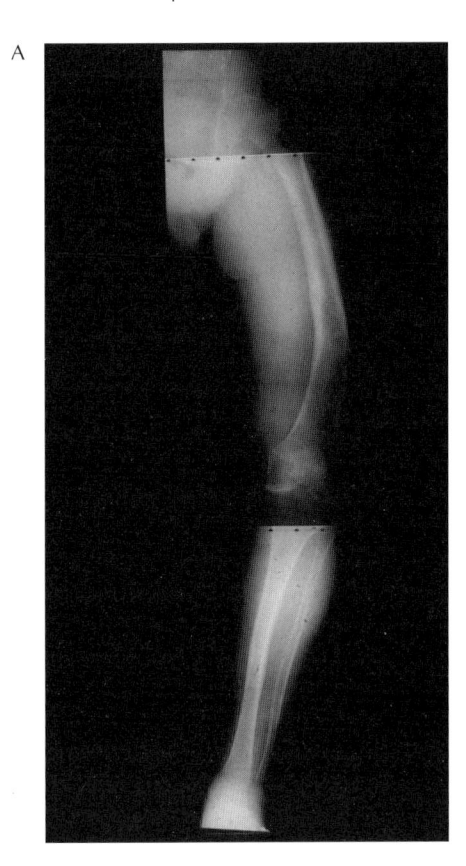

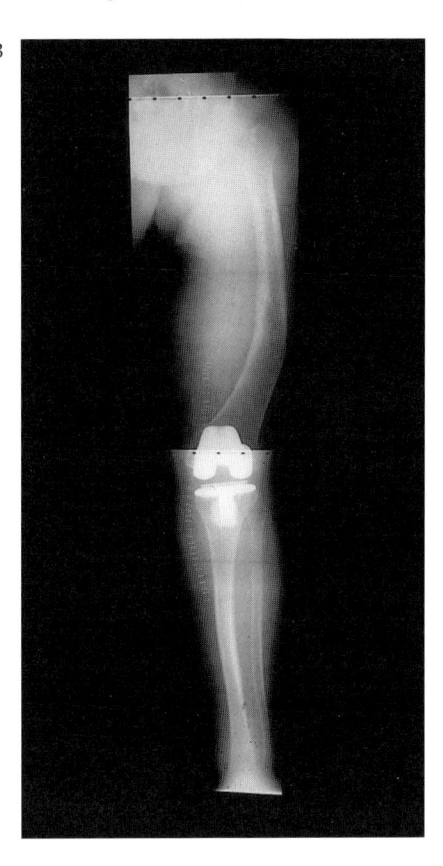

Figure 86.2. (A) Preoperative radiographs of the left lower extremity of a 67-year-old male who sustained bilateral femur fractures treated in traction with resultant malunions and subsequent post-traumatic osteoarthritis of the knees. (B) Postoperative radiographs immediately following surgery that reveal correction of the mechanical axis and the joint line parallel to the floor.

emphasized here that a minimal resection should be made initially so that fine-tuning can be performed to achieve appropriate alignment. The extramedullary alignment rod should again be used after the distal femoral cut is performed to ensure that the appropriate alignment has been attained.

Following the completion of the distal femoral cut, the femur is sized, and the anterior and posterior (AP) femoral condyles are resected. Appropriate rotational alignment of the femoral component is important to normalize patellofemoral tracking and to equalize the flexion and extension spaces. The epicondylar axis and the long axis of the tibia are useful landmarks for determining femoral rotation (chapters 30, 31). The proximal tibia is resected perpendicular to the long axis of the tibial shaft. The flexion and extension spaces are checked with a spacer block and an alignment rod. Once it is determined that the tibial cut is appropriately aligned, any malalignment must come from the distal femur. If recutting the distal femur is required for alignment correction, determination should be made regarding equalization of the flexion and extension gaps prior to repeating the distal cut so that correction of a tight extension gap can be corrected as well. Remember that the collateral ligaments should be balanced prior to repeating the distal femoral cut.

Femoral chamfer cuts are made once correct alignment and soft tissue balance have been obtained and trial components are inserted. The alignment, ligamentous balance, range of motion, and patellofemoral tracking are assessed. If there are any bone defects requiring augmentation or if there is any question regarding stability of the knee, modular components from the CCK system may be used. If augmentation or increased constraint is necessary, it is preferable to use a stemmed component. This may not be possible with a severe diaphyseal deformity unless a custom stem has been made preoperatively (Fig. 86.1). When a custom prosthesis is not available, you may elect to cement the femoral component without a stem extension or to use a shortened stem extension. Following the above preparation, the final implants are cemented in place.

Wound closure is very important in cases of significant angular correction. Care must be taken to close the wounds without tension. If there are multiple incisions about the knee or a severe varus or valgus deformity that may cause tension following correction of the deformity, it may be wise to obtain a preoperative plastic surgery consult. Consideration may be given to the use of a preoperative soft tissue expander or a gastrocnemius rotational flap for wound closure.[7,13]

DISCUSSION

There are no large clinical series of total knee arthroplasty in patients with associated extra-articular angular deformities of the femur. Previous reports have been limited primarily due to the relatively low incidence of this clinical problem. Rand and Franco reported the Mayo Clinic's experience with total knee replacement with associated traumatic angular deformities in only 11 knees of 12000 cases.[4] Certainly all authors agree that one of the primary factors determining the success of knee arthroplasty is achieving proper mechanical alignment.[2,3,7–10,14–17] The surgical approach most prevalent in the orthopedic literature for treatment of osteoarthritis of the knee with extra-articular deformities is correction of the angular deformity at its apex by osteotomy followed by total knee replacement.[1–4] This can be performed with one or two operative procedures. Alternative management of this difficult problem is correction of the angular deformity by altering the joint line resections without additional osteotomy.[4,5] This approach must include appropriate soft tissue releases including sacrificing the posterior cruciate ligament in all cases.

Wolff and Hungerford have reported their results with osteotomy at the apex of the deformity followed by total knee arthroplasty in three cases.[1] Correction of the deformity alone yielded satisfactory results in one additional patient without the need for subsequent total joint replacement. The authors note that the use of a posterior cruciate-retaining prosthesis limits the extent of correction that can be obtained with soft tissue releases about the knee. Soft tissue releases may alter the level of the joint line and place increased tension on the posterior cruciate ligament. Alteration of the joint line could also cause patellar baja and increased stresses at the patellofemoral articulation.

Rand and Franco utilized both joint line resection alone and osteotomy for deformity correction in their series of post-traumatic deformities requiring total knee arthroplasty.[4] There were 6 femoral, 3 tibial, and 2 combined femoral and tibial angular deformities in this series. The deformities ranged in the coronal plane from 8 degrees of valgus to 35 degrees of varus. The range of the sagittal plane deformity was 32 degrees of anterior apex angulation to 18 degrees of posterior apex angulation. Two preexisting nonunions healed following total knee arthroplasty with a long-stem prosthesis. Three deformities were corrected with osteotomy at the time of arthroplasty and the remaining deformities were corrected with alteration of the joint line resection.

The Hospital for Special Surgery (HSS) knee score improved from a preoperative mean of 59 (49 to 69) to a postoperative mean of 74 (45 to 94). Radiographic analysis revealed the limb alignment postoperatively to be 3 degrees of tibiofemoral valgus (4 degrees to 10 degrees valgus). Radiolucent lines were present in all tibial components, but were not progressive in any cases. The complication rate was 55% in this series with two deep infections, one superficial infection, one nonunion of the osteotomy site, one avulsion of the patellar tendon, and one late femur fracture. Due to the high complication rate in this series, these authors recommended osteotomy for deformity correction in the diaphyseal region if the deformity was greater than 10 to 15 degrees of varus or valgus or 20 degrees in the sagittal plane. They noted that most deformities in the metaphyseal area could be corrected by alteration of the joint line resection.

A retrospective review of 18 knees in 16 patients with extra-articular deformities undergoing total knee replacement at our institution included 15 femoral deformities.[5] Correction of the deformity was performed by alteration of the joint line resection with soft tissue releases in each case by the senior author (JNI). There were 10 varus and 3 valgus deformities of the femur. Two additional femoral deformities were due to significant recurvatum from fracture malunions. The etiology of the deformities were as follows: fracture malunions (11), Paget's disease (1), rickets (1), polio (1), and osteomyelitis (1). A posterior cruciate-substituting prosthesis was utilized in all cases. A custom femoral component was employed in two cases due to metaphyseal deformities. The average follow-up was 5 years (2 to 10 years). The mean deformity with relation to the mechanical axis was 14 degrees (5 to 22 degrees), and 17 degrees (6 to 25 degrees) from the anatomic axis (Fig. 86.2). The average deformity in the sagital plane was 16 degrees (5 to 38 degrees) (Fig. 86.2).

The Hospital for Special Surgery Knee Score (HSS) improved from a preoperative mean of 64 to 88 postoperatively. The mean Knee Society and functional scores were 93 (64 to 100) and 83 (55 to 100), respectively. Patient outcomes were graded as excellent (10), good (6), and poor (2) using the HSS grading scale. The two patients with a poor result were graded as failures due to infection requiring implant removal and the need for revision surgery of a failed metal-backed patellar component. It became apparent that not all deformities were fully corrected and radiographic evaluation revealed deformity correction to be within the range of 3 degrees of varus to 4 degrees of valgus with respect to the mechanical axis with a mean of 1 degree of varus alignment. Radiolucent lines of less than 2 mm were seen in five tibial components, but none were progressive. There were no changes of implant position regarding the femoral or tibial components. One patellar component revealed radiographic signs of loosening, but was clinically asymptomatic.

The results of total knee arthroplasty in this group of

patients with extra-articular angular deformity were similar to those of the senior author's long-term results in primary knee replacement surgery using the posterior-stabilized prosthesis with regard to the scoring systems of the Hospital for Special Surgery and the Knee Society.[18–20] Despite the fact that the overall clinical grading of these patients was similar to the experience of primary total knee arthroplasty, the incidence of complications is more comparable to that of revision surgery.[21]

CONCLUSION

Review of the literature certainly does not reveal the most appropriate method for performing total knee arthroplasty in patients with extra-articular angular deformities due to the relative infrequency of this clinical problem. The primary goal of the surgeon should be attaining appropriate mechanical alignment in these difficult cases. The advantages of correction of the angular deformity at the joint line are the avoidance of an additional operative procedure for osteotomy and the risk of nonunion. Thorough preoperative planning is essential and deformity correction by osteotomy prior to arthroplasty should be performed in all femoral deformities that require bony resection above the level of the epicondyles for realignment of the mechanical axis. Attention to detail at the time of surgery should ensure that the bone resection of the distal femur and proximal tibial are perpendicular to the floor for correction of the mechanical axis and to prevent obliquity of the joint line. Posterior cruciate sacrifice and the understanding of appropriate soft tissue releases is mandatory for deformity correction using this method.

References

1. Wolff AM, Hungerford DS, Pepe CL. The effect of extra-articular varus and valgus deformity on total knee arthroplasty. *Clin Orthop.* 1991; 271:35–51.
2. Laskins RS. Angular deformities in total knee replacement. *Orthopaedic Review.* 1981; 10(11):27.
3. Krackow KA. Approaches to planning lower extremity alignment for total knee arthroplasty and osteotomy about the knee. In: *Advances in Orthopaedic Surgery.* Williams & Wilkins; 1983: 69.
4. Rand JA, Franco MG. Revision considerations for fractures about the knee. In: Goldberg, V, ed. *Controversies of Total Knee Arthroplasty.* New York: Raven Press, Ltd.; 1991:235–242.
5. Mann JW, Insall JI, Scuderi G. Total knee replacement with associated extra-articular angular deformities. American Academy of Orthopaedics Annual Meeting. San Francisco, California, February 1997.
6. Jiang C-C, Insall JN. Effect of rotation on the axial alignment of the femur: pitfalls in the use of femoral intramedullary guides in total knee arthroplasty. *Clin Orthop.* 1989; 248:50–56.
7. Insall JN. Surgical techniques and instrumentation in total knee arthroplasty. In: Insall JN, Windsor RD, Scott WN, et al., eds. *Surgery of the Knee.* 2nd ed. New York: Churchill Livingstone, Inc.; 1993:739–804.
8. Insall JN, Ranawat CS, Scott WN, et al. Total condylar knee replacement: preliminary report. *Clin Orthop.* 1976; 120: 149–154.
9. Insall JN, Tria AJ, Scott WN. The total condylar knee prosthesis: the first five years. *Clin Orthop.* 1979; 145:68–77.
10. Clayton ML, Thompson R, Mack RP. Correction of alignment deformities during total knee arthroplasties: staged soft-tissue releases. *Clin Orthop.* 1986; 202:117–124.
11. Garvin KL, Scuderi G, Insall JN. Evolution of the quadriceps snip. *Clin Orthop.* 1995; 321:131–137.
12. Whitesides LA, Ohl MD. Tibial tubercle osteotomy for exposure of the difficult total knee arthroplasty. *Clin Orthop.* 1990; 260:6–9.
13. Gold DA, Scott WN, Scott SA. Soft tissue expanders prior to total knee replacement in the multi-operated knee: a new method to prevent catastrophic skin problems. *J Arthroplasty.* 1996; 11:512–521.
14. Bargren JH, Freeman MAR, Swanson SAV, et al. Arthroplasty in the treatment of arthritic knee. *Clin Orthop.* 1976; 120:65–75.
15. Lotke PA, Ecker ML. Influence of the positioning of prosthesis in total knee replacement. *J Bone Joint Surg.* 1977; 59A:77–82.
16. Bryan RS, Rand JA. Revision total knee arthroplasty. *Clin Orthop.* 1982; 170:116–122.
17. Ritter MA, Faris PM, Keating EM, et al. Postoperative alignment of total knee replacement: its effect on survival. *Clin Orthop.* 1994; 299:153–156.
18. Insall JN. Results of total knee arthroplasty. In: Insall JN, Windsor RD, Scott WN, et al., eds. *Surgery of the Knee.* 2nd ed. New York: Churchill Livingstone, Inc.; 1993:975–982.
19. Stern SH, Insall JN. Posterior stabilized prosthesis: results after follow-up of nine to twelve years. *J Bone Joint Surg.* 1992; 74A:980–986.
20. Colizza WA, Insall JN, Scuderi GR. The posterior stabilized total knee prosthesis: assessment of polyethylene damage and osteolysis after a ten-year minimum follow-up. *J Bone Joint Surg.* 1995; 77A:1713–1720.
21. Haas SB, Insall JN, Montgomery W, et al. Revision total knee arthroplasty with use of modular components with stems inserted without cement. *J Bone Joint Surg.* 1995; 77A:1700–1707.

CHAPTER 87
The Effect of Extra-Articular Deformity on the Femoral Component

David S. Hungerford

INTRODUCTION

It is widely accepted that long-term satisfactory function and survival of both the prosthetic bone interface and the plastic surface of the tibial component requires accurate alignment in total knee arthroplasty. In fact, most patients present with some degree of preoperative malalignment and several chapters in this book deal with problems associated with severe preoperative varus and valgus deformity. However, the majority of these deformities are due to articular cartilage and bone loss of the distal femur, the proximal tibia, or both (Fig. 87.1). Occasionally, the deformity may be due to soft tissue instability with or without intra-articular bone loss. In both situations, the apex of the deformity is at the joint. With these kinds of deformities, ligamentous contractions or laxities may also be present. Regardless of the deformity, the distal femoral and proximal tibial bone cuts are made referencing the anatomical axis of the respective bones. Proper cuts will automatically restore proper alignment. Separate procedures may be necessary to reestablish soft tissue balance but the orientation of the bone cuts to the anatomic axis is not influenced by the direction or degree of the preoperative deformity. Moreover, in *most* instances when the proper bone cuts (level and orientation) have been made, ligamentous stability is reestablished without the need for any supplemental ligamentous balancing procedures (Fig. 87.2).

When patients present with significant *extra-articular* deformities, the foregoing observations concerning alignment and ligament balance no longer apply. First, the anatomical references of the femoral shaft and the tibial shaft no longer apply and second, when the distal femoral and proximal tibial bone cuts result in alignment of the mechanical axis (center of the femoral head to the center of the ankle passing through the center of the knee) ligamentous instability *has been created*. It is the purpose of this and the following chapter to address the implications of extra-articular deformity on the femoral cuts and on the tibial cuts, and the consequences on reestablishing soft tissue stability.

AXIAL ALIGNMENT

The recommended distal femoral and proximal tibial bone cuts for most total knee systems today are perpendicular to the mechanical axis. It is known, however, that the anatomic joint line is not perpendicular to the mechanical axis and that a distal femoral cut perpendicular to the mechanical axis results in an under-resection of the lateral femoral condyle and a compensatory over-resection of the lateral tibial plateau (Fig. 87.3). Kinematic studies on cadaver joints have shown that these minor degrees of malalignment, which are completely offsetting and result in a normally aligned extremity, do not impose a detectable kinematic abnormality in the replaced articulation. However, for purposes of this discussion, we will be using, as examples, the anatomic method of alignment, which results also in an aligned extremity but with *equal* amounts of bone resected from the medial and lateral sides of the joint. Because this anatomic method of achieving both alignment and soft tissue balance results in equal resection of the condyles (medial and lateral) and tibial plateaus, it is easier to visualize the implications of the extra-articular deformity (Fig. 87.4).

Most instrumentation systems for total knee arthroplasty reference the femoral shaft with long intramedullary or extramedullary alignment rods, and either the mechanical axis extraosseously from the center of the knees to the center of the ankle, or the intramedullary tibial shaft. In both instances, the anatomical references (femoral shaft, tibial shaft) presuppose a known and defined relationship to the mechanical axis

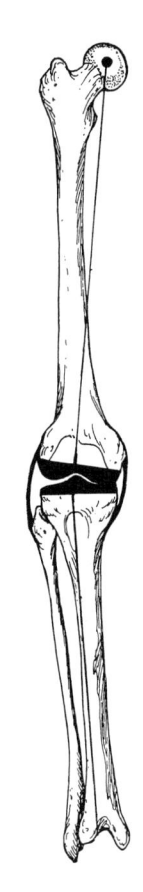

Figure 87.1. Malalignment in most patients presenting for total knee replacement is due to eroded bone and articular cartilage on one side. This diagram shows the orientation of the bone cuts necessary to produce alignment.

(femoral head to center of knee, center of knee to center of ankle). In the case of intra-articular deformity, the degree and orientation of the deformity does not influence these references. However, in the case of extra-articular deformity, the relationship of the anatomical reference to the mechanical axis has been altered and ultimately it is the mechanical axis that must be aligned.

Extra-articular deformities are usually based on one of four conditions—a congenital anomaly, a developmental deformity, a metabolic disease such as Paget's disease and rickets, or an acquired deformity such as a malunited fracture or a prior osteotomy.

IMPLICATIONS OF EXTRA-ARTICULAR DEFORMITY ON THE FEMORAL COMPONENT PLACEMENT

For purposes of this discussion, we are limiting the observation to deformities in the coronal plane (varus, valgus). Deformities may, however, occur in the transverse plane (rotation) or the sagittal plane (flexion, extension). The basic *principles* of the discussion will apply to extra-articular deformities in these other planes.

The accurate orientation of the distal femoral cut to reestablish lower extremity alignment can be determined simply by creating the proper angular relationship of the distal femoral cut to the mechanical axis (center of the knee to the center of the hip). This requires a long-standing film in which the hip is well visualized and the femur is positioned in neutral rotation. Any extra-articular "malalignment" will require an offsetting and compensatory malalignment of the distal femoral cut. The magnitude of this will be influenced by two factors: (1) the absolute magnitude of the axial deformity, and (2) the distance of the deformity from the center of the knee. Figure 87.5 shows a schematic diagram of a distal femoral cut referenced off a mechanical axis to compensate for a 20-degree valgus deformity of the distal femur. Although there is a mathematical formula for calculating the angular relationships that would be required, this can be carried out very simply by templating. Templating demonstrates the magnitude of the required compensatory intra-articular cut. This will help the surgeon to determine the magnitude of the ligamentous imbalance that will be created by this com-

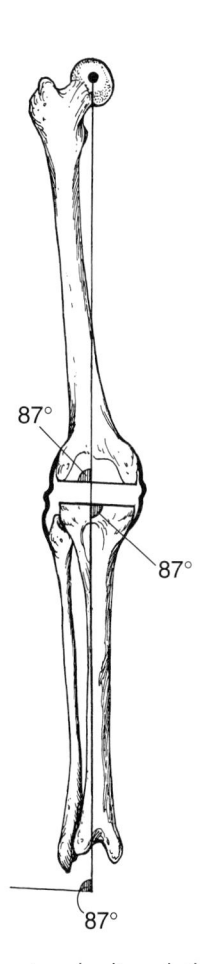

Figure 87.2. With the cut ends aligned, the ligaments are equally balanced and need to be stabilized by filling the gap with sufficient prosthetic material.

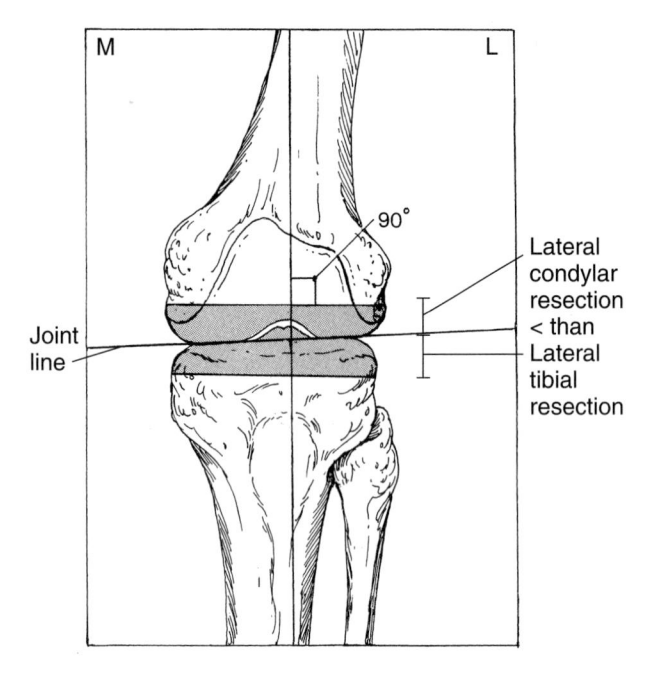

Figure 87.3. Resection of the distal femur and proximal tibia perpendicular to the mechanical axis according to the dictate of the "classical" alignment method results in lateral condylar under-resection, which is compensated for by lateral plateau over-resection.

malunion in the supracondylar region produces the requirement for a dramatic over-resection of the medial femoral condyle to achieve alignment of the knee. In this latter illustration, such a malalignment solved by intra-articular compensation would result in severe medial instability, which in turn would require either a complex major ligamentous reconstruction or the use of a highly constrained prosthesis.

Armed with the knowledge of the required distal femoral compensatory cut, the surgeon can estimate the magnitude and complexity of the soft tissue imbalance that such a compensatory cut would create. The decision must be made whether to resolve the soft tissue issue by ligamentous reconstruction, constrained prosthesis, or simultaneous pre-arthroplasty extra-articular correction of the deformity.

A varus deformity of the femur will require a compensatory over-resection of the lateral femoral condyle. This will produce lateral instability in extension only. Minor degrees of lateral instability are well tolerated because the lateral side of the knee is dynamically stabilized by the iliotibial tract, the biceps tendon, the popliteus, the lateral head of gastroc-soleus muscle, and to a certain extent, by the joint reaction force. Medial compartment instability, however, does not have the same degree of dynamic stabilization because the medial hamstrings are not positioned in a way to provide significant resistance to valgus forces. Therefore, a valgus deformity, requiring a compensatory medially based wedge, is more likely to require an extra-articular correction than a varus deformity of similar magnitude.

The alternative to intra-articular compensation for extra-articular deformity is extra-articular correction. In pensatory cut. Figure 87.6 shows the influence of the location of the deformity on the magnitude of the required compensatory cut. In this illustration it can be seen that a 20-degree valgus malunion of a subtrochanteric fracture has virtually no influence on the orientation of the distal femoral resection, whereas the same degree of

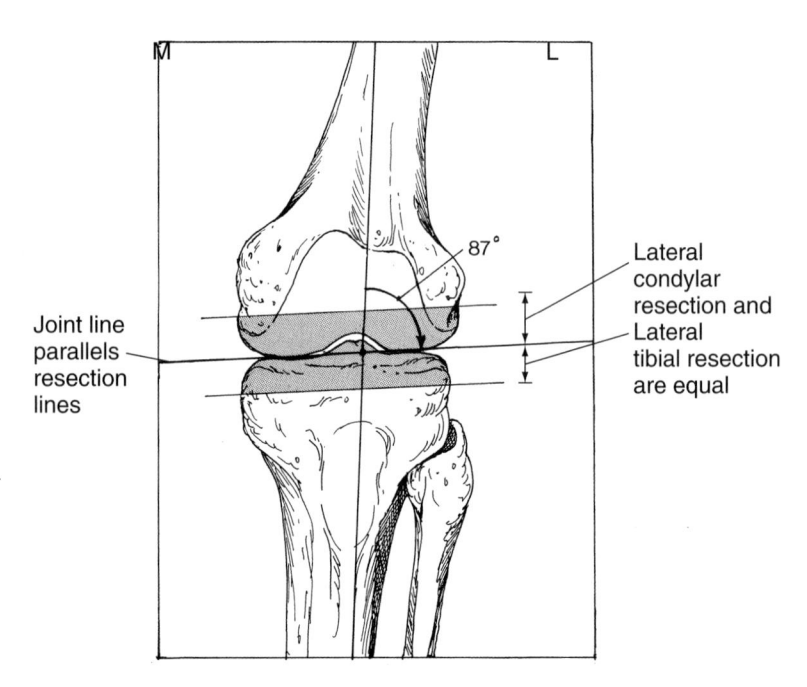

Figure 87.4. Resection of the distal femur at an 87-degree angle (9 degrees to the femoral shaft) and the tibial plateaus also at 87 degrees (3 degrees "varus") to the tibial shaft (which is coincident to the mechanical axis) results in equal resections of the medial and lateral femoral condyles and medial and lateral tibial plateaus.

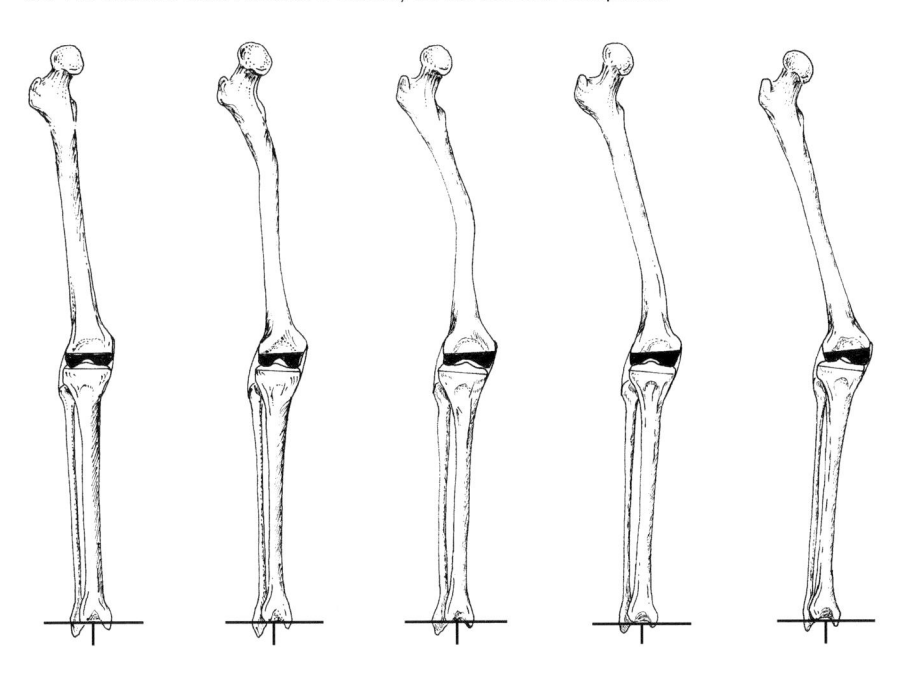

Figure 87.5. Resection level and orientation is shown necessary to correct the malalignment of a 20-degree valgus malunion at the lesser trochanter on the left and proceeding down the femur to the supracondylar region on the right.

most instances, this would consist of a supracondylar osteotomy, which would usually be performed as a separate surgical procedure prior to a total knee replacement. The magnitude of the supracondylar osteotomy would be determined in a very similar way to the orientation of the required distal femoral cut, such as by templating. It must be remembered that the magnitude of the compensatory osteotomy will be a function of the distance of the osteotomy from the actual deformity. That is to say, a 20-degree mid-shaft valgus deformity will not require a 20-degree supracondylar correction. Any deformity is completely corrected only by corrective osteotomy at the apex of the deformity. If a malalignment is complex (i.e., multiplanar), it would be-

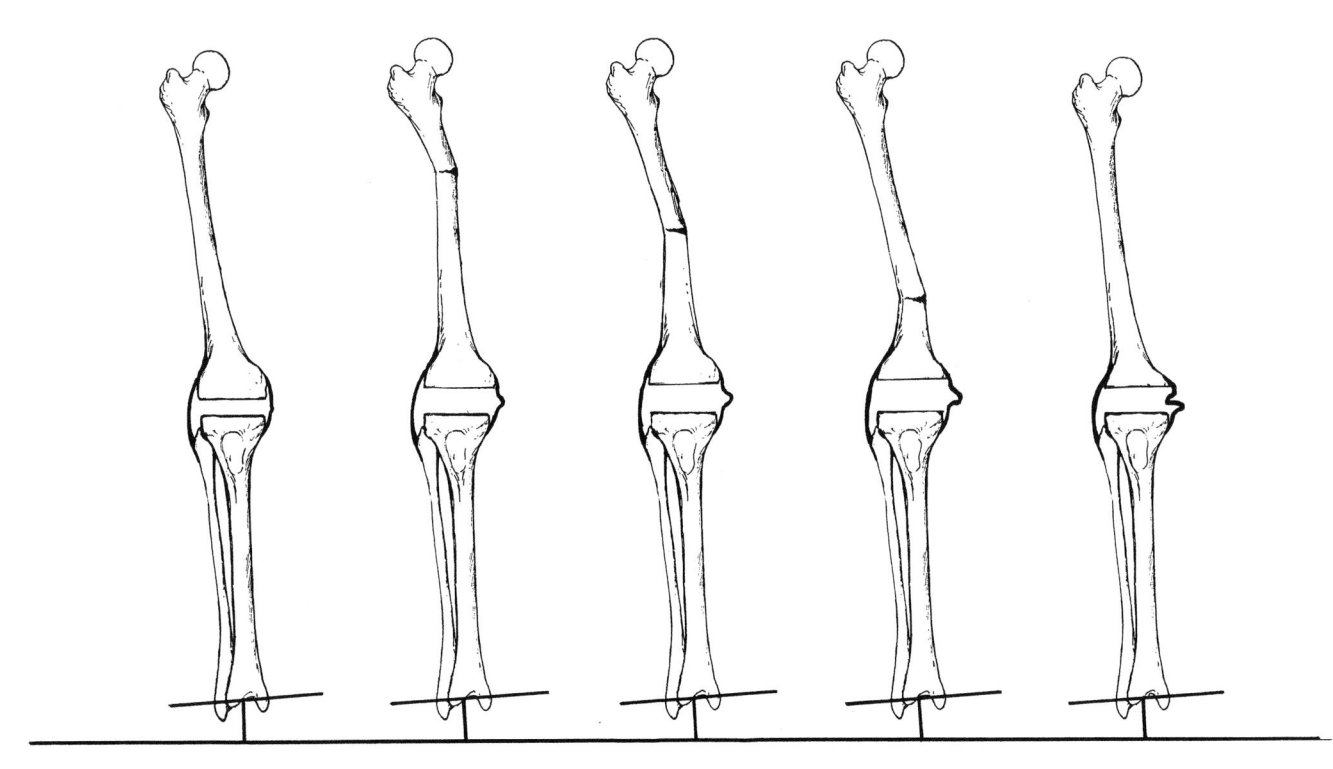

Figure 87.6. Schematic representation of the medial ligament laxity caused by the resections in Figure 87.5.

come more important to attempt a correction of all aspects of the deformity at the apex.

ILLUSTRATIVE CASE

A 63-year-old black woman presented with bilateral severe knee pain of long-standing but leading to severe ambulatory condition over the past 2 years. She had had rickets as a child with severely bowed legs all her life. Knee range of motion bilaterally was limited to 15 to 40 degrees. Both knees were globally unstable, but the varus deformity was not passively correctable.

Long-standing X rays indicated the resection orientation that would be required to produce straight extremities. The required laterally based distal femoral wedge resection would have included the lateral epicondyle creating severe instability. Because of the combination of intra-articular and extra-articular deformity, it was decided to perform a corrective distal femoral supracondylar osteotomy. The intra-articular resections were performed to create equal flexible and extensory gaps, which left a malaligned prosthesis. After the intra-articular cuts were performed, a compensatory supracondylar osteotomy was done. Because of severe limitation of motion, tibial tubercle osteotomies were done to aid exposure. The left knee was done first, followed by the right 2 weeks later. The postoperative X rays show slight under-correction on the left. However, the postop recovery was uneventful and the patient regained 0 to 90-degrees motion and painless stable independent ambulation.

SUMMARY AND CONCLUSION

Extra-articular deformity of the femur is fundamentally different from deformity caused by loss of intra-articular substance. Correction of the latter restores alignment and also usually stability. Extra-articular deformity can be corrected by compensatory intra-articular resections, but to do so introduces instability. The magnitude of the necessary correction can be assessed by templating from the mechanical axis. Although the magnitude of a deformity is obviously important, the distance from the knee also is a determinant in the magnitude of the necessary correction. Because the lateral side of the knee is dynamically stabilized, varus deformities, requiring a laterally based compensatory wedge (producing lateral laxity), will be better tolerated than intra-articular correction of a valgus deformity. Because a compensatory distal femoral cut creates instability only in extension (but not in flexion), the instability pattern is much more complex than a similar degree of tibial deformity. Therefore, the decision to correct an extra-articular femoral deformity by a compensatory extra-articular osteotomy or correction at the site of the deformity will probably be appropriate for a smaller degree of femoral deformity than tibial deformity. Finally, long-standing extra-articular deformity is often the cause of the arthrosis leading to the need for consideration of arthroplasty. In some instances, when the arthrosis is not severe, correction of the extra-articular malalignment will provide sufficient symptomatic relief that arthroplasty can be deferred or avoided altogether.

CHAPTER 88
Total Knee Replacement with Associated Extra-Articular Angular Deformity of the Tibia

John W. Mann III, Giles R. Scuderi, and John N. Insall

INTRODUCTION

Significant extra-articular angular deformity of the tibia with secondary osteoarthritis of the knee is a relatively rare problem. The primary etiology for extra-articular tibial deformities are fracture malunion, failed osteotomies, physeal trauma, osteomyelitis, and metabolic bone disease.[1–3] Regardless of the etiology of the deformity, the primary concern for the reconstructive surgeon is correction of overall limb alignment to increase the longevity of the knee arthroplasty.[4–12] Corrective osteotomy at the site of the deformity has been the primary method of limb realignment prior to or at the time of knee replacement surgery.[1,2,9] Tibial angular deformities may also be corrected by alteration of the joint line resection and soft tissue releases.[2,3] Care must be taken to avoid creating joint line obliquity with this method and a complete understanding of soft tissue releases is crucial when employing this technique. Advantages of this method include the avoidance of an additional procedure for osteotomy and there are no concerns regarding healing of the osteotomy site.

PREOPERATIVE PLANNING

Preoperative planning for total knee arthroplasty in cases with extra-articular angular tibial deformities must include long-standing radiographs of the lower extremity.[1–3,13] Templating should be performed to determine the depth and angle of the proximal tibial resection. The mechanical axis is drawn from the center of the femoral head to the center of the knee joint and extended to determine the desired position for the center of the ankle joint.[13] Radiographic cutouts can be used to determine the degree of proximal tibial joint line resection required for correction of the mechanical axis. Variations from the standard neutral tibial resection are dependent upon the magnitude of the deformity and its proximity to the knee joint.[1] Templating is also done to ensure that, if a stemmed tibial component is utilized, it will seat properly. An offset tibial stem may be required in severe deformities. A modular prosthesis to deal with unanticipated bone deficits and a relatively constrained articulation should also be available.

Evaluation of the soft tissues about the knee should be done prior to angular correction. This is particularly important in the multiply-operated knee or in case of a severe deformity if there is concern regarding the ability to close the soft tissues. A plastic surgery consultation should be obtained and consideration may be given to the use of a tissue expander preoperatively in these cases.[13,14]

SURGICAL TECHNIQUE

A standard anterior midline incision is routinely employed in knee replacement with extra-articular tibial deformities. However, a previous incision is utilized whenever possible and limited soft tissue flaps are developed during the approach to decrease the risk of soft tissue complications. Contractures of the soft tissue from long-standing deformity must be addressed. Medial soft tissue releases in the varus knee are performed to bring the knee to neutral alignment and have been fully described earlier in the book (chapter 25).[13] Subperiosteal dissection of the deep and superficial medial collateral ligaments is performed along the proximal tibia so that a contiguous subperiosteal sleeve is maintained. The semimembranosis and posterior capsule are also routinely released. Valgus releases may be performed at this time, but it is generally easier to do this following the distal femoral and proximal tibial cuts. The valgus release was described in chapter 26. Eversion of the patella may also be limited by tension on the extensor mechanism. In these cases, a quadriceps snip should be performed by releasing the quadriceps tendon from the proximal extent of the medial arthrotomy laterally in an oblique fashion.[15] Occasionally, a tibial tubercle osteotomy is required when the quadriceps snip is not adequate.[16]

It has been our preference to prepare the femur first to aid in the visualization of tibial deformities. The femoral cut is performed in a routine fashion with the valgus resection angle determined from long-standing radiographs.[13] The distal femoral cut should be perpendicular to the mechanical axis. This can be verified intraoperatively with an extramedullary alignment device. Following sizing of the femur and determining the rotational alignment, the anterior and posterior (AP) femoral condyles are resected.

The tibial resection is the key to correction of the deformity. The extramedullary tibial resection guide is oriented so that the alignment rod is centered over the ankle joint. This tends to create an asymmetric resection of the proximal tibia. With severe deformities, there may be no bone resected from one of the tibial plateaus and there may be an obvious bone deficiency, which may require augmentation. Initially it is best to minimize the level of resection and make adjustments later in the case. Spacer blocks are utilized to assess the flexion and extension gaps. The flexion space is checked first. An alignment rod is then attached to ensure that the tibial resection is appropriately aligned. This is also the time when bone deficiencies are quantified. The alignment rod is removed and the extension space and the overall alignment of the extremity is checked. If the knee is appropriately aligned, the degree of augmentation or bone grafting is visualized.

Once the overall alignment and soft tissue balance has been achieved, final preparations for the tibia and femur are made. The sizing and rotational alignment of the tibial component must be determined. If there are any bone defects requiring bone grafting or augmentation, it should be done at this time. Bone grafting techniques have been described elsewhere in the book (chapters 38 and 39). Though it is preferable to use a stem extension with modular tibial augments, this may not be possible in these types of cases because of diaphyseal deformity. Offset stems may be of some benefit. Finally, if there are difficulties with the short stem on the tibial tray, consider an all-polyethylene tibial component, which could be "shaved" to fit the tibial canal (Fig. 88.1).

Wound closure is carried out after implant fixation in a meticulous manner in cases of significant angular correction. Tension-free wound closure is preferable, but not always possible. The preoperative use of soft tissue expansion or a gastrocnemius rotational flap at the time of surgery may aid in a tension-free wound closure.[13,14]

DISCUSSION

There is limited discussion of the treatment of osteoarthritis of the knee in patients with extra-articular tibial deformities in the orthopedic literature. Rand and Franco reviewed 12000 cases of total knee arthroplasty at the Mayo Clinic and found only 11 cases of posttraumatic angular deformities, of which only three cases were isolated to the tibia and two cases were combined femoral and tibial deformities.[2] Wolff and Hungerford described total knee replacement after corrective osteotomy in one case of tibial deformity.[1] Our experience with the correction has been limited to 3 of 18 cases of extra-articular deformities corrected by alteration of the joint line resection and soft tissue releases.[3]

The surgical approach that is chosen for tibial deformity correction should be determined by the experience of the operating surgeon. Alignment correction by osteotomy at the apex of the deformity may be a combined procedure utilizing a long-stemmed tibial prosthesis for stabilization of the osteotomy site or it may be done in a staged fashion.[1,2] Wolff and Hungerford described one case of angular correction in the tibia that alleviated the patient's symptoms without the need for subsequent knee arthroplasty.[1] The advantages of corrective osteotomy prior to, or at the same time as, the total knee arthroplasty are that bony resections are more similar to those routinely performed at the time of arthroplasty. The surgeon may employ either a posterior cruciate-retaining or sacrificing prosthesis. A posterior cruciate-sacrificing prosthesis must be employed if a femoral stem is utilized. Finally, soft tissue releases are in general not as complex if correction is carried out at the apex of the deformity.

Our method of choice for deformity correction has been alteration of the joint line resection at the time of total knee arthroplasty followed by soft tissue releases.[3] Deformity correction by joint line resection alone avoids the need for an additional operative procedure for osteotomy.[2,3] This approach also does not have the inherent risk of nonunion at the osteotomy site. The Mayo Clinic experienced one nonunion at the osteotomy site in three cases requiring osteotomy for angular correction.[2] Finally, surgeons familiar with the use of the posterior cruciate-sacrificing prosthesis will be more familiar with the soft tissue releases required for alignment correction.

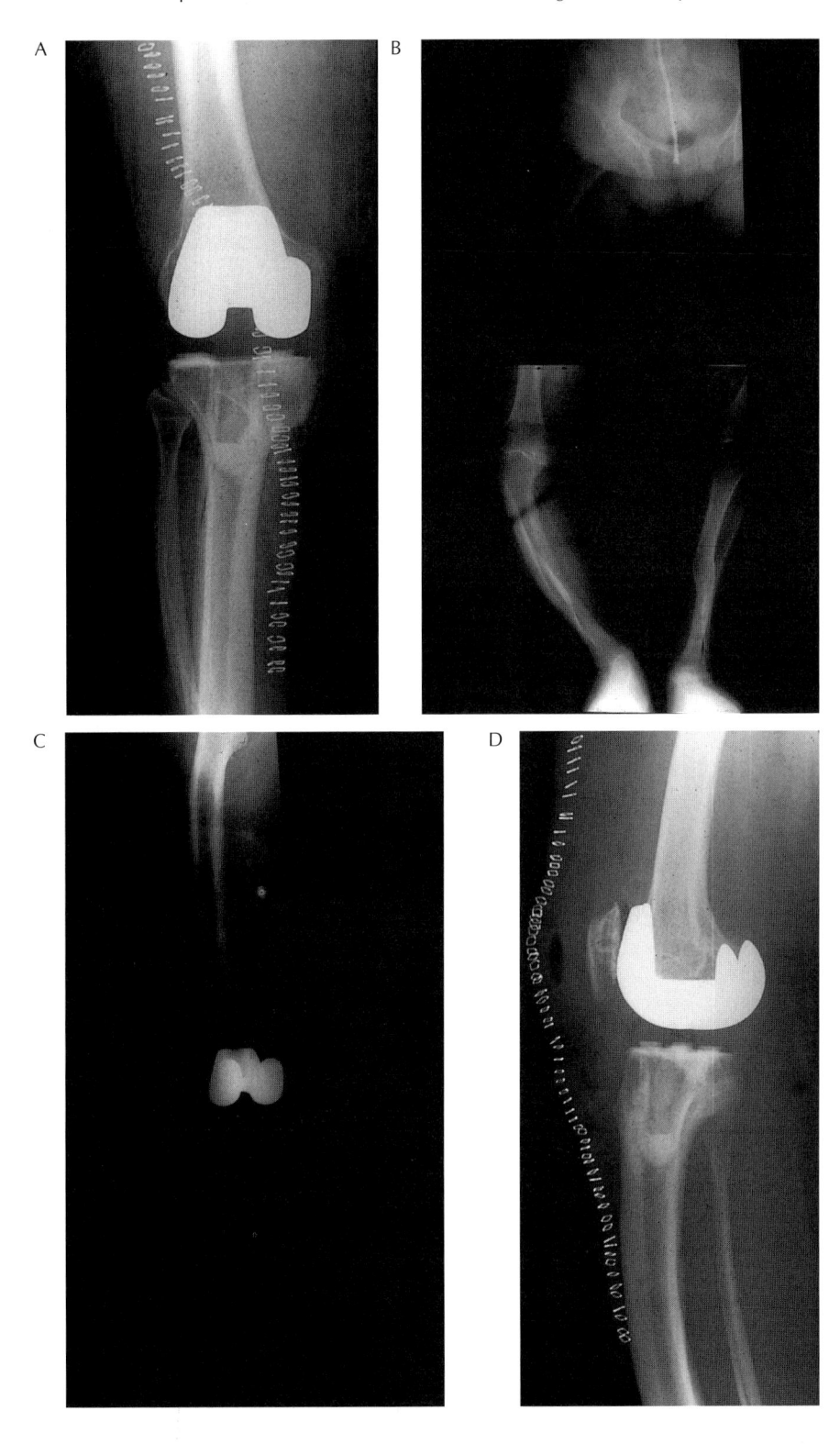

Figure 88.1. Preoperative anteroposterior (A) and lateral radiograph (B). Postoperative anteroposterior (C) and lateral radiograph (D).

Rand and Franco performed angular correction in 6 of 11 cases by joint line resection alone and recommended utilizing this approach in coronal plane deformities of up to 10 to 15 degrees or sagittal plane deformities of up to 20 degrees.[2] Follow-up analysis from their series revealed an improvement of the mean Hospital for Special Surgery (HSS) knee score from 59 (49 to 69) preoperatively to 74 (45 to 94) postoperatively. The overall postoperative limb alignment was 3 degrees of tibiofemoral valgus (4 degrees varus to 10 degrees valgus). All tibial components had nonprogressive radiolucent lines. The complication rate was 55% in this series with two deep infections, one superficial infection, one nonunion of the osteotomy site, one avulsion of the patellar tendon, and one late femur fracture. It was not possible when reviewing this series to determine if the complications were in correction of tibial or femoral deformities.

A retrospective review of 18 knees in 16 patients extra-articular deformities undergoing total knee replacement at our institution included three tibial varus deformities from fracture malunions.[3] Deformity correction was performed by joint line resection in all cases at the time of arthroplasty. The mean tibial deformity was 9 degrees (6 to 15 degrees) in the coronal plane and 6 degrees (5 to 8 degrees) in the sagittal plane. The average follow-up was 5 years (2 to 10 years). The Hospital for Special Surgery Knee Score (HSS) improved from a preoperative mean of 79 to 89 postoperatively. There were two good and one excellent rating according to the HSS grading scale. There were no complications in this group of tibial deformities. Radiographic analysis revealed nonprogressive radiolucent lines in two tibial components.

The results of total knee arthroplasty in this group of patients with extra-articular angular tibial deformities were similar to those of the senior author's (JNI) long-term results in primary knee replacement surgery.[17–19] There were no complications in this group of tibial deformities, but the deformities in this group were not as significant as in the femoral group.

CONCLUSIONS

The primary surgical goal for the treatment of extra-articular angular deformities that require total knee arthroplasty is the correction of limb alignment in these difficult cases. The primary advantage of correction of the angular deformity at the joint line is the avoidance of an additional operative procedure for osteotomy and the risk of nonunion. Thorough preoperative planning is essential to determine the correct degree of joint line resection. Care should be taken at the time of surgery to ensure that the bone resection of the proximal tibia is perpendicular to the floor for correction of the mechanical axis and to prevent obliquity of the joint line. The posterior cruciate ligament must be sacrificed in all significant deformities and appropriate soft tissue releases are mandatory for deformity correction.

References

1. Wolff AM, Hungerford DS, Pepe CL. The effect of extra articular varus and valgus deformity on total knee arthroplasty. *Clin Orthop.* 1991; 271:35–51.
2. Rand JA, Franco MG. Revision considerations for fractures about the knee. In: Goldberg, V, ed. *Controversies of Total Knee Arthroplasty.* New York: Raven Press, Ltd.; 1991:235–242.
3. Mann JW, Insall JI, Scuderi G. Total knee replacement with associated extra-articular angular deformities. American Academy of Orthopaedics Annual Meeting. San Francisco, California, February 1997.
4. Bargen JH, Freeman MAR, Swanson SAV, et al. Arthroplasty in the treatment of arthritic knee. *Clin Orthop.* 1976; 120:65–75.
5. Insall JN, Ranawat CS, Scott WN, et al. Total condylar knee replacement: preliminary report. *Clin Orthop.* 1976; 120: 149–154.
6. Lotke PA, Ecker ML. Influence of the positioning of prosthesis in total knee replacement. *J Bone Joint Surg.* 1977; 59A:77–82.
7. Insall JN, Tria AJ, Scott WN. The total condylar knee prosthesis: the first five years. *Clin Orthop.* 1979; 145:68–77.
8. Bryan RS, Rand JA. Revision total knee arthroplasty. *Clin Orthop.* 1982; 170:116–122.
9. Laskins RS. Angular deformities in total knee replacement. *Orthopaedic Review.* 1981; 10(11):27.
10. Krackow KA. Approaches to planning lower extremity alignment for total knee arthroplasty and osteotomy about the knee. In: *Advances in Orthopaedic Surgery.* Baltimore, MD: Williams & Wilkins; 1983:69.
11. Clayton ML, Thompson R, Mack RP. Correction of alignment deformities during total knee arthroplasties: staged soft-tissue releases. *Clin Orthop.* 1986; 202:117–124.
12. Ritter MA, Faris PM, Keating EM, et al. Postoperative alignment of total knee replacement: its effect on survival. *Clin Orthop.* 1994; 299:153–156.
13. Insall JN. Surgical techniques and instrumentation in total knee arthroplasty. In: Insall JN, Windsor RD, Scott WN, et al., eds. *Surgery of the Knee.* 2nd ed. New York: Churchill Livingston, Inc.; 1993:739–804.
14. Gold DA, Scott WN, Scott SA. Soft tissue expanders prior to total knee replacement in the multi-operated knee: a new method to prevent catastrophic skin problems. *J Arthroplasty.* 1996; 11:512–521.
15. Garvin KL, Scuderi G, Insall JN. Evolution of the quadriceps snip. *Clin Orthop.* 1995; 321:131–137.
16. Whitesides LA, Ohl MD. Tibial tubercle osteotomy for exposure of the difficult total knee arthroplasty. *Clin Orthop.* 1990; 260:6–9.
17. Insall JN. Results of total knee arthroplasty. In: Insall JN, Windsor RD, Scott WN, et al., eds. *Surgery of the Knee.* 2nd ed. New York: Churchill Livingstone, Inc.; 1993:975–982.
18. Stern SH, Insall JN. Posterior stabilized prosthesis: results after follow-up of nine to twelve years. *J Bone Joint Surg.* 1992; 74A:980–986.
19. Colizza WA, Insall JN, Scuderi GR. The posterior stabilized total knee prosthesis: assessment of polyethylene damage and osteolysis after a ten-year minimum follow-up. *J Bone Joint Surg.* 1995; 77A:1713–1720.
20. Haas SB, Insall JN, Montgomery W, et al. Revision total knee arthroplasty with use of modular components with stems inserted without cement. *J Bone Joint Surg.* 1995; 77A:1700–1707.

SECTION 21
Postoperative Management

CHAPTER 89
Rehabilitation

Robert S. Gotlin and Elizabeth A. Becker

INTRODUCTION

Before undergoing total knee arthroplasty (TKA), one must have a thorough understanding of the postoperative commitment to the rehabilitation program. Adapting to the new prosthetic knee involves physical and emotional challenges, both of which have direct effects on one's lifestyle. Although surgery strives to correct the anatomic aberration resulting in disability, the rehabilitation process strives to improve strength and functional performance. TKA is considered one of the most successful procedures for joint disability and the number of cases performed exceeds 230000 per year in the United States. It parallels total hip arthroplasty as one of the most frequently performed joint arthroplasty procedures done today. The most common subjective complaint in those requiring TKA is pain, and the number one handicap is inability to perform one's usual activities of daily living (ADLs). For one person, this could be simple ambulation and for another it could be playing doubles tennis. Because patients differ, rehabilitation strategies must be customized to meet the individual needs of each. Enhancing functional performance is the main concern during the postoperative rehabilitative period. This is accomplished through hard work and adherence to the prescribed rehabilitation program. Beginning with preadmission testing, continuing through surgery and for several months postoperatively, patients are guided through a concise training regime. This is coordinated through the efforts of a dedicated rehabilitation team, which initially convenes at the time of preadmission testing. It is here that a generalized overview of the program is discussed and realistic goals set. Patients are introduced to the assistant devices and training modalities, and are given an overview of the postoperative period. Patient's expectations, anatomic limits of the prosthetic device, and the rehabilitation team's input are carefully integrated for realistic goal setting. It is not surprising and rather common for patients to have unrealistic expectations and goals; however, if one attains a good quality of life with the ability to function relatively pain free, this is acceptable to most. Equally important to reviewing functional expectations is patient education, especially with reference to the financial obligation associated with TKA. Clearing of any potentially stressful financial situations early in the rehabilitation process will ease tensions and direct attention toward functional goals. It is extremely important for the rehabilitation caregivers to establish a positive rapport with each patient, because it is this interaction that will guide recovery for several months and possibly years. Our staff maintains close, open-door contact with patients for several years postop. Patients rely upon our guidance and support for concerns ranging from gait mechanics to level of activity allowed to many other issues related to their new prosthesis. This chapter outlines our rehabilitation program and suggests specific protocols to expedite a safe and sound return to functional performance in those undergoing TKA.

PREOPERATIVE ASSESSMENT

In comparison to recent years, the preoperative assessment now plays a more significant role in TKA postoperative planning. While in the past, this was a time when pertinent laboratory tests were performed and merely a mention made about the postoperative rehabilitation process, now addressed are topics such as home environment, assistant devices used, and vocational support.[1] With cost containment and reduced length of stay (LOS) a significant factor in medical decision making, the preoperative assessment is the time that postoperative planning must be orchestrated. Even though it is our goal to discharge patients directly to the preadmission setting within 3 to 5 postoperative days, complicating issues may prevail that inhibit this from occurring. Potential discharge limiting and postoperative logistic problems are addressed prior to surgery. What has typically been a *consecutive* series of steps from surgery to acute hospitalization to subacute hospitalization or rehabilitation to home therapy to outpatient therapy now must be looked upon as a *concomitant* series of steps and identification of patient needs and rehabilitation timetables preplanned. Although diagnostically related groups (DRGs) still guide acute care LOS, it is anticipated that future guidelines will decrease the recommended LOS. When considering disposition and its related issues, a careful preoperative review could ease the transition from hospital to home or rehabilitation facility. Identification of patients who may ultimately require acute rehabilitation in the immediate postoperative period must occur early. Identifying those individuals potentially requiring transfer to the rehabilitation service should begin before the patient undergoes surgery. If we delay this process until the postoperative phase, unnecessary prolongation of acute LOS will ensue. Although it is obvious that not all those ultimately requiring acute inpatient rehabilitation can be identified early, by isolating a significant number who will, our efficiency as health-care providers improves. Munin noted that patients who subsequently required rehabilitation admission after TKA were those who lived alone, were older in age, have increased number of comorbid conditions, and have greater pain levels.[2] Evans and colleagues concluded that patients who participate in inpatient rehabilitation programs function better at hospital discharge, have a better chance of short-term survival, and return home more frequently than nonparticipants.[44] The act of returning to the home setting may in itself justify the inpatient rehabilitation even though functional performance on long-term follow-up may not differ significantly between control (no inpatient rehabilitation) and inpatient rehabilitation groups. When assessing various outcome studies, we must be critical especially when considering disposition. In doing so, the weighing of financial implications against functional performance is critical and a common ground must be met. As trends move toward independent home exercise programs and away from formal therapy, inpatient rehabilitation can serve as the bridge from acute to independent care. Also, subacute care can achieve similar endpoints with even more potential cost savings. Our experience has mirrored the above authors. The multidisciplinary team continually monitors comorbid and pain factors to prevent untoward complications and setbacks that impede progress. We have credited the multidisciplinary team concept with assuring optimal patient outcomes. One of our key tracking tools is the patient questionnaire. Patients are asked to answer a series of questions prior to and at specified times after surgery (see Tables 89.1, 89.2, and 89.3 at end of chapter). These questionnaires address issues related to the need for TKA and subjective results afterward. It is tools such as these that assist in validating performing TKA and its subsequent rehabilitation.

Favorable outcomes are those that are cost-effective, disability reducing, and successfully achieve significant functional gains. This could be ADL independence or returning to work that was otherwise impossible. Often overlooked but absolutely critical to successful outcome is patient education. This is the major focus of our preadmission testing and its postoperative feedback has been overwhelmingly positive. Most patients have very limited knowledge of the events related to TKA. We extensively review information relative to the surgical procedure and recovery. Patients are given several handouts including those that overview postoperative rehabilitation and others depicting exercises to be familiar with during recovery (see Tables 89.4 and 89.5 at end of chapter). Important information such as potential activation of metal detectors at department stores and/or airports by the prosthesis, requirement of antibiotic prophylaxis for dental work, and prolonged (expected) knee effusion for approximately 6 months postoperatively are all conveyed in these handouts. It is surprising that the majority of patients, if not forewarned, are admitted to the hospital without proper clothing, particularly footwear, for postoperative ambulation. This too is addressed in the handouts. Some patients have multiple premorbid ailments that may interfere with postoperative progress. Medical concerns are addressed by the internal medicine team. This includes baseline laboratory tests and systems review. Physical concerns are addressed by the rehabilitation team. This includes the obese patient who may require a wide walker, the rheumatoid patient who may require a platform walker, and the tall patient who may require a bed extension. Also, those with premorbid contractures (flexion or extension) may have difficulty attaining range of motion postoperatively. We find that flexion contractures greater than 20 degrees are the most difficult to manage. These patients usually receive nighttime extension splints to assist knee extension. By identifying and addressing these associated premorbid ailments in the preoperative assessment, we avoid delays in the rehabilitation process. Historically, the preoperative assessment was not a time for review of the various assistant devices used in the postoperative period. Now we review these at length and educate patients on their proper use. Because patients ambulate on the first postoperative day, it is extremely helpful if there is familiarity with these devices before surgery. This has positive impact on ambulating patients earlier in the postoperative period. The devices typically reviewed are walkers, crutches, and canes. Some centers utilize formal gait analysis prior to surgery[3] but we routinely perform computerized gait analysis several months after surgery.

Although there are certainly benefits derived from this analysis in both the preoperative and postoperative period, we selectively perform it later in the postoperative period. Gait analysis has become an important tool in TKA, and Vaughan and associates propose 10 criteria when considering it.[4] Its contribution is very helpful particularly when analyzing interlimb symmetry. Combined with strength testing, gait analysis allows the clinician to critique functional performance and make necessary training modifications. Another modality commonly used in the recovery phase is the continuous passive motion (CPM) machine (Fig. 89.1), a device that continuously and sequentially flexes and extends the knee. It is a cumbersome but relatively comfortable device that helps expedite recovery in the early postoperative period, which has received extensive literary review.[5-15] Reports of related decreased pain medicine consumption, increased motion, decreased swelling, decreased length of stay, deep vein thrombosis prophylaxis, decreased wound-healing complications, and reduction in the need for postoperative manipulations are replete in the literature. Although its long-term results are not statistically substantiated, its short-term benefits especially as related to reduction in LOS justify its application. In addition to demonstrating the above modalities, inquiry is made about the patient's home environment and physical challenges they will face. Simple tasks such as stair climbing and shower or tub transfers can be challenging in the postoperative period and must be reviewed. The number of staircases and total number of stairs to climb is a significant obstacle in the immediate postoperative period and strategies for negotiating these must be clearly reviewed. Patients are taught to ascend stairs leading with the uninvolved lower limb, followed by the involved lower limb and finally by the assistant device (usually held in the hand opposite the involved lower limb). To descend stairs, one is taught to lead with the assistant device, followed by the involved lower limb, and finally by the uninvolved lower limb (Fig. 89.2). Patients are asked to practice stair climbing with different assistant devices before surgery. It is this time that one can try the various devices in preparation for the challenges ahead. Also at this time issues such as operative anesthesia (general versus epidural) and postoperative pain management are reviewed with the patient by the pain specialist or anesthesiologist. Although the majority of patients at our institution undergo epidural anesthesia, some prefer the general route. After surgery, patient-controlled analgesia (PCA) is utilized for pain control (Fig. 89.3). This delivery system allows patients to actively participate in delivering analgesia. Via the epidural or intravenous route, a predetermined volume of analgesia is delivered from a prefilled chamber by depressing a delivery button (Fig. 89.4). This button is attached directly to the medication chamber. Even though the patient controls the desired frequency of medication administration, the total amount of medication per unit time delivered is regulated by the pain medication specialist. In other words, the patient has unlimited access to attempt medication delivery but many of these may not actually deliver analgesia. To determine optimal dosing, the frequency of chamber activation is tracked on the PCA device. This information is utilized to adjust dosage to assure adequate analgesia without inadvertent overdosing. If a patient has activated the device excessively while still complaining of significant pain and no untoward side effects, the amount of delivered medication may not be sufficient. In contrast, if a patient seems too lethargic, excess medication may have been administered. Although there are documented benefits of epidural anesthesia and analgesia including decreased use of narcotics, facilitated joint mobility and enhanced gait training,[39,40] a persistent drawback to the use of PCA is its untoward side effect of impaired urinary function and patient lethargy. The narcotics typically utilized tend to delay normal micturation. This may prolong the need for urinary catheterization. We try to avoid this via close, continued patient monitoring. In the subsequent days after surgery there is a careful titration of analgesia to allow functional progress with no more than moderate discomfort or lethargy. Our goal is to expedite the transition from PCA to oral analgesia. This usually takes only a few days. We wind up our preadmission session with an outline of the postoperative year. The rehabilitation process is far more lengthy than the operative procedure and preparedness is the key. Because the process is a lengthy one, we ready the patient by describing a series of "sixes." The first series refers to the first 6 postoperative days. During this period patients are depen-

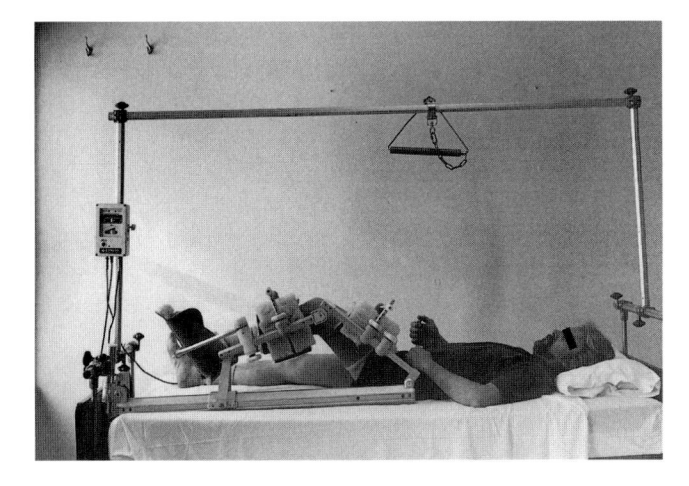

Figure 89.1. CPM machine.

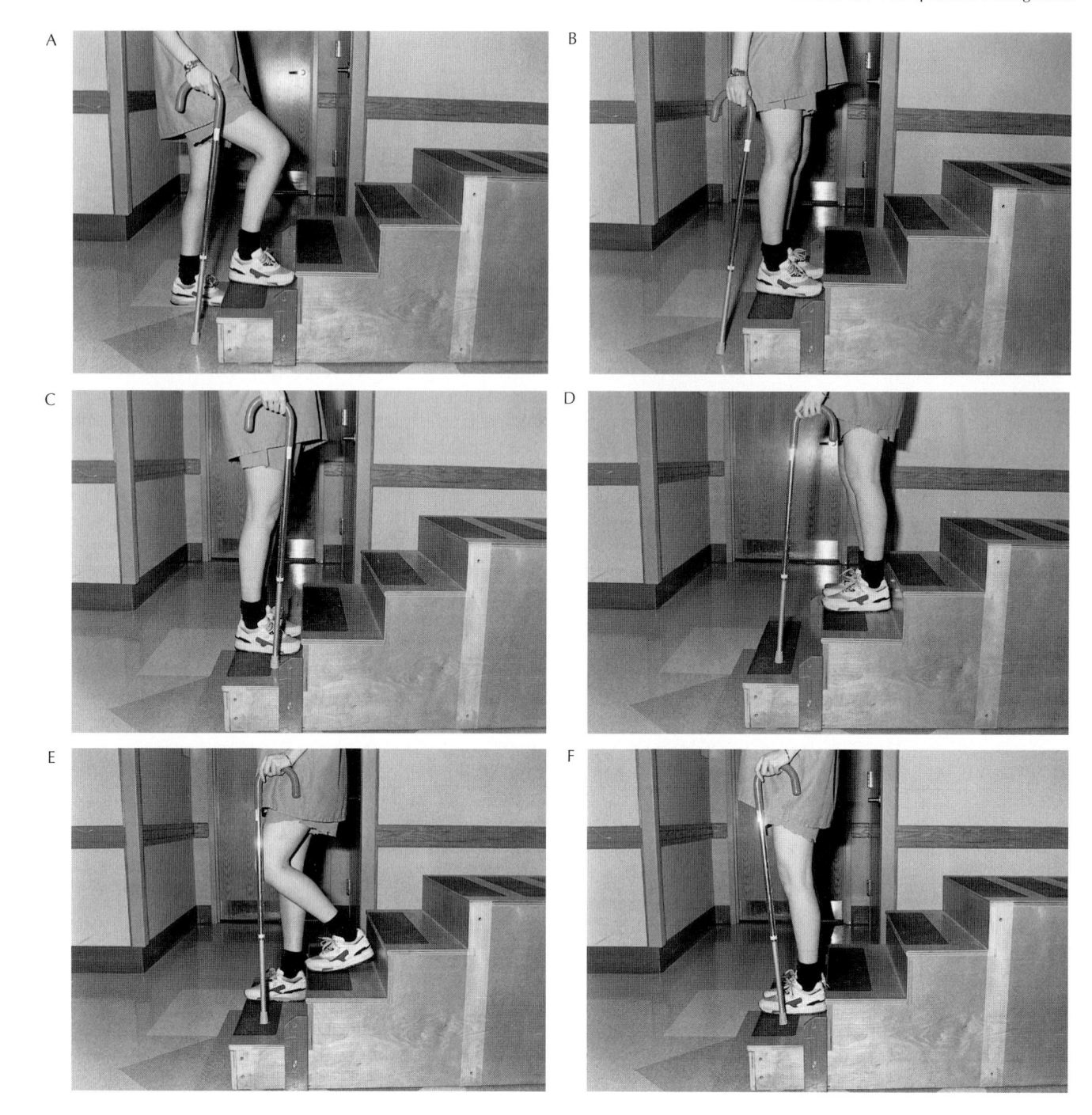

Figure 89.2. Stair-climbing instruction.

dent upon the caregivers for most ADLs and mobility. There is knee discomfort, which is usually moderate in nature. Pain management is extremely important and skillfully managed by the pain service. It is during these days that we strive for ADL independence and gait training. The next series of "sixes" encompasses weeks 2 through 6. Strengthening the lower limbs and mastering the gait cycle is stressed. We emphasize proper gait mechanics and cadence in progressing ambulation using an assistant device to independence without a device (if no other debilitating conditions are present preoperative or postoperative). The last in the series of "sixes" extends through 6 months postoperative. We now focus on functional gains and return to usual ADLs. It is not until completion of this phase that many people experience the outcome they anticipated preoperative.

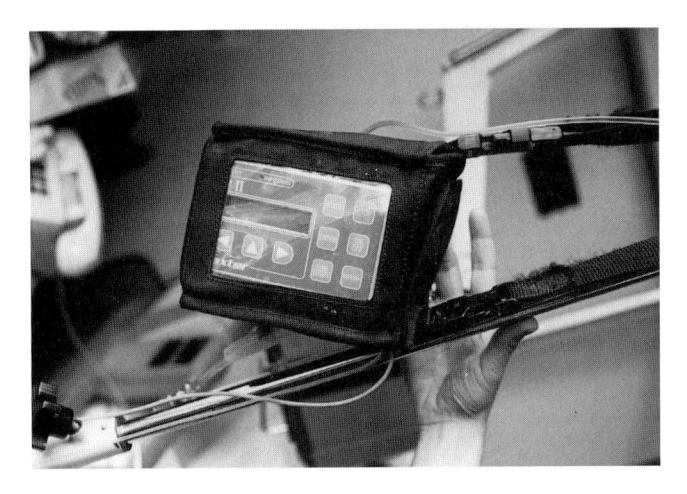

Figure 89.3. PCA: Patient-controlled analgesia.

REHABILITATION

Postoperative rehabilitation begins the day of surgery. A physiatrist with expertise in TKA oversees the rehabilitation program. As a direct extension from the surgeon in the operating room the physiatrist begins the rehabilitation process in the recovery room. Results of the operative procedure are confirmed with the surgical staff and a thorough patient consultation and evaluation is performed. The details of the operative procedure are then reviewed with the patient and treating therapist. A detailed therapeutic prescription plan is written taking into account the patient's medical status and exercise limitations. Any overt aberrations are clearly depicted on the therapy order sheet and verbally communicated to the treating therapist. Daily, the physiatrist updates and/or alters the therapy orders based upon current patient status, both medically and physically. At the same time, postoperative disposition is closely monitored by the physiatrist in close communication with social services.

Phase I

In the recovery room, our goal is to initiate CPM at the maximum tolerable range, usually at least 0 to 60 degrees. Routinely, this is not difficult to achieve in the early hours of recovery. In the immediate postoperative period we see greater ranges than sometimes witnessed on postop day (POD) 1. This is reflective of the postoperative anesthesia effects, which remain for several hours. This is important because the range gains we see early in the recovery phase set the stage for subsequent days. In other words, those who achieve greater ranges during the immediate postoperative period tend to progress ahead of those who achieve lesser ranges. We ask patients to use the CPM machine as much as possible each day and encourage them to sleep with their limb in the machine if desired. Progression is incremental by 5 degrees every few hours and should not produce significant discomfort. We do not recommend progression by greater than 5-degree increments due to potential discomfort. Although the ultimate long-term range of motion after TKA with or without the use of CPM may not differ statistically,[5,6,13] our experience confirms greater early range gains with CPM, which may have direct impact on length of stay. In unpublished data, we have seen a 1 day reduction in length of stay directly related to preadmission education and early range gains with CPM. We continually reinforce the importance of attaining early range of motion. The goal is to attain sufficient range of motion to fruitfully partake in all activities that were impossible prior to TKA. The emphasis on range of motion revolves around the ideal minimal excursion required to master the gait cycle and negotiate stairs. Andriacchi and Wilson, in separate reports, claim that 80 to 90 degrees of knee flexion is required to accommodate these two essential ADLs[16,17] (Fig. 89.5). Shoji claims that 90 degrees of knee flexion is required for many ADLs including arising from a seated position.[18,25] In addition to targeted flexion, we attempt to achieve less than 5 degrees extension deficit (active and passive). We find significant alterations in gait mechanics in those who lack greater than 10 degrees terminal extension. It is also more difficult to compensate for extension than flexion deficits early in the rehabilitation process possibly due to quadriceps weakness. This may be attributed to inefficient eccentric firing of this group if the knee is unable to attain near full extension. Therefore, knee buckling and altered gait mechanics can occur. CPM, although very efficacious in improving flexion range, is less rewarding in achieving extension range. There is great emphasis placed on attaining early range due to a positive correlation between preoperative and postoperative range of motion

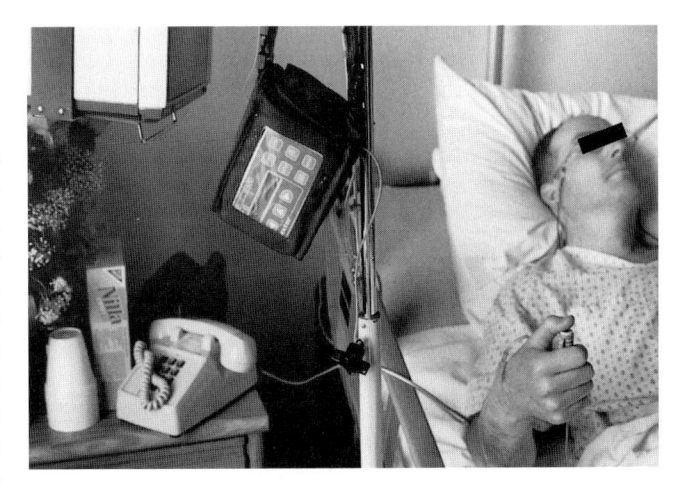

Figure 89.4. PCA device.

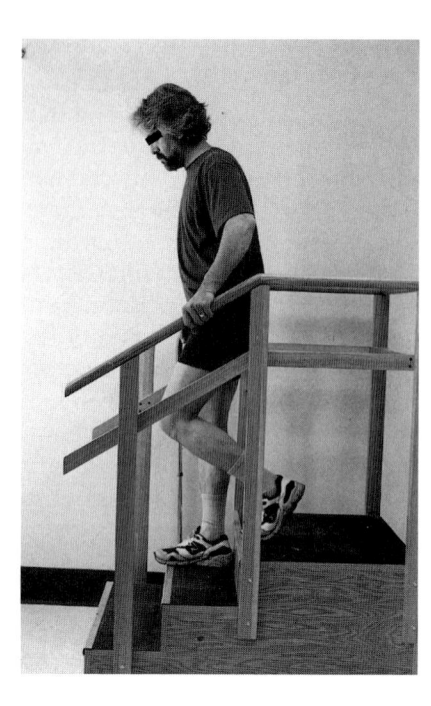

Figure 89.5. Degree of knee flexion on stair descent.

(ROM) as cited by some,[22,23] although disputed by others.[24] We agree with the former, particularly in those patients with a preoperative flexion contracture of greater than 20 degrees. In this group, attaining adequate extension is sometimes difficult. In those with less than a 20-degree flexion contracture, attaining extension is not with much greater effort than in those with minimal to no preoperative contracture. There are many things that lead to potential range limiting factors. One is (postoperative) blood in the knee joint. Education on the potential transformation of copious amounts of blood into motion limiting "scar tissue" is emphasized. The value of early motion inhibiting this process and allowing greater motion gains is stressed. Often patients perceive the therapists as armed forces boot camp drill sergeants. On daily rounds it isn't uncommon to have a patient state "he/she isn't coming back again is he/she? He/she tried to bend my leg like a pretzel." Because it is not without discomfort that early ranges are noted, the transition from operative anesthesia to postoperative analgesia is made very carefully and precisely. In the immediate postoperative period, the pain service begins their very important role in the rehabilitation process. Careful titration of analgesia taking into account potential side effects including drowsiness, bladder or bowel function, respiratory status, GI distress, and hemodynamics, etc., is carried out. An analgesia schedule is created that is coordinated between nursing, rehabilitation therapy, and the pain service to assure appropriate analgesia during the rehabilitation process. Medications are administered at preset times in coordination with scheduled therapy to offer optimal success for each session. Increasing ROM consistently produces the most significant pain in the rehabilitation process so analgesics are prescribed particularly before active assistive ranging by the therapist. Although medication offers pain reduction to assist ranging the knee, other modalities are available as adjuncts in this process. Electrical stimulation (E-stim) can be applied over the ipsilateral quadriceps muscle and acts synergistically during its voluntary contraction to improve knee extension. Its firing coincides with an active quadriceps contraction as regulated by the patient. The use of E-stim has been reported beneficial in improving muscle strength[19,20] and in a related study, to decrease extensor lag (the difference between active and passive motion) while decreasing LOS.[21] Additionally, bracing can be utilized to promote knee extension. Resistive or static splinting (dyna-splint or knee immobilizer respectively) can be applied to assist rather than achieve desired extension range gains. Patients report more discomfort with resistive splinting, but range gains tend to be greater with this technique versus static bracing. In select patients with significant preoperative flexion contractures, fiberglass or plaster casting is applied to maintain and promote extension. Typically this group includes those with greater than 20 degrees flexion contracture and the group with a history of early scar formation (prior surgery with difficulty achieving motion). Some surgeons prefer early static splinting (knee immobilizer) to assist quadriceps function until one is able to safely ambulate while supporting body weight. This usually spans the first few postoperative days. Supportive braces are by no means routine in TKA. Although bracing has a significant presence in orthopedic and musculoskeletal medicine, it has become less popular in the TKA arena. The market is replete with various brace designs. They are categorized as *prophylactic*, *rehabilitative*, and *functional*. All share in common a protective feature to stabilize and/or support the joint braced. Most commonly they are used in ligament injuries either conservatively or postoperative. In 1979, Anderson, Zeman, and Rosenfeld introduced the first *prophylactic* brace, which was used by professional football players.[34] This is a simple brace comprised of a wrap and hinge. A hinged knee sleeve (Fig. 89.6) is an example of such. The efficacy of this design is yet to be substantiated, although its use is widespread.[35] The *rehabilitative* brace (Fig. 89.7) was first introduced by O'Donoghue in 1950.[36] This design was advocated for ligament protection after surgery. Its goal was intended to limit motion and protect the knee against excess load. One pitfall of this design is its potential to promote undue joint stiffness. This is due to the interaction of the knee joint surface with associated proliferative connective tissue.[37] These braces are more

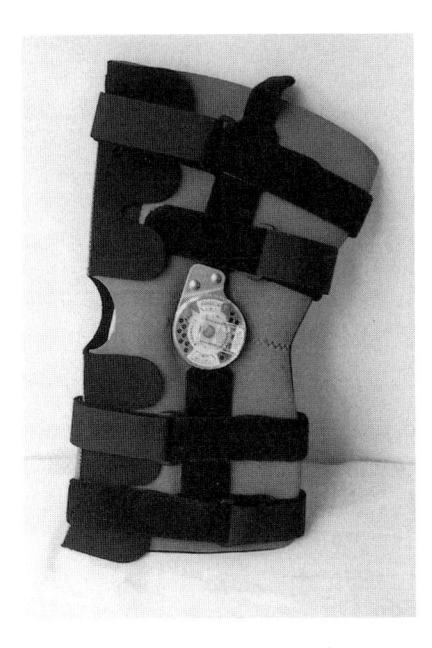

Figure 89.6. Hinged knee sleeve.

complex in design than the prophylactic style often utilizing multiaxis hinges. The *functional* brace (Fig. 89.8) is used when one returns to usual activities of daily living and would benefit from additional joint support. This brace is conforming, and technology aims to adapt it to a low-profile, light-weight design. It too is typically prescribed after ligament injury. As can be seen, these three designs are most commonly used for ligament protection. Their ability to control motion can be shared in the TKA population but for primary TKA they are rarely used. For the average TKA patient, knee stability is adequate and the need for external support rarely required. Although the aforementioned techniques and modalities assist in attaining or stabilizing motion, it should be emphasized that most gains are directly related to the efforts of the patient and therapist. Working in tandem with the pain service, most range gains are achieved by direct active assistive hands on treatment. It is important that a skilled therapist, familiar with TKA, be involved in this treatment. The common denominator related to poor range gains is not overzealous treatment but rather unfamiliarity and "under treatment" by the therapist. As outlined in the TKA protocol (Table 89.6), Phase 1 rehabilitation spans the operative day through POD 5. Encompassing the majority of our first series of "sixes," it is here that early range gains are made. In addition, gait mechanics are stressed along with independence in mobility. Ice is used liberally during this time and its delivery can be via any number of devices. This can be cubes in a plastic bag or a more sophisticated delivery system involving electrical cooling. The main concern is for the system to be effective in delivering "cold." Levy reports decreased blood loss and improvements in early motion and narcotic pain needs with the use of cold compressive dressings.[28] Cold therapy should be administered at the patient's discretion, liberally, with the staff making frequent checks to assure proper icing technique. This includes verification of an intact sensory exam in the area of application. This is to prevent inadvertent

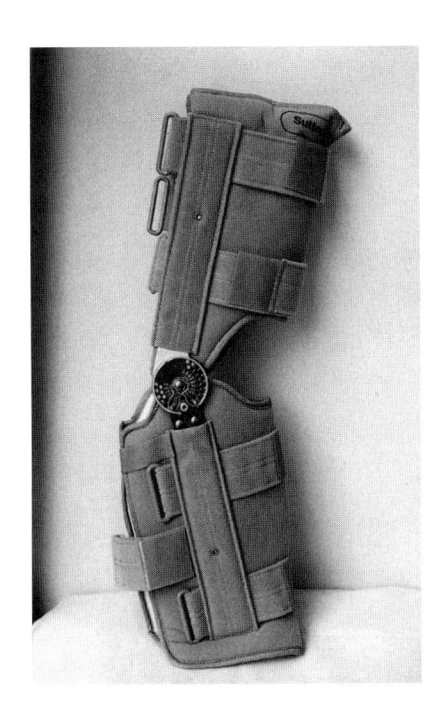

Figure 89.7. Rehabilitative knee brace.

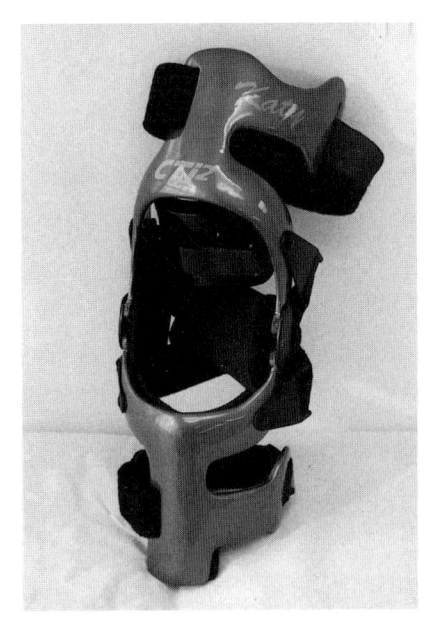

Figure 89.8. Functional knee brace.

freezing or frostbite. In between therapy sessions we advocate independent therapy participation by the patient. If not in the CPM machine or out of bed exercising or consuming a meal, patients are encouraged to perform a series of "bed exercises" (Table 89.7). Instructions for these are placed at each patient's bedside and are to be performed several times each day. Some patients perform these exercises more than the prescribed amount and we encourage this. In addition, we ask patients to perform upper and lower body exercises while in bed and this is accomplished with a device such as Thera-Band (The Hygenic Corporation, Akron, Ohio) (Fig. 89.9). This is a rubber band type substance that is available in different tensions. Each tension grade is specifically color coded and therefore is easily recognized by patients and health-care practitioners. This can be left at the patient's bedside and various resistive exercises performed when patients are not formally in a therapy session. As outlined in the TKA protocol (Table 89.6) emphasis in the immediate postoperative period is on mobility, ROM, and strength gains. Daily goals are reviewed and the rehabilitation team works in tandem with each patient to meet these goals (Fig. 89.10) and demonstrates exercises performed in the early phase of rehabilitation. All exercises are frequently reviewed with the patient by the rehabilitation team. This team includes physicians, therapists, nurses, aids, etc. In addition, patient tracking forms are at the bedside to

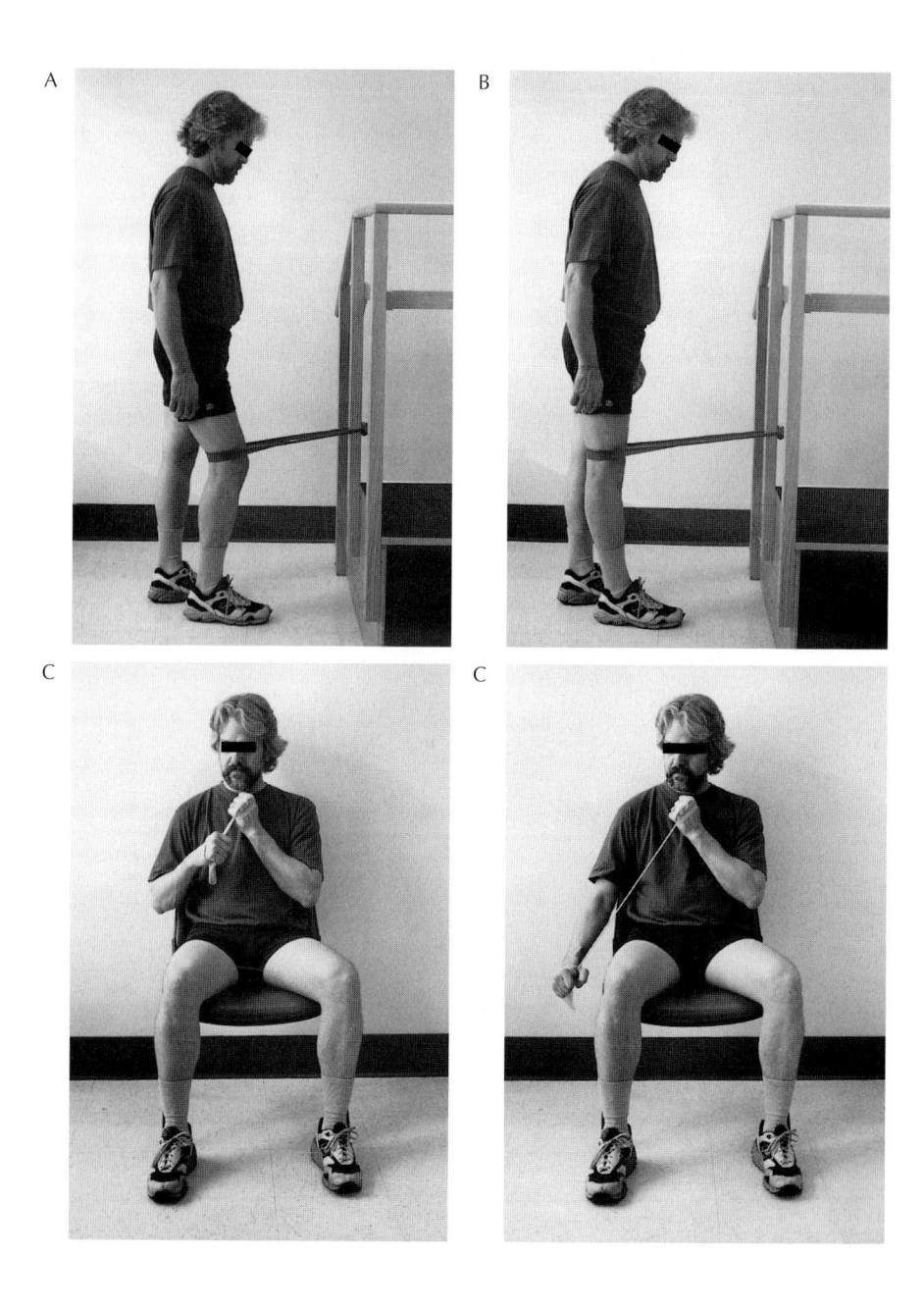

Figure 89.9. Thera Band exercises for the lower and upper extremities.

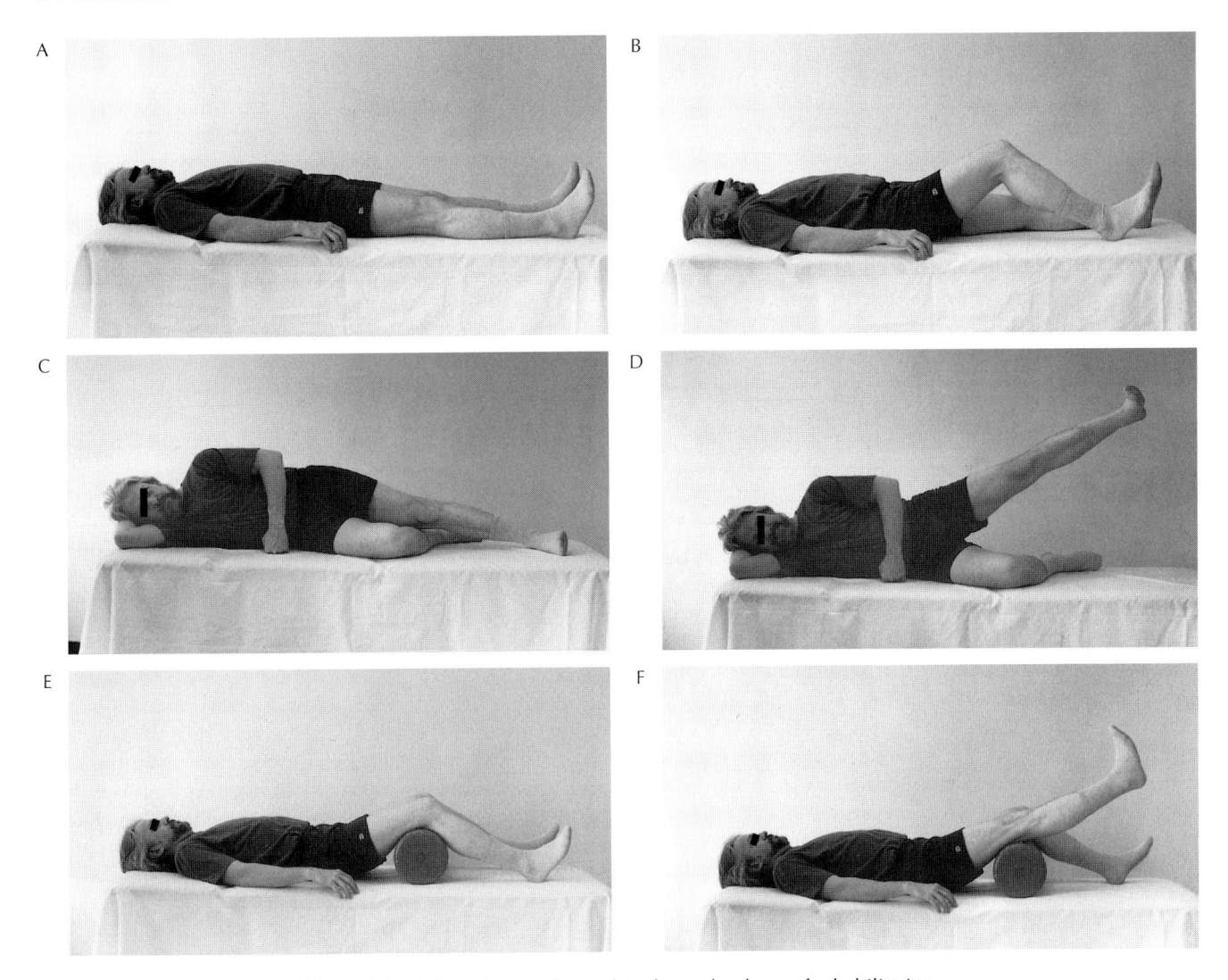

Figure 89.10. Exercises performed in the early phase of rehabilitation.

record daily changes in active range of motion (AROM), passive range of motion (PROM), CPM range, ambulation status, transfer ability, and stair climbing ability (Table 89.8). Patients are often concerned that their assigned therapist may not be "appropriate for them." This can be as simple as male versus female or a concern that the size of the treating therapist is "too small" to handle certain patient morphologies. We try to accommodate patient requests and establish a positive rehabilitation team–patient relationship. We continually assure by word and by action that the rehabilitation team is well staffed and qualified to reach the common goal of maximal performance in the postoperative period. The team approach is ever so critical in this setting. Patient confidence in the rehabilitation team is essential for optimal success. During the hospital stay, patients are seen twice daily Monday through Friday and at least once daily on weekends or holidays. By completion of this phase, independent ambulation with appropriate assistant device, stair climbing (4 to 8 steps), and knee ROM greater than 90 degrees is expected. It is anticipated that patients will be discharged from the hospital to the preadmission setting. Those requiring extended rehabilitation (acute or long-term) hopefully were placed into the appropriate facility by this time. Barring financial restrictions, we attempt to place patients requiring more intensive levels of rehabilitation services into the acute inpatient rehabilitation facility by the second or third postoperative day. For most, this process began during preadmission testing. Keep in mind that most carriers will not approve the rehabilitation admission until the patient begins physical therapy on the acute orthopedic service and has documented acute, inpatient, rehabilitation needs. These commonly relate to ROM, ADL assistance, and ambulation distance. There is no clear consensus about the exact criteria for rehabilitation admission, an issue that complicates the recovery process and potentially prolongs LOS. Dedicated personnel spend many hours engaged in telephone conversation and telecommunication correspondence addressing this matter and to date, confusion prevails. This is a tedious task and often frustrates both the caregivers and patients. Another important criteria for acute rehabilitation admission is the level of confounding comorbid medical conditions. Entities such as rheumatoid arthritis, prior cerebrovascular accident, hypertension, COPD, and multiple sclerosis increase the recovery burden and may complicate discharge planning. It is those with multiple medical entities that usually qualify for acute rehabilitation services because the co-ailments tend to have deleterious effects on recovering from joint arthroplasty. Achieving set goals and improvement in function is not easily achieved in those with confounding medical conditions. A recent review of acute care rehabilitation by Bohannon verified the notion that functional gains influenced discharge disposition, which supports the need for this level of care.[26] In his review, functional measurements were quantified using the functional independence measure system (FIM) (Table 89.9). This reliable system grades one's ability to perform functions such as bed mobility, transfers, locomotion, and stair climbing.[27] Each function is graded 1 (totally dependent) to 7 (totally independent). This is the measure by which most rehabilitation outcomes are tracked. It has a proven record and is easily used. The intensified program offered in the acute rehabilitation setting includes the services of not only daily physical therapy but also daily occupational and recreation therapy along with rehabilitation nursing. Patients focus on functional activities, particularly related to ADLs. More independence in ADLs will decrease the need for home care after discharge. Other functional scales used to assist the planning process for disposition after TKA are the Knee Society Clinical Rating System and SF-36. Kanz and associates concluded that functional deficits specific to the knee in conjunction with general health issues were essential when considering outcome.[37] This information along with the FIM can assist expeditious and appropriate disposition. This can be to home, acute rehabilitation facility, or another center such as sub-acute care, skilled nursing facility, or nursing home. One must not forget the financial implications for expediting the appropriate disposition at the appropriate time. The single greatest expense in TKA (other than implant cost possibly) is the hospital daily charge. A single day decrease in length of stay has significant financial impact on the institution. Responsibility for providing optimal patient care within the economic constraints we face must be shared by all involved.

Phase II

Beginning with the second postoperative week (POW) and continuing through POW 5, rehabilitation emphasizes achievement of maximal knee ROM and independent ambulation with minimal assistance. Activities requiring lateral mobility are introduced including side stepping and carioca (Fig. 89.11). Strengthening of the associated lower extremity muscle groups continues. As the knee effusion begins to abate, greater increases in quadriceps strength will likely be seen. The presence of knee effusion inhibits quadriceps muscle firing[31] and is an important consideration in the rehabilitation process. The presumptive mechanism for effusion related quadriceps inhibition relates to mechanoreceptor sensitivity to capsular strain. The increased intra-articular fluid stresses the encasing capsule stimulating the associated mechanoreceptors to transmit signals to inhibitory interneurons at the spinal level in the central nervous system.[32] These interneurons synapse with alpha motor neurons and inhibit the signals that trigger firing of the quadriceps muscle.[33] The continuous application of ice assists dissipation of the effusion, and to promote quadriceps firing it should remain part of the rehabilitation process for several months. Strength training emphasizes weighted activities as required for ambulation and stair climbing. These include mini step-ups (the height of a conventional step, 6 to 8 inches) (Fig. 89.12), mini knee bends (40 to 50 degrees maximum to avert undue knee stress) (Fig. 89.13), and straight-leg raising (to promote quadriceps strength) (Fig. 89.14). All are done in sets of 10 repetitions, 3 to 5 sets per session.

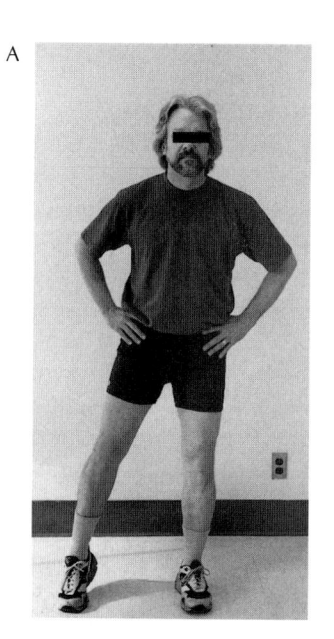

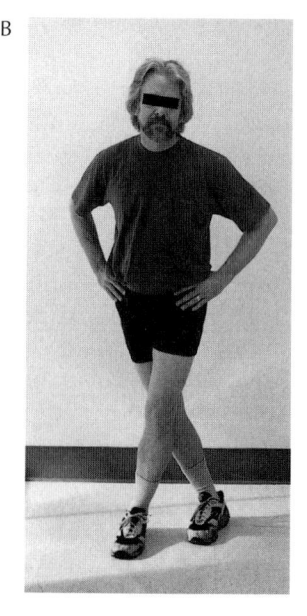

Figure 89.11. Side stepping (A) and carioca (B) exercises.

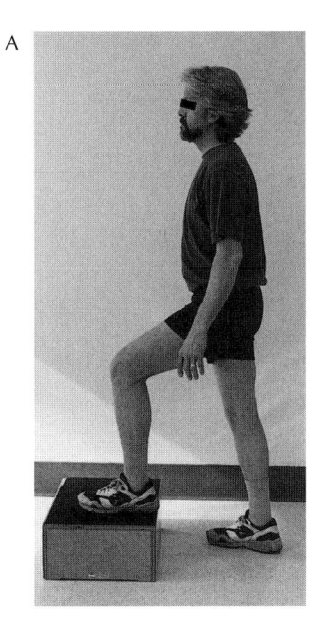

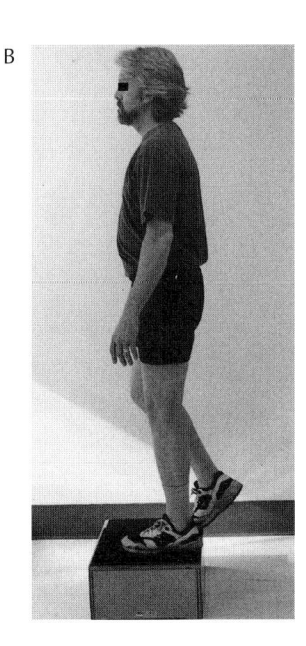

Figure 89.12. The mini step-ups.

During this phase one should not solely focus on strength training but must improve endurance and balance too. Deconditioning is a common sequela after TKA and must be addressed during the rehabilitation process. There is a period of relative immobility surrounding the surgical procedure and stamina is uniformly lacking. Adding to this the fact that a predominantly older population undergoes TKA, one is not surprised that endurance is lacking. However, as the percentage of the elderly population participating in endurance-type activities continues to rise, the stereotype that the older population is "out of shape" probably no longer is accurate. Currently, this age group tends to be in better overall physical condition than in years past. Although endurance may not be as critical in this population as once thought, the overall medical condition still can pose rehabilitation obstacles. In the older population the prevalence of comorbid medical conditions is not uncommon. Being alert to these conditions is essential for a rapid and successful recovery. Taking these factors into account, endurance training may proceed with activities such as riding a stationary bicycle and swimming in a pool. The bicycle exercise begins by adjusting the seat to a low height. This will assist in attaining ROM. The patient should pedal slowly and against minimal resistance. Improving ROM is the only significant goal at this time. As range improves, the seat height is raised to address conditioning and endurance. The reason for the seat height alteration is twofold. The low seat height increases effective ROM of the knee because of the decreased distance between the buttocks and bike pedal. The area for rotary excursion of the involved limb is less now, therefore promoting increased ROM while completing the cycling motion. While efficacious in achieving ROM with the lower seat height, this excess ranging can promote undue patellofemoral stress and possibly lead to anterior knee pain. To avert this, we set the seat height high once satisfactory ROM is achieved. This spares undue patellofemoral forces and allows emphasis on conditioning. The prescription for the stationary bicycle can be determined in several ways. One must first consider complicating medical conditions, particularly cardiac, when setting parameters for this modality. If cardiac disease is present, coordination of care with the patient's cardiologist or primary care physician should be done. This safely determines parameters (resistance, duration, workload, and maximal heart rate) for the cycling exercise. If significant heart disease is present, a coronary stress test may be required to set the above parameters. If no comorbid conditions prevail, we ask patients to begin cycling at very low resistance for 5 minutes, then increase by 5-minute increments. This exercise should be done at least 5 days per week. Most people plateau at 20 to 30 minutes per session 3 to 5 days per week. In addition to the stationary bicycle, swimming activities can begin once the surgical wound is well healed. This typically ranges from 4 days to 4 weeks (barring complications). Surgeon preference usually guides this, but most patients are allowed in the pool within a few weeks postoperative. Initially flutter kicking while supporting the body with the upper extremities on the poolside is recommended. In chest or waist deep water, we begin this exercise by flexing or extending our hips while maintaining extension of the knees. This progresses to flexion or extension of both the hips and knees. "Set

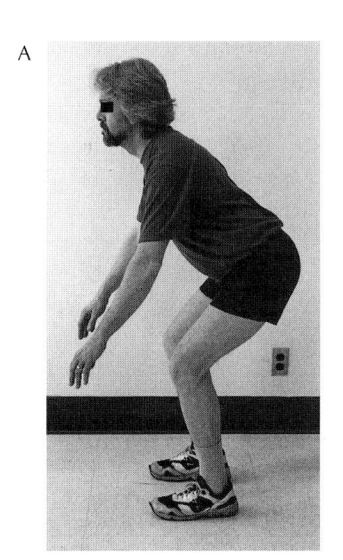

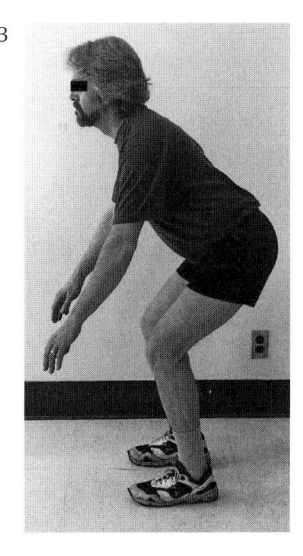

Figure 89.13. The mini knee bends.

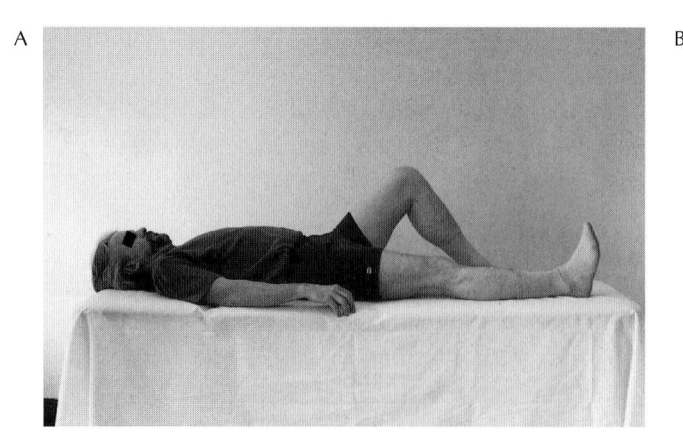

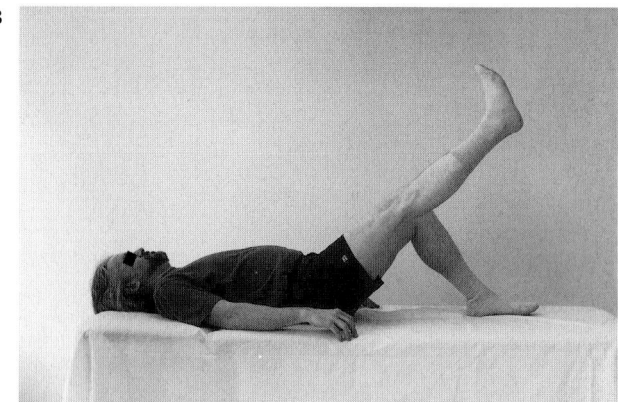

Figure 89.14. Straight leg raise.

number" or "time" guides the exercise prescription. If using "set number," we recommend 10 to 20 repetitions, 3 to 5 sets each. If using "time," the exercise continues for 1 minute and progresses by 30-second intervals. Initially fatigue will guide the workout, but goal setting should incorporate incremental gains on successive sessions. Water exercises can be assisted by utilizing a flotation device. This helps to suspend the body in water and assists underwater exercises such as bicycling, marching in place, jogging, and treading water.[41] The water is an excellent medium to teach balance exercises and stair climbing. Due to the buoyancy effect of water, balance and stair training can be safely and effectively done.[41] Patients have added confidence in the water because a fall due to poor balance in the water does not carry the same sequela as on dry land.

Phase III

This final phase of the rehabilitation program transitions the patient into training from rehabilitating. This usually occurs around 8 weeks postoperative. It should be emphasized that training must continue until at least 6 months postoperative and may continue forever. Training during this phase reemphasizes the essence of Phase II and expands upon strength and functional gains. Our goal is to discard all assistant devices except those required for comorbid conditions. Independence in ADLs and participation in recreational or gainful activities is also anticipated. Again, it must be emphasized that many patients do not subjectively feel significant overall improvement until 6 months postoperative. The body's assimilation of the prosthetic device seems secure at or around this time and directly correlates with patient satisfaction. Although it has been customary to receive "in-home" postoperative rehabilitation for few to several weeks after inpatient discharge, trends now favor decreased post-discharge rehabilitation services particularly in the home setting. More emphasis is placed on independent training or a short course of outpatient therapy. Home videos and improved handouts (with pictorials) now supplement post-discharge care. While this trend continues, the burden of care rests with the health-care provider who must monitor and track outcomes while attempting to create and to enforce revised guidelines in the rehabilitation of this population. It is only through documentation and outcome measurements that guidelines will change reflective of both financial and functional issues. We conclude this phase with a critical assessment of gait mechanics. Performance of video analysis utilizing 3-D digitized kinematic analysis on select patients isolating particular movements that are problematic or biomechanically aberrant is done. This very valuable tool isolates specific kinesiologic parameters that can assist in the detailed analysis and subsequent correction of functional deficits. Although most commonly utilized as a research tool, gait analysis is very effective in isolation of and correction for biomechanical flaws. Entities such as leg length aberrations that are not apparent on static measurements often become apparent on this analysis. The subsequent correction of these discrepancies may reduce the incidence of related mechanical disorders, including low-back pain. Other investigators have likewise utilized gait analysis in assessing functional activities such as stair climbing and gait patterns.[29,30]

CONCLUSION

TKA has given a "new lease on life" to thousands of people afflicted with gait altering and functionally limiting knee pathology. Technology continues to improve prosthetic design, and functional outcomes support the need for further investigation. TKA, once a salvage operation for the painfully degenerative knee, now affords significant improvement of functional ability in those undergoing the procedure. In the not too distant past, all activities requiring impact in excess of simple ambulation was frowned upon in this population. Now, participation in recreational activities such as depicted in Table 89.10 supports the commitment one makes undergoing this procedure. As clearly noted, participation in activities including skiing and tennis are feasible in this population. As research and the dynamics of this procedure improve, postoperative guidelines will also change particularly as the age of those undergoing TKA gets younger. A recent investigation at our institution evaluated activity levels in patients 55 or younger after TKA.[42] One hundred three knees were examined at an average of 8 years postoperatively. The prosthesis was the posterior-stabilized, posterior cruciate-substituting design. Investigative results rated all as good or excellent utilizing the Hospital for Special Surgery and Knee Society scores. Noteworthy was improvement on the Tegner activity score, which showed average improvement from 1.3 preoperatively to 3.5 postoperatively. Twenty-four percent of those evaluated achieved Tegner scores compatible with activities such as tennis, skiing, biking, and heavy farm or construction work. Historically, TKA has not been offered to those of younger age due to several factors. Most important is the anticipation of a subsequent revision TKA in future years due to prosthetic wear. Although earlier designs had shorter longevity, today's designs have expected survivorship of 18 plus years. Modern designs offer flexibility for isolated component alterations, and future designs will undoubtedly have even longer life expectancies. When considering TKA in the younger patient and the potential need for revision surgery, one must ask the question, "Does the associated morbidity and postoperative recovery related to revision TKA outweigh the disability one may experience while postponing TKA for several years to reach an age that will not potentially guarantee the need for such a revision?" In other words, are we justified to ask a person to delay surgery at an earlier age (which is projected to improve function and decrease pain) due to the likelihood of requiring future revision surgery? This issue will continue to be an important factor in TKA planning especially as the age of those undergoing this procedure gets younger. Total joint arthroplasty has afforded many the opportunity to improve function, live with decreased pain, and restore "quality of life." In future years it will continue to play a significant role in musculoskeletal medicine and in doing so, will bridge one from the "world of *disability*" to the "world of *ability*."

References

1. Petty W. Total knee arthroplasty: postoperative care and rehabilitation. In: Petty W, ed. *Total Joint Replacement*. Philadelphia: WB Saunders Company; 1991:533–534.
2. Murin M, Kwok K, Glyn N, et al. Predicting discharge outcome after elective hip and knee arthroplasty. *Am J Phys Med Rehabil*. 1995; 74(4):295.
3. Ganz S. Physical therapy of the knee. In: Insall J, Scott W, Windsor R, et al. *Surgery of the Knee*. 2nd ed. Churchill Livingstone; 1993:1178–1179.
4. Vaughan C, Damiano D, Abel M. How are we doing? Clinical Gait Laboratories. *Biomechanics*. April 1996:69–80.
5. Walker RH, Morris BA, Angulo DC, et al. Postoperative use of continuous passive motion, transcutaneous electrical nerve stimulation, and continuous cooling pad following total knee arthroplasty. *J Arthroplasty*. June 1991; 6(2):151–156.
6. Nadler SF, Malanga GA, Zimmerman JR. Continuous Passive Motion in the Rehabilitation Setting. *Am J Phys Med Rehabil*. June 1993; 72(3):162–164.
7. McInnes J, Larson MG, Daltroy LH, et al. A controlled evaluation of continuous passive motion in patients undergoing total knee arthroplasty. *JAMA*. September 1992; 268(11):1423–1428.
8. Colwell CW, Morris RN. The influence of continuous passive motion on the results of total knee arthroplasty. *Clin Orthop*. March 1992; 276:225–228.
9. Maloney WJ, Schurman DJ, Hangen D, et al. The influence of continuous passive motion on outcome in total knee arthroplasty. *Clin Orthop*. July 1990; 256:162–168.
10. Johnson DP. The effect of continuous passive motion on wound-healing and joint mobility after Knee Arthroplasty. *J Bone Joint Surg*. March 1990; 72-A 3:421–426.
11. McCarthy MR, O'Donoghue PC, Yates JL. The clinical use of continuous passive motion in physical therapy. *JOSPT*. March 1992; 15(3):132–140.
12. Vince KG, Kelly MA, Beck et al. Continuous passive motion after total knee arthroplasty. *J Arthroplasty*. December 1987; 2(4):281–284.
13. Wasilewski SA, Woods LC, Torgerson WR, et al. Value of continuous passive motion in total knee arthroplasty. *Orthopedics*. March 1990; 13(3):291–295.
14. Johnson DP, Deborah DM. Beneficial effects of continuous passive motion after total condylar knee arthroplasty. *Annals of the Royal College of Surgeons of England*. 1992: 74: 412–416.
15. Ververeli PA, Sutton DC, Hearn SL, et al. Continuous passive motion after total knee arthroplasty. *Clin Orthop*. December 1995; 321:208–214.
16. Andriacchi TP, Galante JO, Fermier RW, et al. The influence of total knee replacement design on walking and stair climbing. *J Bone Joint Surg*. 1982; 64A:1328.
17. Wilson SA, McCann PD, Gotlin RS, et al. Comprehensive gait analysis in posterior-stabilized knee arthroplasty. *J Arthroplasty*. 1996; 11(4):359–367.
18. Shoji H, Solomonow M, Yoshino S, et al. Factors affecting postoperative flexion in total knee arthroplasty. *Orthopedics*. June 1990; 13(6):643–649.

19. Balogun JA, Onilari OO, Akeju OA, et al. High voltage electrical stimulation in the augmentation of muscle strength: effects of pulse frequency. *Arch Phys Med Rehabil*. September 1993; 74:910–915.
20. Cheng-Lun Soo, Dean PC, Threlkeld AJ. Augmenting voluntary torque of healthy muscle by optimization of electrical stimulation. *Phys Ther*. March 1988; 68(3):333–337.
21. Gotlin RS, Hershkowitz S, Juris PM, et al. Electrical stimulation effect on extensor lag and length of hospital stay after total knee arthroplasty. *Arch Phys Med Rehabil*. September 1994; 75:957–959.
22. Junnosuke R, Syu S, Kazuki Y, et al. Factors influencing the postoperative range of motion in total knee arthroplasty. *Bulletin Hospital for Joint Diseases*. 1993; 53(3):35–39.
23. Touga S, Kato F, Ito K, et al. Range of motion after total knee replacement. *Japanese Journal of Rheum Joint Surgery*. 1987; 4:559–567.
24. Mullen JO. Range of motion following total knee arthroplasty in ankylosed joint. *Clin Orthop*. 1983; 179:200–203.
25. Ritter MA, Campbell ED. Effect of range of motion on the success of a total knee arthroplasty. *J Arthroplasty*. 1987; 2:95–97.
26. Bohannon RW, Cooper J. Total knee arthroplasty: evaluation of an acute care rehabilitation program. *Arch Phys Med Rehabil*. October 1993; 74:1091–1094.
27. Hamilton BB, Granger CV, Sherwin FS, et al. A uniform national data system for medical rehabilitation. In: Fuhrer MJ, ed. *Rehabilitation Outcomes: Analysis and Measurement*. Baltimore: Paul Brook; 1987.
28. Levy AS, Marmar E. The role of cold compression dressings in the postoperative treatment of total knee arthroplasty. *Clin Orthop*. December 1993; 297:174–178.
29. Skinner HB, Barrack RL, Cook SD, et al. Joint position sense in total knee arthroplasty. *Journal of Orthopedic Research*. 1984; 1:276.
30. Simon SR, Trieshmann HW, Burdett RG, et al. Quantitative gait analysis after total knee arthroplasty for monoarticular degenerative arthritis. *J Bone Joint Surg*. 1983; 65A: 605.
31. McNair PJ, Marshall RN, Maguire K. Swelling of the knee joint: effects of exercise on quadriceps muscle strength. *Arch Phys Med Rehabil*. 1996; 77:896–899.
32. Wood L, Ferrell WR. Response of slowly adapting articular mechanoreceptors in the cat knee joint to alterations in intra-articular volume. *Annals of Rheumatologic Disease*. 1984; 43:327–332.
33. Spencer JD, Hayes KC, Alexander IJ. Knee joint effusion and quadriceps reflex inhibition in man. *Arch Phys Med Rehabil*. 1984; 65:171–177.
34. Anderson G, Zeman S, Rosenfeld R. The Anderson knee stabler. *Physician in Sports Medicine*. 1979; 7:125.
35. Johnston JM, Paulos LE. Prophylactic lateral knee braces. *Medicine and Science in Sports and Exercise*. 1991; 23(7): 787.
36. O'Donoghue DH. Surgical treatment of fresh injuries to the major ligaments of the knee. *J Bone Joint Surg*. 1950; 32A:721.
37. Enneking WF, Horowitz M. The intraarticular effects of immobilization on the human knee. *J Bone Joint Surg*. 1972; 4A:973.
38. Kantz ME, Harris WJ, Levitsky K, et al. Methods for assessing condition-specific and generic functional status outcomes after total knee replacement. *Medical Care*. May, 1992; 30(5):251.
39. McQueen DA, Kelley HK, Wright TF. A comparison of epidural and non-epidural anesthesia and analgesia in total hip or knee arthroplasty patients. *Orthopedics*. February 1992; 15(2):169–173.
40. Pati AB, Perme DC, Trail M, et al. Rehabilitation parameters in total knee replacement patients undergoing epidural vs. conventional analgesia. *JOSPT*. February 1994; 19(2):88–92.
41. Charness AL. Treatment for patients with lower extremity total joint replacement, aquatic therapy. *Biomechanics*. April 1996:63–67.
42. Diduch DR, Insall JN, Scott WN, et al. Total knee replacement in young, active patients: long term follow up and functional outcome. Presented at AAOS Annual Meeting. San Francisco, California, February 1997.
43. deAndrade JR. Activities after replacement of the hip or knee. *Orthopedic Special Edition*. Summer 1995; 1(1):32–33.
44. Evans RL, Connis RT, Hendricks RD, et al. Multidisciplinary rehabilitation versus medical care: a meta-analysis. *Soc Sci Med* 1995; 40(12):1699–1706.

Table 89.1. Total knee arthroplasty—initial patient questionnaire

DATE: _/_/_   MEDICAL RECORD#_____

NAME (LAST, FIRST, MI):_____

EXAMINATION PERIOD: ❑ PRE-OP ❑ 6 MONTHS ❑ 1 YEAR ❑ __YEAR

OPERATED SIDE: ❑ LEFT ❑ RIGHT

Your doctors are carefully evaluating the condition of your knee before and after surgery. Your response to the questions below will help us gather important information that will improve our ability to offer high quality care to patients with knee arthritis. *Questions about your knee refer to the knee that was or will be operated on.* If you have already had knee replacement surgery on this knee, please complete sections 1 and 2 of the questionnaire. If you have not had your knee replaced just complete section 1.

<u>NOTE</u>: PLEASE INDICATE ONLY ONE (1) ANSWER FOR EACH QUESTION

SECTION #1—*All patients should complete this section.*

1. On a scale of 0 to 10 with 0 meaning "no pain" and 10 meaning "severe pain" please indicate the degree of knee pain that you <u>regularly</u> experience. (**Analog**)

   No Pain   Severe Pain
   ❑ 0 ❑ 1 ❑ 2 ❑ 3 ❑ 4 ❑ 5 ❑ 6 ❑ 7 ❑ 8 ❑ 9 ❑ 10

2. Do you experience any knee pain when you are walking? (**Walking**)
   ❑ None/Or you ignore it
   ❑ Mild/Occasional or intermittent
   ❑ Mild/Stairs only
   ❑ Mild Stairs and level walking
   ❑ Moderate/Pain comes and goes
   ❑ Moderate/Pain each day
   ❑ Severe/Constant, disabling pain

3. Do you experience any knee pain when you are at rest? (**Resting**)
   ❑ None
   ❑ Mild
   ❑ Moderate
   ❑ Severe

4. If you have pain in your knee, where do you feel it? (You may choose more than one.)
   ❑ In the front on the knee
   ❑ In the inner side of the knee (medial)
   ❑ In the outer side of the knee (lateral)
   ❑ In the back of the knee
   ❑ In the entire knee area
   ❑ Not applicable/No pain

5. Which is your current activity level? (**Activity**)
   ❑ I am bedridden or confined to a wheelchair.
   ❑ I am sedentary with minimal capacity for walking or other activity.
   ❑ I perform light labor such as house cleaning, yardwork, assembly line work, light sports.
   ❑ I perform moderate manual labor with lifting heavy weight, and participate in moderate sports such as walking or bicycling.
   ❑ I participate in heavy manual labor, I frequently lift heavy weights and participate in vigorous activity such as tennis and racquetball.

6. Do you need assistance in getting out of bed? (**Transfer**)
   ❑ I can get out of bed on my own.
   ❑ I need the assistance of another person.

7. What is your current work capacity? (**Work Capacity**)
   ❑ 100% of normal
   ❑ 75% of normal
   ❑ 50% of normal
   ❑ 25% of normal
   ❑ 0% of normal

8. How do you put on shoes and socks? (**Shoes/Socks**)
   ❑ With no difficulty
   ❑ With slight difficulty
   ❑ With extreme difficulty
   ❑ I am unable to do it without assistance.

9. How do you go up and down stairs? (**Stairs**)
   ❑ Normally (one foot on each step).
   ❑ Normally but require use of the rail when going down.
   ❑ I require use of the rail while going up and down.
   ❑ I can go up the stairs by using the rail but I am unable to go down.
   ❑ I am unable to go up and down stairs.

(Continued)

Table 89.1. (Continued)

10. How do you stand up from a sitting position? **(Sit to Stand)**
    - ❏ I can arise from a chair without using my arms.
    - ❏ I have to use my arms to help me get up from a chair.
    - ❏ I cannot get up from a chair without assistance from another person.
11. Do you need support when walking? **(Walking Support)**
    - ❏ I walk without any support
    - ❏ I use one cane when I go on a long walk
    - ❏ I use one cane most of the time
    - ❏ I use one crutch
    - ❏ I use two canes
    - ❏ I use two crutches
    - ❏ I use a walker
    - ❏ I am unable to walk
12. How long can you walk <u>without</u> support? (i.e., a cane, or crutches, etc.) **(Time Walked/ No Support)**
    - ❏ I can walk an unlimited amount of time, more than 60 minutes, without support.
    - ❏ I can only walk 31–60 minutes without support.
    - ❏ I can only walk 11–30 minutes without support.
    - ❏ I can only walk 2–10 minutes without support.
    - ❏ I can only walk less than 2 minutes without support.
    - ❏ I am unable to walk without support.
13. How long can you walk <u>with</u> support? **(Time Walked/With Support)**
    - ❏ Unlimited, greater than 60 minutes
    - ❏ 31–60 minutes
    - ❏ 11–30 minutes
    - ❏ 2–10 minutes
    - ❏ Less than 2 minutes
    - ❏ I am unable to walk
    - ❏ Not applicable/I walk without support
14. How far can you walk without stopping because of knee pain? **(Distance)**
    - ❏ I can walk unlimited distances
    - ❏ I can walk more than 10 blocks
    - ❏ I can walk 5–10 blocks
    - ❏ I can walk less than 5 blocks
    - ❏ I can only walk short distances within my home
    - ❏ I am confined to a wheelchair or a bed
15. How long can you sit in a chair? **(Sitting)**
    - ❏ I am comfortable sitting in any chair one hour or longer.
    - ❏ I am only comfortable sitting in a high chair for 30 minutes or less.
    - ❏ I am unable to sit comfortably in a chair.
16. How do you get in and out of a car? **(Car)**
    - ❏ It is easy
    - ❏ It is difficult
    - ❏ I am unable to sit comfortably in any chair
17. Could you utilize public transportation such as a bus or subway if you wanted to use it? **(Public Transportation)**
    - ❏ Yes
    - ❏ No
18. Does this knee interfere with sleeping? **(Sleep)**
    - ❏ Yes
    - ❏ No
19. Does this knee interfere with sexual activity? **(Sex)**
    - ❏ Yes
    - ❏ No
20. What medications are you currently taking <u>for your knee</u>? (You may choose more than one answer) **(Medication)**
    - ❏ None
    - ❏ Anti-inflammatory medicine such as aspirin, Advil, ibuprofen, etc.
    - ❏ Steroid medication
    - ❏ Narcotic medication
    - ❏ Other medication
21. Do you <u>often</u> have pain in any joints besides your operative knee? (You may choose more than one answer) **(Other Joint Pain)**
    - ❏ None
    - ❏ Low Back Pain
    - ❏ Operative Side: ❏ Hip   ❏ Shoulder   ❏ Ankle/Foot
    - ❏ Other Side: ❏ Hip   ❏ Shoulder   ❏ Ankle/Foot   ❏ Knee

Source: From Summit Medical Systems, Inc., 1993, Minneapolis, MN.

Table 89.2. Physical medicine and rehabilitation physical therapy discharge questionnaire

The Department of Physical Medicine and Rehabilitation strives to provide the highest quality care to those undergoing joint replacement surgery and rehabilitation. Our staff continually analyzes and critiques protocols attempting to assure optimal outcome. It would benefit all if you would be kind enough to complete the following survey prior to your discharge.

1) Who was your surgeon? _____
2) What procedure did you have? _____ Date _____
3) Did you receive preoperative physical therapy?   ❏ Yes   ❏ No
4) If yes, did you find it: ❏ very beneficial   ❏ beneficial   ❏ not beneficial
5) How many times/day did you receive physical therapy?   ❏ 1   ❏ 2   ❏ 3
    Approximately how long was each session?   ❏ 1–15 min   ❏ 16–30 min   ❏ >30 min
6) Were you given your bed exercises on your first day after surgery?   ❏ Yes   ❏ No
7) How many times/day did you perform these exercises?   ❏ 1   ❏ 2   ❏ 3   ❏ >3
8) What was most difficult in arising from bed the first day postop? _____
   _____
9) Did the pain medication help your participation in therapy?   ❏ Yes   ❏ No
10) How many times/day did you use the CPM?   ❏ None   ❏ 1×   ❏ 2×   ❏ 3×   ❏ >3×
11) Who most often assisted you getting into the CPM? _____
12) How many times/day did you sit up in the chair? _____ For approximately how
    long each time?   ❏ 1–5 min   ❏ 6–15 min   ❏ 16 min–30 min   ❏ >30 min
13) Did you sit in the chair for meals?   ❏ Yes   ❏ No
14) Which staff members most often assisted you back into bed?
    ❏ Physical Therapist   ❏ Nurse   ❏ Physical Therapy Aide   ❏ Nursing Assistant
    ❏ Other _____
15) What day after surgery did you start walking to the bathroom?
    ❏ 1st   ❏ 2nd   ❏ 3rd   ❏ 4th
16) Did you use the ❏ bedpan or ❏ bathroom more in the hospital?
17) Did other staff members assist your ambulation besides the physical therapist?
    ❏ Yes   ❏ No
18) On what day did you attempt stair climbing? _____
19) Did you attend any group sessions?   ❏ Yes   ❏ No   If so, how many? _____
20) Did the therapist review a home exercise program with you?   ❏ Yes   ❏ No
    Were written instructions given?   ❏ Yes   ❏ No

Additional Comments: (if you need more space please use the back of the sheet)
_____
_____

Name: (optional) _____ Today's date _____

Table 89.3. Total knee arthroplasty—F/U questionnaire

DATE: __/__/__ MEDICAL RECORD# _____
NAME (LAST, FIRST, MI): _____
EXAMINATION PERIOD: ❏ PRE-OP ❏ 6 MONTHS ❏ 1 YEAR ❏ __ YEAR
OPERATED SIDE: ❏ LEFT ❏ RIGHT

Your doctors are carefully evaluating the condition of your knee before and after surgery. Your response to the questions below will help us gather important information that will improve our ability to offer high quality care to patients with knee arthritis. *Questions about your knee refer to the knee that was or will be operated on.*

NOTE: PLEASE INDICATE ONLY ONE (1) ANSWER FOR EACH QUESTION

1. On a scale of 0 to 10 with 0 meaning "no pain" and 10 meaning "severe pain" please indicate the degree of knee pain that you <u>regularly</u> experience. **(Analog)**
    No Pain   Severe Pain
    ❏ 0 ❏ 1 ❏ 2 ❏ 3 ❏ 4 ❏ 5 ❏ 6 ❏ 7 ❏ 8 ❏ 9 ❏ 10
2. Do you experience any knee pain when you are walking? **(Walking)**
    ❏ None/Or you ignore it
    ❏ Mild/Occasional or intermittent
    ❏ Mild/Stairs only
    ❏ Mild Stairs and level walking
    ❏ Moderate/Pain comes and goes
    ❏ Moderate/Pain each day
    ❏ Severe/Constant, disabling pain
3. Do you experience any knee pain when you are at rest? **(Resting)**
    ❏ None
    ❏ Mild
    ❏ Moderate
    ❏ Severe
4. Do you need assistance in getting out of bed? **(Transfer)**
    ❏ I can get out of bed on my own.
    ❏ I need the assistance of another person.
5. How do you go up and down stairs? **(Stairs)**
    ❏ Normally (one foot on each step).
    ❏ Normally but require use of the rail when going down.
    ❏ I require use of the rail while going up and down.
    ❏ I can go up the stairs by using the rail but I am unable to go down.
    ❏ I am unable to go up and down stairs.
6. Do you need support when walking? **(Walking Support)**
    ❏ I walk without any support
    ❏ I use one cane when I go on a long walk
    ❏ I use one cane most of the time
    ❏ I use one crutch
    ❏ I use two canes
    ❏ I use two crutches
    ❏ I use a walker
    ❏ I am unable to walk
7. How far can you walk without stopping because of knee pain? **(Distance)**
    ❏ I can walk unlimited distances
    ❏ I can walk more than 10 blocks
    ❏ I can walk 5–10 blocks
    ❏ I can walk less than 5 blocks
    ❏ I can only walk short distances within my home
    ❏ I am confined to a wheelchair or a bed

Source: Summit Medical Systems, Inc., 1993, Minneapolis, MN.

Table 89.4. Beth Israel Medical Center Department of Physical Medicine and Rehabilitation, Preoperative information for total knee arthroplasty candidates

The following packet is a general overview of the physical therapy program you will receive after your surgery. It may be altered by your doctor or therapist according to your individual needs. We are available to help you get back on your feet. The physical therapist will:

1. help you become independent getting in and out of bed.
2. help you become independent walking with the necessary assistive device (walker, crutches or cane).
3. help you walk up and down stairs.
4. help you bend and straighten your knee.
5. educate you on the use of the CPM (continuous passive motion) machine, a device that will slowly bend and straighten your knee. This device will be attached to or placed on your bed for use while you are in bed.
6. educate you on proper leg positioning, i.e., when in bed and not in the CPM machine, your knee should be straight with a **towel or blanket under your ankle**.

You will be scheduled for physical therapy twice per day Monday through Friday and once per day on the weekends.

On the day of surgery, the CPM machine will be started in the recovery room.

On the morning after your surgery, physical therapy will begin. You will:

1. perform the knee bedside exercises (see attached sheet).
2. be assisted to sit up and dangle your legs at the edge of the bed.
3. be assisted to walk using a walker or other assistive device.
4. continue the use of the CPM machine.

From this point, physical therapy will progress. You will be encouraged to walk longer distances and bend your knee further. As your walking improves, you will be progressed to crutches or a cane. Your goals for discharge (3–5 days after surgery) will include the following:

1. independent ambulation on level surfaces and stairs with assistive device.
2. bending your knee to a right angle.
3. safely demonstrating your home exercise program (HEP).

It is important that you do the bedside exercises on your own, at least five times per day. This will help strengthen your lower extremity and achieve the goals for discharge.

Icing your knee is also very important and should be done frequently throughout the day. To get ice, you must ask your nurse, nurse's aide, or physical therapist.

As soon as you can walk with assistance to the bathroom, we encourage you to do so instead of using the bedpan. A nurse, or nurse's aide or physical therapist can assist you to the bathroom. You should eat your meals while sitting in a chair with your legs dangling. At times, you may not feel like getting up for meals, but please try to do so. It will speed your recovery. If the meal is delivered while you are in bed, just call the nurse and someone will come to assist you to the chair.

Please bring soft rubber soled shoes for ambulating.

On behalf of the Department of Physical Medicine and Rehabilitation at Beth Israel Medical Center we look forward to working with you. If you have any questions, please contact us at (212) 870-9221 for the North Division, or (212) 420-2750 at the Petrie Campus.

Table 89.5. Beth Israel Medical Center Department of Physical Medicine and Rehabilitation, home exercise programs

TOTAL KNEE ARTHROPLASTY HOME EXERCISE PROGRAM

The home exercise program will assist your recovery and improve strength. It is important that you take time to exercise every day. The exercise program will take approximately 30 minutes to complete and should be done two times per day. If you are having any problems with the exercises, please call Beth Israel Medical Center, Dept. of Physical Medicine and Rehabilitation at (212) 870-9221 for the North Division, or (212) 420-2750 for the Petrie Campus.

Recovering from a total knee replacement and returning to a more active lifestyle will take time. It is important to be patient, to be an active participant in your exercise program, and to strictly follow the guidelines outlined in the enclosed packet.

Important Information

Now that you are home, you must keep working on bending and straightening your leg, as well as help increase the range of motion of your knee. This will enable you to walk, climb stairs and curbs, and sit on chairs or on the toilet.

1. It will take approximately six months for the swelling in your knee to go down. Therefore, it is important to ice your knee 3–4 times per day for at least the first six weeks after surgery. This should be done for 10–20 minutes at a time. The best time to ice is after you exercise or do a lot of walking. To ice, you can use storage sized Ziplock bags filled with ice, or two large (10″ × 14″) gel packs, which can be purchased at a surgical supply store. The best way for icing your knee is with the knee extended, i.e., straight with a towel rolled under your ankle.
2. Try not to sit for more than 45 minutes at any given time because your knee may become stiff and/or swelling of the entire leg may occur. If you wish to sit for longer periods of time, i.e., watching a movie or T.V., you should stand and walk a short distance and attempt to bend and straighten your knee several times.
3. Do not sleep or sit with anything under your knee, i.e., a pillow.
4. If at anytime you notice persistent fever, swelling, pain, or drainage from your wound, immediately call your surgeon.
5. It is important that all physicians and dentists caring for you to know that you have a joint prosthesis. You will require antibiotics before and after any invasive procedures or dental work to protect against infection. You will be given a "medical alert" card.
6. Your new knee may activate metal detectors in airports and department stores. This is noted on your "medical alert" card.

HOME EXERCISE PROGRAM FOLLOWING TOTAL KNEE REPLACEMENT (TKR)

PLEASE DO EACH EXERCISE 30 TIMES, TWO TIMES A DAY
DO NOT HOLD YOUR BREATH WHILE EXERCISING
THESE EXERCISES ARE MOST IMPORTANT FOR YOUR KNEE

1- ANKLE PUMPS:
While lying flat on your back with your knee straight, bend ankle up and down as far as possible in both directions. Repeat with other leg.

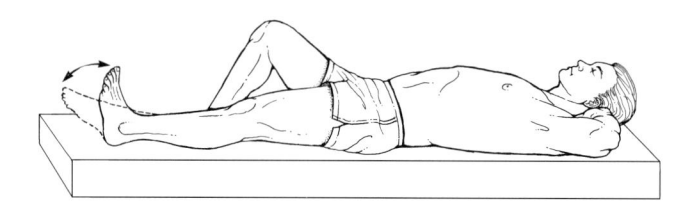

**2- HEEL SLIDES:
While lying flat on your back with your knees straight, slowly slide your heel in toward your buttocks. You should then straighten to the starting position. Please keep your foot on the surface at all times. Repeat with other leg.

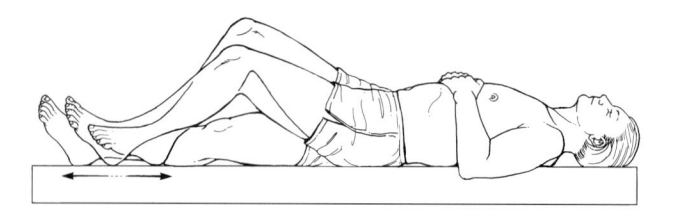

Table 89.5. (Continued)

3- KNEE PRESS:
With your legs straight and a towel rolled up <u>under your ankle</u>, press knee down for contracting your thigh muscle.
Hold for 5 seconds and then relax. Repeat with other leg.

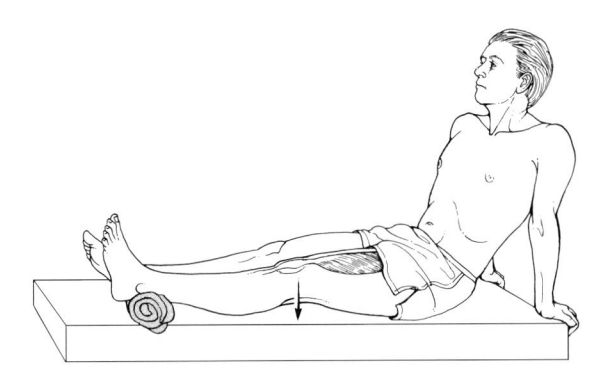

4- STRAIGHT LEG RAISE:
While lying flat on your back with your uninvolved leg bent and your foot flat on the surface, **tighten** your thigh and lift your involved leg. Keep your knee straight. Only lift to the height of the uninvolved knee. Repeat with other leg.

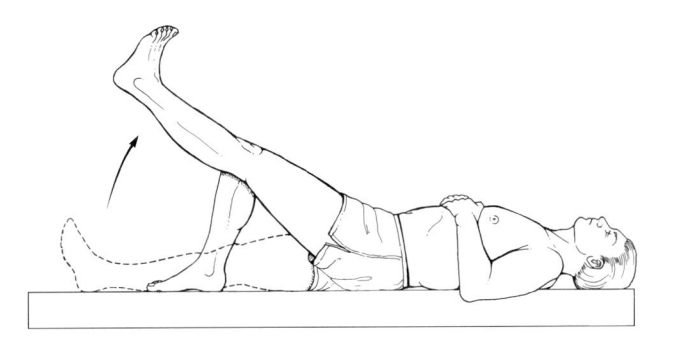

5- SIDE LYING ABDUCTION:
While lying on your uninvolved side bend your uninvolved leg forward.
Raise involved leg about five inches and then lower to the starting position.
Do Not allow your toes or knee to turn upward. Repeat with other leg.

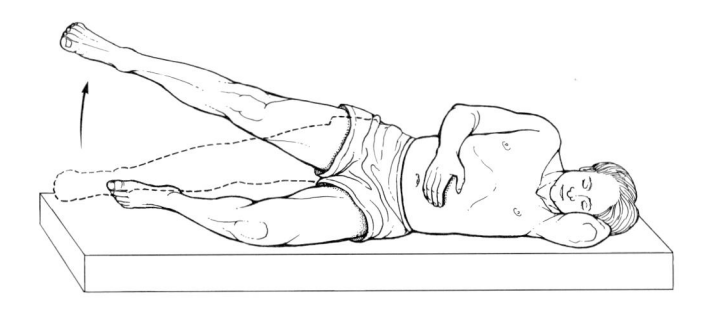

(Continued)

Table 89.5. (Continued)

6- SITTING KNEE EXTENSION:
While sitting in a chair, straighten your involved knee as far as you can.
Hold for 5 seconds. Repeat with other leg.

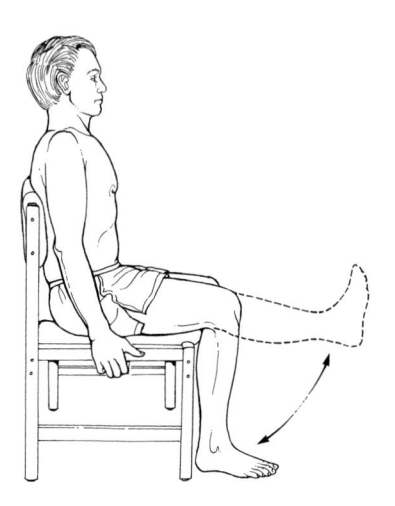

FOR ALL STANDING EXERCISES, BE SURE TO MAINTAIN UPRIGHT POSTURE.

7- STANDING KNEE BENDING:
While holding on to a supportive surface, i.e. a counter top, bend your involved knee so that your foot rises toward your buttock.
Do not twist your leg inward or outward.
Then perform with your uninvolved leg.

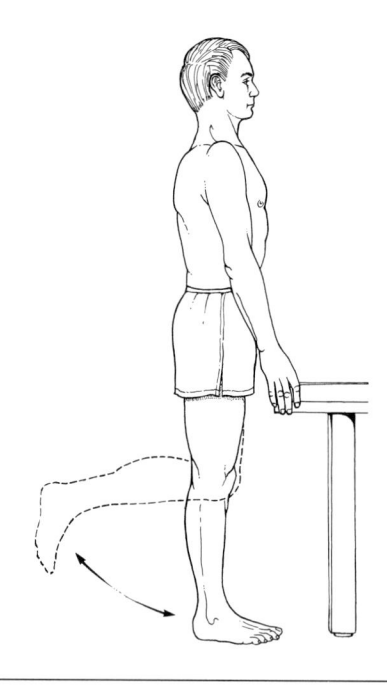

Table 89.5. (Continued)

8- STANDING HIP BENDING:
While holding on to a supportive surface, lift your knee up toward your shoulder by bending at the hip and knee.
Then perform with your uninvolved leg.

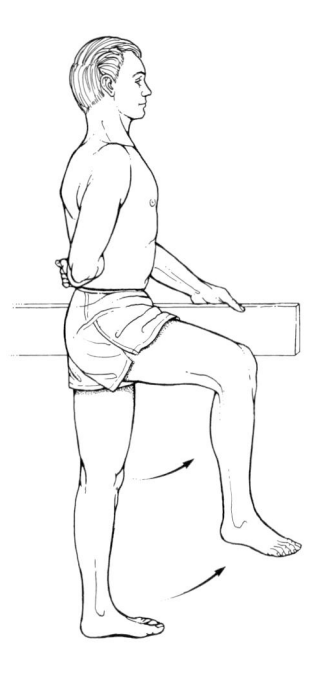

9- STANDING HIP ABDUCTION:
While holding on to a supportive surface, bring your involved leg out to the side keeping your toes pointing forward.
Then perform with your uninvolved leg.

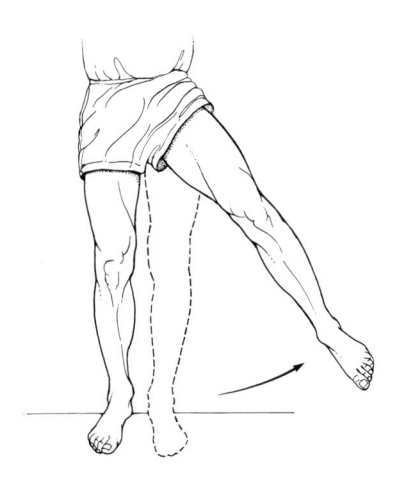

(Continued)

Table 89.5. (Continued)

10- STANDING HIP EXTENSION:
   While holding on to a supportive surface, bring your involved leg back keeping your knee straight. Then perform with your uninvolved leg.

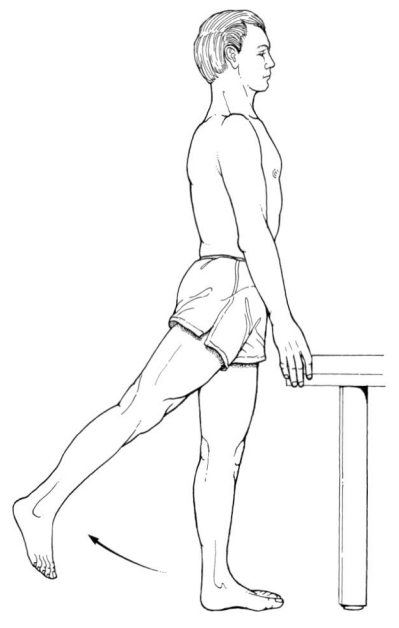

11- STANDING TERMINAL KNEE EXTENSION:
   While holding on to a supportive surface, bend your involved knee slightly. Gently pull back your knee by tightening your thigh muscles, straightening your knee.
   Hold for 5 seconds. Do not over extend your knee.

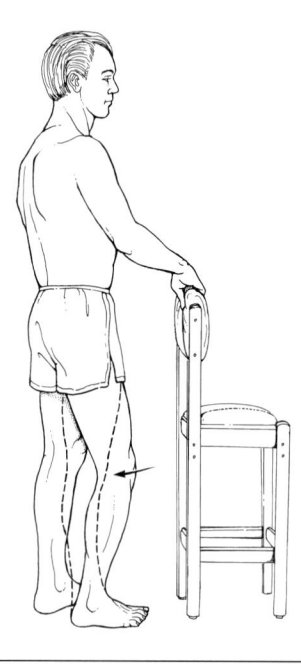

Table 89.5. (Continued)

12- HEEL RAISES:
   While holding on to a supportive surface, lift both heels off the ground toward the ceiling.
   Hold for 5 seconds and then slowly return to the starting position.

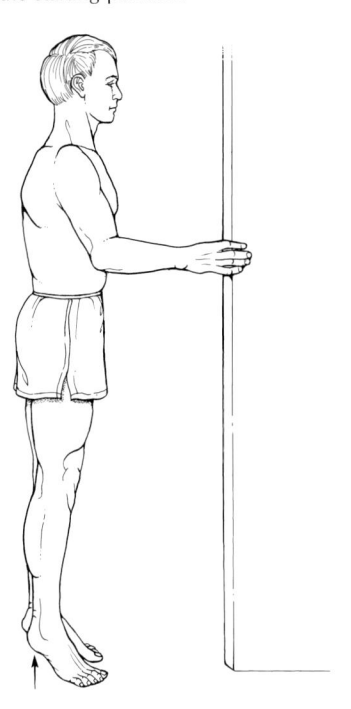

**13-SITTING ASSISTED KNEE BEND:
   While sitting in a chair with your uninvolved leg crossed in front of your involved ankle, push your involved foot backwards, assisting with the bending of the knee.
   Hold for 5 seconds.

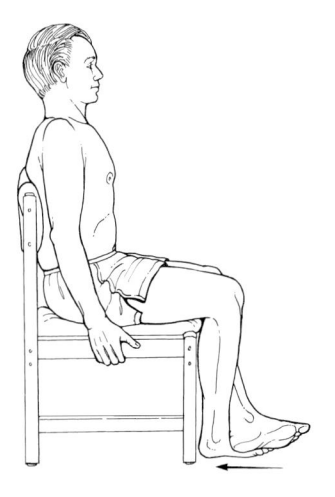

September 13, 1996

Table 89.6. Beth Israel Medical Center Department of Physical Medicine and Rehabilitation TKA protocol

TOTAL KNEE ARTHROPLASTY (TKA) POSTOPERATIVE REHABILITATION PROTOCOL

Phase I–Early Function (Week 1)

GOALS:
1. Demonstrate home exercise program (HEP), proper ambulation, continuous passive motion (CPM) use, icing, and range of motion (ROM).
2. Independence in getting in and out of bed and transfers between various surfaces.
3. Independent ambulation with appropriate assistant device.
4. Stair negotiation with supervision.
5. Early balance control.
6. Attain full extension and 90 degrees flexion of the involved knee.

Preoperative Physical Therapy

The patient is seen for a preoperative physical therapy session which includes:
- review of the hospital TKR protocol.
- review of all bedside exercises.
- instruction for CPM use and ROM exercises.
- ambulation training with a standard walker on level surfaces.
- stair training.
- importance of frequent icing.
- goals for discharge from the hospital.
- review of the financial obligation for home ambulation device.

Day of Surgery
- CPM 0–60 started in Recovery Room for greater than 4 hours total.
- Ice for 20 minutes every 1–2 hours.
- Passive extension: when not in CPM, a bolster should be under your ankle to help attain knee extension without hyperextension of the knee.

POD #1
- Increase CPM approximately 10 degrees (more if tolerated). Continue daily until attaining 90 degrees <u>active</u> knee flexion.
- Review and perform bedside exercises:
  - ankle pumps
  - gluteal sets
  - heel slides
- Dangle with necessary assistance.
- Ambulate with a standard walker 15′ with moderate assistance.
- Sit out of bed for 15 minutes.
- Active range of motion (AROM) 0–60.

POD #2
- Continue as above.
- Emphasis is on gaining ROM, proper gait pattern with assistive device, decreasing pain and effusion, and promoting independence with functional activities.
- Perform bed exercises independently 5×/day.
- Transfers and bed mobility performed with minimum assistance to the involved leg.
- Perform straight leg raise and terminal knee extension.
- Ambulate with standard walker 50′ with minimal assistance.
- Ambulate into the bathroom and practice sitting on the toilet.
- Sit out of bed for 45 minutes twice per day, in addition to all meals. Limit sitting to 45 minutes at a time.
- AROM 0–70.

POD #3
- Continue as above.
- Transfers and bed mobility performed with contact guarding to the involved leg.
- Ambulate with standard walker 100–150′ with supervision.
- Attempt ambulation with wide base quad cane (WBQC) with necessary assistance.
- Begin standing hip flexion and knee flexion exercises.
- Out of bed for most of the day, including all meals. Limit standing to 45 minutes at a time.
- Use bathroom with assistance for all toileting needs.
- AROM 0–80.

POD #4
- Continue as above.
- Bed mobility and transfers performed with supervision.
- Ambulate 200′ with WBQC and supervision.
- Negotiate 4 steps with a WBQC, a single rail, and necessary assistance for safety.

Table 89.6. (Continued)

- Perform home exercise program with contact guard and verbal cues.
- Out of bed most of the day walking and sitting.
- AROM 0–90.

POD #5
- Continue as above.
- Bed mobility and transfers performed independently.
- Ambulate with a WBQC 200′ independently.
- Negotiate 4–8 steps with a WBQC and a single rail independently.
- Perform home exercise program independently.
- AROM 0–90.
- Discharge from the hospital to home.

Phase II Progressive Function (Weeks 2–5)

GOALS:
1. Progress from WBQC to straight cane.
2. Improve involved lower extremity strength and proprioception.
3. Maximize function in the home environment.
4. Attain 0–110 active knee motion.

Weeks 2–3
- Continue with HEP, increase sets to 30/ 2× day.
- Monitor incision site and swelling.
- Progress ambulation distance (increase 1/2 block to 1 block every day) with WBQC.
- Begin stationary bicycle with supervision for 5–7 minutes.
- Begin standing wall slides.
- Incorporate static and dynamic balance exercises.
- AROM 0–100.

Weeks 3–4
- Continue as above.
- Practice with straight cane indoors.
- Increase stationary bicycle endurance to 7–8 minutes/2× day.
- Attempt unilateral stance on the involved leg, side stepping.
- Incorporate gentle knee-bends concentrating on eccentric control of quadriceps.
- Attain AROM 0–105.

Weeks 4–5
- Continue as above.
- Ambulate with straight cane only.
- Increase bicycle to 10 minutes/2× day.
- Progress with gentle lateral activities, i.e., lateral stepping, carioca.
- Attain AROM 0–110.

Phase III Advanced Function (Weeks 6–8)

GOALS:
1. Eliminate straight cane.
2. Attain full ROM (0–120).
3. Master functional tasks within the home environment.

Weeks 6–7
- Continue as above.
- Ambulate indoors <u>without</u> device.
- Focus exercises on strength and eccentric control of muscles (add cuff weights to exercise regimen).
- Focus on unilateral balance activities.

Weeks 7–8
- Continue as above.
- Devise exercise program for patient to follow including strength and endurance training.
- Eliminate straight cane.

The above time frames are goals for achievement. Each patient should be considered individually. Activity may be progressed sooner if previous week's goals have been achieved.

If you have any questions or need additional information, contact:

North Division	Petrie Division
Robert S. Gotlin, D.O., at (212) 870-9028	Jeff Young, M.D., at (212) 844-8676
Coleen Baquero, P.T., at (212) 870-9221	Mary Fischer, P.T., at (212) 420-2750

Table 89.7. Beth Israel Medical Center Department of Physical Medicine and Rehabilitation, bedside exercises

---

KNEE BEDSIDE EXERCISES

Do 10 of each exercise. Do not hold your breath.

Repeat these exercises 5 times per day.
1. Bend ankles up and down.
2. Tighten thigh muscles by pushing the back of your knee into the bed. Hold for 5 seconds, then relax.
3. Tighten buttock muscles by squeezing them together. Hold for 5 seconds, then relax.
4. Slowly bend your knee by sliding your heel toward your buttock. Then straighten it and repeat again.

*Place towel roll **under your ankle** when not in CPM machine.

Table 89.8. Patient tracking form

PATIENT: _____ PHYSICIAN: _____
DATE SURG: _____ P.T.: _____
PRE-OP: YES   NO
Flex: measured in sitting
Ext: measured in supine, towel roll under ankle.

date/POD#	Bed Mobility	Transfers	Ambulation	Stairs	ROM/CPM
			AM: PM:		CPM: PROM: AROM:
			AM: PM:		CPM: PROM: AROM:
			AM: PM:		CPM: PROM: AROM:
			AM: PM:		CPM: PROM: AROM:
			AM: PM:		CPM: PROM: AROM:
			AM: PM:		CPM: PROM: AROM:

Date of Discharge: _____ Discharge to: _____

Table 89.9. Functional independence measure (FIM)

LEVELS	7 Complete Independence (Timely, Safely) 6 Modified Independence (Device)	NO HELPER

	Modified Dependence
	  5 Supervision
	  4 Minimal Assist (Subject = 75%+)
	  3 Moderate Assist (Subject = 50%+)
	Complete Dependence
	  2 Marginal Assist (Subject = 25%+)
	  1 Total Assist (Subject = 0%+)
		HELPER

☐ Self Care	ADMIT	DISCH
A. Eating	☐	☐
B. Grooming	☐	☐
C. Bathing	☐	☐
D. Dressing-Upper Body	☐	☐
E. Dressing-Lower Body	☐	☐
F. Toileting	☐	☐
Sphincter Control		
G. Bladder Management	☐	☐
H. Bowel Management	☐	☐
Mobility Transfer:		
I. Bed, Chair, Wheelchair	☐	☐
J. Toilet	☐	☐
K. Tub, Shower	☐	☐
Locomotion		
L. Walk/Wheelchair	☐	☐
M. Stairs	☐	☐
Communication		
N. Comprehension	☐	☐
O. Expression	☐	☐
Social Cognition		
P. Social Interaction	☐	☐
Q. Problem Solving	☐	☐
R. Memory	☐	☐
TOTAL FIM		

Table 89.10. Recreational activities

ACTIVITIES AFTER TOTAL KNEE ARTHROPLASTY	
Highly recommended:	stationary bicycle, calisthenics, ballroom dancing, square dancing, golf, skiing (stationary), swimming, walking
Recommended:	bowling, jazz dancing, fencing, nautilus, rowing, skiing (cross country), speed walking, table tennis, weightlifting
Only with prior expertise:	bicycling, canoeing, horseback riding, ice skating, rock climbing, roller/inline skating, skiing (downhill)
Only with physician approval:	aerobics, tennis (doubles)
Avoid:	baseball, softball, football, handball, hockey, jogging, lacrosse, racquetball/squash, soccer, tennis (singles), volleyball

CHAPTER 90
Postoperative Pain Management

Nigel E. Sharrock

INTRODUCTION

Total knee arthroplasty (TKA) is one of the most painful operations performed and the majority of patients having TKA are over the age of 65 with multiple medical comorbidities.[1] Thus, the stress of the pain and the potential side effects of the analgesic regimes in this high-risk population make optimal pain control an issue of vital importance in their perioperative care.

The common comorbidities in these elderly patients include hypertension, obesity, ischemic heart disease, pulmonary hypertension, and chronic obstructive lung disease. Perioperatively, the patients lose blood, and may develop hypotension or shock, require transfusions, and sustain intraoperative pulmonary emboli from thrombi and/or bone marrow.[2,3] Any of these factors may perturb the cardiopulmonary system, which in turn can alter sensitivities to various analgesic regimes.

CHARACTER OF PAIN

The pain is usually severe for 2 to 3 days and is aggravated by distension of the knee and movement. The pain is usually relieved somewhat by elevating the limb, reducing the swelling by local cooling, and limiting motion. Early ambulation aggravates the pain. Although the severe pain lasts only 3 days, analgesia is usually required for some time to facilitate aggressive physical therapy.

TECHNIQUES

For many years, subcutaneous or intramuscular narcotics were the sole form of postoperative analgesia for most operations. The quality of analgesia was usually suboptimal and side effects from too little or too much narcotic were not uncommon.[4] In recent years, a more complex approach to pain management has developed with the incorporation of epidural analgesia with narcotics alone, narcotics plus local anesthetics, or local anesthetic by itself. In addition, patient-controlled analgesia (PCA) systems and constant infusion systems have become commercialized. The use of peripheral nerve blocks to augment analgesia has been promoted and the concept of multimodal analgesia formalized.

Multimodal analgesia entails utilizing a number of different agents or techniques to blunt the pain or pain-triggering mechanisms at several sites.[5] In total knee arthroplasty, this may include the concurrent use of epidural analgesia with an infusion of local anesthesia, oral nonsteroidal anti-inflammatory drugs (NSAIDS), and systemic narcotics on demand. Thus the pain is suppressed peripherally somewhat with the NSAIDs, the nerve root and/or spinal cord pain transmission is affected with the epidural anesthetic and the central nervous system integration of pain is interrupted with the narcotics. Additional modalities such as restricting motion and local cooling can also be included. The theoretical benefits of this approach are that the side effects of any particular technique are minimized enabling synergy between regimens to develop. Nowadays, most patients benefit from some form of multimodal analgesia.

Rather than describe each technique in detail, the essence of each technique is provided in Tables 90.1, 90.2, and 90.3. The rest of the narrative deals with a variety of issues and controversies relating to analgesia following TKA.

REHABILITATION

The type of analgesia has a major impact on how patients rehabilitate following TKA. It is important that the physical therapists be aware of the type of analgesia employed and interaction with physical therapists should be established to determine the best mode of analgesia at different phases of rehabilitation. Systemic narcotics in the early postoperative period provide insufficient pain relief for continuous passive motion (CPM). On the

Table 90.1. Techniques and quality of analgesia

	Technique	Quality of analgesia
Intramuscular Narcotics	I.M. injections of morphine etc., 3–4 hourly by nursing staff.	Suboptimal
Intravenous PCA	Intravenous PCA-patient demand doses of morphine 1–2 mg provides intermittent IV boluses.	Fair analgesia but improves after 24–36 hours.
Epidural Infusion	Infusion of local anesthesia ± narcotic via epidural catheter. Rate adjusted by staff.	Very good analgesia with correct doses.
Epidural PCA	Adds option of patient adding bolus doses as required. Local anesthetic bupivacaine 0.12% + fentanyl 5 μg/mL or morphine.	Better than infusion alone—more flexible.
Intrathecal Narcotics	Single dose of subarachnoid morphine 0.2–0.3 mg with spinal anesthetic.	Acceptable analgesia for 8–24 hours, thereafter inadequate.
Sciatic + Femoral Blocks	Preoperatively inject with aid of nerve stimulator bupivacaine 0.25 or 0.5% plus epinephrine combined with general or spinal anesthesia.	Total analgesia for 8–12 hours but thereafter little.
Continuous Femoral Block	Insert catheter into femoral sheath. Infusion of 0.25% bupivacaine 2–3 days postoperatively. Augment analgesia with systemic narcotics.	Very good analgesia for the anterior knee but not posterior.

other hand, patients do not tend to develop hypotension upon standing with systemic narcotics, therefore early ambulation can be encouraged with patients on an intravenous patient-controlled analgesia (IV PCA) modality. With epidural analgesia, concentrations of bupivacaine over 0.2% and possibly even over 0.1% lead to a degree of muscle weakness and/or postural hypotension that limits efforts to ambulate patients.[6] Thus, if these concentrations are used for the first 24 to 48 hours, ambulation should be delayed yet rehabilitation can proceed by advancing CPM. If early ambulation is required, the dose of bupivacaine can be reduced to 0.05% when patients can ambulate with these weaker local anesthetic-containing solutions.

If the primary goal is to establish a range of motion, epidural analgesia provides excellent analgesia for this purpose. This may be particularly helpful in the revision or complex cases.

In a randomized trial comparing epidural with general anesthesia for total knee arthroplasty, we noted that a number of indices of enhanced rehabilitation were observed in the group receiving epidural anesthesia and epidural analgesia.[7] By contrast, the general anesthesia patients received systemic narcotics. More of the patients receiving epidural analgesia could negotiate stairs before discharge. The mean time to negotiate stairs was 1.5 days earlier in patients receiving epidural analgesia. In addition, patients achieved 90 degrees of flexion about 1 day earlier with epidural analgesia. Thus, epidural analgesia provides not only superior analgesia but also enhanced early recovery. These observations have recently been confirmed in another center.[8]

Table 90.2. Duration, technical support, and cost of analgesia

	Duration	Technical support	Cost
IM Narcotics	No limitations	None (by nursing staff)	Cheap
IV PCA	No limitations. Requires intravenous.	Pharmacy, nursing, and physician support.	Costs of pumps, disposables ± physician oversight.
Epidural Infusion	2–5 days. Limited by catheter disconnect, concern of epidural infection and ambulation.	Requires pain services with anesthesiologist, pharmacy, nursing input. Skill with placing epidurals.	Pharmacy costs, pumps, disposables, plus physician oversight.
Epidural PCA	Same as above	Same as above	Same as above
Intrathecal Narcotics	Limited to 12–18 hours.	Little. Use with spinal. Perhaps requires overnight respiratory monitoring.	Cheap
Sciatic + Femoral Block	Limited to 8–12 hours.	None postoperative. Requires skilled anesthesiologist.	Cheap
Continuous Femoral Blocks	2–5 days. Limited by catheter displacement, injection risk and ambulation.	Require skilled anesthesiologist plus comprehensive pain service, pumps, etc.	Expensive: kits, infusion pump, physician service.

Table 90.3. Major advantages and disadvantages of analgesia regimes

	Advantages	Disadvantages
IM Narcotics	Cheap. No nursing or pharmacy in-service or change in systems.	Poor analgesia, probably contributes to poor medical outcome—respiratory, GI dysfunction, and rehabilitation.
PCA	Better way to administer narcotics. Patient satisfaction higher. Increased nursing acceptance.	Suffers same disadvantage as IM narcotics.
Epidural Technique	Best-quality analgesia. Flexible over time with varying rates and concentrations of agents. PCA mode makes the technique more flexible. Patients can ambulate with lower concentrations of local anesthetic. Concern for infections risk limits use to 3–4 days.	Risk of epidural hematoma with anticoagulation. Expensive (MD costs). Require pain service. Early ambulation *may* be delayed. Tendency to hypotension. Interpretation of compartment syndrome impaired.
Intrathecal Morphine Sulfate	Simple. Good analgesia.	Short-lived—then requires systemic narcotics. Nausea, vomiting, pruritus, respiratory depression.
Sciatic Femoral Block	Excellent analgesia 8–12 hours.	Thereafter requires systemic narcotics. Requires time and skilled anesthesiologist.
Continuous Femoral Nerve Block	Very good analgesia, especially if combined with IV PCA	Cost, complex, requires skill plus pain service.

DOES THE TYPE OF ANALGESIA AFFECT THE RATE OF DEEP VEIN THROMBOSIS?

The rate of deep vein thrombosis (DVT) following TKA is about 50% with general anesthesia and 40% with epidural anesthesia.[9] The mechanism for this difference is unknown. To determine whether epidural analgesia, by prolonging the effect of the epidural postoperatively, could lower the rate of DVT even further, we retrospectively investigated the rate of DVT following TKA in patients who had epidural anesthesia, but who thereafter had epidural analgesia or systemic narcotics. The rates were similar: 41% (108 of 266) with epidural analgesia and 43% (78 of 182) with systemic narcotics.[10] Thus, even though this was not a randomized study, it seems unlikely that epidural analgesia reduces DVT per se.

IS EPIDURAL ANALGESIA SAFE TO USE WITH ANTICOAGULANTS?

The use of aspirin and NSAIDs is ubiquitous in orthopedic patients and studies have shown no increased incidence of perioperative bleeding or epidural hematoma when performing regional anesthesia in patients receiving these agents.[11] In spite of claims that it is safe to use epidural anesthesia in patients receiving low molecular weight heparin (LMWH),[12] there appears to be an increased risk of epidural hematoma with both the insertion and removal of epidural catheters in patients who are anticoagulated.[13,14] Isolated case reports of epidural hematoma continue to appear using LMWH in epidural or spinal anesthesia.[15] Of more concern, is the fact that at least 30% of cases with epidural hematoma associated with epidural analgesia in Germany occurred following the removal of the epidural catheters in those patients who were on LMWH. This led to the recommendation that the catheter be withdrawn several hours after the injection of LMWH. However, in our experience, at least 10% of epidural catheters become dislodged spontaneously and there is no control over this timing. In the USA, at least six cases of epidural hematoma have been reported to the FDA in association with LMWH prompting a warning regarding the concurrent use of epidural anesthesia or analgesia with LMWH.

The author believes that if LMWH is to be used, IV PCA should be used in place of epidural analgesia. Unfortunately, this regimen provides poor analgesia, delayed rehabilitation, and the prospect of an increased risk of wound hematoma. We prefer to use epidural analgesia combined with aspirin and a mechanical device such as boots[16] or foot pumps[17] and early ambulation. With this regime, low rates of DVT can be achieved without the risk of bleeding complications while preserving the beneficial effects of epidural analgesia.

COMPLEXITIES OF A PAIN SERVICE

The type of analgesia used in a hospital is largely dependent upon the type of support services available, as well as the preparedness of hospital administration, nursing, pharmacy, and anesthesia departments to cooperate to establish a service.[18] Lack of enthusiasm from any department can prevent the establishment of a service. Without it, the only modes of analgesia are either short-term nerve blocks or systemic narcotics; neither providing optimal pain relief. To function effectively, ongoing interface between departments to resolve issues is important. Incorporation of surgeon's concerns as well as input from the physical therapists further augment the success of the program.

There are significant initiation costs that include the in-servicing of nurses, buying pumps, etc., but once established, the ongoing costs are not high. At the Hospital for Special Surgery, the cost of the entire program that treats over 3000 patients annually is just over $100,000. This program is no more expensive than nurses giving intermittent injections of narcotics when one takes into account the time taken, storage of emesis basis, etc.

CONTRAINDICATIONS TO EPIDURAL ANALGESIA

Apart from the concurrent use of LMWH, there are a number of situations in which epidural analgesia is not suitable. Patients with hemophilia are best managed with general anesthesia and IV PCA following surgery. Intramuscular narcotics are also ill-advised in these patients. Patients with prior spine surgery can have effective epidural analgesia,[19] but from time to time, spread patterns of local anesthetics within the epidural space are suboptimal. Patients addicted to narcotics preoperatively have altered drug sensitivity and often prefer IV PCA or intramuscular narcotics, although epidural analgesia provides better pain relief. In our experience, patients with preoperative reflex sympathetic dystrophy of the knee also have markedly altered drug requirements requiring high infusion rates of concentrated local anesthetic (e.g., 15 mL/hr of 0.25% bupivacaine) to obtain satisfactory analgesia. Finally, it is safe to perform epidural analgesia in patients with infected knees because the risk of epidural abscess does not increase in this setting.

CAN EPIDURAL ANALGESIA REDUCE THE RATE OF POSTOPERATIVE MEDICAL COMPLICATIONS?

Apart from pulmonary embolism, the most common complications following TKA include myocardial infarction, delirium or confusion, congestive heart failure, atrial fibrillation, ileus, hypoxia of unknown cause, and respiratory depression. In a randomized trial of epidural versus general anesthesia, no differences in these complications were observed between analgesic regimens.[1] In a separate trial reviewing the effect of epidural analgesia versus systemic narcotics after bilateral total knee arthroplasty, we found no difference in the frequency of delirium nor other hematological variables between analgesia regimes.[20] Our conclusion is that many of these complication are due to metabolic injury in at-risk individuals, and optimal analgesia of any type does not alter the rates significantly. However, excessive narcotic administration can contribute to respiratory depression, as well as cognitive and gastrointestinal dysfunction.[21] The easiest way to minimize narcotic administration is to use epidural analgesia.

WHAT DO YOU DO IF THE EPIDURAL CATHETER PULLS OUT?

Epidural catheters are taped in and are apt to become dislodged when patients move, bed linens are changed, or merely when the tape loosens from the back. When this occurs, a pragmatic approach is to see how well the patient tolerates systemic narcotics. If the response is adequate, IV PCA can be used; if not, an epidural catheter should be reinserted. If the catheter becomes dislodged after 36 hours, there is usually little reason to reinsert it. However, if the catheter becomes dislodged in the first 24 hours, it is usually better to reinsert it because this limits the dosage of narcotics and provides significantly better analgesia. Upon reinsertion of the catheter, patients are universally grateful, which tells you something about the comparative analgesic effects of systemic narcotics and epidural analgesia. If the patients have been given Coumadin and their prothrombin time is elevated, the author would not recommend replacing the catheter.

LIMITATIONS WITH NARCOTICS

For the first 48 hours, pain relief with systemic narcotics, whether administered by IV PCA or intramuscularly is inferior to epidural analgesia.[22] For the first 24 hours in particular, narcotic requirements are very high, the analgesia is suboptimal (especially with any movement) and the risk of airway obstruction, hypoxia, or respiratory depression significant. Thereafter, tissue levels of narcotic increase and pain scores stabilize.[6]

Whether the accumulated dose of morphine predisposes to cognitive impairment or ileus is unknown, but it probably does if excessive doses are used.

PHYSIOLOGICAL EFFECTS OF EPIDURAL INFUSIONS IN PATIENTS FOLLOWING TKA

Excessive narcotics can cause respiratory depression leading to hypoxia, tachycardia, pulmonary hypertension, and arterial hypertension. Epidural analgesia, by providing pain relief and a degree of vasodilatation, lowers heart rate, blood pressure, and pulmonary artery pressure providing an improved physiological state. This can be particularly beneficial to patients with compromised cardiopulmonary function.

However, the vasodilatation (or inability to reflexly vasoconstrict) means that these patients cannot vasoconstrict when assuming the upright posture or in response to acute blood loss. Thus, the incidence of acute hypotension tends to be increased using epidural infusions containing local anesthetic.[7] These physiological effects should be understood when patients are bleeding from their wounds or when early ambulation is planned. Lower concentrations of bupivacaine cause less vasodilatation, which can be helpful. However, lower concentrations of local anesthetic provide less effective analgesia, so that higher doses of narcotics are required.

COMPARTMENT SYNDROME AND EPIDURAL ANALGESIA

Patients who undergo complex revision TKA in which the anterior compartment is entered may develop compartment syndrome (CS) following surgery. The ability to diagnose CS early depends upon recognition of excessive pain, altered sensation over the dorsum of the foot, and weakness in the extensors of the ankle or toes. Epidural analgesia with local anesthetics can interfere with these signs thereby delaying the diagnosis. Thus, if there is any likelihood of developing CS, epidural analgesia is best avoided. Options include use of IV PCA or epidural analgesia with narcotics alone (without local anesthetic).

RISK OF PERONEAL PALSY FOLLOWING TKA

Patients who have a preoperative flexion contracture or a valgus deformity or in whom a hematoma develops in the back of the knee are apt to have stretch placed on the peroneal nerve perioperatively.[23] If peroneal nerve dysfunction develops following surgery, the splints should be removed, and the knee flexed to relieve tension from the nerve. Because epidural analgesia can delay the diagnosis of peroneal nerve dysfunction, it is preferable to verify normal return of peroneal function following surgery prior to starting the epidural infusion in high-risk cases. Alternatively, patients can be placed on IV PCA, if there is any risk of subsequent development of peroneal nerve dysfunction.

If patients develop peroneal nerve dysfunction on an epidural infusion, the infusion should be stopped and the patient reexamined. If there is any question about the integrity of the nerve, the knee should be examined and placed in flexion. Patients with severe spinal stenosis may conceivably develop compression of the L4 or L5 nerve roots if they are kept supine with their lumbar spine in extension. One approach may be to sit these patients up partially following surgery in order to flex the spine.

HOW LONG SHOULD THE EPIDURAL CATHETER BE LEFT IN?

The main disadvantage of leaving the catheter in too long is the potential risk of infection. When placed aseptically in surgical patients, the risk of infection is small. At the Hospital for Special Surgery, we have had no epidural infections after total hip arthroplasty (THA) or TKA following a policy of withdrawing catheters within 72 hours. By this time, most patients are ambulating and the pain is manageable with oral narcotics. Some centers leave epidural catheters in for a longer period of time but this must increase the risk of infection to some degree.

LIMITATIONS OF OTHER TECHNIQUES

Subarachnoid narcotics such as Duramorph® (0.2 to 0.5 mg) provide sufficient analgesia following THA but are generally insufficient following TKA. With higher doses (0.3 mg or greater), pruritus, nausea, and vomiting as well as late respiratory depression become limitations. The duration of analgesia is limited to 12 to 18 hours and in many centers, these patients require monitoring in special care areas for 24 hours, which limits its use.

Peripheral nerve blocks provide excellent analgesia but the blocks last less than 24 hours. Thereafter, narcotics are necessary. These techniques also require time to administer and a skilled anesthesiologist. They are, however, useful in environments in which acute pain programs have not been established. With complex knee surgery, it may be ill-advised to use sciatic blocks, which could delay the diagnosis of compartment syndrome or peroneal nerve injury. Techniques for inserting catheter in the femoral sheath have been developed that enable continuous femoral nerve blocks providing significant analgesia.[24,25]

DOES EPIDURAL ANALGESIA INCREASE THE RATE OF URINARY TRACT INFECTION?

With epidural analgesia, a urinary catheter should be inserted to prevent retention. As long as retention is avoided, and catheters removed in 48 to 72 hours, urinary infection is uncommon. Epidural or spinal anesthesia does not increase the risk of urinary infection over general anesthesia.[26] With the routine use of urinary catheters inserted under epidural anesthesia, rates of urinary infection are low and do not present a reason to avoid epidural analgesia. In patients with renal dysfunction, prostatic hypertrophy or a history of urinary infection, we prefer to place a urinary catheter under antibiotic coverage, prevent urinary retention, and remove the catheter several days later when the patient is ambulating.

COMPLICATIONS OF ANALGESIA REGIMES

The complications of the analgesic regimes have been mentioned throughout the chapter and are tabulated under disadvantages in Table 90.3. A number of specific complications will be discussed further.

The major problem with system narcotics is respiratory depression. This is apt to occur in patients prone to snoring who develop episodic hypoxia when sedated with narcotics.[27] With excessive pain, excessive narcotics are administered leading to inadequate ventilation. Excessive narcotics probably do have an effect on cognition and gastrointestinal dysfunction. It is unknown whether the inadequate analgesia predisposes patients with cardiac disease to myocardial infarction.[28]

Intravenous PCA systems can malfunction, although rarely, leading to excessive intravenous narcotics if the pumps are held above the patient. Epidural catheters offer too high a resistance so that excessive doses do not occur with pump failure. Of course, false programming can lead to problems with IV as well as epidural analgesia.

The major problem with intrathecal narcotics is respiratory depression, which is likely to occur up to 8 to 10 hours later.[29,30] Thus these patients require additional surveillance. In addition, this technique causes a high incidence of nausea, vomiting, and pruritus limiting its appeal.

The major complication with nerve blocks is neuropraxia, although this is less common when nerve stimulators are utilized by skilled anesthesiologists. The other concern is to avoid sciatic blocks if there is any risk to the peroneal nerve.

The complications of epidural analgesia are mentioned elsewhere. The major problem is epidural hematoma. This is a rare complication but occurs in severe situations—in patients with underlying hematologic disorders (e.g., hemophilia or von Willebrand disease), patients on anticoagulants (especially LMWH), and when there is technical difficulty placing the epidural. Case reports suggest that 50% of cases of epidural hematoma occurred when there was technical difficulty placing the epidural catheter.[15]

The initial symptom of epidural hematoma is usually back pain, which proceeds neurologic signs in the legs. Back pain during epidural infusions may also occur in patients with spinal stenosis when they bolus themselves with the patient-controlled analgesia (PCA) mode. Early diagnosis of epidural hematoma is therefore often delayed until neurologic sequelae occurs. If decompression is delayed, neurologic recovery may be incomplete.

Epidural abscess is extremely unusual if catheters are removed within 72 hours. However, experience with longer periods of infusion in cancer patients demonstrates that infections may occur, and the rate increases with the length of time the catheters are left in place.

Nausea, itching, and urinary retention are manageable side effects of epidural analgesia.

SUMMARY

There are a variety of approaches to pain relief following TKA. This is partly due to the fact that the pain is very severe and no technique is perfect. Of the currently available technique, epidural analgesia offers the best analgesic modality over an extended period of time. The limitations of epidural analgesia as well as a number of issues necessary to optimally manage this technique were discussed. The limitations of systemic narcotics and other regimens were also discussed.

References

1. Williams-Russo P, Sharrock NE, Mattis S, et al. Cognitive effects after epidural vs general anesthesia in older adults. A randomized trial. *JAMA*. 1995; 274:44–50.
2. Parmet JL, Berman AT, Horrow JC, et al. Thromboembolism coincident with tourniquet deflation during total knee arthroplasty. *Lancet*. 1993; 341:1057–1058.
3. Parmet JL, Horrow JC, Singer R, et al. Echogenic emboli upon tourniquet release during total knee arthroplasty: pulmonary hemodynamic changes and embolic composition. *Anesth Analg*. 1994; 79:940–945.
4. Austin KL, Stapleton JV, Mather LE. Relationship between blood meperidine concentrations and analgesic response: a preliminary report. *Anesthesiology*. 1980; 53:460–466.
5. Moiniche S, Hjortso NC, Hansen BL, et al. The effect of balanced analgesia on early convalescence after major orthopaedic surgery. *Acta Anaesthesiol Scand*. 1994; 38:328–335.
6. Turner G, Blake D, Buckland M, et al. Continuous extradural infusion of ropivacaine for prevention of postoperative pain after major orthopaedic surgery. *Br J Anaesth*. 1996; 76:606–610.
7. Williams-Russo P, Sharrock NE, Haas SB, et al. Randomized trial of epidural versus general anesthesia. Outcomes after primary total knee replacement. *Clin Orthop*. 1996; 331:199–208.
8. Singelyn FJ, Deyaert M, Joris D, Pendeville E, et al. Effects of intravenous patient-controlled analgesia with morphine, continuous epidural analgesia, and continuous three-in-one block on postoperative pain and knee reha-

bilitation after unilateral total knee arthroplasty. *Anaesth Analg.* 1998; 87:88–92.
9. Sharrock NE, Brien WW, Salvati EA, et al. The effect of intravenous fixed-dose heparin during total hip arthroplasty on the incidence of deep-vein thrombosis. A randomized, double-blind trial in patients operated on with epidural anesthesia and controlled hypotension. *J Bone Joint Surg Am.* 1990; 72-A:1456–1461.
10. Sharrock NE, Hargett MJ, Urquhart B, et al. Factors affecting deep vein thrombosis rate following total knee arthroplasty under epidural anesthesia. *J Arthroplasty.* 1993; 8:133–139.
11. Horlocker TT, Wedel DJ, Schlichting JL. Postoperative epidural analgesia and oral anticoagulant therapy. *Anesth Analg.* 1994; 79:89–93.
12. Bergqvist D, Lindblad B, Mätzsch T. Low molecular weight heparin for thromboprophylaxis and epidural/spinal anaesthesia—is there a risk? *Acta Anaesthesiol Scand.* 1992; 36:605–609.
13. Modig J. Spinal or epidural anaesthesia with low molecular weight heparin for thromboprophylaxis requires careful postoperative neurological observation. *Acta Anaesthesiol Scand.* 1992; 36:603–604.
14. Vandermeulen EP, Van Aken H, Vermylen J. Anticoagulants and spinal-epidural anesthesia. *Anesth Analg.* 1994; 79:1165–1177.
15. Sternlo J-E, Hybbinette C-H. Spinal subdural bleeding after attempted epidural and subsequent spinal anaesthesia in a patient on thromboprophylaxis with low molecular weight heparin. *Acta Anaesthesiol Scand.* 1995; 39: 557–559.
16. Haas SB, Insall JN, Scuderi GR, et al. Pneumatic sequential-compression boots compared with aspirin prophylaxis of deep-vein thrombosis after total knee arthroplasty. *J Bone Joint Surg Am.* 1990; 72-A:27–31.
17. Westrich GH, Sculco TP. Prophylaxis against deep venous thrombosis after total knee arthroplasty: pneumatic plantar compression and aspirin compared with aspirin alone. *J Bone Joint Surg Am.* 1996; 78-A:826–834.
18. Ready LB, Oden R, Chadwick HS, et al. Development of an anesthesiology-based postoperative pain management service. *Anesthesiology.* 1988; 68:100–106.
19. Sharrock NE, Urquhart B, Mineo R. Extradural anaesthesia in patients with previous lumbar spine surgery. *Br J Anaesth.* 1990; 65:237–239.
20. Williams-Russo PG, Urquhart BL, Sharrock NE, et al. Postoperative delirium: predictors and prognosis in elderly orthopedic patients. *J Am Geriatr Soc.* 1992; 40:759–767.
21. Liu SS, Carpenter RL, Mackey DC, et al. Effects of perioperative analgesic technique on rate of recovery after colon surgery. *Anesthesiology.* 1995; 83:757–765.
22. Raj PP, Knarr DC, Vigdorth E, et al. Comparison of continuous epidural infusion of a local anesthetic and administration of systemic narcotics in the management of pain after total knee replacement surgery. *Anesth Analg.* 1987; 66:401–406.
23. Horlocker TT, Cabanela ME, Wedel DJ. Does postoperative epidural analgesia increase the risk of peroneal nerve palsy after total knee arthroplasty? *Anesth Analg.* 1994; 79:495–500.
24. Singelyn FJ, Contreras V, Gouverbeur JM. Epidural anesthesia complicating continuous 3-in-1 lumbar plexus blockade. *Anesthesiology.* 1995; 83:217–220.
25. Edwards ND, Wright EM. Continuous low-dose 3-in-1 nerve blockade for postoperative pain relief after total knee replacement. *Anesth Analg.* 1992; 75:265–267.
26. Michelson JD, Lotke PA, Steinberg ME. Urinary-bladder management after total joint-replacement surgery. *N Engl J Med.* 1988; 319:321–326.
27. Rosenberg J, Dirkes WE, Kehlet H. Episodic arterial oxygen desaturation and heart rate variations following major abdominal surgery. *Br J Anaesth.* 1989; 63:651–654.
28. de Leon-Casasola OA, Lema MJ, Karabella D, et al. Postoperative myocardial ischemia: epidural versus intravenous patient-controlled analgesia. A pilot project. *Reg Anesth.* 1995; 20:105–112.
29. Bernards CM, Hill HF. Physical and chemical properties of drug molecules governing their diffusion through the spinal meninges. *Anesthesiology.* 1992; 77:750–756.
30. Bromage PR, Camporesi EM, Durant PAC, et al. Rostral spread of epidural morphine. *Anesthesiology.* 1982; 56:431–436.

CHAPTER 91
The Stiff Knee

Van P. Stamos and James V. Bono

INTRODUCTION

The ultimate goal of total knee arthroplasty is to achieve a stable painless knee with an excellent range of motion allowing for maximum function. A normal knee should have a range of motion from 0 degrees to approximately 140 degrees, although functional demands for most activities of daily living such as walking, sitting, driving, and climbing stairs can be easily accomplished with motion from 10 degrees to 95 degrees. The uncomplicated total knee arthroplasty usually results in a range of motion of 0 to 5 degrees to 115 to 120 degrees, which, although not as full as a normal knee, allows greater motion than is needed for basic function.[1] Recalling this basic information is critical when evaluating a knee with a limited range of motion.

Stiffness following total knee arthroplasty can be extremely disappointing to both patient and surgeon. It can also be one of the most difficult complications to remedy. When faced with a stiff knee, the surgeon must remember that the best predictors of postoperative motion are preoperative motion and the passive motion achieved at surgery with the patella reduced and the joint capsule closed.[2-7] This fact is particularly important when evaluating a patient who has been operated on by another surgeon; if only 60 degrees of flexion was achieved at surgery and the patient has 60 degrees two weeks postoperatively, he is doing quite well. However, if 125 degrees of flexion was achieved at surgery and two weeks later the patient has only 60 degrees of flexion, he is doing quite poorly. The treating surgeon must consider the passive range of motion at the time of surgery when assessing the stiff knee; one should not be influenced by arbitrarily defined numbers!

Knee stiffness can be the result of a myriad of causes with some being more easily remedied than others. It is imperative that the surgeon fully evaluate the stiff knee and properly identify the cause so that appropriate treatment can be administered. Differentiating the stiff painful knee from the stiff painless knee can be particularly helpful.

CAUSES

Infection

Infection following total knee arthroplasty may present in many ways. Fortunately, it is the rare patient who presents with systemic signs of sepsis such as fever, chills, and/or shock. Far more common is the patient who is slow to progress following total knee arthroplasty despite aggressive physical therapy and other modalities. Flexion goals are not met, and the knee is insidiously painful and stiff. Constitutional symptoms as well as local wound problems are often absent, leaving pain and stiffness as the only signs of infection. It is therefore imperative that sepsis be excluded when presented with the stiff knee. The evaluation and treatment of infected total knee arthroplasties is fully discussed elsewhere in this book.

Associated Conditions

Knee stiffness may not be directly attributable to the knee itself. Disorders of the hip and spine may present as pain in the knee. Evaluation of both areas should be performed when assessing the stiff knee to exclude hip or spine pathology.[8] A flexion contracture of the hip may contribute to a flexion contracture of the knee. Ideally, hip abnormalities should be corrected prior to addressing disorders of the knee.

A wide array of nerve or muscular disorders must also be considered when evaluating the stiff knee.[29] Diseases of the central nervous system that result in spasticity will markedly affect motion and impede physical therapy. Because revision surgery is rarely helpful in this patient group, they must be identified to prevent the surgeon from proceeding with surgery that will almost certainly not achieve its intended goals.

Reflex Sympathetic Dystrophy

Reflex sympathetic dystrophy is a particularly troublesome disorder that results in knee pain and stiffness. It is often difficult to diagnose and may be extremely difficult to treat. Any additional insult such as trauma or surgery to a limb exhibiting this condition will usually aggravate symptoms. Therefore, it is critical that the surgeon identify this disorder prior to any surgical intervention.

Commonly described as a disorder of the upper extremity, lower extremity involvement is often overlooked. The incidence following total knee arthroplasty has been reported as 0.8%,[9] so the surgeon must have a high index of suspicion to make the appropriate diagnosis. Diagnostic tests are seldom useful; the diagnosis is made on clinical grounds. Pain out of proportion to objective findings on physical examination is the classic sign, but the patient usually also exhibits delayed functional recovery, vasomotor disturbances, and trophic changes.[9-11] Physical examination may reveal skin hypersensitivity, decreased temperature, edema, and hyperhydrosis. In late stages, atrophy of the skin may be present. Limitation of motion affects flexion more commonly than extension, and the patellofemoral joint is often quite sensitive.

Treatment should be instituted immediately once the diagnosis is made. If symptoms have been present for less than 6 weeks, nonsteroidal anti-inflammatory medication and physical therapy for range of motion and desensitization are the mainstays of treatment.[10] The patient should be encouraged to bear weight and use the limb as much as possible. If the duration of symptoms has been more than 6 weeks, lumbar sympathetic block may be required. Blockade of the sympathetic nervous system to the lower extremities is both therapeutic and diagnostic. It should alleviate symptoms, at least initially. When it does not, the diagnosis of reflex sympathetic dystrophy becomes suspect. Usually, several sequential blocks are required to provide lasting relief. Critical to success is the institution of aggressive physical therapy immediately following blockade. Some authors have reported success rates as high as 80% with this regimen.[12] The key factors for a positive outcome are early recognition, aggressive treatment, and the avoidance of additional surgery or trauma to the extremity.[10]

Heterotopic Ossification

Occasionally, heterotopic ossification can be identified following total knee arthroplasty. Most commonly it is seen in the quadriceps muscle or anterior supracondylar region of the femur but other locations have also been reported (Fig. 91.1). Historically, its incidence following knee arthroplasty was considered low.[13] It was also con-

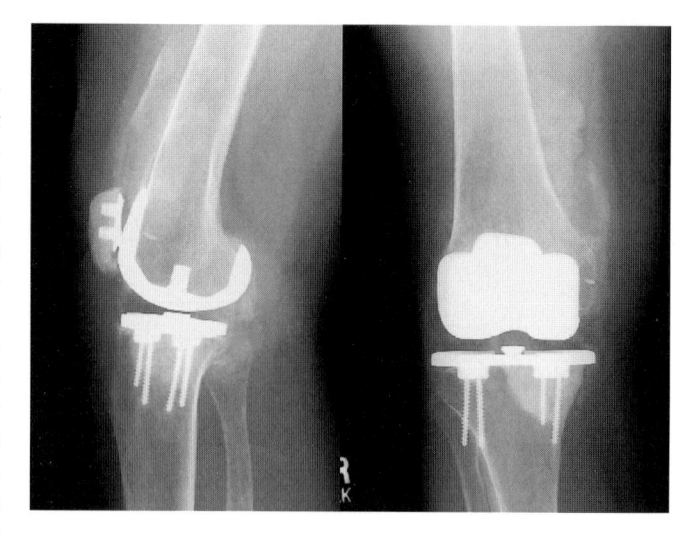

Figure 91.1. A 72-year-old woman with chronic pain and stiffness 9 years following total knee replacement. Anteroposterior and lateral radiographs reveal abundant heterotopic ossification.

sidered a rare cause of knee stiffness. One case report described a patient who developed severe myositis ossificans following knee replacement with a porous ingrowth prosthesis.[14] The diagnosis of hypertrophic osteoarthritis was felt to be a predisposing factor when combined with extensive surgical exposure of the distal femur at the time of surgery and postoperative manipulation of the knee. In addition, the authors noted difficulty managing the dosage of coumadin in the postoperative period in this patient.

However, a recent retrospective review of 98 primary knee arthroplasties in 70 patients demonstrated an incidence of heterotopic ossification of 26%.[15] The authors identified significantly elevated lumbar spine mineral bone density in those patients who developed heterotopic ossification as compared to a matched control group of patients who did not develop ectopic bone. Based on these findings they identified increased lumbar spine bone mineral density as an indicator of patients at risk for the development of postoperative heterotopic ossification.

Treatment consists of excision of ectopic bone followed by prevention of recurrence with either radiotherapy or pharmacologic means. The response to this treatment is not entirely predictable so it should be reserved for cases in which there is severe limitation of motion and extensive heterotopic ossification.

Arthrofibrosis

Arthrofibrosis is probably the most common cause of knee stiffness in patients with mechanically sound reconstruction.[3] These patients develop adhesions or dense scar within the joint or extensor mechanism that either act to tether or mechanically impede full joint motion. Attempts to identify predisposing factors for the development of arthrofibrosis have been largely unsuccessful. Thus, preventive measures are limited. Prolonged periods of immobilization is certainly a causative factor. Currently, most joint surgeons implement aggressive rehabilitation in the postoperative period in an attempt to decrease the incidence of this complication. At many institutions this often includes the use of continuous passive motion, the efficacy of which is uncertain. Several studies have concluded that continuous passive motion has no effect on range of motion when measured at 3 months and 1 year.[5,7,16] These studies do, however, demonstrate significantly greater flexion in the early postoperative period for patients who were treated with continuous passive motion.

TECHNICAL CONSIDERATIONS

The etiology of stiffness following knee arthroplasty is often technique related, which often can be elucidated on radiographs or by physical examination. These patients can be distinguished from patients with arthrofibrosis by comparing their postoperative motion with that achieved at surgery. Limitation of motion, if technique related, will be present at the time of surgery. Prior to attributing these imperfections to surgical error, one must consider a few points. Although it should be the goal of every surgeon to implant prosthetic components in anatomic position and perfect alignment to allow full range of motion, this is not achievable in all cases due to variations in anatomy and technical limitations available. Because there are limits to the sizes and configurations of implants used and the variations in anatomy are infinite, compromises are often necessary after considering the alternatives.

Five broad categories of technical imperfections can lead to knee stiffness. These are retained bone or osteophytes of the posterior femoral condyles, malalignment, imbalance of the extension gap and flexion gap, improperly sized components, and improper reconstruction of the patellofemoral joint.

At the time of primary knee arthroplasty, bone or osteophytes along the posterior femoral condyles and femur should be removed, if possible. This is best accomplished in the following fashion. With a trial femoral component in position, a curved osteotome is used to resect any excess posterior bone. The trial component is used as a template so the surgeon can precisely remove the correct amount of bone and often includes the removal of a small portion of normal posterior femoral condyle. If resection of posterior bone is incomplete, the remaining bone can impinge on the posterior edge of the tibial component or tibia resulting in a mechanical impediment to full flexion. Residual posterior bone can be identified on a lateral radiograph and should be looked for when a patient presents with a stiff knee (Fig. 91.2).

Restoration of proper mechanical alignment is critical to assure both proper function and longevity of a knee implant.[17] This includes alignment in sagittal, coronal, and rotational planes. Significant malalignment in any of these planes can result in decreased range of motion. Standing 3-feet anteroposterior and lateral radiographs are most helpful in assessing alignment and should be obtained for any patient in whom revision surgery is being considered. In the coronal plane, it is not uncommon to see errors of up to 3 degrees on either the femoral or tibial component.[1] It would be highly unusual for this amount of malalignment to result in motion limitation.[1,17] However, when measurements exceed 5 degrees, the likelihood of resultant loss of motion increases dramatically. In the sagittal plane, excessive flexion or extension of the femoral component can lead to limitation of motion, but the degree of error must be quite large and is rarely seen as the cause. This is not the case with the tibial component at which a relatively small degree of malalignment in this plane can significantly affect motion. The slope of the tibial prosthesis relative to the long axis of the tibia should be carefully evaluated. Excessive posterior slope may result in lack

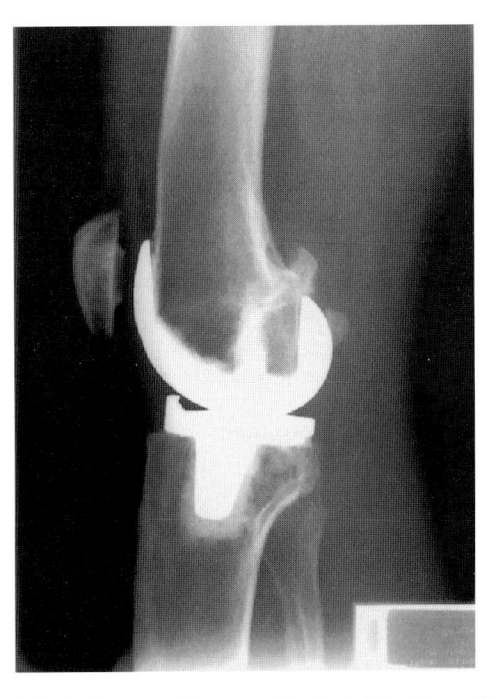

Figure 91.2. A 66-year-old man with diminished knee flexion resulting from retained posterior osteophytes.

of full extension and instability in flexion. Anterior slope (i.e., hyperextension of the tibial component) is likely to lead to recurvatum deformity and lack of full flexion. Of course, the amount of posterior slope designed into the particular component implanted must be taken into account when evaluating the radiograph.

Improper balance of the extension and flexion gaps can clearly lead to stiffness following knee arthroplasty. This includes both asymmetry of the individual gap as well as mismatch between gaps. If the extension gap is tight relative to an appropriate flexion gap, lack of full extension is the result. Conversely, if the flexion gap is tight relative to an appropriate extension gap, limited flexion is observed.

Incorrect sizing of the implant will affect knee motion. For both the femoral and tibial components, appropriate anteroposterior dimension is most important for restoration of knee mechanics. Oversizing of the femoral component results in tightening of the collateral ligaments in flexion. The resultant flexion-extension gap mismatch leads to incomplete flexion. Undersizing of the tibial tray, when combined with excessive anterior placement on the tibia, will also affect motion. In this situation, the uncovered posterior cortex of the tibia leads to a mechanical block from contact between the posterior femur and tibia as the knee is flexed. Finally, oversizing of the composite thickness of the tibial component and liner will result in a knee that is globally too tight, limiting both flexion and extension.

Complications associated with reconstruction of the patellofemoral joint can result in decreased flexion.[18] Maltracking or tilting of the patella can have an effect on motion by both mechanical and pain-medicated pathways. Patients with these findings often demonstrate an unwillingness to fully flex their knees. If the reconstructed patella is too thick, increased forces across the patellofemoral joint may impede flexion.

Identification of technical imperfections when presented with the stiff knee is relatively straightforward. The difficulty lies in whether those findings are the actual cause of stiffness. The surgeon must remember that technical imperfections can be identified in many well-functioning total knee replacements.

MISCELLANEOUS

Anecdotal cases of loose bodies within the joint have been described. In one case report, an intra-articular fragment of methylmethacrylate was identified.[19] Knee motion was restored after arthrotomy and removal of the offending loose body. Fracture of the polyethylene should also be considered when determining the cause of knee stiffness.

TREATMENT
General

Treatment should be directed at the causative factor. The previous section addressed the treatment of infection, reflex sympathetic dystrophy, and heterotopic ossification. This section discusses treatments for stiffness related to arthrofibrosis or technical errors. Included are some associated with significant complications of which the surgeon and patient must be aware prior to embarking on these courses of action. Manipulation and arthroscopy are directed toward the treatment of arthrofibrosis. These modalities should be reserved for patients who originally had adequate motion but have lost it over time. The patient who never had adequate motion is unlikely to benefit from arthroscopy or manipulation.

Manipulation

Although controversy exists regarding its use and effectiveness, manipulation of the stiff total knee arthroplasty can be a useful treatment if used appropriately. Timing is probably the most critical element if manipulation is to be successful. The surgeon must remember that manipulation is theoretically designed to produce disruption of immature, early adhesions. It is not designed to disrupt solidly formed adhesions or to stretch tendon or muscle. Therefore its effectiveness is markedly diminished beyond 6 weeks postoperatively when adhesions are nearing maturity. Beyond this time, the increased risk of complications such as femur fracture, patellar fracture, or rupture of the extensor mechanism should discourage the surgeon from performing a manipulation. The most effective time to perform a manipulation is within 6 weeks of surgery, so patients need to be identified and treated early if one is to be successful.

The current prevailing opinion of most joint replacement surgeons is that manipulation does not affect ultimate range of motion after knee arthroplasty. This conclusion is based on studies that compared patients who underwent manipulation under anesthesia to those who did not.[2,13] These investigations found the ultimate motion at one year after surgery to be the same in these two groups. On the surface, one might then conclude that manipulation has no influence on ultimate motion. However, because of inherent bias, these two groups are not matched making such a conclusion suspect. The patients who underwent manipulation were chosen because they were slow to progress as compared to the unmanipulated group. Ultimately, motion was comparable in both groups. Manipulation allowed the slower patients to, in effect, catch up to the other, rapidly progressing patients. Based on studies to date, it is extremely difficult to determine the true long-term influence of manipulation. Regardless of the actual influences on ultimate range of motion, one cannot deny the very positive benefits, particularly psychological, of a successful manipulation on the patient, therapist, and surgeon.

In order to be effective, manipulation, like any procedure, needs to be performed correctly. General or regional anesthesia is mandatory to provide adequate muscle relaxation and control of pain thereby decreasing the risk of fracture or extensor mechanism rupture. Once under anesthesia, passive range of motion should be measured with the patient supine. Extension is assessed by supporting the heel with the hip slightly flexed. The amount of extension is recorded. Flexion is measured by supporting the lower extremity from the thigh with the hip flexed to 90 degrees. The knee is allowed to bend passively to maximum flexion with gravity. Once the arc of motion has been determined, manipulation is performed. With the patient's leg supported by both hands around the calf and the ankle in the surgeon's axilla, a gentle steady flexion force is applied. As the adhesions are torn, the surgeon will feel a sensation of crepitus and flexion of the knee will gradually increase. Alternatively, the leg may be allowed to free fall from full extension into flexion. This maneuver is repeated several times; the weight of the limb itself is used to disrupt adhesions. With the knee in extension, an attempt at mobilization of the patella should be performed by applying inferior and medially directed forces, which assists in lysis of adhesions in the suprapatellar pouch. These maneuvers should be repeated until the motion attained at surgery is reproduced or no further progress is made. Post-manipulation motion is then measured in the manner described previously. Continuous passive motion should be instituted immediately and set to the maximum extension and flexion achieved with manipulation. Following the procedure, adequate analgesia must be given so the patient does not experience pain and resist the motion that has been achieved. An epidural catheter maintained for 24 to 48 hours following the manipulation is often beneficial. An aggressive physical therapy program is then instituted to avoid losing the motion gained with manipulation.

Arthroscopy

Arthroscopic treatment of disorders of the knee is the most common procedure in orthopedic practice. Its use in the treatment of problematic knee arthroplasty, however, is relatively uncommon.[20,21] When contemplating the use of arthroscopy for the stiff knee, the indications and prerequisites are similar to those for manipulation; that is, the motion of the knee is less than that attained at surgery, rehabilitation is slow to progress, and the etiology is thought to be arthrofibrosis. Arthroscopy, though, can be attempted after the 6-week postoperative time period in which manipulation is most effective. Because the adhesions are lysed directly, even mature secondary scar can be removed safely. Intuitively, one might think arthroscopic lysis of adhesions followed by aggressive therapy would be a highly effective treatment of arthrofibrosis. In reality this approach has yielded limited success.[22–25,27,35] The most promising results have been in patients treated for tethered patella syndrome in which the fibrous bands of secondary scar are isolated to the patellofemoral joint. These patients have a reproducible pattern of symptoms characterized by painful patellar grinding and crunching when actively extending the knee and some limitation of motion. There is a consistent pattern of fibrous band formation with the most common occurring at the superior border of the patellar component. Less common are bands that tether the patella or fat pad to the intercondylar notch region. In patients with these constellations, long-term results have been excellent following arthroscopic removal of these "tethering bands."

One might also reasonably consider the use of the arthroscope for the removal of a foreign body that is impeding motion. Although no series have been reported, one would expect a positive outcome if used to treat the case described earlier of an intra-articular fragment of methylmethacrylate limiting joint motion. In knee replacements in which the posterior cruciate ligament is thought to be too tight, and therefore restrict motion, one may consider arthroscopic release of the PCL.

Revision Surgery

Ultimately, the surgeon must address the stiff knee that is the result of technical imperfections.[28,30] Attempts to improve motion in these patients require revision knee arthroplasty and the potential complications associated with such an undertaking. Therefore, prior to embarking on such a potentially hazardous course, the potential benefit must be clearly demonstrated. This benefit should be determined in the context of the functional range of knee motion described in the introductory section of this chapter and the true functional requirements of the patient. When contemplating revision surgery for knee stiffness, the surgeon and patient must have reasonable expectations and goals. The surgeon must have experience in revision surgery and have a clear surgical plan.[32,33,36,37] The patient must understand that the outcome with revision surgery may not be improved and may in fact be worsened. Both must be prepared for complete revision of all components. As the saying goes, "Hope for the best, prepare for the worst."

Techniques used for revision of total knee replacements are described in detail in Chapter 51. What follows is merely an overview of revision surgery as it pertains to treatment of the stiff knee.

Revision of the stiff knee arthroplasty requires attention to detail that begins with the skin incision and surgical approach. Previous incisions should be used whenever possible. Because the skin is often contracted and tenuous in this group of patients, excision of hypertrophic scar is strongly discouraged because it may not allow a tension-free closure at the completion of the procedure. In addition, closure may require rotational flaps or grafts so the surgeon must be prepared by using appropriate incisions and handling all tissues carefully. Nearly all cases will require an extensile approach to avoid the disastrous complication of avulsion of the patellar tendon. Favored approaches include the quadriceps snip,[31] V-Y quadriceps turndown, and tibial tubercle osteotomy, all of which are thoroughly described in Section 4: Surgical Approaches.

Next, the suprapatellar pouch and medial and lateral gutters are examined. All scar and fibrous tissue in these areas is excised, and the undersurface of the quadriceps tendon is debrided. The knee is then flexed, and the components are examined for evidence of loosening or abnormal polyethylene wear. Patellar tracking and function of the extensor mechanism are assessed. If the patellar has been resurfaced, the composite thickness should be measured with a caliper. Measurements greater than 26 mm in males and 24 mm in females may indicate resection at time of patellar reconstruction.[18] As described earlier in this chapter, the resultant overly thick patella can be a cause of limited flexion. Range of motion is then assessed once thorough debridement of scar and mobilization of the extensor mechanism are complete. Occasionally, adequate motion will have been restored. More commonly, however, further evaluation is required.

Overall static alignment and symmetry of the extension and flexion gaps are then assessed. If abnormalities are observed, one must determine if correction can be achieved with exchange of the polyethylene and soft tissue releases. Custom-designed angled bearing inserts have been described for use in these situations.[26] If present, the modular tibial insert is then removed, and attention is directed posteriorly. Dense scar and residual bone along the posterior femur is excised. Adequacy of removal is assessed by finger palpation. Subsequently, range of motion is checked after replacement of the tibial insert. If it is considered inadequate, revision of the femoral and/or tibial components is performed if a technical imperfection has been identified.

Flexion of the knee is evaluated both with the patella everted and with the patella reduced. Diminished flexion with the patella reduced compared with the patella everted indicates extrinsic tightness of the extensor mechanism due to scarring and fibrosis. In this setting, lengthening of the quadriceps mechanism may be accomplished by creating several relaxing incisions in the tendon with a #11 knife blade.

Prior to closure, patellar tracking is reevaluated carefully. Lateral release and/or revision of the patellar component to decrease its thickness may be required. The surgical wound is then closed utilizing meticulous surgical technique and cautious handling of the tissues.

CONCLUSION

The knee that is stiff following total knee arthroplasty presents a difficult problem to the surgeon. Prior to embarking on a treatment regimen that may include revision surgery, which is fraught with complications, one must be certain the benefits to the individual patient outweigh the risks. Knee motion from 10 to 95 degrees may be perfectly adequate for some and unacceptable for others. Similarly, the cause of limitation of knee motion and corrective treatment with acceptable risk must be identified. Revision surgery should be pursued only after these factors are considered.

References

1. Krackow KA. Postoperative period. In: *The Technique of Total Knee Arthroplasty*. St. Louis: The C.V. Mosby Company; 1990:385–424.
2. Fox JL, Poss R. The role of manipulation following total knee replacement. *J Bone Joint Surg*. 1981; 63-A:357–362.
3. Harvey JA, Barry K, Kirby SP, et al. Factors affecting the range of movement of total knee arthroplasty. *J Bone Joint Surg*. 1993; 75-B:950–955.
4. Kim JM, Moon MS. Squatting following total knee arthroplasty. *Clin Orthop*. 1995; 313:177–186.
5. Maloney WJ, Schurman DJ, Hangen D, et al. The influence of continuous passive motion on outcome in total knee arthroplasty. *Clin Orthop*. 1990:162–166.
6. Menke W, Schmitz B, Salm S. Range of motion after total condylar knee arthroplasty. *Arch Orth Traum Surg*. 1992; 11:280–281.
7. Wasilewski SA, Woods LC, Torgerson WR, et al. Value of continuous passive motion in total knee arthroplasty. *Orthopedics*. 1990; 13:291–296.
8. Vince KG, Eissmann E. Stiff total knee arthroplasty. In: *Knee Surgery*. Baltimore: Williams and Wilkins; 1994:1529–1538.
9. Katz MM, Hungerford DS. Reflex sympathetic dystrophy affecting the knee. *J Bone Joint Surg*. 1987; 69-B:797–801.
10. Cooper DE, DeLee JC. Reflex sympathetic dystrophy of the knee. *J Am Acad Orthop Surg*. 1994; 2:79–86.
11. Katz MM, Hungerford DS, Krackow KA. Reflex sympathetic dystrophy as a cause of poor results after total knee arthroplasty. *J Arthroplasty*. 1986; 2:117–122.

12. Ogilvie-Harris DJ, Roscoe M. Reflex sympathetic dystrophy of the knee. *J Bone Joint Surg*. 1987; 69-B:804–809.
13. Daluga D, Lombardi AV, Mallory TH, et al. Knee manipulation following total knee arthroplasty: Analysis of prognostic variables. *J Arthroplasty*. 1991; 6:119–128.
14. McClelland SJ, Rudolf LM. Myositis ossificans following porous-ingrowth TK replacement. *Orthop Rev*. 1986; 15: 223–227.
15. Furia JP, Pellegrini VD. Heterotopic ossification following primary total knee arthroplasty. *J Arthroplasty*. 1995; 10: 413–419.
16. Ververeli PA, Sutton DC, Hearn SL, et al. Continuous passive motion after total knee arthroplasty. Analysis of cost and benefits. *Clin Orthop*. 1995; 321:208–215.
17. Hungerford DS. Alignment in total knee replacement. *Instr Course Lectures*. 1995; 44:455–468.
18. Barnes CL, Scott RD. Patellofemoral complications of total knee replacement. *Instr Course Lectures*. 1993; 42:303–307.
19. Robins PR. Internal derangement of the knee caused by a loose fragment of methylmethacrylate following total knee arthroplasty. A case report. *Clin Orthop*. 1977; 4:208–210.
20. Johnson DR, Friedman RJ, McGinty JB, et al. The role of arthroscopy in the problem total knee replacement. *Arthroscopy*. 1990; 6:30–32.
21. Lintner DM, Bocell JR, Tullos HS. Arthroscopic treatment of intraarticular fibrous bands after total knee arthroplasty. A follow-up note. *Clin Orthop*. 1994; 309:230–233.
22. Bocell JR, Thorpe CD, Tullos HS. Arthroscopic treatment of symptomatic total knee arthroplasty. *Clin Orthop*. 1991; 271:125–134.
23. Campbell ED. Arthroscopy in total knee replacements. *Arthroscopy*. 1987; 3:31–35.
24. Sprague NF, O'Connor RL, Fox JF. Arthroscopic treatment of postoperative knee fibroarthrosis. *Clin Orthop*. 1982; 166:165–172.
25. Thorpe CD, Bocell JR, Tullos HS. Intra-articular fibrous bands. Patellar complications after total knee replacement. *J Bone Joint Surgery*. 1990; 72-A:811–814.
26. Shaw JA. Angled bearing inserts in total knee arthroplasty. A brief technical note. *J Arthroplasty*. 1992; 7:211–216.
27. Beight JL, Yao B, Hozack WJ, et al. The patellar "clunk" syndrome after posterior stabilized knee arthroplasty. *Clin Orthop*. 1994; 299:139–142.
28. Blesier RB, Matthews LS. Complications of prosthetic knee arthroplasty. In: *Complications in Orthopaedic Surgery*. New York, N.Y. SCP Communications, Inc. 1994:1075–1086.
29. Dellon AL, Mont MA, Krackow KA. Partial denervation for persistent neuroma pain after total knee arthroplasty. *Clin Orthop*. 1995; 316:145–150.
30. Dorr LD, Boiardo RA. Technical considerations in total knee arthroplasty. *Clin Orthop*. 1986; 205:5.
31. Garvin KL, Scuderi G, Insall JN. Evolution of the quadriceps snip. *Clin Orthop*. 1995; 321:131–137.
32. Jacobs MS, Hungerford DS. Revision total knee arthroplasty of aspetic failure. *Clin Orthop*. 1988; 226:78–89.
33. Nichols DW, Dorr LD. Revision surgery for stiff total knee arthroplasty. *J Arthroplasty*. 1990; 5:573–577.
34. Sculco TP, Faris PM. Total knee replacement in the stiff knee. *Techn Orthop*. 1988; 8:45–49.
35. Vernace JV, Rothman RH, Booth RE. Arthroscopic management of the patellar clunk syndrome following posterior stabilized total knee arthroplasty. *J Arthroplasty*. 1989; 4:179–182.
36. Vince KG. Revision knee arthroplasty. In: *Operative Orthopaedics*. Philadelphia: J.B. Lippincott Company; 1993: 1988–2010.
37. Vince KG. Revision knee arthroplasty technique. *Instr Course Lectures*. 1993; 42:325–339.

# CHAPTER 92
Deep Vein Thrombosis (DVT) and Total Knee Arthroplasty

Gilbert B. Cushner, Fred D. Cushner, and Michael A. Cushner

Deep vein thrombosis (DVT) formation following total knee arthroplasty (TKA) remains a proverbial thorn in the side of orthopedic surgeons. In spite of ever-improving surgical techniques, deep vein thrombosis and its associated risks of pulmonary embolism remains a serious complication of total knee arthroplasty.[1,2] Without prophylaxis and depending on the prophylaxis technique utilized, the prevalence of DVT may be as high as 84%.[3] This chapter will review current treatment options most commonly used today. Efficacy as well as limitations will also be discussed.

This chapter will concentrate on data obtained from studies involving TKA because DVT incidence varies between total hip arthroplasty and total knee arthroplasty procedures. In contrast to total knee arthroplasty, total hip arthroplasty (THA) has more femoral vein occlusion (proximal vein), a higher incidence of occurrences on the nonoperative side (40%), and more fatal pulmonary emboli.[4,5]

WHO'S AT RISK?

Because of the risk, although remote, of fatal pulmonary emboli and the morbidity of possible chronic venous insufficiency, efforts have been made to try to identify patients who might be prone to develop DVT and its sequelae. In contrast to medical and other surgical patients, there appears to be no relationship to age, ischemic heart disease, congestive heart failure, smoking, hypertension, existing carcinoma, or duration of anesthesia.[6] Kim[7] has suggested that obesity may play a role, but Sharrock[6] did not find this association. Underlying disease (rheumatoid versus osteoarthritis) did not influence the incidence of DVT.[7] Anders and colleagues[3] found a 50% reduction of DVT in patients who had autologous blood donations prior to total knee arthroplasty. Perhaps changes in blood viscosity could explain this reduction of morbidity, but this was not measured. Kim[7] found no increase incidence of thrombosis in patients with anatomic venous variation or in patients with more than five venous valves in the thigh as suggested by Liu.[8] Virchow's triad states that thrombosis is related to vessel wall changes, blood flow, and coagulability.[9] Venostasis and tissue hypoxia with resulted endothelial changes are certainly present during total knee arthroplasty but local factors alone cannot explain the 10 to 20% clot incidence in the nonoperative leg. Based on the above studies, it can be seen that selective preoperative prophylaxis is not an option because it is difficult to identify only those patients at risk for DVT formation. It should be noted that there are some factors in which the surgeon does have control. Sharrock[6] had reviewed risk factors of DVT formation and noticed that there was an inter-surgeon difference in clot formation. This difference could be due to changes in postoperative course between surgeons as well as the failure to use Esmarch bandages at tourniquet reinflation thus leading to stasis of blood remaining in the venous system.

PATHOGENESIS

Thrombin is a key enzyme in the pathogenesis of intravascular clotting. It is inhibited by a naturally occurring antiproteinase (antithrombin III), with formation of a complex of thrombin-antithrombin III (TAT). Before thrombin is inhibited, it can initiate fibrin formation by cleaving fibrinopeptides A and B from fibrinogen. Levels of TAT and fibrinopeptide are circulating measures of thrombin generation. Tissue plasminogen activator (t-PA) is released from epithelial cells and promotes formation of plasmin from circulating plasminogen. Plasmin cleaves fibrin into fibrin degradation products including D-dimer.[4] T-PA and D-dimer are measures of clot dissolution.

Ginsberg and associates[10] found a tendency for higher preoperative TAT levels in patients with thrombosis after total knee arthroplasty and total hip arthroplasty. However, the number in this study was small, and the total knee arthroplasty patients were not separated from those with total hip arthroplasty. No absolute value was noted under which thrombosis did occur and the group received heparin postoperatively. TKA patients had a 22% rate of DVT, lower than most series without prophylaxis.[10] Lower antithrombin III levels repeated by Stulberg[11] were not confirmed by Kim.[7] Sharrock and colleagues[4] found a significant increase in fibrinopeptide A, TAT, and D-dimer following surgery with tourniquet deflation. These were not correlated with patients who developed significant thrombosis. In fact, nonrandomized studies have shown no consistent change in coagulation or fibrinolytic activity that can be linked to DVT formation.[5] From the proceeding, it is obvious that DVT is multifactorial, and there is no screened procedure to absolutely identify those at increased risks; therefore, the approach must be for universal prophylaxis.

DIAGNOSIS OF DVT

Even with the best attempts at preventing deep vein thrombosis some failures occur and it becomes important to diagnose DVT in the lower extremities. Physical exam of the patient is the first step in diagnosis, but unlike other ailments, clinical findings may be quite subtle with the patients often symptomatic. Unfortunately, in many instances, pulmonary embolism is the first presentation of a DVT, especially proximal thrombosis.[12] The classic signs and symptoms of DVT include pain in the calves at rest and foot dorsi flexion, pitting edema 3 cm above the medial malleoli, and a palpable difference in temperature between the legs. Also as a measure of girth, calf and thigh circumference should be compared to detect differences in size. Because half of those who get pulmonary embolism do not exhibit any clinical signs, other diagnostic tests are necessary for detection of DVT.[13]

Venography is the gold standard and often noted to be the most reliable method to which other methods are tested.[12] Not only is the method expensive, but it is invasive and with the improved results there also exists increased morbidity including contrast allergy, delayed limb edema, contrast nephropathy, phlebitis, and a 4% incidence of causing a DVT.[14–16]

Transcutaneous Doppler flow test is inexpensive, noninvasive, and readily available. Comparing results to venography, sensitivities range from 40 to 96%.[12–15] These varied results show the operator dependence that exists with this tool and diminishes its usefulness as a screening tool. The method also is less accurate in detecting thrombosis in calf veins and early thrombus. It is unable to examine proximal to the profunda femoris vein and thus misses pelvic thrombi as well.

Compression Duplex Ultrasonography is another alternative, but like Doppler studies it is highly operator dependent and is distorted by hematoma or soft tissue masses, which distort the venous system.[12] It also is unable to accurately diagnose thrombi less than 1 cm in the deep venous system of the lower extremity.[17]

Nuclear medicine studies using either radioactive iodine (^{125}I) or technetium (^{99}mTc) have also been attempted as a way to accurately and noninvasively diagnose DVT. It is up to 83% sensitive,[18] but is less accurate in areas close to the operative wound where the labeled fibrinogen has been incorporated into the wound, creating confusing background radiation.[19] It is a poor screening tool due to expense, delay in results, and the requirement of nuclear medicine capabilities.

A less-used, but interesting method is the use of electrical signals, or impedance plethysmography (IPG). This method takes advantage of the fact that blood is a good conductor of electricity, and by applying Ohm's Law (voltage = current $\times$ resistance) one can use a weak electrical current, measure voltage in areas of the extremity, and indirectly assess local blood volume. Venous blood volume in the leg normally varies with pressure changes during respiration but these changes are diminished when thrombosis is present.[20] Other methods use cuff occlusion and deletion to measure vein engorgement and the presence of thrombi.[12] IPG requires patient cooperation with complete relaxation of the leg muscles and no motion of the leg. IPG is painless, noninvasive, portable, and safe. Sensitivity ranges from 83 to 97% in the proximal leg but are 17% sensitive in the calf.[12] Both legs must be examined to compare differences and a bilateral abnormal IPG is an indeterminate study.

SIGNIFICANCE OF CALF CLOTS

Debate over the significance of calf clots remains unanswered. Lotke and associates[21] studied 175 patients who underwent TKA and were examined postoperatively by venography, plethysmography, fibrinogen scans, and ventilation-perfusion lung scans to detect thrombosis. One hundred twenty-six (72%) of the patients had small or large clots in the calf. Seventy-one (41%) of the patients had small thrombi in the calf and 55 (31%) had large thrombi in the calf. Only two patients (1%) had a clinically significant pulmonary emboli, while six (3%) patients had asymptomatic pulmonary emboli not associated with calf thrombi. The authors concluded that there is a high possibility of development of DVT after total knee arthroplasty and most of these thrombi in the calf were with low risk of a clinically significant pulmonary embolism. These authors recommended that DVT prophylaxis be implemented for patients who have proximal thrombi.

This view is not held by all authors. Haas and colleagues[22] reviewed the records of 1625 TKAs and found that those patients with calf thrombi were found to have a significantly greater risk for symptomatic and asymptomatic pulmonary emboli. These authors concluded that calf clots should be treated or undergo follow-up studies to detect proximal propagation.

One last point of concern in deciding to treat calf clots is the prevention of post-phlebitis syndrome on chronic venous insufficiency (CVI). In patients with symptomatic DVT, up to 90%[23] may develop CVI, whereas in asymptomatic DVTs, the incidence is similar to an uninvolved limb.[24] This may be secondary to valve damage that may occur with symptomatic DVTs. It has been suggested that the development of symptomatic CVI is uncommon. Warwick and associates[25] reviewed 134 limbs following THA 14 to 21 years after the indicated procedure and found a 2% incidence of CVI from the THA procedure. The incidence of CVI in the TKA population remains to be proven.

PROPHYLAXIS AGENT— WHAT ARE THE OPTIONS?

Aspirin

Aspirin is most likely the oldest synthetic drug known to man. This natural salicylate found in the bark of the white willow was a common folk remedy in the 1700s. Later the synthetic version was developed in Europe in the 1800s. The modern-day version, acetylsalicylic acid (ASA), was manufactured by the Bayer Company and given the trademark named aspirin.[27] For most of its existence it was known as a pain and fever medication and only later were the antithrombotic properties recognized.

Certain antibiotics, cardiovascular drugs, anesthetics, and narcotics may alter platelet function. Even large amounts of ginger, onion, garlic, and chinese black tree fungus may disrupt platelet aggregation and cause bleeding.[28] Craven[29] first noted the bleeding side effects of aspirin suggesting its role as an antithrombotic agent. Investigations continued[30,31] throughout the 1960s and in 1971 Vane first described aspirin's role in the inhibition of prostaglandin synthesis for which he was later awarded the Nobel Prize.[31] Much of the work with thromboembolism and aspirin looked at the arterial side of circulation and the effect with myocardial infarct and stroke. It was once believed that DVT formation resulted from fibrin deposits forming a net and catching erythrocytes while arterial thrombi were the result of platelets.[32] Further anatomic studies revealed the presence of platelets in venous thrombi and aspirin's role in preventing venous clots by disrupting platelet aggregation.[33]

Aspirin interrupts the formation of thromboxane by irreversibly binding and inactivating the cyclooxygenase. Cyclooxygenase is part of the PGH synthase enzyme. Aspirin interrupts the formation of thromboxane by irreversibly binding and inactivating the cyclooxygenase in platelets. Cyclooxygenase is also present in the endothelial cells where it is necessary for the production for prostacyclin. Cyclooxygenase in the platelet is more sensitive to aspirin than the vascular cyclooxygenase present in endothelial cells. This combined with the differential distribution of the cyclooxygenase enzyme results in a greater decrease in thromboxane and overall decrease in platelet aggregation.

Platelets are unable to synthesize new proteins and cannot repair the damage caused by aspirin. Therefore, cyclooxygenase activity is restored 8 to 10 days after stopping aspirin when platelet turnover takes place.[34] The platelet PG synthesis is ten times more sensitive to oral doses of aspirin than other tissues, and thus the 600 to 1000 mg dose for antipyretic and analgesic effects are much higher than those needed to inhibit platelets.[35,36] A daily dose of as little as 30 to 50 mg of aspirin results in complete suppression of platelet thromboxane biosynthesis after 7 to 10 days.[34]

Aspirin treatment is inexpensive, readily available, and does not require lab testing. These factors made it an attractive alternative to consider for the prophylaxis of DVT formation.

Aspirin Studies

Most studies have concentrated on hip surgery and DVT prophylaxis due to the greater incidence of problems with thrombi above the knee. McKenna has two of the few studies that have examined DVT prophylaxis in knee replacements. In 1976 McKenna and associates published[37] a prospective study that examined the incidence of postoperative DVTs in knee replacement patients. All patients had clinical examinations, I^{125} fibrinogen scanning, and those with suspected DVT also had venography. Sixteen of the 30 patients (53%) had confirmed thrombi; nine in the operated limb only, four bilaterally, and three with pulmonary embolism. No patients were placed on aspirin for DVT prophylaxis, but nine took aspirin for their rheumatoid arthritis preoperatively and continued on the same dose postoperatively. The doses ranged from 1.6 to 5.7 grams daily. Only one of these nine patients on aspirin (11%) had thrombosis. The incidence of thromboembolism in the patients who did not take aspirin or any other antiplatelet drug was 88%. It should be noted that the number of patients was small, not randomized, and the dose of aspirin was variable.

In 1980, McKenna and associates[38] published another paper looking at the use of aspirin versus intermittent calf and thigh compression. Forty-three patients over the age of 40 undergoing total knee arthroplasty were enrolled in the study. Patients were randomly assigned to one of four groups: group one received a placebo, group two received 1.3 grams of aspirin three times daily, group three received 325 mg three times, and group four had intermittent low-pressure compression devices (IPCD). The patients were monitored using I^{125} fibrinogen scanning and venography with ventilation perfusion scans in those suspected of having pulmonary emboli. The placebo group had a 75% incidence of DVT, the low-dose aspirin group—78%, the high-dose aspirin group—8%, and the IPCD group—10%. This study concludes that high-dose aspirin and low-pressure IPCD were effective in preventing thrombolism. Unfortunately, this low rate of DVT formation has not been reproduced in other studies using aspirin as prophylaxis.

Haas and colleagues[39] published a comparison on the effectiveness of pneumatic sequential compression devices versus aspirin for the prevention of DVTs after total knee arthroplasty. This prospective randomized study assigned patients to one of these two modalities. One hundred nineteen patients completed the study with 72 undergoing a unilateral arthroplasty and 47 with bilateral knees operated on at the same operation. Those in the mechanical compression group had a boot that was placed on the uninvolved leg preoperatively and on both legs postoperatively. These boots remained on the extremities continuously except for when the patient was washing or walking. The aspirin group received 650 mg of aspirin twice a day until the day of discharge and starting the day before the operation. The patients had a bilateral venogram performed between the fourth and sixth postoperative days. In the unilateral group, the incidence of DVT formation was 26 versus 47% in the aspirin group. In the bilateral group the incidence of DVT was 48% in those using compression boots and 68% in the patients taking aspirin. This study confirms the effectiveness of the compression boots and the importance of increased incidence of DVT in those undergoing bilateral operations. The low DVT rate using aspirin as prophylaxis was not reproduced in this study.

Lotke and colleagues[21] examined the effectiveness of aspirin and warfarin after total joint arthroplasty in the hip and the knee. Three hundred eighty-eight patients were assigned randomly to one of the two groups. The patients taking aspirin were given 325 mg twice daily begun the day before surgery. Warfarin treatment consisted of a 10 mg dose on the night of surgery, none on postoperative day one and then adjusted doses to keep the prothrombin time between 1.2 and 1.5 times controlled values. All patients received a venogram and ventilation profusion scan prior to discharge. The results were no different with regard to size or location of DVTs in the aspirin or warfarin group. The venogram was positive in 55.5% of the patients: 28% had small calf clots (less than 3 cm), 16% had large calf clots (greater than 3 cm), 3.9% had popliteal clots, and 6.7% had femoral clots. The patients with total knee procedures performed had 2.6 times greater incidence of calf DVT than total hip arthroplasty patients. There is no difference between the two groups with respect to changes in the ventilation profusion scans, both groups having an 18.9% incidence of changes and only 0.5% had clinical evidence of pulmonary embolism. There was no difference between the two groups with respect to bleeding complications. The authors concluded that both aspirin and warfarin are equally effective prophylaxis against DVT. With a 55.5% DVT formation rate, perhaps this should be reworded that both aspirin and Warfarin are equally *ineffective* in a prophylaxis against DVT.

Recently, Westrich and associates[40] used ASA prophylaxis as a control for a study evaluating the efficacy of the pneumatic plantar compression. Overall, the ASA control group had a DVT rate of 59%. When separating unilateral TKA from the bilateral TKAs, DVT rates of 67% and 52% were noted, respectively. The study results above, once again, approach those rates seen when no prophylaxis is utilized.

Warfarin

Mechanism

Often viewed as a gold standard for DVT prophylaxis, warfarin therapy has been used for this purpose in lower limb surgery for over 40 years. It disrupts coagulation by acting as a vitamin K antagonist inhibiting vitamin K epoxide and possibly vitamin K reductase. Vitamin K is an essential part of the coagulation cascade serving as a cofactor for the synthesis of a number of vital proteins responsible for calcium bonding. These include predominantly the prothrombin complex: factor II (prothrombin), factor VII (proconvertin), factor IX (Christmas factor), and factor X (Stuart-Prower factor). Warfarin also disrupts a formation of the vitamin K-dependent proteins (C and S) by limiting the carboxylation process interrupting their natural anticoagulant effect.

Warfarin is almost always administered orally and is rapidly absorbed in the intestine and reaches maximal blood concentrations in 90 minutes, but the observed anticoagulant effects are not seen for 24 to 36 hours and the full effect probably does not occur until 72 to 96 hours when complete replacement of the normal prothrombin complex takes place. Factor VII and protein C have similarly short half-lives at 6 to 7 hours. The inhibition of these competing proteins (coagulation versus anticoagulation) leads to a homeostasis in the coagulation pathway and precludes any net anticoagulation or coagulation early effect. It is not until later when the remaining decarboxylated factors accumulate and overall anticoagulation takes place.[41] Warfarin dose response is influenced by pharmokinetic factors such as differences in absorption or clearance as well as technological factors including inaccuracies and laboratory testing and reporting, poor patient compliance, and poor doctor-to-patient communication. Initial daily prothrombin times, and later weekly values, are necessary to avoid underdosing or overdosing of the drug because many factors can either inhibit or increase warfarin's effect.

Warfarin's anticoagulant effect is enhanced by low vitamin K intake and reduced vitamin K absorption. Liver disease and drugs that limit warfarin's clearance on the liver will also potentiate the effects. Hypermetabolic conditions such as hyperthyroidism or patients with fever may have a faster response to warfarin due to increased metabolism of vitamin K factors.

Warfarin's anticoagulant effect is counteracted by increased vitamin K intake, and reduced absorption of warfarin secondary to the use of cholestyramine. Drugs that increase the activity of hepatic mixed oxidases (barbiturates, rifamain, penicillin and others) will also decrease the effect of warfarin. Alcohol has the potential to increase clearance of warfarin through increased hepatic enzymes. Studies have shown that this is not always the case.[41,42]

A hereditary resistance to warfarin has been reported.[43] The condition requires a five-fold to twenty-fold increase in dose to achieve an anticoagulant effect. This is likely due to an altered affinity because plasma levels are higher than average.[41]

Warfarin, with its complicated pharmacokinetics, delay of onset, and close monitoring, is not a drug that should be administered with standard dosing. There is a 1 to 5% prevalence of systemic side effects including major bleeding or prolonged anticoagulant effects secondary to an idiosyncratic reaction.[44,45] Local reactions include wound drainage and late healing secondary to increased swelling and hematoma formation.[45] Warfarin also has many drug interactions. An example of this is a combination of a nonsteroidal anti-inflammatory pain medication, which results in thirteen-fold increase in hemorrhagic peptic ulcer formation in patients over 65.[46] This is a special concern to the many degenerative joint disease patients with multiple joint disorders who rely on NSAIDS for their other joint pain while recovering from knee arthroplasty.

Warfarin Study Results

An examination of low-dose warfarin was performed by Laflamme and associates[47] patients undergoing total knee arthroplasty. One hundred ten patients were enrolled in the study and started on 10 mg of warfarin on the evening prior to surgery and 5 mg were given the night of surgery. The remaining doses were adjusted to keep prothrombin time between 1.2 and 1.5 times control. These patients had venograms performed on an average of the ninth postoperative day. DVTs occurred in 24 (21.4%) and no pulmonary emboli were reported. There was one episode of major bleeding (0.9%), one episode of minor bleeding (0.9%), and no episodes of wound problems or infection. The authors conclude that warfarin prophylaxis in total knee arthroplasty was safe and effective in preventing DVT.

Kaempffe and colleagues[48] did a study with 49 consecutive patients undergoing lower extremity joint replacement, hip and knee, either with warfarin-treated or pneumatic compression as a form of DVT prophylaxis. The presence of DVT was determined by venography, venous doppler, or impedance plethysmography. A warfarin dose of 10 mg was given the evening prior to surgery and followed by a 5 mg dose the night of surgery for those in the warfarin group. Dosing was then based on maintaining a prothrombin time of 15 seconds. The pneumatic compression was applied at the time of surgery and consisted of both thigh and calf compression. An equal percentage of patients undergoing total knee arthroplasty and total hip arthroplasty (25%) developed DVT. IPC was more effective than warfarin following hip arthroplasty (16 versus 24% incidence of DVT). Warfarin was more effective than IPC following knee arthroplasty (19 versus 32% incidence of DVT). The authors conclude that warfarin and IPC are safe and effective in the prevention of DVTs. Once again, conclusions are limited based on the small sampling of patients available in this study.

Hodge[49] also examined warfarin and pneumatic calf compression (PCC) for DVT prophylaxis in one group of 35 patients undergoing total knee arthroplasty versus those on warfarin prophylaxis. These patients received 10 mg of warfarin the night before surgery and subsequently were dosed to keep prothrombin time between 1.3 and 1.5 times the control. The second group of 66 patients were treated with PCC boots starting on the opposite leg during surgery and the operative leg after wound closure. Bilateral venograms were performed during the eighth and tenth postoperative days. The overall incidence of DVT in the warfarin group was 30% with 29% having calf thrombi and 6% having thigh thrombi. In the PCC boot group there was a 31% evidence of DVT with 27% having calf thrombi and 6% with thigh thrombi. Neither group had treatment related complications. Interestingly, a cost analysis was performed comparing the two groups. The warfarin group was approximately 50% more expensive than PCC boots. The author concluded that both forms of therapy are safe and effective in reducing DVT but economical factors may make compression devices a more favorable option.

Warfarin has fallen out of favor at some institutions. Review of several studies show that the efficacy of Coumadin is poor. Data from five large multicenter studies have become available[50] showing a reported DVT rate of 38 to 55% for warfarin with a proximal clot formation noted in the 7 to 12% range. These were large clinical trials with Coumadin as a control arm. Venograms were used to diagnose a clot so even under the most ideal of circumstances, a high DVT formation rate was noted.

Mechanical Compression

Many nonpharmalogical methods of DVT prophylaxis have been used as both sole prophylaxis as well as an adjuvant to other therapy. Intermittent pneumatic compression is the most effective of the mechanical compression devices with the others, early ambulation, elastic stockings, and elevation of limbs with mixed results and modest benefits not suitable for those at high risk.[51] Intermittent pneumatic compression became popular due to their ease of administration and lack of side effects. These devices work by reducing stasis and intermittently increasing the velocity of venous blood flow and enhancing endogenous fibrinolytic activity.[52,53]

There exists a balance between thrombin (clot formation) and plasmin (clot-dissolving action) on fibrinogen, which researchers have postulated being an important determinant of thrombosis. Examination of thrombin and plasmin by-products shows that calf compression alters thrombin and plasmin activity thus modifying coagulation and fibrinolytic pathways. Those who did not receive mechanical compression as DVT prophylaxis had an increase in thrombin activity and decrease in plasmin activity resulting in a greater ratio of clot-forming activity compared to clot-dissolving activity thus having a theoretical greater risk of DVT formation. Those using calf compression have a minor rise in thrombin activity but also increased plasmin activity with the overall result of similar ratios in their thrombin-plasmin by-products as their preoperative values.

In summary, the fibrinolytic system is stimulated by the mechanical calf compression and can overcome the increase in thrombin activity, thus preventing DVT. It is unclear if these protective changes are solely the result of the increase of venous blood flow or if an unidentified "activator" is released with compression.[52,53]

The most-common compression devices are the calf and thigh and lower extremity compression devices. In 1983 Gardener and Fox[54] describe a physiologic pumping mechanism in the foot, which activates upon weightbearing. With this principle in mind, venous "foot" pumps have been developed as a form of mechanical compression. These devices have been shown to maintain venous blood flow and decrease the incidence of DVT in postoperative patients and are believed to be as effective as calf and thigh compression.[55]

Wilson and colleagues[56] who noted a high DVT rate in their postoperative total knee arthroplasty patients designed a postoperative randomized study to compare the efficacy of mechanical compression with an arterial venous impulse foot pump compared to a control group. Fifty-nine patients were randomly placed in one of two groups. The foot pump was applied for 10 postoperative days. Both groups had a venogram performed after 10 postoperative days. The number of major thrombosis (major calf or proximal vein) in the control group was 59.4%, whereas in the foot pump group the number was significantly smaller at 17.8%. The total number of thrombosis (minor and major) was 68.7% in the control group and 50% in the foot pump group. The authors are unclear in their definition of what constitutes a major versus minor thrombosis and conclude that, with respect to major life-threatening clots, a foot pump is an effective method of DVT prophylaxis.

Westrich and associates[40] recently reported their results with pneumatic plantar compression (PPC) devices. Using venograms prior to discharge, DVT rates of 27% were noted for unilateral TKA and 28% for the bilateral groups. It is interesting to note that in the group that was negative for DVT formation, the PPC devices were in place for a mean of 19.2 hours per day, whereas those positive for DVT formation utilized these devices for a mean of 13.4 hours per day. Unfortunately, when not in a prospective study, achieving 19.2 hours of daily use may be difficult to achieve.

Low Molecular Weight Heparin

New to the arena of DVT prophylaxis is low molecular weight heparin (LMWH). Many of the initial studies of LMWH were used in total hip arthroplasty patients with little information available on the efficacy of LMWH in the total knee arthroplasty patient. Mechanism of action, risks and benefits, and study results will be discussed in the following section.

Mechanism of Action

Low molecular weight heparins are available in many forms (see Table 92.1). Although unfractionated heparin has a molecular weight of 12 to 15,000 daltons, using depolymerization procedures lower molecular weight heparin between 3 K and 10 K daltons can be achieved.[57] All LMWH are not equally created and numerous forms of LMWH have been studied.

The mechanism of action of LMWH rests in its ability to inhibit factor XA of the clotting cascade. Although all LMWH have certain anti-XA properties, with rela-

Table 92.1. Characteristics of several low molecular weight heparins available

Agent	Molecular weight (mean daltons)	Plasma half-life (hours)	Anti Xa– anti IIA ratio
Heparin	15,000	0.5–1	1 ≤ 1
Enoxaparin	4,500	3–4.5	2.7–1
RD Heparin	6,000	3–4	2.0–1
Fragmin	5,000	2–3	2.0–1
Logiparin	4,500	1.5–2	1.9–1

tively little anti-thrombin (anti-IIA) properties. Anti-IIA is important in obtaining surgical hemostasis and LMWH can be compared by their anti-XA to anti-IIA ratio. Ratios from 3 to 1 to 5 to 1 have been reported.[58] It has been noted that the anti-XA effect is inversely proportioned to the molecular weight of the heparin. Therefore, the lower molecular weight LMWHs have a higher anti-XA effect. Standard heparin inhibits its anticoagulant effects by forming a bridge between thrombin and anti-thrombin III. LMWH are effective by their anti-XA activity. Other mechanism actions of LMWH includes anti-platelet aggregation but the LMWH have less anti-platelet aggregation than unfractionated Heparin.

The RD Heparin Arthroplasty Group[58] evaluated the efficacy of Ardeparin in the prevention of DVT in total hip arthroplasty as well as total knee arthroplasty patients. This was the first study that compared LMWH to low-dose warfarin anticoagulation. DVT formation was studied with venograms prior to hospital discharge and these authors noted 46% risk reductions with LMWH usage. Bleeding events were studied and by evaluating the number of clinically significant bleeding events, as well as by comparison of the blood loss index (preop hemoglobin minus postop hemoglobin plus number of units PRBC transfused). Although the blood loss index was higher in the LMWH group (0.5 mg/dl), there was no difference in the number of clinical significant bleeding events. Work with Ardeparin was repeated by the Ardeparin arthroplasty study group of which we were investigators. Once again, a risk reduction rate of 27% with low molecular weight heparin usage (27% versus 30%) was noted.[59]

Hull and colleagues[60] found similar results when using the LMWH Logiparin. Despite only using once-a-day dosing, once again, LMWH was superior to Coumadin in preventing DVTs.

Levine and associates[61] studied Ardeparin in a double-blind randomized trial versus graduated compression stockings. Once again, venograms were used to evaluate DVT formation. Results showed 29.8% positive clots in the Ardeparin group compared to 58.3% in the placebo group. Bleeding events were similar with a 2.5% occurrence rate in the Ardeparin group versus 2.4% in the placebo group. Proximal DVTs were reduced in the Ardeparin group with 2.1% occurrence in the Ardeparin group versus 15.5% in the control group.

LeClerc and associates[62] compared the Enoxaparin in patients who were undergoing total knee arthroplasty or a tibial osteotomy and clot formation was compared to a placebo group. Patients received 30 mg subcutaneously every 12 hours starting the morning of postoperative day number one. Clot formation was detected by venogram with 58% DVT formation noted in the placebo group versus 17% in the Enoxaparin group. There were no proximal clots in the Enoxaparin group versus 19% in the placebo group. It is interesting to note that the DVT formation rate in the placebo group is similar to the values seen when warfarin is used for prophylaxis. Bleeding complications were similar between these two groups.

LeClerc and associates[63] performed a follow-up study comparing Enoxaparin to warfarin. As with the previous study, patients were dosed with 30 mg subcutaneously every 12 hours while those on warfarin had dose adjustments with a goal of an INR of 2 to 3. Results showed a DVT rate of 51.7% (10.4% proximal) for the warfarin group with a 36.9% (11.7% proximal) rate for the Enoxaparin group. Bleeding events were similar for the two groups. It should be noted that the clot formation rate for this study was increased compared to the previous study by these same authors. This may be due to a smaller sample and a smaller number of investigator sites that may have put some bias for the data.

Spiro and colleagues[64] also compared Enoxaparin to warfarin in prevention of DVT following total knee arthroplasty. Once again, lower DVT rates were noted in the Enoxaparin group (25.4%) versus the Warfarin group (45.4%). Proximal clots were also much lower in the Enoxaparin group with 1.7% versus 11.4% in the warfarin group. It should be noted that the overall incidence of hemorrhage complications observed in the Enoxaparin group was increased (6.9% versus 3.4%). This may be related to the fact that prophylaxis was initiated in the recovery room. It appears that prophylaxis with the Enoxaparin early may lower the overall clot formation rate as compared with the LeClerc data, but this may be at the expense of more bleeding complications seen in this study, which had its dosing starting in the immediate postoperative period.

CHOOSING THE CORRECT PROPHYLAXIS AGENT

The 1995 report from the Fourth American College of Physicians consensus conference updated the previous guidelines for DVT prophylaxis.[51] This conference reviewed clinical data and treatment recommendations (Table 92.2). Although this group concluded that aspirin, low dose heparin and warfarin provided only marginal efficacy for DVT prophylaxis, this panel went on to suggest that intermittent pneumatic compression as well as low molecular weight heparin are the prophylaxis methods of choice[50] (Table 92.3). It should be noted that these suggestions are based on clinical trials utilizing the above modalities. More data is needed to determine the overall DVT rate when prophylaxis methods are stacked (i.e., both intermittent pneumatic compression and low molecular weight heparin are utilized). It should be noted that of the five LMWH studies reviewed, two studies showed an overall increase in blood loss, incidence of hemorrhage, or transfusion requirements. This area deserves further discussion because it is the risk of bleeding complications that may deter the surgeon from utilizing the more effective prophylaxis agent.

Bleeding complications do not start with the use of LMWH because it is a known complication of the total knee arthroplasty procedure. In fact, bleeding has been reported as often as 6% of cases even when a placebo is utilized. Stulberg and colleagues[65] evaluated 638 total knees and evaluated a variety of prophylaxis methods. A wound complication rate of 18.1% was noted within this study group and did not vary on the agents utilized. From this study 10.6% of the patients had culture negative drainage from this study and 8.3% showed a delayed recovery secondary to the wound problems. Warfarin in itself is not without risks. Sutherland and associates[66] evaluated the complication rate with warfarin and found a 4% systemic complication rate with 12% requiring discontinuation of the prophylaxis agent. This complication rate occurred in the setting of a goal prothrombin time of 1.5 times normal.

The bleeding rates of these trials were difficult to compare due to the difference in bleeding definitions, dosage of low molecular weight heparin, concurrent medications, sample size as well as timing of dosage. For example, the RD Heparin Arthroplasty Group noticed a higher blood loss index, but when clinic significant bleeding were examined, there was no difference between the Ardeparin and warfarin group.[58] Similar results can be seen in the bleeding complications noted by Heit and colleagues. In this study group an overall complication rate of 7.9% was noted, but if one looked at only the clinically significant events that required an invasive diagnostic or therapeutic procedure or study withdrawal, then this number drops to 3%.

The above discussion is not meant to trivialize the bleeding events following a total knee arthroplasty for wound problems can be disastrous in this study population. What must be remembered is that bleeding problems are multifactorial and perhaps some of these wound complications could be avoided with changes in surgical technique. Careful hemostasis, meticulous closure as well as proper dosing of the medications may be able to decrease bleeding occurrences with low molecular weight heparins. Proper dosing includes starting the initial dose in 12 to 24 hours after the end of the case as well as a 12-hour dosing (not bid). Use of other agents such as aspirin or nonsteroidal anti-inflammatories should also be avoided during this prophylaxis period as well as the immediate preoperative period. Further studies are ongoing at our institution to evaluate the bleeding complication rate when the above guidelines are utilized.

Table 92.2. Studies reviewed by ACCP conference

Regimen	Number of trials	DVT incidence
Placebo	4	61%
Low dose heparin	1	34%
LMWH	7	30%
Warfarin	5	47%
ASA	1	79%
IPC	4	11%

Table 92.3. 1995 ACCP consensus recommendations (orthopedic)

	Knee replacement
Stockings	NR
Intermittent pneumatic compression	Yes Grade A-1
Aspirin	NR
Low dose UFH	NR
Adjusted dose UFH	NR
Warfarin	NR
LMWH	Yes (q12h postoperatively, fixed dose) Grade A-1
Vena cava filter	Last resort Grade C-4

Letter grades A to C indicate conclusiveness ratings, with grade A being conclusive.
Number grades 1 to 3 indicate the abundance of clinical trials, with grade 1 involving the most trials.
INR—international normalized ratio; LMWH—low molecular weight heparin; NR—not recommended; UFH—unfractionated heparin

IS DVT PROPHYLAXIS NEEDED?

Although it is commonly thought that by lowering DVT formation a reduction in fatal pulmonary emboli would also occur, this is a difficult hypothesis to test because it is estimated that due to the low incidence of fatal pulmonary emboli, 40,000 patients would be needed to achieve a suitable powered clinical trial.[67]

Despite the above, Haas and associates[22] were able to demonstrate a reduction in asymptomatic and symptomatic pulmonary embolism rate when a DVT was not present. Using venogram data, the pulmonary embolism rate was 6.9% in the presence of calf thrombi compared to 2% in the absence of DVT. Vresilovic and colleagues[68] noted pulmonary embolism in 5.6% despite warfarin prophylaxis.

Recently, Ansari and colleagues[67] evaluated the rate of fatal pulmonary emboli in 1390 TKAs performed without routine prophylactic anticoagulation. Results showed a 0.22% fatal pulmonary embolism rate for unilateral TKA compared to 0.7% in the bilateral TKA group. The question remains about how many of these deaths could have been prevented.

TREATMENT OF DVT

The goals in treatment of deep vein thrombosis include (1) immediate inhibition of the growth of the thrombus, (2) promotion of the thromboembolic resolution, and (3) prevention of recurrence.[70] This is initially accomplished by intravenous administration of heparin, which inhibits growth of the DVT. It also allows fibrinolytic dissolution to begin, but does not guarantee prevention or recurrence. The standard treatment regiment calls for substituting oral warfarin for IV heparin once an appropriate PT valve is maintained. This takes usually 3 to 5 days of combined warfarin and heparin treatment until adequate anticoagulation is achieved by the warfarin, and heparin may be discontinued. The length of treatment on warfarin varies depending on the risk of further DVT or PE. Length of treatment is controversial with recommendations varying from a minimum of 6 weeks up to 6 months or 1 year.[71]

Plasminogen is the inactive precursor of plasmin the active fibrinolytic enzyme. Thrombolytic therapy either with streptokinase (SK) or urokinase (UL) act by transforming plasminogen to plasmin. The use of thrombolytic therapy for treatment of deep vein thrombosis has been limited due to side effects including major bleeding, febrile reactions, and anaphylactic shock. Thrombolytic therapy is indicated for treatment of deep vein thrombosis in selected patients with large proximal clots and a low risk of bleeding complications.

Mechanical venous interruption such as Greenfield filters are used in patients in whom anticoagulation is contraindicated or when recurrent PE exists even with anticoagulation therapy. The most serious complications occur with migration of the devices through the vasculature and heart. Other complications include hemorrhage, perforation of the duodenum, and the ureter as well as formation of a thrombus proximal to the filter. The rates of these complications are unknown. Previously direct removal of venous thrombi was advocated, but it is now rarely done because of high incidence of recurrent thrombosis postoperatively.[71]

CONCLUSION

As orthopedic surgeons, we are all biased by our personal opinions and experiences. This is very evident when looking at the DVT prophylaxis patterns used by individual surgeons. Although comparing 30 years of DVT data is similar to comparing apples to oranges (or perhaps the entire fruit basket!), some trends have become evident. Recent well-designed studies discussed above cast doubt on the previous confidence in ASA and warfarin. Although no prophylaxis method is ideal, mechanical compression devices and low molecular weight heparin appear promising. Further studies are needed to evaluate this true DVT rate when these modalities are both utilized. Together, as is done at many institutions, the length of therapy required must also be better defined.

References

1. Le Clerc JR, Geerts WH, Des Jardins L, La Flamme GH, L'Esperance BL, Demers C, Kassis J, Cruickshank M, Whitmore L, Delorme F. Prevention of venous thromboembolism after knee arthroplasty a randomized double blind trial comparing Enoxaparin with warfarin. *ANN Intern Med*. 1996; 124:619–626.
2. Pidala MJ, Donovan DL, Kepley RF. A prospective study on intermittent pneumatic compression in the prevention of deep vein thrombosis in patients undergoing total hip or total knee replacement. *Surg-General-Obstet*. 1992; 175: 47–51.
3. Anders MJ, Lifeso RM, Landis M, Mikulsky J, Meinking C, McCracken KS. Effect of preoperative donation of autologous blood on deep-vein thrombosis following total joint arthroplasty of the hip or knee. *J Bone Joint Surg*. 1996; 78-A:574–580.
4. Sharrock NE, Sculco TP, Ranawat CS, Maynard MJ, Harpel PC. Changes in circulatory indices of thrombosis and fibrinolysis during total knee arthroplasty performed under tourniquet. *J Arthroplasty*. 1995; 10:523–526.
5. Stulberg BN, Francis CW, Pellegrini VD, Miller ML, Shull S, DeSwart R, Easley K, Totterman S, Marden VJ. Antithrombin III/low dose heparin in the prevention of deep vein thrombosis after total knee arthroplasty. *Clin Orthop*. 1989; 248:152–157.
6. Sharrock NE, Hargett MJ, Urquhart B, Peterson MGE, Ranawat C, Insall J, Windsor R. Factors affecting deep vein thrombosis rate following total knee arthroplasty under epidural anesthesia. *J Arthroplasty*. 1993; 8:133–139.
7. Kim YH. The incidence of deep vein thrombosis after cementless and cemented knee replacement. *J Bone Joint Surg*. 1990; 72:779–783.

8. Liu GC, Ferris EJ, Reifsteck JR, et al. Effect of anatomical variations on deep vein thrombosis of the lower extremity. *Am J Roentgenol*. 1986; 146:845–848.
9. Virchow R. Neuer Fall von Todticher, Embolie der Lungenarterien 1856. *Arch Pathol Anat*. 10:225–228.
10. Ginsberg JS, Brill-Edwards P, Panju A, Patel A, McGinnis J, Smith F, Dale I, Johnston M, Ofosu F. Preoperative plasma levels of thrombin–antithrombin II complex correlate with the development of venous thrombosis after major hip or knee surgery. *Thrombosis and Haemostasis*. 1995; 74:602–605.
11. Stulberg BW, Lucas FV, Belhobek GU. Anti-thrombin III as a marker of venous thromboembolism: a preliminary report. *Trans Orthop Res Soc*. 1984; 9:100.
12. Morrey BF. *Joint Replacement Arthroplasty*. New York: Churchill Livingston; 1991:67–82.
13. Lambie JM, et al. Diagnostic accuracy in venous thrombosis. *Br Med J*. 1970; 2:142–143.
14. Canale ST. *Campbell's Operative Orthopaedics*. St. Louis: Mosby; 1998:270–285.
15. Albrechtsson U, Olsson CG. Thrombotic side effects of lower limb venography. *Lancet*. 1976; 1:723–724.
16. Thomas ML, MacDonald LM. Complications of ascending phlebography of the leg. *Br Med J*. 1978; 2:317–318.
17. Borris LC, Christiansen HM, Lassen MR, et al. Comparison of real time B-mode ultrasonography and bilateral ascending phlebography for detection of postoperative deep vein thrombosis following elective hip surgery. *Thromb Haemost*. 1989; 61:363–365.
18. Sadler DA. Diagnosis of deep-vein thrombosis comparison of clinical evaluation, ultrasound, plethysmography and venoscan with x-ray venogram. *Lancet*. 1984;716–719.
19. Harris WH, Athanasoulis C, Waltman AC, Salzman EW. Cuff-impedance phlebography and ^{125}I fibrinogen scanning versus roentenographic phlebography for diagnosis of thrombophlebitis following hip surgery. *J Bone Joint Surg. Am*. 1976; 58(7):938–944.
20. Mullick SC, Wheeler HB, Songser GF. Diagnosis of deep venous thrombosis by measurement of electrical impedance. *Am J of Surg*. 1970; 119:417–423.
21. Lotke PQ, Palevsky H, Keenan AM, Meranze S, Steingerg ME, Ecker ML, Kelly MA. Aspirin and warfarin for thromboembolic disease after total joint arthroplasty. *Clin Orthop*. 1996; 324:251–258.
22. Haas SB, Tribos CB, Insall JN, Becker MW, Windsor RE. The significance of calf thrombi after total knee arthroplasty. *J Bone Joint Surg Br*. 1992; 74(B)-6:799–802.
23. Philbrick T, Becker DM. Calf deep venous thrombosis—a wolf in sheep's clothing? *Arch Intern Med*. 1988; 148:2131–2138.
24. Mudge M, Hughes LE. The long-term sequelae of deep vein thrombosis. *Br J Surg*. 1978; 65:692–694.
25. Warwick D, Perez J, Vicker C, Bannister G. Does total hip arthroplasty predispose to chronic venous insufficiency. *J Arthrop*. 1996; II(5):529–533.
26. Hedner T, Everts B. The early clinical history of salicylates in rheumatology and pain. *Clin Rheumatol*. 1998; 17(1):17–25.
27. Mann CC, Plummer ML. *The Aspirin Wars: Money, Medicine and 100 Years of Ramant Competition*. New York: Knopf; 1991.
28. George JN, Shattil SJ. The clinical importance of acquired abnormalities of platelet function. *NEJM*. 1991; 324(I):27–35.
29. Craven LL. Experiences with aspirin (acetylsalicylic acid) in the nonspecific prophylaxis of coronary thrombosis. *Mississippi Valley Med J*. 1953; 75:38–42.
30. Weiss HJ, Aledort LM, Kockwa S. The effect of salcylates on the hemostatic properties of platelets in man. *J Clin Invest*. 1986; 47:2169–2180.
31. Mustard JF, Packham MA. Factors influencing platelet function: adhesion, release and aggregation. *Pharmacol Rev*. 1970; 22:97–187.
32. DeLee JC, Rockwood CA. The use of aspirin in thromboemboli disease. *J Bone Joint Surg* 1980; 62(A):149–152.
33. Salzman EW, Harris WH, DeSanctis RW. Reduction in venous thromboembolism by agents affecting platelet function. *NEJM*. 1971; 284:1287–1292.
34. Patrono C. Aspirin as an antiplatelet drug. *NEJM*. 1994; 330(18):1287–1294.
35. Roth GJ, Calverley DC. Aspirin, platelets and thrombosis: theory and practice. *Blood*. 1994; 83(4):885–989.
36. Campbell WB. Lipid-derived autocoids: eicosanoids and platelet activation factor. In: *Goodman and Gilman's The Pharmacological Basis of Therapeutics*. 8th ed. New York: Pergamon Press; 1990.
37. McKenna R, Bachmann F, Kaushal SP, Galante JO. Thromboembolic disease in patients undergoing total knee replacement. *J Bone Joint Surg*. 1976; 58-A:928–932.
38. McKenna R, Galante J, Bachmann F, et al. Prevention of venous thromboembolism after total knee replacement by high-dose aspirin or intermittent calf and thigh compression. *Br Med Journal*. 1980; 280:514–517.
39. Haas SB, Insall JB, Scuderi GR, Windsor RE, Ghelman B. Pneumatic sequential-compression boots compared with aspirin prophylaxis of deep-vein thrombosis after total knee arthroplasty. *J Bone Joint Surg*. 1990; 72-A:27–31.
40. Westrich GH, Sculco TP. Prophylaxis against deep venous thrombosis after total knee arthroplasty. *J Bone Joint Surg*. 78A(6):826–834.
41. Hirsh J, Dalen JE, Deykin E, et al. Oral anticoagulants: mechanism of action, clinical effectiveness and optimal therapeutic range. *Chest*. 1992; 102(supp 4):312S–326S.
42. O'Reilly RA. Lack of effect of fortified wine injested during fasting and anticoagulant therapy. *Arch Intern Med*. 1981; 141:458–459.
43. O'Reilly, Aggeler PM, Hoag MS, et al. Hereditary transmission of exceptional resistance to coumadin anticoagulant drugs. *NEJM*. 1983; 308:1229–1230.
44. Lieberman JR, Gererts WH. Prevention of venous thromboembolism in orthopaedic patients. *J Bone Joint Surg*. 1976; 58(A) (7):903–913.
45. Sutherland CJ, Schurman JR. Complications associated with warfarin prophylaxis in total knee arthroplasty. *Clin Orthop*. 1987; 219:158–162.
46. Shorr RI, Ray WA, Daugherty JR, Griffin MR. Current use of nonsteroidal anti-inflammatory drugs and oral anticoagulants places elderly persons at high risk for hemorrhagic peptic ulcer disease. *Arch Inter Med*. 1993; 153:165–170.
47. Laflamme GH, Laflamme GE, Paiment, Beaumont P. Effi-

cacy and safety of low dose warfarin prophylaxis in cemented total knee prosthesis. *Ann Chir*. 1994; 48(8):717–722.
48. Lotke PQ, Palevsky H, Keenan MA, Meranze S, Steingerg ME, Ecker ML, Kelly MA. Aspirin and warfarin for thromboembolic disease after total joint arthroplasty. *Clin Orthop*. 1996; 324:251–258.
49. Hodge WA. Prevention of deep vein thrombosis after total knee arthroplasty. *Clin Orthop*. 1991; 271:101–105.
50. Clasett TP, Anderson FA Jr, Heit J, et al. Prevention of venous thromboembolism. *Chest*. 1995; 108(suppl):312S–334S.
51. Salzman EW, Harris WH. Prevention of venous thromboembolism in orthopaedic patients. *J Bone Joint Surg*. 1976; 58A(7):903–913.
52. Allenby F, Boardman L, Pflug J, Calnan J. Effects of external pneumatic intermittent compression on fibrinolysis in man. *Lancet*. 1973; 2:1412–1414.
53. Weitz J, Michelsen J, Gold K, Owen J, Carpenter D. Effects of intermittent pneumatic calf compression on postoperative thrombin and plasmin activity. *Thromb and Haemost*. 1986; 56:198–201.
54. Gardner AM, Fox RH. The venous pump of the human foot: preliminary report. *Bristol Med Chir J*. 1983; 98:109–114.
55. Wilson NV, Das SK, Maurice H, et al. Thrombosis prophylaxis in total knee replacement. *Br J Surg*. 1992; 74(1):50–52.
56. Wilson NV, Das SK, Smibert MG, Thomas EM, Kakkar VV. Thrombosis prophylaxis in total knee replacement: does a simple mechanical method help? *Br J Surg*. 1992; 77(12):1417.
57. Zimlich RH, Fulbright M, Friedman RJ. Current status on anticoagulation therapy after total hip and total knee arthroplasty. *JAAOS*. 1996; 4(1):54–62.
58. RD Heparin Arthroplasty Group. RD heparin compared with warfarin for the prevention of venous thromboembolic disease following total hip or knee arthroplasty. *J Bone Joint Surg Am*. 1994; 76:1174–1185.
59. Heit J, Berkowitz S, Bona R, Comp P, Corson J, Cushner F, Ellio G, Garino J, Lyons R, Ohar J, Holloway S, Zacquis L. Efficacy and safety of Normiflo (A LMWH) compared to warfarin for prevention of venous thromboembolism following total knee replacement: a double-blind dose-ranging study. *Thromb Haemost*. 1997; 77(1):32–38.
60. Hull R, Raskob G, Brant R. A comparison of subcutaneous low-molecular weight heparin with warfarin for prophylaxis against deep-vein thrombosis after hip or knee implantation. *N Engl J Med*. 1993; 329(19):1370–1376.
61. Levine MN, Gent M, Hirsh J, Wertz J, et al. Ardeparin (low molecular weight heparin) vs. graduated compression stockings for the prevention of venous thromboembolism. A randomized trial in patients undergoing knee surgery. *Arch Intern Med*. 1996; 156:851–856.
62. Leclerc JR, Geerts WH, DesJardins L, et al. Prevention of deep vein thrombosis after major knee surgery: a randomized double blind trial comparing a low molecular weight heparin fragment (enoxaparin) to placebo. *Thromb Haemost*. 1992; 67:417–423.
63. Leclerc JR, Geerts WN, DesJardins L, I'Esporance B, Cruikshank M, et al. Prevention of venous thromboembolism (WTE) after knee arthroplasty—a randomized double-blind trial comparing a low molecular-weight heparin fragment (enoxaparin) to warfarin. *Ann Int Med*. 1996; 124(7):619–626.
64. Spiro TE, Fitzgerald RH, Trowbridge AA, et al. Enoxaparin a low molecular weight heparin and warfarin for the prevention of venous thromboembolic disease after elective knee replacement surgery. *Blood*. 1993; 82:410A (abstract).
65. Stulberg BN, Insall JN, Williams GW, Ghelman B. Deep vein thrombosis following total knee replacement. *J Bone Joint Surg*. 1984; 66A(2):194–201.
66. Sutherland CJ, Schurman JR. Complications associated with warfarin prophylaxis in total knee arthroplasty. *Clin Orthop*. 1987; 219:158–162.
67. Ansari S, Warwick D, Ackroyd CE, Newman MA. Incidence of fatal pulmonary embolism after 1390 knee arthroplasties without routine prophylactic anticoagulation except in high risk cases. *J Arthrop*. 1997; 12(C):599–602.
68. Uresilovic EJ, Hozack WJ, Booth RE, Rothman RN. Incidence of pulmonary embolism after total knee arthroplasty with low dose coumadin prophylaxis. *Clin Orthop*. 1993; (286):27–31.
69. Petersdorf RG. *Harrison's Principles of Internal Medicine*. Aukland: McGraw-Hill; 1983:1565.
70. Sabiston DC. *Textbook of Surgery: The Biological Basis of Modern Surgical Practice*. 15th ed. W.B. Saunders Co.; 1997: 1602–1606.

Glossary of Implants

Product Name

AGC Cruciate Retaining

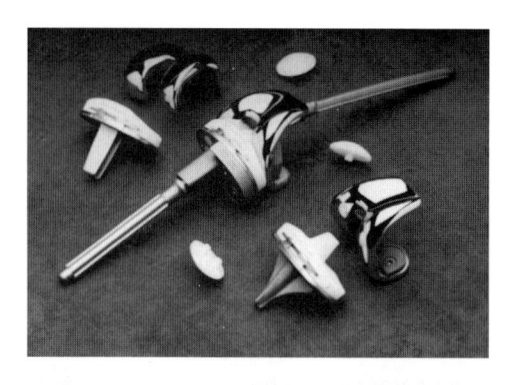

Company

Biomet, Inc.
Airport Industrial Park
Warsaw, IN 46581-8137
(219) 267-6639

Constraint Features

PCL Retaining

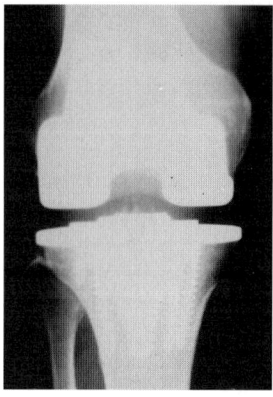

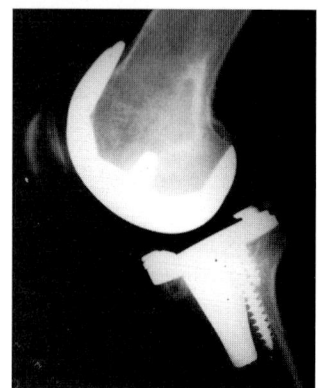

Product Name

AGC Posterior Stabilized

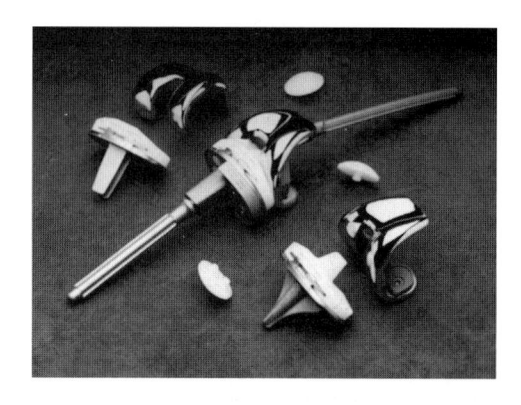

Company

Biomet, Inc.
Airport Industrial Park
Warsaw, IN 46581-8137
(219) 267-6639

Constraint Features

PCL Substituting

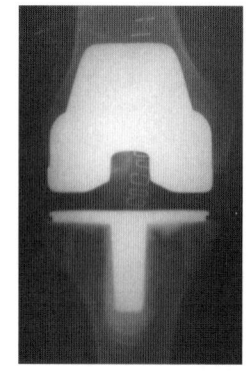

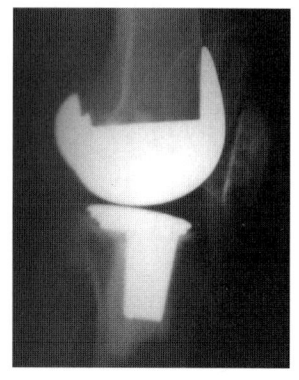

Glossary of Implants

Product Name

Finn

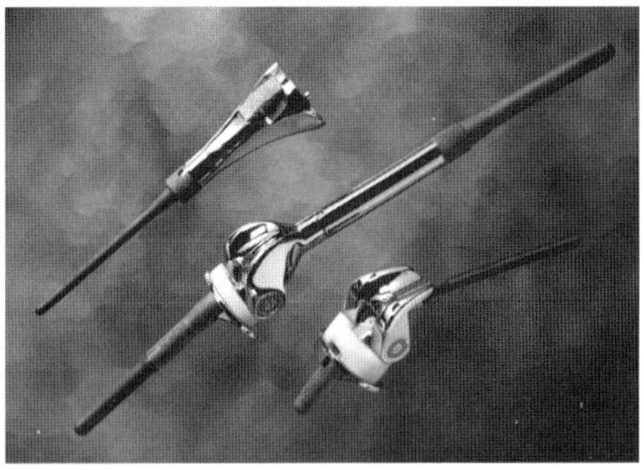

Company

Biomet, Inc.
Airport Industrial Park
Warsaw, IN 46581-8137
(219) 267-6639

Constraint Features

PCL Substituting
Varus/Valgus Constrained
Linked Constrained

Product Name

Maxim Complete Knee System

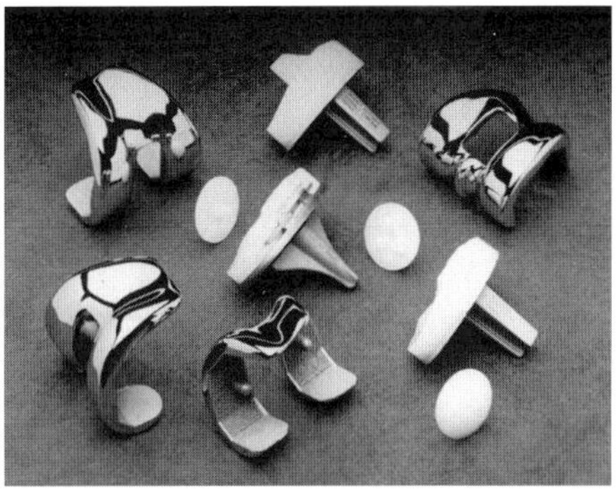

Company

Biomet, Inc.
Airport Industrial Park
Warsaw, IN 46581-8137
(219) 267-6639

Constraint Features

PCL Retaining
PCL Substituting
Varus/Valgus Constrained

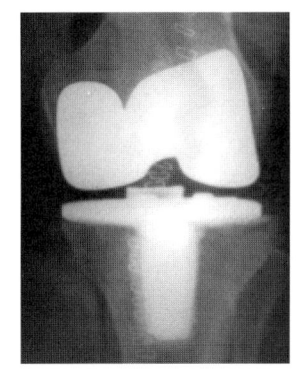

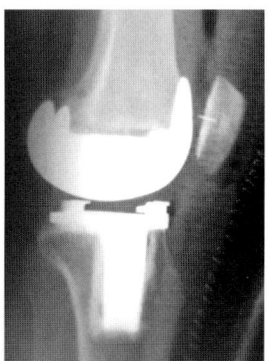

Product Name

Performance Cruciate Retaining

Company

Biomet, Inc.
Airport Industrial Park
Warsaw, IN 46581-8137
(219) 267-6639

Constraint Features

PCL Retaining

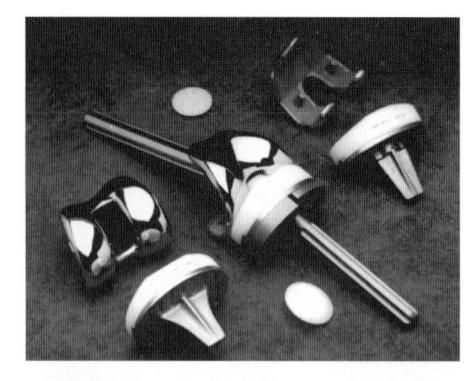

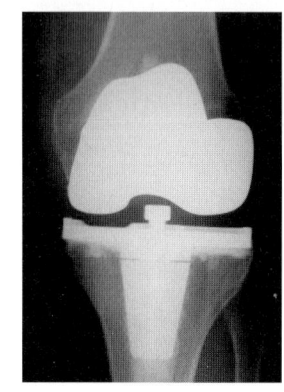

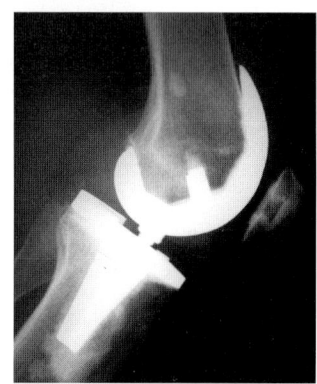

Product Name

Performance Posterior Stabilized

Company

Biomet, Inc.
Airport Industrial Park
Warsaw, IN 46581-8137
(219) 267-6639

Constraint Features

PCL Substituting

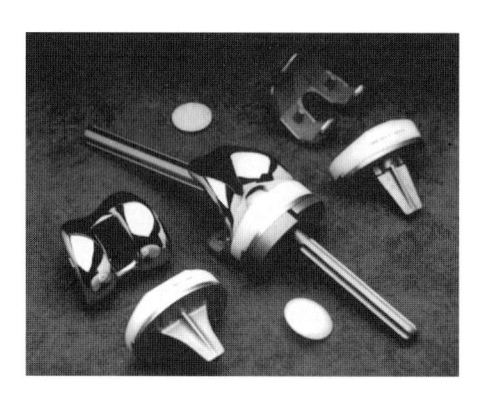

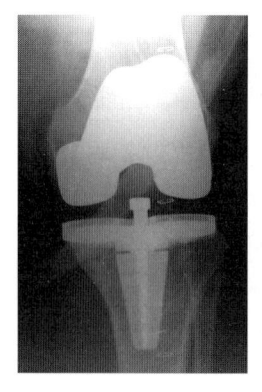

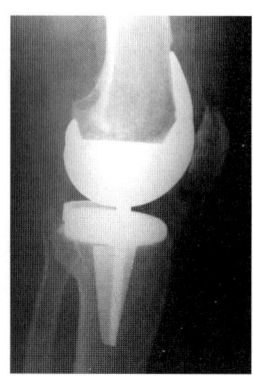

Product Name
Townley TKO System

Company
Biopro
17 17th Street
Port Huron, MI 48060
(810) 982-7777

Constraint Features
PCL Retaining

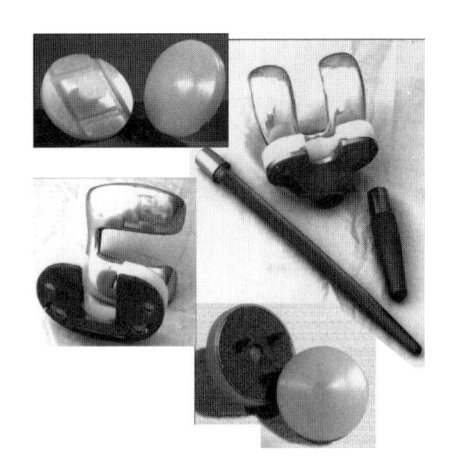

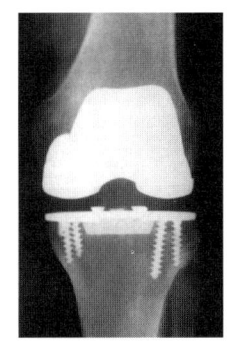

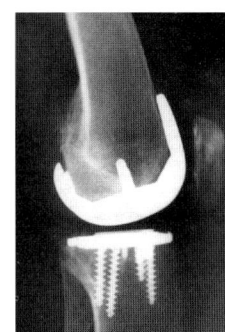

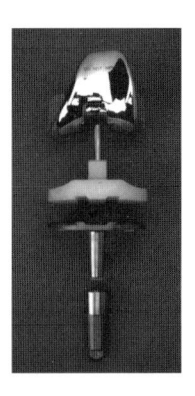

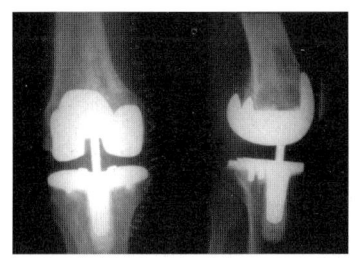

Product Name
AMK

Company
DePuy Orthopaedics, Inc.
700 Orthopaedic Dr.
Warsaw, IN 46581-0988
(800) 366-8143

Constraint Features
PCL Substituting

Product Name
AMK CR

Company
DePuy Orthopaedics, Inc.
700 Orthopaedic Dr.
Warsaw, IN 46581-0988
(800) 366-8143

Constraint Features
PCL Retaining

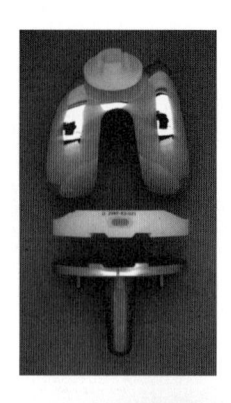

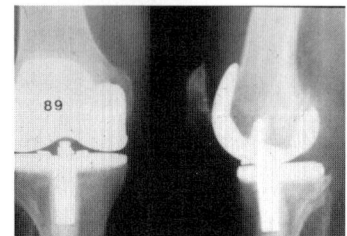

Product Name
Coordinate

Company
DePuy Orthopaedics, Inc.
700 Orthopaedic Dr.
Warsaw, IN 46581-0988
(800) 366-8143

Constraint Features
PCL Substituting
Varus/Valgus Constrained

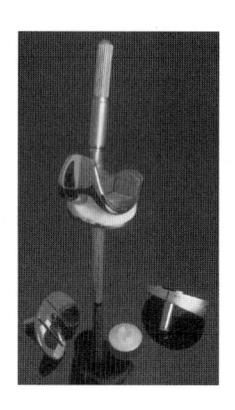

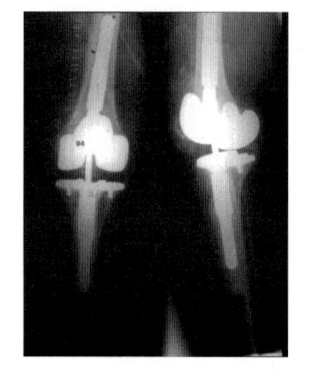

Product Name
New Jersey LCS

Company
DePuy Orthopaedics, Inc.
700 Orthopaedic Dr.
Warsaw, IN 46581-0988
(800) 366-8143

Constraint Features
PCL Retaining
PCL Substituting

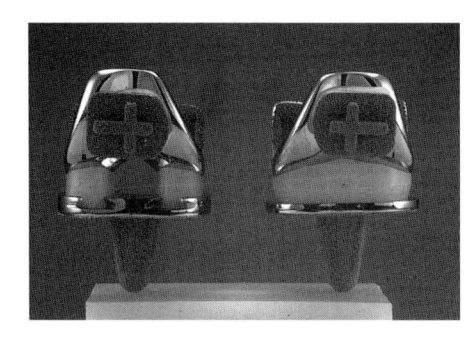

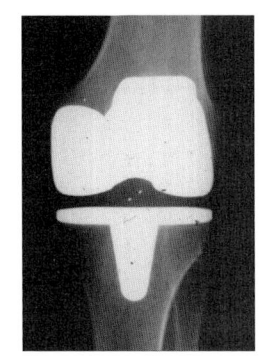

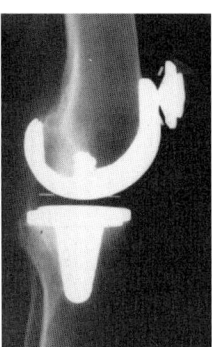

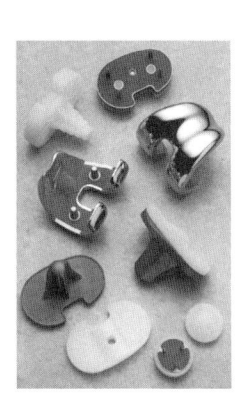

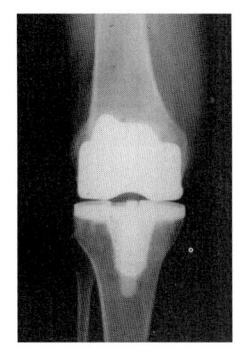

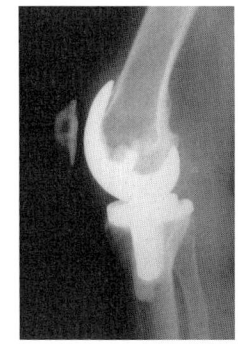

Product Name
The Foundation

Company
Encore Orthopaedics, Inc.
9800 Metrix Boulevard
Austin, TX 78758
(800) 456-8696

Constraint Features
PCL Retaining

Product Name
The Foundation

Company
Encore Orthopaedics, Inc.
9800 Metrix Boulevard
Austin, TX 78758
(800) 456-8696

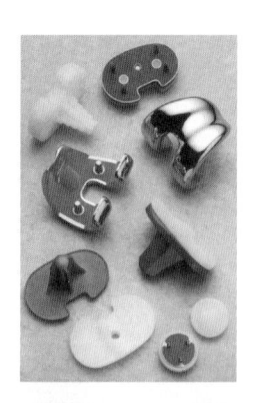

Constraint Features
PCL Substituting

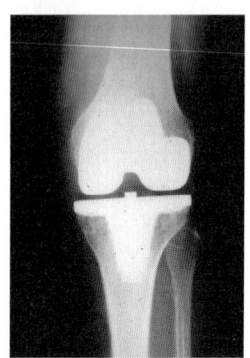

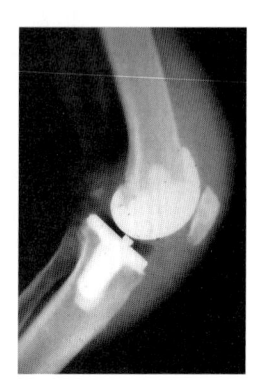

Product Name
Optetrak

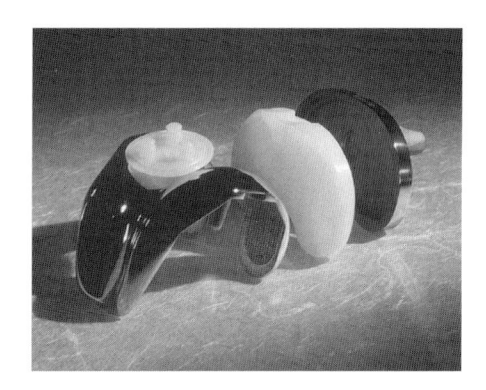

Company
Exactech, Inc.
4613 NW 6th Street
Gainesville, FL 32609
(800) 392-2832

Constraint Features
PCL Retaining
PCL Substituting
Varus/Valgus Constrained

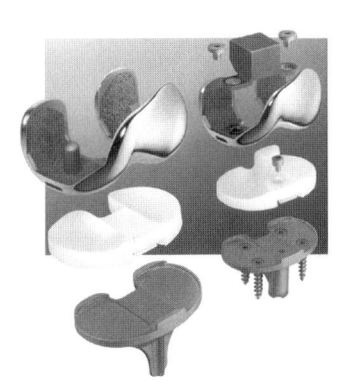

Product Name
Duracon

Company
Howmedica Worldwide, Inc.
301 Route 17 N. 9th Floor
Rutherford, NJ 07070
(201) 507-7300

Constraint Features
PCL Retaining
PCL Substituting

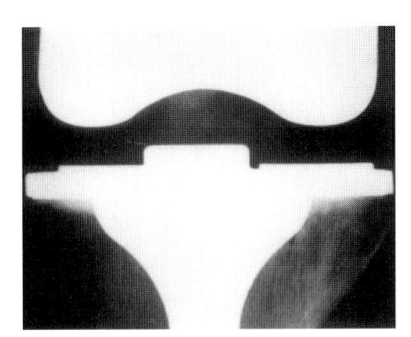

Product Name
Kinemax Plus

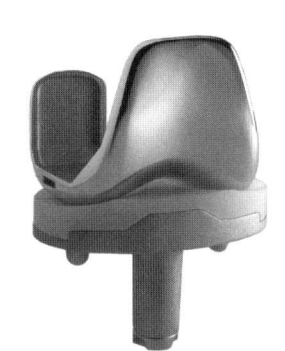

Company
Howmedica Worldwide, Inc.
301 Route 17 N. 9th Floor
Rutherford, NJ 07070
(201) 507-7300

Constraint Features
PCL Retaining
PCL Substituting
Varus/Valgus Constrained

Product Name
PCA Modular

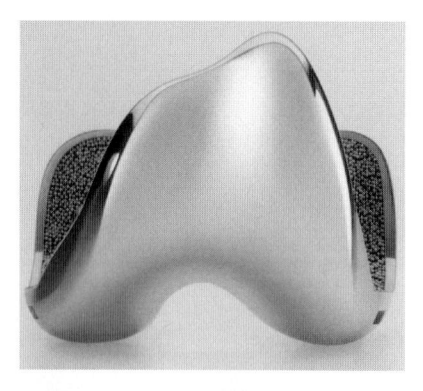

Company
Howmedica Worldwide, Inc.
301 Route 17 N. 9th Floor
Rutherford, NJ 07070
(201) 507-7300

Constraint Features
PCL Retaining

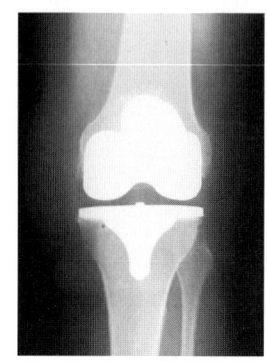

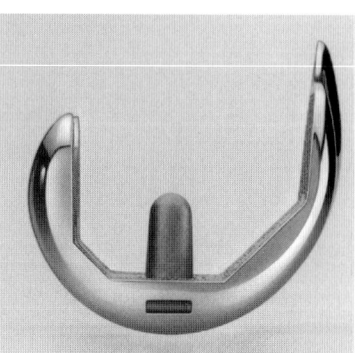

Product Name
PCA Primary

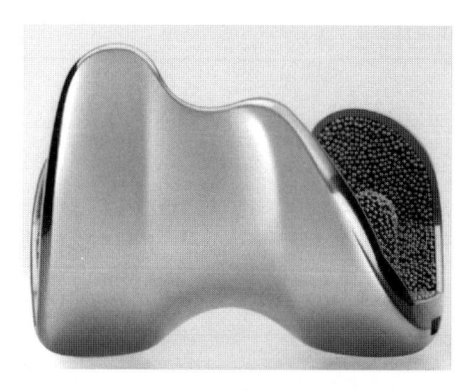

Company
Howmedica Worldwide, Inc.
301 Route 17 N. 9th Floor
Rutherford, NJ 07070
(201) 507-7300

Constraint Features
PCL Retaining

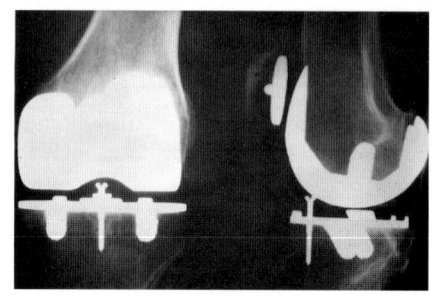

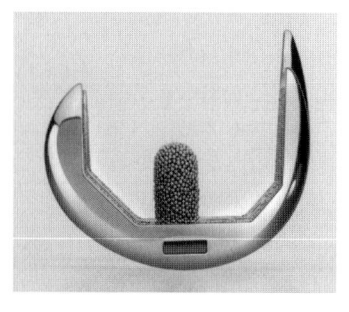

Product Name
Continuum CR

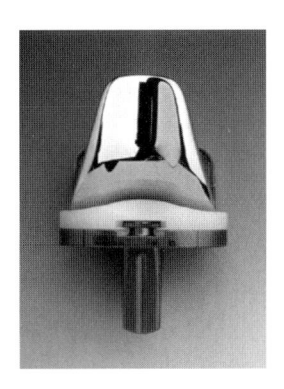

Company
Implex Corp.
80 Commerce Dr.
Allendale, NJ 07401-1600
(201) 818-1800

Constraint Features
PCL Retaining

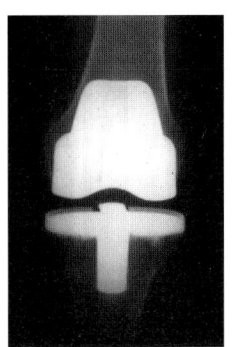

Product Name
Continuum PS

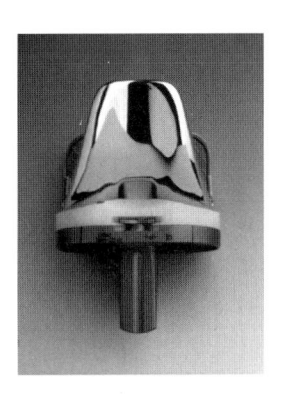

Company
Implex Corp.
80 Commerce Dr.
Allendale, NJ 07401-1600
(201) 818-1800

Constraint Features
PCL Substituting

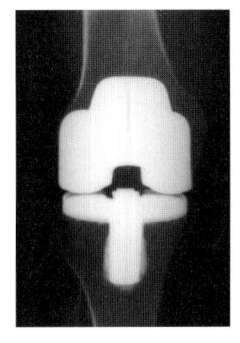

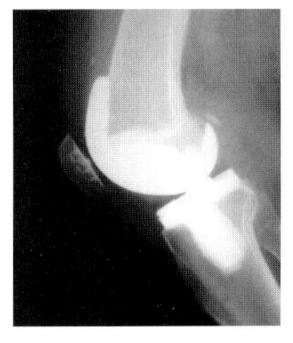

Product Name
Continuum Revision

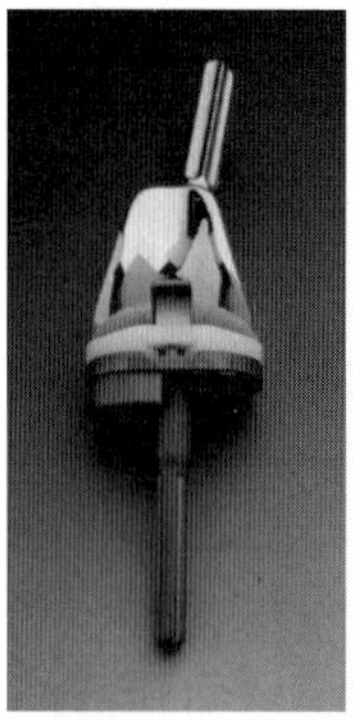

Company
Implex Corp.
80 Commerce Dr.
Allendale, NJ 07401-1600
(201) 818-1800

Constraint Features
PCL Substituting

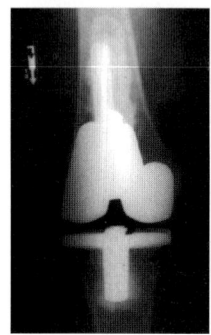

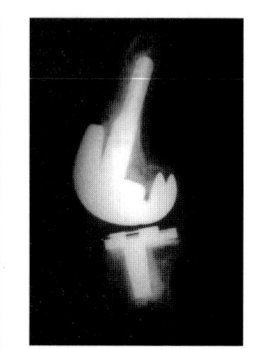

Product Name
Insall Burstein PS All Poly

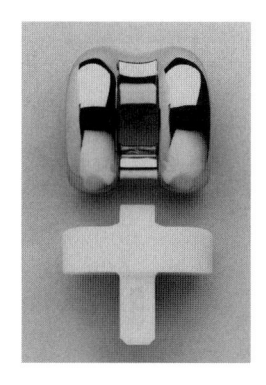

Company
Johnson & Johnson Professional, Inc.
325 Paramount Dr.
Raynham, MA 02767
(800) 451-2006

Constraint Features
PCL Substituting

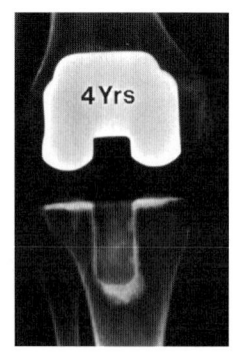

Product Name
Insall Burstein PS Metal Back Tibia

Company
Johnson & Johnson Professional, Inc.
325 Paramount Dr.
Raynham, MA 02767
(800) 451-2006

Constraint Features
PCL Substituting

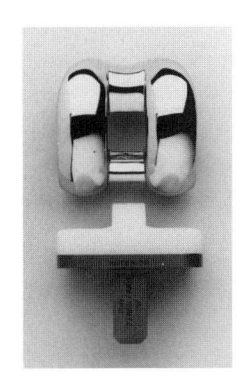

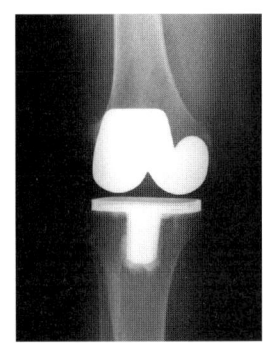

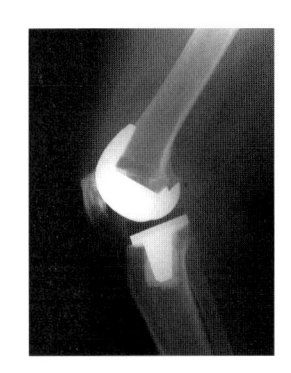

Product Name
P.F.C. Modular TC3

Company
Johnson & Johnson Professional, Inc.
325 Paramount Dr.
Raynham, MA 02767
(800) 451-2006

Constraint Features
PCL Substituting

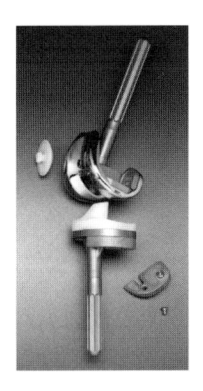

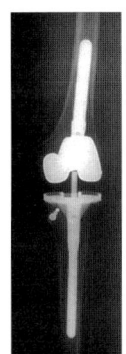

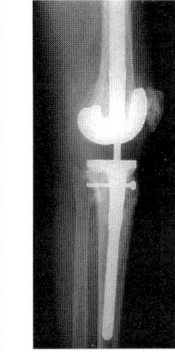

Product Name

P.F.C. Modular Total Knee
 System—CR

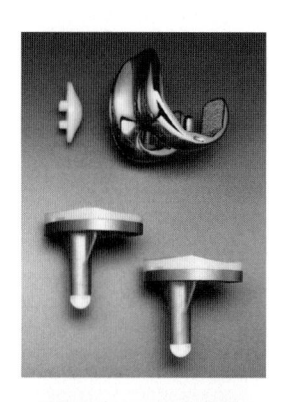

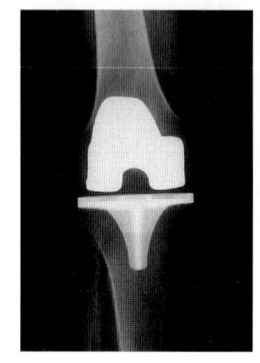

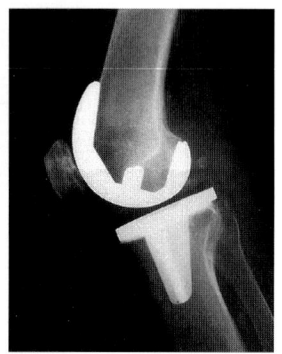

Company

Johnson & Johnson Professional,
 Inc.
325 Paramount Dr.
Raynham, MA 02767
(800) 451-2006

Constraint Features

PCL Retaining

Product Name

P.F.C. Modular Total Knee
 System—PS

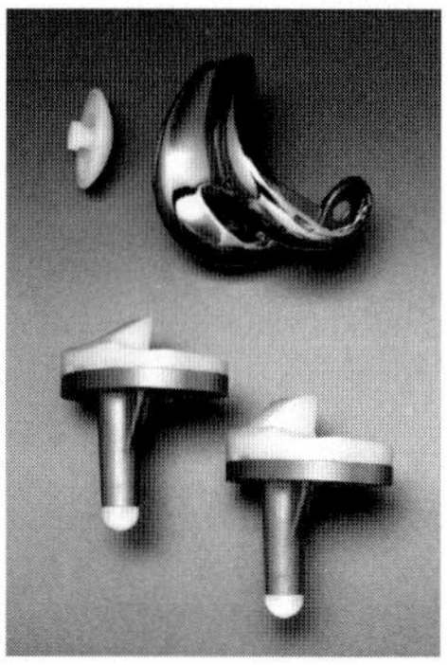

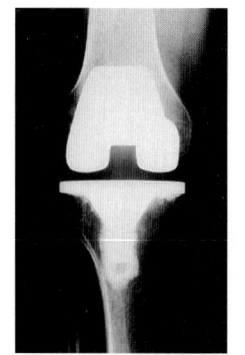

Company

Johnson & Johnson Professional,
 Inc.
325 Paramount Dr.
Raynham, MA 02767
(800) 451-2006

Constraint Features

PCL Substituting

Product Name
P.F.C. Sigma Cruciate Retaining

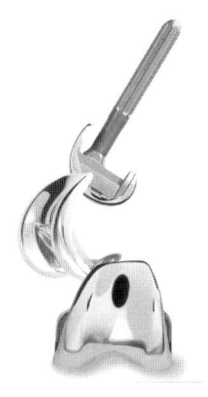

Company
Johnson & Johnson Professional, Inc.
325 Paramount Dr.
Raynham, MA 02767
(800) 451-2006

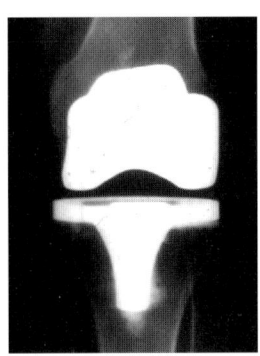

Constraint Features
PCL Retaining
PCL Substituting
Varus/Valgus Constrained

Product Name
P.F.C. Sigma Posterior Stabilized

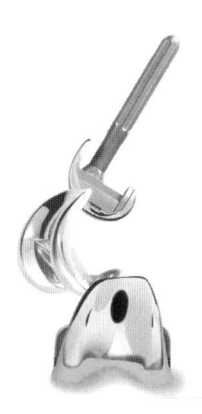

Company
Johnson & Johnson Professional, Inc.
325 Paramount Dr.
Raynham, MA 02767
(800) 451-2006

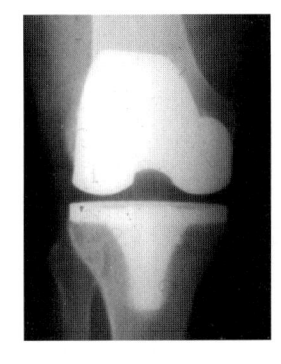

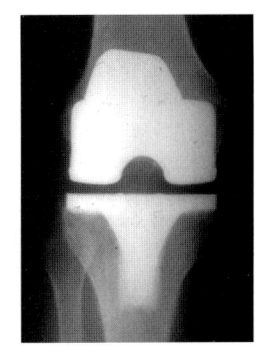

Constraint Features
PCL Retaining
PCL Substituting
Varus/Valgus Constrained

Product Name
S-Rom

Company
Johnson & Johnson Professional, Inc.
325 Paramount Dr.
Raynham, MA 02767
(800) 451-2006

Constraint Features
PCL Substituting
Varus/Valgus Constrained
Linked Constrained

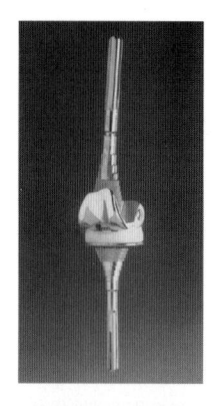

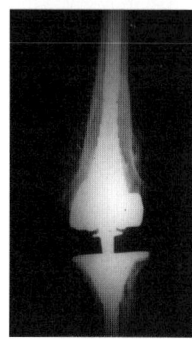

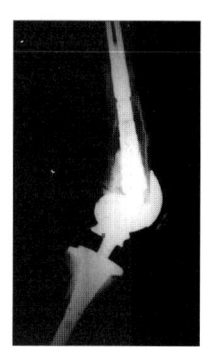

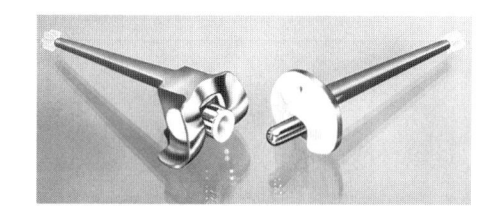

Product Name
Endo-Model

Company
Link America, Inc.
321 Palmer Rd.
Denville, NJ 07834-9708
(800) 932-0616

Constraint Features
Varus/Valgus Constrained
Linked Constrained

Product Name
Series 3000

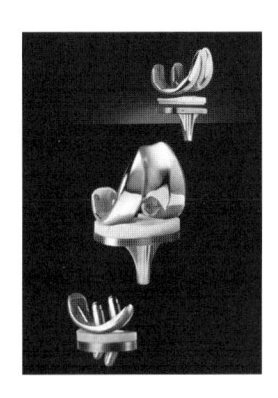

Company
Osteonics Corp.
59 Rte. 17
Allendale, NJ 07401-1677
(800) 447-7836

Constraint Features
PCL Retaining
PCL Substituting
Constrained

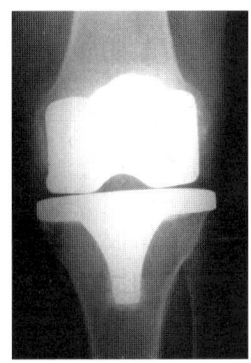

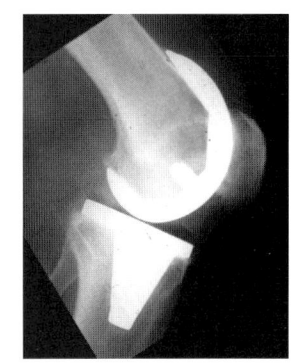

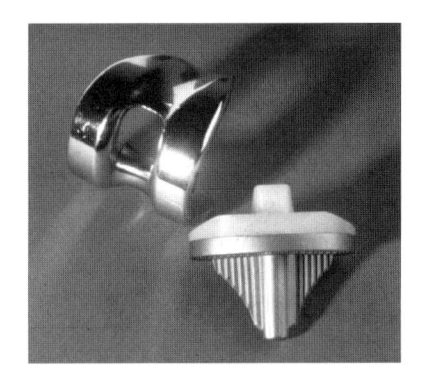

Product Name
Series 7000

Company
Osteonics Corp.
59 Rte. 17
Allendale, NJ 07401-1677
(800) 447-7836

Constraint Features
PCL Retaining
PCL Substituting
Varus/Valgus Constrained

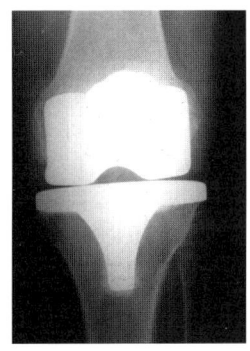

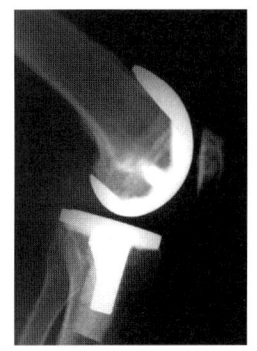

Product Name

Genesis I

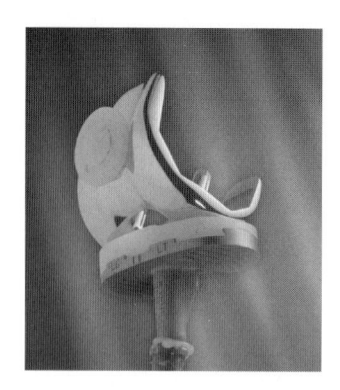

Company

Smith & Nephew Richards, Inc.
1450 Brooks Road
Memphis, TN 38116
(800) 821-5700

Constraint Features

PCL Retaining
PCL Substituting
Varus/Valgus Constrained

Product Name

Genesis II

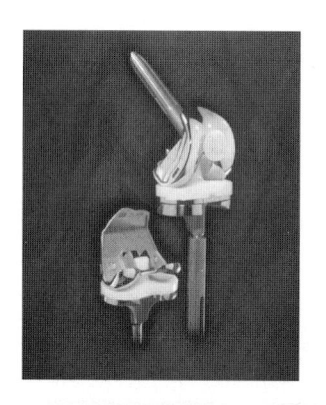

Company

Smith & Nephew Richards, Inc.
1450 Brooks Road
Memphis, TN 38116
(800) 821-5700

Constraint Features

PCL Retaining
PCL Substituting
Varus/Valgus Constrained

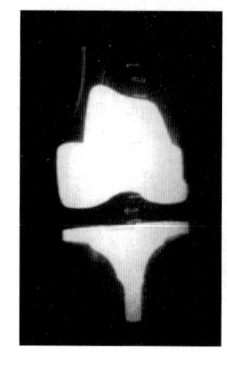

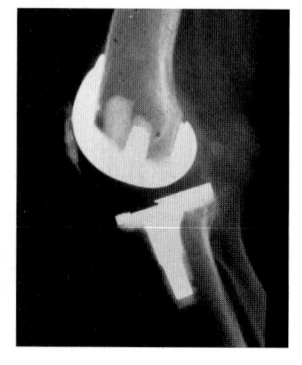

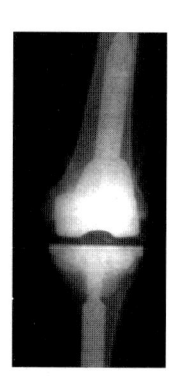

Product Name

Profix

Company

Smith & Nephew Richards, Inc.
1450 Brooks Road
Memphis, TN 38116
(800) 821-5700

Constraint Features

PCL Retaining
PCL Substituting
Varus/Valgus Constrained

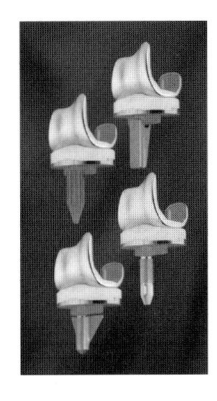

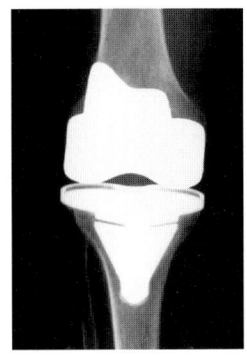

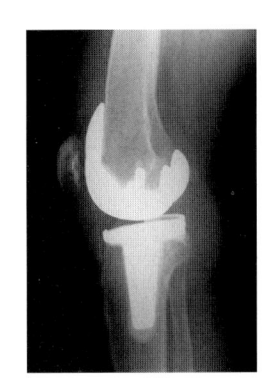

Product Name

Profix Cruciate Retaining Revision Prosthesis

Company

Smith & Nephew Richards, Inc.
1450 Brooks Road
Memphis, TN 38116
(800) 821-5700

Constraint Features

PCL Retaining
PCL Substituting
Varus/Valgus Constrained

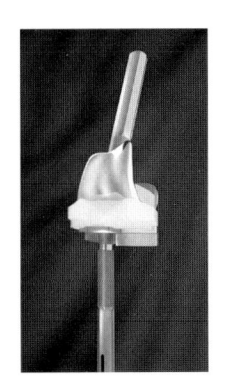

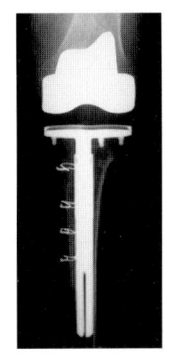

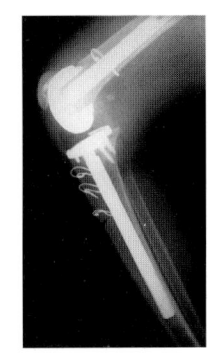

Product Name
Profix with Tibial Stem

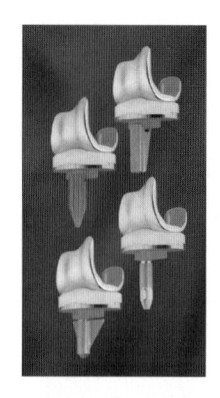

Company
Smith & Nephew Richards, Inc.
1450 Brooks Road
Memphis, TN 38116
(800) 821-5700

Constraint Features
PCL Retaining
PCL Substituting
Varus/Valgus Constrained

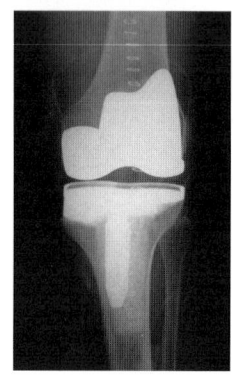

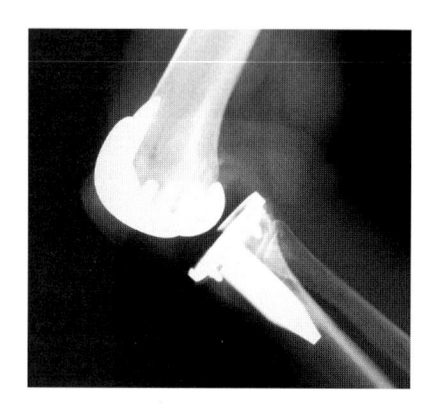

Product Name
Apollo

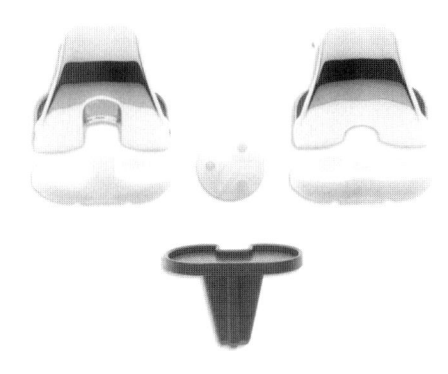

Company
Sulzer Orthopedics, Inc.
9900 Spectrum Dr.
Austin, TX 78717
(800) 888-4676

Constraint Features
PCL Retaining
PCL Substituting
Varus/Valgus Constrained

Glossary of Implants

Product Name
Apollo PS

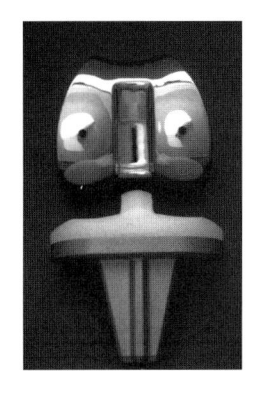

Company
Sulzer Orthopedics, Inc.
9900 Spectrum Dr.
Austin, TX 78717
(800) 888-4676

Constraint Features
PCL Substituting

Product Name
Natural-Knee II

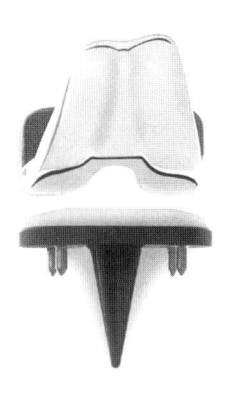

Company
Sulzer Orthopedics, Inc.
9900 Spectrum Dr.
Austin, TX 78717
(800) 888-4676

Constraint Features
PCL Retaining
PCL Substituting
Varus/Valgus Constrained

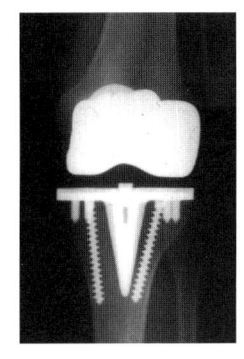

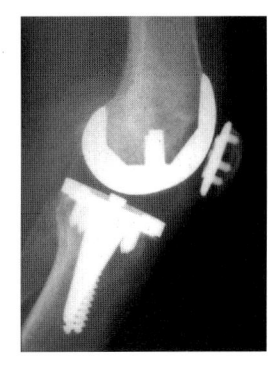

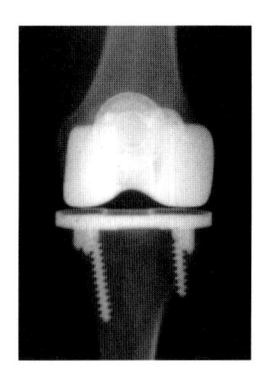

Product Name
Advance

Company
Wright Medical Technology, Inc.
5677 Airline Rd.
Arlington, TN 38002-9501
(800) 238-7188

Constraint Features
PCL Retaining
PCL Substituting

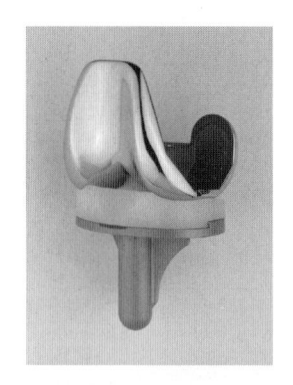

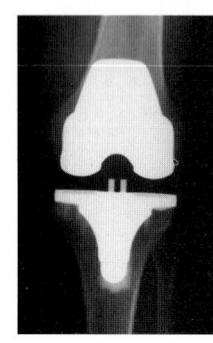

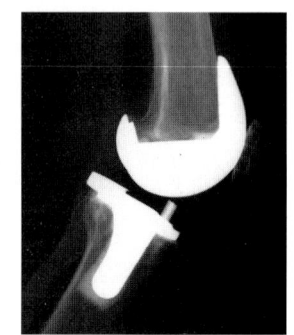

Product Name
Advantim Revision PS

Company
Wright Medical Technology, Inc.
5677 Airline Rd.
Arlington, TN 38002-9501
(800) 238-7188

Constraint Features
PCL Substituting
Constrained

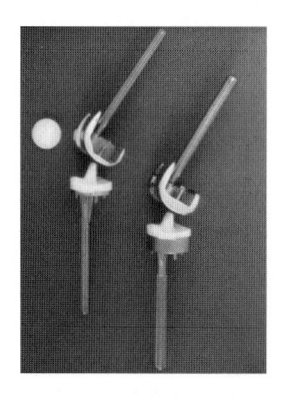

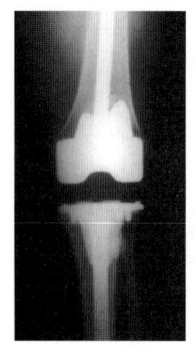

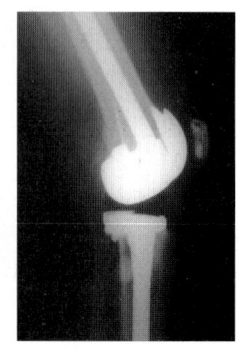

Glossary of Implants

Product Name
Advantim TC CR with All Poly Tibia

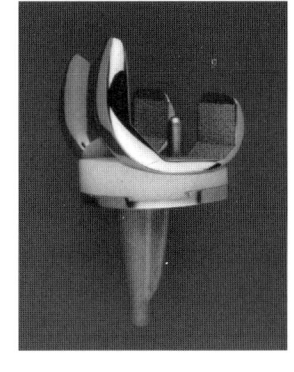

Company
Wright Medical Technology, Inc.
5677 Airline Rd.
Arlington, TN 38002-9501
(800) 238-7188

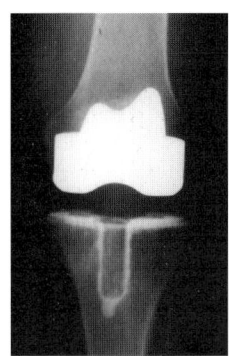

Constraint Features
PCL Retaining
Constrained

Product Name
Advantim TC CR with CF Tibia

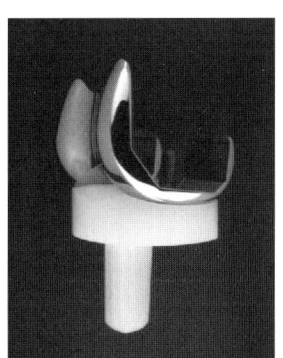

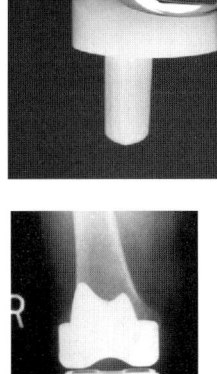

Company
Wright Medical Technology, Inc.
5677 Airline Rd.
Arlington, TN 38002-9501
(800) 238-7188

Constraint Features
PCL Retaining

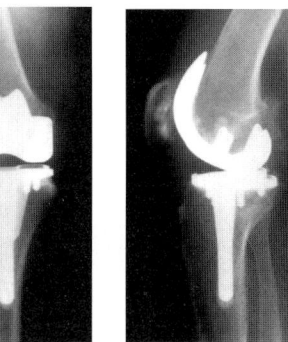

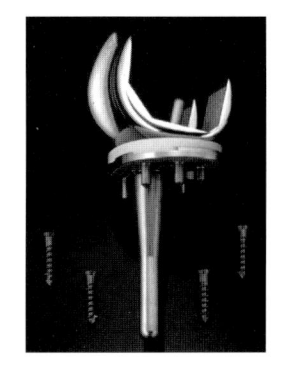

Product Name
Advantim TC PS

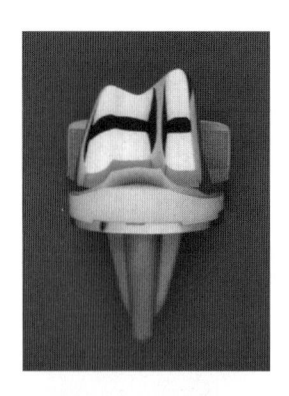

Company
Wright Medical Technology, Inc.
5677 Airline Rd.
Arlington, TN 38002-9501
(800) 238-7188

Constraint Features
PCL Substituting

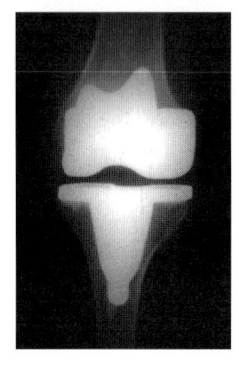

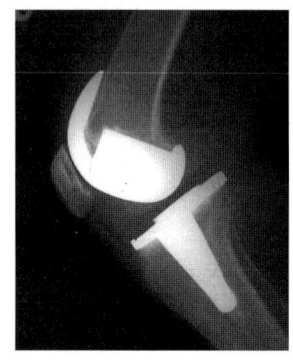

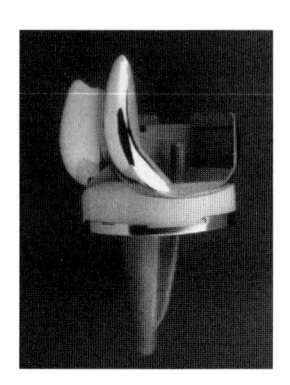

Product Name
Axiom Cruciate Retaining Primary

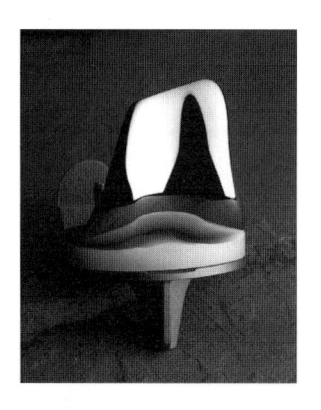

Company
Wright Medical Technology, Inc.
5677 Airline Rd.
Arlington, TN 38002-9501
(800) 238-7188

Constraint Features
PCL Substituting

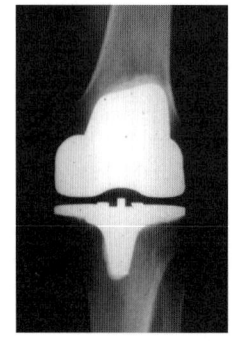

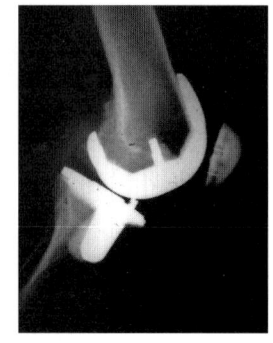

Glossary of Implants

Product Name

Axiom PS Primary

Company

Wright Medical Technology, Inc.
5677 Airline Rd.
Arlington, TN 38002-9501
(800) 238-7188

Constraint Features

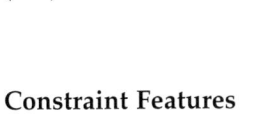

PCL Retaining

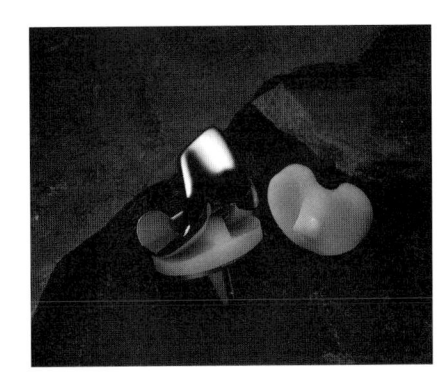

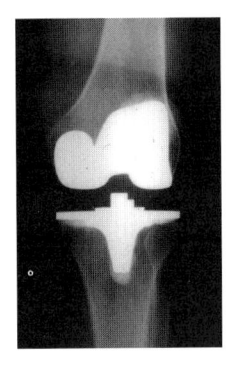

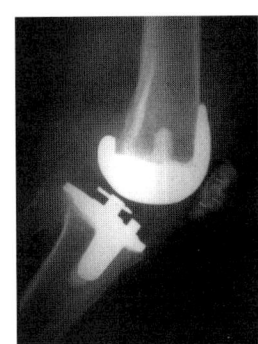

Product Name

Axiom Revision Prosthesis

Company

Wright Medical Technology, Inc.
5677 Airline Rd.
Arlington, TN 38002-9501
(800) 238-7188

Constraint Features

PCL Substituting
Constrained

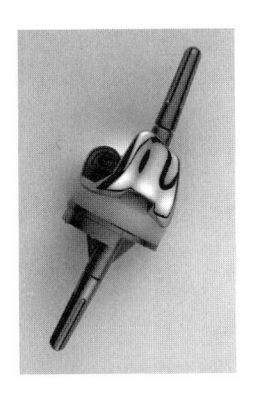

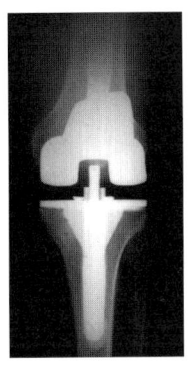

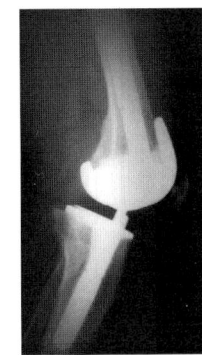

Product Name
TCP III

Company
Zimmer, Inc.
P.O. Box 708
Warsaw, IN 46581-0708
(800) 613-6131

Constraint Features
PCL Substituting

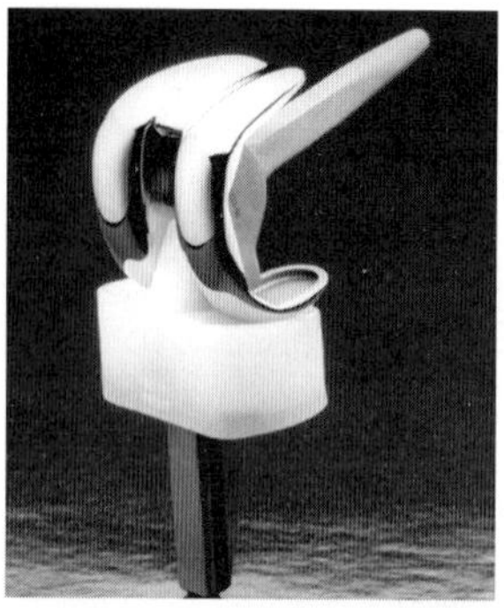

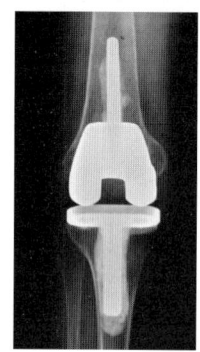

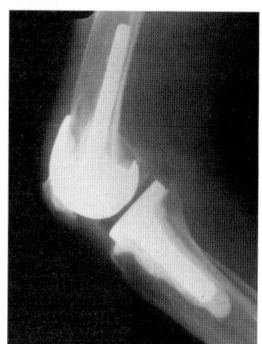

Product Name
Insall Burstein I All Poly Tibia

Company
Zimmer, Inc.
P.O. Box 708
Warsaw, IN 46581-0708
(800) 613-6131

Constraint Features
PCL Substituting

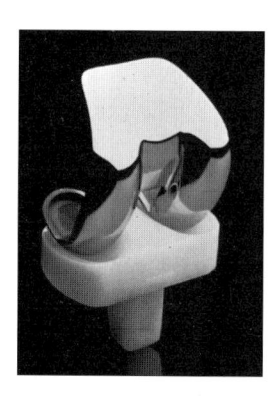

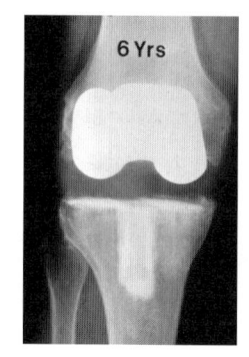

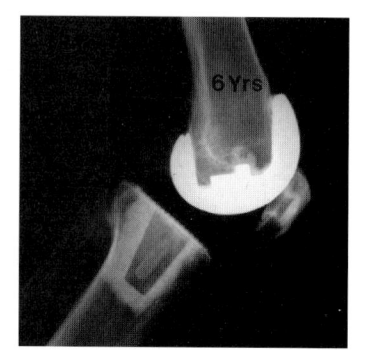

Product Name
Insall/Burstein I Metal Back Tibia

Company
Zimmer, Inc.
P.O. Box 708
Warsaw, IN 46581-0708
(800) 613-6131

Constraint Features
PCL Substituting

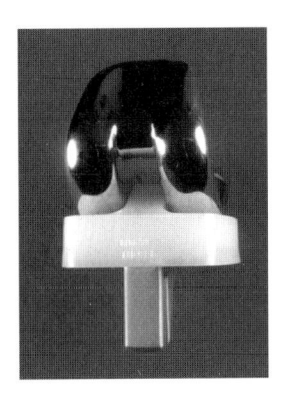

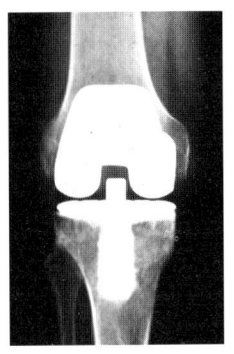

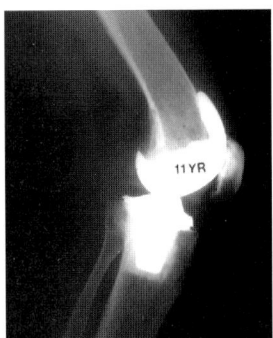

Product Name
Insall/Burstein II

Company
Zimmer, Inc.
P.O. Box 708
Warsaw, IN 46581-0708
(800) 613-6131

Constraint Features
PCL Substituting
Varus/Valgus Constrained

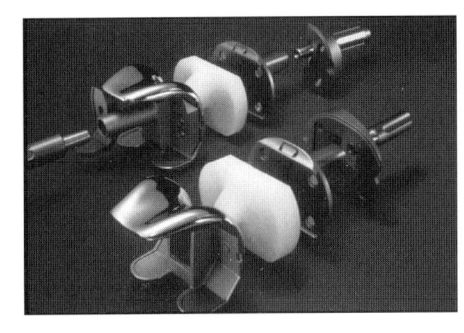

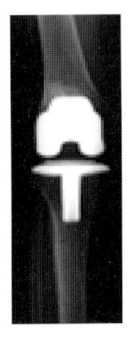

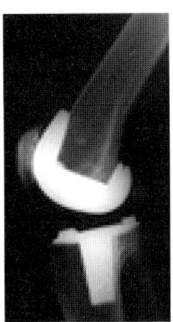

Product Name
Insall/Burstein II CCK

Company
Zimmer, Inc.
P.O. Box 708
Warsaw, IN 46581-0708
(800) 613-6131

Constraint Features
PCL Substituting
Varus/Valgus Constrained

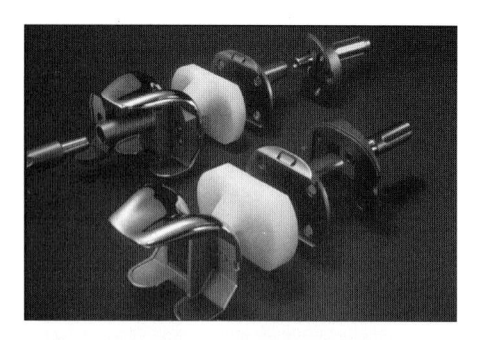

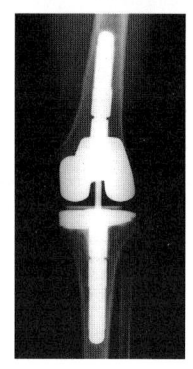

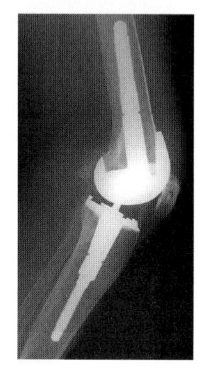

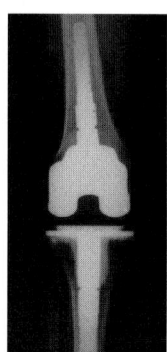

Product Name
MG II

Company
Zimmer, Inc.
P.O. Box 708
Warsaw, IN 46581-0708
(800) 613-6131

Constraint Features
PCL Retaining

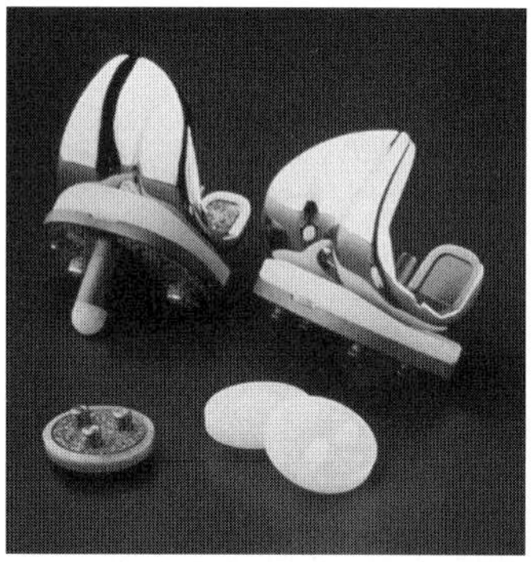

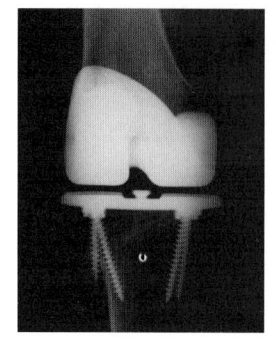

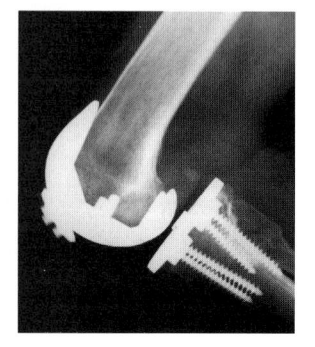

Product Name
NexGen Cruciate Retaining

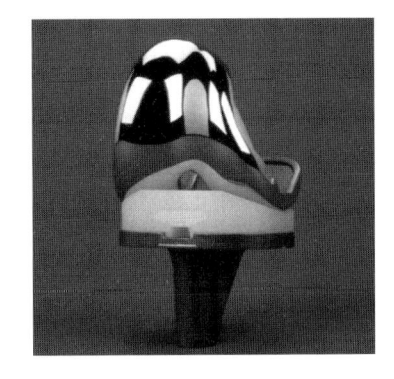

Company
Zimmer, Inc.
P.O. Box 708
Warsaw, IN 46581-0708
(800) 613-6131

Constraint Features
PCL Retaining

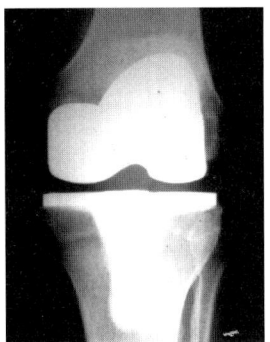

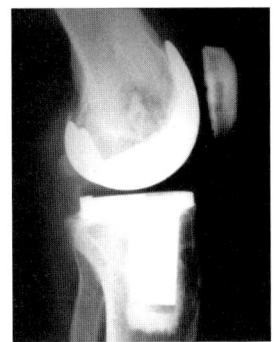

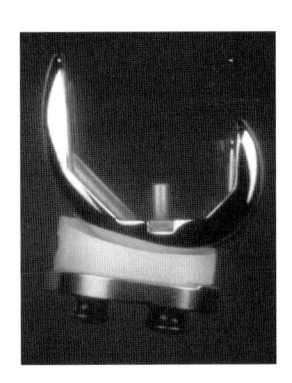

Product Name
NexGen PS

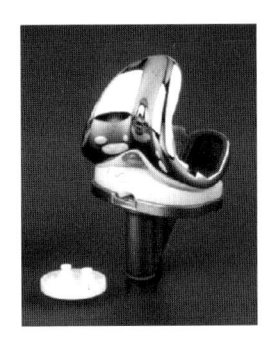

Company
Zimmer, Inc.
P.O. Box 708
Warsaw, IN 46581-0708
(800) 613-6131

Constraint Features
PCL Substituting

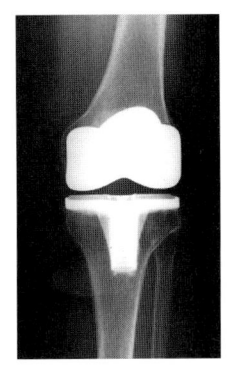

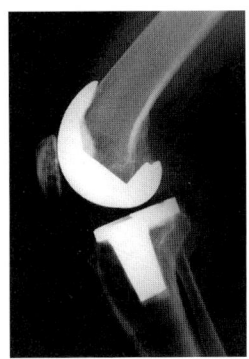

Product Name
NexGen Legacy PS

Company
Zimmer, Inc.
P.O. Box 708
Warsaw, IN 46581-0708
(800) 613-6131

Constraint Features
PCL Substituting

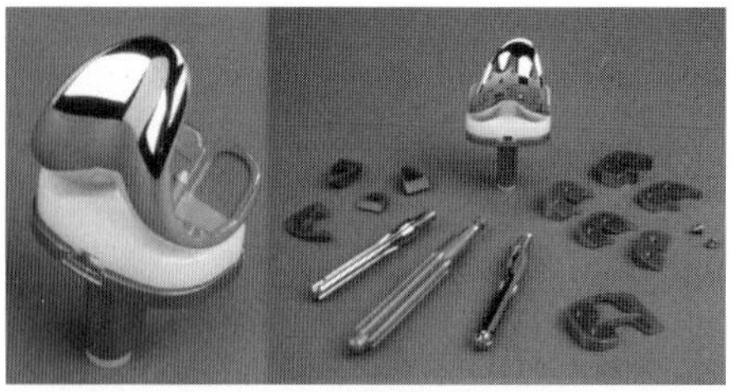

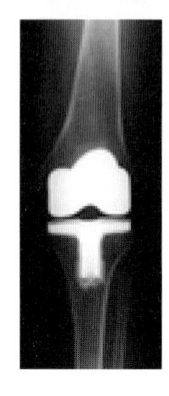

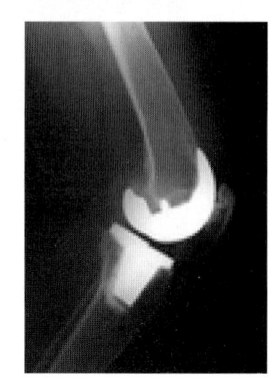

Product Name
NexGen Legacy CCK

Company
Zimmer, Inc.
P.O. Box 708
Warsaw, IN 46581-0708
(800) 613-6131

Constraint Features
PCL Substituting
Constrained

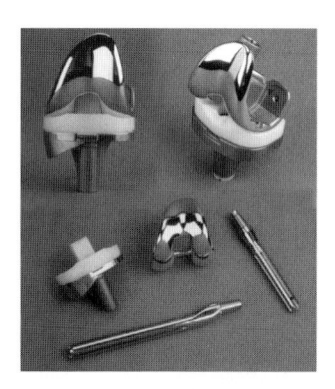

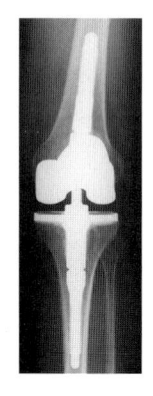

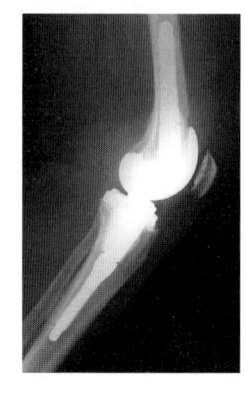

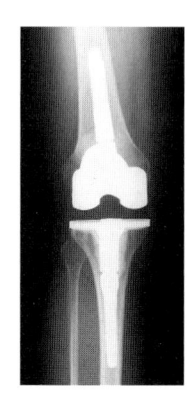

Product Name
MBK

Company
Zimmer, Inc.
P.O. Box 708
Warsaw, IN 46581-0708
(800) 613-6131

Constraint Features
PCL Retaining

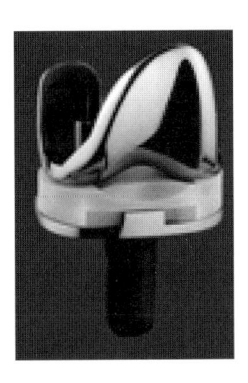

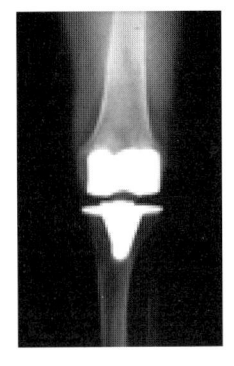

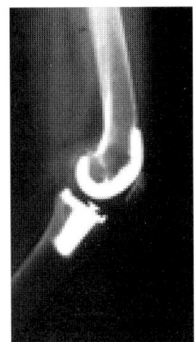

Index

Page numbers followed by *f* or *t* denote figures or tables, respectively.

A

AAOS (American Academy of Orthopaedic Surgeons), outcomes assessment by, 40–41, 43
Abscess, epidural, 685
Access disease, osteolysis with, cementing as seal against, 274
Acetabular reamers, in femoral allografting, 425, 426*f*
Acetylsalicylic acid. *See* Aspirin
ACL. *See* Anterior cruciate ligament
Active range of motion, assessment of
 in painful total knee arthroplasty, 349
 preoperative, 6
Activities of daily living (ADL)
 as goals in continuous passive motion, 655
 inability to perform, patient complaints about, 651
 rehabilitation and, 653–654, 660
Activity levels
 and patellar fracture, 507
 in patients 55 or younger, evaluation of, after total knee arthroplasty, 663
Advance prosthesis, 726
Advantim Revision PS prosthesis, 726
Advantim TC CR with All Poly Tibia prosthesis, 727
Advantim TC CR with CF Tibia prosthesis, 727
Advantim TC PS prosthesis, 728
Adverse outcomes, predictors of, patient information on, 4
AGC Cruciate Retaining prosthesis, 706
AGC knee system, 53, 706
AGC Posterior Stabilized prosthesis, 706
Age considerations, 3, 663
 in cementless total knee arthroplasty, 262, 271
Agency for Health Policy and Research, 37
AIMS (Arthritis Impact Measurement Scales), 43
Airflow, in operating room, 168, 465, 534

Albumin levels, preoperative measurement of, 5
Algorithmic diagnostic model, 346
Alignment. *See also specific components, alignment of*
 anatomic, 177, 178*f*
 assessment of
  in general physical examination, 6
  in Knee Society Score, 34*f*, 35
  radiographic, 9–10, 12, 14*f*
  for total knee arthroplasty following high tibial osteotomy, 601
 in cementless total knee arthroplasty, 263–267
 ideal, 189
 in painful total knee arthroplasty, 349
 supine and standing, preoperative assessment of, 6
Allografting
 with arthrodesis, for infected total knee replacement, 499
 in cementless revision arthroplasty, 440–450
  bone preparation technique for, 441–442, 441*f*–444*f*
  grafting technique for, 442–444
  graft preparation and placement in, 444
  in infected knee, 446–448
  pain score analysis after, 445, 445*t*
  results of, since 1984, 444–446, 446*f*–448*f*
 for extensor mechanism reconstruction, following total knee arthroplasty, 516–518
 femoral, 398, 424–431
  advantages and disadvantages of, 424
  for bicondylar defects, 425, 428*f*
  clinical results of, 429–430
  common clinical conditions requiring, 424
  complications in, 398, 429–430
  contraindications to, 425
  cost-effectiveness of, 424
  fixation in, 425, 428, 429*f*

Allografting (*continued*)
  graft incorporation in, 425–428
  indications for, 424–425
  ligamentous reattachment with, 428–429, 430*f*
  postoperative management in, 429
  preoperative planning for, 425
  selection of structural allograft for, 425
  surgical technique for, 425–429, 426*f*–429*f*
  for unicondylar defects, 425, 427*f*
  using acetabular reamers for defect preparation and reconstruction, 425, 426*f*
  versatility of, 424
 immunocompatibility in, 449
 for patellar tendon repair, 521–523, 522*f*–523*f*
  radiographic findings of double patella with, 523, 523*f*
  technique of, 522–523
 press-fit stem fixation in, 451, 452, 454*f*–455*f*, 457–460, 459*f*
 in revision arthroplasty, 385, 386*t*, 415–431
 in supracondylar fractures, 566–567, 574–575
 tibial, 396–397, 406–408, 415–423
  allograft availability for, ensuring, 418
  case studies of, 419–422
  for combined defects, 420–422, 421*f*
  complications in, 419
  for contained defects, 416–417, 418–419, 419–420, 420*f*
  contraindications to, 416
  fixation in, 417, 419
  graft healing in, 416
  graft incorporation in, 416
  impaction approach in, 417
  important technical considerations in, 418
  indications for, 416
  operative timing in, 418
  perioperative infection in, 418

737

Allografting (*continued*)
    postoperative rehabilitation in, 418
    radiographic assessment for, 419–422, 420*f*–423*f*
    results of, 418–419
    soft tissue management in, 418
    SPECT scan of, 416
    success in, measurement of, 416
    techniques for, 416–418
        in tibial fractures, 590, 590*f*, 594, 595*f*, 597
        for uncontained defects, 418–419, 422, 422*f*
        for uncontained or combined defects, 417–418
ALOS. *See* Average length of stay
Alternatives, to total knee arthroplasty, 4–5
Ambulatory aids
    discarding of, after rehabilitation, 662
    need for, as subtraction in knee scores, 32*f*, 33, 34*f*, 35
    patient education on, 652–653
    after unicondylar replacement, 110
Ambulatory treatment, of supracondylar fractures, 546–548
American Academy of Orthopaedic Surgeons (AAOS), outcomes assessment by, 40–41, 43
AMK CR prosthesis, 710
AMK prosthesis, 709
Amputation, for infected total knee replacement, 491, 499
Anaerobic infection, in painful total knee arthroplasty, 350
Analgesia
    complications with specific regimes of, 682*t*, 685
    cost of, 681*t*
    and deep vein thrombosis, 682
    duration of, 681*t*
    major advantages and disadvantages in specific regimes of, 682*t*
    multimodal, 680
    patient-controlled (PCA), 653, 655*f*, 680
        complications of, 682*t*, 685
        cost of, 681*t*
        duration of, 681*t*
        major advantages and disadvantages of, 682*t*
        patient education on, 653
        and patient lethargy, 653
        quality of, 681*t*
        during rehabilitation, 681
        technical support for, 681*t*
        technique for, 681*t*
        transition from, to oral analgesia, 653
        and urinary function, 653
    after posterior cruciate ligament-sacrificing procedure, 65
    after posterior cruciate ligament-sparing procedure, 59
    quality of, 681*t*
    during rehabilitation, 653, 656, 680–681
    technical support for, 681*t*
    techniques, 681*t*
Anatomic alignment, 177, 178*f*
    in cementless total knee arthroplasty, 264, 265*f*
Anatomic measured resection, 243–244, 245*f*
    in cementless total knee arthroplasty, 265–268

Anderson Orthopaedic Research Institute (AORI), bone loss classification system of, 402–408, 404*f*
    prerequisites for, 402, 402*f*
Anesthesia, 115, 168
    difficulties with, patient history of, 5
    for manipulation of stiff knee, 691
    patient education on, 653
Anesthesiologist fees, 23
Anesthetics, local, 680
    for patients with preoperative reflex sympathetic dystrophy, 683
Angular deformity, preoperative assessment of, 6
Ankle(s)
    assessment of, 5–6
    in painful total knee arthroplasty, 349
    orientation of tibial rotation and alignment to, in total knee replacement after Maquet osteotomy, 615
    radiographic assessment of, 12
    transmalleolar axis of, as landmark for tibial component position, 253
Ankle pumps, 670*t*
Ankylosed knee. *See also* Arthrodesis
    prior, total knee arthroplasty for patients with, 627–631
Ankylosing spondylitis, and patient difficulty with anesthesia, 5
Anspach instrument, in component removal, 379–380
Anterior cruciate ligament
    absent, as contraindication to unicondylar replacement, 107
    attrition of, with unicondylar replacement, 106
    blood supply to, 326
    in combined deformities, 217
    deficiency of, in varus deformity, 189
    division of
        in medial release, for varus deformity correction, 190
        in subvastus approach, 125, 125*f*
    preoperative assessment of, 6
    retention of
        in meniscal-bearing knees, 82, 86–87, 87*f*
        in total knee arthroplasty after patellectomy, 623
        in unicondylar replacement, 106
    sacrifice of
        and femoral rollback, 50
        with meniscal-bearing knees, 82, 87*f*
Anterior drawer sign
    in painful total knee arthroplasty, 349
    in preoperative assessment, 6
Anterior femoral notching, 166
    and supracondylar fracture, 563–564, 564*f*
Anterior recurrent tibial artery, 326–327, 327*f*
Anterior surgical approach, 115–118
    arthrotomy in, 117*f*, 118
    closure in, 117*f*, 118
    for medial release, for varus deformity correction, 189–190
    patient positioning for, 115–116
    preparation for, 115–116
    skin and superficial dissection in, 116*f*, 116–118
Anteroposterior axis, 230*f*
    for femoral component rotation, 230–231

Anteroposterior axis (*continued*)
    as secondary landmark, to epicondylar axis, 232–233, 233*f*
    measurement of, sex and, 231*t*
Anteroposterior radiographic view, 6–7, 9, 10*f*
    of bone defects
        F2A femoral, 404
        F2B femoral, 405
    of component loosening, 353, 354*f*–355*f*, 356
    in degenerative joint disease, 15*f*
    of flexion contracture, 211–212, 212*f*
    in osteonecrosis, 16*f*
    of painful total knee arthroplasty, 351, 352*f*, 365
    of patella, 317
    of patellar instability, 332
    of problematic total knee arthroplasty, 368
    semiflexed weight-bearing, 10–12, 13*f*–14*f*
    supine, 9, 10*f*
    for total knee arthroplasty following high tibial osteotomy, 601–602
    for total knee replacement after Maquet osteotomy, 615, 615*f*
    weight-bearing, 9, 10*f*
        preoperative, for medial release, for varus deformity correction, 189
Antibiotic(s)
    with debridement, for infected total knee replacement, 493
    discontinuation of, before revision, for determination of infective agent, 467–468
    elution of
        from antibiotic-loaded cement, 477*f*, 477–478
        from PROSTALAC, 487–488
    preoperative, for revision arthroplasty in infected knee, 440
    prophylaxis, 4, 465
    resistance to, development of, in antibiotic suppression in infected total knee replacement, 492
    spacer impregnated with, in two-stage arthroplasty, 3, 471
    treatment with
        for infected knee, 467
        in interval between two phases of two-stage revision arthroplasty, 466–467
Antibiotic-loaded cement, 258, 259, 440, 466–468, 471
    and bacterial bioadherence, 478
    elution of antibiotic from, 477*f*, 477–478
    properties of, 477–478
    prosthesis with (PROSTALAC), 471, 473–490 (*See also* PROSTALAC)
    role of, 476–477
    strength of, 478
Antibiotic suppression alone, for infected total knee replacement, 491, 492–493
    complications with, 492
    prerequisites for, 492
Anticoagulants
    in deep vein thrombosis prophylaxis, 696–700
    in deep vein thrombosis treatment, 702
    epidural analgesia with, safety of, 682, 685

Antithrombin III, in deep vein thrombosis, 694–695
AORI (Anderson Orthopaedic Research Institute), bone loss classification system of, 402f, 402–408, 404f
Apollo prosthesis, 62, 724
Apollo PS prosthesis, 725
Approaches, surgical, 113–162. *See also specific surgical approaches*
AP view. *See* Anteroposterior radiographic view
Arcuate ligament, in valgus deformity, 138, 139f, 197
  release of, in lateral release, 199, 200f
Arthritis. *See* Osteoarthritis; Rheumatoid arthritis
Arthritis Impact Measurement Scales (AIMS), 43
Arthrodesis
  for infected total knee replacement, 465, 469, 475, 483, 491, 494–499, 496f–498f
    bone grafting with, 495, 499
    compression, 496f–497f, 496–499
    contraindications to, 494
    disabilities and compensations from, 494–495
    fixation in, 496–499
      biplanar external, 496, 496f
      dual plating in, 496, 497f
      external, 496, 496f
      internal, 496–499, 497f–498f
      intramedullary rods for, 496–499, 498f
    indications for, 494
    maximizing bone surface contact in, 495
    positioning in, 495
    success rates of, 495
    techniques for, 495–499
  prior, total knee arthroplasty for patients with, 627–631
    alignment in, 629
    complications in, 630
    incision for, 628
    indications for, 627
    ligament stability in, 629, 630f
    osteotomies in, 629, 629f
    postoperative care in, 630–631
    prosthetic choice for, 627–628
    results of, 627
    surgical technique in, 627–630, 629f–630f
    trial reduction in, 629–630
  for supracondylar fracture, 566–567
Arthrofibrosis
  arthroscopic management of, 368–369, 373, 691
  with constrained prostheses for revision arthroplasty, 103t
  stiff knee with, 688–689
    treatment of, 690–692
Arthrography
  of component loosening, 355–356
  of painful total knee arthroplasty, 351, 355–356, 357, 358f
  of polyethylene wear, 357, 358f
Arthroscopic debridement
  as alternative to total knee arthroplasty, 4–5
  in patellar fracture, 510
  for soft tissue impingement, 368–371, 370f–372f

Arthroscopic diagnosis, in problematic total knee arthroplasty, effectiveness of, 368
Arthroscopic management
  of arthrofibrosis, 368–369, 373, 691
  of high tibial osteotomy symptoms, 602
  of hypertrophic synovitis, 369–371, 371f
  of loose bodies, 369
  of patella clunk, 368–369, 368–370, 370f–371f
  of patellar component loosening, 368, 369, 372f, 372–373
  of patellar instability, 368, 372
  of patellar subluxation, 368, 372
  of patellar tracking, 368, 372
  of problematic total knee arthroplasty, 368–374
    complications in, 373
    effectiveness of, 368, 373–374
    indications for, 369
    postoperative management in, 373
    technique in, 369
  of prosthetic wear, 368–369, 371–372, 372f
  of retained posterior cruciate ligament stump, 369, 371, 372f
  of soft tissue impingement, 368–371, 370f–372f
  of stiff knee, 691
Arthrosis, patellofemoral, Maquet osteotomy for, 613, 614f
  total knee replacement after, 613–620
Arthrotomy, 118
  lateral parapatellar (*See* Lateral parapatellar arthrotomy)
  medial parapatellar (*See* Medial parapatellar arthrotomy)
  trivector-retaining (*See* Trivector-retaining arthrotomy)
Articular surfaces, radiographic assessment of, 9–10
Ascending parapatellar artery, 326
Aspiration, of knee
  in evaluation for patellar revision, 533
  in infected knee replacement
    with antibiotic suppression, 492–493
    before revision arthroplasty, 471
  in problematic total knee arthroplasty, 368
Aspirin
  in deep vein thrombosis prophylaxis, 696, 702
    studies on, 696–697
  epidural analgesia with, safety of, 682
Assessment, preoperative, of patient, 5–7
Augmentation, bone
  modular, 396
    for femoral deficiency, 295–296
    for tibial deficiency, 409–414
      alignment of, 411, 411f
      cost-benefit ratio of, 413
      in primary total knee arthroplasty, 409–411
      stems and stem extensions in, 409–412, 411f–413f
      and third-body wear, 413
      types of, 409–411, 411f
  in total knee arthroplasty following high tibial osteotomy, 606
  wedges for, 393
    biomechanics of, 395
    cementing of, 395
    femoral, 398
    full, 409, 410f, 411

Augmentation, bone (*continued*)
    half, 409, 410f, 411
    mini, 411
    modular, 396, 409–414
    shapes of, 395
    size of, 395
    tibial, 289, 290f, 406–407, 409–414
      metallic, 395–396
      with plateau fracture, 293f, 294
Autogenous bone grafting
  with arthrodesis, for infected total knee replacement, 499
  distal femoral condyle as graft source in, 290f, 290–295, 296f
  for femoral deficiency, 295–297
    after prior supracondylar osteotomy or fracture, 296–297, 297f
  posterior femoral condyle as graft source in, 293
  in supracondylar fractures, 566–567, 569, 574–575
    with blades plate fixation, 570
  for tibial deficiency, 289–294
    fixation in, 291, 291f
    after plateau fracture, 293f, 294
    reconstitution of upper tibial surface in, 291, 291f
    results of, 292f, 292–294
    technique of, 289–291, 290f–291f
Autografts. *See* Autogenous bone grafting
Autologous blood donation
  patient information on, 4
  and reduction in deep vein thrombosis, 694
Autologous bone chips, as biologic cement, in cementless total knee arthroplasty, 263, 264f
  implantation of, 269, 269f
Average length of stay (ALOS), and hospital costs, 20t, 21–22, 23–24
Axiom Cruciate Retaining Primary prosthesis, 728
Axiom PS Primary prosthesis, 729
Axiom Revision prosthesis, 729

B

Baha location, drift of patella into, minimizing, in anterior approach, 117f, 118
Balancing, of flexion-extension gap
  basic principles for, 165–167, 166f
  in cementless total knee arthroplasty, 266
  in correction of combined deformities, 220–221
  femoral component rotation and, 227, 238
  in flexion contracture correction, 210, 211f, 213, 213f–214f, 221–222
  instruments for, 183–184, 184f
  in lateral release for valgus deformity, 199, 199f, 202
  in ligament advancement, 207
  in medial release, for varus deformity correction, 193, 193f
  problems in, and stiff knee, 689–690
  in revision arthroplasty, for tibial fractures, 595–596
  in revision arthroplasty for stiff knee, 692
  in total knee arthroplasty following high tibial osteotomy, 607
  in total knee replacement with femoral extra-articular deformity, 637

Barium sulfate, in cement, 257
Bayesian diagnostic model, 345–346
Beam hardening, in computed tomography of metallic implants, 363
Bedside exercises, in rehabilitation, 658, 678t
Benefits, of total knee arthroplasty, 4
Beth Israel Medical Center
 patient education by, 669t
 rehabilitation protocol of, 676f–677f
 standard protocol of, for radiographic evaluation, 6–7
Bias, in outcomes assessment, 42
Biceps femoris, in valgus deformity, 138, 139f
 release of, in lateral release, 199, 200f, 201
Bicycle, stationary
 in rehabilitation, 661
 seat height of, 661
Bidding, competitive, and prosthesis cost, 25
Bilateral disease, sequential or simultaneous arthroplasty for, 4
Biologic fixation
 autologous bone chips in, in cementless total knee arthroplasty, 263, 264f, 269, 269f
 calcium phosphate ceramics in, 277–286
 successful long-term, prerequisites for, 284
Blade plates fixation
 in high tibial osteotomy, removal of, in subsequent total knee arthroplasty, 603–605, 605f
 of supracondylar fractures, 561f, 562, 567–570, 570f
Bleeding, with constrained prostheses for revision arthroplasty, 103t, 104
Bleeding disorders, and patient outcome, 5
Blood, in knee joint, and postoperative range of motion, 656
Blood clots. See also Deep vein thrombosis
 calf, significance of, 695–696
Blood donation, autologous
 patient information on, 4
 and reduction in deep vein thrombosis, 694
Blood flow, and deep vein thrombosis, 694
Blood recovery drains, patient information on, 4
Bone
 eburnated, as contraindication to unicondylar replacement, 107
 retained, and stiff knee, 689, 689f
Bone augmentation
 modular, 396
  for femoral deficiency, 295–296
  for tibial deficiency, 409–414
   alignment of, 411, 411f
   cost-benefit ratio of, 413
   in primary total knee arthroplasty, 409–411
   stems and stem extensions in, 409–412, 411f–413f
   and third-body wear, 413
   types of, 409–411, 411f
  in total knee arthroplasty following high tibial osteotomy, 606
 wedges for, 393
  biomechanics of, 395
  cementing of, 395
  femoral, 398

Bone augmentation (continued)
 full, 409, 410f, 411
 half, 409, 410f, 411
 mini, 411
 modular, 396, 409–414
 shapes of, 395
 size of, 395
 tibial, 289, 290f, 406–407, 409–414
  metallic, 395–396
  with plateau fracture, 293f, 294
Bone block, and flexion contracture, 210, 211f
Bone-cement interface
 assessment of, in painful total knee arthroplasty, 352
 bone necrosis at, 258–259
 exposure of, in component removal, 379
 take down of, in component removal, 379–381, 380f
Bone chips, autologous, as biologic cement, in cementless total knee arthroplasty, 263, 264f
 implantation of, 269, 269f
Bone deformities, developmental, in valgus deformity, 138f, 139
Bone grafting, 385, 386t, 393
 with arthrodesis, for infected total knee replacement, 495, 499
 in cementless revision arthroplasty, 440–450
  bone preparation technique for, 441–442, 441f–444f
  grafting technique for, 442–444
  graft preparation and placement in, 444
  in infected knee, 446–448
  pain score analysis after, 445, 445t
  results of, since 1984, 444–446, 446f–448f
 distal femoral condyle as graft source in, 290f, 290–295, 296f
 for femoral deficiency, 398
  allografting in, 398, 424–431
  autogenous, 295–297
  after prior supracondylar osteotomy or fracture, 296–297, 297f
 posterior femoral condyle as graft source in, 293
 press-fit stem fixation in, 451, 452, 454f–455f, 457–460, 459f
 in supracondylar fractures, 566–570, 574–575
 techniques of, 396
 with tendon allografting, for patellar tendon repair, 522–523
 for tibial deficiency, 396–397
  advantages and disadvantages of, 396
  allografting in, 396–397, 406–408, 415–423
  autogenous, 289–291, 289–294, 290f–291f, 406
  fixation in, 291, 291f
  after plateau fracture, 293f, 294
  reconstitution of upper tibial surface in, 291, 291f
  results of, 292f, 292–294
  technique of, 289–291, 290f–291f
 in tibial fractures, 577–578, 579f, 580f, 590, 590f, 594, 595f, 597–598
 in total knee arthroplasty following high tibial osteotomy, 606
 in total knee replacement with tibial extra-articular deformity, 646

Bone ingrowth fixation, calcium phosphate ceramics for, 277–286
Bone loss/defects, 274, 287–297. See also Femoral deficiency; Patellar deficiency; Tibial deficiency
 asymmetric, 393
 as cause of component loosening, 356–357, 356f–357f
 cavitary, 401
 cement as seal against, 274–275
 central, 401
 classification of, 385, 393, 401–408, 415–416, 424
  Anderson Orthopaedic Research Institute system of, 402–408, 404f
   prerequisites for, 402, 402f
  in borderline cases, 403
  comprehensive, 401–402
  Dorr's, 401
  historical review of schemes for, 401–402
  Insall's, 401
  postrevision radiographs in, 402
  radiographic assessment in, 401, 402
  Rand's, 401
  using system of, 408
 combined type of, 385, 393, 415–416
 with component loosening, 393, 406–408, 409, 410f
 computed tomography of, 357, 357f
 contained, 385, 393, 415–416, 424
 discontinuity, 401
 etiology of, 393
 intercalary, 401
 management of
  general concepts in, 393–400
  options for, 393–394
  in primary total knee arthroplasty, 393–394
   tibial modularity in, 409–411
  in revision arthroplasty, 385, 391–431
   cementless, 440–450
   femoral allografting for, 424–431
   simple approach to, 385, 386f
   tibial allografting for, 415–423
   tibial modularity for, 412
 modular augments for, tibial, 409–414
 pathologic fracture with, 356f, 357
 peripheral, 384, 393, 401
 preoperative planning for, 394
 radiographic evaluation of, 356f, 357
 segmental, 401
 size of, 393
 symmetric, 393
 type 2 (damaged metaphyseal bone), 403
 type 3 (deficient metaphyseal segment), 403
 type 1 (intact metaphyseal bone), 403
 uncontained, 385, 415–416, 424
 and use of constrained prostheses in revision arthroplasty, 97–98
 with valgus deformity, 289, 295, 409, 410f
 with varus deformity, 289, 295, 409, 410f
Bone marrow scan, in infection, 360–361, 362f
Bone necrosis (osteonecrosis)
 advanced, 17f
 at cement-bone interface, 258–259
 early, 16f
 of femoral condyle, autogenous bone grafting for, 296, 296f
 as indication for total knee arthroplasty, 3

Bone necrosis (osteonecrosis) (continued)
  magnetic resonance imaging in, 16–17, 16f–17f
  radiographic evaluation of, 16–17, 16f–17f
  radionuclide bone scan in, 16
Bone-prosthesis interface
  exposure of, in component removal, 379
  radiolucent line at, as sign of component loosening, 353–356
  stresses at, retention of posterior cruciate ligament and, 51–53
  take down of, in component removal, 379–381, 380f
  violation of, in patellar revision, 528
Bone resection. *See also specific bones, cutting/resection of*
  anatomic alignment and, 177, 178f
  anatomic measured, 243–244, 245f
    in cementless total knee arthroplasty, 265–268
  basic principles of, 165–167, 166f–167f
    in cementless total knee arthroplasty, 265–266, 267–268
  compensatory, in extra-articular deformity, 640–644, 641f–643f, 646
  in correction of combined deformities, 220–221
  in flexion contracture correction, 212–214
  increased, for tibial defects, 394
  in lateral release for valgus deformity, 198–199, 198f–199f
  and ligament balancing, 210, 211f
  mechanical axis and, 177, 178f
  and prosthetic fit/instability, 194f, 194–195
Bone resorption, with infection, in painful total knee arthroplasty, 357–358, 359f
Bone scan
  of component loosening, 356–357
  of degenerative joint disease, 12–14
  in infection, 358–361, 365, 368
    incongruent, 360, 361f, 365
  of patella, to assess viability after total knee arthroplasty, 506
  of periprosthetic fracture, 364
  of reflex sympathetic dystrophy, 364–365
  of spontaneous osteonecrosis, 16
Bone stock deficiency. *See Bone loss/defects*
Brace(s)
  cast, for supracondylar fractures, 546–547, 546f–547f
  functional, 656–657, 657f
  hinged, for supracondylar fractures, 547f, 547–548
    displacement with, 547–548, 547f–548f
    with rush rods, 556
  postoperative, in rehabilitation, 656–657
  prophylactic, 656, 657f
  rehabilitative, 656–657, 657f
Bulk purchasing, and prosthesis cost, 24–25
Bunnell-type repair, of patellar tendon rupture, 520–521
Bupivacaine
  delay of ambulation with, 681
  for patients with preoperative reflex sympathetic dystrophy, 683
Bursal tenderness, preoperative assessment of, 6

C
Calcium phosphate ceramics
  basic science of, 277–278
  in biologic fixation, 277–286
  environmental conditions and methods in manufacture of, 277
  implant coatings of
    animal investigations of, 278–281
    application of, 278
    and bone formation on perimeter and internal surface lengths, 280–281, 281f–282f
    in cancellous bone environment, 278–281
    clinical experience with, 281–284
    concerns about, 284
    and lamellar bone formation, 281, 283f
    versus non-coated fiber-metal implants, 278–284, 279f–283f
    and pore volume filled with bone, 279f, 280
    and pull-out strength, 280, 280f
    radiographic evaluation of, 284
    scanning electron microscopy backscatter analysis of, 281, 282f
    separation of, from titanium substrate, 284
  long-term stability of, 278
  solubility and bioresorption of, 278
Calf, assessment of, 6
Calf circumference, in deep vein thrombosis, 695
Calf clots, significance of, 695–696
Calf compression, for deep vein thrombosis prophylaxis, 699
  warfarin *versus*, 698–699
Canes, 652–653
Capitated payment, 19
Capsule
  anterior, attenuation of, flexion contracture and, 210–211
  lateral, in valgus deformity, 197
  medial
    elevation of
      in subvastus approach, 122–123, 123f
      from tibia, in subvastus approach, 122, 122f
    tightening of, in proximal patellar realignment, 333
  in midvastus approach, 127–128
  preservation of, in subvastus approach, 121, 121f
  of suprapatellar pouch, division of, in subvastus approach, 121, 122f
Capsulotomy, in flexion contracture correction, 221
Carioca, in rehabilitation, 660, 660f
Cartilage thinning. *See also Joint-space narrowing*
  radiographic evaluation of, 10–12
Cast brace, for supracondylar fractures, 546–547, 546f–547f, 566
Casting
  after allografting for extensor mechanism reconstruction, 517
  after allografting for patellar tendon repair, 523
  of patellar fractures, 509
  for patellar tendon rupture, 520
  postoperative
    in flexion contracture correction, 214
    in rehabilitation, 656

Casting (continued)
  preoperative, of flexion contracture, 212
  in resection arthroplasty, 494
  for supracondylar fractures, 546, 565
  for tibial fractures, 578–579, 580f, 582, 584–586, 585f, 588
Caveats, 4–5
Cavitary bone defect, 401
CEA (cost-effectiveness analysis), 26t, 26–27
Ceiling price, of prosthesis, 25
Cellulitis, as contraindication to single-stage revision, for infected knee, 468
Cement/cementing
  in allografting, 417, 428
  antibiotic-loaded, 258, 259, 440, 466–468, 471
    and bacterial bioadherence, 478
    elution of antibiotic from, 477f, 477–478
    properties of, 477–478
    prosthesis with (PROSTALAC), 471, 473–490 (*See also PROSTALAC*)
    role of, 476–477
    strength of, 478
  in autogenous bone grafting, for tibial deficiency, 291, 291f
  biologic, autogenous bone chips as, 263, 264f
  implantation of, 269, 269f
  in blades plate fixation of supracondylar fracture, 570
  bone penetration of, 258–259
  versus cementless fixation, 84–87, 88f, 260, 262, 269–270, 273
  and component removal, 380–381, 381f, 381–382
  of femoral component, 259
    in hybrid total knee arthroplasty, 273–276
  for filling bone defects, 394–395, 424
    femoral, 405
    reinforcement of, with screws, 395
    tibial, 394–395, 407–408
  formation/preparation of
    centrifugation in, 258, 259, 478
    doughy material phase in, 257–258
    initial liquid period in, 257–258
    phases of, 257
    transition from doughy state to solid in, 257–258
    in vacuum, 258–259, 478
  humidity and, 257–258
  in hybrid total knee replacements, 260
  interface of
    with bone
      assessment of, in painful total knee arthroplasty, 352
      bone necrosis at, 258–259
      exposure of, in component removal, 379
      take down of, in component removal, 379–381, 380f
    with prosthesis
      assessment of, in painful total knee arthroplasty, 352
      violation of, in patellar revision, 527–528, 527f–528f
  mantle of, fracture of, in painful total knee arthroplasty, imaging of, 353
  in meniscal-bearing knees, survivorship of, *versus* cementless replacements, 84–87, 88f

Cement/cementing (*continued*)
  modulus of, 259
  monomer, polymer, and polymerization in, 257–259
  of onset patella, 301–302
  of patella component, 259
  in patellar revision, 529
  of patellar rotating patella implant, 311, 313
  in posterior cruciate ligament-sacrificing procedure, 64
  in posterior cruciate ligament-sparing procedure, 58, 260
  in posterior-stabilized condylar knee, 259–260
  in presence of femoral deficiency, 398
  in presence of tibial defects, 397
  in primary total knee arthroplasty, 257–261
  in revision arthroplasty, 435–439
    implant selection for, 436
    results of, 436–439
  as seal against bone loss, 274–275
  of stems, 451–452
    in constrained prostheses, 79–80
  technique in, 259–260
  temperature and, 257–258
    effect of power instruments on, 258–259
  thickness of, around prosthesis, 258
    on femoral side, 258
    ideal, in total hip arthroplasty, 258
    on tibial side, 258
  of tibial component, 259–260
    design of tibial tray and, 260
    extension maneuver in, 260
    in hybrid total knee arthroplasty, 273–276
    pressurized, 259–260
  in tibial modular augmentation, 413
  in total knee replacement after Maquet osteotomy, 618
  unique properties in various manufacturings of, 258
  viscosity of, 258
Cementless revision arthroplasty, 440–450
  bone grafting in, 440–450
    bone preparation technique for, 441–442, 441f–444f
    grafting technique for, 442–444
    graft preparation and placement in, 444
  in infected knee, 440, 446–448
  pain score analysis after, 445, 445t
  results of, 440
  since 1984, 444–446, 446f–448f
Cementless total knee arthroplasty, 262–272
  age and, 262, 271
  anatomic alignment in, 263–264, 265f
  autologous bone chips as biologic cement in, 263, 264f
    implantation of, 269, 269f
  bone resection in, 267
  versus cementing, 84–87, 88f, 260, 262, 269–270, 273
  classical alignment in, 263–264, 265f
  clinical results of, 262, 269–270, 270f
  femoral component design in, 262–263
  hydroxyapatite and tricalcium phosphate in enhancement of, 277–286
  implant alignment and kinematics in, 263–267

Cementless total knee arthroplasty (*continued*)
  implant design in, 262–263
    biologic considerations in, 262–263
    geometry of, 263
  instruments for, 177
  measured resection in, 265–268
  patella medialization in, 266–268, 268f
  patellar component design in, 263, 264f
  patient selection for, 262
  porous coating in, 262–263
  posterior cruciate ligament retention in, 266–267
  radiographic evaluation of, 270, 270f, 273
  restoration of anatomy in, 265–266
  restoration of normal alignment in, 263–265, 265f
  surgical approach in, 267
  surgical techniques in, 267–269
  tibial component design in, 263
  tibial sizing in, 268
  trial reduction in, 268–269
  ultracongruent polyethylene insert in, 266, 266f
Central bone defect, 401, 415
Centrifugation, of cement, 258–259, 478
Cervical instability, and patient difficulty with anesthesia, 5
Chief complaint, in painful total knee arthroplasty, establishment of, 347
Chondrocalcinosis, as contraindication to unicondylar replacement, 107
Chondromalacia, and unicondylar replacement, 107
Christmas factor (factor IX), in coagulation, warfarin and, 697–698
Chronic venous insufficiency, prevention of, 696
Classical alignment, in cementless total knee arthroplasty, 264, 265f
Clindamycin, elution of, 477
Clinical evaluation, 29–45
Closure(s)
  in anterior approach, 117f, 118
  in femoral allografting, 429
  in lateral approach, for valgus deformity correction, 146f, 146–147
  in lateral retinacular release, 329
  in midvastus approach, 129
  in total knee arthroplasty for patients with prior arthrodesis, 630
  in total knee arthroplasty with tibial extra-articular deformity, 646
  in total knee replacement with femoral extra-articular deformity, 637–638
  in trivector-retaining arthrotomy, 132
CMW cement, 258
Coagulability, and deep vein thrombosis, 694
Cobalt chrome, for porous coating, in cementless total knee arthroplasty, 262–263
Codivilla technique, of quadriceps lengthening, 514, 515f–516f
Codman, E. A., 43
Cold flow, with constrained prosthesis, 75, 76f
Cold patella, in lateral retinacular release, 329–330, 506
Cold therapy
  in postoperative pain management, 680
  in rehabilitation, 657–658, 660

Collateral ligaments. *See also* Lateral collateral ligament; Medial collateral ligament
  balancing of, 189
  blood supply to, 326
  contracture of, with persistent flexion contracture, 210
  incompetent/deficient, constrained prosthesis with, 77–78, 102
  in revision arthroplasty, 386, 388
  rotational alignment of femoral component and, 178–179
Combined deformities
  correction of, 216–223, 217f
    bone resection in, 220–221
    postoperative treatment in, 222
  definition of, 216
  incidence of, 216
  lateral release for, 219–220, 219f–220f
  medial release for, 218f, 218–219
  preoperative planning for, 217–218
  radiographic evaluation of, 217
  surgical approach in, 218
  surgical pathology of, 216–217
Compartment syndrome, epidural analgesia and, 684
Compere patellectomy, 622f, 622–623
Competitive bidding, and prosthesis cost, 25
Complication(s)
  medical, 4
  patient information on, 4
  rheumatoid arthritis and, 5
  surgical, 4
Component(s). *See also* Femoral component; Patellar component; Tibial component
  loosening of
    with antibiotic suppression in infected total knee replacement, 492
    arthrography of, 355–356
    bone loss/defects as cause of, 356–357, 356f–357f
    bone loss with, 393, 406–408, 409, 410f
    with constrained prostheses for revision arthroplasty, 103t, 104
    infection and, 357–358, 359f–360f
    osteolysis and, 356–357, 356f–357f
    in painful total knee arthroplasty, 352–357, 353f, 353–357
    radiographic assessment of, 353f–356f, 353–357
    with posterior-stabilized condylar knee, 69, 72
    radionuclide bone scan of, 356–357
    subsidence with, 353, 354f
  position of, 225–253
  removal of
    bone loss with, 393
    exposure of failed prosthesis in, 378–379, 378f–379f
    instruments for, 377, 379–382, 380f, 382f
    in revision arthroplasty, 377–383, 494
    preoperative assessment and planning for, 377–378
    preoperative templating for, 377–378, 378f
    successful, points central to, 383
    in two-stage exchange arthroplasty, 481

Compression, mechanical, for deep vein thrombosis prophylaxis, 699, 701t, 701–702
 aspirin *versus*, 697
 warfarin *versus*, 698–699
Compression arthrodesis, 496f–497f, 496–499
Compression Duplex Ultrasonography, in deep vein thrombosis diagnosis, 695
Computed tomography
 in degenerative joint disease, 15, 16f
 of femoral component rotation, 238f, 363, 363f, 365
 metallic implants and beam hardening in, 363
 of osteolysis, 356f, 357
 of osteophytes, 16f
 in painful total knee arthroplasty, 349, 351, 363
 of patellar instability, 332–333, 333f
 of periprosthetic fracture, 364
 of tibial component rotation, 249–250, 252f, 363, 365
 for total knee arthroplasty following high tibial osteotomy, 602
 ultra-fast cine technique, for femoral rollback assessment, 50
Condylar buttress plate, for supracondylar fracture fixation, 567, 570
Confidentiality, data collection/outcomes assessment and, 40–41
Consent, informed, 4
Constrained condylar prosthesis, 69, 70f, 75, 76f
 in lateral release for valgus deformity, in elderly, low-demand patients, 197–198
 versus total condylar III prosthesis, 69–70
Constrained intercondylar prostheses, limitations of, as premise for ligament advancement, 205–206
Constrained prostheses, 69, 70f, 75–80
 background and design of, 75
 cold flow with, 75, 76f
 in collateral ligament incompetence, 77–78
 current models of, 75–77
 designs of, 97–101, 98f–101f
 disadvantages of, 75
 in extra-articular deformity correction, 633, 635–636
 with flexion-extension gap mismatch, 77–78
 hyperextension stops in, 77
 indications for, 77–78, 101–102
 in lateral release for valgus deformity, 203
 in elderly, low-demand patients, 197–198
 linked (hinged), 75–80, 97
 linked *versus* nonlinked, 77, 80
 medullar stem extensions for, 78–79, 79f
 modes of restraint in, 75–76, 77t
 nonlinked, 75
 for revision arthroplasty, 97–105, 436, 437f
  complications with, 103t, 104
  results of, 102t, 102–104
 rotating hinge, 75, 76f
 selection of, clinical setting and, 98–101
 in supracondylar femur fracture, 101f, 102

Constrained prostheses (*continued*)
 surgical technique for, 78–79, 79f
 versus total condylar III prosthesis, 69–70
 for total knee arthroplasty after patellectomy, 624
 for total knee arthroplasty following high tibial osteotomy, 607
 for total knee arthroplasty for patients with prior arthrodesis, 627–629, 630f
Contact areas, of meniscal-bearing knees, 92–93
Contact points, tibiofemoral, posterior shift of. *See* Femoral rollback
Contained bone defects, 385, 393, 415–416, 424
Continuous passive motion (CPM)
 after manipulation of stiff knee, 691
 in postoperative management, 653, 653f, 655–656
  analgesia during, 680–681
  in arthroplasties with tibial defects, treated with bone grafting, 291
  in lateral release for valgus deformity, 201
  and length of stay, 653, 655
  maximum tolerable range of, 655–656
  and peroneal nerve tension, 201
  in posterior cruciate ligament-sparing procedure, 58–59
  in supracondylar fracture fixation, with retrograde intramedullary nail, 559
  in total knee arthroplasty for patients with prior arthrodesis, 630
  in unicondylar replacement, 110
Continuum CR prosthesis, 715
Continuum PS prosthesis, 715
Continuum Revision prosthesis, 716
Contractures, flexion. *See* Flexion contracture(s)
Contraindications, to total knee arthroplasty, 3–4
Coonse-Adams V-Y quadricepsplasty. *See also* V-Y quadricepsplasty
 for patellar revision, 526, 526f
Coordinate prosthesis, 710
Cost(s), 19–27
 of analgesia, 681t
 analysis of, 20–23
 average of length of stay (ALOS) and, 20t, 21–24
 of cementless fixation, 275
 fixed *versus* variable, 22, 22f
 health-care
  exponential rise in, 19
  increase in, *versus* consumer price index, 20f
 Hermann Hospital study of, 20t, 22–23
 historical issues in, 19–20
 hospital, 20t, 20–22, 21f–22f
 Lahey Clinic study of, 20t, 20–21, 21f
 Northwestern Memorial Hospital study of, 20t, 21f–22f, 21–23
 operating room, 20t, 21f, 21–22
 outcome assessment and, 37
 posthospitalization, 22–23
 prehospitalization, 23
 of professional fees, 23
 of prosthesis, 20t, 21f, 21–22, 22, 24–25
  awareness of issues associated with, 24
  ceiling price and, 25

Cost(s) (*continued*)
  competitive bidding and, 25
  volume discounting and, 24–25
 of rehabilitation, 22–23, 651–652, 659–660
 third-party payers and, 19–20
Cost containment, 23–26
Cost-effectiveness analysis (CEA), 26t, 26–27
Cost-shifting, 23
Coumadin. *See* Warfarin
CPM. *See* Continuous passive motion
C-reactive protein
 in painful total knee arthroplasty, 358
 in problematic total knee arthroplasty, 368
Crepitation
 in painful total knee arthroplasty, 349
 preoperative assessment of, 6
Criterion validity, 41
Crosslinks, from validated instruments, for outcomes assessment, 43
Cruciate ligament. *See* Anterior cruciate ligament; Posterior cruciate ligament
Crutches, 652–653
Crystalline deposits, as contraindication to unicondylar replacement, 107
CT. *See* Computed tomography
Curved medial parapatellar incision, 116
Curved stems, for constrained prostheses, 79, 79f
Curvilinear arthrotomy, 118
Custom implants, 98
 for femoral deficiency, 398
 for tibial deficiency, 397
 in total knee arthroplasty following high tibial osteotomy, 605–606, 605f–606f
 in total knee replacement with femoral extra-articular deformity, 635–636, 636f, 637
Cutting blocks, 181, 181f, 182
 femoral, in femoral component rotation, 241f, 241–242
Cutting guides
 femoral, 182f, 182–183, 237
  in posterior cruciate ligament-sparing procedure, 54–55
 patellar, 301, 302f, 507, 507f
 tibial, 181–182, 182t, 244–245
  inadvertent external rotation of, 246, 248f
  medial displacement of, 245, 246f
  for modular augmentation, 411, 411f
  in posterior cruciate ligament-sparing procedure, 55
  in total knee replacement after Maquet osteotomy, 616–618, 616f–618f
Cutting instruments, 181, 181f
Cutting slots, 181
Cybex testing
 after quadriceps snip, 150–151, 153t
 after V-Y quadricepsplasty, 157
Cyclooxygenase, aspirin and, 696
Cyst formation, in degenerative joint disease, 12, 15f

D

Dangling stems, for constrained prostheses, 78–79, 79f
Data
 collection of
  disruption of patient flow with, 40

Data (*continued*)
  expense, hassle, and complexity of, 40
  instruments for, 41–42
  medicolegal risk and confidentiality in, 40–41
  for outcome assessment, 39–45
  reasons for, 40–41
  essential elements of, in outcomes assessment, 41
  overload of, 40
D-dimer, in deep vein thrombosis, 694–695
Dead bone sandwich, avoidance of, in revision arthroplasty, for tibial fractures, 596
Debilitated, minimally ambulatory patient, supracondylar fracture in, treatment of, 551, 551f
Debridement
  arthroscopic
    as alternative to total knee arthroplasty, 4–5
    in patellar fracture, 510
    for soft tissue impingement, 368–371, 370f–372f
  for infected total knee replacement, 491
    with antibiotic, 493
  in patellar revision, 535
Deconditioning, 661
Deep vein thrombosis, after total knee arthroplasty, 694–704
  analgesia type and, 682
  classic signs and symptoms of, 695
  diagnosis of, 695
  inter-surgeon difference in, 694
  obesity and, 694
  pathogenesis of, 694–695
  and patient outcome, 5
  patients at risk for, 694
  physical findings in, 695
  prevalence of, 694
  prevention of chronic venous insufficiency with, 696
  prophylaxis against
    agents for, 696–700
    aspirin for, 696–697, 702
    aspirin *versus* mechanical compression for, 697
    aspirin *versus* warfarin for, 697
    guidelines of Fourth American College of Physicians for, 700–701, 701t
    low molecular weight heparin for, 699–702, 701, 701t
    low molecular weight heparin *versus* compression stockings for, 700
    low molecular weight heparin *versus* warfarin for, 700
    mechanical compression for, 699, 701t, 701–702
    need for, 701–702
    selection of agent for, 700–701
    stacking of methods for, 701
    warfarin for, 697–699, 702
    warfarin *versus* mechanical compression for, 698–699
  reduction in, autologous blood donation and, 694
  significance of calf clots in, 695–696
  treatment of, 702
Deformities. *See also specific deformities*
  combined
    correction of, 216–223
    definition of, 216
  correction of, 187–223

Deformities. (*continued*)
  retention of posterior cruciate ligament and, 51
  preoperative assessment of, 6
  as subtraction in knee scores, 32f, 33
Degenerative joint disease
  computed tomography in, 15, 16f
  magnetic resonance imaging in, 14–15, 15f
  radiographic assessment of, 12–15, 14f–15f
  radionuclide bone scan of, 12–14
Diabetes mellitus
  and painful total knee arthroplasty, 348
  and patient outcome, 5
Diagnosis
  associated with successful total knee arthroplasty, 3
  principles of, 346–347
Diagnosis-related groups (DRGs), 19–20, 23, 652
Diagnostic categories, in painful total knee arthroplasty, 346f, 346–347
Diagnostic findings, in painful total knee arthroplasty, 348
Diagnostic models
  algorithmic, 346
  Bayesian, 345–346
  linear, 345
  in painful total knee arthroplasty, 345–346
DiGioia-Rubash classification system, of supracondylar fractures, 565
Disability, functional, as indication for total knee arthroplasty, 3
Discharge planning, 23
Discharge questionnaire, 667t
Disclosure, to patient, 4–5
Discoloration, of skin, in reflex sympathetic dystrophy, 350
Discontinuity bone defect, 401
Disease process, as indication for total knee arthroplasty, 3
Disease-specific instruments, for outcomes assessment, 42
Distal patellar realignment
  clinical cases of, between January 1980 and January 1994, 340
  Hauser procedure for, 341
  materials and methods for, 337–340
  medial tibial tubercle transfer in, 337, 339–340, 340f
  medial transfer of medial one-half of patellar tendon in, 338–339, 339f
  modified Roux-Goldthwait procedure for, 337–338, 338f, 342
  for patellar dislocation/subluxation, 540
  for patellar instability, 337–342
  results of, 341
  Roux-Goldthwait procedure for, 341
  surgical procedure for, 337–340
DJD. *See* Degenerative joint disease
Doppler flow test, transcutaneous, in deep vein thrombosis diagnosis, 695
Dorr's classification, of bone defects, 401
Double patella, radiographic findings of, after allografting for patellar tendon repair, 523, 523f
Draping technique, 168–173, 169f–172f
  for anterior approach, 116
Drawer sign
  anterior, in preoperative assessment, 6
  in painful total knee arthroplasty, 349
  posterior, in posterior cruciate ligament-sacrificing procedure, 61

DRGs (diagnosis-related groups), 19–20, 23, 652
Drop and dangle routine, after posterior cruciate ligament-sacrificing procedure, 65
Drumstick appearance, in combined deformities, with rheumatoid arthritis, 217
Duracon prosthesis, 713
DVT. *See* Deep vein thrombosis, after total knee arthroplasty
Dynamic compression screw plates, for supracondylar fracture fixation, 567, 569

E
Eburnated bone, as contraindication to unicondylar replacement, 107
Effective joint space, cementing as limitation of, 274–275
Effusion
  preoperative assessment of, 6, 601
  and quadriceps inhibition, 660
Elderly patients
  comorbid conditions in, 680
  debilitated, minimally ambulatory, supracondylar fracture in, treatment of, 551, 551f
  deconditioning in, and rehabilitation, 661
  lateral release for valgus deformity in, constrained condylar knee for, 197–198
  pain management in, 680
  total condylar III prosthesis in, 104
Electrical signals, in deep vein thrombosis diagnosis, 695
Electrical stimulation, in rehabilitation, 656
Electrocautery, 181
  in anterior surgical approach, 116
Electron microscopy backscatter analysis
  of autologous bone chips, as biologic cement, 263, 264f
  of calcium phosphate ceramic implant coatings, 281, 282f
Endocarditis, with antibiotic suppression in infected total knee replacement, 492
Endo-Model prosthesis, 720
End Result System, 43
Epicondylar axis, 230f
  of distal femur, 178
  for femoral component rotation, 177–178, 179f, 227–235, 236, 238–239, 242, 332, 361–363
    in correction of combined deformities, 221
    in lateral release for valgus deformity, 198–199, 198f–199f, 202
    and patellar tracking, 321–322, 322f
    in revision arthroplasty, 387
    surgical technique in, 232–234, 232f–234f
    theoretical arguments supporting, 231–232
  interobserver variation in defining, 242
  measurement of, sex and, 231t
  relationship of
    to longitudinal axis of lower extremity, in flexion and extension, 236, 238
    with posterior condylar axis, 177–178, 179f, 183, 198

Epicondyle(s)
　identification of
　　in femoral component rotation, 232, 232f–233f
　　in implantation of meniscal-bearing knees, 93–96
　　as reference for femoral component alignment, 177–178
Epidural abscess, 685
Epidural analgesia, 680
　with anticoagulants, safety of, 682, 685
　and compartment syndrome, 684
　complications of, 682t, 685
　contraindications to, 683
　and deep vein thrombosis, 682
　delay of ambulation with, 681
　infusion, 681t
　　cost of, 681t
　　duration of, 681t
　　quality of, 681t
　　technical support for, 681t
　　technique for, 681t
　major advantages and disadvantages of, 682t
　after manipulation of stiff knee, 691
　patient-controlled
　　cost of, 681t
　　duration of, 681t
　　quality of, 681t
　　technical support for, 681t
　　technique for, 681t
　patient education on, 653
　and peroneal palsy, 684
　physiological effects of, 683–684
　and reduction in postoperative medical complications, 683
　during rehabilitation, 681
　versus systemic narcotics, 683
Epidural anesthesia, 115, 168
Epidural catheter
　dislodged, management of, 683
　and urinary tract infection, 684–685
　use of, duration of, 684
Epidural hematoma, 682, 685
Erythrocyte sedimentation rate
　in painful total knee arthroplasty, 358
　in problematic total knee arthroplasty, 368
Erythromycin-cement complex, 476
Esmarch bandage, 116, 694
Examination, physical
　general, in patient assessment, 5–6
　of knee, preoperative, 6
　in painful total knee arthroplasty, 348–350
　preoperative, for revision arthroplasty, 377
　in problematic total knee arthroplasty, 368
　for total knee arthroplasty following high tibial osteotomy, 601–602
Exchange arthroplasty
　evolution of, 473–474
　single-stage, 474–475
　　caution with, 475
　　contraindications to, 468
　　for infected total knee replacement, 465–470, 466f
　　length of interval between two halves of procedure in, 466–467
　　operative procedure in, 468
　　outcome of, 469
　　postoperative management in, 468

Exchange arthroplasty (continued)
　　preoperative considerations in, 467–468
　　rationale for, 466–467
　　versus two-stage revision, 466–467, 469–470
　two-stage, 471–472, 473–474, 475–476
　　clinical results in, 472, 475f, 475–476
　　for infected total knee arthroplasty, 471–476
　　operative technique for, 471–472
　　phases of, 471
　　PROSTALAC in, 471, 473, 479–488
　　rationale for, 466–467
　　spacer blocks for
　　　antibiotic-loaded, 466, 471, 476–477, 478–480
　　　articulated, 479–480
　　　methylmethacrylate, 476, 478–479
Exercises. See also Rehabilitation
　bedside, in rehabilitation, 658, 678t
　home, in rehabilitation, 652, 662, 670t–675f
Exposure
　anterior approach for, 115–118
　for arthrodesis, in infected total knee replacement, 495
　basic tenets of, 115
　for femoral allografting, 425
　medial parapatellar arthrotomy for, 115–118, 131, 132f
　for meniscal-bearing knees, 81–82, 84f
　minimizing skin and soft tissue tension in, 115
　for patellar revision, 526, 526f, 534f, 534–535
　for patellectomy, 622–623
　for posterior cruciate ligament-sparing procedure, 54
　proximal, extension of, for prevention of tibial tubercle avulsion, 519–520
　for proximal patellar realignment, 540, 542f
　quadriceps snip for, 149–154
　for revision arthroplasty, 378–379, 378f–379f, 435–436, 692
　for stiff knee, options for, 155, 156f, 692
　subvastus approach for, 119–126
　　difficulties in, maneuvers for, 123–125, 124f
　surgical approaches for, 113–162
　for tibial fracture revision, 594
　tibial tubercle osteotomy for, 159–162
　for total knee arthroplasty after supracondylar femoral osteotomy, 610–611
　for total knee arthroplasty following high tibial osteotomy, 603–605, 603f–605f
　for total knee arthroplasty for patients with prior arthrodesis, 628
　for total knee replacement after Maquet osteotomy, 615–616
　for total knee replacement with femoral extra-articular deformity, 636
　for total knee replacement with tibial extra-articular deformity, 645–646
　trivector-retaining arthrotomy for, 131–137
　for unicondylar replacement, 107
　V-Y quadricepsplasty for, 155–158
Extension
　femoral rollback in, 49–50

Extension (continued)
　preoperative assessment of, 6
　range of, continuous passive motion and, 655–656
　stabilization of knee in, in revision arthroplasty, 384, 385t, 387–388, 388f
Extension gap
　balance of, with flexion gap (See Flexion-extension gap, balance of)
　mismatch of, with flexion gap (See Flexion-extension gap, mismatch of)
Extensor lag
　flexion contracture and, 210–211
　patellar fracture and, 509
　PROSTALAC and, 485
　quadriceps tendon repair and, 514
　as subtraction/deduction, in knee scores, 32f, 33, 34f, 35
　tibial tubercle osteotomy and, 151–152
　in total knee arthroplasty after patellectomy, 625
　V-Y quadricepsplasty and, 156
Extensor mechanism
　alignment of, 315–342
　attenuation of, flexion contracture and, 210–211
　calcification of, following patellectomy, 622
　complications in
　　with constrained prostheses for revision arthroplasty, 104
　　femoral component rotation and, 361–363
　　patients with increased risk for, 519
　　with posterior-stabilized condylar knee, 69, 71–72
　　trivector-retaining arthrotomy and, 134–135
　disruption of, 519 (See also Patellar tendon, rupture of; Quadriceps tendon, rupture of; Tibial tubercle avulsion)
　　in painful total knee arthroplasty, 363–364, 364f
　　with tibial fractures, 589–590
　dissection down to, in anterior surgical approach, 116–118
　dysfunction of, 503–542
　　management of, general guidelines for, 525
　insufficiency of, as indication for total knee arthroplasty, 3
　in painful total knee arthroplasty, assessment of, 349
　patella and, 621, 622f
　performance of, patellar preparation and, 167
　preoperative assessment of, 6
　reconstruction of
　　allografting for, following total knee arthroplasty, 516–518
　　in partial patellectomy, 510–511
　tension of, and patellar fracture, 507
　tension on, minimizing, in anterior surgical approach, 118
Extra-articular deformity. See also Valgus deformity; Varus deformity
　causes of, 632, 635, 640, 641f, 645
　correction of
　　alteration of joint line resection for, 635, 638–639, 645, 646–648

Extra-articular deformity (*continued*)
    axial alignment in, 640–641, 642f
    compensatory bone resection in, 640–644, 641f–643f
    creation of instability in, 632, 640, 642
    extra-articular, 642–644
    joint line obliquity with, 645
    options in, 632
    osteotomy at apex of deformity for, 635, 638, 645, 646
    primary surgical goal in, 648
    supracondylar osteotomy for, 642–644
    templating for, 632, 635, 645
  effect on femoral component, 640–644
  effect on tibial component, 632–634
    determination of, 632–634, 633f
  femoral, total knee replacement with, 635–639
    preoperative planning for, 635–636
    radiographic evaluation in, 635
    results of, 638–639
    surgical technique in, 636f–637f, 636–638
  tibial, total knee replacement with, 645–648
    preoperative planning for, 645
    results of, 646–648
    surgical technique in, 645–646, 647f
  tibial *versus* femoral, 634
Extra-articular layer, in valgus deformity, 137–138, 138f–139f
Extraction devices, in component removal, 380f, 380–382, 382f
Extraction punch, in femoral component removal, 380f, 380–381
Extramedullary guides
  for femoral cuts, 182f, 182–183
    in femoral component rotation, 237
  for tibial cuts, 181–182, 182t, 244–245

F

Fabello-fibular ligament, in valgus deformity, 138, 139f
Face validity, 41
Factor II (prothrombin), in coagulation, warfarin and, 697–698
Factor IX (Christmas factor), in coagulation, warfarin and, 697–698
Factor VII (proconvertin), in coagulation, warfarin and, 697–698
Factor X (Stuart-Prower factor), in coagulation, warfarin and, 697–698
Family, and postoperative care and rehabilitation, 5
Fat emboli
  prevention of, in cutting femur, 54–55
  in sequential or simultaneous arthroplasty for bilateral disease, 4
Fatigue, in meniscal-bearing knees, 90–91
Fat pad(s)
  incision of, in lateral approach, for valgus deformity correction, 142, 142f
  patellar
    excision of, blood supply disruption in, and patellar fracture, 505
    reduction of, in subvastus approach, 124f, 125
Fee-for-service, 19
Feet. *See* Foot
Femoral artery, 327f

Femoral component
  alignment of, 177–179
    anterior cortex as reference for, 177–178
    anteroposterior, in revision arthroplasty, 386
    axial, and patellar tracking, 319f, 322
    epicondyles as reference for, 177–178
    flexion-extension gap as reference for, 177–179, 180f
    ideal, 189
    intramedullary canal as reference for, 177–178
    posterior condylar axis as reference for, 177–178, 179f
    problems in, and stiff knee, 689–690
    rotational (*See* Femoral component, rotation of)
  basic principles for, 165
  cementing of, 259
  cementless fixation of, in hybrid total knee arthroplasty, 273–276
    indications for, 274–275
  in cementless total knee arthroplasty
    alignment of, 263–265
    design of, 263
      bimetal, 262–263
      porous coating of, 262–263
    survivorship of, 270
  custom, in total knee replacement with femoral extra-articular deformity, 635–636, 636f, 637
  design of, and patellar fracture, 507
  evaluation of, in patellar revision, 526–527
  extra-articular deformity and, 640–644
  loosening of
    as contraindication to use of Rush rods for supracondylar fracture, 554
    in painful total knee arthroplasty, 353–357, 354f
    with posterior-stabilized condylar knee, 72
    radiographic assessment of, 353–356, 354f
    radionuclide bone scan of, 356–357
  matching of, to anteroposterior dimension of femur, 166–167
  in meniscal-bearing knees, 91–92, 91f–92f
  migration of, with F3 defects, 405–406
  in painful total knee arthroplasty, radiographic evaluation of, 351, 352f
  in PROSTALAC, 481–482, 482f
  realignment of, in patellar instability, 341
  removal of
    in failed arthroplasty, 379–381, 380f–381f
    instruments for, 379–380, 380f
    with minimal damage to bone stock, 381, 381f
    well-fixed cemented stem and, 380–381, 381f
  rotation of
    alternatives for, 240–242
    anatomic landmarks for, 229–232, 230f
    anteroposterior axis for, as secondary landmark, to epicondylar axis, 232–233, 233f
    computed tomography of, 238f, 363, 363f, 365

Femoral component (*continued*)
    epicondylar axis for, 177–178, 179f, 227–235, 236, 238–239, 242, 321–322, 322f, 332, 361–363
      in correction of combined deformities, 221
      in lateral release for valgus deformity, 198–199, 198f–199f, 202
      posterior condylar axis for, 387
      surgical technique in, 232–234, 232f–234f
      theoretical arguments supporting, 231–232
    external, 167, 227–229, 539
      in revision arthroplasty, 387
    and flexion-extension gap balance, 227
    flexion gap technique for, 229
    goal of, 240
    importance of, 227–229, 236
    internal
      adverse effects of, 227, 337, 349, 361–363, 363f–364f, 539
      avoidance of, 167, 332
      in lateral release for valgus deformity, 198–199, 198f–199f
    lateral retinacular release in, 237
    malalignment of, in painful total knee arthroplasty, 349, 361–363, 363f–364f, 365
    methods of, 229–232
    and need for patellar revision, 527
    and patellar tracking, 167, 178–179, 227, 233–234, 236, 237, 238, 239, 240, 245, 247f, 301, 317, 320–322, 322f, 328, 332, 539
    posterior condylar axis for, 229, 236, 317, 361–363
      in revision arthroplasty, 387
      as secondary landmark, to epicondylar axis, 232–233
    with posterior cruciate-substituting knee replacement, 240–242
    technique in, 240–241, 241f
    in revision arthroplasty, 387–388, 387f–388f
    in revision surgery for patellar instability, 333, 333f
    tibial component and, 243–244, 250–251
    tibial resection and, 240–241, 245
    tibial shaft axis for, 229, 236–239
      clinical results in, 237–238, 238f, 238t
      versus posterior condylar axis, 237–238, 238f
      surgical technique in, 236–237, 237f
    in total knee replacement with femoral extra-articular deformity, 637
    and trochlear groove, 227, 228f
    trochlear groove as reference for, 229–230, 242
  sizing of
    incorrect, and stiff knee, 689–690
    and instability, 194f, 194–195
    oversizing in, avoidance of, 55
    in revision arthroplasty, 385t, 385–387, 386f
  stemmed
    press-fit, in revision arthroplasty, 451–461
    in total knee arthroplasty after supracondylar femoral osteotomy, 610, 611f

Index

Femoral component (*continued*)
    in total knee replacement with femoral extra-articular deformity, 635–636, 636f, 637
    translation of, and patellar tracking, 322, 322f
    in unicondylar replacement, 108, 109
    valgus angle of, 177–179
Femoral condyle
    distal, as source for autogenous bone grafts
        for more involved femoral condyle, 295, 296f
        for tibia, 290f, 290–294
    osteonecrosis of, autogenous bone grafting for, 296, 296f
    posterior, as source for autogenous bone grafting, in tibial deficiency, 293
Femoral deficiency
    bone grafting for, 398
        allografting in, 398, 424–431
            advantages and disadvantages of, 424
            for bicondylar defects, 425, 428f
            clinical results of, 429–430
            common clinical conditions requiring, 424
            complications in, 398, 429–430
            contraindications to, 425
            cost-effectiveness of, 424
            fixation in, 425, 428, 429f
            graft incorporation in, 425–428
            indications for, 424–425
            ligamentous reattachment with, 428–429, 430f
            postoperative management in, 429
            preoperative planning for, 425
            selection of structural allograft for, 425
            surgical technique for, 425–429, 426f–429f
            for unicondylar defects, 425, 427f
            using acetabular reamers for defect preparation and reconstruction, 425, 426f
            versatility of, 424
        allografts for, 398
            complications with, 398
        autogenous, 295–297
    in cementless total revision arthroplasty, 441, 441f–443ff
    cavitary, 401
    classification of, 401–402, 401–406, 404t, 424
    complex, differentiation of, landmarks for, 402
    custom component for, 398
    discontinuity, 401
    F2A defects in (one condyle involvement), 404, 404f
    F2B defects in (involvement of both condyles), 404–405, 405f
    F1 defects in, 403, 403f, 404t
    F2 defects in, 403f–404f, 403–405, 404t
    F3 defects in, 404t, 405f, 405–406
    implant fixation in presence of, 398
    intercalary, 401
    management of, 397–398
    metallic augmentation for, 398
    segmental, 401
    small, methylmethacrylate as filler for, 295
    with valgus deformity, 409, 410f

Femoral fractures
    intraoperative, with PROSTALAC, 486t, 487
    periprosthetic, 545–575
        blade plates fixation, 561f, 562, 567–570, 570f
        evaluation of, 564
        nonoperative treatment of, 545–552
        retrograde intramedullary nail for internal fixation of, 558–562
        revision arthroplasty for, 565–566, 568, 573–575
        rush rods for, 553–557, 573
        supracondylar (*See* Supracondylar fractures)
Femoral nerve block
    cost of, 681t
    duration of, 681t
    major advantages and disadvantages of, 682t
    quality of, 681t
    technical support for, 681t
    technique for, 681t
Femoral notching, 166, 178
    anterior, and supracondylar fracture, 557, 563–564, 564t
    avoidance of, in subvastus approach, 126
Femoral osteotomy
    as alternative to total knee arthroplasty, 4–5
    supracondylar (SCFO)
        for extra-articular deformity correction, 642–644
        failed, incidence of, 610
        prior, autogenous bone grafting after, 296–297, 297f
        results of, 610
        total knee arthroplasty after, 610–612
            clinical results of, 611
            preoperative planning in, 610, 611f
            removal of previous hardware in, 610, 611f
            surgical approach in, 610–611
Femoral rollback, 49
    definition of, 49
    with posterior-stabilized condylar knee, 67, 69, 71
    retention of posterior cruciate ligament and, 50, 55f–56f
    sacrifice of posterior cruciate ligament and, 62–63
    in total knee arthroplasty after patellectomy, 624, 624f
    in total knee replacement after Maquet osteotomy, 617
Femoral sleeve release, in lateral approach, for valgus deformity correction, 144, 145f
Femur
    anterior
        cutting/resection of
            and flexion space, 165
            and patellofemoral joint, 165
        exposure of, in subvastus approach, 125f, 126
    bone loss or defect in (*See* Femoral deficiency)
    complications in, with constrained prostheses for revision arthroplasty, 103t, 104
    cutting/resection of (*See also* Femoral osteotomy)
        anatomic alignment and, 177, 178f

Femur (*continued*)
    in anatomic measured resection, 243
    basic principles of, 165–167, 166f–167f
    in cementless total knee arthroplasty, 265–266, 267
    compensatory, in extra-articular deformity, 640–644, 641f–643f
    in correction of combined deformities, 220–221
    extramedullary *versus* intramedullary jigs for, 182f, 182–183
    in femoral component rotation, 233, 236–237, 237f, 240–242, 241f
    guides for, 55–56, 182f, 182–183, 237
    and instability, 194f, 194–195, 202
    instruments for, 182f, 182–183
    in lateral approach, for valgus deformity correction, 145–146, 146f
    in lateral release for valgus deformity, 198–199, 198f–199f
    mechanical axis and, 177, 178f
    in medial release, for varus deformity correction, 192f, 192–193
    for meniscal-bearing knees, 93
    over-resection, in flexion-extension gap technique, 243
    in posterior cruciate ligament-sparing procedure, 54–55, 55f–56f
    and prosthetic fit, 194f, 194–195
    in total knee arthroplasty after supracondylar femoral osteotomy, 611
    in total knee arthroplasty following high tibial osteotomy, 606–607
    in total knee arthroplasty for patients with prior arthrodesis, 629
    in total knee replacement with femoral extra-articular deformity, 635–636, 636–637
    in total knee replacement with tibial extra-articular deformity, 646
    cysts of, and supracondylar fracture, 564
    distal, cutting/resection of, basic principles for, 165–167
    extra-articular deformity of
        versus tibial extra-articular deformity, 634
        total knee replacement with, 635–639
            preoperative planning for, 635–636
            radiographic evaluation in, 635
            results of, 638–639
            surgical technique in, 636f–637f, 636–637
    lesions of, incidentally discovered, in radiographic evaluation, 12
    ligament advancement on
        distal, abandonment of, 208
        proximal, 206–208
    posterior, cutting/resection of, basic principles for, 165–167
    preparation of, for bone grafting in cementless revision arthroplasty, 441, 441f–443f
    subluxation of, in tibial deficiency, 289, 290f
    in valgus deformity, 139
Fibrin, in deep vein thrombosis, 694–695
Fibrinogen, in deep vein thrombosis, 694–695, 699
52-inch radiographic view, 7
    standing, 12, 14f
Finn prosthesis, 707

Fixation, 255–286
    in allografting, 417, 419, 425, 428, 429f
    in arthrodesis, for infected total knee
        replacement, 496–499
    biologic
        autologous bone chips in, 263, 264f,
            269, 269f
        calcium phosphate ceramics in,
            277–286
        successful long-term, prerequisites for,
            284
    cement in, 257–261 (See also
        Cement/cementing)
        in revision arthroplasty, 435–439
    cementless, 262–272
        in revision arthroplasty, 440–450
    of fractures (See specific fractures)
    in hybrid total knee arthroplasty,
        273–276
    of onset patella, 301–302
    in presence of femoral deficiency, 398
    in presence of tibial defects, 397
    press-fit stem, in revision arthroplasty,
        451–461
        operative technique for, 456–459,
            456f–459f
        preoperative planning and templating
            for, 452–453, 452f–455f
        results of, 459–460
    in revision arthroplasty, 384–386, 433–461
    in total knee replacement after Maquet
        osteotomy, 618
Flexion
    femoral rollback in, 49–50
    preoperative assessment of, 6
    range of, continuous passive motion
        and, 655
    sacrifice of posterior cruciate ligament
        and, 62
    stability in, sacrifice of posterior cruciate
        ligament and, 62–63, 63f–64f
    stabilization of knee in, in revision
        arthroplasty, 384–388, 385t,
        386f–387f
Flexion contracture(s)
    assessment of
        in Hospital for Special Surgery Knee
            Score, 32f, 33
        in Knee Society Score, 34f, 35
    bone block and, 210, 211f
    causes of, 210, 211f
    combined with varus or valgus
        deformity, 216
        correction of, 216–223, 217f
        lateral release for, 219–220, 219f–220f
        medial release for, 218f, 218–219
        preoperative planning for, 217–218
        surgical pathology of, 216–217
    correction of, 221f, 221–222
        complications in, 214
        ligament balancing in, 210, 211f, 213,
            213f–214f, 221–222
        postoperative casting in, 214
        postoperative management of, 214
        results of, 214–215
        surgical technique for, 212–214,
            213f–214f
    in total knee arthroplasty, 210–215
    preoperative casting of, 212
    preoperative evaluation of, 211–212
    radiographic evaluation of, 211–212,
        211f–212f
    small, correction not required for, 215

Flexion contracture(s) (continued)
    soft tissue, 210, 211f
    in varus deformity, 189, 190f
Flexion-extension gap
    balance of
        basic principles for, 165–167, 166f
        in cementless total knee arthroplasty,
            266
        in correction of combined deformities,
            220–221
        femoral component rotation and, 227,
            238
        in flexion contracture correction, 210,
            211f, 213, 213f–214f, 221–222
        instruments for obtaining, 183–184,
            184f
        in lateral release for valgus deformity,
            199, 199f, 202
        in ligament advancement, 207
        in medial release, for varus deformity
            correction, 193, 193f
        problems in, and stiff knee, 689–690
        in revision arthroplasty for stiff knee,
            692
        in revision arthroplasty for tibial
            fractures, 595–596
        in total knee arthroplasty following
            high tibial osteotomy, 607
        in total knee replacement with femoral
            extra-articular deformity, 637
        evaluation of, in lateral approach, for
            valgus deformity correction,
            144–145, 144f–145f
    mismatch of
        constrained prostheses in, 77–78
        in revision arthroplasty, 386–387
        as reference for femoral component
            alignment, 177–179, 180f
Flexion-extension gap technique, 243, 244f
    disadvantages of, 243, 245f
    femoral component rotation in, 229
    inadequate tibial resection in, 248–249,
        250f–251f
    tibial position in, 243, 244f
Flexion-extension plane, tibial component
    position in, 244–246, 246f
Flexion space, cutting/resection of anterior
    femur and, 165
Fluoroscopic radiographic views, of
    component loosening, in painful
    total knee arthroplasty, 353, 355f
Foot, assessment of
    in painful total knee arthroplasty, 349
    preoperative, 5–6
Foot pump, for deep vein thrombosis
    prophylaxis, 699
Foreign body reaction, and component
    loosening, 356–357, 356f–357f
The Foundation prosthesis, 711–712
Four-bar linkage system, of knee, 621, 622f,
    623
Fourth American College of Physicians for,
    guidelines of, for deep vein
    thrombosis prophylaxis, 700–701,
    701t
Fracture(s). See also specific types and
    anatomic sites
    patient history of, 5
Frames, for cutting, 181, 181f
Freedom
    linear, 97
    rotational, 97
    meniscal-bearing knees and, 90

Freeman-Samuelson implant, 49, 304
Function, assessment of
    in Hospital for Special Surgery Knee
        Score, 32f, 33
    in Knee Society Score, 34f, 35–36
    in Western Ontario and MacMallister
        Osteoarthritis Index, 36
Functional brace, 656–657, 657f
Functional disability, as indication for total
    knee arthroplasty, 3
Functional independence measure, in
    rehabilitation, 660, 679t
Functional status, of patient, in painful
    total knee arthroplasty, 348

G
Gait
    assessment of
        in painful total knee arthroplasty,
            349
        postoperative, in rehabilitation,
            652–653, 662
        preoperative, 5–6
        for total knee arthroplasty following
            high tibial osteotomy, 601
        video analysis for, 662
    extension deficits and, 655
    flexion required in, as goal in continuous
        passive motion, 655
    retention of posterior cruciate ligament
        and, 51, 91
Gallium scanning, in infection, 368
Gap theory, 227
Gas, intra-articular, with infection, in
    painful total knee arthroplasty,
    357–358, 360f
Gastrocnemius muscle, lateral head of
    release or lengthening of
        in flexion contracture correction, 213,
            214f, 221f
        in lateral approach, for valgus
            deformity correction, 144
        in lateral release for valgus deformity,
            199–201, 200f, 203
        in lateral release for valgus deformity
            combined with flexion
            contracture, 219
        in medial parapatellar arthrotomy, for
            valgus deformity, 139
    in valgus deformity, 138, 139f
General anesthesia, 115
    patient education on, 653
Genesis I, 722
Genesis II, 722
Genesis total knee prosthesis, 304, 307,
    722
Genicular arteries, 326–327, 327f
    disruption of, in lateral retinacular
        release
        and need for patellar revision, 525
        and patellar fracture, 505–506
    inferior lateral, preservation of, in
        quadriceps snip, 151
    in midvastus approach, 129
    preservation of, in lateral retinacular
        release, 329f, 329–330, 335
    in proximal patellar realignment, 333
Gentamicin
    addition of, to cement, 468, 474, 476
    elution of, 477
Genu valgum, 189, 190f, 203
Geomedic knee, loosening of, and tibial
    fracture, 576

Gerdy's tubercle
  elevation of, in lateral approach, for valgus deformity correction, 142f, 143, 147
  in valgus deformity, 137–138, 139f
Gigli saw, in femoral component removal, 380, 380f
Gold standard, in criterion validity, 41
Gonarthrosis, unicondylar replacement in, 110
Goniometer, for range of motion assessment, 6
Gout, and patient outcome, 5
Graduated blocks, in posterior cruciate ligament-sparing procedure, 56, 58f
Greenfield filters, for deep vein thrombosis treatment, 702
GUEPAR implant, 75, 257

H

Hamstring
  lateral
    lengthening of, in medial parapatellar arthrotomy, for valgus deformity, 139
    release or lengthening of, in lateral approach, for valgus deformity correction, 144
    in valgus deformity, 138, 139f
  strength of, after quadriceps snip, 150–152, 153t
Hauser procedure, for distal patellar realignment, 341
Health maintenance organizations (HMOs), 20
Health status instruments, general, for outcomes assessment, 43
Healy, William, 207
Heel raises, 675t
Heel slides, 670t
Hemarthroses, with constrained prostheses for revision arthroplasty, 104
Hematoma, epidural, 682, 685
Hemophilia
  as indication for total knee arthroplasty, 3
  pain management in patients with, 683
Heparin
  for deep vein thrombosis treatment, 702
  low molecular weight
    for deep vein thrombosis prophylaxis, 699–702, 701, 701t
    compression stockings *versus*, 700
    warfarin *versus*, 700
    epidural analgesia with, safety of, 682, 685
    formulations of, characteristics of, 700t
    mechanism of action, 699–700
Herbert prosthesis, 75
Hermann Hospital, cost analysis by, 20t, 22–23
Heterotopic ossification
  with PROSTALAC, 486t, 486–487
  and stiff knee, 688, 688f
  treatment of, 688
High tibial osteotomy
  decreased posterior or anterior slope with, 602, 602f
  and extra-articular deformity, 632
  pain with, management of, 601–602
  total knee arthroplasty following, 601–609

High tibial osteotomy (*continued*)
  custom-made components in, 605–606, 605f–606f
  existing hardware in, and implant selection, 602–603, 603f
  indications for and contraindications to, 601–602
  patella infera in, 602, 605–607
  patient evaluation for, 601–602
  poor prognostic factors in, 601, 608
  postoperative management of, 607
  preoperative radiographic evaluation for, 601–602, 602f
  preoperative templating for, 605–606, 605f–606f
  removal of hardware in, 603–605, 605f
  results of, 607–608
  soft tissue condition in, 603
  staple retention or removal in, 603, 603f–604f
  techniques in, 602–607, 603f–606f
Hinged knee braces, for supracondylar fractures, 547f, 547–548
  displacement with, 547–548, 547f–548f
  with rush rods, 556
Hinged knee sleeve, 656, 657f
Hinge prostheses, 75–80, 76f, 97
  in lateral release for valgus deformity, 203
  lessons learned from, 75
  for revision arthroplasty, results of, 102
Hip(s), assessment of
  in painful total knee arthroplasty, 349
  preoperative, 5–6
  radiographic, 7, 12
  with stiff knee, 687
  for total knee arthroplasty following high tibial osteotomy, 601–602
Hip center-femoral shaft angle, in femoral component rotation, 229, 230f
History
  in clinical evaluation of painful total knee arthroplasty, 345, 347
  general medical, of patient, in preoperative assessment, 5
  preoperative
    for revision arthroplasty, 377
    for total knee arthroplasty following high tibial osteotomy, 601–602
  in problematic total knee arthroplasty, 368
  social, of patient, 5
  in total knee arthroplasty following high tibial osteotomy, 601
HMOs (health maintenance organizations), 20
Hohmann retractor, in medial release, for varus deformity correction, 190, 191f
Home exercises, in rehabilitation, 652, 662, 670t–675f
Hospital(s), reimbursement of, 19–20
Hospital costs
  analysis of, 20t, 20–22, 21f–22f
  average length of stay and, 20t, 21–24
  Lahey Clinic study of, 20t, 20–21, 21f
  Northwestern Memorial Hospital study of, 20t, 21f–22f, 21–23
Hospital for Special Surgery
  development of posterior-stabilized condylar knee at, 67–70
  posterior cruciate ligament-sacrificing procedure at, 61

Hospital for Special Surgery Knee Score, 31–33, 32f, 42
  versus other outcome measures, 36–37
  for patient self-assessment, 7
  questionnaire adaptation of, 43
Humidity, and cement, 257–258
Hybrid total knee arthroplasty, 260, 273–276
  cost of, 275
  indications for, 274–275
  published results of, 273
  radiographic evaluation of, 275f
  results of, 274–275, 274f–275f
Hydroxyapatite
  basic science of, 277–278
  in biologic fixation, 277–286
  environmental conditions and methods in manufacture of, 277
  implant coatings of
    animal investigations of, 278–281
    application of, 278
    and bone formation on perimeter and internal surface lengths, 280–281, 281f–282f
    in cancellous bone environment, 278–281
    clinical experience with, 281–284
    concerns about, 284
    and lamellar bone formation, 281, 283f
    versus non-coated fiber-metal implants, 278–284, 279f–283f
    and pore volume filled with bone, 279f, 280
    radiographic evaluation of, 284
    scanning electron microscopy backscatter analysis of, 281, 282f
    separation of, from titanium substrate, 284
    versus titanium implants, 278–279
  long-term stability of, 278
  optimal thickness of, 278
  solubility and bioresorption of, 278
Hyperextension stops, 77
Hypotension, with epidural analgesia, 683–684
Hypotheses, generation of, in painful total knee arthroplasty, 345–347, 346f

I

Ice, postoperative use of, 657–658
Iliotibial band (I-T band)
  contracture of, in valgus deformity, 197, 217
  reattachment of, in lateral approach, for valgus deformity, 147
  release or lengthening of
    in lateral approach, for valgus deformity, 140, 141f
    in lateral release for valgus deformity, 199–200, 200f, 202–203
    in lateral release for valgus deformity combined with flexion contracture, 219, 219f
    in medial parapatellar arthrotomy, for valgus deformity, 139
    in total knee arthroplasty following high tibial osteotomy, 607
  in valgus deformity, 137–138, 139f
Imaging. *See also specific imaging modalities*
  of painful total knee arthroplasty, 348, 351–367
Immobilization devices, for supracondylar fractures, 546–548, 546f–548f, 565, 567–568

Impedance plethysmography, in deep vein thrombosis diagnosis, 695
Importance, as diagnostic principle, 346
Incision(s)
  for anterior approach, 116f, 116–118
  for arthrodesis, in infected total knee replacement, 495
  basic tenets for, 115
  curved medial parapatellar, 116
  for exposure of failed prosthesis, 378–379, 378f–379f
  for insertion of Rush rods, in supracondylar fracture, 555
  for lateral approach, in valgus deformity correction, 140–141, 140f–141f
  for medial release, for varus deformity correction, 189–190
  for meniscal-bearing knees, 81–82, 84f, 93
  for midvastus approach, 127
  old, preoperative assessment of, 6
  for patellar revision, 526, 526f
  for patellectomy, 622–623
  prior, and patellar revision, 525
  prior lateral, and new incision, 115, 116
  prior vertical, and new incision, 115, 116
  for proximal patellar realignment, 540, 542f
  for quadriceps snip, 149
  retinacular, 117f, 118
    lateral, 140–141, 141f
  for retrograde intramedullary nail, in supracondylar fracture fixation, 559
  for revision arthroplasty for stiff knee, 692
  sham, 378
  straight midline, 116
  in subvastus approach, 119, 120f
  for tibial fracture revision, 594
  for tibial tubercle osteotomy, 159–160, 160f
  for total knee arthroplasty after supracondylar femoral osteotomy, 610–611
  for total knee arthroplasty following high tibial osteotomy, 603–605, 603f–605f
  for total knee arthroplasty for patients with prior arthrodesis, 628
  for total knee replacement after Maquet osteotomy, 615–616
  for total knee replacement with femoral extra-articular deformity, 636
  for total knee replacement with tibial extra-articular deformity, 645–646
  in trivector-retaining arthrotomy, 132
  for unicondylar replacement, 107
  in V-Y quadricepsplasty, 155, 157f
Indications, for total knee arthroplasty, 3–8
Indium-labeled leukocyte scan, in infection, 358–361, 361f–362f, 365
  false-positive, marrow scan for detection of, 360–361, 362f
Indomethacin, suppository, after posterior cruciate ligament-sparing procedure, 59
Infected total knee replacement
  alternative procedures for management of, 491–501
  amputation for, 491, 499
  antibiotic suppression alone for, 491, 492–493
    complications with, 492
    prerequisites for, 492

Infected total knee replacement (*continued*)
  arthrodesis for, 465, 469, 475, 483, 491, 494–499, 496f–498f
  debridement for, 491
    with antibiotic, 493
  decision making in
    complex, 491–492
    utilities analysis in, 492
  deep infection in, prevalence of, 491
  drainage and antibiotic treatment of, 467
  early, assessment of, 467
  heroic attempts in, 491–492
  resection arthroplasty for, 491, 494, 495f
  revision arthroplasty for, 357, 463–490, 493–494
    antibiotic-impregnated cement in, 440, 466–468, 471, 473–490
    antibiotic treatment before, 440
    cementless fixation and bone grafting in, 440, 446–448
    historical perspective on, 465
    prosthesis of antibiotic loaded acrylic cement (PROSTALAC) IN, 471, 473–490 (*See also* PROSTALAC)
    single-stage, 465–470, 466f
      contraindications to, 468
      length of interval between two halves of procedure in, 466–467
      operative procedure in, 468
      outcome of, 469
      postoperative management in, 468
      preoperative considerations in, 467–468
      rationale for, 466–467
      versus two-stage revision, 466–467, 469–470
    surgical prerequisites for, 493–494
    two-stage, 471–472, 473–474, 475–476
      clinical results in, 472, 475f, 475–476
      operative technique for, 471–472
      phases of, 471
      PROSTALAC in, 471, 473, 479–488
      rationale for, 466–467
      spacer blocks for, 466, 471, 476–477, 478–479, 478–480, 479–480
  stiff knee with, 687
  treatment of, prime objective in, 491
Infection
  antibiotic prophylaxis against, 465
  deep
    with constrained prostheses for revision arthroplasty, 103t, 104
    overall incidence of, 357
  epidural catheters and, 684–685
  in painful total knee arthroplasty, 357–361
    bone resorption with, 357–358, 359f
    diagnosis of, 350, 358
    false-positive bone scans in, detection of, 360–361, 362f
    incongruent bone scans in, 360, 361f, 365
    indium-labeled leukocyte scan in, 358–361, 361f–362f, 365
    intra-articular gas with, 357–358, 360f
    nuclear imaging of, 358
    nuclear imaging with inflammatory-specific agents in, 358–361
    periosteal reaction with, 357–358, 359f
    radiographic assessment of, 357–358, 359f–360f

Infection (*continued*)
    scintigraphy of, 358
    sinography of, 361, 363f
    technetium 99m-sulfur colloid marrow scan in, 360–361, 362f
    three-phase bone scan in, 358–361, 365
  perioperative, in tibial allografting, 418
  in problematic total knee arthroplasty, assessment for, 368
  in total knee arthroplasty (*See* Infected total knee replacement)
Inferolateral genicular artery, 326–327, 327f
  disruption of, in lateral retinacular release, and patellar fracture, 505–506
Inferomedial genicular artery, 326–327, 327f
Inflammation
  as contraindication to unicondylar replacement, 107
  two-stage arthroplasty in, 3
Inflammatory arthritis, as indication for total knee arthroplasty, 3
Informed consent, 4
Infusion systems, for pain management, 680
Inlay patella, 301, 304–309
  all polyethylene, uncemented, 306
  all polyethylene biconvex, cemented, 307
  biomechanical studies on, 304–305, 305f
  clinical studies of, 306–308
  historical development of, 304
  and intraosseous vascular supply, 308
  metal-backed polyethylene, uncemented, 306–307
  versus onset patella, 306, 307–308
  in patellar bone loss, severe cases of, 308
  patellar fracture with, pattern of, 305
  surgical technique for, 305–306
  weakening of reamed-out bone with, 308
Insall Burstein I All Poly Tibia prosthesis, 730
Insall Burstein I Metal Back Tibia prosthesis, 731
Insall-Burstein® posterior-stabilized condylar knee prosthesis, 62, 67–74, 95, 730–732
  in correction of combined deformities, 218–219
  development of, history of, 67–70
  dislocation of, 69
  extensor mechanism complications with, 69, 71–72
  femoral loosening with, 72
  femoral rollback with, 67, 69, 71
  in hybrid total knee replacement, 274f
  Insall-Burstein I, 67, 68f, 730–731
  Insall-Burstein II, 69, 731–732
  long-term results of, 72–73
  metal-backed tibial component in, 68–69, 73
  patellar complications and fractures with, 67–68, 71–72
  posterior cruciate ligament-substituting mechanism in, 67, 69, 71–72
  short-term results with, 70–72
  survivorship of, 67, 72–73
  tibial loosening with, 69, 72
  versus total condylar knee, 67, 71, 73
  in total knee arthroplasty after patellectomy, 623–624, 624f
Insall Burstein PS All Poly prosthesis, 716
Insall Burstein PS Metal Back Tibia, 717
Insall-Salvati ratio, for patellar height assessment, 9, 11f, 351

Insall's classification, of bone defects, 401
Inset patella. *See* Inlay patella
Instability
  anteroposterior
    and residual pain with patellectomy, 623
    in total knee arthroplasty after patellectomy, 625
  assessment of
    in Hospital for Special Surgery Knee Score, 32f, 33
    in Knee Society Score, 34f, 35
    preoperative, 6
  creation of, in correction of extra-articular deformity, 632, 640, 642
  femoral resection and, 194f, 194–195, 202
  with flexion contracture correction, 214
  with lateral release for valgus deformity, 202
  ligamentous, constrained prostheses and, 97, 101–102
  medial release and, 194f, 194–195
  in painful total knee arthroplasty, 349, 352–353, 354f
  patellar (*See* Patella, instability of)
  with PROSTALAC, 480, 485, 486, 486t
  size of femoral component and, 194f, 194–195
  in valgus deformity, 197
Instrument(s)
  for balancing knee, 183–184, 184f
  for component removal, 377, 379–382, 380f, 382f
  cutting, 181, 181f
  design of, 181
  for femoral preparation, 182–183
  on Mayo stands, 172f, 173
  for patellar preparation, 183, 183f
  for patellar revision, 527–528, 527f–528f
  power, and temperature, 258–259, 267
  for revision arthroplasty, 384
  for tibial preparation, 181–182
Instrumentation, 175–185
  advances in, dichotomy of, with prostheses development, 177
  principles of, 177–181
  tibiofemoral alignment and, 177, 178f
Intercalary bone defect, 401
Intercalary graft, for supracondylar fracture, 574–575
Intercondylar fossa radiographic view, 10, 12f–13f
Intercondylar notch, radiographic evaluation of, 10, 12f–13f
Intermittent compression devices, for deep vein thrombosis prophylaxis, 699
Intermittent low-pressure compression devices, for deep vein thrombosis prophylaxis, aspirin *versus*, 697
Intra-articular layer, in valgus deformity, 138–139, 139f
Intramedullary canal, as reference for femoral component alignment, 177–178
Intramedullary guides
  for femoral cuts, 182f, 182–183, 220–221
    in femoral component rotation, 236–237, 237f
    in posterior cruciate ligament-sparing procedure, 54–55
  for tibial cuts, 181–182, 182t, 244–245
    in posterior cruciate ligament-sparing procedure, 55

Intramedullary rods
  in arthrodesis fixation, 496–499, 498f
  for supracondylar fracture fixation, 573–575
Intramuscular narcotics
  cost of, 681t
  duration of, 681t
  major advantages and disadvantages of, 682t
  quality of, 681t
  technical support for, 681t
  technique for, 681t
Intrathecal narcotics
  complications of, 682t, 685
  cost of, 681t
  duration of, 681t
  major advantages and disadvantages of, 682t
  quality of, 681t
  technical support for, 681t
  technique for, 681t
Iodine scanning, in deep vein thrombosis diagnosis, 695
Isolation drape, 169, 171f

J
Joint line
  elevation of, in repair of F2B femoral defects, 405
  maintenance of, in management of bone loss, 393
  reestablishment of, in revision arthroplasty, 387, 387f
  transmission of force away from, stems for, 451
Joint line obliquity, with extra-articular deformity correction, 645
Joint space
  effective, cementing as limitation of, 274–275
  in flexion contracture, radiographic evaluation of, 211–212, 212f
  in painful total knee arthroplasty, radiographic evaluation of, 351
  radiographic assessment of, 9–10
Joint-space narrowing
  in degenerative joint disease, 12, 15f
  radiographic evaluation of, 10–12

K
Kessler stitch, in patellectomy, 511
Kinematic rotating hinge prosthesis, 75, 76f, 97, 99f
  in lateral release for valgus deformity, 203
  for revision arthroplasty, results of, 102
  in supracondylar femur fracture, 101f
Kinematics, in cementless total knee arthroplasty, 263–267
Kinemax Plus prosthesis, 713
Kissing osteophytes, 108
Knee(s)
  aspiration of
    in evaluation for patellar revision, 533
    in infected knee replacement
      with antibiotic suppression, 492–493
      before revision arthroplasty, 471
    in problematic total knee arthroplasty, 368
  preoperative examination of, 6
Knee bends
  mini, 660, 661f
  sitting-assisted, 675t

Knee Function Score, in Knee Society Score, 34f, 35–36
Knee press, 671t
Knee Score, in Knee Society Score, 34f, 35
Knee scores, 31–38, 42
  comparison of measures for, 36–37
  crosslinks to, from validated instruments, 43
  Hospital for Special Surgery Knee Score, 31–33, 32f, 42
  Knee Society Score, 33–36, 34f, 42
  questionnaire adaptations of, 42–43
  uses of, 37
  validity of, 41–42
  Western Ontario and MacMallister Osteoarthritis Index, 36
Knee Society Clinical Rating System, 660
Knee Society Radiographic Scoring System, 352–353, 353f
Knee Society Score, 33–36, 34f, 42
  versus other outcome measures, 36–37
  for patient self-assessment, 7
  in preoperative assessment, 6
Krackow stitch
  in allografting for extensor mechanism reconstruction, 516–517, 517f
  in patellectomy, 511
KSS. *See* Knee Society Score

L
Lachman's test, in preoperative assessment, 6
Lahey Clinic, cost analysis by, 20t, 20–21, 21f
Lamellar bone formation, calcium phosphate ceramic-coated implants and, 281, 283f
Laminar flow, in operating room ventilation, 168, 465, 534
Laminar spreaders
  in flexion contracture correction, 221, 221f
  in lateral release for valgus deformity, 198
  in medial release, for varus deformity correction, 192, 192f
Lasers, 181
Lateral approach, 137–148
  versus medial parapatellar arthrotomy, 140
  for patellar rotating prosthesis implantation, 310
  preserving surgical option of tibial tubercle osteotomy in, 143
  for valgus deformity, 137–148, 203
    bone resections in, 145–146, 145f–146f
    femoral sleeve release in, 144, 145f
    flexion-extension gap evaluation in, 144–145, 144f–145f
    iliotibial band release or lengthening in, 140, 141f
    instrumentation in, 145f, 145–146
    lateral arthrotomy-coronal Z-plasty in, 140–141, 141f–142f
    patella dislocation/joint exposure for, 143, 143f
    rationale for, 139–140
    results of, 147f, 148
    soft tissue management in, 147–148
    soft tissue (prosthetic) closure in, 146f, 146–147
    steps in, 140
    surgical technique in, 140–147
    tibial sleeve release in, 143–144, 144f

Lateral collateral ligament
  contracture of, in valgus deformity, 197
  release of
    in lateral approach, for valgus
      deformity correction, 144
    in lateral release for valgus deformity,
      199–200, 200f, 203
    in lateral release for valgus deformity
      combined with flexion
      contracture, 219, 219f
    in total knee arthroplasty following
      high tibial osteotomy, 607
    in revision arthroplasty, 388
  in valgus deformity, 138, 139f
Lateral compartment, in degenerative joint
  disease, 12, 15f
Lateral epicondyle, intraoperative
  identification of, 232, 233f
Lateral femoral periosteum, contracture of,
  in valgus deformity, 197
Lateral ligament advancement, 205–206,
  208, 208f–209f
  after care in, 208–209
Lateral ligament complexes, preoperative
  assessment of, 6
Lateral meniscus, separation of, from
  anterior attachment, in subvastus
  approach, 125f, 125–126
Lateral mobility, rehabilitation and, 660,
  660f
Lateral parapatellar arthrotomy
  in total knee arthroplasty following high
    tibial osteotomy, 604, 606
  in total knee replacement after Maquet
    osteotomy, 615–616
Lateral radiographic view, 6–7, 9, 11f
  of bone defects, 402
    F2A femoral, 404
  in degenerative joint disease, 15f
  in osteonecrosis, 16f
  of painful total knee arthroplasty, 351,
    352f, 365
  of patella, 317, 318f
  of patellar instability, 332
  preoperative, for medial release, for
    varus deformity correction, 189
  of problematic total knee arthroplasty,
    368
  for total knee arthroplasty following
    high tibial osteotomy, 601–602,
    602f
  for total knee replacement after Maquet
    osteotomy, 615
Lateral release
  benefits and pitfalls of, 326–331
  and patellar tracking, 326–331
  for valgus deformity, 197–204
    bone resection in, 198–199, 198f–199f
    combined with flexion contracture,
      219–220, 219f–220f
    complications of, 197, 201–203
    implant selection for, 197–198
    instability with, 202
    with knee in extension, 219
    patellar instability with, 202
    peroneal nerve palsy with, 201, 220
    postoperative management in, 201
    results of, 202–203
    soft tissue releases in, 199–201,
      199f–201f
      order of, 199, 200f
    surgical techniques for, 197–201,
      197f–201f

Lateral retinaculum
  contracture of, in valgus knee, and
    patellar tracking, 328
  release of
    all-inside technique for, 328–329, 330
    benefits and pitfalls of, 326–331
    blood supply disruption in, 327,
      329–330, 335, 505–506, 525
    closure in, 329
    debate over, 329–330
    in femoral component rotation, 237
    not recommended, in patellar
      dislocation, 539
    and patellar fracture, 505–507
    in patellar realignment, 335, 337
    in patellar revision, 535
    and patellar tracking, 237, 266–267,
      301, 319–320, 323, 326–331
    preservation of genicular arteries in,
      329f, 329–330, 335
    for prevention of tibial tubercle
      avulsion, 520
    in proximal patellar realignment, 333
    in quadriceps snip, 149
    quadriceps tendon rupture with, 514
    reasons for, 327–328
    results of, 330
    stepwise approach to, 328–329
    surgical approach in, 327
    technique of, 327–329
    in two-stage exchange arthroplasty,
      with PROSTALAC, 482, 483f
    for valgus deformity, 199, 200f, 201,
      202–203
    for valgus deformity combined with
      flexion contracture, 219, 219f
    in V-Y quadricepsplasty, 155
  in valgus deformity, 137–138, 139f
Lateral superior genicular artery, in
  proximal patellar realignment, 333
Legal risks, of data collection/outcomes
  assessment, 40–41
Leg length, radiographic assessment of, 12,
  14f
Length of stay
  average (ALOS), and hospital costs, 20t,
    21–22, 23–24
  continuous passive motion and, 653, 655
  reduced, and rehabilitation, 651–652
Lethargy, patient-controlled analgesia and,
  653
Leukocyte count
  in infection, 368
  in painful total knee arthroplasty, 358
Leukocyte scan
  indium-labeled, in infection, 358–361,
    361f–362f, 365
  technetium 99m-labeled, in infection,
    358–359
Lifestyle alteration, as alternative to total
  knee arthroplasty, 4–5
Ligament(s), preoperative assessment of, 6
Ligament advancement, 205–209
  applicability of techniques for, premises
    for, 205–206
  after care in, 208–209
  experiences with, critical review of, 205
  in extra-articular deformity correction,
    634
  on femur
    distal, abandonment of, 208
    proximal, 206–208
    lateral, 205–206, 208, 208f–209f

Ligament advancement (continued)
    medial, 205–206, 206–208, 206f–208f, 607
    proximal, on femur, 206–208
    suturing in, 207–208, 207f–208f
  of vastus lateralis, in patellectomy, 622
  of vastus medialis
    in patellar realignment, 333, 337
    in patellectomy, 622, 622f
Ligament balancing. See also Flexion-
  extension gap
  in anatomic measured resection, 243
  in cementless total knee arthroplasty, 266
  in femoral component rotation, 241
  in flexion contracture correction, 210,
    211f, 213, 213f–214f, 221–222
  in medial release, for varus deformity
    correction, 193, 193f
  in meniscal-bearing total knee
    arthroplasty, 82, 84f–86f
  with retention of posterior cruciate
    ligament, 51, 55–57, 58f
  in revision arthroplasty, 388
Ligament release. See also specific ligaments,
  release of
  basic principles of, 165
Limb salvage, in management of infected
  total knee replacement, 491–501
Linear diagnostic model, 345
Linear freedom, 97
Local anesthetics, 680
  for patients with preoperative reflex
    sympathetic dystrophy, 683
Locking loop ligament fixation suture,
  207f, 207–208
London Hospital, single-stage revision for
  infected knee at, 465–470
Long radiographic view, 7
  standing, 12, 14f
  preoperative, for medial release, for
    varus deformity correction, 189
  for total knee arthroplasty following
    high tibial osteotomy, 601–602
Loose bodies
  arthroscopic management of, 369
  in degenerative joint disease, 15f
  magnetic resonance imaging of, 14–15,
    15f
  radiographic evaluation of, tunnel
    (intercondylar fossa) view for, 10,
    13f
  and stiff knee, 690
Loosening, of components
  with antibiotic suppression in infected
    total knee replacement, 492
  arthrography of, 355–356
  bone loss/defects as cause of, 356–357,
    356f–357f
  bone loss with, 393, 406–408, 409, 410f
  with constrained prostheses for revision
    arthroplasty, 103t, 104
  femoral
    as contraindication to use of Rush
      rods for supracondylar fracture,
      554
    in painful total knee arthroplasty,
      353–357, 354f
    with posterior-stabilized condylar
      knee, 72
    radiographic assessment of, 353–356,
      354f
    radionuclide bone scan of, 356–357
  infection and, 357–358, 359f–360f
  osteolysis and, 356–357, 356f–357f

Loosening, of components (*continued*)
  in painful total knee arthroplasty,
      352–357, 353*f*
    radiographic assessment of, 353*f*–356*f*,
        353–357
  patellar
    arthroscopic management of, 368–369,
        372*f*, 372–373
    femoral component rotation and, 227
    in painful total knee arthroplasty, 352,
        353–357, 355*f*
    and patellar fracture, 507, 509–510, 512
    revision of, 524–532
  radionuclide bone scan of, 356–357
  tibial
    bone loss with, 406–408
    in painful total knee arthroplasty,
        353–357, 353*f*–357*f*
    with posterior-stabilized condylar
        knee, 69, 72
    radiographic assessment of, 353–356,
        353*f*–356*f*
    radionuclide bone scan of, 356–357
    subsidence with, 353, 354*f*
Low-Contact-Stress total knee system, 81,
    83*f*, 90, 711
  cemented
    bicruciate-retaining, survivorship of,
        86–87
    unicompartmental, survivorship of,
        85–86
  cemented rotating platform,
      survivorship of, 87
  contact areas of, 92
  contraindications to, 86
  in lateral release for valgus deformity, 203
  mid- and long-term results with, 90
Low molecular weight heparin
  for deep vein thrombosis prophylaxis,
      699–702, 701, 701*t*
    compression stockings *versus*, 700
    warfarin *versus*, 700
  epidural analgesia with, safety of, 682
  formulations of, characteristics of, 700*t*
  mechanism of action, 699–700
L-plates, in high tibial osteotomy, removal
    of, in subsequent total knee
    arthroplasty, 603–605
L-shaped arthrotomy, in subvastus
    approach, 119–120
Lumbar spine, assessment of, in painful
    total knee arthroplasty, 349
Lumbar sympathetic block, for reflex
    sympathetic dystrophy, 364, 688
Lumbosacral spine, assessment of, in painful
    total knee arthroplasty, 349–350

M
MacIntosh interpositional arthroplasty, 257
Magnetic resonance imaging
  in degenerative joint disease, 14–15, 15*f*
  for femoral rollback assessment, 50
  of loose bodies, 14–15, 15*f*
  in osteochondritis dissecans, 14–15, 15*f*
  in osteonecrosis, 16–17, 16*f*–17*f*
  of painful total knee arthroplasty,
      limitations on, from metallic
      artifacts, 351, 363, 365
  for total knee arthroplasty following
      high tibial osteotomy, 602
Malpractice, exposure to, data
      collection/outcomes assessment
      and, 40–41

Managed care, 20
Manipulation, of stiff knee, 690–691
  anesthesia for, 691
  timing of, 690
Maquet osteotomy
  for patellofemoral arthrosis, 613, 614*f*,
      618–619
  total knee replacement after, 613–620
    clinical evaluation for, 615
    common problems encountered in,
        620*t*
    posterior cruciate ligament retention
        or substitution in, 615, 617, 618,
        619*f*
    preoperative planning for, 615
    radiographic evaluation for, 615, 615*f*
    results of, 618
    surgical approach for, 615–616
    surgical technique in, 615–618,
        616*f*–618*f*
    tibial internal/external rotation in,
        617–618, 618*f*
    tibial resection in, 616–618, 616*f*–618*f*
      in anteroposterior plane, 616*f*,
          616–617
      saw blade length for, 618, 618*f*
      in varus/valgus plane, 617, 617*f*
    tibial sizing and fixation in, 618
Mark II prosthesis, 94–95
Mark I prosthesis, 94–95
Marrow scan, in infection, 360–361, 362*f*
Maxim Complete Knee System, 707
Mayo Clinic
  periprosthetic tibial fracture classification
      of, 576, 577*f*, 578*t*, 587
  V-Y quadricepsplasty modification of,
      155, 157*f*
    results of, 156–157
Mayo stands
  creation of pocket from operating table
      to, 169, 171*f*–172*f*
  instruments placed on, 172*f*, 173
MBK prosthesis, 90–96, 735
  contact areas of, 92–93
  design of, 91–92, 91*f*–93*f*
  implantation of, surgical technique for,
      93–94, 94*f*
  preliminary results of, 94–95
  radiographic evaluation of, 95, 95*f*
Measured resection, 243–244, 245*f*
  in cementless total knee arthroplasty,
      265–268
Mechanical angle, in femoral component
    rotation, 229, 231*f*
Mechanical axis, 177, 178*f*
Mechanical compression, for deep vein
    thrombosis prophylaxis, 699, 701*t*,
    701–702
  aspirin *versus*, 697
  warfarin *versus*, 698–699
Mechanical venous interruption, for deep
    vein thrombosis treatment, 702
Medial collateral ligament
  advancement of, 205–206, 206–208,
      206*f*–208*f*
    after care in, 208–209
    suturing in, 207, 207*f*–208*f*
  in total knee arthroplasty following
      high tibial osteotomy, 607
  incompetence of, constrained prostheses
      with, 77–78
  release of
    basic principles of, 165

Medial collateral ligament (*continued*)
    in total knee replacement with femoral
        extra-articular deformity, 636
    in total knee replacement with tibial
        extra-articular deformity, 645–646
    for varus deformity, 189–196
      approach for, 189–190
      combined with flexion contracture,
          218*f*, 218–219
      complications of, 194–195
      instability with, 194*f*, 194–195
      patellar instability with, 195
      preoperative planning for, 189
      results of, 193–194
      technique for, 189–193, 190*f*–193*f*
      tibial tubercle avulsion with, 195
  in revision arthroplasty, 388
Medial compartment, in degenerative joint
    disease, 12, 15*f*
Medial epicondyle
  intraoperative identification of, 232, 233*f*
  in ligament advancement, 206–207
Medial epicondyle sulcus, as reference for
    femoral component alignment,
    198–199, 199*f*
Medial ligament advancement, 205–206,
    206–208, 206*f*–208*f*, 607
  after care in, 208–209
  suturing in, 207, 207*f*–208*f*
Medial ligament complexes, preoperative
    assessment of, 6
Medial parapatellar arthrotomy, 115–118,
    131, 132*f*
  blood supply disruption in, and patellar
      fracture, 505
  conversion of
    to quadriceps snip, 190
    to V-Y quadricepsplasty, 190
  in correction of combined deformities,
      218
  for exposure of failed prosthesis, 378–379
  versus lateral approach, 140
  in lateral release for valgus deformity, 198
  in lateral retinacular release, 327, 329
  in medial release, for varus deformity
      correction, 189–190
  versus midvastus approach, 129–130
  modified, in V-Y quadricepsplasty, 155
  in patellar revision, 525–526
  in proximal patellar realignment, 333
  versus subvastus approach, 119
  for total knee arthroplasty after
      supracondylar femoral osteotomy,
      611
  for total knee arthroplasty following
      high tibial osteotomy, 606
  for total knee replacement after Maquet
      osteotomy, 615–616
  for total knee replacement with femoral
      extra-articular deformity, 636
  versus trivector-retaining arthrotomy,
      131–132
  for valgus deformity, 147
    disadvantages of, 139
    failure rates of, 137
    surgical technique in, 139
Medial release
  in femoral component rotation, 241
  for varus deformity, 189–196
    combined with flexion contracture,
        218*f*, 218–219
Medial retinaculum, repair of, rupture of,
    and patellar tracking, 328

Medial skin flap, in subvastus approach, 119, 120f
Medial surgical approach, for patellar rotating prosthesis implantation, 310, 312f–313f
Medical complications, 4
Medical management, as alternative to total knee arthroplasty, 4–5
Medical Outcomes Study, 43
Medicare
  cost control measures of, 19–20, 23
  professional fees allowed by, 23
Medullary canal, obliterated, patient history of, 5
Membrane arthroplasties, 257
Meniscal-bearing knees, 81–96, 82f
  bicruciate retaining, 82, 86–87, 87f
  closure in procedure for, 83
  contact areas of, 92–93
  cruciate sacrificing, 82, 87f
  implantation of, 84
  incision for, 81–82, 84f
  knee exposure for, 81–82, 84f
  in lateral release for valgus deformity, 203
  ligament balancing for, 82, 84f–86f
  New Jersey Low-Contact-Stress, 81–90, 83f, 92, 203, 711
  posterior cruciate retaining, 82, 87f
  preoperative radiographic assessment for, 81, 83f
  preparation for, 81
  principles of, 90–91
  prosthetic design in, 91–92, 91–93, 91f–93f
  radiographic evaluation of, 95, 95f
  results of, preliminary, 94–95
  surgical technique for, 81–83, 93–94, 94f
  survivorship of, cemented versus cementless, 84–87, 88f
Meniscal tears, magnetic resonance imaging of, 16–17
Meniscus
  lateral, separation of, from anterior attachment, in subvastus approach, 125f, 125–126
  patellar, 308
Merchant radiographic view, 6–7, 9–10, 11f
  in painful total knee arthroplasty, 351–352, 353f
  of patella, 317, 318f
  of patellar instability, 332
  of problematic total knee arthroplasty, 368
  for total knee arthroplasty following high tibial osteotomy, 601–602
  for total knee replacement after Maquet osteotomy, 615
Merkel-Johnson treatment algorithm, for supracondylar fractures, 565–566
Metallic artifacts, and limitation on magnetic resonance imaging of painful total knee arthroplasty, 351, 363, 365
Metallosis, with polyethylene wear, 357, 358f, 533, 534f
Metaphyseal bone, in AORI classification of bone defects, 402f, 402–403
Methylene blue, for marking patellar peg holes, 64
Methylmethacrylate
  as filler for bone defects, 289, 295
  for fixation, in autogenous bone grafting, 291, 291f, 294
  fragments of, and stiff knee, 690, 691
  in preparation of cement, 257–258

Methylmethacrylate spacer blocks, in two-stage revision, for infected total knee arthroplasty, 476, 478–479
MG II prosthesis, 732
Midas Rex, in component removal, 379–380
Middle-age patients, osteoarthritic, unicondylar replacement in, 107
Middle genicular artery, 326–327, 327f
Midvastus approach, 127–130, 128f
  evolution of, 129–130
  indications for and contraindications to, 127
  versus medial parapatellar arthrotomy, 129–130
  for revision surgery, 127
  surgical experience with, 130
  surgical technique in, 127–129
  vastus medialis neurovascular anatomy and, 129
Miller-Galante prosthesis, 269, 533, 535–538
  using hybrid fixation, results with, 273
Mini knee bends, 660, 661f
Mini step-ups, 660, 661f
Miyakawa patellectomy, 622
Modular augmentation, 396
  for femoral deficiency, 295–296
  for tibial deficiency, 409–414
    alignment of, 411, 411f
    cost-benefit ratio of, 413
    in primary total knee arthroplasty, 409–411
    stems and stem extensions in, 409–412, 411f–413f
    and third-body wear, 413
    types of, 409–411, 411f
Modular PFC posterior cruciate-substituting knee replacement, femoral component rotation in, 240–242
Modular total knee systems, 98, 100f
  in lateral release for valgus deformity, 198
Monomer, in cement preparation, 257–259
Morphine pump, after posterior cruciate ligament-sparing procedure, 59
Morphine sulfate, intrathecal, major advantages and disadvantages of, 682t
Morse-taper, in tibial modular augmentation, 409, 413
Motor block, 115
MRI. See Magnetic resonance imaging
Multimodal analgesia, 680
Muscle strength, assessment of
  in Hospital for Special Surgery Knee Score, 32f, 33
  questionnaire adaptation of knee score for, 43
Myositis ossificans, 688

N

Nail(s)
  intramedullary, in arthrodesis fixation, 496–499, 498f
  retrograde intramedullary, for supracondylar fracture fixation, 558–562
    aftercare with, 559–560
    designs of, 558, 559f
    fit of, intercondylar distances of commonly used femoral prosthesis for determination of, 558, 559t

Nail(s) (continued)
  versus open reduction with plate fixation, 558
  patient positioning for, 558, 560f
  preoperative planning for, 558
  technique for, 558–559, 560f
Narcotics, in pain management, 680
  complications of, 682t, 685
  excessive, physiological effects of, 683
  intramuscular
    contraindications to, 683
    cost of, 681t
    duration of, 681t
    major advantages and disadvantages of, 682t
    quality of, 681t
    technical support for, 681t
    technique for, 681t
  intrathecal
    cost of, 681t
    duration of, 681t
    major advantages and disadvantages of, 682t
    quality of, 681t
    technical support for, 681t
    technique for, 681t
  limitations of, 684
  patients addicted to, analgesia for, 683
  and respiratory depression, 683
  systemic
    complications of, 682t, 685
    and deep vein thrombosis, 681
    versus epidural analgesia, 683
    limitations with, 683
    during rehabilitation, 680–681
    and respiratory depression, 685
    switch to, with dislodged epidural catheter, 683
Natural-Knee™, 264f, 269–270, 725
Neer classification system, of supracondylar fractures, 545. 564–565
  treatment guidelines based on, 567
Nerve blocks, 680
  complications of, 682t, 685
  cost of, 681t
  duration of, 681t
  limitations of, 684
  major advantages and disadvantages of, 682t
  quality of, 681t
  technical support for, 681t
  technique for, 681t
Neurologic disorders, and painful total knee arthroplasty, 348–350
Neuromata, local, 349–350
Neuropathic arthropathy, as indication for total knee arthroplasty, 3
Neurovascular compromise, 4
New Jersey Low-Contact-Stress prosthesis, 81–90, 83f, 92, 203, 711
NexGen Cruciate Retaining prosthesis, 733
NexGen Legacy CCK prosthesis, 734
NexGen Legacy PS prosthesis, 734
NexGen PS prosthesis, 733
Noiles knee prosthesis, 97, 100f
Nonambulatory treatment, of supracondylar fractures, 548–549, 548f–550f
Nonsteroidal anti-inflammatory drugs
  epidural analgesia with, safety of, 682
  interaction of, with warfarin, 698
  in pain management, 680
  for reflex sympathetic dystrophy, 688

Northwestern Memorial Hospital, cost
    analysis by, 20t, 21f–22f, 21–23
Notch radiographic view, 10, 12f–13f
Notch view, for total knee replacement
    after Maquet osteotomy, 615
No-thumb test, of patellar tracking, 57, 167,
    195, 318, 342, 529
NSAIDs. See Nonsteroidal anti-
    inflammatory drugs
Nuclear imaging
    in deep vein thrombosis diagnosis, 695
    of infection, 358
    with inflammatory-specific agents, in
        infection, 358–361
    in painful total knee arthroplasty, 351,
        358–361, 365
    for total knee arthroplasty following
        high tibial osteotomy, 602
Nutrition, patient, preoperative assessment
    of, 5

O
Obese patients
    advisability of total knee arthroplasty in,
        4
    deep vein thrombosis in, 694
    extensor mechanism disruption in, 519
    midvastus approach in, 129
    patellar fracture in, 507
    patellar tracking in, limited subfascial
        dissection of skin and
        subcutaneous tissue for, 323
Oblique prepatellar artery, 326
Occult neuropathia, patient history of, 5
Octogenarians, osteoarthritic, unicondylar
    replacement in, 107
Offset stems, 452f
    for constrained prostheses, 79, 79f
    for total knee arthroplasty following
        high tibial osteotomy, 605f,
        605–606
    for total knee replacement with femoral
        extra-articular deformity, 635, 636f
    for total knee replacement with tibial
        extra-articular deformity, 645–646
One-stage exchange arthroplasty. See
    Single-stage revision
One-stitch test, of patellar tracking,
    318–319, 320f
Onset patella, 301–303, 304
    fixation of, 301–302
    versus inlay patella, 306, 307–308
    patella preparation for, 301, 302f
    patellar osteotomy for, 301, 302f
    placement of, 301, 302f
Open reduction with internal fixation
    (ORIF)
    of periprosthetic tibial fractures, 587–591,
        590f, 594
    of supracondylar fractures, 565–570
Operating room
    cost of, 20t, 21f, 21–22, 22
    humidity of, and cement, 257–258
    preparation of, 7
    temperature of, and cement, 257–258
    ventilation of, 168, 465, 534
Optetrak prosthesis, 712
ORIF. See Open reduction with internal
    fixation
Osteoarthritis
    combined deformities with, 216–217
    cost-effectiveness analysis of total knee
        arthroplasty for, 26–27, 27t

Osteoarthritis (continued)
    and flexion contracture, 211f, 215
    as indication for total knee arthroplasty,
        3
    patellar fracture after total knee
        arthroplasty in, 505
    unicondylar replacement for, 106–111
Osteochondral fracture, magnetic
    resonance imaging of, 14–15
Osteochondritis dissecans
    magnetic resonance imaging of, 14–15,
        15f
    radiographic evaluation of, tunnel
        (intercondylar fossa) view for, 10,
        13f
Osteolysis, 274, 393. See also Bone
    loss/defects
    cement as seal against, 274–275
    and component loosening, 356–357,
        356f–357f
    computed tomography of, 357, 357f
    with femoral defects, 405
    pathologic fracture with, 356f, 357
    with posterior-stabilized condylar knee,
        73
    radiographic evaluation of, 356f, 357
    in bone defect classification, 402
    with tibial defects, 406–408
    with tibial fractures, 577
    tibial modular augmentation and, 413
Osteomyelitis, in painful total knee
    arthroplasty, 358–361, 359f–360f
Osteonecrosis
    advanced, 17f
    at cement-bone interface, 258–259
    early, 16f
    of femoral condyle, autogenous bone
        grafting for, 296, 296f
    as indication for total knee arthroplasty,
        3
    magnetic resonance imaging in, 16–17,
        16f–17f
    radiographic evaluation of, 16–17,
        16f–17f
    radionuclide bone scan in, 16
Osteonics Omnifit prosthesis,
    hydroxyapatite-coated, 283–284
Osteopenia
    and patellar fracture, 507
    with reflex sympathetic dystrophy, 364
    and supracondylar fracture, 545
Osteoperiosteal release, in lateral approach,
    for valgus deformity correction,
    143–144, 144f–145f
Osteophyte(s)
    computed tomography of, 16f
    in degenerative joint disease, 12, 15f
    kissing, 108
    radiographic evaluation of, tunnel
        (intercondylar fossa) view for, 10,
        13f
    removal of
        in cementless total knee arthroplasty,
            267, 268
        in flexion contracture correction, 213,
            213f, 221, 221f
        in lateral release for valgus deformity,
            198
        in medial release, for varus deformity
            correction, 191–193, 193f
        in meniscal-bearing total knee
            arthroplasty, 82
        in patellar inlay technique, 305

Osteophyte(s) (continued)
    in posterior cruciate ligament-sparing
        procedure, 55, 57
    in subvastus approach, 123, 123f
    in unicondylar replacement, 107–108
    retained, and stiff knee, 689, 689f
Osteotome
    caution with, in tibial fracture revision,
        594–595
    in component removal, 379, 380f
    stacking technique with, 381, 383, 383f
    in flexion contracture correction, 213,
        213f
    in medial release, 218
    for varus deformity correction,
        190–191, 191f, 193, 193f
    in patellar revision, 527, 527f, 535, 535f
    and tibial plateau fracture, 581
    in total knee arthroplasty following high
        tibial osteotomy, 606
    in total knee arthroplasty for patients
        with prior arthrodesis, 629, 629f
Osteotomy. See specific anatomic sites and
    procedures
Outcome(s)
    adverse, patient information on, 4
    medical conditions affecting, 5
    versus result, 39
Outcomes assessment, 39–40
    bias in, 42
    crosslinks from validated instruments
        for, 43
    current approach to, 41–42
    data collection for, 39–45
    data overload in, 40
    disruption of patient flow with, 40
    essential data elements of, 41
    establishing uniformity in, 40
    expense, hassle, and complexity of, 40
    Hospital for Special Surgery Knee Score
        for, 31–33, 32f, 42
    instruments for, 41–42
        disease-specific, 42
        general health status, 43
        reproducibility or reliability of, 41–42
        responsiveness of, 41–42
        selection of, 42–43
        validation of, 41–42
        validity of, 41–42
    knee scores for, 31–38, 42
        comparison of measures of, 36–37
        uses of, 37
    Knee Society Score for, 33–36, 34f, 42
    medicolegal risk and confidentiality in,
        40–41
    patient focus of, 39–40
    patient self-assessment for, 7, 43
    questionnaires adaptations of knee
        scores for, 42–43
    reasons for, 40–41
    in rehabilitation, 652, 665t–668t
    Western Ontario and MacMallister
        Osteoarthritis Index for, 36
Overstuffing, of patellofemoral joint, with
    posterior-stabilizing condylar
    knee, 67–68, 72
Oxford meniscal knee, 85, 90
    contact areas of, 92
Oxidative degradation, 90

P
Paget's disease, radiographic assessment
    of, 12

Pain
    assessment of
        in Hospital for Special Surgery Knee Score, 31, 32f
        in Knee Society Score, 34f, 35
        in Western Ontario and MacMallister Osteoarthritis Index, 36
    with high tibial osteotomy, treatment in, 601–602
    as indication for total knee arthroplasty, 3
    as most common subjective complaint after total knee arthroplasty, 651
    patellofemoral, due to arthrosis, tibial tubercle osteotomy for, 613, 614f, 618–619
    patellofemoral complications and, 332
    persistent
        in infected total knee replacement, amputation in, 499
        with PROSTALAC, 486, 486t
    postoperative, character of, 680
    preoperative evaluation of, for total knee arthroplasty following high tibial osteotomy, 601–602
    referred, in painful total knee arthroplasty, 347–348
    in reflex sympathetic dystrophy, 350
    residual, with patellectomy, anteroposterior instability and, 623
Painful total knee arthroplasty
    arthrography of, 351, 355–356
    chief complaint in, establishment of, 347
    clinical evaluation of, 345–350
    complications of total knee arthroplasty in, 352–361
        necessitating revision surgery, 352–353
    component loosening, 353–357
        femoral, 353–357, 354f
        infection and, 357–358, 359f–360f
        osteolysis and, 356–357, 356f–357f
        patellar, 352, 353–357, 355f
        radiographic assessment of, 353f–356f, 353–357
        radionuclide bone scan of, 356–357
        tibial, 352–357, 353f–357f
    computed tomography of, 349, 351, 363
    diagnostic categories in, 346f, 346–347
    diagnostic findings in, 348
    diagnostic models for, 345–346
    diagnostic principles in, 346–347
    differential diagnosis of, 345–347, 346f
    establishing degree of disability and severity of complaint in, 345
    evaluation of, 343–374
    exploration of, without adequate preoperative diagnosis, 345
    extensor mechanism disruption in, 363–364, 364f
    functional status of patient in, 348
    history in, 345, 347
    hypothesis generation in, 345–347, 346f
    imaging of, 348, 351–367
    infection in, 357–361
        bone resorption with, 357–358, 359f
        diagnosis of, 350, 358
        false-positive bone scans in, detection of, 360–361, 362f
        incongruent bone scans in, 360, 361f, 365
        indium-labeled leukocyte scan in, 358–361, 361f–362f, 365
        intra-articular gas with, 357–358, 360f

Painful total knee arthroplasty (continued)
        nuclear imaging of, 358
        nuclear imaging with inflammatory-specific agents in, 358–361
        periosteal reaction with, 357–358, 359f
        radiographic assessment of, 357–358, 359f–360f
        scintigraphy of, 358
        sinography of, 361, 363f
        technetium 99m-sulfur colloid marrow scan in, 360–361, 362f
        three-phase bone scan in, 358–361, 365
    inspection of knee in, 348
    magnetic resonance imaging of, limitations on, from metallic artifacts, 351, 363, 365
    malposition/malrotation of components in, 361–363, 363f–364f, 365
    nature of pain in, 347
    nuclear imaging of, 351, 358–361, 365
    other musculoskeletal pain with, 347–348
    in painful total knee arthroplasty, radiographic assessment of, 357–358, 359f–360f
    pain out of proportion to physical findings in, 350
    pain radiation in, 347
    palpation in, 349
    patellar fracture in, 363, 364f
    periprosthetic fractures in, 364–365
    physical examination in, 348–350
    polyethylene wear in, 357, 358f
    radiographic evaluation of
        conventional, in routine assessment, 351–352, 352f–353f, 365
        Knee Society scoring system for, 352–353, 353f
    reflex sympathetic dystrophy in, 350, 364–365
    sleep patterns of patient in, 348
    stability in, 348
    symptoms in, 347–348
    tendon tears in, 351, 363–364
    time course of complaint in, 347
Pain management
    and deep vein thrombosis, 682
    in elderly patients, 680
    in hemophiliacs, 683
    multimodal analgesia in, 680
    patient-controlled (PCA), 653, 655f, 680
        complications of, 682t, 685
        cost of, 681t
        duration of, 681t
        major advantages and disadvantages of, 682t
        patient education on, 653
        quality of, 681t
        during rehabilitation, 681
        technical support for, 681t
        technique for, 681t
    transition from, to oral analgesia, 653
    in patients addicted to narcotics, 683
    in patients with preoperative reflex sympathetic dystrophy, 683
    in patients with prior spine surgery, 683
    after posterior cruciate ligament-sacrificing procedure, 65
    after posterior cruciate ligament-sparing procedure, 59
    postoperative, 680–686
        complications of specific regimes in, 682t, 685
        patient education on, 653

Pain management (continued)
    specific analgesics in
        cost of, 681t
        duration of, 681t
        major advantages and disadvantages of, 682t
        quality of, 681t
        technical support for, 681t
        technique for, 681t
    techniques of, 680
    PROSTALAC and, 485
    during rehabilitation, 653, 656, 680–681
Pain service, complexities of, 682–683
Palacos cement, 258, 468, 474, 477–478, 481, 484
Palpation, in painful total knee arthroplasty, 349
Parkinson's disease, as indication for total knee arthroplasty, 3
Particulate disease, and component loosening, 356–357, 356f–357f
Passive range of motion, assessment of
    in painful total knee arthroplasty, 349
    preoperative, 6
Patella
    arthrosis of, refractory pain with, tibial tubercle osteotomy for, 613, 614f, 618–619
    avascular necrosis of, 506
    blood supply of, 326–327, 327f
        disruption of
            in lateral retinacular release, 327, 329–330, 335, 505–506
            and patellar fracture, 505–506
    bone loss in, inlay patellar component in severe cases of, 308
    bone loss or defect in (See Patellar deficiency)
    bone scans of, to assess viability after total knee arthroplasty, 506
    circumferential border of, identification of, in patellar revision, 526, 527f
    clinical importance of, 621
    cold, in lateral retinacular release, 329–330, 506
    cutting/resection of, 180–181
        in cementless total knee arthroplasty, 267–268
        excessive, and patellar fracture, 506–507
        eyeball technique for, 301
        guides for, 301, 302f, 507, 507f
        inadequate, and patellar fracture, 506–507
        instruments for, 183, 183f
        level of, 301, 302f
        in onset technique, 301, 302f
        for patellar rotating prosthesis, 310–311, 312f–313f
    dislocations of, with PROSTALAC, 485–486, 486t
    double, radiographic findings of, after allografting for patellar tendon repair, 523, 523f
    drift of, into baha location, minimizing, in anterior approach, 117f, 118
    elevation of, in total knee arthroplasty for patients with prior arthrodesis, 628
    enucleation of, in patellectomy, 622f, 622–623
    evaluation of existing components in, 526–527

Patella (continued)
  eversion of
    in anterior surgical approach, 118
    in cementless total knee arthroplasty, 267
    in correction of combined deformities, 218
    in lateral approach, for valgus deformity correction, 142–143, 148
    in medial release, for varus deformity correction, 190
    in midvastus approach, 128–129
    in patellar revision, 526
    for patellar rotating patella implantation, 310, 311f
    in quadriceps snip, 149
    in revision arthroplasty for stiff knee, 692
    in subvastus approach, 122–125, 123f, 124f
    in total knee arthroplasty following high tibial osteotomy, 606
    in total knee replacement with femoral extra-articular deformity, 636
    in total knee replacement with tibial extra-articular deformity, 646
    in trivector-retaining arthrotomy, 133
    in V-Y quadricepsplasty, 155
  fat pad of
    excision of, blood supply disruption in, and patellar fracture, 505
    reduction of, in subvastus approach, 124f, 125
  functional anatomy of, 621, 622f
  height of
    in allografting for patellar tendon repair, 522–523
    assessment of, 9, 11f
    and impingement complications with posterior-stabilized condylar knee, 71–72
    in painful total knee arthroplasty, 351, 352f–353f, 363
  high point of, preoperative assessment of, 317, 318f
  instability of
    arthroscopic management of, 368, 372
    avoidance of, key to, 332
    common causes of, following total knee arthroplasty, 131
    computed tomography of, 332–333, 333f
    distal patellar realignment for, 337–342
      clinical cases of, between January 1980 and January 1994, 340
      Hauser procedure in, 341
      materials and methods for, 337–340
      medial tibial tubercle transfer in, 337, 339–340, 340f
      medial transfer of medial one-half of patellar tendon in, 338–339, 339f
      modified Roux-Goldthwait procedure in, 337–338, 338f, 342
      results of, 341
      Roux-Goldthwait procedure in, 341
      surgical procedure for, 337–340
    evaluation of, 332–333, 333f
    incidence of, 332
    internal rotation of tibial component and, 249–253, 252f
    with medial release, for varus deformity correction, 195

Patella (continued)
    muscle imbalance and, 332
    in painful total knee arthroplasty, 348
    physical findings in, 332
    with PROSTALAC, 482, 485–486
    proximal patellar realignment for, 332–336
      complications in, 335
      postoperative management in, 333
      results of, 334–335
      surgical technique in, 333, 334f
    radiographic evaluation of, 332–333
    surgical technique and, 332
    symptoms of, 332
    time of onset, 332
  medialization of
    in cementless total knee arthroplasty, 266–268, 268f
    in inlay technique, 305
    in onset technique, 301, 302f
    and patellar tracking, 321, 321f, 328
    in painful total knee arthroplasty, assessment of, 349
  preoperative assessment of, 6, 332
  preparation of, 299–314
    basic principles for, 167
  radiographic assessment of, 9–10, 11f
  reduction of, with meniscal-bearing knees, 83
  resurfacing of
    complications in, 317, 324, 326, 332
    controversy over, 317
    inlay technique for, 301, 304–309
    onset technique for, 301–303, 304
    in posterior cruciate ligament-sparing procedure, 58
  rotating. See Rotating patella
  symmetry of, and patellar tracking, 321, 321f
  thickness of
    diminished, adverse effects of, 301
    in inlay technique, 305–306
    normal, restoration of, 301, 302f, 506–507
    and patellar tracking, 320–321, 321f, 328, 328f
  tracking of (See Patellar tracking)
  trivector anatomy of quadriceps tendon acting on, surgical approach retaining, 131–137
  in valgus deformity, 139, 317, 319f
  visualization of, in anterior surgical approach, 116
Patella alta, 139, 351, 363
Patella baja, 317, 318f, 329, 341, 351, 363, 378, 521
Patella infera, in total knee arthroplasty following high tibial osteotomy, 602, 605–607
Patellar arthrosis, Maquet osteotomy for, 613, 614f, 618–619
  total knee replacement after, 613–620
Patellar clunk syndrome, 236, 349, 368
  arthroscopic management of, 368–370, 370f–371f
  evaluation for and correction of, in patellar revision, 526
  nonoperative management of, 370
  patient evaluation for, 368–369
  with posterior-stabilized condylar knee, 68, 71–72, 370
Patellar component
  alignment of, 180–181
  all-polyethylene, revision of, 525, 527, 527f

Patellar component (continued)
  assessment of, in painful total knee arthroplasty, 351–352, 353f
  button position of, and patellar tracking, 321, 321f
  cementing of, 259
    in hybrid total knee arthroplasty, 273–276
  in cementless total knee arthroplasty
    design of, 263, 264f
    survivorship of, 270
  design of, and patellar fracture, 507
  extraction of, in failed arthroplasty, 382–383, 383f
  facetted, alignment of, 180–181
  implantation of, in patellar revision, 529
  inlay/inset, 301, 304–309
    all polyethylene, uncemented, 306
    all polyethylene biconvex, cemented, 307
    biomechanical studies on, 304–305, 305f
    clinical studies of, 306–308
    historical development of, 304
    and intraosseous vascular supply, 308
    metal-backed polyethylene, uncemented, 306–307
    versus onset patella, 306, 307–308
    in patellar bone loss, severe cases of, 308
    patellar fracture with, pattern of, 305
    surgical technique for, 305–306
    weakening of reamed-out bone with, 308
  loosening of
    arthroscopic management of, 368–369, 372f, 372–373
    femoral component rotation and, 227
    in painful total knee arthroplasty, 352, 353–357, 355f
    and patellar fracture, 507, 509–510, 512
    revision of, 524–532
  metal-backed
    goal of, 533
    introduction of, 533
    premature failing of, 533
    removal of, 535t, 535f–536f, 535–538
      prying technique for, 535, 535f
      wedge-platform technique for, 535, 535f
    revision of, 525, 528, 528f, 533–538
      evaluation and preoperative planning for, 533–534
      indications for, 533, 534t
      polyethylene wear and, 533, 534f
      surgical techniques for, 534f–537f, 534–538
  onset, 301–303, 304
    fixation of, 301–302
    versus inlay patella, 306, 307–308
    patella preparation for, 301, 302f
    patellar osteotomy for, 301, 302f
    placement of, 301, 302f
  patellar rotating, 310–314, 311f–312f
    final implantations of, 313
    lateral approach in resection for, 310
    medial approach in resection for, 310, 312f–313f
    patellar preparation for, 311
    postoperative rehabilitation with, 313
    surgical technique for, 310, 312f–313f
    survivorship of, 313
    trial in implantation of, 310–311
  single-peg, in patellar revision, 528–529, 530f, 533–535, 536f

Patellar component (continued)
   three-peg, in patellar revision, 528–529, 529f–530f, 533–534
Patellar deficiency
   cavitary, 401
   classification of, 401
      exclusion of, in AORI system, 403
   discontinuity, 401
   inlay patellar component in severe cases of, 308
   management of, in revision arthroplasty, 403
   segmental, 401
Patellar dislocation/subluxation, 539–542
   arthroscopic management of, 368, 369, 372
   with constrained prostheses for revision arthroplasty, 103t, 104
   determining need for surgical intervention in, 525
   distal realignment technique for, 540
   evaluation of and preoperative planning in, 539
   factors in, 524
   femoral component rotation and, 361–363, 363f, 539
   in lateral approach, for valgus deformity correction, 143, 143f
   with patellar rotating patella, 313
   predisposing factors to, 539, 540t
   with PROSTALAC, 486, 486t
   prosthetic design and, 539
   proximal realignment for, 539–540, 541f–542f
   radiographic evaluation of, 539, 540f
   traumatic, 539
   treatment of, 539–540, 540t
   with trivector-retaining arthrotomy, 134, 134f
   valgus deformity and, 137
Patellar fracture-dislocation, 508
Patellar fractures
   activity level and, 507
   arthroscopic debridement in, 510
   blood supply disruption and, 505–506
   classification of, 508
      based on clinical outcome and treatment, 508
   clinical presentation of, 508–509
   comminuted, treatment of, 509, 511–512
   component design and, 507
   component loosening and, 507, 509–510, 512
   component malalignment and, 507
   with constrained prostheses for revision arthroplasty, 103t, 104
   diagnosis of, 508–509
   displaced
      and failure of metal-backed patellar component, 533
      treatment of, 509–510, 511–512
   extensor mechanism tension and, 507
   femoral component rotation and, 227, 361–363
   fixation of, 509–511
   horizontal, 508
   incidental, 509
   with inlay prosthesis, pattern of, 305
   management of, 509–510
   nondisplaced, treatment of, 509, 512
   nonoperative treatment of, 509–511, 512
   obesity and, 507
   operative treatment of, 509–512

Patellar fractures (continued)
   in painful total knee arthroplasty, 363, 364f
   with patellar rotating patella, 313
   patellar thickness and, 301
   patellectomy for, 509
      partial, 510f, 510–511
      results of, 511–512
      total, 511–512
      total knee arthroplasty after, 623
   periprosthetic, determining need for surgical intervention in, 524–525
   with posterior-stabilizing condylar knee, 67–68, 71–72
   postoperative timing of, 505
   radiographic evaluation of, 509
   range of motion, increased, and, 507
   removal of peripheral bone and, 507
   resection technique and, 506–507
   stress or fatigue, 508, 508f
      treatment of, 509
   after total knee arthroplasty, 505–513
      etiology of, 505–507
      incidence of, 505, 506t
      minimizing risk of, recommendations for, 507
   traumatic, 508, 508f
   with trivector-retaining arthrotomy, 134, 134f
   type I, 508
   type II, 508
   type III, 508
   type IV, 508
   vertical
      through fixation hole, 508, 508f
      treatment of, 509
   weak bone and, 507
Patellar ligament, suturing and repair of, in patellectomy, 511
Patellar meniscus, 308
Patellar revision
   of all-polyethylene component, 525, 527, 527f
   circular versus ovoid component in, 525
   clinical experience with, 529
   determining need for, 524–525
   dome-shaped versus sombrero component in, 525
   evaluation of remaining bone stock in, 528–529
   identification of circumferential border of patellar in, 526, 527f
   implantation of component in, 529, 535, 536f
   instruments for, 527–528, 527f–528f
   of loose component, 524–532
   of metal-backed components, 525, 528, 528f, 533–538
      evaluation and preoperative planning for, 533–534
      indications for, 533, 534t
      polyethylene wear and, 533, 534f
      surgical techniques for, 534f–537f, 534–538
   nonresurfacing of patella in, 528–529
   polyethylene wear and, 525, 533, 534f
   postoperative treatment in, 529
   preoperative planning for, 525
   scar excision in, 526, 527f
   selecting implant for, 525
      algorithm for, 529, 530f
   single-peg component in, 528–529, 530f, 533–535, 536f
   in stiff knee, 526, 526f

Patellar revision (continued)
   surgical approach in, 525–526, 526f
   three-peg implant in, 528–529, 529f–530f, 533–534, 535, 536f
Patellar subluxation. See Patellar dislocation/subluxation
Patellar tendon
   avulsion of, 155
      protection against, in total knee arthroplasty following high tibial osteotomy, 606
      from tibial tubercle, 519–520
         avoidance of, preventive measures for, 519–520
         with medial release, for varus deformity correction, 195
   blood supply to, 326
   distal realignment of, 337–342
   elevation of, in total knee arthroplasty following high tibial osteotomy, 606
   medial one-half of, medial transfer of, in distal patellar realignment, 338–339, 339f
   in midvastus approach, 128
   patellectomy and, 621
   protection of, in component removal, 379, 381
   risk to, in distal patellar realignment, 341
   rupture of, 520–522, 522f
      allografting for, 521–523, 522f–523f
         radiographic findings of double patella with, 523, 523f
         technique of, 522–523
      Bunnell-type repair of, 520–521
      in close proximity to tibial tubercle insertion, 521
      direct repair of, 520
      end-to-end repair of, 520
      etiology of, 520
      at inferior pole of patella, 520–521
      Kelikian technique for, 521, 521f
      management of, 519–523
      in painful total knee arthroplasty, 351, 363–364
      postoperative timing of, 520
      with PROSTALAC, 486, 486t
      after proximal patellar realignment, 335
      repair techniques for, 520–522
      semitendinous tendon in repair of, 521, 521f
   separation of, from anterior tibia, in subvastus approach, 122, 123f
   visualization of, in anterior surgical approach, 116
Patellar tracking, 180–181
   in cementless total knee arthroplasty, 266–267
   femoral axial alignment and, 319f, 322
   femoral component rotation and, 167, 178–179, 227, 233–234, 236, 237, 238, 239, 240, 245, 247f, 301, 317, 320–322, 322f, 328, 332, 539
   femoral translation and, 322, 322f
   intraoperative assessment of, 317–325, 327
      alternative techniques for, 318–319, 320f
      checklist for, 320–323
      preferred technique for, 318, 319f
   in lateral release for valgus deformity, 198, 201, 202

Patellar tracking (continued)
    lateral retinacular contracture in valgus knee and, 328
    lateral retinacular release and, 237, 266–267, 301, 319–320, 323, 326–331
    limited subfascial dissection of skin and subcutaneous tissue for, 323
    in medial release, for varus deformity correction, 195
    no-thumb test of, 58, 167, 195, 318, 342, 529
    one-stitch test of, 318–319, 320f
    with onset prosthesis, 302
    in painful total knee arthroplasty, 349, 352
    patella button position and, 321, 321f
    patellar anatomy and, 328
    in patellar revision, 529
    patella symmetry and, 321, 321f
    patella thickness and, 320–321, 321f, 328, 328f
    in posterior cruciate ligament-sacrificing procedure, 62–64, 64f
    in posterior cruciate ligament-sparing procedure, 58
    preoperative assessment of, 317, 318f–319f
        for medial release, for varus deformity correction, 189
    problems in
        adverse effects of, 317
        arthroscopic management of, 368, 372
        causes of, 327–328
        distal patellar realignment for, 337–342
        intraoperative, significance of, 319–320
        proximal patellar realignment for, 332–336
        as red flag for surgeon, 319
        and stiff knee, 689–690
        with PROSTALAC, 485–486
    prosthesis shape and, 328
    in revision arthroplasty for stiff knee, assessment of, 692
    rupture of medial retinacular repair and, 328
    soft-tissue releases and, 323
    tenaculum clamp in testing of, 195
    tibial component position and, 328, 328f, 332
    tibia position and, 320, 322–323, 323f
    in total knee arthroplasty following high tibial osteotomy, 607
    in total knee replacement after Maquet osteotomy, 615, 618
    towel clip test of, 318, 320f
    in unicondylar replacement, 108, 108f
    valgus deformity and, 137
Patellar turndown, 149, 150f, 152–153
Patellectomy
    as contraindication to posterior cruciate ligament sacrifice, 61
    indications for, 621
    mechanical disadvantage of, 621
    for patellar fracture
        partial, 510f, 510–511
        results of, 511–512
        total, 511–512
    total knee arthroplasty after, 623
    for refractory pain, due to arthrosis, 613
    residual pain with, anteroposterior instability and, 623
    techniques of, 510f, 510–511, 622f, 622–623

Patellectomy (continued)
    Compere, 622f, 622–623
    Miyakawa, 622
    total knee arthroplasty after, 621–626
        femoral rollback in, 624, 624f
        patient selection for, 623
        posterior-stabilized condylar knee in, 72–73, 623–624, 624f
        postoperative management in, 625–626
        results of, 625
        surgical technique in, 623–624, 624f
Patellofemoral arthroplasty, 613
Patellofemoral articulation, 180–181
Patellofemoral compartment, in degenerative joint disease, 12, 15f
Patellofemoral complications, 131, 524, 539. See also specific patellar complications
    component design and, 524
    determining need for surgical intervention in, 524–525
    in painful total knee arthroplasty, 351–352, 353f
    patient risk factors for, 524
    and stiff knee, 689–690
    trivector-retaining arthrotomy and, 131, 134–135
    valgus deformity and, 137
Patellofemoral compression, in painful total knee arthroplasty, assessment for, 349
Patellofemoral joint
    cutting/resection of anterior femur and, 165
    overstuffing of, with posterior-stabilizing condylar knee, 67–68, 72
    radiographic assessment of, 9–10, 11f
Patient(s)
    appropriate rehabilitation therapist for, concerns about, 659
    disclosure to and informed consent of, 4
    expectations of, for total knee arthroplasty, 651
    focus on, in outcomes assessment, 39–40
    general medical history of, 5
    perceptions of, about rehabilitation therapists, 656
    preoperative assessment of, 5–7
    questionnaires for, in rehabilitation planning and assessment, 652, 665t–668t
    rapport with, in rehabilitation, 651
    selection of, 3–8
    self-assessment by, 7, 43
    social history of, 5
Patient classification, in Knee Society Score, 36
Patient-controlled analgesia (PCA), 653, 655f, 680
    complications of, 682t, 685
    cost of, 681t
    duration of, 681t
    major advantages and disadvantages of, 682t
    patient education on, 653
    and patient lethargy, 653
    quality of, 681t
    during rehabilitation, 681
    technical support for, 681t
    technique for, 681t
    transition from, to oral analgesia, 653
    and urinary function, 653

Patient education
    on in-home rehabilitation, 662
    on outline of postoperative year, 653–654
    on postoperative pain management, 653
    on rehabilitation, 652–654, 669t–675f
    on total knee arthroplasty, 651
Patient flow, disruption of, with outcomes assessment, 40
Patient Outcome Research Team, 31, 37
Patient positioning
    for anterior surgical approach, 115–116
    for supracondylar fracture fixation, with retrograde intramedullary nails, 558, 560f
Patient preparation, 168
    draping technique in, 168–173, 169f–172f
Patient tracking forms, in rehabilitation, 658–659, 678t
PCA. See Patient-controlled analgesia
PCA Modular prosthesis, 714
PCA Primary prosthesis, 714
PCL. See Posterior cruciate ligament
Penicillin-cement complex, 476
Penicillin G, in PROSTALAC, 484
Peptic ulcers, and patient outcome, 5
Performance Cruciate Retaining prosthesis, 708
Performance evaluation, knee scores for, 31–38
Performance Posterior Stabilized prosthesis, 708
Periarticular tendinitis, in painful total knee arthroplasty, 349
Periosteal elevator
    in flexion contracture correction, 213, 221, 221f
    in medial release, for varus deformity correction, 190, 191f, 218, 218f
Periosteal reaction, with infection, in painful total knee arthroplasty, 357–358, 359f
Peripheral bone defect, 401, 415
Peripheral nerve blocks, 680
    complications of, 682t, 685
    cost of, 681t
    duration of, 681t
    limitations of, 684
    major advantages and disadvantages of, 682t
    quality of, 681t
    technical support for, 681t
    technique for, 681t
Peripheral neuropathy, 349–350
Peripheral vascular disease, and patient outcome, 5
Periprosthetic fractures
    bone scan of, 364
    computed tomography of, 364
    femoral, 545–575
        blade plates fixation, 561f, 562, 567–570, 570f
        evaluation of, 564
        nonoperative treatment of, 545–552
        retrograde intramedullary nail for internal fixation of, 558–562
        revision arthroplasty for, 565–566, 568, 573–575
        rush rods for, 553–557, 573
    management of, 543–598
    in painful total knee arthroplasty, 364–365
    patellar, determining need for surgical intervention in, 524–525

Periprosthetic fractures (*continued*)
  tibial
    anatomic fracture patterns of, 576, 577f
    bone grafting for, 577–578, 579f, 579f–580f, 580f, 590, 590f, 594, 595f, 597–598
    classification of, 576–583, 577f, 578t, 587
    clinical presentation of, 592
    fixation techniques for, 590–591
    incidence of, 587, 592
    nonoperative treatment of, 584–586, 585f, 587, 588–589, 588f–589f
    open reduction with internal fixation of, 587–591, 590f, 594
    operative treatment of, technical considerations in, 590
    predisposing factors for, 587
    radiographic evaluation of, 594
    review of literature on, 592
    revision arthroplasty for, 584, 588, 590–591, 592–598
      avoidance of dead bone sandwich in, 596
      objectives in, 594
      operative technique for, 594–597, 596f
      postoperative protocols in, 597
      preoperative planning for, 594
      results of, 597–598
    treatment algorithms for, 582–583, 583f, 588, 588f, 592–593
    treatment goals in, 587–588, 592
    treatment options for, 592–594
Peroneal nerve
  preoperative assessment of, 6
  surgical decompression of, 201
Peroneal nerve palsy
  epidural analgesia and, 684
  with flexion contracture correction, 214
  with lateral release for valgus deformity, 201, 220
  risk of, following total knee arthroplasty, 684
Pes anserinus tendons
  contracture of, in varus deformity, 189, 190f
  release of, in varus deformity correction, 190–191
Pes bursitis, tibial component medial overhang and, 268
PFC Modular TC3 prosthesis, 717
PFC Modular Total Knee System—CR, 718
PFC Modular Total Knee System—PS, 718
PFC Sigma Cruciate Retaining prosthesis, 719
PFC Sigma Posterior Stabilized prosthesis, 719
Physical examination
  general, in patient assessment, 5–6
  in painful total knee arthroplasty, 348–350
  preoperative, for revision arthroplasty, 377
  in problematic total knee arthroplasty, 368
  for total knee arthroplasty following high tibial osteotomy, 601–602
Piecrusting technique, in valgus deformity correction
  in lateral release, 200, 200f
  for lengthening iliotibial band, in lateral approach, 140, 141f

Plain film
  of degenerative joint disease, 12
  of painful total knee arthroplasty, 351–352, 352f–353f
  of spontaneous osteonecrosis, 16, 16f–17f
Planovalgus deformity, assessment for, 6
Plantar compression, pneumatic, for deep vein thrombosis prophylaxis, 697, 699
Plasma flame-spraying technique, for application of calcium phosphate ceramics, 278
Plasmin, in deep vein thrombosis, 694–695, 699, 702
Plastic surgery consultation, for total knee replacement with tibial extra-articular deformity, 645
Platelet aggregation, aspirin and, 696
Plating
  in arthrodesis, for infected total knee replacement, 496, 497f
  in high tibial osteotomy, removal of, in subsequent total knee arthroplasty, 603–605, 605f
  for supracondylar fractures, 558, 561f, 562, 567–570, 570f, 573
  for tibial fractures, 590, 596–597
PMMA. *See* Polymethylmethacrylate
Pneumatic calf compression, for deep vein thrombosis prophylaxis, warfarin *versus*, 698–699
Pneumatic compression devices, for deep vein thrombosis prophylaxis, 699, 701t, 701–702
  aspirin *versus*, 697
  warfarin *versus*, 698–699
Pneumatic plantar compression, for deep vein thrombosis prophylaxis, 697, 699
Polio
  arthritis associated with, as indication for total knee arthroplasty, 3
  patient history of, 5
Polycentric knee, 31
  loosening of, and tibial fracture, 576, 578f
Polyethylene, ultrahigh-molecular-weight, maximum permissible compressive stress limit of, 81
Polyethylene debris
  contamination with, in component removal, 379, 379f
  in problematic total knee arthroplasty, 368
  reaction to, and component loosening, 356–357
Polyethylene implants. *See also specific components and prostheses*
  fracture of, and stiff knee, 690
  implantation of, in posterior cruciate ligament-sparing procedure, 58–59
  in meniscal-bearing knees, 92, 93f
  overhang of, 248, 249f
  quality of, 90
  removal of, in failed arthroplasty, 381–383, 382f
  in tibial component, size and thickness of, 248, 249f–250f
  ultracongruent, in cementless total knee arthroplasty, 266, 266f
  in unicondylar replacement, 109
Polyethylene wear
  arthrography of, 357, 358f
  arthroscopic management of, 371–372, 372f
  in constrained prosthesis, 76

Polyethylene wear (*continued*)
  metallosis with, 357, 358f, 533, 534f
  in painful total knee arthroplasty, 352, 357, 358f
  and patellar revision, 525, 533, 534f
  in posterior-stabilized condylar knee, 73
  retention of posterior cruciate ligament and, 52
  and supracondylar fracture, 564
Polymer, in cement preparation, 257–259
Polymerization, of cement, 257–259
Polymethylmethacrylate (PMMA)
  alternatives to, 277
  antibiotic additives to, 471
  in blades plate fixation of supracondylar fracture, 569
  development of, 257
  femoral cysts filled with, and supracondylar fracture, 564
  for filling bone defects, 424
  formation/preparation of, 257–259
  modulus of, 259
  in patellar revision, 529
  properties of, 259
  removal of, in patellar revision, 527–528, 527f–528f
  thermal necrosis from, and patellar fracture, 507
  toxicity and leaching of, 258
Popliteal cyst, preoperative assessment of, 6
Popliteus tendon
  contracture of, in valgus deformity, 197
  preserving integrity of, in correction of varus deformity, 165
  release of
    in lateral approach, for valgus deformity correction, 144
    in lateral release for valgus deformity, 199–200, 200f, 203
    in lateral release for valgus deformity combined with flexion contracture, 219, 219f
    in total knee arthroplasty following high tibial osteotomy, 607
  in valgus deformity, 138, 139f
Porous coatings
  calcium phosphate ceramics for, 277–286
  application of, 278
  in cementless total knee arthroplasty, 262–263
  cost of, 275
  removal of components with, 381–382
Posterior condylar axis, 230f
  for femoral component rotation, 229, 236, 317, 361–363
  in revision arthroplasty, 387
  as secondary landmark, to epicondylar axis, 232–233
  versus tibial shaft axis, 237–238, 238f
  measurement of, sex and, 231t
  as reference for femoral component alignment, 177–178, 179f, 198
  relationship of, with epicondylar axis, 177–178, 179f, 183, 198
Posterior cruciate ligament
  in combined deformities, 217
  deficiency of, in varus deformity, 189
  in flexion contracture, 210
  instability of, and patellar revision, 533
  preoperative assessment of, 6
  release of
    in arthroscopic management of stiff knee, 691

Posterior cruciate ligament (*continued*)
    in lateral approach, for valgus deformity correction, 143
    in lateral release for valgus deformity, 199, 200*f*, 220
    in medial parapatellar approach, for valgus deformity, 139
    in meniscal-bearing knees, 91, 93–95
    retained stump of, arthroscopic management of, 369, 371, 372*f*
    retention of, 49–60, 91
        cementing in procedures with, 57–58, 260
        in cementless total knee arthroplasty, 266, 267
        and correction of deformity, 51
        cutting femur in procedure with, 54–55, 56*f*
        cutting tibia in procedure with, 55, 57*f*
        exposure of knee for procedure with, 54
        in extra-articular deformity correction, 638, 646
        and femoral rollback, 49–50, 55*f*–56*f*
        in flexion contracture correction, 214–215
        and function, 53
        and gait, 51, 91
        implantation of definitive components in procedure with, 57–58
        in lateral release for valgus deformity, 197, 202, 220
        ligament balancing with, 51, 55–57, 58*f*
        in meniscal-bearing knees, 82, 86–87, 87*f*
        patella resurfacing and tracking with, 57
        postoperative care and rehabilitation in, 58–59
        preparation of patient for, 54
        and proprioception, 53, 91
        and range of motion, 49, 52, 59
        in revision arthroplasty, 389
        and stability, 50–51, 91
        stresses at bone-prosthesis interface and wear with, 51–52
        survival of prosthesis with, analysis of, 53
        technique of, 54–59, 55*f*–57*f*
        and tibial component position, 245–246
        in total knee arthroplasty after patellectomy, 623–624
        in total knee arthroplasty following high tibial osteotomy, 606–607, 607
        in total knee replacement after Maquet osteotomy, 615, 617, 618, 619*f*
        in unicondylar replacement, 106
        in varus deformity correction, 51, 192, 194
    sacrifice of, 61–66
        in cementless total knee arthroplasty, 269
        contraindications to, 61
        design of components in procedure with, 62
        in extra-articular deformity correction, 635, 636, 639, 648
        and femoral rollback, 62–63
        and flexion, 62
        in flexion contracture correction, 221
        indications for, 61

Posterior cruciate ligament (*continued*)
        in lateral release, for valgus deformity, 197, 202–203
        in medial release
            for varus deformity, 189, 192, 194
            for varus deformity combined with flexion contracture, 218–219
        with meniscal-bearing knees, 82, 87*f*
        patellar tracking in, 62, 64*f*
        postoperative care and rehabilitation in, 65
        and stability, 61, 62–63, 63*f*–64*f*
        surgical principles of, 61–62
        surgical technique in, 62–65, 63*f*–64*f*
        with total condylar knee, 67
        in total knee arthroplasty following high tibial osteotomy, 606
    stabilizing function of, 621, 622*f*
    substitution for, 61–62, 95
        in cemented revision arthroplasty, 436
        in cementless total knee arthroplasty, 266
        in correction of combined deformities, 217–218
        and femoral component rotation, 240–242
        in lateral release for valgus deformity, 197
        in posterior-stabilized condylar knee, 67, 69, 71–72
        in revision for supracondylar fracture, 574
        in total knee arthroplasty after patellectomy, 626
        in total knee arthroplasty following high tibial osteotomy, 606–607
        in total knee replacement after Maquet osteotomy, 617, 618, 619*f*
        in total knee replacement with femoral extra-articular deformity, 636
        in varus deformity correction, 189, 192, 194
    tight, with inadequate tibial resection, 248, 250*f*
Posterior drawer sign
    in painful total knee arthroplasty, 349
    in posterior cruciate ligament-sacrificing procedure, 61
Posterior oblique ligament, 206
Posterior-stabilized condylar knee, 62, 67–74, 95
    cementing in, 259–260
    in correction of combined deformities, 218–219
    development of, history of, 67–70
    dislocation of, 69
    extensor mechanism complications with, 69, 71–72
    in extra-articular deformity correction, 634, 636
    femoral loosening with, 72
    femoral rollback with, 67, 69, 71
    in hybrid total knee replacement, 274*f*
    Insall-Burstein, 62, 67–74, 68*f*, 69, 95, 730–732
    in lateral release for valgus deformity, 197, 202–203
    long-term results of, 72–73
    metal-backed tibial component in, 68–69, 73
    patella clunk syndrome with, 68, 71–72, 370

Posterior-stabilized condylar knee (*continued*)
    patellar complications and fractures with, 67–68, 71–72
    posterior cruciate ligament-substituting mechanism in, 67, 69, 71–72
    in revision arthroplasty, 389, 436
    short-term results with, 70–72
    survivorship of, 67, 72–73
    tibial loosening with, 69, 72
    versus total condylar knee, 67, 71, 73
    in total knee arthroplasty after patellectomy, 72–73, 623–624, 624*f*
    in total knee arthroplasty after supracondylar femoral osteotomy, 611*f*
    in total knee arthroplasty following high tibial osteotomy, 606
Posterior tibial artery, 326–327, 327*f*
Posteroanterior radiographic view, 6–7
Posthospitalization costs, 22–23
Postoperative management, 649–704
    in allografting for extensor mechanism reconstruction, 517
    in allografting for patellar tendon repair, 523
    in arthroplasties with tibial defects, treated with bone grafting, 291
    in arthroscopy, for problematic total knee arthroplasty, 373
    in correction of combined deformities, 222
    in distal patellar realignment, with medial tubercle transfer, 340
    family and, 5
    in femoral allografting, 429
    in flexion contracture correction, 214
    in lateral release for valgus deformity, 201
    in ligament advancement, 208–209
    in meniscal-bearing knees, 83–84
    in patellar revision, 529
    in patellar rotating patella, 313
    in posterior cruciate ligament-sacrificing procedure, 65
    in posterior cruciate ligament-sparing procedure, 58–59
    in PROSTALAC system, 482
    in proximal patellar realignment, 333
    in quadriceps tendon repair, 514
    in single-stage revision, for infected knee, 468
    in supracondylar fracture fixation
        with retrograde intramedullary nail, 559–560
        with Rush rods, 556
    in tibial allografting, 418
    in tibial tubercle osteotomy, 161
    in total knee arthroplasty after patellectomy, 625–626
    in total knee arthroplasty following high tibial osteotomy, 607
    in total knee arthroplasty for patients with prior arthrodesis, 630–631
    in trivector-retaining arthrotomy, 133
    in unicondylar replacement, 110
    in V-Y quadricepsplasty, 156
Post-phlebitis syndrome, on chronic venous insufficiency, prevention of, 696
Post-traumatic arthritis, as indication for total knee arthroplasty, 3

Povidone-iodine
  in patient preparation, 168, 169f
  swabs soaked in, packing knee with, in single-stage revision for infected knee, 467–468
PPS (prospective payment system), 19–20
Pre-cut maneuver, in lateral approach, for valgus deformity correction, 143
Prehospitalization costs, 23
Preoperative planning, 1–27
  for medial release, for varus deformity correction, 189
  for rehabilitation, 651–654
Preoperative radiographic evaluation, 6–7, 9–18
  Beth Israel Medical Center standard protocol for, 6–7
  for medial release, for varus deformity correction, 189
  for patellar revision, 533
  of patellar tracking, 317, 318f
  for total knee arthroplasty following high tibial osteotomy, 601–602, 602f
  for total knee replacement after Maquet osteotomy, 615, 615f
  for total knee replacement with femoral extra-articular deformity, 635
Press-fit condylar knee arthroplasty, published results of, 273
Press-fit stem fixation
  for constrained prostheses, 78, 79f
  in revision arthroplasty, 451–461
    operative technique for, 456–459, 456f–459f
    preoperative planning and templating for, 452–453, 452f–455f
    results of, 459–460
  for tibial fractures, 577, 579f, 594
Pressurized technique, for cementing tibial component, 259–260
Price, ceiling, of prosthesis, 25
Primary total knee arthroplasty
  bone loss management in, 393–394
    tibial modularity for, 409–411
  cement in, 257–261
  goal of, 165
  principles of, 163–173, 166f
  quadriceps snip in, 149–150
  tibial tubercle osteotomy for, 160–161
  trivector-retaining arthrotomy in, 133–134, 134f
Principles
  basic, of surgical technique, 165–167, 166f
  of diagnosis, 346–347
  of instrumentation, 177–181
  of primary total knee arthroplasty, 163–173, 166f
Probability, as diagnostic principle, 346
Problematic total knee arthroplasty
  arthroscopic diagnosis in, effectiveness of, 368
  arthroscopic management of, 368–374
    complications in, 373
    effectiveness of, 368, 373–374
    indications for, 369
    postoperative management in, 373
    technique in, 369
  infection in, assessment for, 368
  patient evaluation in, 368–369
  radiographic evaluation of, 368
Proconvertin (factor VII), in coagulation, warfarin and, 697–698

Professional fees, 23
Profix Cruciate Retaining Revision Prosthesis, 723
Profix prosthesis, 723
Profix with Tibial Stem, 724
Prophylactic brace, 656, 657f
Proprioception
  ligament balancing and, 56
  retention of posterior cruciate ligament and, 52–53, 91
Prospective payment system (PPS), 19–20
PROSTALAC, 471, 480–488
  advantages and disadvantages of, 487
  antibiotic elution from, 487–488
  clinical results with, 483–485
  complications with, 486t, 486–487
  design and evolution of, 480–481
  and extensor lag, 485
  and knee score, 486
  and knee stability, 480, 485
  in management of infected total knee prosthesis, 473–490
  and pain relief, 485
  and patellar instability, 485–486
  patients excluded from series with, 483, 483f
  postoperative management of, 482
  and range of motion, 485
  and recurrent infection, 486f, 487
  removal of, 482–483
  surgical technique for, 481–482, 482f–483f
Prostheses. See also specific types of prostheses
  cost of, 20t, 21, 21f, 22, 24–25
    awareness of issues associated with, 24
    ceiling price and, 25
    competitive bidding and, 25
    volume discounting and, 24–25
  design of, 47–110
  development of, dichotomy of, with instrumentation advances, 177
  failed
    exposure of, 378–379, 378f–379f
    removal of, 377–383
  fit of, bone resections and, 194f, 194–195
  glossary of, 705–735
  history of, 31
  interface of
    with bone
      exposure of, in component removal, 379
      radiolucent line at, as sign of component loosening, 353–356
      stresses at, retention of posterior cruciate ligament and, 51–52
      take down of, in component removal, 379–381, 380f
      violation of, in patellar revision, 528
    with cement
      assessment of, in painful total knee arthroplasty, 352
      violation of, in patellar revision, 527–528, 527f–528f
  wear of
    arthrography of, 357, 358f
    arthroscopic management of, 371–372, 372f
    in constrained prosthesis, 76
    in meniscal-bearing knees, 81, 84–87, 90–91
    with metallosis, 357, 358f
    metallosis with, 357, 358f, 533, 534f

Prostheses (continued)
  in painful total knee arthroplasty, 352, 357, 358f
  and patellar revision, 525, 533, 534f
  in posterior-stabilized condylar knee, 73
  retention of posterior cruciate ligament and, 52–53
  sacrifice of posterior cruciate ligament and, 62
  and supracondylar fracture, 564
  in unicondylar replacement, 109f, 109–110
Prosthesis of antibiotic-loaded acrylic cement. See PROSTALAC
Prosthetic notch plasty, 574
Protein C, in coagulation, warfarin and, 697–698
Prothrombin (factor II), in coagulation, warfarin and, 697–698
Proximal-distal position, of tibial component, 244, 246f, 248–249, 249f–251f
Proximal patellar realignment
  complications in, 335
  for patellar dislocation/subluxation, 539–540, 541f–542f
  for patellar instability, 332–336
  postoperative management in, 333
  results of, 334–335
  surgical technique in, 333, 334f
Prying technique, for removal of metal-backed patellar component, 535, 535f
Pseudoarthrosis, for infected total knee replacement, 494, 495f
Psoriasis, and patient outcome, 5
Pulmonary embolism, with total knee arthroplasty, 694–695
  association of, with calf clots, 695–696
  deep vein thrombosis prophylaxis and, 701–702
  and patient outcome, 5
Pulse, distal, preoperative assessment of, 6

Q
Q-angle incision, for lateral approach, 140, 140f
Quadriceps mechanism, distal realignment of, for patellar instability, 337–342
Quadriceps muscle
  in combined deformities, 217
  function of
    flexion contracture and, 210–211
    midvastus approach and, 129–130
  heterotopic ossification of, 688
  imbalance of, proximal patellar release and, 335
  inhibition of, effusion and, 660
  malalignment of, and patellar instability, 131
  in painful total knee arthroplasty, assessment of, 349
  patella and, 621
  redirecting resultant force vector of, in proximal patellar realignment, 333
  strength of
    assessment of, in Hospital for Special Surgery Knee Score, 33
    after quadriceps snip, 150–152, 153t
Quadricepsplasty, V-Y, 155–158
  in component removal, 379
  conversion of medial parapatellar arthrotomy to, 190

Quadricepsplasty (*continued*)
  conversion of quadriceps snip to, 152
  in correction of combined deformities, 218
  evolution of, 155, 157f
  for excessive tension on tibial tubercle, 195
  Mayo Clinic modification of, 155, 156–157, 157f
  operative procedure in, 155, 157f–158f
  in patellar revision, 526, 526f, 529
  postoperative rehabilitation in, 156
  versus quadriceps snip, 155
  results of, 156–157
  in revision arthroplasty for stiff knee, 692
  versus tibial tubercle osteotomy, 155
  in total knee arthroplasty following high tibial osteotomy, 606
  in total knee arthroplasty for patients with prior arthrodesis, 628
Quadriceps snip, 149–154
  in component removal, 379, 381, 383
  conversion of, to V-Y quadricepsplasty, 152
  conversion of medial parapatellar arthrotomy to, 190
  in correction of combined deformities, 218
  for excessive tension on tibial tubercle, 195
  Insall modification of (patellar turndown), 149, 150f, 151
  in meniscal-bearing total knee arthroplasty, 82
  in midvastus approach, 127, 129
  original approach described by Coonse and Adams, 149, 150f, 151
  in patellar revision, 535
  patient selection for, 149–150
  for prevention of tibial tubercle avulsion, 519–530
  in revision arthroplasty for stiff knee, 692
  in stiff knee, 155, 156f
  surgical outcome in, 150–152, 152f, 153t
  surgical technique in, 149, 151f
  tibial tubercle osteotomy as alternative to, 151–152
  in total knee arthroplasty following high tibial osteotomy, 606
  in total knee replacement with femoral extra-articular deformity, 636
  versus V-Y quadricepsplasty, 155
Quadriceps tendon
  for allograft, in patellar tendon repair, 523
  fibrous tissue accumulating in, with posterior-stabilizing condylar knee, 68
  lengthening of, in V-Y quadricepsplasty, 155, 158
  in midvastus approach, 127, 128f, 129–130
  reconstruction of, with extensor mechanism allograft, 516–518, 517f
  rupture of, 516
    causes of, in total knee arthroplasty, 514
    direct repair of, 514–515, 515f–516f
    with lateral retinacular release, 514
    in painful total knee arthroplasty, 351, 363–364
  suturing and repair of, in patellectomy, 511

Quadriceps tendon (*continued*)
  trivector anatomy of, surgical approach retaining, 131–137
  visualization of, in anterior surgical approach, 116
Quadriceps torque, decreased, with total knee arthroplasty after patellectomy, 625
Quadriceps turndown. *See* Quadricepsplasty, V-Y
Quality Adjusted Life Years (QALYs), in cost-effectiveness analysis of total knee arthroplasty, 26–27, 27t
Questionnaire(s)
  adapted from knee scores, 42–43
  general health status, for outcomes assessment, 43
  for patient self-assessment, 7, 43
  for rehabilitation planning and assessment, 652, 665t–668t
  validated, crosslinks from, for outcomes assessment, 43

R

Radiographic evaluation
  of bone defects
    for allograft planning, 419–422, 420f–423f
    for classification, 401, 402, 408
    F2A femoral, 404
    F2B femoral, 405
    F1 femoral, 403
    F2 femoral, 403
    F3 femoral, 405–406
    T2A tibial, 406
    T2B tibial, 407
    T1 tibial, 406
    T2 tibial, 406
    T3 tibial, 408
  of cementless total knee arthroplasty, 270, 270f, 273
  of combined deformities, 217
  of component loosening, 353–357, 354f–356f
  of degenerative joint disease, 12–15, 14f–15f
  of double patella, after allografting for patellar tendon repair, 523, 523f
  of femoral component placement, 182–183
  of flexion contracture, 211–212, 211f–212f
  of hybrid total knee replacement, 275f
  of hydroxyapatite-coated implants, 284
  of infection, 357–358, 359f–360f
  Knee Society scoring system for, 352–353, 353f
  in meniscal-bearing knees, 81, 83f, 95, 95f
  of osteolysis, 356f, 357
  of osteonecrosis, 16–17, 16f–17f
  of painful total knee arthroplasty, in routine assessment, 351–352, 352f–353f, 365
  of patellar fracture, 509
  of patellar instability, 332–333
  of periprosthetic fractures
    femoral, 564
    tibial, 594
  preoperative, 6–7, 9–18
    Beth Israel Medical Center standard protocol for, 6–7
    for medial release, for varus deformity correction, 189
    for patellar revision, 533

Radiographic evaluation (*continued*)
  of patellar tracking, 317, 318f
  for total knee arthroplasty following high tibial osteotomy, 601–602, 602f
  for total knee replacement after Maquet osteotomy, 615, 615f
  for total knee replacement with femoral extra-articular deformity, 635
  of problematic total knee arthroplasty, 368
  of reflex sympathetic dystrophy, 364
  standard distance for, 7
  of supracondylar fractures, 545, 568
  of tibia defects, 394
Radiographic views. *See also specific radiographic views*
  anteroposterior, 6–7, 9, 10f
    in degenerative joint disease, 15f
    in osteonecrosis, 16f
    supine, 9, 10f
    weight-bearing, 9, 10f
  lateral, 6–7, 9, 11f
    in degenerative joint disease, 15f
    in osteonecrosis, 16f
  long (52-inch), 7
    standing, 12, 14f
  Merchant, 6–7, 9–10, 11f
  posteroanterior, 6–7
  semiflexed weight-bearing AP, 10–12, 13f–14f
  standard, 9–10
  supplemental, 10–12
  tunnel (intercondylar fossa), 10, 12f–13f
Rand's classification, of bone defects, 401
Range of motion
  assessment of
    in Hospital for Special Surgery Knee Score, 32f, 33
    in Knee Society Score, 34f, 35
    in painful total knee arthroplasty, 349
    preoperative, 6
    questionnaire adaptation of knee score for, 43
  increased, and patellar fracture, 507
  in normal knee, 687
  posterior-stabilized condylar knee and, 67, 69–71
  PROSTALAC and, 485
  quadriceps snip and, 151–152, 152f, 153t
  rehabilitation and, 655–660
    limiting factors in, 656
    poor gains in, under treatment and, 657
  retention of posterior cruciate ligament and, 49, 52, 59
  in stiff knee, 687
    manipulation and, 690–691
  tibial tubercle osteotomy and, 161
  in uncomplicated total knee arthroplasty, 687
RD Heparin Arthroplasty Group, 700–701
Reamers
  acetabular, in femoral allografting, 425, 426f
  in press-fit stem fixation, 455, 456f
Recreational activities, participation in, after total knee arthroplasty, 663, 679t
Rectus snip
  in midvastus approach, 127
  for patellar revision, 526, 526f, 529

Recurvatum deformity
  and stiff knee, 690
  in total knee arthroplasty after patellectomy, 625
Referred pain, in painful total knee arthroplasty, 347–348
Reflex sympathetic dystrophy
  cardinal signs of, 350
  classical clinical presentation of, 364
  incidence of, following total knee arthroplasty, 688
  lumbar sympathetic blockade for, 364, 688
  osteopenia with, 364
  in painful total knee arthroplasty, 350, 364–365
  patient information on, 4
  physical findings in, 688
  as poor prognostic factor, for total knee arthroplasty following high tibial osteotomy, 601–602, 608
  positive outcome in, key factors in, 688
  preoperative, analgesia for patients with, 683
  radiographic findings in, 364
  radionuclide bone scan of, 364–365
  scintigraphy of, 364
  and stiff knee, 350, 688
  treatment of, 688
Rehabilitation, 651–664
  acute, preoperative identification of patients requiring, 652
  admission approval for, 659–660
  in allografting for extensor mechanism reconstruction, 517
  in allografting for patellar tendon repair, 523
  as alternative to total knee arthroplasty, 4–5
  analgesia during, 653, 656, 680–681
  appropriate therapist for patient in, concerns about, 659
  in arthroplasties with tibial defects, treated with bone grafting, 291
  in arthroscopy, for problematic total knee arthroplasty, 373
  bedside exercises in, 658, 678t
  Beth Israel Medical Center protocol for, 676f–677f
  bracing in, 656–657, 657f
  continuous passive motion in, 653, 653f, 655–656
  in correction of combined deformities, 222
  customized, 651
  daily goals in, 658
  disposition in, planning process for, 659–660
  in distal patellar realignment, with medial tubercle transfer, 340
  electrical stimulation in, 656
  family and, 5
  in femoral allografting, 429
  financial considerations in, 22–23, 651–652, 659–660
  in flexion contracture correction, 214
  functional independence measures in, 660, 679t
  goals of, 651
  home exercises in, 652, 662, 670t–675f
  ice/cold therapy in, 657–658, 660
  in lateral release for valgus deformity, 201
  in ligament advancement, 208–209

Rehabilitation (continued)
  in meniscal-bearing knees, 83–84
  multidisciplinary team approach in, 652, 659
  in patellar revision, 529
  in patellar rotating patella, 313
  patient education on, 652–654, 669t–675f
  patient expectations and, 651
  patient perceptions of therapists in, 656
  patient questionnaires in, 652, 665t–668t
  patient tracking forms in, 658–659, 678t
  phase III of, 662
  phase II of, 660–662, 660f–662f
  phase I of, 655–660, 659f
  in posterior cruciate ligament-sacrificing procedure, 65
  in posterior cruciate ligament-sparing procedure, 59–60
  preoperative assessment and planning for, 651–654
    identifying premorbid conditions in, 652
  prescription plan for, 655
  in PROSTALAC system, 482
  in proximal patellar realignment, 333
  in quadriceps tendon repair, 514
  rapport with patients in, 651
  series of sixes in, 653–654, 657
  in single-stage revision, for infected knee, 468
  stair climbing instruction in, 653, 654f
  stationary bicycle in, 661–662
  in supracondylar fracture fixation
    with retrograde intramedullary nail, 559–560
    with Rush rods, 556
  swimming in, 661–662
  Thera Band exercises in, 658, 658f
  in tibial allografting, 418
  in tibial tubercle osteotomy, 161
  in total knee arthroplasty after patellectomy, 625–626
  in total knee arthroplasty following high tibial osteotomy, 607
  in total knee arthroplasty for patients with prior arthrodesis, 630–631
  transition from, to training, 662
  in trivector-retaining arthrotomy, 133
  in unicondylar replacement, 110
  in V-Y quadricepsplasty, 156
Rehabilitative brace, 656–657, 657f
Reliability, of outcomes assessment measures, 41–42
Removal, of components
  bone loss with, 393
  exposure of failed prosthesis in, 378–379, 378f–379f
  instruments for, 377, 379–382, 380f, 382f
  in revision arthroplasty, 377–383, 494
    preoperative assessment and planning for, 377–378
    preoperative templating for, 377–378, 378f
  successful, points central to, 383
  in two-stage exchange arthroplasty, 481
Reproducibility, of outcomes assessment measures, 41–42
Resection arthroplasty, for infected total knee replacement, 491, 494, 495f
Respiratory depression, narcotics and, 683, 685
Responsiveness, of outcomes assessment measures, 41–42
Result, versus outcome, 39

Retinacular arthrotomy, 117f, 118
Retinacular incision, 117f, 118
  lateral, 140–141, 141f
Retrograde intramedullary nail, for supracondylar fracture fixation, 558–562
  aftercare with, 559–560
  designs of, 558, 559f
  fit of, intercondylar distances of commonly used femoral prosthesis for determination of, 558, 559t
  versus open reduction with plate fixation, 558
  patient positioning for, 558, 560f
  preoperative planning for, 558
  technique for, 558–559, 560f
Retropatellar bursa, entry into, in midvastus approach, 128
Revision arthroplasty, 375–389
  bone loss management in, 385, 391–431
    cementless, 440–450
    femoral allografting for, 424–431
    general concepts for, 393–400
    simple approach to, 385, 386f
    tibial allografting for, 415–423
    tibial modularity for, 412
  cemented, 435–439
    implant selection for, 436
    results of, 436–439
  cementless, 440–450
  complications in, 438–439
  component removal in, 377–383, 494
    exposure of failed prosthesis in, 378–379, 378f–379f
    femoral, 379–381, 380f–381f
    instruments for, 377, 379–382, 380f, 382f
    patellar, 382–383, 382f–383f
    preoperative assessment and planning for, 377–378
    preoperative templating for, 377–378, 378f
    successful, points central to, 383
    tibial, 381–382, 381f–382f
  constrained prostheses for, 97–105, 436, 437f
    complications with, 103t, 104
    implant designs of, 97–101, 98f–101f
    results of, 102t, 102–104
  failure in, defining, 435
  femoral component in, selecting size of, 385t, 385–387, 386f
  femoral component rotation in, 387–388, 387f–388f
  fixation techniques in, 384–386, 433–461
  flexion-extension gap in, 386–387
  hinge prosthesis for, 102
  for infected knee replacement, 357, 463–490, 493–494
    antibiotic-impregnated cement in, 440, 466–468, 471, 473–490
    antibiotic treatment before, 440
    cementless fixation and bone grafting in, 440, 446–448
    historical perspective on, 465
    prosthesis of antibiotic loaded acrylic cement (PROSTALAC) in, 471, 473–490 (See also PROSTALAC)
    single-stage, 465–470, 466f
      contraindications to, 468
      length of interval between two halves of procedure in, 466–467
      operative procedure in, 468

Revision arthroplasty (*continued*)
    outcome of, 469
    postoperative management in, 468
    preoperative considerations in, 467–468
    rationale for, 466–467
    versus two-stage revision, 466–467, 469–470
  surgical prerequisites for, 493–494
  two-stage, 471–472, 473–474, 475–476
    clinical results in, 472, 475f, 475–476
    operative technique for, 471–472
    phases of, 471
    PROSTALAC in, 471, 473, 479–488
    rationale for, 466–467
    spacer blocks for, 466, 471, 476–477, 478–479, 478–480, 479–480
  instruments for, 384
  lack of bone for reference in, 384
  midvastus approach for, 127
  need for, in patients receiving primary arthroplasty at younger age, 663
  organized approach needed in, 384, 385f
  in painful total knee arthroplasty, complications of total knee arthroplasty necessitating, 352–353
  patellar
    of all-polyethylene component, 525, 527, 527f
    circular *versus* ovoid component in, 525
    clinical experience with, 529
    determining need for, 524–525
    dome-shaped *versus* sombrero component in, 525
    evaluation of remaining bone stock in, 528–529
    identification of circumferential border of patellar in, 526, 527f
    implantation of component in, 529, 535, 536f
    instruments for, 527–528, 527f–528f
    of loose component, 524–532
    of metal-backed components, 525, 528, 528f, 533–538
      evaluation and preoperative planning for, 533–534
      indications for, 533, 534t
      polyethylene wear and, 533, 534f
      surgical techniques for, 534f–537f, 534–538
    nonresurfacing of patella in, 528–529
    polyethylene wear and, 525, 533, 534f
    postoperative treatment in, 529
    preoperative planning for, 525
    scar excision in, 526, 527f
    selecting implant for, 525
      algorithm for, 529, 530f
    single-peg component in, 528–529, 530f, 533–535, 536f
    in stiff knee, 526, 526f
    surgical approach in, 525–526, 526f
    three-peg implant in, 528–529, 529f–530f, 533–534, 535, 536f
  for patellar instability
    distal patellar realignment in, 337–342
    proximal patellar realignment in, 332–336
  for periprosthetic femoral fractures, 565–566, 568, 573–575
  posterior-stabilized implants in, 389, 436
  preoperative assessment of, 435
  press-fit stem fixation in, 451–461

Revision arthroplasty (*continued*)
  operative technique for, 456–459, 456f–459f
  preoperative planning and templating for, 452–453, 452f–455f
  results of, 459–460
  problems in, diagram of, 385f
  quadriceps snip in, 149–150
  reestablishment of joint line in, 387, 387f
  reestablishment of tibia platform in, 384–385, 385t, 386f–387f
  soft tissue balancing in, 388
  stabilization of knee in extension in, 384, 385t, 387–388, 388f
  stabilization of knee in flexion in, 384–388, 385t, 386f–387f
  for stiff knee, 691–692
  success in, 439
  success rates, 435
    factors affecting, 435
  for supracondylar fractures, 565–566, 568, 573–575
  technique for, 435–436
    three-step, 384–389, 385t
  for tibial periprosthetic fractures, 584, 588, 590–591, 592–598
    avoidance of dead bone sandwich in, 596
    objectives in, 594
    operative technique for, 594–597, 596f
    postoperative protocols in, 597
    preoperative planning for, 594
    results of, 597–598
  tibial tubercle osteotomy for, 160–161
  trivector-retaining arthrotomy in, 133–134, 134f
  in unicompartmentally replaced knee, 106
Revision knee arthroplasty, cemented, 435–439
Rheumatoid arthritis
  combined deformities with, 217
  combined deformity in, 216
  and complications, 5
  and flexion contracture, 211f, 214–215
  as indication for total knee arthroplasty, 3
  patellar fracture after total knee arthroplasty in, 505
  and patient difficulty with anesthesia, 5
  and patient outcome, 5
  and valgus deformity, 137–138, 138f
Risks, of total knee arthroplasty, 4
Robotic arms, 181
Rotaglide knee, 90, 92
Rotary blades, 181, 183f
Rotating hinge prosthesis, 75, 76f, 77
Rotating patella, 310–314, 311f–312f
  final implantations of, 313
  lateral approach in resection for, 310
  medial approach in resection for, 310, 312f–313f
  patellar preparation for, 311
  surgical technique for, 310, 312f–313f
  survivorship of, 313
  trial in implantation of, 310–311
Rotation
  of femoral component (*See* Femoral component, rotation of)
  of tibial component (*See* Tibial component, rotation of)

Rotational freedom, 97
  constrained prostheses and, 97
  meniscal-bearing knees and, 90
Roux-Goldthwait procedure
  modified, in distal patellar realignment, 337–338, 338f
  quadriceps tendon rupture with, 514
RSD. *See* Reflex sympathetic dystrophy
Rush rods, for supracondylar fractures, 553–557, 573
  complications with, 557
  contraindications for use of, 554
  fracture reduction before insertion of, 554, 555f
  indications for use of, 553, 554f
  operative technique for, 554–556, 555f–556f
  positioning of, 555f, 555–556
  postoperative care with, 556
  relative indications for use of, 553–554
  results with, 553, 556–557, 566
  stress relief in, 555, 555f

S
S. A. L. knee, 90
Salvage procedures, in management of infected total knee replacement, 491–501
Saphenous nerve, in midvastus approach, 129
Scar(s)
  excision of, in patellar revision, 526, 527f
  and postoperative range of motion, 656
  preoperative assessment of, for revision arthroplasty, 377, 435
  previous, identification of, for total knee arthroplasty following high tibial osteotomy, 601
SCFO. *See* Supracondylar femoral osteotomy
Sciatic nerve block
  cost of, 681t
  duration of, 681t
  major advantages and disadvantages of, 682t
  quality of, 681t
  technical support for, 681t
  technique for, 681t
Scintigraphy
  in infection, 358
  in reflex sympathetic dystrophy, 364
  for total knee arthroplasty following high tibial osteotomy, 602
Scores, knee. *See* Knee scores
Screw fixation, in tibial tubercle osteotomy, 161–162
Screw reinforcement, of cement fill, for tibial defects, 395
Screw-washer element
  in lateral release, for combined deformities, 220
  in ligament advancement, 207–208, 208f
Scuderi turndown technique, for direct repair of quadriceps tendon rupture, 514, 515f–516f
Segmental bone defect, 401, 415
Self-assessment, patient, 7, 43
Semiflexed weight-bearing AP radiographic view, 10–12, 13f–14f
Semimembranosus muscle
  contracture of, in varus deformity, 189, 190f
  elevation of, in medial release, for varus deformity correction, 191, 191f

Semimembranosus muscle (*continued*)
  release of
    in total knee replacement with femoral extra-articular deformity, 636
    in total knee replacement with tibial extra-articular deformity, 645–646
Semitendinous tendon, for patellar tendon repair, 521, 521f
Sepsis
  as contraindication to total knee arthroplasty, 3
  with infected total knee replacement, 491
    amputation in, 491, 499
    arthrodesis in, 494, 496, 499
    stiff knee in, 687
  in painful total knee arthroplasty, 350
  quadriceps snip in, 149
Septicemia, with antibiotic suppression in infected total knee replacement, 492
Series 3000 prosthesis, 721
Series 7000 prosthesis, 721
SF-12, 40, 43
SF-36, 7, 40, 43, 660
Sham incision, 378
Shaving, in patient preparation, 168
Shower curtain isolation drape, 169, 171f
Side lying abduction, 671t
Side stepping, in rehabilitation, 660, 660f
Simplex cement, 258, 259, 479–480, 484
Single photon emission computerized tomography (SPECT), for allograft assessment, 416
Single-stage revision, for infected total knee replacement, 465–470, 466f, 474–475
  caution with, 475
  contraindications to, 468
  length of interval between two halves of procedure in, 466–467
  operative procedure in, 468
  outcome of, 469
  postoperative management in, 468
  preoperative considerations in, 467–468
  rationale for, 466–467
  versus two-stage revision, 466–467, 469–470
Sinography, of infection, 361, 363f
Sitting-assisted knee bends, 675t
Sitting knee extension, 672t
Sixes, series of, in rehabilitation, 653–654, 657
Skin
  discoloration of, in reflex sympathetic dystrophy, 350
  dissection of (*See* Incision(s))
  preoperative assessment of, 6
    for revision arthroplasty, 377
    for total knee arthroplasty following high tibial osteotomy, 601
  preparation/marking of, 168–169, 170f
    for posterior cruciate ligament-sparing procedure, 54
  tension of, minimizing, in exposure, 115
Skin flap, medial, in subvastus approach, 119, 120f
Skin necrosis, 115, 119
Skin ulcerations, and patient outcome, 5
Sleep patterns, of patient, in painful total knee arthroplasty, 348

Social history, of patient, 5
  assessment of, for total knee arthroplasty following high tibial osteotomy, 601
Social Security Amendments of 1983, 19
Soft tissue
  balancing, 183–184, 184f (*See also* Flexion-extension gap, balance of)
  contracture of, and flexion contracture, 210, 211f
  coverage
    expanders to obtain, 4
    inadequate, as contraindication to total knee arthroplasty, 3–4
  impingement of
    arthroscopic management of, 368–371, 370f–372f
    patient evaluation for, 368–369
  management of
    in lateral approach, for valgus deformity correction, 147–148
    in revision arthroplasty, 388
    in tibial allografting, 418
  release of (*See specific ligamentous releases*)
  tension of, minimizing, in exposure, 115
SONC. See Spontaneous osteonecrosis
Spacer blocks
  in posterior cruciate ligament-sacrificing procedure, 61
  in two-stage revision, for infected total knee replacement
    antibiotic-loaded, 466, 471, 476–477, 478–480
    methylmethacrylate, 476, 478–479
    articulated, 479–480
    PROSTALAC, 471, 473, 479–488
Spasticity, stiff knee with, 687
Special situations, 599–648
SPECT (single photon emission computerized tomography), for allograft assessment, 416
Spinal anesthesia, 115
  patient difficulty with, 5
Spine, assessment of, 5–6
  in painful total knee arthroplasty, 349–350
  with stiff knee, 687
  for total knee arthroplasty following high tibial osteotomy, 601
Spine surgery, prior, analgesia for patients with, 683
Splinting
  postoperative, in rehabilitation, 656–657
  in postoperative management, in ligament advancement, 208–209
Spontaneous osteonecrosis (SONC)
  magnetic resonance imaging in, 16–17, 16f–17f
  radiographic evaluation of, 16–17, 16f–17f
  radionuclide bone scan in, 16
S-Rom prosthesis, 720
Stability/instability
  anteroposterior
    flexion-extension gap and, 165–166
    patella and, 621, 622f
    and residual pain with patellectomy, 623
  in total knee arthroplasty after patellectomy, 625
  assessment of
    in Hospital for Special Surgery Knee Score, 32f, 33

Stability/instability (*continued*)
  in Knee Society Score, 34f, 35
  preoperative, 6
  for total knee arthroplasty following high tibial osteotomy, 601
  correction of extra-articular deformity and, 632, 640, 642
  femoral component rotation and, 227
  femoral resection and, 194f, 194–195, 202
  with flexion contracture correction, 214
  with lateral release for valgus deformity, 202
  ligamentous
    constrained prostheses and, 97, 101–102
    in total knee arthroplasty for patients with prior arthrodesis, 629, 630f
  medial release and, 194f, 194–195
  in painful total knee arthroplasty, 348, 349, 352–353, 354f
  patellar (*See* Patella, instability of)
  posterior-stabilized condylar knee and, 67, 71–72
  with PROSTALAC, 480, 485, 486, 486t
  retention of posterior cruciate ligament and, 50–51, 91
  sacrifice of posterior cruciate ligament and, 61, 62–63, 63f–64f
  size of femoral component and, 194f, 194–195
  in valgus deformity, 197
Stabilization, of knee
  in extension, in revision arthroplasty, 384, 385t, 387–388, 388f
  in flexion, in revision arthroplasty, 384–388, 385t, 386f–387f
Stair climbing
  assessment of, in Knee Society Score, 34f, 36
  epidural anesthesia and, 681
  flexion required for, 655, 656f
  in painful total knee arthroplasty, 348
  posterior-stabilized condylar knee and, 67, 70–71
  in rehabilitation
    as goal in continuous passive motion, 655
    independent, 659
    instruction for, 653, 654f
    strength training for, 660–661, 661f
  retention of posterior cruciate ligament and, 51
Standardization, and cost containment, 25
Standing alignment, preoperative assessment of, 6
Standing AP radiographic view, 9, 10f
Standing hip abduction, 673t
Standing hip bending, 673t
Standing hip extension, 674t
Standing knee bending, 672t
Standing long radiographic view, 12, 14f
  preoperative, for medial release, for varus deformity correction, 189
Standing terminal knee extension, 674t
Staphylococcus aureus infection, in total knee replacement, 493
Staples, from previous high tibial osteotomy, in subsequent total knee arthroplasty, 603, 603f–604f
Stationary bicycle
  in rehabilitation, 661
  seat height of, 661

Stem(s)
  cemented, 451–452
  flutes or spines on, 452, 452f
  geometries of, 452
  insertion of, traditional methods of, 451–452
  offset, 452f
    for constrained prostheses, 79, 79f
    for total knee arthroplasty following high tibial osteotomy, 605f, 605–606
    for total knee replacement with femoral extra-articular deformity, 635, 636f
    for total knee replacement with tibial extra-articular deformity, 645–646
  operative technique for, 456–459, 456f–459f
  press-fit
    for constrained prostheses, 78, 79f
    in revision arthroplasty, 451–461
      operative technique for, 456–459, 456f–459f
      preoperative planning and templating for, 452–453, 452f–455f
      results of, 459–460
    for tibial fractures, 577, 579f, 594–597
  purpose of, 451
  size/length of, determination of, 452–453, 455f
  in tibial fracture revision, 577–578, 579f, 581, 590, 590f, 593f, 593–595, 596f
  in tibial modularity, 409–412, 411f–413f
  for total knee replacement with tibial extra-articular deformity, 645
  uncemented, 451–452
Stem extensions
  cemented versus non-cemented, 79–80
  for constrained prostheses, 78–79, 79f
  in tibial modularity, 409–412, 411f–413f
Steroid therapy
  as alternative to total knee arthroplasty, 4–5
  and patellar fracture, 507
Stiff knee, 687–693
  arthrofibrosis and, 688–689
  arthroscopic management of, 691
  assessment of, in Western Ontario and MacMallister Osteoarthritis Index, 36
  associated conditions in, 687
  causes of, 687–689
  exposure in, options for, 155, 156f
  flexion-extension gap imbalance and, 689–690
  heterotopic ossification and, 688, 688f
  infection and, 687
  malalignment of components and, 689–690
  manipulation of, 690–691
    anesthesia for, 691
    timing of, 691
  patellar revision in, 526, 526f
  quadriceps snip in, 149–154
  reflex sympathetic dystrophy and, 350, 688
  retained bone or osteophytes and, 689, 689f
  revision arthroplasty for, 691–692
  sizing of components and, 689–690
  stress of, and femoral periprosthetic fracture, 573
  technical considerations in, 689–690

Stiff knee (continued)
  tibial tubercle osteotomy in, 159–162
  treatment of, 690–692
    general, 690
  V-Y quadricepsplasty in, 155–158
Stockinette, 168, 169f
Straight-leg raise, 671t
Straight-leg raises, 660, 661f
Straight midline incision, 116
Strength training, in rehabilitation, 660–661, 661f
Streptokinase, for deep vein thrombosis, 702
Stresses, at bone-prosthesis interface, retention of posterior cruciate ligament and, 51–53
Stress shielding, 351, 352f, 393, 438, 452, 460
Stroke, patient history of, 5
Stuart-Prower factor (factor X), in coagulation, warfarin and, 697–698
Subchondral sclerosis, in degenerative joint disease, 12, 15f
Subsidence
  with femoral defects, 403–405
  with tibial defects, 406–407
  with tibial loosening, 353, 354f
Subtractions, in Hospital for Special Surgery Knee Score, 32f, 33
Subvastus approach, 119–126
  anterior cruciate ligament division in, 125, 125f
  arthrotomy in
    lower limb of, 121–122, 122f
    L-shaped, 119–120
    medial limb of, 120, 121f
  in cementless total knee arthroplasty, 267
  cutaneous landmarks in, 119, 120f
  difficult, maneuvers for, 123–125, 124f
  dividing capsule of suprapatellar pouch in, 121, 122f
  elevation of medial capsule from tibia in, 122, 122f
  elevation of medial capsule in, 122–123, 123f
  exposure of anterior femur in, 125f, 126
  final steps in, with scalpel and forceps, 124f–125f, 125–126
  incision in, 119, 120f
  lifting up vastus medialis in, 119, 121f
  versus medial parapatellar arthrotomy, 119
  medial skin flap in, 119, 120f
  patellar eversion in, 122–125, 123f, 124f
  patellar fat pad reduction in, 124f, 125
  preserving capsule in, 121, 121f
  removal of medial osteophytes in, 123, 123f
  separation of patellar tendon from anterior tibia in, 122, 123f
  steps in, 119–126
  versus trivector-retaining arthrotomy, 135
Sulfur colloid marrow scan, in infection, 360–361, 362f
Superior genicular artery, in midvastus approach, 129
Superior lateral genicular artery, 326–327, 327f
  disruption of, in lateral retinacular release, and patellar fracture, 505–506

Superior lateral genicular artery (continued)
  localization of, in lateral retinacular release, 329
  preservation of, in lateral retinacular release, 329f, 329–330, 335
Supine alignment, preoperative assessment of, 6
Supine AP radiographic view, 9, 10f
Supracondylar femoral osteotomy (SCFO)
  for extra-articular deformity correction, 642–644
  failed, incidence of, 610
  prior, autogenous bone grafting after, 296–297, 297f
  results of, 610
  total knee arthroplasty after, 610–612
    clinical results of, 611
    preoperative planning in, 610, 611f
    removal of previous hardware in, 610, 611f
    surgical approach in, 610–611
Supracondylar fractures
  above total knee arthroplasty, 553, 563
    anterior femoral notching and, 557, 563–564
    blades plate fixation of, 567–570, 570f
    bone grafting in, 566–569, 570, 574–575
    cast brace for, 546–547, 546f–547f, 566
    classification of, 564–565
      clinically significant, criteria for, 564
      DiGioia-Rubash system of, 565
      Neer system of, 564–565
      Neer system of, treatment guidelines based on, 567
    closed treatment/reduction of, 545–552, 568
    constrained prostheses in, 101f, 102
    in debilitated, minimally ambulatory patient, 551, 551f
    definition of, 563
    displaced, 545
      controversy over treatment of, 545, 558
    general treatment principles for, 545–546
    hinged knee braces for, 547f, 547–548
      displacement with, 547–548, 547f–548f
    historical overview of, 563
    immobilization devices for, 546–548, 546f–548f, 565, 567–568
    incidence of, 553, 558, 563
    internal fixation of, 546
    malunion of, 546, 547f, 549, 566, 573
    management of, 568–569
      competing principles of fracture immobilization and joint mobility in, 573–574
      goals of, 563
      Merkel–Johnson treatment algorithm for, 565–566
    nondisplaced, 545
    nonoperative treatment of, 545–552
      ambulatory, 546–548
      complications of, 550
      meta-analysis of literature on, 549–550
      methods of, 546–549
      nonambulatory, 548–549, 548f–550f
      results of, 549–550, 565–568
    open reduction with internal fixation for, 565–570
    polyethylene wear and, 564
    postoperative timing of, 545

Supracondylar fractures (*continued*)
    presentation and initial evaluation of, 545
    radiographic evaluation of, 545
    retrograde intramedullary nail for fixation of, 558–562
        aftercare with, 559–560
        designs of, 558, 559f
        fit of, intercondylar distances of commonly used femoral prosthesis for determination of, 558, 559t
        versus open reduction with plate fixation, 558
        patient positioning for, 558, 560f
        preoperative planning for, 558
        technique for, 558–559, 560f
    review of literature on, 565–568
    revision arthroplasty for, 565–566, 568, 573–575
    risk factors for, 557, 563–564, 564t
    Rush rods for, 553–557, 573
        complications with, 557
        contraindications for use of, 554
        fracture reduction before insertion of, 554, 555f
        indications for use of, 553, 554f
        operative technique for, 554–556, 555f–556f
        positioning of, 555f, 555–556
        postoperative care with, 556
        relative indications for use of, 553–554
        results with, 553, 556–557, 566
        stress relief in, 555, 555f
    skeletal traction for, 548–549, 548f–550f, 565–567
    tibial pin traction in balanced suppression for, 548f–550f, 549
    treatment algorithm for, 568f
    treatment options in, 545–546
    valgus alignment in treatment of, 556, 556f
    varus alignment and, 556, 556f
    classification of, 545
        degenerative or rheumatoid cysts and, 564
        Neer system of, 545
    prior, autogenous bone grafting after, 296–297, 297f
Supracondylar notches, avoidance of, in subvastus approach, 126
Supracondylar region, anterior, heterotopic ossification of, 688
Suprapatellar pouch
    capsular folds of, release of, in midvastus approach, 128–129
    capsule of, division if, in subvastus approach, 121, 122f
    hypertrophy of, in valgus deformity, 139
Supreme genicular artery, 326–327, 327f
Surgeon fees, 23
Surgeon standardization, and cost containment, 25
Surgery, preparation for, 7
Surgical approaches, 113–162. *See also specific surgical approaches*
    anterior, 115–118
    lateral, 137–148
    medial parapatellar, 115–118, 131, 132f
    midvastus, 127–130, 128f
    subvastus, 119–126
    trivector-retaining, 131–137

Surgical attire, and infection, 465
Surgical complications, 4
Surgical technique. *See also specific procedures and techniques*
    basic principles of, 165–167, 166f
Survivorship analysis, 3
    of cementless total knee arthroplasty, 269–270
    of medial release, for varus deformity correction, 193
    of meniscal-bearing knees, cemented *versus* cementless, 84–87, 88f
    of patellar rotating patella, 313
    of posterior-stabilized condylar knee, 67, 72–73
    retention of posterior cruciate ligament and, 52–53
    of tricompartmental replacement, 107
Suturing
    in allografting for extensor mechanism reconstruction, 516–517, 517f
    in anterior approach, 117f, 118
    in lateral approach, for valgus deformity, 146–147
    in lateral release, for combined deformities, 220, 220f
    in ligament advancement, 207–208, 207f–208f
    in patellar tendon repair, 520–521
    in patellectomy, 511
    in trivector-retaining arthrotomy, 132
Swedish Knee Arthroplasty Register, 53
Swelling
    with infection, in painful total knee arthroplasty, 357–358
    preoperative assessment of, 6
    reduction of, before revision in infected knee, 467
    in reflex sympathetic dystrophy, 350
Swimming, in rehabilitation, 661–662
Symptomatology, as indication for total knee arthroplasty, 3
Synovectomy
    in patellar revision, 535, 535f
    in trivector-retaining arthrotomy, 133
Synovial fluid, analysis of, in painful total knee arthroplasty, 358
Synovial proliferation, as contraindication to unicondylar replacement, 107
Synovial thickening, preoperative assessment of, 6
Synovitis
    in component removal, 379, 379f
    as contraindication to unicondylar replacement, 107
    hypertrophic, arthroscopic management of, 369–371, 371f

T

T. A. C. K. knee, 90
Tangential axial radiographic view, 6–7, 9–10, 11f
    in painful total knee arthroplasty, 351–352, 353f, 365
    of patella, 317, 318f
    of patellar instability, 332
    of problematic total knee arthroplasty, 368
    for total knee arthroplasty following high tibial osteotomy, 601–602
    for total knee replacement after Maquet osteotomy, 615

Tax Equity and Fiscal Responsibility Act of 1982 (TEFRA), 19
TCP III prosthesis, 730
Technetium bone scans, for assessing patellar viability, after total knee replacement, 506
Technetium 99m-labeled leukocyte scan, in infection, 358–359
Technetium 99m-sulfur colloid marrow scan, in infection, 360–361, 362f
Technetium scanning, in deep vein thrombosis diagnosis, 695
TEFRA (Tax Equity and Fiscal Responsibility Act of 1982), 19
Temperature
    and cement, 257–258
    power instruments and, 258–259, 267
Templating
    for component removal, in revision arthroplasty, 377–378, 378f
    for extra-articular deformity correction, 632, 635, 645
    for press-fit stem fixation, in revision arthroplasty, 452–453, 452f–455f
    for total knee arthroplasty following high tibial osteotomy, 605–606, 605f–606f
Tensing devices, 184, 184f
Tethered patella syndrome, 691
Tetracycline labeling, of autologous bone chips, as biologic cement, 263, 264f
Thera Band exercises, 658, 658f
Thermal necrosis, and patellar fracture, 507
Thigh, assessment of, 6
Thigh circumference
    in deep vein thrombosis, 695
    in painful total knee arthroplasty, measurement of, 349
Thigh compression, for deep vein thrombosis prophylaxis, 699
Third-body wear, modularity and, 413
Third-party payers
    and health-care costs, 19–20
    outcome assessment and, 37
3-D digitized kinematic analysis, of gait, 662
Three-joint radiographic view, 12, 14f
Three-point fixation stems, for constrained prostheses, 78–79
Thrombin, in deep vein thrombosis, 694–695, 699
Thrombin-antithrombin III (TAT), in deep vein thrombosis, 694–695
Thrombolytic therapy, for deep vein thrombosis, 702
Thrombosis. *See* Deep vein thrombosis, after total knee arthroplasty
Thromboxane, aspirin and, 696
Tibia
    bone loss or defect in (*See* Tibial deficiency)
    complications in, with constrained prostheses for revision arthroplasty, 104
    cutting/resection of (*See also* Tibial osteotomy)
        anatomic alignment and, 177, 178f
        in anatomic measured resection, 243–244, 245f
        in autogenous bone grafting for tibial deficiency, 289–290
        basic principles of, 165–167, 166f–167f

Tibia (continued)
    in cementless total knee arthroplasty, 266, 267
    compensatory, in extra-articular deformity correction, 632–634, 633f, 640–644, 641f–643f, 646
    in coronal plane, 179
    in correction of combined deformities, 221
    extramedullary versus intramedullary jigs for, 181–182, 182t, 242–245
    and femoral component rotation, 240–241, 245
    guides for, 55, 181–182, 182t, 244–245, 411, 411f, 616–618, 616f–618f
        inadvertent external rotation of, 246, 248f
        medial displacement of, 245, 246f
    inadequate, 248–249, 250f–251f
    increased, for tibial defects, 394
    instruments for, 181–182
    in knee with 3-degree varus transverse axis, methods of, 227–228, 228f
    in lateral approach, for valgus deformity correction, 145, 145f
    in lateral release for valgus deformity, 199
    mechanical axis and, 177, 178f
    in medial release, for varus deformity correction, 193
    for meniscal-bearing knees, 93–94
    for modular augmentation, 411, 411f
    over-resection of, 248–249
    in posterior cruciate ligament-sacrificing procedure, 61
    in posterior cruciate ligament-sparing procedure, 55, 57f
    in sagittal plane, 179–180
    and tibial component position, 243–253
    in total knee arthroplasty following high tibial osteotomy, 606
    in total knee arthroplasty for patients with prior arthrodesis, 629
    in total knee replacement after Maquet osteotomy, 616–618, 616f–618f
    varus, inadvertent or error, 243, 245, 245f, 246f, 251–253
  elevation of medial capsule from, in subvastus approach, 122, 122f
  extra-articular deformity of
    versus femoral extra-articular deformity, 634
    total knee replacement with, 645–648
        preoperative planning for, 645
        results of, 646–648
        surgical technique in, 645–646, 647f
  lesions of, incidentally discovered, in radiographic evaluation, 12
  posterior slope of, recreation of, 245–246, 247f
  preparation of
    in allografting for patellar tendon repair, 522f, 522–523
    for bone grafting in cementless revision arthroplasty, 441–442, 443f–444ff
  proximal
    allografting of, in revision arthroplasty, 415–423
    bulky, with tibial tubercle osteotomy, 614
    cutting/resection of, basic principles for, 165–167

Tibia (continued)
    external rotation deformity of, in valgus deformity, 197
    skeletonized, in medial release, for varus deformity correction, 191, 192f
    in valgus deformity, 139
Tibia component
    rotation of
        meniscal-bearing knees and, 90
Tibial arteries, 326–327, 327f
Tibial component
    alignment/position of, 179–180, 243–253
        in anatomic measured resection, 243–244, 245f
        anteroposterior, 244, 246f, 247, 248f–249f
        effects of, 243
        and femoral component rotation, 243–244
        in flexion-extension gap technique, 243, 244f
        in flexion-extension plane, 244–246, 246f
        ideal, 189
        mediolateral, 244, 246f, 247, 248f–249f
        orientation of, to ankle, in total knee replacement after Maquet osteotomy, 615
        problems in, and stiff knee, 689–690
        rotational (See Tibial component, rotation of)
    basic principles for, 165
    cementing of, 259–260
        design of tibial tray and, 260
        extension maneuver in, 260
        pressurized, 259–260
    in cementless total knee arthroplasty
        design of, 263
        position of, 263–265
        size of, 268
        survivorship of, 270
    collapse of, failure of arthroplasty with, 378f
    extra-articular deformity and, 632–634
        determination of, 632–634, 633f
    fixation of, in total knee replacement after Maquet osteotomy, 618
    lateral overhang of, 247
    loosening of
        bone loss with, 406–408
        in painful total knee arthroplasty, 353–357, 353f–357f
        with posterior-stabilized condylar knee, 69, 72
        radiographic assessment of, 353–356, 353f–356f
        radionuclide bone scan of, 356–357
        subsidence with, 353, 354f
    medial overhang of, 247, 248f, 268
    in meniscal-bearing knees, 92–93, 93f
    metal-backed, with posterior-stabilized condylar knee, 68–69, 73
    in painful total knee arthroplasty, radiographic evaluation of, 351, 352f–353f
    in patellar revision, evaluation of, 527
    polyethylene size and thickness in, 248, 249f–250f
    positional freedom of, 244, 246f
    posterolateral overhang of, 247, 249f
    in PROSTALAC, 481–482, 482f
        failure of, 487
    removal of
        with cemented stem that is not smooth, 382

Tibial component (continued)
    circumferential exposure in, 381, 381f
    in failed arthroplasty, 381–382, 381f–382f
    instruments for, 381–382, 382f
    with uncemented distally porous-coated stem, 382
  rotation of, 244, 246f, 249–253
    anatomic landmarks for, 250–253
    clinical methods of determining, 250–253
    computed tomography of, 249–250, 252f, 363, 365
    external, 244, 246f
    femoral component and, 250–251
    floating trial of, 250–253
    internal, 244, 246f, 349
        avoidance of, 332
        problems with, 249, 252f, 363
    orientation of, to ankle, in total knee replacement after Maquet osteotomy, 615
    in painful total knee arthroplasty, 349, 365
    and patellar tracking, 320, 322–323, 323f, 328, 328f, 332
    proximal-distal, 244, 246f, 248–249, 249f–251f
    rotational (See Tibial component, rotation of)
    in total knee replacement after Maquet osteotomy, 617–618, 618f
    in translational planes, 244, 246f
    in varus-valgus plane, 244–245, 246f
  sizing of
    incorrect, and stiff knee, 689–690
    optimal, 247
    in total knee replacement after Maquet osteotomy, 618
  stemmed, 452f–453f, 457f–458f
    press-fit, in revision arthroplasty, 451–461
    for tibial fracture revision, 577–578, 579f, 581, 590, 590f, 593f, 593–597, 596f
    for total knee arthroplasty following high tibial osteotomy, 605f, 605–606
    for total knee replacement with tibial extra-articular deformity, 645–646
  translation of, for tibial defects, 394
  in unicondylar replacement, 108, 109–110
  varus angle of, 179
Tibial deficiency
  bone grafting for
    advantages and disadvantages of, 396
    allografting in, 396–397, 406–408, 415–423
      allograft availability for, ensuring, 418
      case studies of, 419–422
      for combined defects, 420–422, 421f
      complications in, 419
      for contained defects, 416–417, 418–419, 419–420, 420f
      contraindications to, 416
      fixation in, 417, 419
      graft healing in, 416
      graft incorporation in, 416
      impaction approach in, 417
      important technical considerations in, 418
      indications for, 416

Tibial deficiency (*continued*)
    operative timing in, 418
    perioperative infection in, 418
    postoperative rehabilitation in, 418
    results of, 418–419
    soft tissue management in, 418
    SPECT scan of, 416
    success in, measurement of, 416
    techniques for, 416–418
      for uncontained defects, 418–419, 422, 422f
      for uncontained or combined defects, 417–418
  autogenous (autograft), 289–294, 396, 406
    distal femoral condyle as graft source in, 290f, 290–294
    reconstitution of upper tibial surface in, 291, 291f
    results of, 292f, 292–294
    technique of, 289–291, 290f–291f
    in cementless total revision arthroplasty, 441–442, 443f–444ff
    indications for, 415
    in tibial fractures, 577–578, 579f, 579f–580f, 580f, 590, 590f, 594, 595f, 597–598
  causes of, with total knee arthroplasty, 415
  cavitary, 401, 415
  cement fill for, 394–395
    reinforcement of, with screws, 395
  central, 397, 415
  classification of, 401–402, 401–403, 404t, 406–408, 415–416
  combined defects in, 385, 415–416
  complex, differentiation of, landmarks for, 402
  component translation for, 394
  contained defects in, 385, 415–416
  custom components for, 397
  discontinuity, 401
  femoral subluxation in, 289, 290f
  implant fixation in presence of, 397
  increased bone resection for, 394
  intercalary, 401
  intraoperative evaluation of, 394
  management of, 394–397
  modular augmentation for, 409–414
    alignment of, 411, 411f
    cost-benefit ratio of, 413
    in primary total knee arthroplasty, 409–411
    in revision arthroplasty, 412
    stems and stem extensions in, 409–412, 411f–413f
    and third-body wear, 413
    types of, 409–411, 411f
  peripheral, 394–397, 415
  in plateau fracture, 294
    management of, 293f, 294
  radiographic assessment of, 394
  segmental, 401, 415
  small, methylmethacrylate for filling, 289
  T2A defects in (one plateau), 406, 407f
  T2B defects in (both plateaus), 407, 407f
  T1 defects in, 404t, 406, 406f
  T2 defects in, 404t, 406–407, 407f
  with tibial fractures, 593
    postoperative
      type I, 577, 578f–579f
      type II, 577–578, 580f
  tibial rim destruction in, 289, 290f

Tibial deficiency (*continued*)
  uncontained defects in, 385, 415–416
  with varus deformity, 409, 410f
  wedge augmentation for, 289, 290f, 293f, 294, 406–407
    metallic, 395–396
    modular, 409–414
Tibial epiphysis, blood supply to, 326
Tibial fractures
  atraumatic, 584
  displaced, 589–590
  intraoperative, 581–582
    mechanisms in, 581
    type I, 581, 581f–582f
    type II, 581–582, 582f
    type III, 582
    type IV, 582
  with loose prosthesis, 576–577, 577, 578f, 583, 587, 588, 588f, 590–591, 593
  nondisplaced, 588–589, 588f–589f
  nonunion, malunion, or delayed union of, 593f, 593–594, 597
  periprosthetic
    anatomic fracture patterns of, 576, 577f
    bone grafting for, 577–578, 579f, 579f–580f, 580f, 590, 590f, 594, 595f, 597–598
    classification of, 576–583, 577f, 578t, 587
    clinical presentation of, 592
    fixation techniques for, 590–591
    incidence of, 587, 592
    nonoperative treatment of, 584–586, 585f, 587, 588–589, 588f–589f
    open reduction with internal fixation of, 587–591, 590f, 594
    operative treatment of, technical considerations in, 590
    predisposing factors for, 587
    radiographic evaluation of, 594
    review of literature on, 592
    revision arthroplasty for, 584, 588, 590–591, 592–598
      avoidance of dead bone sandwich in, 596
      objectives in, 594
      operative technique for, 594–597, 596f
      postoperative protocols in, 597
      preoperative planning for, 594
      results of, 597–598
    treatment algorithms for, 582–583, 583f, 588, 588f, 592–593
    treatment goals in, 587–588, 592
    treatment options for, 592–594
  postoperative, 576–581
    type I, 576–577, 578f–579f
    type II, 577–578, 579f–580f
    type III, 578–579, 580f
    type IV, 579–581, 581f
  proximal, 588, 588f
  stress, 584f, 584–586, 587, 589f, 592
  with tibial tubercle osteotomy, 161–162, 576, 579–581, 581f, 584–586, 585f
  timing of, intraoperative *versus* postoperative, 576
  traumatic, 577, 578, 584–586, 585f, 587, 592
  with well-fixed prosthesis, 576, 577–578, 583, 588, 588f, 590–591, 593
Tibial medullary canal, tibial tubercle osteotomy and, 614
Tibial metaphysis, blood supply to, 326

Tibial osteotomy
  as alternative to total knee arthroplasty, 4–5
  compensatory, in extra-articular deformity correction, 632–634, 633f, 640–644, 641f–643f, 646
  high
    decreased posterior or anterior slope with, 602, 602f
    and extra-articular deformity, 632
    pain with, management of, 601–602
    total knee arthroplasty following, 601–609
      custom-made components in, 605–606, 605f–606f
      existing hardware in, and implant selection, 602–603, 603f
      indications for and contraindications to, 601–602
      patella infera in, 602, 605–607
      patient evaluation for, 601–602
      poor prognostic factors in, 601, 608
      postoperative management of, 607
      preoperative radiographic evaluation for, 601–602, 602f
      preoperative templating for, 605–606, 605f–606f
      removal of hardware in, 603–605, 605f
      results of, 607–608
      soft tissue condition in, 603
      staple retention or removal in, 603, 603f–604f
      techniques in, 602–607, 603f–606f
Tibial pin traction in balanced suppression, for supracondylar fractures, 548f–550f, 549
Tibial plateau
  fractures of, 576
    intraoperative, 581, 581f–582f
    with osteolysis, 356f
    postoperative, 576–577, 578f–579f
  tibial bone loss in, 294
    management of, 293f, 294
  transverse axis of, as landmark for tibial component position, 253
Tibial plateau-tibial shaft angle, in femoral component rotation, 229, 231f
Tibial platform, reestablishment of, in revision arthroplasty, 384–385, 385t, 386f–387f
Tibial shaft, fracture of, 578–579, 580f
Tibial shaft axis, for femoral component rotation, 229, 236–239
  clinical results in, 237–238, 238f, 238t
  versus posterior condylar axis, 237–238, 238f
  surgical technique in, 236–237, 237f
Tibial sleeve release, in lateral approach, for valgus deformity correction, 143–144, 144f
Tibial tray, design of, and cementing of tibial component, 260
Tibial tubercle
  anteriorization of, in patellectomy, 623
  appearance and position of, conditions altering, 253
  avoidance of, in subvastus approach incision, 119
  distortion of, with tibial tubercle osteotomy, 613–614, 614f, 617–618
  elevation of, in tibial tubercle osteotomy, 162

Tibial tubercle (*continued*)
  fractures of, 588, 588*f*
    intraoperative, 582
    postoperative, 579–581, 581*f*
  as landmark for tibial component position, 253
  medial, transfer of, in distal patellar realignment, 337, 339–340, 340*f*
  medialization of, in distal patellar realignment, 540
  protection of, at insertion site, for avulsion prevention, 519
  as reference for tibial rotational alignment, 180
  transfer of, in tibial tubercle osteotomy, 162
Tibial tubercle avulsion, 519–520
  avoidance of, preventive measures for, 519–520
  with medial release, for varus deformity correction, 195
Tibial tubercle osteotomy, 159–162
  as alternative to quadriceps snip, 151–152
  clinical results of, 160–161
  for component removal, 379, 382, 383
  for distal patellar realignment, 540
  fixation of, screw *versus* wire, 161–162
  Maquet, total knee replacement after, 613–620
    clinical evaluation for, 615
    common problems encountered in, 620*t*
    posterior cruciate ligament retention or substitution in, 615, 617, 618, 619*f*
    preoperative planning for, 615
    radiographic evaluation for, 615, 615*f*
    results of, 618
    surgical approach for, 615–616
    surgical technique in, 615–618, 616*f*–618*f*
    tibial internal/external rotation in, 617–618, 618*f*
    tibial resection in, 616–618, 616*f*–618*f*
    tibial sizing and fixation in, 618
  for patellar revision, 526, 526*f*, 529
  for patellofemoral pain due to arthrosis, 613, 614*f*, 618–619
  postoperative rehabilitation in, 161
  preserving surgical option of, in lateral approach, 143
  for prevention of tibial tubercle avulsion, 520
  reattachment of, 160
  for revision arthroplasty, 160–161
  for revision arthroplasty for stiff knee, 692
  in stiff knee, 155, 156*f*
  surgical procedure in, 159–160, 160*f*
  tibial fractures with, 161–162, 576, 579–581, 581*f*, 584–586, 585*f*
  for total knee arthroplasty after supracondylar femoral osteotomy, 611
  for total knee arthroplasty following high tibial osteotomy, 604, 606
  for total knee arthroplasty for patients with prior arthrodesis, 628
  for total knee replacement with femoral extra-articular deformity, 636
  for total knee replacement with tibial extra-articular deformity, 646
  unique features of, 613–614, 614*f*
  versus V-Y quadricepsplasty, 155

Tibiofemoral contact areas, posterior shift of. *See* Femoral rollback
Tinel's sign, 349
Tissue plasminogen activator (tPA), in deep vein thrombosis, 694–695
Titanium
  versus hydroxyapatite-coated implants, 278–279
  hydroxyapatite or tricalcium phosphate coatings on, 279, 284
  for porous coating, in cementless total knee arthroplasty, 262–263
Tobramycin
  addition of, to cement, 259, 471, 476, 479–480
  elution of, 477, 477*f*, 487–488
  in PROSTALAC, 481, 483–484
Total condylar III prosthesis, 69–70, 71*f*, 75, 76*f*, 77, 97, 98*f*
  in complex knee reconstruction, 104
  versus constrained condylar prosthesis, 69–70
  in elderly patients, 104
  in revision arthroplasty, results with, 102–104, 436–439
  for total knee arthroplasty for patients with prior arthrodesis, 627–629
Total condylar knee, 61–65, 62, 68*f*
  as gold standard, 67, 73
  versus posterior-stabilized condylar knee, 67, 71, 73
Total hip arthroplasty, patient history of, 5
Total knee arthroplasty
  age considerations in, 3, 262, 271, 663
  alternatives to, 4–5
  benefits of, 4
  contraindications to, 3–4
  historical perspective on, 3, 31
  indications and patient selection for, 3–8
  risks of, 4
Total knee replacement scores, 31–38
Tourniquet
  in posterior cruciate ligament-sparing procedure, 54
  in total knee arthroplasty following high tibial osteotomy, 606
Towel clip test, of patellar tracking, 318, 320*f*
Townley TKO System, 709
Traction, skeletal, for supracondylar fractures, 548–549, 548*f*–550*f*, 565–567
Training, transition to, from rehabilitation, 662
Transcondylar angle, in femoral component rotation, 229, 230*f*
Transcutaneous Doppler flow test, in deep vein thrombosis diagnosis, 695
Transepicondylar axis. *See* Epicondylar axis
Translational planes, tibial component position in, 244, 246*f*
Transmalleolar axis, of ankle, as landmark for tibial component position, 253
Transverse infra-patellar artery, 326–327
Trauma, prior, radiographic assessment of, 12
Tricalcium phosphate
  basic science of, 277–278
  in biologic fixation, 277–286
  environmental conditions and methods in manufacture of, 277
  implant coatings of
    animal investigations of, 278–281

Tricalcium phosphate (*continued*)
  application of, 278
  and bone formation on perimeter and internal surface lengths, 280–281, 281*f*–282*f*
  in cancellous bone environment, 278–281
  clinical experience with, 281–284
  concerns about, 284
  and lamellar bone formation, 281, 283*f*
  versus non-coated fiber-metal implants, 278–284, 279*f*–283*f*
  and pore volume filled with bone, 279*f*, 280
  and pull-out strength, 280, 280*f*
  scanning electron microscopy backscatter analysis of, 281, 282*f*
  long-term stability of, 278
  solubility and bioresorption of, 278
Tricompartmental total knee arthroplasty
  all polyethylene, uncemented inset patellar implant in, 306
  survivorship analysis of, 107
  unicondylar replacement *versus*, 106–107, 110
Tricon-M prosthesis, 269, 304
Tricon-P prosthesis, 304
Trillat procedure, 540
Trivector-retaining arthrotomy, 131–137
  complications of, 134, 134*f*
  materials and methods for, 132–133
  versus medial parapatellar arthrotomy, 131
  and patellofemoral stability, 131, 134–135
  postoperative management in, 133
  in primary total knee replacement, 133–134, 134*f*
  results of, 133–134, 134*f*
  in revision surgery, 133–134, 134*f*
  subjects for, 133
  versus subvastus approach, 135
  surgical technique in, 132, 132*f*, 133*f*
  in unicondylar knee replacement, 133–134, 134*f*
Trochlear groove
  in cementless total knee arthroplasty, 263, 266
  femoral component rotation and, 227, 228*f*
  as reference for femoral component rotation, 229–230, 242
Trochlear line, 230*f*
Tunnel radiographic view, 10, 12*f*–13*f*
  modified, 10–12, 13*f*–14*f*
2 + 2 design, of posterior-stabilized condylar knee, 69
Two-stage arthroplasty, in inflammatory conditions, 3
Two-stage revision, for infected total knee replacement, 471–472, 473–474, 475–476
  clinical results in, 472, 475*f*, 475–476
  operative technique for, 471–472
  phases of, 471
  PROSTALAC in, 471, 473, 479–488
  rationale for, 466–467
  spacer blocks for
    antibiotic-loaded, 466, 471, 476–477, 478–480
    articulated, 479–480
    methylmethacrylate, 476, 478–479

U

Ulcer(s)
  peptic, and patient outcome, 5
  skin, and patient outcome, 5
Ultracongruent polyethylene insert, in cementless total knee arthroplasty, 266, 266f
Ultra-Drive thin osteotome, 527
Ultrasound
  in deep vein thrombosis diagnosis, 695
  for tendon assessment, in painful total knee arthroplasty, 363–364
Uncontained bone defects, 385, 415–416, 424
Unicondylar replacement, 106–111
  contraindications to, 107
  controversy over, 106, 110
  implant design for, 108–110
  in middle-aged osteoarthritic patients, as first arthroplasty, 107
  in osteoarthritic octogenarian, as first and last arthroplasty, 107
  versus osteotomy, 106–107, 110
  patient selection for, 106–107
  proper sizing of components in, 108
  rehabilitation after, 110
  results of, 106
  surgical procedure for, 107–108, 108f
  versus tricompartmental replacement, 106–107, 110
  trivector-retaining arthrotomy in, 133–134, 134f
  wear patterns in, 109f, 109–110
University of Indiana, Patient Outcome Research Team of, 31
Urinary function, patient-controlled analgesia and, 653
Urinary tract infection, epidural catheter and, 684–685
Urokinase, for deep vein thrombosis, 702
Utilities analysis, for decision making, in infected total knee replacement, 492
Utilization review, 21

V

Vacuum, cement preparation in, 258–259, 478
Valgus alignment
  in painful total knee arthroplasty, 349
  radiographic assessment of, 12, 14f
  in supracondylar fracture treatment, 556, 556f
Valgus angle, of femoral component, 177–179
  anterior cortex as reference for, 177–178
  epicondyles as reference for, 177–178
  intramedullary canal as reference for, 177–178
  posterior condylar axis as reference for, 177–178, 179f
Valgus deformity
  bone loss in, 289, 295, 409, 410f
  combined with flexion contracture, 216
    correction of, 216–223, 217f
    lateral release for, 219–220, 219f–220f
    preoperative planning for, 217–218
    surgical pathology of, 216–217
  and complications with posterior-stabilized condylar knee, 69
  developmental bone deformities in, 138f, 139
  extra-articular layer in, 137–138, 138f–139f

Valgus deformity (*continued*)
  and femoral component, 640–644
  fixed, 137, 138f, 197
  frequency of, *versus* varus deformity, 197
  intra-articular layer in, 138–139, 139f
  lateral approach for, 137–148, 203
    bone resections in, 145–146, 145f–146f
    femoral sleeve release in, 144, 145f
    flexion-extension gap evaluation in, 144–145, 144f–145f
    iliotibial band release or lengthening in, 140, 141f
    instrumentation in, 145f, 145–146
    lateral arthrotomy-coronal Z-plasty in, 140–141, 141f–142f
    patella dislocation/joint exposure for, 143, 143f
    rationale for, 139–140
    results of, 147f, 148
    soft tissue management in, 147–148
    soft tissue (prosthetic) closure in, 146f, 146–147
    steps in, 140
    surgical technique in, 140–147
    tibial sleeve release in, 143–144, 144f
  lateral release for, 197–204
    bone resection in, 198–199, 198f–199f
    complications of, 197, 201–203
    implant selection for, 197–198
    instability with, 202
    patellar instability with, 202
    peroneal nerve palsy with, 201, 220
    postoperative management in, 201
    results of, 202–203
    soft tissue releases in, 199–201, 199f–201f
      order of, 199, 200f
    surgical techniques for, 197–201, 197f–201f
  lateral retinacular contracture in, and patellar tracking, 328
  ligament advancement in correction of, 205–206, 207–208
  medial parapatellar arthrotomy for, 147
    disadvantages of, 139
    failure rates of, 137
    surgical technique in, 139
  meniscal-bearing knees in, 81–82, 84f, 93
  midvastus approach in, 127
  over-release of, 167
  patella in, 317, 319f
  patellar complications in correction of, 137
  pathologic anatomy of, 137, 138f
  pathophysiology of, 197
  piecrusting technique in, 140, 141f, 200, 200f
  posterior condylar axis in, 177–178, 179f
  posterior cruciate ligament in correction of, 52
  preoperative assessment of, 6
  subvastus approach in, 119
  supracondylar femoral osteotomy for, 610
  and tibial component, 632–634
  types of, based on soft tissue integrity, 147
Valgus stability/instability
  assessment of, in Hospital for Special Surgery Knee Score, 33
  femoral component rotation and, 227
  preoperative assessment of, 6

Valgus stress, and constrained prosthesis, 76–77
Validation, of outcomes assessment measures, 41–42
Validity, of outcomes assessment measures, 41–42
Vancomycin
  addition of, to cement, 471, 476
  elution of, 477, 477f, 487–488
  in PROSTALAC, 481, 483
Varus alignment
  in painful total knee arthroplasty, 349
  radiographic assessment of, 12, 14f
  and success/longevity of total knee arthroplasty, 189
  and supracondylar fracture, 556, 556f
  of tibial component, 179
Varus cut, tibial, inadvertent or error, 243, 245, 245f, 246f, 251–253
Varus deformity
  bone loss in, 289, 295, 409, 410f
  combined with flexion contracture, 216
    correction of, 216–223
    medial release for, 218f, 218–219
    preoperative planning for, 217–218
    surgical pathology of, 216–217
  femoral, total knee replacement with, 635
  and femoral component, 640–644
  fixed, 189
  frequency of, *versus* valgus deformity, 197
  ligament advancement in, 208, 209f
  ligament advancement in correction of, 205–206
  ligament release in, basic principles of, 165
  medial release for, 189–196
    approach for, 189–190
    complications of, 194–195
    instability with, 194f, 194–195
    patellar instability with, 195
    preoperative planning for, 189
    results of, 193–194
    technique for, 189–193, 190f–193f
    tibial tubercle avulsion with, 195
  meniscal-bearing knees in, 81–82, 84f
  midvastus approach in, 127
  posterior condylar axis in, 177–178, 179f
  posterior cruciate ligament in correction of, 51, 189, 192, 194
  subvastus approach in, 119, 121–122
  and tibial component, 632–634
  unicondylar replacement in, 107–108
Varus stability/instability
  assessment of, in Hospital for Special Surgery Knee Score, 33
  femoral component rotation and, 227
  preoperative assessment of, 6
Varus stress, and constrained prosthesis, 76–77
Varus-valgus plane, tibial component position in, 244–245, 246f
Vascular claudication, 348
Vascular disorders, and painful total knee arthroplasty, 348–350
Vascular insufficiency
  with infected total knee replacement, amputation in, 499
  patient history of, 5
Vasodilatation, with epidural analgesia, 683–684
Vastus intermedialis, stabilizing force of, preservation of, in trivector-retaining arthrotomy, 131

Vastus lateralis
    advancement of, in patellectomy, 622
    stabilizing force of, preservation of, in trivector-retaining arthrotomy, 131
Vastus medialis
    advancement of
        in patellar realignment, 333, 337
        in patellectomy, 622, 622f
    lifting up, in subvastus approach, 119, 121f
    maintaining integrity of, in quadriceps snip, 149, 151
    neurovascular anatomy of, 129
    splitting of, in midvastus approach, 127–130
    stabilizing force of, preservation of, in trivector-retaining arthrotomy, 131
Vastus medialis oblique
    enhancing strength of, in physiotherapy for patellar subluxation or dislocation, 525
    transection of, in trivector-retaining arthrotomy, 132
Venography, in deep vein thrombosis diagnosis, 695
Ventilation, of operating room, 168, 465, 534
Vessel wall changes, and deep vein thrombosis, 694
Video analysis, of gait, 662
Virchow's triad, 694
Vitamin K, in coagulation, warfarin and, 697–698
Volume discounting, and prosthesis cost, 24–25
V-Y quadricepsplasty, 155–158
    in component removal, 379
    conversion of medial parapatellar arthrotomy to, 190
    conversion of quadriceps snip to, 152
    in correction of combined deformities, 218
    evolution of, 155, 157f
    for excessive tension on tibial tubercle, 195
    Mayo Clinic modification of, 155, 156–157, 157f
    operative procedure in, 155, 157f–158f
    for patellar revision, 526, 526f, 529
    postoperative rehabilitation in, 156
    versus quadriceps snip, 155
    results of, 156–157
    in revision arthroplasty for stiff knee, 692
    versus tibial tubercle osteotomy, 155
    in total knee arthroplasty following high tibial osteotomy, 606

V-Y quadricepsplasty (continued)
    in total knee arthroplasty for patients with prior arthrodesis, 628

W

Walkers, 652–653
Walking. See also Gait
    assessment of, in Knee Society Score, 34f, 35–36
    flexion contracture and, 210
    in painful total knee arthroplasty, 348
Warfarin
    for deep vein thrombosis prophylaxis, 697–699, 702
        aspirin versus, 697
        low molecular weight heparin versus, 700
        mechanical compression versus, 698–699
        study results on, 698–699
    for deep vein thrombosis treatment, 702
    drug interactions of, 698
    hereditary resistance to, 698
    mechanism of action, 697–698
    side effects of, 698
Wear, prosthetic
    arthrography of, 357, 358f
    arthroscopic management of, 371–372, 372f
    in constrained prosthesis, 76
    in meniscal-bearing knees, 81, 84–87, 90–91
    metallosis with, 357, 358f, 533, 534f
    in painful total knee arthroplasty, 352, 357, 358f
    and patellar revision, 525, 533, 534f
    in posterior-stabilized condylar knee, 73
    retention of posterior cruciate ligament and, 51–52, 53
    sacrifice of posterior cruciate ligament and, 62
    and supracondylar fracture, 564
    in unicondylar replacement, 109f, 109–110
Wedge augmentation, for bone loss/defects, 393
    biomechanics of, 395
    cementing of, 395
    femoral, 398
    full wedges in, 409, 410f, 411
    half-wedges in, 409, 410f, 411
    mini-wedges in, 411
    modular, 396, 409–414
    shapes of, 395
    size of, 395
    tibial, 289, 290f, 406–407, 409–414
        metallic, 395–396

Wedge augmentation, for bone loss/defects (continued)
    with plateau fracture, 293f, 294
Wedge-platform technique, for removal of metal-backed patellar component, 535, 535f
Weight-bearing AP radiographic view, 9, 10f
    preoperative, for medial release, for varus deformity correction, 189
    semiflexed, 10–12, 13f–14f
Weight-bearing as tolerated, in trivector-retaining arthrotomy, 133
Western Ontario and MacMallister Osteoarthritis Index (WOMAC), 7, 31, 36
    crosslinks from, for outcomes assessment, 43
    versus other outcome measures, 36–37
White blood cell count, in infection, 368
White blood cells, radiolabeled imaging of, in infection, 358–361, 361f–362f
Whiteside's line, 93
Wire fixation, in tibial tubercle osteotomy, 161–162
WOMAC. See Western Ontario and MacMallister Osteoarthritis Index
Worker's Compensation cases, in total knee arthroplasty following high tibial osteotomy, 601, 608
Wound healing
    albumin levels and, 5
    in anterior approach, 118
    in bone grafting for tibial deficiency after plateau fracture, 293f, 294
    failure of, in painful total knee arthroplasty, 350
Wound infection
    with constrained prostheses for revision arthroplasty, 103t, 104
    in painful total knee arthroplasty, 350
Wright Advance prosthesis, 726
Wright Axiom Cruciate Retaining Primary prosthesis, 728
Wright Axiom PS Primary prosthesis, 729
Wright Axiom Revision prosthesis, 729

Y

Younger patients, total knee arthroplasty in, 663

Z

Zimmer Regular cement, 258
Z-plasty, in lateral approach, for valgus deformity, 140–141, 141f–142f, 146–147